ANNUAL REVIEW OF
IMMUNOLOGY

ANNUAL REVIEW OF IMMUNOLOGY

VOLUME 19, 2001

WILLIAM E. PAUL, *Editor*
National Institutes of Health, Bethesda, Maryland

C. GARRISON FATHMAN, *Associate Editor*
Stanford University, Stanford, California

LAURIE H. GLIMCHER, *Associate Editor*
Harvard University School of Public Health

www.AnnualReviews.org   science@AnnualReviews.org   650-493-4400

ANNUAL REVIEWS
4139 El Camino Way • P.O. BOX 10139 • Palo Alto, California 94303-0139

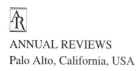

ANNUAL REVIEWS
Palo Alto, California, USA

International Standard Serial Number: 0732-0582
International Standard Book Number: 0-8243-3019-6

Annual Review and publication titles are registered trademarks of Annual Reviews.

∞ The paper used in this publication meets the minimum requirements of American
National Standards for Information Sciences—Permanence of Paper for Printed Library
Materials, ANSI Z39.48-1992.

Annual Reviews and the Editors of its publications assume no responsibility for the
statements expressed by the contributors to this *Annual Review*.

TYPESET BY TECHBOOKS, FAIRFAX, VA
PRINTED AND BOUND IN THE UNITED STATES OF AMERICA

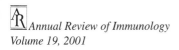Annual Review of Immunology
Volume 19, 2001

CONTENTS

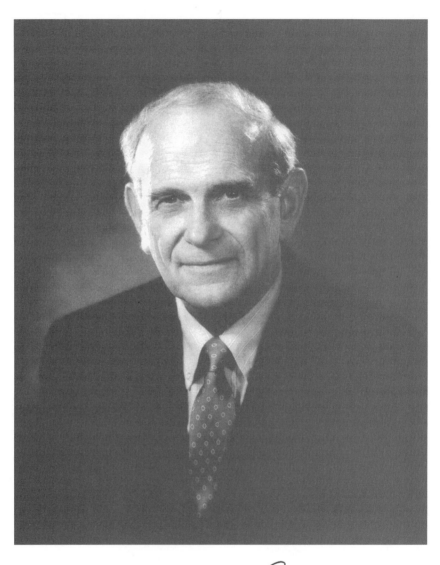

Herman N. Eisen

Annu. Rev. Immunol. 2001. 19:1–21

SPECIFICITY AND DEGENERACY IN ANTIGEN RECOGNITION: Yin and Yang in the Immune System

Herman N. Eisen

Center for Cancer Research and Department of Biology, Massachusetts Institute of Technology, Cambridge, Massachusetts 02139; e-mail: hneisen@mit.edu

Key Words antibodies, T cell receptors, peptide-MHC complexes, epitope density, affinity maturation

■ **Abstract** One of the hallmarks of the immune system is specificity, a concept based on innumerable observations that antibodies react with the substance that elicited their production and only a few other structurally similar substances. The study of T cells has begun to suggest, however, that in responses mediated by their antibody-like receptors (T cell receptor or TCR) an individual T cell, expressing a singular TCR, can discriminate as exquisitely among antigens as the most specific antibodies but also exhibit "degeneracy": i.e., it can react with many disparate antigens (peptide-MHC complexes). An explanation for this duality (specificity and degeneracy) can be found in (i) the powerful amplifying signal transduction cascades that allow a T cell to respond to the stable engagement of very few TCR molecules, initially perhaps only one or two out of around 100,000 per cell, by their natural ligands (peptide-MHC complexes or epitopes on antigen-presenting cells—or APC) and (ii) the inverse relationship between TCR affinity for epitopes and epitope density (the number of copies of an epitope per APC). Older observations on the excess of total globulin production over specific antibody production in response to conventional immunization procedures suggest that B cells also exhibit degeneracy, as well as specificity. These views are developed against a backdrop describing how the author became interested in the immune system and has pursued that interest.

> "... a concept of science drawn from ... [textbooks] ... is no more likely to fit the enterprise that produced them than an image of a national culture drawn from a tourist brochure."
>
> Thomas Kuhn, *Structure Of Scientific Revolutions*

INTRODUCTION

Sometime around 1960 Rene Dubos, a distinguished microbiologist, visited Washington University School of Medicine in St. Louis to talk about special bacterial cultures as sources of novel enzymes. I was his official host and expected

0732-0582/01/0407-0001$14.00

1

us to discuss similarities and differences between adaptive enzymes, as they were then called, and antibodies. Instead, he kept wanting to know how I had become interested in immunology. I remember being much annoyed by his persistent interest and ignored it. But I never forgot it and I address it now, not because the answer is especially interesting, but because his question was reasonable, for when my interests had developed there were virtually no textbooks or courses in immunology, and only a few days were devoted to it in medical school curricula. The attempt to answer the question also provides a convenient starting point for this anecdote-driven approach to the principal theme of this chapter—how the idea of specificity in immune reactions, grounded in a century of experience with antibodies, is likely to be significantly modulated by evidence that a T cell, expressing a singular antibody-like receptor, can respond to many disparate antigens (generally, short peptides associated with major histocompatibility complex (MHC) proteins.

EARLY VIEWS AND ACTIVITIES

To begin with some personal notes, it seems to me that my early views and activities were much influenced by two circumstances: First, I grew up in a large Jewish community in Brooklyn, a part of New York City that at the time (the 1920s) seemed suburban. My father, as a 12-year-old accompanied only by his younger brother, had migrated from what was then part of the Austro-Hungarian Empire to New York in 1895. They joined my grandfather, who had migrated several years before, and my mother, who, as a child, had similarly arrived in the United States with her parents at about the same time from eastern Europe. With that background it should not be surprising that I grew up with a sense that antisemitism in the world around us was pervasive. Though certainly not as overt as in eastern Europe, in the United States it was nevertheless regarded as a fact of life, like birth and death. When chemistry in high school was the only subject I found interesting and I expressed an interest in becoming a chemist or chemical engineer, my father argued that this was not a realistic choice because of dismal employment possibilities: Large companies in the chemicals industry did not hire Jews. In medicine, however, a somewhat related field, one's destiny was in one's own hands. So, because my father was persuasive and I was not yet 16 when I entered college, I enrolled as a premedical student.

The other circumstance that may be worth mentioning is that while in high school I was suspected of having pulmonary tuberculosis. The diagnosis became firmer after one year of college and led to a year's enforced bed-rest. I read extensively and remember being particularly affected by Sinclair Lewis's *Arrowsmith*, with its idealistic physician-scientist as the main protagonist, and by Darwin's *Origin of Species*, with its powerful but simple idea expressed in chapter after chapter of magnificent prose. (But Darwin's *On the Descent of Man* I found impenetrable and never finished.)

At New York University (NYU), as an undergraduate, I happened to attend a seminar on the synthesis of some epinephrine-like molecules and their physiologic effects. The speaker, a graduate student in organic chemistry named Morris Ziff, who later became a distinguished rheumatologist, described how small changes in structure, such as shifting an OH group from one carbon in a benzene ring to an adjacent carbon, led to dramatic effects on a cat's blood pressure. The fascination of seeing, as an impressionable teenager, the connection between molecular structure and biologic function made a deep impression and must have left me especially receptive to the chemically oriented immunology I would shortly after encounter in papers from the Landsteiner and Pauling laboratories.

The medical school I attended from 1939 to 1943 (New York University, usually called Bellevue after its great teaching hospital) bore no resemblance to its counterparts in the following decades or now. Teaching in the clinical departments depended upon a part-time faculty who earned their livelihood in solo private practice. The preclinical departments were remarkably small. For instance, the biochemistry department had, I think, four faculty members and about the same number of graduate students; grants to support research were pitifully meager. There was nevertheless a sense that serious research was being carried out, especially in certain fields, among them infectious diseases. The latter was marked later by the triumphs of Jonas Salk and Albert Sabin (both of whom had graduated a few years previously) in developing the vaccines against poliovirus that may well now be on the way to eliminating this pathogen from the world.

In contrast, the research environment at Columbia University's College of Physicians and Surgeons, where I subsequently served as a resident in pathology, was vastly larger and more impressive. It listed a large and illustrious faculty, especially in biochemistry, many of them Jewish refugees from Nazi Germany. It had an impressive group of bright graduate students, some also refugees, like Kurt Bloch, and many drawn from New York's City College and destined to become leading figures in biochemistry–David Shemin, Seymour Cohen, and Boris Magasanik to name some. It was, however, to Michael Heidelberger's laboratory in the Department of Medicine that I was particularly drawn. Heidelberger, proud of his training as an organic chemist, had, together with Oswald Avery, discovered that the major antigens of pathogenic pneumococci were polysaccharides. One of the consequences of this momentous discovery was that antibodies were finally and unambiguously shown to be proteins (in immune precipitates made with purified polysaccharide antigen). It also led to quantitative precipitation assays to measure antibody concentrations in serum, in weight units, in contrast to the prevailing methods of determining titers by serial dilution. Titers could be determined rapidly and easily and, in the hands of skillful analysts and with appropriate sera, could yield unambiguous results. This was the case, for example, in all of Landsteiner's elegant work in determining the structural basis for antibody specificity. But titer determinations could also be subjective and misleading, as was soon demonstrated in a study I carried out with Manfred Mayer, a graduate student in the Heidelberger lab at the time and later a leading figure in the study of complement proteins.

A series of papers had appeared showing that when adrenal cortical steroids were injected along with antigen into rats, the resulting antibody titers substantially exceeded those found after injecting the antigen alone, indicating that these hormones, involved in general stress responses, enhanced antibody production. When we repeated the work, measuring serum antibodies by quantitative precipitin reactions, we could find no effect from the adrenal hormones. The results brought to an abrupt halt a line of investigation that was receiving wide attention because of its implications for enhancing human immune responses.

Following a return to Bellevue Hospital and a medical residency, I served during an extended vacation as a ship's surgeon on a boat carrying cargo down the west coast of South America and bananas back to New York. Though intermittently busy treating injuries resulting from loading and unloading of cargo and administering bismuth or arsenicals to treat crewmen with syphilis, I had much free time for reading in solitude on the uppermost hurricane deck. I had brought along the revised edition of Landsteiner's monograph on the "Specificity of Serological Reactions" and read most of it. Published at the time of Landsteiner's death in 1943, it was a superb summary of what was known about immunology at the time, and the final chapter, by Linus Pauling, was a wonderful description of noncovalent molecular interactions. Though it was largely addressed to Landsteiner's work on the reactions of antisera with small organic molecules (haptens), the view it provided of molecular complementarity as the basis for antigen recognition by antibodies doubtless helped cement my interest in the immune system, and particularly in the use of structurally well-defined small molecules as substitutes for more complex antigens, such as the red blood cells and bacteria then (and subsequently) commonly used as antigens to study immune responses. There was, however, no obvious way to pursue that interest, for opportunities to engage in research were then limited.

At the time, the academically inclined physicians I knew carried out research in a few hours taken away from busy practices, using all sorts of make-shift arrangements. But all of this was shortly to change as the federal government became committed to support research in universities, including medical schools. The change was due largely to World War II when, as described in Daniel Kevles' superb article (*Daedalus* 121:195–235 [1992]), "Physics won (the war) with microwave radar, proximity fuses, and solid-fuel rockets, and ... ended it with the atomic bomb." Before the war, biomedical research was almost entirely dependent on a few philanthropists and philanthropic institutions who distributed their largess to a small number of highly selected, elite institutions. NYU was definitely not one of them. After the war, however, federal funds became more widely distributed—not only to physics and chemistry, of obvious interest to the defense establishment, but to biomedical research as well. The National Institutes of Health (NIH) expanded and devoted a sizeable proportion of its funds to support research fellowships for "promising young biomedical scientists and for basic and applied biomedical research conducted in universities and medical schools."

As an early beneficiary of that commitment, I received a senior NIH fellowship in 1948. A forerunner of today's physician-scientist awards, it could not have come at a better time. I was then about to make the most important move in my life in marrying Natalie Aronson and starting to raise a family that would ultimately include five children. The fellowship facilitated this momentous step by providing a generous stipend ($3600/yr), allowing me to devote myself full-time to research for two years. My official mentor at NYU was William Tillett, chairman of the Department of Medicine who, fortunately, seemed not interested in what I did or where I did it. As I was drawn to chemistry, I spent time in the Department of Biochemistry, and the chairman, R. Keith Canaan, a courtly Englishmen who enjoyed a considerable reputation for his early work on the acid-base titration of ovalbumin, graciously provided me with bench space in his lab. There I was completely free to pursue whatever interests I had. That freedom, which I then took for granted, was an extraordinary opportunity, now only available in rare special postdoctoral fellowships, like those at the Whitehead Institute at Massachusetts Institute of Technology: the several remarkably accomplished young scientists who have emerged from that program in recent years testify to the power of early independence for young scientists.

In Canaan's lab I was bent on using low mol. wt. molecules—haptens—to study immune reactions of medical interest. I visualized taking advantage of them to study hypersensitivity reactions and so turned to sulfonamides. These antibacterial drugs were revolutionizing the treatment of many infectious diseases, but one major drawback was that they occasionally caused severe allergic reactions. The attractiveness of using such well-defined molecules was enhanced by the controversies surrounding studies of hypersensitivity reactions to conventional protein antigens, such as diphtheria toxin. Later, at meetings of the American Association of Immunologists, Elvin Kabat's criticisms of work with purified bacterial toxins led to unwary victims of his formidable verbal skills being referred to as having been "kabatized," rather than baptized, by the their first public encounter with a scientific controversy. With low mol. wt. antigenic surrogates, however, critical reactants could be unambiguously identified by specific inhibition with other, structurally related simple molecules, e.g., using hapten inhibition in vivo, paralleling its established use in vitro, to define the specificity of hypersensitivity reactions.

BINDING OF HAPTENS TO ANTIBODIES

The plan to study immune reactions was put in motion but then set aside temporarily in favor of another that grew from the work being done by Fred Karush, another postdoctoral fellow with whom I happened to share bench space in Canaan's lab. Karush was using equilibrium dialysis to study the reversible binding of dodecyl sulfates to bovine serum albumin while I was learning how to generate and purify antibodies to diazotized small molecules. We decided to join forces, using equilibrium dialysis to study the binding of small dialyzable molecules (haptens) to purified antibodies. Fred had received a PhD in physical chemistry from the University of Chicago, spent a year in physics of MIT, and then gone to work as a paint chemist at DuPont to support his family. But, eager to return to academia and to study proteins, he obtained a three-year National Research Council fellowship, starting in Canaan's lab at NYU. By sheer luck, our disparate interests and backgrounds were joined in a collaborative study that marked a turning point for each of us. From Fred I learned to appreciate the elegance of physical chemistry; he may have learned a bit of biology and medicine from me; and we both came away from the collaboration with a lifelong friendship that involved as well our respective families.

To study the binding of an azodye to antibody, we turned to azobenzenearsonate (called R) because it was being extensively used by Pauling, Pressman, and Campbell to analyze antibody reactions with polyvalent azodyes. Anti-R antibodies were purified from rabbit antisera (raised against Razo-protein conjugates) with the aid of insoluble adsorbants made by coupling the Razo group to red blood cell stroma, in a primitive form of what was later called affinity chromatography. With conventional dialysis membranes, which were permeable to small azo dyes but not to antibodies, it was clear from the first experiment that when one started with a colorless antibody solution on one side of the membrane and a solution of a red Razo-phenol dye on the other side, the red dye became obviously concentrated on the side containing the antibody. More than the exciting visual effect, by varying the initial dye concentration and thereby the amount of hapten bound, it was a straightforward matter to determine both the equilibrium binding constant of the binding reaction (the antibody's affinity for the dye) and the number of binding sites per antibody molecule.

ANTIBODY VALENCE: The Number of Binding Sites Per Antibody Molecule

The number of binding sites was much debated at the time, in part because of its implications for how antibodies are generated. From the ability of some immune precipitates to bind additional antigen (proteins or polysaccharides), Heidelberger and Kendall inferred that antibodies had multiple binding sites for antigen. Focusing on precipitin reactions in which conventional high mol. wt. antigens were replaced by azodyes having multiple haptenic groups per molecule, Pauling considered the results in his lab to justify his preference for two sites per antibody molecule, the simplest form of multivalency. Heidelberger, who evidently preferred more than two sites (to fit the view of the immune precipitate as a 3-dimensional lattice, formed by linking antibodies and antigens in widely varying ratios), mentioned, with obvious satisfaction in one of his many reminiscences, having observing evidence for trivalent antibody in one of Pauling's lectures. Felix Haurowitz differed from both, however, and insisted that there was a single binding site per antibody molecule.

Why the insistence on univalence? Haurowitz, while living temporarily in Constantinople as a refugee from Hitler's Germany, had initially proposed, with Breinl, the antigen-template theory of antibody formation. In the theory's refined form advanced about 10 years later by Pauling, the antibody molecule was viewed as a single polypeptide chain that, as a newly synthesized nascent molecule, folded up around an antigen template, thereby acquiring two binding sites complementary in shape to antigenic sites (now called epitopes, after Jerne). Since antigens characteristically have many different epitopes per molecule—assume two for simplicity, A and B—some bivalent antibodies would have two anti-A sites and others two anti-B sites, but the majority would be bispecific, i.e. with one anti-A site and the other, on the same molecule, being anti-B (the ratio of their frequencies being 1:1:2, according to Pauling). Aware of this possibility, Haurowitz had searched for antibodies with two different specificities but could not find them. Therefore, being totally wed to the antigen-template theory (as was everyone else at the time), he maintained that antibodies had to be univalent.

When Karush and I published our evidence for two anti-R sites per antibody molecule (in the *J. Am. Chem. Soc.*, where papers on antibodies from the Pauling lab had been regularly appearing), the response was mostly gratifying. Pauling sent us a congratulatory letter, noting especially his pleasure at seeing the idea of bivalency confirmed. Haurowitz ignored the results and continued to maintain for years that antibodies are univalent.

BIVALENCE VS. BISPECIFICITY

We returned to the issue of antibody bispecificity shortly afterwards, analyzing antibodies produced in response to 2,4-dinitrophenyl-bovine gamma globulin (DNP-BGG): The antisera contained abundant levels of anti-DNP antibodies and even more anti-BGG antibodies, but, as found previously by Haurowitz, there was no evidence for bispecific antibodies–e.g., there were no anti-BGG molecules that had anti-DNP activity. That antibodies are bivalent but not bispecific was disquieting, but few remarked about it. Kabat (not known for commenting favorably about other people's work) was one of the few. Yet, neither he nor I nor anyone else at the time was sufficiently motivated by this apparent disconnect between theory and observation to think seriously about alternatives to the antigen-template hypothesis. To those not active in immunology at the time it is probably impossible to imagine the powerful hold this hypothesis had for over 20 years, until the publication of Burnet's monograph on clonal selection and independent powerful evidence from Anfinsen and colleagues that a protein's conformation, including the shape of its binding sites, is dictated by its amino acid sequence.

Having experienced the excitement of laboratory research, I was not ready to leave it for the private practice of medicine, then the only obvious means for supporting a family. Karush had moved to a temporary position at the Sloan Kettering Institute in David Pressman's group, and I was then also offered a job in

Pressman's program, which involved the tissue localization in mice of radioiodinated antibodies raised against tissue antigens, a foreshadowing of modern efforts for the immunotherapy of cancer. I was not excited by the program and after 10 months accepted a position back at NYU in a newly formed Department of Industrial Medicine.

DELAYED-TYPE HYPERSENSITIVITY SKIN REACTIONS

The Department had received a gift from the Standard Oil Company of NJ to set up a lab to study diseases of significance for the company. I was not sure what they had in mind or why the position was offered to me, but it provided a total of $10,000/yr to start up a new lab, hire a technician, and pay me a salary that would have to be augmented by part-time private practice. I had no difficulty in deciding to focus on allergic skin reactions to dinitrobenzenes, to take advantage of both Landsteiner's early work on delayed type hypersensitivity (DTH) to these compounds and Fred Sanger's landmark use of 2,4-dinitrophenyl (DNP) amino acids to establish that proteins are linear polymers of amino acids joined in alpha peptide bonds, a concept that at the time was still being debated. As a postdoctoral fellow, I had heard Sanger's seminar a couple of years before, describing how he attached DNP to the N-terminal amino acid of an insulin chain and to its various proteolytic fragments; then, after hydrolysis, he identified the released DNP-amino acids by silica gel chromatography. Intending to apply this approach to purified antibodies, I had synthesized 2,4-dinitrofluorobenzene (DNFB was used to prepare DNP-amino acids and peptides but was not then available commercially). I abandoned the project when I become sensitized to DNFB, evidently by handling it carelessly, and developed severe contact dermatitis. Thus, when I started the study of DTH reactions to dinitrobenzenes a few years later, I had my own skin reactions to turn to for experimental purposes, as well as those of deliberately sensitized guinea pigs.

A large number of 2,4-dinitrobenzene derivatives, including DNFB, were tested on both DNFB-sensitized guinea pigs and on my own skin, using the simple patch tests commonly used by dermatologists. From hydrolysates of skin from guinea pigs painted with some dinitrobenzenes, DNP-amino acid could be identified using Sanger's chromatographic systems. The results confirmed Landsteiner's conclusion, drawn from the use of phenol at high pH as a model protein: 2,4-dinitrobenzenes having good "leaving" groups in the carbon-1 position reacted well with protein and elicited the delayed-type hypersensitivity skin reaction. This property divided the dinitrobenzenes distinctly into those that could or could not elicit these allergic reactions; with one exception, the results with the guinea pigs and my own skin were entirely concordant.

The exception, 2,4-dinitrobenzesulfonic acid (DNBSO3), was inactive on the sensitized guinea pigs but elicited responses on my skin. As the sulfonate derivative was water soluble, it seemed that the difference could have been due to the presence of sweat ducts in human skin and their absence in guinea pig skin. (The idea was, incidentally, supported by applying a patch test on my skin at the edge of an old vaccination scar and seeing the typical DTH allergic skin reaction develop on the normal skin but not on the contiguous scar, presumably because scars lack sweat ducts.) The reaction on human skin indicated that DNBSO3 formed DNP-proteins in situ, and we showed that it was indeed a highly effective reagent for preparing water soluble DNP-proteins; it also had the added advantage over DNFB of reacting almost exclusively with lysine side chains.

WASHINGTON UNIVERSITY MEDICAL SCHOOL IN ST. LOUIS

The arrangement made initially with the Industrial Medicine Department was that I would spend half-time in research, allowing the other half for medical practice. Instead, I came to spend increasingly long days in the lab and to see patients only in the evening. This was fine for research, but unfair to patients, and even more unfair to our growing family. The publications, however, were not unnoticed, and one day in the lab I received a phone call from W. Barry Wood who wanted to know if I would be interested in a position in the Department of Medicine, of which he was chairman, at Washington University's medical school in St. Louis. He had persuaded the Rockefeller Foundation to endow a chair in Dermatology, within his department, arguing that research on skin disease, traditionally carried out within Departments of Dermatology, were languishing, unlike the vigorous research being carried out in many departments of internal medicine on diseases of the kidney, cardiovascular system, etc. I was thus offered an endowed chair as Professor of Medicine and head of the dermatology service of Barnes Hospital, the medical school's great teaching hospital, even though I had had no training in dermatology. With a generous salary and liberal lab space, it meant not only enhanced research opportunities but an end to exhausting moonlighting in private medical practice. Before I could accept the offer, Wood let me know that he was returning to Johns Hopkins, where he had previously spent many years, and that he would be succeeded as department chief by Carl Moore. Part of the offer's attraction was Woods great reputation as a charismatic leader in academic medicine. But Moore was also enormously respected for his intellect and character, and once I had met him any doubts I may have had vanished. I accepted the offer enthusiastically.

Moore proved to be a wonderful colleague and in time a close friend. Though Wood had moved to Johns Hopkins we became close collaborators when, with Benard Davis (Harvard), Harry Ginsberg (University of Pennsylvania), and Renato Dulbecco (Salk Institute), we wrote a new textbook of microbiology. I was responsible for the immunology chapters. Intended to differ from traditional textbooks, it sought to describe not only what was known at the time, but how we got to know it. The effort was initially exhilarating; the first edition came to be widely used; and the Immunology section was subsequently published as a series of separate volumes. After an equally satisfactory second edition, the later ones suffered from my lack of first-hand experience with the emerging new information about cellular immunology, which had to be incorporated. The comments about textbooks in general in Thomas Kuhn's quotation at the beginning of this article could well apply to the final edition, appearing about 20 years after the first one. It was a relief to end the series.

When we first arrived in St. Louis renovations for my lab were still underway and would not be completed for about six months. Arthur Kornberg, head of Microbiology, generously offered me space in a lab where all of the department's graduate students worked, clustered together by design, rather than in their mentors' individual labs. The department was small and populated by a young and extraordinarily talented faculty and group of postdoctoral fellows, and a daily journal club at the communal lunch added to the general level of excitement about science.

QUENCHING ANTIBODY FLUORESCENCE

To analyze antigen recognition by antibodies in greater detail than had previously been possible, we wanted to measure differences in free energies of binding of various haptens to purified antibodies. When DNBSO3 was used to produce highly substituted, water soluble DNP-proteins as antigens, which were administered in complete Freund's adjuvant, the resulting rabbit antisera contained suprisingly abundant amounts of anti-DNP antibodies, often around 50 times more than we had previously obtained with different immunization procedures, and the antibody could be easily isolated in highly purified form. I told Sidney Velick about these wonderful antibodies, and he in turn told me about the wonderful procedure he was using to analyze the binding of pyridine nucleotides to a dehydrogenase enzyme: The procedure was based on the transfer of energy emitted by UV light-activated tryptophan residues of the protein to bound ligand. The resultant quenching of the tryptophan's fluorescence emission depended in large measure on spectral overlap between the ligand's absorption spectrum and the tryptophan's emission spectrum. It took some time for me grasp the power of that approach, and I suspect that Velick was at first skeptical about the ready availability and purity of the isolated antibodies. But once the spectral overlap between tryptophan fluorescence emission and the absorption spectrum of the principal DNP ligands was appreciated, Velick carried out the first fluorometric titration of anti-DNP antibodies with e-DNP-lysine. The quenching of the antibodies' fluorescence by the bound DNP-hapten was dramatic, and it was immediately evident that the antibody we were dealing with had exceptionally high affinity for the DNP ligand, about 10,000-fold higher than the affinity of the anti-DNP antibodies (and the anti-benzenearsonate antibodies) we had analyzed previously in New York. Those antibodies had been elicited by immunization procedures then in vogue, which relied on injections of large amounts of alum-precipitated DNP (or Razo-) proteins.

AFFINITY MATURATION

Because fluorescence-quenching titrations required small amounts of antibody and could be carried out rapidly, it was possible for Gregory Siskind, who later came as a visitor to the lab, to analyze many samples of antibody isolated at different times after injecting rabbits with various quantities of antigen. The results revealed clearly that over time, after small amounts of antigen were injected, there was a progressive increase in the antibodies' affinity for ε-DNP-lysine, the ideal surrogate for the principal epitope of the immunizing protein.

It had long been known that after immunization antisera increased in "avidity" over time, i.e., in the stability of the complexes they formed with the antigen. But with conventional protein antigens, having various epitopes per molecule, increasing stability of the antibody-antigen complexes formed with antisera could come about for a variety of reasons, such as increasing diversity of the recognized epitopes. This complexity had led some to recommend that the term avidity be abandoned altogether because it could not be clearly defined. Even in Jerne's classic study of antisera neutralization of diphtheria toxin, where increasing stability over time was evident, the binding was complicated, the number and variety of epitopes per molecule of antigen (toxin) were unknown, and the antitoxin molecules were also not univalent. With small ligands such as ε-DNP-lysine, however it was clear that the antibodies' intrinsic affinities were measured. That the antibodies appearing initially and those appearing later differed in intrinsic affinity for the same ligand thus provided unambiguous evidence that the antibody binding sites changes over time. The progressive changes, later termed affinity maturation by Siskind and Benacerraf, were subsequently seen to occur with antibodies made against various other haptenic groups. The changes, together with the later finding of somatic hypermutation of antibody genes by Milstein, Berek, Rajewsky and others, provided a coherent (though still gross) view of how antigen recognition, as reflected in affinity for epitopes, can serve as a potent driving force for immune responses.

When clonal selection was first advanced it rested, many of us thought, on pretty skimpy evidence. Several direct attempts to "falsify" it (in the sense used by Hans Popper)—by determining whether single antibody-forming cells could produce two (or more) distinctly different antibodies—had yielded contradictory results. Affinity maturation did not really distinguish between this and the antigen template theory, which, for a very short time, could be viewed as a competing paradigm. Clonal selection provided an obvious explanation for affinity maturation, with progressively diminishing levels of antigen after immunization leading to increasingly selective stimulation of cells ("clones") making the higher affinity antibody. However, the serum antibody changes could also be explained by a treadmill mechanism, in which the affinities of the antibodies synthesized over time did not really change—it may have been that only the average affinity of serum antibodies increased as the levels of free antigen available to selectively bind and remove high affinity antibodies diminished over time. The treadmill possibility was ruled out when Lisa Steiner joined the lab and showed that the antigen-binding activity of antibodies synthesized by isolated lymph node cells, collected at various times after immunization, paralleled changes in the intrinsic affinity of serum antibodies. Her additional finding that antibodies synthesized promptly in a secondary (memory) response to the antigen had the same high affinity as those made many months after the primary response was initiated were especially telling: They could be easily explained by clonal selection but not by the template theory.

Although cellular immunologists embraced clonal selection without a second thought, some immunochemists fought a rearguard action against it, finding the supporting evidence too skimpy. One of the battlegrounds was the heterogeneity of serum antibodies: Though an "average" intrinsic affinity could be assigned to purified anti-hapten antibodies, innumerable experiments had shown that virtually all preparations behaved as though they were mixtures of molecules having different affinities for a common ligand. According to clonal selection, the mixtures were obviously the polyclonal products of diverse antibody-producing clones responding to the same antigen. But to many immunochemists this heterogeneity was seen to reflect sloppiness in the folding of nascent antibody molecules (around an antigen-template), or even as an artefact, the result of inhomogeneity in the hapten-protein conjugates used to elicit antibody production (i.e., with haptenic groups substituted in diverse amino acid residues of the carrier protein). We had found earlier that, even with a homogeneous DNP-protein as antigen [having a single DNP group attached to a specified residue (lysine 41) in bovine pancreatic ribonuclease], the elicited anti-DNP antibodies were just as heterogeneous in affinity for DNP-lysine as were the antibodies raised against conventional heterogeneous DNP-proteins antigens. Our results were published only in a Harvey Lecture, and we naively assumed they would settle the matter. But, as they were not in a peer-reviewed journal, they may have been overlooked. In any case, some skilled immunochemists subsequently wasted much effort ingeniously constructing homogeneous antigens.

MYELOMA PROTEINS AS HOMOGENEOUS (MONOCLONAL) ANTIBODIES

If the polyclonal explanation were correct, the antibody molecules produced by a single clone should bind the antigen with uniform affinity. The only candidates available at the time for such a test were myeloma proteins. Secreted by myeloma (plasma cell) tumors, they had the same basic heavy- and light-chain structure as antibodies, but even so, many, even Rod Porter, the astute discoverer of the multichain structure of immunoglobulins, regarded them as abnormal "paraproteins" because they were made by abnormal (cancer) cells. Given the enormous number of different antigens and the prevailing idea that an antibody recognizes a single epitope, or a few similar ones, the chances of finding a myeloma protein that specifically bound any particular epitope were expected to be extremely small. We nevertheless undertook the search because an attractive means for rapidly screening serum samples from individuals carrying myeloma tumors could be visualized.

DNP amino acids undergo a prominent "red" spectral shift when bound to anti-DNP antibodies, probably because of so-called charge-transfer complexes formed by the bound ligand with a tryptophan residue in or very close to the antibody binding site. The shift appeared to be a distinctive marker for anti-DNP antibody binding sites in general, since we had consistently seen it with these antibodies from diverse sources (rabbits, guinea pigs, chickens, etc). When, however, a DNP amino acid bound to serum albumin, the abundant serum protein that binds (weakly) a great many different ligands, the absorption spectrum shifted in the opposite direction (to the "blue"). Thus, it seemed that simple spectrophotometric readings of myeloma serum samples to which DNP-lysine had been added would quickly reveal whether this ligand was bound to a myeloma protein that behaved like an antibody.

The opportunity to test this screening procedure turned up unexpectedly when Arthur Kornberg and the entire faculty in the Department of Microbiology moved from Washington University to Stanford. I was offered the chairmanship of the Washington Department with the tough mandate to rebuild it, but I welcomed the chance to move from a clinical to a preclinical department. One of the unexpected rewards of making the move was that I inherited a number of instruments that the former department members had chosen not to take with them, including an elegant double-beam Cary spectrophotometer. With the aid of that instrument and specially constructed cuvettes, it was possible to test a myeloma serum in a couple of minutes. The screening required a large number of serum samples, of course, and fortunately these were generously made available by Kurt Osterland, who had for years been collecting them from patients with myeloma tumors. When the screening got underway, we anticipated, as noted above, that we would be lucky to find one out of perhaps a thousand with the desired properties. Instead, one turned up within the first twenty tested. The active serum, called BRY (after the patient's family name) came from a patient who had left the hospital and was gone without a trace, and only three ml of her serum was available in Osterland's collection. That was sufficient to isolate enough of the myeloma protein (an IgG1 molecule) to show that it had two binding sites per molecule, one in each Fab fragment, and that DNP lysine bound to it in the same way as to conventional anti-DNP antibodies. It differed however in one important respect: The binding affinity was clearly homogeneous, unlike the heterogeneity that characterized all of the innumerable samples of anti-DNP antibodies isolated from immunized animals. The results supported other mounting evidence for the "one cell-one antibody" rule, the keystone of the clonal selection hypothesis.

AN EMBARRASSING ERROR

When the results with the human myeloma protein were presented at the 1967 Cold Spring Harbor Symposium (the first one devoted to immunology), Mike Potter offered to provide our screening program with serum from mice, in his large collection, carrying diverse myeloma tumors. Out of the first approximately 100 sera tested, two anti-DNP myeloma proteins were identified. The first one, MOPC-315, bound e-DNP-lysine strongly, and as the tumor was readily transplantable into normal BALB/c mice, large amounts of this monoclonal antibody could be expected and indeed were eventually produced. The paper describing its properties carried a triumphal note, but it was disturbing to realize shortly after publication that it had a couple of significant errors. I describe these in some detail below because they illustrate the self-correcting character that is inherent in the scientific enterprise. This aspect of science seems at times to be utterly incomprehensible to journalists, politicians, and the public at large—as I was to find out painfully many years later when enmeshed in the notorious case of alleged scientific fraud involving David Baltimore and Theresa Imanishi-Kari.

Based on peptide fingerprints, MOPC-315 was reported to have a kappa light chain. The error came about because Potter, a coauthor, had previously prepared fingerprints of several lambda light chains and seen that they were all were similar to each other but were distinctly unlike MOPC-315's light chain; hence the latter was considered to be a kappa chain, the only other light chain type known at the time. Ultimately this protein's light chain proved to be the first example of an uncommon lambda chain type, designated lambda-2. The other error was mine and less forgivable. To determine MOPC-315's affinity for DNP-lysine we had used especially small plastic chambers designed to carry out equilibrium dialysis with extremely small (50 μl) volumes and fabricated in our department's machine shop. Using the new chambers we found that the amount of radiolabeled ligand bound at saturation corresponded consistently to about 1.2 moles ligand per mole myeloma protein (antibody). As the number of sites had to be an integral number and was definitely not two, we concluded that it was one, i.e., that this ostensibly monoclonal antibody was univalent! The result was especially disconcerting because of the role Karush and I had played in establishing that antibodies are bivalent, which by then (about 15 years later) was universally accepted. But to some skeptics the apparent univalency confirmed their suspicion that myeloma proteins were indeed "paraproteins" and differed from conventional antibodies. That there really were two binding sites per molecule of myeloma protein, however, and not one as reported, became clear some time later when higher concentrations of MOPC-315 and of another anti-DNP myeloma protein had to be used in the small plastic chambers (to measure the equilibrium binding of weakly bound ligands), and the new results clearly pointed to two sites per molecule for each of these proteins. It then became apparent that some protein (with its bound ligand) was lost by adsorption to the chambers' plastic walls during the equilibration period. Though small in amount, the proportion of adsorbed protein was significant when low concentrations of protein were introduced (as in the initial report) but negligible when high protein concentrations were used. To have been unaware that proteins bind to many plastic surfaces was particularly embarassing because "solid phase" assays for antibodies and antigens were being introduced at about that time and their effectiveness was known to derive from the firm binding of trace amounts of proteins to plastic surfaces.

What was done about the errors, once they were discovered? They were not publicized with great fanfare as errata or by letters of correction to the journals, as was later indignantly demanded by critics of the senior authors in the Baltimore case. Instead, the corrections were simply incorporated into later publications, along with other findings, as part of the normal self-correcting process.

IDIOTYPES OF MYELOMA PROTEINS AS TUMOR-SPECIFIC ANTIGENS

Since each myeloma protein was expected to have a unique antigen-binding site or idiotype, the question arose as to whether MOPC-315, which had its origin in a BALB/c mouse, could stimulate the other mice of this genetically uniform strain to produce antibodies to protein 315's idiotype. At the time Stitaya Sirishina was traveling in the United States on a Rockefeller Foundation fellowship with a view toward reorganizing the Department of Microbiology at the Mahidol University in Thailand. He became interested in the idiotype question and turned what was to be a brief visit into a prolonged stay, during which he showed that mice injected with anti-DNP myeloma proteins produced antibodies that were evidently specifically "anti-idiotypes," since their reactivity with the corresponding myeloma protein was blocked by DNP-compounds.

A myeloma protein's idiotype corresponds literally to a tumor-specific antigen, since it is uniquely a product of the tumor that produces it. But the protein is copiously secreted by the tumor cells, and it was not clear that enough of it was present on the surface of tumor cells to result in their destruction by the anti-idiotypic antibodies. Despite the uncertainty, Dick Lynch, then a postdoc in the lab, injected MOPC-315 cells into mice that had been immunized with purified protein 315. In nearly all mice, tumors failed to grow out. And in the few animals in which the tumors eventually appeared, they proved to be idiotype negative because they had ceased to produce the myeloma protein's heavy chain. Similar results were obtained with another hapten-specific myeloma protein, MOPC-460 (but not to a third one, of unknown specificity). Kristian Hannestad, who came as a sabbatical visitor, studied the problem further; on returning to Tromso, Norway, he and his colleagues continued to analyze the rejection mechanism. It is far more complex than was originally visualized: They have shown that T cells recognize peptides from a segment of light chain that contributes to the myeloma protein's ligand-binding site and that these T cells seem to be responsible for tumor cell destruction. The anti-idiotype approach was later extended by others to humans with B cell lymphomas, evidently with some occasional benefits.

THE FREQUENCY OF LIGAND-BINDING MYELOMA PROTEINS

The finding of several myeloma proteins with considerable affinity for nitrophenyl groups among the small number of myeloma sera screened was (and is) not expected because of the general view that (i) each individual produces an enormous number of different antibodies, and (ii) the reactivity of each antibody appears to be highly restricted to one antigen (and a few similar ones). To test the alternative possibility—that an antibody can bind more promiscuously to a variety of disparate epitopes—we chose, more or less at random, a large number of organic molecules (the aim was 57, the number appearing in a popular advertisement for the Heinz food company) to determine if any of them could inhibit the binding of a radiolabeled DNP ligand to MOPC-315. Several competitors were found by Maria Michaelides, the most active being menadione or vitamine K3 (2-methyl-1,4-naphthaquinone). It turned out that this ligand was also bound by several conventionally produced polyclonal antibodies to various dinitrophenyl- and trinitrophenyl-protein antigens, indicating a vague match in structure, corresponding to what was later labeled molecular mimicry by Oldstone. Several others examples of such "strange" cross reactions by antibodies, usually encountered serendipitously, have been noted. But with the advent of Milstein's and Kohler's powerful procedure for generating monoclonal antibodies, the extent to which individual myeloma proteins and conventional antibodies react with many disparate epitopes ceased to be of interest. Whether individual antibody-producing cells, B cells, can react with diverse antigens is an issue we revisit at the end of this chapter.

One of the unexpected benefits of studying hapten-specific myeloma proteins emerged from the efforts of David Givol and colleagues at the Weizmann Institute. While analyzing a pepsin digest of MOPC-315 with its bound ligand (a yellow DNP amino acid), they found an unusually small yellow fragment, its color indicating that it retained the ligand. The fragment proved to consist only of noncovalently associated variable domains of the light and heavy chains ($V_L + V_H$). Called Fv, it accounted for all the hapten-binding activity of the intact protein. Single chain Fv recombinant proteins, made with V_L and V_H linked covalently by a flexible, short polypeptide chain, were subsequently prepared by many others from various monoclonal antibodies for use as potential therapeutic agents (e.g., linked to a toxic protein in so-called immunotoxins).

A MOVE TO MIT AND T CELLS

I joined the Center for Cancer Research at the Massachusetts Institute of Technology (MIT) when it opened in 1973. Salvator Luria, its founding director and guiding spirit, had written to me about a role for immunology in the Center and our correspondence led to an offer to join it. This came at a time when I was having to spend much time and energy on medical school administrative affairs and was eager to become again more fully immersed in the laboratory. The offer was attractive moreover because MIT was close to Woods Hole (on Cape Cod), where our family had enjoyed summer vacations for many years. And so, after having experienced academic life only in medical schools for over 30 years, and having particularly enjoyed it at Washington University, I found myself transplanted into a totally different academic scene. At MIT science was everywhere. The Cancer Center was an integral part of the Biology Department, and both were populated by a remarkable group of talented and energetic faculty. And in the Harvard-MIT Program for Health Sciences and Technology, with which I was associated for a time, interesting interactions with colleagues in physics and chemistry and the engineering sciences were commonplace. MIT seemed a form of scientific heaven. And, reinforced by the opening of the closely affiliated Whitehead Institute a few years ago, it still does as I write this 27 years later.

At MIT our interests in antigen recognition gradually shifted from antibodies to T cells. When the distinction between B and T cells first became apparent (in the early 1960s), it greatly excited cellular immunologists. The excitement was not shared by most chemically-minded immunologists, who initially were disdainful of what they perceived as a lack of rigor. A prominent immunochemist friend once asked me gleefully if I was aware that B and T were the first and last letters of b ... t, the ubiquitous barnyard substance. It was clear, nevertheless, that T cells could transfer delayed type hypersensitivity (DTH) skin reactions from sensitized to normal recipient animals, indicating that T cells expressed antigen-specific receptors (T cell receptors or TCR) and that T cell–mediated reactions could be as specific as those due to antibodies. For example, I had been sensitized by 2,4-dinitrofluorobenzene, as noted above, and I responded to patch tests on my own skin to various nitrobenzenes only if they formed 2,4-dinitrophenyl derivatives of skin proteins in situ (in guinea pigs), but not if the derivatives were 2, 6-dinitrophenyl or 2,4,6-trinitrophenyl.

T CELL CLONES

When procedures became available for generating mouse T cell clones and growing them in culture with retention of normal function for prolonged periods, the temptation to study antigen recognition by these cells became irresistible. We concentrated on CD8 T cells primarily because they could kill cancer cells rapidly in test tube assays. For a time each new postdoctoral fellow coming to the lab was asked to generate T cell clones. Many were produced, and we concentrated on those clones that grew readily and could be maintained in culture for years.

One of the better clones was called 2C. Generated initially by Mischa Sitkovsky, then a recent immigrant from the Soviet Union, it was nurtured and developed by

David Kranz, who also generated a monoclonal antibody that reacted exclusively with the TCR on 2C cells. These cells served as the basis for a collaborative effort with Susumu Tonegawa that resulted in cloning the genes for the α and β subunits of the clone's TCR, shortly after genes for TCR β subunits had been cloned independently by Mark Davis and Tak Mak. The initial paper describing the complete primary structure of the 2C TCR was written rapidly with Tonegawa et al and appeared in print (in *Nature*) around a month after the manuscript was started. Carrying a triumphal note as the first complete sequence of both the α and β subunits of a TCR (the 2C TCR), the paper could serve as a model for how speed, borne of unrestrained competiveness, can lead to major errors: What the paper called the α gene turned out to code for a subunit (γ) of what was soon realized to be part of the $\gamma\delta$ TCR on a special small T cell subset, called $\gamma\delta$ T cells, having quite different functions. The β gene described was also not the correct one for the 2C TCR. Eventually, however, the correct α and β genes for the TCR on the 2C clone were established with Kranz's help when Sha, in Dennis Loh's lab at Washington University Medical School, expressed them as transgenes in mice.

ANTIGEN RECOGNITION BY A T CELL

What does the 2C TCR recognize? Following the Zinkernagle and Doherty finding that MHC proteins "restrict" antigen recognition by T cells, and the findings by Unanue and Townsend and others that short peptides arising as proteolytic fragments from proteins, intracellular or other, associate with the MHC, it was evident that TCR generally recognize peptide-MHC complexes in which the MHC component restricts recognition of the peptide. When the 2C clone was first derived, it was readily apparent that its TCR recognized Ld, a non-self (or allogeneic) class I MHC protein present on the cells used to immunize mice that lacked this particular protein. But identification of the peptide associated with Ld required the heroic efforts of Keiko Udaka and Ted Tsomides, who systematically analyzed the myriad of peptides in mouse spleen extracts, separating them chromatographically (by HPLC) and painstakingly identifying active fractions by the cytolytic responses of 2C cells. From spleens of around 1000 mice they ultimately purified two peptides. Their overlapping amino acid sequences led to the identity of their source, which turned out to be a mitochondrial "housekeeping" protein (α keto-glutarate dehydrogenase), expressed in all cells.

As with virtually all T cells, the 2C TCR also has to recognize an indigenous (self) MHC protein in order to complete its maturation in the thymus. For T cells expressing the 2C TCR, this self-MHC was shown to be Kb in breeding experiments with 2C transgenic mice. This TCR can thus recognize peptide-Kb as well as peptide-Ld complexes, including those in which the same peptide (from α keto-glutarate dehydrogenase) is associated with Ld and Kb. Some years later, Tallquist and Pease identified another peptide, from a different mitochondrial protein, that is recognized by the 2C TCR in association with Kb.

DEGENERACY IN ANTIGEN RECOGNITION BY 2C T CELLS

How many other peptide-MHC complexes do 2C cells recognize? The recognition of complexes by a TCR is easily evaluated from the responses of CD8 T cells to target cells that express a restricting MHC protein and are incubated with various synthetic peptides. By binding to the MHC, the peptides form peptide-MHC complexes on the target cells. If the complexes are recognized by cytolytic T cells the target cells are destroyed. Simple cytolytic assays of this kind have determined that the 2C TCR can recognize a great many different peptide-MHC complexes involving at least 12 peptides (some with overlapping sequences) in association with two restricting MHC proteins (Kb and Ld). They also respond to another MHC protein, from a third MHC locus (H-2^r), probably in association with still other peptides. It also appears from the maturation of these cells in mice lacking classical class I MHC proteins that they can recognize a class I MHC of the so-called nonclassical type, which possibly binds some glycolipids instead of short peptides in its binding groove. The ability to recognize and respond to so many different structures warrants a distinct term and degeneracy seems appropriate. Degeneracy has been seen previously to various extents, as in reactions attributed to molecular mimicry by Oldstone and in Wucherpfenig's and Strominger's elegant study with T cells that react with a peptide from myelin basic protein as well as many viral peptides. There is no good reason to doubt that many other TCR would exhibit similar degrees of degeneracy if examined thoroughly.

T CELLS CAN DISCRIMINATE SHARPLY BETWEEN SIMILAR STRUCTURES

Although 2C T cells exhibit much degeneracy, they can also display exquisite specificity in discriminating between very similar epitopes. For example, these T cells lyse target cells presenting a particular peptide-MHC complex, call it A, but not the same target cells that present the same number of a slightly different complex, call it A', where A and A' bind equally well to the MHC molecule and where the difference between A and A' is a single O atom resulting from a phenylalanine-tyrosine substitution in the peptide. This sharp selectivity by the TCR matches the high degree of specificity seen in the most discriminating reactions of antibodies or enzymes.

SPECIFICITY VERSUS DEGENERACY

How can a single TCR display exquisite specificity in some reactions and such extensive degeneracy in others? An explanation for specificity is not hard to discern. Specificity, the capacity to discriminate between two similar structures, depends not only on the difference in strength (call it affinity) of the two reactions but on how they are detected. Since all detection systems have a threshold, below which reactions cannot be detected, a pair of ligands whose strengths of reaction straddle the threshold can be sharply distinguished. This, in fact, is the situation with the above cited example of the A and A' epitopes that differ only by a phenylalanine-tyrosine substitution (i.e., by 1 O atom): Epitope (A), which elicits target cell lysis, has the lowest affinity measureable for a TCR-epitope reaction (about $3 \times 10^3 \text{ M}^{-1}$), which is probably at the threshold, and for epitope A' the affinity is probably just below the threshold.

Degeneracy is more intriguing because of its implications for the hypothesis that has served as the guiding paradigm for immunology over the past 40 years. The degenerate and specific reactions we are referring to here have been detected primarily by cytolytic assays. The extent of target cell destruction in these assays depends not only upon their displaying a peptide-MHC complex (epitope) that is recognized by the TCR, but upon the number of copies of epitope per target cell ("epitope density"). It also depends upon the affinity of the TCR for the epitope (i.e., on the equilibrium constant for the TCR-epitope reaction). And from studies carried out with Yuri Sykulev, Richard Cohen, and Ted Tsomides, it appears that high epitope densities are required for low-affinity reactions while low epitope densities suffice for high-affinity reactions, where affinity refers explicitly to the equilibrium constant for the binding of a peptide-MHC complex (epitope) to the TCR. This inverse relationship calls to mind the law of mass action, the fundamental rule for reversible chemical reactions in solution, although the application of this law to reactions between the TCR and peptide-MHC complexes, each embedded in a cell surface membrane, requires assumptions that are doubtless overly simplistic.

ONE CELL—MANY SPECIFICITIES

The central principle of the clonal selection hypothesis, the "1 cell–1 antibody" rule, has been repeatedly confirmed. It has been extended, almost subliminally, to mean "1 cell–1 specificity" because an antibody molecule characteristically reacts, as ordinarily measured, with a single antigen and a few structurally similar ones. For T cells, the corresponding 1 cell–1 TCR rule is also correct (although some T cells can have two TCR owing to the absence of allelic exclusion for the α subunit of $\alpha\beta$ TCR). However, the responsiveness of T cells to diverse epitopes indicates that the "1 cell–1 specificity" rule for these cells is inappropriate. A more reasonable slogan would be "1 cell–many specificities," with the magnitude of "many" still to be determined.

WHY T CELLS EXHIBIT MORE DEGENERACY THAN ANTIBODIES

Given the great structural similarity between antibodies and TCR, why should T cells, via their TCR, display so much more degeneracy than antibodies? The likely answer (aside from the possibility that TCR binding sites are more flexible and conformationally adaptable to ligands than are antibody binding sites) is that very few of the many TCR molecules on a T cell's surface (perhaps only one or two out of around 100,000) have to be initially engaged in a stable TCR-epitope complex to trigger a T cell response. This great sensitivity stems from powerful amplification effects of signal transduction. Moreover, the capacity to recognize— i.e., to respond to—so many different epitopes reflects the importance of epitope density on antigen presenting cells. At a sufficiently high epitope density, even a very weakly recognized epitope can generate enough stable complexes with the TCR to trigger a T cell response.

ARE B CELLS SIMILARLY DEGENERATE?

The foregoing view may also apply to B cells. An indication that they can exhibit degeneracy can be seen in the levels of serum proteins following injections of antigens in conventional immunization procedures. It has been observed that antisera have elevated levels of total globulin that greatly exceed the levels of the antibodies that react specifically, in conventional assays, with the administered antigen. It may be that Jerne, in proposing the anti-idiotype network, was influenced by this difference. A more likely explanation than an anti-idiotypic network is that B cell responses in vivo are substantially degenerate, as are the T cell responses considered above. Thus, administration of an antigen (call it X) results in stimulating not only those B cells whose secreted Igs function as recognizable anti-X antibodies, but probably also many other B cells, whose secreted Ig molecules have too low an affinity for X to qualify as anti-X antibodies. When normal B cell clones become available, it may be feasible to test this possibility.

We have been told intermittently over the past thirty years that the end of the quest to understand the immune system is in sight. A distinguished immunologist was recently quoted in the *New York Times* as having said that we are within "a whisper" of understanding the immune system. The current level of understanding is indeed truly impressive. Monumental is not too much of an exaggeration, compared to the level of understanding in evidence at the first meeting of the American Immunologists I attended in 1949: There were about 50 or 60 people in attendance out of the total membership at that time of about 250. Yet, current efforts to engage the immune system to protect against cancers or the AIDS pandemic or malaria or tuberculosis, or to suppress the often devastating effects of autoimmunity, are still glaringly ineffectual. They stand as a stark reminder of how much more remains to be understood and effectively applied.

References were omitted here to conserve space. Anyone interested in the publications referred to in this article can find them at the following web site: http://web.mit.edu/biology/www/Ar/eisen.html (click on References).

Annu. Rev. Immunol. 2001. 19:23–45

IN VIVO ACTIVATION OF ANTIGEN-SPECIFIC CD4 T CELLS

Marc K. Jenkins[1], Alexander Khoruts[2], Elizabeth Ingulli[3], Daniel L. Mueller[2], Stephen J. McSorley[1], R. Lee Reinhardt[1], Andrea Itano[1], and Kathryn A. Pape[1]

[1]*Department of Microbiology, Center for Immunology, University of Minnesota Medical School, Minneapolis, MN 55455; e-mail: marcj@mail.ahc.umn.edu, mcsor001@tc.umn.edu, reinhard@lenti.med.umn.edu, itano001@c.umn.edu, pape001@tc.umn.edu*

[2]*Department of Medicine, Center for Immunology, University of Minnesota Medical School, Minneapolis, MN 55455; e-mail: khoru001@tc.umn.edu, dmuell@lenti.med.edu*

[3]*Department of Pediatrics, Center for Immunology, University of Minnesota Medical School, Minneapolis, MN 55455; e-mail: ingul001@tc.umn.edu*

Key Words CD4 T cells, in vivo immune response, immunological memory, dendritic cells

■ **Abstract** Physical detection of antigen-specific CD4 T cells has revealed features of the in vivo immune response that were not appreciated from in vitro studies. In vivo, antigen is initially presented to naïve CD4 T cells exclusively by dendritic cells within the T cell areas of secondary lymphoid tissues. Anatomic constraints make it likely that these dendritic cells acquire the antigen at the site where it enters the body. Inflammation enhances in vivo T cell activation by stimulating dendritic cells to migrate to the T cell areas and display stable peptide-MHC complexes and costimulatory ligands. Once stimulated by a dendritic cell, antigen-specific CD4 T cells produce IL-2 but proliferate in an IL-2–independent fashion. Inflammatory signals induce chemokine receptors on activated T cells that direct their migration into the B cell areas to interact with antigen-specific B cells. Most of the activated T cells then die within the lymphoid tissues. However, in the presence of inflammation, a population of memory T cells survives. This population is composed of two functional classes. One recirculates through nonlymphoid tissues and is capable of immediate effector lymphokine production. The other recirculates through lymph nodes and quickly acquires the capacity to produce effector lymphokines if stimulated. Therefore, antigenic stimulation in the presence of inflammation produces an increased number of specific T cells capable of producing effector lymphokines throughout the body.

0732-0582/01/0407-0023$14.00

INTRODUCTION

The adaptive immune response is the result of interactions between foreign substances and the host's antigen receptor–bearing lymphocytes and antigen-presenting cells (APC). These interactions take place in several complex microenvironments within the body and play out over a period of several weeks, with the end result being elimination of the foreign substance. The complexity of the immune response is so daunting that reductionist approaches have been necessary to understand the interacting parts. In vitro culture systems, cloned cell lines, purified lymphokines, and synthetic peptide antigens have contributed to our current understanding that CD4 T cells produce lymphokines and proliferate when their T cell antigen receptors bind to an APC displaying the appropriate peptide–class II MHC molecule and costimulatory ligands (1, 2).

However, reductionist approaches may now be limiting our ability to understand and manipulate the in vivo immune response. The long-term T cell clones and transformed cells lines often used in vitro may not behave like naïve or memory T cells that participate in the in vivo immune response. Disruption of lymphoid tissues to produce the single cell suspensions required for in vitro cultures destroys the spatial relationships between T cells and APC that exist in vivo and separates the cells from factors produced by the lymphoid stroma. In vitro cultures cannot be used to study the critically important process whereby T cells migrate from lymphoid sites of initial activation to nonlymphoid sites of antigen deposition. Perhaps the greatest limitation of in vitro culture systems, however, is that they do not replicate the effect that inflammation has on the in vivo T cell response. It has been known for many years that adjuvants, and the inflammatory mediators that they induce, influence the quality of the T cell response to foreign antigen. Injection of foreign antigen with an adjuvant induces robust humoral and cell-mediated immune responses, whereas injection of foreign antigen alone does not (3). Furthermore, injection of purified foreign antigen in the absence of inflammation induces a state of unresponsiveness to subsequent immunization with antigen plus adjuvant (4, 5). To date, the fundamental capacity of inflammation to dictate T cell immunity or tolerance cannot be replicated in vitro.

Recently, several approaches have been developed that allow the physical tracking of T cells of known peptide-MHC specificity within the body during in vivo immune responses. These approaches have shed light on in vivo antigen presentation, T cell proliferation, death, migration, tolerance induction, and memory cell generation. This review focuses on these new findings with an emphasis on unique features of the in vivo response that were not appreciated in cell culture studies. In addition, the steps in the in vivo CD4 T cell activation process that are regulated by inflammation are discussed.

METHODS FOR TRACKING ANTIGEN-SPECIFIC CD4 T CELLS IN VIVO

Past attempts to study the T cell response in vivo relied on functional tests to enumerate the number of cells present. Limiting dilution analyses of antigen-driven proliferation or cell-mediated cytotoxicity produced estimates of the frequency of antigen-specific T cells present at various times after introduction of antigen into the host (6). The limitation of this approach is that T cells must undergo many cell divisions and survive for several weeks in culture to be scored in the assay. Furthermore, the cells must perform the function being measured. Antigen-specific T cells that do not survive well in vitro, or are not, for example, cytotoxic, are missed with this type of assay. The frequency with which antigen-specific T cells produce a given lymphokine in response to in vitro stimulation with antigen has been determined by the enzyme-linked immunospot assay (7). The sensitivity of this assay is comparable to flow cytometric detection of antigen-specific T cells using fluorochrome-labeled peptide-MHC multimers when the T cells under study have been primed in a such a way that all antigen-specific T cells produce the lymphokine being measured (8). However, this is not always the case, and in these situations, enzyme-linked immunospot assay underestimates the frequency of antigen-specific T cells (9).

The solution to this problem has come from methods that allow physical detection of T cells based solely on TCR specificity. The most direct method relies on fluorochrome-labeled, multimeric peptide-MHC complexes. One version of this approach involves refolding soluble, empty, class I MHC molecules with a single antigenic peptide. The peptide-MHC complex is then biotinylated and mixed with a streptavidin-labeled fluorochrome to produce a tetramer (10). This tetramer binds to CD8 T cells that express an appropriate TCR. The strength of this approach is that it can theoretically measure all potentially responsive T cells in the normal repertoire. A weakness is that the frequency of T cells specific for most peptide-MHC complexes in naïve individuals is below the limit of detection of flow cytometry (8, 11, 12). Thus, peptide-MHC multimers cannot currently be used to study the immune response before clonal expansion occurs. Another weakness is that peptide–class II MHC tetramers are more difficult to prepare because the peptide must be covalently attached to the class II MHC molecule (13).

A second method is based on the knowledge that ~70% of the CD4 T cells that respond to the pigeon cytochrome c peptide 81-104 in mice that express H-2 I-E^k possess a TCR containing a characteristic TCR-Vα chain and CDR3 region on the TCR-Vβ chain (14). Because the system is used to track the normal T cell repertoire, it has the same strengths and weaknesses as peptide-MHC multimer-based detection: The entire repertoire of pigeon cytochrome c peptide-I-E^k-specific CD4 T cells can theoretically be tracked but, because of the infrequency of naïve precursors, only after clonal expansion.

One way to solve the technical problem of the infrequency of naïve T cells with a single specificity is adoptive transfer of naïve TCR transgenic T cells into syngeneic normal recipients (15). This maneuver produces a traceable naïve T cell population of known peptide-MHC specificity within the recipient, comprising 0.5–1% of cells in the secondary lymphoid organs. The transferred cells can be distinguished from those of the recipient with antibodies specific for the TCR clonotype or an allelic marker such as Thy 1 or CD45. One advantage of this method is that the earliest events in T cell activation in vivo can be studied because the antigen-specific T cells are abundant enough to be detected by flow cytometry or immunohistology before clonal expansion. A potential disadvantage is that even though only a small number of T cells is transferred, the resulting frequency of antigen-specific T cells is still higher than normal. Although all of the effects of this elevated frequency are unknown, the kinetics and relative magnitude of clonal expansion and loss reported for transferred T cells after in vivo exposure to antigen are identical to those described for endogenous T cells tracked by the two methods described above (15).

LOCATION OF NAÏVE T CELLS

Most studies of the earliest events in the T cell activation process in vivo have focused on the secondary lymphoid organs (lymph nodes, spleen, and Peyer's patches) because a variety of methods have shown that naïve CD4 T cells are found primarily, if not exclusively, in these tissues (16–18). Naïve CD4 T cells are further restricted within secondary lymphoid organs to the T cell–rich areas known as the paracortex in the lymph nodes and Peyer's patches, and the periarteriolar lymphoid sheath (PALS) in the spleen (19) (Figure 1). The restriction to lymph nodes is explained by the fact that naïve T cells express a unique set of receptors, which bind ligands that are only expressed on the specialized blood vessels of the lymph nodes known as high endothelial venules (HEV). For example, naive T cells use CD62L for rolling on vessel walls, and CC chemokine receptor (CCR) 7 for integrin activation and extravasation (20). HEV are the only blood vessels in the body that display the ligands for these receptors (Glycam-1, CD34, SLC, and ELC) (20). Naïve T cells move from the blood into the spleen because all blood contents are emptied directly from terminal branches of the central arteriole into marginal sinuses and then the red pulp (19). The T cells then move from the red pulp into the PALS by a poorly understood CD62L-independent, G protein–dependent mechanism (21). Once in the PALS or paracortex, naïve T cells remain there in part because they express CCR7 and sense the SLC and ELC chemokines that are produced in the T cell areas (22). After spending about one day in the T cell areas, naïve T cells leave the lymphoid tissue in which they reside and return to blood to enter a different lymphoid tissue.

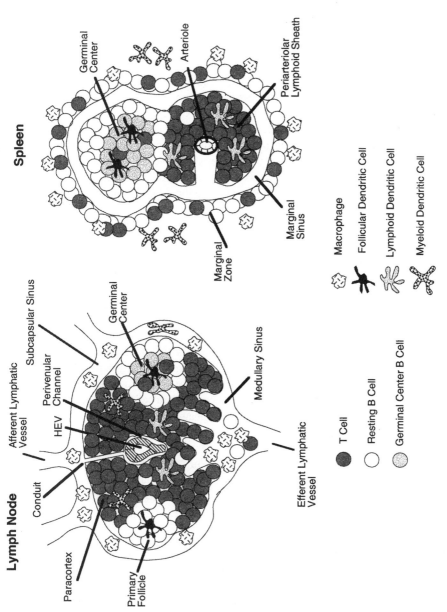

Figure 1   Schematic views of cross-sections through a lymph node and one splenic white pulp cord.

IN VIVO ANTIGEN PRESENTATION TO NAÏVE T CELLS

The restriction of naïve T cells to the T cell areas of secondary lymphoid organs implies that the APC that initiate the primary immune response must also be located there. This contention is supported by the finding that the earliest signs of activation in naïve T cells in vivo can be detected within an hour of antigen injection (23), a time when the cells are still in the T cell area (24). By far the most abundant class II MHC-expressing cell type in the T cell area is the dendritic cell (25). The other potential class II MHC-expressing APC for CD4 T cells, B cells, and macrophages are located outside of the T cell areas; B cells reside in follicles and macrophages in the subcapsular and medullary sinuses of lymph nodes and the red pulp and marginal zone of the spleen (19). Thus, the anatomy, and a wealth of in vitro experiments demonstrating their potency as APC for naïve T cells (25), suggests that dendritic cells are the APC that initiate in vivo T cell responses.

We obtained physical evidence supporting this hypothesis by staining lymph node sections from recipients of ovalbumin peptide-I-A^d-specific TCR transgenic T cells with a pan-dendritic cell-specific anti-CD11c antibody and an anti-clonotypic antibody specific for the transferred T cells, each labeled with a different fluorochrome (26). In the absence of ovalbumin, the transferred T cells were intermingled with dendritic cells in the paracortex of the lymph node, and many of the T cells were in physical contact with a dendritic cell. Within 16 h of subcutaneous injection of ovalbumin, the number of contacts and the average size of the contact area between the transferred T cells and dendritic cells increased three- to fourfold over the basal level. Antigen-dependent increases in interaction between the antigen-specific T cells and macrophages or B cells were not observed at these early times because these cells were not present in the T cell areas. Similarly, MacLennan and colleagues found that antigen-stimulated CD4 T cells first entered the cell cycle when associated with dendritic cells in the T cell areas (27). These results are consistent with the hypothesis that the initial antigen presentation to naïve CD4 T cells in vivo is carried out exclusively by dendritic cells. In vitro studies where cells from dissociated splenic tissue are used as APC do not replicate this phenomenon because B cells are by far the most abundant APC under these conditions.

Dendritic Cell Migration

The dendritic cells that were found interacting with antigen-specific T cells in the paracortex could have acquired soluble antigen from incoming lymph. Anatomic evidence suggests that this is probably not the case, however. Lymph is carried from tissues via afferent lymphatic vessels into the subcapsular sinus of a connected lymph node (19) (Figure 1). Cells appear to be capable of squeezing between the cells that make up the floor of this sinus and entering the regions occupied by T and B cells (28). Surprisingly, however, soluble molecules do not easily flow from the subcapsular sinus into the lymphocyte-rich areas of the lymph node. Tracers injected into afferent lymphatic vessels appear in the subcapsular sinus and in thin conduits that run through the lymphocyte-rich areas but not in the lymphocyte-rich areas themselves (28).

The inaccessibility of the T cell area to lymph-borne antigen raises the possibility that antigen is carried from the site of antigen deposition into the T cell area by a migrating dendritic cell. The T cell areas of the lymph nodes are occupied by two types of dendritic cells, one that expresses CD11b and is derived from the myeloid lineage and another that expresses DEC-205 and CD8α and is derived from the lymphoid lineage (29). Both types of dendritic cells probably originate in nonlymphoid tissues as one of several immature precursors. For example, the skin contains epidermal Langerhans cells and monocytes, both of which have been shown to migrate from nonlymphoid tissues into the T cell areas of the draining lymph node (30, 31). Langerhans cells express DEC-205 (32), whereas monocytes that migrate to the T cell areas acquire some of the phenotypic characteristics of dendritic cells, including high-level expression of MHC and B7, but lack DEC-205 and CD8α (31). These markers and results from several gene-targeting experiments (33, 34) indicate that lymphoid dendritic cells are derived from migrating Langerhans cells, whereas myeloid dendritic cells are derived from migrating monocytes. The finding that cells with the phenotype of myeloid dendritic cells can be grown in vitro from monocyte precursors in the presence of GM-CSF and IL-4 further supports the latter possibility (35). Preliminary results from our studies suggest that the dendritic cells that are interacting with antigen-specific CD4 T cells early after subcutaneous injection of intact ovalbumin are myeloid dendritic cells. This could be related to the fact that monocytes have better access to antigen in the subcutaneous tissue than do Langerhans cells or dermal dendritic cells. In contrast, antigens that enter the epidermis are probably carried to the T cell area and presented by Langerhans cells.

In contrast to the lymph nodes, tracer studies have shown that the T and B cell areas of the spleen are freely accessible to soluble antigen shortly after intravenous injection. Staining with a monoclonal antibody specific for a peptide-class II MHC complex derived from hen egg lysozyme (HEL) showed that most B cells in the follicles produced peptide-MHC complexes from HEL within several hours (36). However, peptide-MHC complexes were not detected on most of the dendritic cells in the T cell areas at this early time. Such complexes appeared eventually, first in the outer PALS and then throughout the PALS by 24 hr after HEL injection. This process is greatly enhanced in the presence of LPS-induced inflammation (37), as is the migration of myeloid dendritic cells from the marginal zone into the PALS (38). Therefore even in the absence of a physical barrier to free antigen, antigen presentation in the splenic T cell areas may be carried out by dendritic cells that acquire antigen outside of the T cell area. This implies that the resident lymphoid dendritic cells of the spleen are inefficient at antigen uptake or processing, perhaps as a result of prior maturation (39). However, antigen presentation by resident lymphoid dendritic cells cannot be ruled by this approach because it is unlikely that peptide-MHC-specific antibodies can detect the low number of peptide-MHC complexes that can trigger a T cell.

Dendritic Cell Maturation

The movement of dendritic cell precursors from nonlymphoid tissues or the marginal zone into the T cell areas is greatly enhanced by inflammation (38). Dendritic cell migration in the context of inflammation is associated with a functional maturation process involving changes in antigen processing and T cell stimulation potential (40). Freshly isolated Langerhans cells, or monocyte-derived dendritic cells grown in vitro with GM-CSF and IL-4, efficiently engulf particles including dying cells and large volumes of extracellular fluid and store the ingested material in unprocessed form in MIIC vesicles. Exposure to inflammatory mediators, such as LPS, causes these immature dendritic cells to produce peptide–class II MHC complexes and shuttle these complexes into CIIV vesicles that eventually fuse with the plasma membrane (41). Inflammation also reduces the turnover of peptide–class II MHC complexes on the surface of dendritic cells (42). This maturation process is likely a mechanism of adjuvant action. Inflammation caused by adjuvants would lead to much greater antigen presentation because many immature dendritic cells would migrate from the tissue of antigen deposition into the T cell area, and in the process mature to display more stable and abundant peptide-class II MHC complexes.

CLONAL EXPANSION

Naïve CD4 T cells proliferate in the T cell areas shortly after recognition of peptide-MHC complexes on dendritic cells (24, 27). This proliferation is evidenced by an increase in the number of antigen-specific CD4 T cells within the relevant secondary lymphoid organs, 3–7 days after antigen injection (14, 27, 43, 44). The magnitude of the clonal expansion is much greater if antigen is administered with an adjuvant (43). For example, naïve antigen-specific T cells increase 10–20-fold in number in the lymphoid tissue 3 days after subcutaneous injection of soluble ovalbumin, and 20–100-fold after injection of ovalbumin plus LPS (45) or unmethylated CpG-containing DNA (46).

Role of CD28

The effect of adjuvant-induced inflammation on T cell proliferation correlates with a preceding effect on lymphokine production. Approximately three times as many antigen-specific naïve CD4 T cells produce IL-2 in vivo 10 hr after subcutaneous injection of antigen plus LPS as do so after injection of antigen alone (47). The antigen-stimulated T cells must express CD28 to experience the enhancing effect of LPS on early IL-2 production and later clonal expansion (47). The requirement for CD28 is probably related in part to the capacity of LPS to stimulate B7 expression in dendritic cells (38) and to direct B7 molecules into the

CIIV vesicles containing peptide-MHC complexes (41), ensuring that the TCR and CD28 ligands are localized on the surface.

Role of IL-2

The correlation between clonal expansion and IL-2 production made it reasonable to suspect that the in vivo proliferation of antigen-stimulated T cells would be critically dependent on IL-2. This hypothesis was also supported by the finding that T cells from IL-2-deficient mice proliferate much less well in vitro than do T cells from normal mice in response to optimal TCR stimulation (48). Surprisingly, however, the TCR-driven clonal expansion of CD4 T cells lacking IL-2 (49) or components of the IL-2 receptor (50, 51) is minimally or not at all impaired in vivo. Moreover, the ability of LPS to enhance clonal expansion of naïve antigen-specific CD4 T cells is preserved in the absence of IL-2 (47). Therefore, other signals or growth factors must be capable of driving CD4 T cell proliferation in vivo, although IL-2 may contribute. As noted below, IL-2 plays an important role in the elimination of activated T cells. The dual function of IL-2, as both a T cell growth factor early in the response and a death factor later, may make it difficult to reveal the growth factor activity of IL-2 in IL-2-deficient animals.

Role of Inflammatory Cytokines

IL-1 or TNF-α mimic the enhancing effect of LPS on the in vivo expansion of antigen-stimulated T cells (45). These inflammatory cytokines may mediate this effect indirectly through CD28. Adjuvant molecules are recognized by pattern recognition receptors (52) on cells of the innate immune system, for example macrophages, at the antigen injection site, causing the release of TNF-α and IL-1. These cytokines may stimulate B7 expression on antigen-presenting dendritic cells, resulting in a greater level of CD28 signaling in interacting T cells. Anti-CD40 antibodies may mediate adjuvant effects by a similar B7-dependent mechanism (53). However, it is also likely that CD28 costimulation is involved in a direct effect of IL-1 or TNF-α on CD4 T cells. Support for this possibility comes from in vitro experiments that show that the proliferation of highly purified CD4 T cells in response to plastic surfaces coated with TCR and CD28 ligands is augmented by IL-1 (54, 55). Since IL-1 could not act on an APC in this experiment, it must have acted directly on the T cells.

FOLLICULAR MIGRATION

One of the most important functions of CD4 T cells is to recognize peptide-MHC complexes on antigen-specific B cells and provide help for antibody production. Because naïve T and B cells are anatomically separated from each other in the secondary lymphoid organs, one or both cell types must move if interaction is to take place. Recent work suggests that T and B cells specific for epitopes from the same antigen both move from their starting locations to meet at the border between the T and B cell areas (24, 56, 57). Nahm and coworkers provided the first evidence for the T cell movement by showing that CD4 T cells expressing MBP-specific TCR V segments appeared in the follicles of mice immunized with MBP (58). The basis for this phenomenon was identified in several tracking studies that showed that antigen-specific CD4 T cells migrate from the T cell area into the B cell–rich follicles, after first proliferating in the T cell area (43, 44, 59). The migration of activated CD4 T cells into follicles only occurred in mice that were injected with antigen and adjuvant (43, 45). This phenomenon is explained by regulated expression of chemokine receptors. Naïve T cells express CCR7, which is specific for chemokines produced by stromal cells in the T cell areas (SLC and ELC), but not CXCR5, which is specific for BLC produced by follicular stromal cells (22). Cyster and coworkers showed that CXCR5 expression is induced on antigen-specific T cells several days after in vivo exposure to antigen and adjuvant, but not antigen alone (60). The requirement for adjuvant may be explained by the findings of Lane and colleagues that CXCR5 induction and follicular migration are dependent on signals through CD28 and OX40, the ligands for which (B7 and OX40 ligand) are induced on dendritic cells by inflammation (61). Induction of CXCR5 on antigen-specific CD4 T cells correlates with a gain in the ability to migrate in response to BLC and loss of responsiveness to SLC and ELC (60). The predicted effect of these changes in chemokine receptor expression would be loss of retention in the T cell areas and directed movement toward the follicles.

ELIMINATION OF ACTIVATED T CELLS

The number of antigen-specific T cells in the lymphoid tissues falls dramatically after the peak of clonal expansion. Much of the loss must be due to cell death because the body would soon fill up with lymphocytes if this were not the case. However, there is confusion about the molecular basis for death because of conflicting results on the effects of death receptors and survival proteins. For example, the loss of antigen-stimulated T cells from the lymphoid tissue after the peak of clonal expansion has been shown to be Fas-dependent, bcl-2-insensitive in some studies (62) and Fas-independent, bcl-2-sensitive in others (63). Abbas and colleagues have proposed that these discrepancies are explained by the duration of antigen presentation (64). If antigen is presented transiently, perhaps because only a single antigen injection was given or the antigen under study has a short in vivo half-life, then the loss is caused by growth factor withdrawal. This type of apoptosis occurs via a Fas-independent, caspase-9-dependent pathway, which is antagonized by bcl-2 (65). This is a reasonable scenario because in vivo lymphokine production ceases at least one day before the beginning of the loss phase (47). If antigen is presented chronically, because of repeated injection or expression by the host, then Abbas and colleagues propose that activation-induced cell death occurs (64). This type of apoptosis is dependent on Fas and is poorly inhibited by bcl-2 (65). This scenario is plausible because chronic activation causes expression of Fas on T cells (66). In addition, a death pathway involving Fas could explain the paradoxical death-promoting effects of IL-2 because IL-2 prevents the activation of FLICE inhibitor protein, which normally inhibits Fas signaling (67).

It should be noted that agreement on these scenarios has not been reached. Using an ex vivo assay, Marrack and coworkers showed that superantigen-stimulated T cells die by a mechanism that involves internal production of reactive oxygen species, but not Fas, TNF receptors, or caspases (68). These investigators argue that reactive oxygen species damage mitochondrial membranes, leading to metabolic dysfunction and death.

The loss phase of the response is another site of adjuvant action. In the absence of adjuvant-induced inflammation, the loss of antigen-specific T cells from the lymphoid tissues after the peak of clonal expansion is nearly complete. In contrast, many more cells survive the loss phase after injection of antigen or superantigen plus adjuvants such as LPS or IL-1 (43, 45, 69). This sparing effect can be induced by injection of LPS 24 hr after superantigen injection (69) and induced equally well in normal and CD28-deficient mice (70). Because lymphokine production by antigen-stimulated T cells is CD28-dependent (47), it is unlikely that this is the target of this late adjuvant effect. It is possible that LPS promotes survival by protecting T cells from the toxic effects of reactive oxygen species by some unknown mechanism.

GENERATION OF MEMORY CELLS

Affinity Maturation

The antigen-specific T cells that survive the loss phase after exposure of the host to antigen and adjuvant are responsible for immunological memory (71). In several systems where endogenous CD4 T cells were tracked, the antigen-specific cells from the secondary response expressed a restricted set of TCRs compared with those that participated in the primary response (14, 72). In this case, T cells from the secondary response possessed higher TCR affinities for peptide-MHC complexes derived from the immunogen than cells from the primary response (73). These results have led to the conclusion that the T cell response undergoes affinity maturation as T cells with the highest-affinity TCRs survive preferentially over T cells with lower affinities.

Acquisition of Effector Lymphokine Production Potential

The antigen-specific CD4 T cells that remain in the lymphoid tissues several weeks after exposure to antigen and adjuvant or microbes have phenotypic characteristics of memory T cells (74). They have divided many times and express low levels of CD45RB and high levels of CD44 and LFA-1. In addition, the antigen-experienced

CD4 T cells produce lymphokines more rapidly than naïve T cells and at lower doses of antigen. Antigen-experienced CD4 T cells also produce a broader set of lymphokines than do naïve T cells. Naïve CD4 T cells produce large amounts of IL-2 and TNF-α when stimulated by antigen in vivo but little or no effector lymphokines such as IFN-γ, IL-4, or IL-5. In contrast, antigen-experienced T cells from immunized hosts acquire the capacity to produce effector lymphokines depending on the cytokines present during the period of initial stimulation. In vitro studies have shown that naïve T cells that are stimulated with antigen in the presence of IL-12 or IFN-α differentiate into cells capable of producing the Th1 lymphokines IFN-γ and lymphotoxin upon recall, whereas cells that are stimulated in the presence of IL-4 become cells that produce the Th2 cytokines IL-4, IL-5, IL-6, and IL-10 (75). In vitro, this differentiation process can be driven to an extreme in which the T cells produce only the Th1 set or the Th2 set (76). Memory T cells resembling polarized Th1 or Th2 cells are induced in vivo in some immune responses usually involving chronic infections. For example, antigen-specific CD4 T cells from Leishmania-infected C57BL/6 mice produce primarily Th1 lymphokines, whereas cells from infected BALB/c mice produce Th2 lymphokines (77). However, in most immune responses including those in humans, memory T cells display complex patterns of lymphokine production that are not easily categorized as Th1- or Th2-type (78). The degree of heterogeneity in effector lymphokine production exhibited by memory T cells probably reflects the mixture of inflammatory cytokines produced by the innate immune system in response to the adjuvant present during the primary response. For example, naïve CD4 T cells are likely to acquire the capacity to produce IFN-γ in response to priming with antigen plus LPS or during Gram-negative bacterial infections because LPS is a strong inducer of IL-12 production in vivo (79, 80). Other microbial adjuvants may stimulate cells of the innate immune system to produce IL-12 and IL-4, causing the population of memory T cells to acquire Th1 and Th2 lymphokine production potential.

The important role that inflammatory cytokines play in T cell proliferation and differentiation may help explain why administration of antigen in the absence of inflammation induces immune tolerance. The few antigen-specific CD4 T cells that remain in the lymphoid tissues several weeks after initial exposure to antigen without inflammation also have phenotypic characteristics of memory T cells (23), and have divided in the past (23, 81). However, unlike memory cells produced by priming with antigen plus adjuvant, these antigen-experienced T cells do not produce IL-2 or effector lymphokines (23, 81, 82), with the possible exception of IL-10 (83), when challenged with antigen. The IL-2 production defect may be related to antigen presentation by the B7^{low} dendritic cells that are present in uninflamed lymphoid tissues. The T cells might receive signals through CTLA-4 under these conditions because CTLA-4 has a higher affinity for B7 than CD28. CTLA-4 signaling has been shown to be critical for the induction of T cell anergy in vivo (82). This may come about because CTLA-4 inhibits T cell proliferation. In vitro experiments have shown that T cells are unable to produce IL-2 shortly after stimulation through the TCR, and that proliferation is required for recovery from this defect (84–86). CTLA-4-mediated inhibition of proliferation would be expected to prevent this recovery, leaving the T cells in a hyporesponsive state. The effector lymphokine production defect observed in CD4 T cells after exposure to antigen in the absence of adjuvant is almost certainly related to the fact that the T cells recognized antigen in an environment devoid of IL-12 or other differentiating cytokines.

Migration

Memory T cells also differ from naïve T cells in their tissue distribution and circulation pattern (74). Mackay and colleagues found that most of the T cells that enter afferent lymphatic vessels express surface molecules typical of memory cells (87). Because lymphatic vessels receive cells from nonlymphoid tissues, this result suggests that some memory T cells reside in these sites. In addition, Lefrancois and coworkers showed that many antigen-stimulated CD8 T cells enter the lamina propria of the gut during the primary response and remain there in an activated state for many days (88). Recent work from our group, in which antigen-specific CD4 T cells were tracked by whole-body immunohistology, showed that nonlymphoid tissues (especially liver, lungs, and gut) are the major reservoir of antigen-experienced T cells after the loss phase of the primary response induced by intravenous injection of antigen plus adjuvant (18). The movement of antigen-experienced T cells into nonlymphoid tissues is another site of adjuvant action because very few antigen-stimulated T cells moved into nonlymphoid tissues in response to antigen alone. The antigen-experienced CD4 T cells that were present in nonlymphoid tissues after immunization with antigen plus adjuvant produced more IFN-γ after in vivo rechallenge with antigen than did the cells present in the lymph nodes of the same animals. Together these results are consistent with a model in which the antigen-specific CD4 T cells that achieve the highest level of differentiation (defined by IFN-γ production potential) leave the secondary lymphoid organs and enter the nonlymphoid tissues. This movement is probably facilitated by the induction of adhesive ligands on vascular endothelial cells by inflammatory cytokines produced in response to the adjuvant (89, 90). Because acquisition of IFN-γ production potential is related to prior exposure to IL-12 (75) and cell division history (91), it is possible that the T cells that enter the nonlymphoid tissues are those that experienced the highest IL-12 concentration and/or divided the most in the lymphoid tissues.

Evidence for the existence of a nonlymphoid tissue–seeking memory T cell population in humans has also been reported. Lanzavecchia and coworkers showed that CD45RA-negative, and thus antigen-experienced, T cells in the blood are comprised of two populations, one expressing CCR7 and the other lacking CCR7 (92). The CD45RA−, CCR7+ cells express high levels of CD62L and low levels of cutaneous lymphocyte antigen, LFA-1, and $\alpha4\beta1$ integrin. In contrast the CCR7− cells express low or variable levels of CD62L and high levels of cutaneous lymphocyte antigen, LFA-1, and $\alpha4\beta1$ integrin. These expression patterns suggest that CD45RA−, CCR7+ cells circulate through lymph nodes, whereas CCR7− cells are excluded from lymph nodes and circulate through nonlymphoid tissues. The CCR7− cells produced IFN-γ, IL-4, and IL-5 rapidly when stimulated with anti-CD3 in vitro, whereas the CD45RA−, CCR7+ cells did not. However, CD45RA−, CCR7+ cells lost CCR7 after 10 days of in vitro stimulation with anti-CD3 and acquired the capacity to produce effector lymphokines. This result, and the finding that CCR7− cells had shorter telomeres (and thus had divided more often), suggest that CD45RA−, CCR7+ cells give rise to CCR7− cells. Together, these results suggest a scenario in which naïve T cells give rise to CD45RA−, CCR7+ cells that retain lymph node homing, which upon further stimulation give rise to CCR7− cells that circulate between blood and nonlymphoid tissues. Support for this idea comes from Bell and colleagues who identified two functionally distinct memory cell subsets in the rat (93).

CCR7 may also play a role in T cell migration within the lymphoid tissues in the mouse. Chaplin and colleagues reported that in vitro–differentiated Th2 cells migrated to the border between the T and B cell areas, whereas Th1 cells localized to the T cell areas of the spleen after adoptive transfer and immunization with antigen (94). Th1 cells expressed CCR7 and Th2 cells did not, and this difference played a role in migration behavior because transduction of the Th2 cells with CCR7 caused them to localize to the T cell areas. These results suggest that Th2 cells are good B cell helpers in part because they are not tethered by CCR7 in the T cell area and can migrate to the B cell areas. However, this model does not account for the capacity of Th1 cells to help B cells switch to IgG2a production (95) nor explain the fact that human IFN-γ-producing memory cells do not express CCR7 (92).

Persistence of the Memory Phenotype

The temporal stability of the phenotypic changes that occur in antigen-experienced CD4 T cells is controversial. On the one hand, in vitro–differentiated Th1 and Th2 cells retain their original lymphokine production patterns for months after transfer into naïve recipients (96). Similarly, Stockinger and coworkers found that antigen-specific CD4 T cells retained the CD44[high] phenotype and the capacity to produce IFN-γ for months under conditions where antigen was only presented for a brief period (97). On the other hand, work by other investigators has shown that CD45RB[low] cells revert to the naïve CD45RB[high] phenotype (98, 99) and that the enhanced helper function of CD4 memory T cells is lost over time (100). We found that naïve antigen-specific CD4 T cells became LFA-1[high] within several days of immunization with antigen plus adjuvant but reverted to an LFA-1[low] phenotype 10 weeks later, or within one week after transfer into naïve recipients, and reverted to some of the functional behaviors of naïve T cells (101). These results are consistent with the possibility that the expression of memory-phenotype homing receptors, and the nonlymphoid tissue-homing pattern determined by these receptors, are retained in CD4 T cells only as long as antigen is present. This may be a major difference between T cell subsets because the memory phenotype and function of CD8 T cells are maintained in the absence of antigen (102, 103).

MODEL OF THE PRIMARY CD4 T CELL RESPONSE

Figure 2 shows a speculative model for the series of events that occur in naïve T cells during a primary immune response in the lymph nodes after subcutaneous injection of antigen plus adjuvant. This is the type of response that generates effector lymphokine-producing memory cells and is induced by microbes because they contain foreign proteins and molecules with adjuvant properties.

Adjuvant molecules are recognized by pattern recognition receptors on cells of the innate immune system at the antigen injection site, causing the release of TNF-α and IL-1. These cytokines signal the local tissue dendritic cells or monocytes to leave the tissue and migrate via an afferent lymphatic vessel to the draining lymph node after first ingesting antigen. During the migration process, these cells mature to produce peptide-MHC complexes from the ingested antigen and deliver these to the cell surface along with newly synthesized B7 molecules. After arriving at the lymph node, the dendritic cells crawl through the floor of the subcapsular sinus and present peptide-MHC complexes to naïve antigen-specific CD4 T cells in the T cell area. The T cells produce high levels of IL-2 and an unknown T cell growth factor, and they proliferate. This proliferation occurs in an IL-12-rich environment due to IL-12 produced by dendritic cells in response to the adjuvant. Many of the proliferating T cells die in the T cell area, but the anti-apoptotic effect of the adjuvant ensures that some survive. Of the survivors, those that divided the most and experienced the highest concentration of IL-12 lose CCR7, gain P-selectin ligand, and acquire the capacity for rapid IFN-γ production. Antigen-activated T cells that do not achieve this threshold number of cell divisions, or IL-12 concentration, remain CCR7+ and acquire rapid IL-2 production potential, but not the capacity for IFN-γ production. After leaving the lymphoid tissues during the primary response, the CCR7+ cells recirculate through lymphoid tissues like naïve T cells. In contrast, the CCR7− cells are excluded from lymph nodes and remain in the blood or enter nonlymphoid tissues that express P-selectin. As long as residual antigen is present to drive the survival of CCR7− cells, then a second exposure to antigen will result in rapid production of effector lymphokines at the site of antigen entry either by CCR7− cells that happen to reside in that tissue or by CCR7− cells that are rapidly recruited from blood. As antigen is cleared from the body, CCR7− cells die or revert to the CCR7+ phenotype; in either case only CCR7+ memory cells remain. If antigen enters the body during this phase, then CCR7+ cells will be activated in the lymphoid organs and rapidly differentiate into CCR7−, effector lymphokine-producing cells capable of migrating to the site of antigen deposition. This process would be more efficient than the primary response because CCR7+ memory cells could achieve effector lymphokine production faster than naïve T cells, and extrinsic factors such as antibodies from the primary response would facilitate antigen presentation (101, 104).

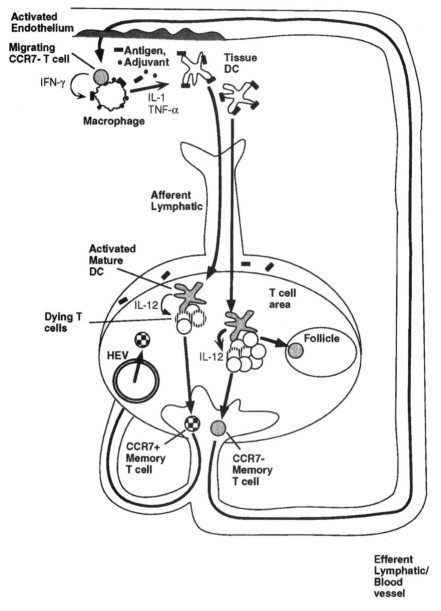

Figure 2 Diagrammatic representation of a productive primary CD4 T cell response to antigen in the presence of adjuvant-induced inflammation.

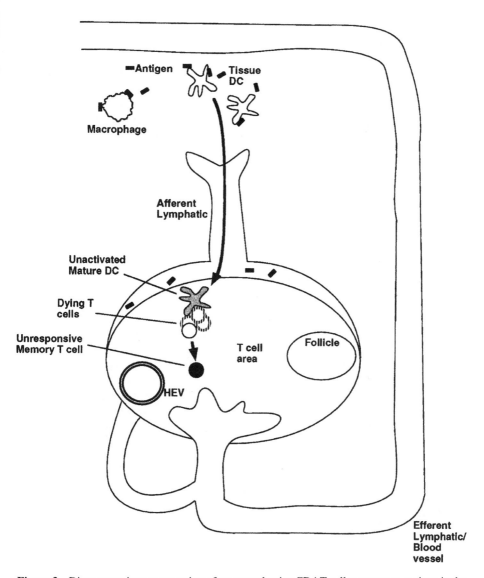

Figure 3   Diagrammatic representation of an unproductive CD4 T cell response to antigen in the absence of inflammation.

A very different outcome would result from antigen presentation in the absence of inflammation (Figure 3). Based on the aforementioned model, presentation of an injected antigen would be relatively inefficient because it would depend on the low level of dendritic cell migration that occurs under noninflammatory conditions, or the small amount of antigen that leaks across the subcapsular barrier to be taken up by lymphoid–tissue resident dendritic cells. In either case, antigen presentation would be carried out by dendritic cells that do not express high levels of costimulatory ligands. Lack of the anti-apoptotic effects of inflammatory cytokines would cause most of the T cells to die. The minimal signaling through CD28, IL-1 receptor, and receptors for differentiating cytokines such as IL-12 and IL-4, experienced in the primary response would limit IL-2 and effector lymphokine production potential in any memory cells that survived. The combination of death of most of the expanded antigen-specific T cell population and the functional defects in the survivors could explain the induction of peripheral tolerance by antigen administration in the absence of inflammation.

Visit the Annual Reviews home page at www.AnnualReviews.org

LITERATURE CITED

1. Mueller DL, Jenkins MK, Schwartz RH. 1989. Clonal expansion versus functional clonal inactivation: a costimulatory signalling pathway determines the outcome of T cell antigen receptor occupancy. *Annu. Rev. Immunol.* 7:445–90

2. Davis MM, Boniface JJ, Reich Z, Lyons D, Hampl J, Arden B, Chien Y. 1998. Ligand recognition by alpha beta T cell receptors. *Annu. Rev. Immunol.* 16:523–44

3. Dresser DW. 1961. Effectiveness of lipid and lipidophilic substances as adjuvants. *Nature* 191:1169–71

4. Dresser DW. 1962. Specific inhibition of antibody production. II. Paralysis induced in adult mice by small quantities of protein antigen. *Nature* 191:1169–71

5. Chiller JM, Habicht GS, Weigle WO. 1971. Kinetic differences in unresponsiveness of thymus and bone marrow cells. *Science* 171:813–15

6. Dozmorov I, Eisenbraun MD, Lefkovits I. 2000. Limiting dilution analysis: from frequencies to cellular interactions. *Immunol. Today* 21:15–18

7. Taguchi T, McGhee JR, Coffman RL, Beagley KW, Eldridge JH, Takatsu K, Kiyono H. 1990. Analysis of Th1 and Th2 cells in murine gut-associated tissues. Frequencies of CD4+ and CD8+ T cells that secrete IFN-gamma and IL-5. *J. Immunol.* 145:68–77

8. Murali-Krishna K, Altman JD, Suresh M, Sourdive DJ, Zajac AJ, Miller JD, Slansky J, Ahmed R. 1998. Counting antigen-specific CD8 T cells: a reevaluation of bystander activation during viral infection. *Immunity* 8:177–87

9. Zajac AJ, Blattman JN, Murali-Krishna K, Sourdive DJ, Suresh M, Altman JD, Ahmed R. 1998. Viral immune evasion due to persistence of activated T cells without effector function. *J. Exp. Med.* 188:2205–13

10. Altman JD, Moss PAH, Goulder JR, Barouch DH, McHeyzer-Williams MG, Bell JI, McMichael AJ, Davis MM. 1996. Phenotypic analysis of antigen-specific T lymphocytes. *Science* 274:94–96

11. Busch DH, Pilip IM, Vijh S, Pamer EG. 1998. Coordinate regulation of complex T cell populations responding to bacterial infection. *Immunity* 8:353–62

12. Kotzin BL, Falta MT, Crawford F, Rosloniec EF, Bill J, Marrack P, Kappler J. 2000. Use of soluble peptide-DR4 tetramers to detect synovial T cells specific for cartilage antigens in patients with rheumatoid arthritis. *Proc. Natl. Acad. Sci. USA* 97:291–96

13. Kozono H, White J, Clements J, Marrack P, Kappler J. 1994. Production of soluble MHC class II proteins with covalently

bound single peptides. *Nature* 369:151–54

14. McHeyzer-Williams MG, Davis MM. 1995. Antigen-specific development of primary and memory T cells in vivo. *Science* 268:106–11

15. Pape KA, Kearney ER, Khoruts A, Mondino A, Merica R, Chen Z, Ingulli E, White J, Johnson J, Jenkins MK. 1997. Use of adoptive transfer of T-cell-antigen-receptor-transgenic T cells for the study of T-cell activation in vivo. *Immunol. Rev.* 156:67–78

16. Bradley LM, Watson SR. 1996. Lymphocyte migration into tissue: the paradigm derived from CD4 subsets. *Curr. Opin. Immunol.* 8:312–20

17. Mackay CR, Andrew DP, Briskin M, Ringler DJ, Butcher EC. 1996. Phenotype, and migration properties of three major subsets of tissue homing T cells in sheep. *Eur. J. Immunol.* 26:2433–39

18. Reinhardt RL, Khoruts A, Merica R, Jenkins MK. 2000. Whole body tracking of individual CD4 T cells reveals that non-lymphoid tissue is the major reservoir of immunological memory. Submitted

19. Picker LJ, Siegelman MH. 1993. Lymphoid tissues and organs. In *Fundamental Immunology*, ed. W. E. Paul, 145–97. New York: Raven

20. Campbell JJ, Butcher EC. 2000. Chemokines in tissue-specific and microenvironment-specific lymphocyte homing. *Curr. Opin. Immunol.* 12:336–41

21. Cyster JG, Goodnow CC. 1995. Pertussis toxin inhibits migration of B and T lymphocytes into splenic white pulp cords. *J. Exp. Med.* 182:581–86

22. Cyster JG. 1999. Chemokines and cell migration in secondary lymphoid organs. *Science* 286:2098–2102

23. Pape KA, Merica R, Mondino A, Khoruts A, Jenkins MK. 1998. Direct evidence that functionally impaired CD4+ T cells persist in vivo following induction of peripheral tolerance. *J. Immunol.* 160:4719–29

24. Garside P, Ingulli E, Merica RR, Johnson JG, Noelle RJ, Jenkins MK. 1998. Visualization of specific B and T lymphocyte interactions in the lymph node. *Science* 281:96–99

25. Steinman RM, Pack M, Inaba K. 1997. Dendritic cells in the T-cell areas of lymphoid organs. *Immunol. Rev.* 156:25–37

26. Ingulli E, Mondino A, Khoruts A, Jenkins MK. 1997. In vivo detection of dendritic cell antigen presentation to CD4+ T cells. *J. Exp. Med.* 185:2133–41

27. Luther SA, Gulbranson-Judge A, Acha-Orbea H, MacLennan ICM. 1997. Viral superantigen drives extrafollicular and follicular B cell differentiation leading to virus-specific antibody production. *J. Exp. Med.* 185:551–62

28. Ebnet K, Kaldjian EP, Anderson AO, Shaw S. 1996. Orchestrated information transfer underlying leukocyte endothelial interactions. *Annu. Rev. Immunol.* 14:155–77

29. Shortman K, Vremec D, Corcoran LM, Georgopoulos K, Lucas K, Wu L. 1998. The linkage between T-cell and dendritic cell development in the mouse thymus. *Immunol. Rev.* 165:39–46

30. Silberberg-Sinakin I, Thorbecke GJ, Baer RL, Rosenthal SA, Berezowsky V. 1976. Antigen-bearing langerhans cells in skin, dermal lymphatics and in lymph nodes. *Cell. Immunol.* 25:137–51

31. Randolph GJ, Inaba K, Robbiani DF, Steinman RM, Muller WA. 1999. Differentiation of phagocytic monocytes into lymph node dendritic cells in vivo. *Immunity* 11:753–61

32. Inaba K, Swiggard WJ, Inaba M, Meltzer J, Mirza A, Sasagawa T, Nussenzweig MC, Steinman RM. 1995. Tissue distribution of the DEC-205 protein that is detected by the monoclonal antibody NLDC-145. I. Expression on dendritic cells and other subsets of mouse leukocytes. *Cell. Immunol.* 163:148–56

33. Wu L, D'Amico A, Winkel KD, Suter M, Lo D, Shortman K. 1998. RelB is

essential for the development of myeloid-related CD8alpha– dendritic cells but not of lymphoid-related CD8alpha+ dendritic cells. *Immunity* 9:839–47

34. Sato N, Ahuja SK, Quinones M, Kostecki V, Reddick RL, Melby PC, Kuziel WA, Ahuja SS. 2000. CC Chemokine receptor (CCR)2 is required for Langerhans cell migration and localization of T helper cell type 1 (Th1)-inducing dendritic cells. Absence of CCR2 shifts the leishmania major-resistant phenotype to a susceptible state dominated by Th2 cytokines, B cell outgrowth, and sustained neutrophilic inflammation. *J. Exp. Med.* 192:205–18

35. Sallusto F, Lanzavecchia A. 1994. Efficient presentation of soluble antigen by cultured human dendritic cells is maintained by granulocyte/macrophage colony-stimulating factor plus interleukin 4 and downregulated by tumor necrosis factor alpha. *J. Exp. Med.* 179:1109–18

36. Zhong G, Sousa CR, Germain RN. 1997. Antigen-unspecific B cells and lymphoid dendritic cells both show extensive surface expression of processed antigen-major histocompatibility complex class II complexes after soluble protein exposure in vivo or in vitro. *J. Exp. Med.* 186:673–82

37. Reis e Sousa C, Germain RN. 1999. Analysis of adjuvant function by direct visualization of antigen presentation in vivo: endotoxin promotes accumulation of antigen-bearing dendritic cells in the T cell areas of lymphoid tissue. *J. Immunol.* 162:6552–61

38. DeSmedt T, Pajak B, Muraille E, Lespagnard L, Heinen E, Baetselier PD, Urbain J, Leo O, Moser M. 1996. Regulation of dendritic cell numbers and maturation by lipopolysaccharide in vivo. *J. Exp. Med.* 184:1413–24

39. de St Groth BF. 1998. The evolution of self-tolerance: a new cell arises to meet the challenge of self-reactivity. *Immunol. Today* 19:448–54

40. Banchereau J, Briere F, Caux C, Davoust J, Lebecque S, Liu YJ, Pulendran B, Palucka K. 2000. Immunobiology of dendritic cells. *Annu. Rev. Immunol.* 18:767–811

41. Turley SJ, Inaba K, Garrett WS, Ebersold M, Unternaehrer J, Steinman RM, Mellman I. 2000. Transport of peptide-MHC class II complexes in developing dendritic cells. *Science* 288:522–27

42. Cella M, Engering A, Pinet V, Pieters J, Lanzavecchia A. 1997. Inflammatory stimuli induce accumulation of MHC class II complexes on dendritic cells. *Nature* 388:782–87

43. Kearney ER, Pape KA, Loh DY, Jenkins MK. 1994. Visualization of peptide-specific T cell immunity and peripheral tolerance induction in vivo. *Immunity* 1:327–39

44. Gulbranson-Judge A, MacLennan I. 1996. Sequential antigen-specific growth of T cells in the T zones and follicles in response to pigeon cytochrome c. *Eur. J. Immunol.* 26:1830–37

45. Pape KA, Khoruts A, Mondino A, Jenkins MK. 1997. Inflammatory cytokines enhance the in vivo clonal expansion and differentiation of antigen-activated CD4+ T cells. *J. Immunol.* 159:591–98

46. Sun S, Kishimoto H, Sprent J. 1998. DNA as an adjuvant:capacity of insect DNA and synthetic oligodeoxynucleotides to augment T cell responses to specific antigen. *J. Exp. Med.* 187:1145–50

47. Khoruts A, Mondino A, Pape KA, Reiner SL, Jenkins MK. 1998. A natural immunological adjuvant enhances T cell clonal expansion through a CD28-dependent, interleukin (IL)-2-independent mechanism. *J. Exp. Med.* 187:225–36

48. Schorle H, Holtschke T, Hunig T, Schimpl A, Horak I. 1991. Development and function of T cells in mice rendered interleukin-2 deficient by gene targeting. *Nature* 352:621–24

49. Kneitz B, Herrmann T, Yonehara S, Schimpl A. 1995. Normal clonal expansion but impaired Fas-mediated cell death

and anergy induction in interleukin-2-deficient mice. *Eur. J. Immunol.* 25:2572–77

50. Leung DT, Morefield S, Willerford DM. 2000. Regulation of lymphoid homeostasis by IL-2 receptor signals in vivo. *J. Immunol.* 164:3527–34

51. Lantz O, Grandjean I, Matzinger P, Di Santo JP. 2000. γ chain required for naïve CD4⁺ T cell survival but not for antigen proliferation. *Nature Immunol.* 1:54–58

52. Medzhitov R, Janeway C, Jr. 2000. Innate immune recognition: mechanisms and pathways. *Immunol. Rev.* 173:89–97

53. Maxwell JR, Campbell JD, Kim CH, Vella AT. 1999. CD40 activation boosts T cell immunity in vivo by enhancing T cell clonal expansion and delaying peripheral T cell deletion. *J. Immunol.* 162:2024–34

54. Joseph SB, Miner KT, Croft M. 1998. Augmentation of naive, Th1 and Th2 effector CD4 responses by IL-6, IL-1 and TNF. *Eur. J. Immunol.* 28:277–89

55. Curtsinger JM, Schmidt CS, Mondino A, Lins DC, Kedl RM, Jenkins MK, Mescher MF. 1999. Inflammatory cytokines provide a third signal for activation of naive CD4⁺ and CD8⁺ T cells. *J. Immunol.* 162:3256–62

56. Cyster JG, Goodnow CC. 1995. Antigen-induced exclusion from follicles and anergy are separate and complementary processes that influence peripheral B cell fate. *Immunity* 3:691–701

57. Fulcher DA, Lyons AB, Korn SL, Cook MC, Koleda C, Parish C, Fazekas de St. Groth B, Basten A. 1996. The fate of self-reactive B cells depends primarily on the degree of antigen receptor engagement and availability of T cell help. *J. Exp. Med.* 183:2313–28

58. Fuller KA, Kanagawa O, Nahm MH. 1993. T cells within germinal centers are specific for the immunizing antigen. *J. Immunol.* 151:4505–12

59. Zheng B, Han S, Kelsoe G. 1996. T helper cells in murine germinal centers are antigen-specific emigrants that downregulate Thy-1. *J. Exp. Med.* 184:1083–91

60. Ansel KM, McHeyzer-Williams LJ, Ngo VN, McHeyzer-Williams MG, Cyster JG. 1999. In vivo-activated CD4 T cells upregulate CXC chemokine receptor 5 and reprogram their response to lymphoid chemokines. *J. Exp. Med.* 190:1123–34

61. Brocker T, Gulbranson-Judge A, Flynn S, Riedinger M, Raykundalia C, Lane P. 1999. CD4 T cell traffic control: in vivo evidence that ligation of OX40 on CD4 T cells by OX40-ligand expressed on dendritic cells leads to the accumulation of CD4 T cells in B follicles. *Eur. J. Immunol.* 29:1610–16

62. Van Parijs L, Peterson DA, Abbas AK. 1998. The Fas/Fas ligand pathway and Bcl-2 regulate T cell responses to model self and foreign antigens. *Immunity* 8:265–74

63. Petschner F, Zimmerman C, Strasser A, Grillot D, Nunez G, Pircher H. 1998. Constitutive expression of Bcl-xL or Bcl-2 prevents peptide antigen-induced T cell deletion but does not influence T cell homeostasis after a viral infection. *Eur. J. Immunol.* 28:560–69

64. Refaeli Y, Van Parijs L, Abbas AK. 1999. Genetic models of abnormal apoptosis in lymphocytes. *Immunol. Rev.* 169:273–82

65. Lenardo M, Chan KM, Hornung F, McFarland H, Siegel R, Wang J, Zheng L. 1999. Mature T lymphocyte apoptosis–immune regulation in a dynamic and unpredictable antigenic environment. *Annu. Rev. Immunol.* 17:221–53

66. Hiromatsu K, Aoki Y, Makino M, Matsumoto Y, Mizuochi T, Gotoh Y, Nomoto K, Ogasawara J, Nagata S, Yoshikai Y. 1994. Increased Fas antigen expression in murine retrovirus-induced immunodeficiency syndrome, MAIDS. *Eur. J. Immunol.* 24:2446–51

67. Refaeli Y, Van Parijs L, London CA, Tschopp J, Abbas AK. 1998. Biochemical mechanisms of IL-2-regulated Fas-mediated T cell apoptosis. *Immunity* 8:615–23

68. Hildeman DA, Mitchell T, Teague TK, Henson P, Day BJ, Kappler J, Marrack PC. 1999. Reactive oxygen species regulate activation-induced T cell apoptosis. *Immunity* 10:735–44

69. Vella AT, McCormack JE, Linsley PS, Kappler JW, Marrack P. 1995. Lipopolysaccharide interferes with the induction of peripheral T cell death. *Immunity* 2:261–70

70. Vella AT, Mitchell T, Groth B, Linsley PS, Green JM, Thompson CB, Kappler JW, Marrack P. 1997. CD28 engagement and proinflammatory cytokines contribute to T cell expansion and long-term survival in vivo. *J. Immunol.* 158:4714–20

71. Antia R, Pilyugin SS, Ahmed R. 1998. Models of immune memory: on the role of cross-reactive stimulation, competition, and homeostasis in maintaining immune memory. *Proc. Natl. Acad. Sci. USA* 95:14926–31

72. McHeyzer-Williams LJ, Panus JF, Mikszta JA, McHeyzer-Williams MG. 1999. Evolution of antigen-specific T cell receptors in vivo: preimmune and antigen-driven selection of preferred complementarity-determining region 3 (CDR3) motifs. *J. Exp. Med.* 189:1823–38

73. Savage PA, Boniface JJ, Davis MM. 1999. A kinetic basis for T cell receptor repertoire selection during an immune response. *Immunity* 10:485–92

74. Dutton RW, Bradley LM, Swain SL. 1998. T cell memory. *Annu. Rev. Immunol.* 16:201–23

75. Murphy KM, Ouyang W, Farrar JD, Yang J, Ranganath S, Asnagli H, Afkarian M, Murphy TL. 2000. Signaling and transcription in T helper development. *Annu. Rev. Immunol.* 18:451–94

76. Mosmann TR, Cherwinski H, Bond MW, Giedlin MA, Coffman RL. 1986. Two types of murine helper T cell clone. I. Definition according to profiles of lymphokine activities and secreted proteins. *J. Immunol.* 136:2348–57

77. Reiner SL, Locksley RM. 1995. The regulation of immunity to Leishmania major. *Annu. Rev. Immunol.* 13:151–77

78. Picker LJ, Singh MK, Zdraveski Z, Treer JR, Waldrop SL, Bergstresser PR, Maino VC. 1995. Direct demonstration of cytokine synthesis heterogeneity among human memory/effector T cells by flow cytometry. *Blood* 86:1408–19

79. Flesch IE, Hess JH, Huang S, Aguet M, Rothe J, Bluethmann H, Kaufmann SH. 1995. Early interleukin 12 production by macrophages in response to mycobacterial infection depends on interferon gamma and tumor necrosis factor alpha. *J. Exp. Med.* 181:1615–21

80. Skeen MJ, Miller MA, Shinnick TM, Ziegler HK. 1996. Regulation of murine macrophage IL-12 production. *J. Immunol.* 156:1196–1206

81. Lanoue A, Bona C, von Boehmer H, Sarukhan A. 1997. Conditions that induce tolerance in mature CD4$^+$ T cells. *J. Exp. Med.* 185:405–14

82. Perez VL, Van Parijs L, Biuckians A, Zheng XX, Strom TB, Abbas AK. 1997. Induction of peripheral T cell tolerance in vivo requires CTLA-4 engagement. *Immunity* 6:411–17

83. Buer J, Lanoue A, Franzke A, Garcia C, von Boehmer H, Sarukhan A. 1998. Interleukin 10 secretion and impaired effector function of major histocompatibility complex class II-restricted T cells anergized in vivo. *J. Exp. Med.* 187:177–83

84. Beverly B, Kang S, Lenardo MJ, Schwartz RH. 1992. Reversal of in vitro T cell clonal anergy by IL-2 stimulation. *Int. Immunol.* 4:661–71

85. DeSilva DR, Urdahl KB, Jenkins MK. 1991. Clonal anergy is induced in vitro by T cell receptor occupancy in the absence of proliferation. *J. Immunol.* 147:3261–67

86. De Mattia F, Chomez S, Van Laethem F, Moulin V, Urbain J, Moser M, Leo O, Andris F. 1999. Antigen-experienced T cells

undergo a transient phase of unresponsiveness following optimal stimulation. *J. Immunol.* 163:5929–36

87. Mackay C, Marston W, Dudler L. 1990. Naive and memory T cells show distinct pathways of lymphocyte recirculation. *J. Exp. Med.* 171:801–17

88. Kim SK, Schluns KS, Lefrancois L. 1999. Induction and visualization of mucosal memory CD8 T cells following systemic virus infection. *J. Immunol.* 163:4125–32

89. van Oosten M, van de Bilt E, de Vries HE, van Berkel TJ, Kuiper J. 1995. Vascular adhesion molecule-1 and intercellular adhesion molecule-1 expression on rat liver cells after lipopolysaccharide administration in vivo. *Hepatology* 22:1538–46

90. Arvilommi AM, Salmi M, Jalkanen S. 1997. Organ-selective regulation of vascular adhesion protein-1 expression in man. *Eur. J. Immunol.* 27:1794–1800

91. Bird JJ, Brown DR, Mullen AC, Moskowitz NH, Mahowald MA, Sider JR, Gajewski TF, Wang CR, Reiner SL. 1998. Helper T cell differentiation is controlled by the cell cycle. *Immunity* 9:229–37

92. Sallusto F, Lenig D, Forster R, Lipp M, Lanzavecchia A. 1999. Two subsets of memory T lymphocytes with distinct homing potentials and effector functions. *Nature* 401:708–12

93. Bunce C, Bell EB. 1997. CD45RC isoforms define two types of CD4 memory T cells, one of which depends on persisting antigen. *J. Exp. Med.* 185:767–76

94. Randolph DA, Huang G, Carruthers CJ, Bromley LE, Chaplin DD. 1999. The role of CCR7 in TH1 and TH2 cell localization and delivery of B cell help in vivo. *Science* 286:2159–62

95. Stavnezer J. 2000. Molecular processes that regulate class switching. *Curr. Top. Microbiol. Immunol.* 245:127–68

96. Swain S. 1994. Generation and in vivo persistence of polarized Th1 and Th2 memory cells. *Immunity* 1:543–52

97. Garcia S, DiSanto J, Stockinger B. 1999. Following the development of a CD4 T cell response in vivo: from activation to memory formation. *Immunity* 11:163–71

98. Bell EB, Sparshott SM. 1990. Interconversion of CD45R subsets of CD4 T cells in vivo. *Nature* 348:163–66

99. Tough DF, Sprent J. 1994. Turnover of naive- and memory-phenotype T cells. *J. Exp. Med.* 179:1127–35

100. Gray D, Matzinger P. 1991. T cell memory is short-lived in the absence of antigen. *J. Exp. Med.* 174:969–74

101. Merica R, Khoruts A, Pape KA, Reinhardt RL, Jenkins MK. 2000. Antigen-experienced CD4 T cells display a reduced capacity for clonal expansion in vivo that is imposed by factors present in the immune host. *J. Immunol.* 164:4551–57

102. Lau LL, Jamieson BD, Somasundaram T, Ahmed R. 1994. Cytotoxic T-cell memory without antigen. *Nature* 369:648–52

103. Hou S, Hyland L, Ryan KW, Portner A, Doherty PC. 1994. Virus-specific CD8+ T-cell memory determined by clonal burst size. *Nature* 369:652–54

104. Hamano Y, Arase H, Saisho H, Saito T. 2000. Immune complex and Fc receptor-mediated augmentation of antigen presentation for in vivo Th cell responses. *J. Immunol.* 164:6113–19

Annu. Rev. Immunol. 2001. 19:47–64

CROSS-PRESENTATION, DENDRITIC CELLS, TOLERANCE AND IMMUNITY

William R. Heath[1] and Francis R. Carbone[2]

[1]Immunology Division, The Walter and Eliza Hall Institute, Post Office Royal Melbourne Hospital, Parkville, Victoria 3052, Australia; e-mail: heath@wehi.edu.au
[2]Department of Microbiology and Immunology, University of Melbourne, Parkville, Victoria 3050, Australia; e-mail: f.carbone@microbiology.unimelb.edu.au

Key Words   cross-priming, antigen presentation, cytotoxic T lymphocytes, CD8, T cells

■ **Abstract**   This review examines the role of cross-presentation in tolerance and immunity. We discuss (*a*) the antigenic requirements for cross-presentation, (*b*) the phenotype of the antigen presenting cell (APC), (*c*) the cellular interactions and molecular signals involved in cross-priming, and (*d*) the factors that direct the immune system toward tolerance or immunity. A large part of this review is dedicated to summarizing our current knowledge of the cross-presenting APC.

WHAT IS CROSS-PRESENTATION?

Early experiments examining the nature of MHC-restriction during T cell priming showed that minor histocompatibilty antigens were capable of being transferred from those cells expressing these antigens to host antigen-presenting cells (APC) (1). Priming involving this type of antigen transfer was termed cross-priming to differentiate it from direct T cell activation by the actual cells expressing the minor antigens. In recent times, such presentation has been given the term cross-presentation (2).

According to this simple definition, cross-presentation can involve either class I– or class II–restricted antigens, although this term has often been associated solely with class I–restricted antigens. This association is partly historical because the original cross-priming experiments involved class I–restricted cytotoxic T lymphocyte (CTL) priming to minor antigens. Unlike the situation with class I, where contention remains regarding the nature and extent of exogenous antigen presentation (for discussion, see 3), there is little debate that transfer of antigen from one cell to another can readily occur in the context of class II–restricted presentation. That exogenous antigens have ready access to the class II processing pathway has long been accepted. Thus, a special term for this type of class II–restricted

0732-0582/01/0407-0047$14.00

antigen presentation is not necessary. However, given that the same professional APC can present transferred antigen to both helper and killer T cells (4), we believe that the single term of cross-presentation is appropriate for both class I– and class II–restricted presentation of cell-associated antigens.

Finally, we should note that T cell activation resulting from cross-presentation could, on the basis of our definition, lead to T cell priming (cross-priming) or T cell tolerance (cross-tolerance). Indeed, this decision between tolerance and immunity has increasingly become the focus of attention in this field. Based on the definition of cross-presentation as the transfer from antigen-bearing cell to antigen-presenting cell, we attempt to review cross-presentation's role in tolerance and immunity. We discuss (*a*) the antigenic requirements for cross-presentation, (*b*) the phenotype of the APC, (*c*) the cellular interactions and molecular signals involved in cross-priming, and (*d*) factors that direct the immune system toward tolerance or immunity. A large part of this review is dedicated to summarizing our current knowledge of the cross-presenting APC, with the intention of advertising our view that this cell is yet to be identified.

ANTIGENIC REQUIREMENTS FOR CROSS-PRESENTATION

Cross-presentation of cellular antigens is involved in many different responses, including those to tumors (5), viruses (6), graft tissues (1) and even self (7). Such studies have included minor histocompatibility antigens (1) and many viral proteins, including poliovirus antigens (6), influenza hemagglutinin (8), influenza nucleoprotein (9), and SV40 t antigen (10). Soluble antigens like ovalbumin (OVA) (11) and β-galactosidase (11) can also be cross-presented if they are injected in a cell-associated form by simple cell adsorption. At present, there is no limitation on the type of antigen that can be cross-presented, with membrane-associated, secreted, and nuclear antigens all represented in the above studies. However, several studies primarily using the nucleoprotein or glycoprotein of lymphocytic choriomeningitis virus (12, 13) have failed to observe class I–restricted cross-presentation. Whether these latter proteins are resistant to cross-presentation or simply never reach levels of expression sufficient to achieve cross-presentation is yet to be clarified.

This brings us to the important issue of antigen expression levels and their influence on cross-presentation. We believe antigen expression levels are one of the major factors determining the outcome of several types of immunity. It is also the primary reason for three areas of contention in the literature with respect to the role of cross-presentation in (*a*) DNA vaccination, (*b*) tumor immunity and (*c*) tolerance to peripheral self antigens. In the case of DNA vaccination, some groups claim that DNA-encoded antigens are cross-presented and that this leads to CTL induction (14). Other groups provide evidence that DNA priming is initiated only by transfected professional APC (15). For tumor responses, there is clear evidence that tumor antigens can induce responses by cross-priming (5), but some researchers fail to observe this in their models (12). Finally, cross-presentation of self-antigens has been reported to induce peripheral tolerance (16), but some peripherally expressed antigens are ignored (13, 17), which suggests that they are not cross-presented.

We think there is a simple explanation for all three areas of controversy, i.e. the level of antigen expressed by a cell must be above a certain threshold for cross-presentation to occur (18). At first, this explanation seems obvious; antigens always need to be above a certain threshold concentration before they will be seen by the immune system. But cross-presentation is a little more complicated. Because a cell expresses enough antigen to be recognized directly by an effector CTL does not mean that it will provide sufficient antigen for cross-presentation by professional APC. This simple point is often overlooked. Many researchers assume that if a transfectant expresses sufficient antigen to be recognized by CTL, then it will be appropriate for studies determining the role of cross-presentation in immunity. We have clearly shown that islet cells directly presenting endogenous antigen may be killed by activated CTL when they express as little as 0.03 ng OVA per μg of protein, but constitutive cross-presentation of islet OVA is only detected when β cells express greater than this amount (18, 19). Whether the different concentration requirements simply reflect an inherent inefficiency in the transfer of antigen from the antigen-expressing cell to the APC remains unclear. Regardless, because an islet cell expresses enough antigen to be killed does not mean that it will express enough for cross-presentation.

If, as we argue, antigen expression needs to be higher for cross-presentation than for direct presentation, then the contradictory observations with DNA vaccination can be easily explained. DNA vaccines that express lower levels of antigen will only prime when professional APC are directly transfected, whereas more efficient expression vectors will provide enough antigen for cross-presentation. Thus, in the latter case, cross-presentation will be seen to have a role in vaccination, whereas in the former, it will not.

Similarly, tumors transfected with model tumor antigens, or even those expressing real tumor antigens, will only cross-prime if the level of antigen expression is sufficiently high. Lower levels may enable tumor killing by activated CTL and, as reported by Zinkernagel and coworkers (12), may even allow tumors to prime when injected into lymphoid organs. However, tumors with lower antigen expression levels will not be able to cross-prime. Thus, failure to demonstrate cross-priming with a tumor is not sufficient evidence to conclude that this tumor cannot cross-prime, unless it is clear that the antigen expression levels are appropriately high.

Finally, with respect to peripheral tolerance, we have recently shown that OVA expressed in the pancreas below a certain threshold concentration (0.03 ng OVA per μg of islet protein) will not be cross-presented and is therefore ignored by the immune system. In contrast, when OVA is expressed above this threshold, it provides sufficient antigen for cross-presentation and is able to induce tolerance (18).

One important question raised by our studies with OVA expressed in the pancreas was whether the relatively high dose of antigen required for cross-presentation was physiological. There are two main reasons to conclude that this is the case. First, many naturally expressed antigens have been shown to induce CTL by cross-priming, e.g. minor histocompatibility antigens (1), SV40 t antigen (10), and poliovirus antigens (6). Although it could be argued that each of these examples measured cross-priming under conditions that did not occur naturally, the second, and more substantial, reason to argue that we are within physiological limits stems from the observation that 1.0 μg OVA per mg of islet protein was sufficient to induce activation of CD8 T cells by cross-presentation (19). After a brief search of the literature, we suggest that this antigen concentration is at the higher range of protein expression levels, but not unphysiological. Numerous antigens are expressed at this level and even higher, e.g. insulin in a whole murine pancreas is at 0.73 μg/mg protein (21). Because islets only contribute approximately 1% of the pancreas mass, the amount of insulin within islets (100 $\times$ 0.73 = 73 μg/mg protein) is considerably higher than the OVA in our model. The following further illustrate this point: S-100 protein in rat adipose tissue is at 1.3 μg/mg protein (22); thiol-protein disulfide oxidoreductase in rat liver is at 4 μg/mg protein (23); kallikrein in whole rat pancreas is at 1.3 μg/mg protein (24); annexin II, V, and VI in human heart tissue are at 2.5, 3.7, and 14 μg/mg protein, respectively (25), and metallothionin in rat liver is at 4.3 μg/mg protein (26). Thus, the 1.0 μg OVA per mg protein required to observe cross-presentation in transgenic mice (19) appears to be within the physiological dose range, though it may be at the higher end.

Two additional questions stem directly from our understanding that antigen dose is critical for cross-presentation. First, is the antigen dose threshold the same for all tissues, and second, are there other factors that determine the efficiency of cross-presentation? Although it is yet to be addressed whether thresholds vary from cell-type to cell-type, there is evidence that the level of antigen expression required for cross-presentation varies with circumstance. For example, transgenic mice expressing less than 0.03 μg OVA per mg of protein in their islets did not show cross-presentation of OVA under normal conditions, but if activated CTL were injected into these mice to kill the islet cells, then OVA was efficiently cross-presented in the draining pancreatic lymph node (18, 19). This observation implied that destruction of islet cells could increase the efficiency of cross-presentation of islet antigens. The basis for the improved presentation is unknown, but several recent studies suggest that it may be because apoptotic cells are a favorite target captured by the cross-priming APC (27–29). Albert and colleagues (28) showed that apoptotic macrophages infected with influenza virus in vitro could be captured by dendritic cells and their antigens cross-presented to class I–restricted CTL. Thus, in the OVA-expressing model, destruction of islet cells by activated CTL (which would have led to the generation of apoptotic islet cells) probably increased the amount of available antigen for cross-presentation. This observation somewhat alters our earlier conclusion that cross-presentation requires antigen expression levels in the higher physiological range because in this case

<0.03 μg/mg protein, a moderate physiological dose by conservative standards, was sufficient to cause cross-presentation. It therefore seems reasonable to conclude that numerous self- or infection-derived proteins will be expressed at levels capable of cross-presentation, but that the extent of cross-presentation will depend on factors such as the health of the cells expressing the antigen.

Although apoptotic cells have been strongly implicated as targets for the cross-priming APC, there is no evidence to exclude the possibility that live cells are also targets. Certainly, when islet OVA was cross-presented in unmanipulated transgenic mice, there was no evidence for the presence of apoptotic islet cells. However, small numbers of apoptotic cells might have been overlooked.

Both macrophages (27) and dendritic cells (28) have been reported to cross-present antigens from apoptotic cells. However, only dendritic cells are able to induce naïve CTL to respond via cross-priming (30). This result is presumably because dendritic cells are the only cells capable of supplying costimulatory signals. It is interesting that dendritic cells were shown to cross-present both apoptotic and necrotic cells to class II–restricted T cells (31, 32), but only apoptotic cells provided a source of class I–restricted determinants (28). The reason for a discrepancy between the antigenic requirements for the class I versus class II pathways of cross-presentation is unclear; perhaps it is simply a matter of efficiency. Given the capacity of heat shock proteins (HSPs) to induce CTL by cross-priming (33–35), and the abundance of HSPs in the cytosol, necrotic cell material should possess the capacity to be cross-presented in the context of class I. In support of this view, Pardoll and colleagues (36) recently reported that cell debris could be cross-presented on class I molecules in vitro. Such debris was not generated by apoptosis and consisted largely of membrane-associated material. Because most of the analysis of the cellular requirements for class I–restricted cross-presentation has been performed in vitro, extension of these studies in vivo may reveal other less efficient pathways of antigen access to class I. Indeed, it has yet to be demonstrated that apoptosis or necrosis are essential for cross-presentation in vivo.

Although macrophages have a number of receptors for apoptotic cells, dendritic cells appear to use $\alpha_v\beta_5$ and CD36 (29). These two receptors may function together with thrombospondin to form a molecular bridge linking the dendritic cell to its apoptotic target (37). Analysis of whether the absence of any of these molecules can prevent cross-presentation in vivo will be of great interest.

In addition to antigen dose and tissue damage, at least two other factors influence cross-presentation in vivo. These are (a) the age of the host and (b) the tissue examined. It has been reported that the age of onset of cross-priming is delayed somewhat compared to that of direct priming (38). Cross-priming was not evident until about day five of life, whereas mice as young as three days old could respond by direct priming with adult APC. In other studies (8, 39), cross-presentation of three different islet antigens (two transgenic and one natural) was only detectable in the pancreatic node when mice reached approximately three weeks of age. It is interesting that cross-presentation of renal antigens in the same mice was detected at the earliest time examined (day 10), suggesting that the age of onset of cross-presentation is differentially regulated in each tissue. Why cross-presentation might be switched off in the pancreas of young mice is a matter for speculation; perhaps it relates to the extensive remodelling and associated apoptosis of the pancreatic islets that occur during this time (40–43). Remodeling might otherwise supply dangerously high amounts of self-antigens to the cross-presentation pathway, if this pathway were operative.

In summary, several factors appear to strongly influence the degree of cross-presentation in vivo: (*a*) antigen dose, (*b*) tissue damage (possibly due to targeting of apoptotic cells or release of HSPs), (*c*) age of the host, and (*d*) tissue type.

THE PHENOTYPE OF THE APC

So far we have reviewed some of the antigenic requirements for cross-presentation; in the next section we address the phenotype of the cross-priming APC. We need to emphasize two important points before we begin. First, it is possible that several different types of APC are capable of cross-presentation. Second, demonstration in vitro that a cell can cross-present antigens does not prove that it is the cell responsible for cross-presentation in vivo. This latter point needs particular emphasis, as repeated in vitro demonstration of class I–restricted presentation of exogenous antigens by cultured dendritic cells has led many researchers to assume that conventional dendritic cells are capable of cross-presentation in vivo, despite the paucity of evidence.

Macrophages were the first cell-type reported capable of class I–restricted exogenous presentation (44); some studies even implicated them in cross-presentation (45, 46). However, there is a great deal of evidence indicating that macrophages are poor stimulators of naïve T cells (47), which questions their role in cross-priming. Furthermore, when we consider the data that previously implicated macrophages as the cross-priming APC, we must remember that these conclusions were based on the incorrect assumption that dendritic cells were incapable of phagocytosis (48). This assumption was only recently clarified when dendritic cells were shown to be phagocytic during their immature stage, and to downregulate phagocytosis and upregulate antigen-processing when signaled to mature (49). Thus, in the past, the cross-priming APC may have been inappropriately identified as a macrophage by virtue of its phagocytic activity (45).

There are numerous in vitro studies that show dendritic cells, macrophages, and even B cells are capable of class I–restricted presentation of exogenous antigens(27–29, 36, 50–59). These studies have used soluble antigens (50–53, 55, 60), antigens attached to beads (52, 56), immune complexes (54), and pathogens (57, 58), but very few have examined exogenous presentation of cellular material, i.e. cross-presentation (27–29, 36, 59). The studies that have examined exogenous presentation of cellular material have reported that both dendritic cells (28, 29, 36, 59), and macrophages (27) perform cross-presentation, though only when given apoptotic cells or cell debris as an antigen source. B cells, on the other hand, were found to be unnecessary for cross-presentation in vivo (61). These studies provide strong evidence that bone marrow–derived or splenic dendritic cell preparations can cross-present cellular antigens, apoptotic cells in particular. The role of macrophages is less clear. Bhardwaj and colleagues (28) claim that macrophages cannot cross-present apoptotic material. They also suggest that Bellone's data supporting a role for macrophages (27) may be explained by the contamination of dendritic cells in their macrophage preparations (59).

Although the above models provide strong evidence that dendritic cells are capable of cross-presentation in vitro, it is unclear whether these cells truly reflect the cell responsible for cross-priming in vivo. It is surprising that there is very little in vivo evidence to implicate conventional dendritic cells in cross-priming. Other than the observations that the APC responsible for cross-presentation is bone marrow–derived (5, 7) and phagocytic (45), there are very few reports of phenotypical analysis of the cross-priming APC in vivo (46, 62, 63). When we consider that the first description of cross-priming was a quarter of a century ago (1), this seems to be an inordinately small number of reports. Furthermore, if we examine the three cases of identification of the cross-priming APC in vivo, there appears to be a common theme that suggests (*a*) that the cross-priming APC can only be isolated under conditions of inflammation and (*b*) that there might be more than one type of cross-priming APC.

Pulaski and colleagues were the first to isolate a cross-priming APC (46). They used a spontaneous lung carcinoma transfected with the genes for OVA and IL-3 to show that cells infiltrating the tumor could cross-present tumor-associated antigens. In antibody depletion studies using APC-T cell cluster formation as a measure of cross-presentation, they were able to characterize the cross-priming APC as a macrophage-like cell, although notably it did not express F4/80. This was adherent in 2 h; did not express CD4, CD8, F4/80, DEC205, 33D1, and B220; but did express class I, class II, FcR, Mac-1, and B7-1. Given our current knowledge of the diversity of dendritic cell populations (64), we can now say that this APC was quite likely a dendritic cell.

In similar studies, Chiodoni et al (63) reported that CD11c-expressing dendritic cells infiltrating tumors transfected with the genes for GM-CSF and CD40 ligand were able to cross-present tumor antigens. We must be somewhat cautious when interpreting this as evidence for isolation of the cross-priming APC from in vivo, because in this study, similar to the in vitro studies of others (28, 36), tumor debris and infiltrating dendritic cells were co-incubated for long periods in vitro as a consequence of the purification process. In the report by Pulaski et al discussed earlier (46), the APC isolation procedure was not specified, which raises the possibility that they also inadvertently allowed antigen-loading of the APC during isolation in vitro.

The third report to have isolated the cross-priming APC showed that APC from the pancreas of mice transgenically expressing TNF-α in their islet β cells were able to present islet antigens to CD8 T cells (62). These authors reported that the presenting population contained CD11c$^+$ cells (dendritic cells), but they did not prove that these cells were responsible for cross-presentation of the islet antigens. The three reports described above (46, 62, 63) provide evidence that the cross-priming APC (with antigen) can be isolated from mouse tissues, and they suggest that this cell is of dendritic origin. However, we must note that in all three examples the APC was isolated from inflammatory tissues, with no evidence of isolation from tissues such as the spleen or lymph nodes. This raises the important question of why there are no reported isolations of this APC from lymphoid tissues, particularly when this is exactly where most examples of cross-priming or cross-tolerance would expect to find the APC. Such failure is certainly not for lack of looking, because we and many others have examined lymphoid tissues without success. Failure to isolate the APC in lymphoid tissue suggests that the APC responsible for cross-presentation in these tissues is different from that found in inflammatory tissues. Furthermore, because conventional dendritic cells can be isolated from lymphoid tissues, failure to isolate the cross-priming APC from this site suggests that it is not a conventional dendritic cell. Failure to isolate this cell could be either because it dies during isolation or because it presents antigen very poorly when isolated. To assume that the cross-priming APC is a member of the dendritic cell family seems reasonable when we consider its ability to prime naïve CTL, but until the cross-priming APC can be identified, this issue must remain an open question. There is a growing number of dendritic cell subsets, with at least three in the spleen and perhaps up to five in the lymph nodes (K Shortman, personal communications). There is also plenty of reason to expect identification of yet other subsets. Perhaps the most encouraging data in the race to identify the cross-priming APC has come from MacPherson's laboratory, where they study rat dendritic cell subsets (65). In a recent report, two different types of dendritic cells were found in the afferent lymph draining the gut mucosa. An advantage of the rat model is that it is possible to collect afferent lymph by surgically removing the mesenteric lymph nodes and allowing regrowth of the lymphatic drainage vessels. By collecting lymph from the thoracic duct of such rats, MacPherson's group (65) was able to identify two CD11c$^+$ dendritic cell populations based on their expression of CD4 and OX41. What was special about the CD4$^-$OX41$^-$ subset was that they contained apoptotic bodies that were derived from gut epithelial cells. Although there is no definitive evidence that these dendritic cells can cross-present such epithelial cell antigens, their presence is consistent with reports that apoptotic cells are excellent sources of antigen for cross-presentation (28, 29). These dendritic cells may be the rat equivalent of the constitutively trafficking mouse APC responsible for cross-tolerance (7, 16). This supposition is supported by the observed constitutive trafficking of these dendritic cells to T cell areas of lymphoid tissues. Furthermore, these dendritic cells, compared to their CD4+OX41+ counterparts, appear to survive poorly in vitro and to be relatively weak stimulators of T cell proliferation. These findings may explain why such cells have been difficult to identify in the mouse. Determining the capacity of these cells to cross-present epithelial antigens, as well as the direction of the immune responses they induce, i.e. immunity or tolerance, will be very important.

It is interesting that rat dendritic cells have also been reported to be cytolytic. Josien and colleagues (66) provided evidence that a subset of rat dendritic cells that expressed the natural killer cell receptor protein 1 were able to kill NK-sensitive targets (YAC-1) but were not able to kill an insensitive target (P815). More recently, this dendritic cell subset was shown to be CD4⁻OX41⁻ (R Josien, personal communications), the same phenotype as that reported by Macpherson's group to contain apoptotic bodies (65). The observation that dendritic cells can kill cells expressing low levels of MHC molecules raises the interesting possibility that this subset functions by scanning the periphery for cells with defective MHC expression (because they are either cancerous or infected). They could then kill the defective cells, engulf their apoptotic bodies, and cross-present their antigens in the draining lymph nodes. Interesting evidence suggests that the killer dendritic cells do phagocytose their targets (R Josien, personal communications).

CELLULAR INTERACTIONS AND MOLECULAR SIGNALS FOR CROSS-PRIMING

As analysis of the cellular interactions and molecular signals required for cross-priming has been extensively reviewed recently (67, 68), we here only highlight some of the more salient points and discuss the latest findings. Three cell types appear to be essential for cross-priming. The first is the APC, which as we have indicated above is largely uncharacterized. The second is the CTL precursor. The third is a CD4⁺ helper T cell (44). We are not certain if cross-priming always requires CD4⁺ T cell help because a response is difficult to define as dependent on cross-priming. But, so far, all examples of cross-priming that have been examined for their helper requirements are CD4 T cell dependent (4, 61, 69). These examples include responses to minor antigens (69), OVA-loaded spleen cells (4), and tumors (61). However, not all CTL responses are CD4 dependent; many viruses, for example, are able to induce CTL immunity in the absence of CD4 T cells (70–72). In this respect, it will be interesting to see whether cross-priming to poliovirus (6) is helper dependent.

CD4 T cells appear to help by modifying the APC, which licenses it to become fully competent for CTL priming (reviewed in 67). Evidence for this was first provided by the observation that CD4 and CD8 T cells need to interact with the same APC in order to generate CTL immunity (73), including CTL immunity by cross-priming (4). The requirement for co-recognition of the same APC suggested two possibilities: (a) the CD4 T cells help by delivering short-range cytokine signals (74), or (b) helper cells are needed to modify the APC into a form capbable of CTL priming (75). Three reports, two of which examined cross-priming, provided strong evidence for the second alternative by showing that a CD40-specific monoclonal antibody could replace the need for CD4 T cells during priming (61, 76, 77). Because CD40 is expressed by APC, and CD40-ligand (CD154) is expressed by CD4 T cells, this observation suggested that CD4 T cells normally provide help by signaling CD40 on the cross-priming APC. These studies also indicated that there could be a temporal separation between the CD4-APC interaction and CD8-APC interaction. Demonstration that CD154 signaling of CD40 was the help provided by CD4 T cells meant that the two T cell subsets did not need to meet on the same APC but could simply interact sequentially with the APC. In this way, CD4 T cells could act like catalysts, moving from APC to APC, licensing each for CTL priming. Later, CD8 T cells could find one of these licensed APC and receive the signals necessary for full maturation into functional CTL.

As usual, things are never as simple as they first seem. Since CD154 was shown to act as a helper signal, other alternative molecular interactions have been implicated in CTL generation. Bachmann and colleagues (78) provided evidence that priming CTL to lymphocytic choriomeningitis virus or vesicular stomatitis virus was CD40 independent, and that unknown factor(s) supplied by CD8 T cells could license the dendritic cells for effective priming. These studies were, however, not strictly cross-priming. In a separate series of experiments, Pardoll and associates (36) revealed three separate forms of help for CTL generation. They confirmed that CD40 signaling could contribute to CTL priming, this time in response to vaccinia virus. Using an in vitro model of cross-priming, they also provided evidence for two CD40 independent forms of CD4 T cell help, one soluble and the other mediated by contact with the APC. So far, however, neither form of help has been specifically defined.

A number of other potential molecular interactions between T cells and APC may be important for cross-priming. These include TRANCE/TRANCE-ligand, OX40/OX40L, CD28/B7, ICOS/B7RP, and 4-1BB/4-1BB-ligand. Preliminary findings indicate that B7 molecules are involved in cross-priming (S Schoenberger, personal communications), but none of the other interactions has been examined.

As far as cytokine requirements are concerned, IL-12 is the most likely cytokine to have an essential role in signaling between the APC and T cells. Like B7-1 and B7-2 (79, 80), this cytokine is upregulated upon CD40 stimulation (81). Furthermore, it is essential for some (82, 83), but not all (84, 85), examples of CTL priming, which include responses to exogenous antigens (83). However, whether IL-12 has a role in cross-priming remains to be determined.

In summary, although we know there are three important cell types involved in cross-priming and that there must be downstream products of CD40 signaling that are critical for CTL activation, there is very little knowledge of the exact molecules involved in this process.

FACTORS THAT DIRECT THE IMMUNE SYSTEM TOWARD TOLERANCE OR IMMUNITY

Cross-presentation has two different sides, traditionally known as cross-priming and cross-tolerance. As discussed above, cross-priming involves the activation of CD4 and CD8 T cells in the generation of CTL immunity to cell-derived antigens.

Cross-priming is involved in responses to virus infection, cancer cells, and transplanted histoincompatible tissues. On the other side of the cross-presentation coin is cross-tolerance, which involves the induction of T cell tolerance via the cross-presentation of cellular antigens, usually derived from normal healthy tissues. Cross-tolerance has been reported to induce CD4 and CD8 T cell tolerance by either deletion (16, 86) or anergy (87).

The ability of the cross-presentation process to induce either immunity or tolerance can be explained in two alternative ways: either (a) there are two different types of APC, one that targets foreign antigens and is responsible for cross-priming, and another that targets self-antigens and induces cross-tolerance; or (b) there is only one type of cross-presenting APC, which can be switched from tolerogenic to immunogenic depending on the nature of the antigen. We favor the second scenario because it is difficult to explain how foreign and self-antigens can be differentially targeted for cross-presentation when both are associated with self-tissue. However, an argument for the first scenario may be that the cross-priming APC is only interested in antigen when there is damage associated with infection, whereas the cross-tolerance APC continuously samples healthy tissue and induces tolerance. This argument is problematic because it would preclude responses to many tumors and nonlytic viruses, and it would favor cross-priming during tissue trauma associated with injury. The observation that mice respond to the same antigen, OVA, by either cross-priming or cross-tolerance, depending on whether it is foreign (OVA-loaded spleen cells) or self (OVA expressed in the pancreas of transgenic mice), clearly indicates that the antigen itself cannot dictate the type of response. Therefore, the circumstances in which the antigen is seen must dictate the response. But, how could this work?

Two main models provide possible solutions to this problem. Janeway and colleagues (88) suggest that APCs have pattern-recognition receptors that they use to identify characteristic molecules unique to pathogens. This idea led Janeway's group to discover the Toll-like receptors in mammalian cells (89–91). In this model, the APCs are not capable of priming until they receive a signal through their pattern-recognition receptors, as for example may occur when lipopolysaccharide interacts with TLR-4 (92). If we translate this model into the cross-presentation process, then pathogen products would convert the APC from its normal tolerogenic state to an activated state capable of cross-priming. In this way, normal body tissues could be continuously sampled by the cross-presenting APC. Antigens from these tissues would be cross-presented in the draining lymph nodes and, in the absence of infection, would induce cross-tolerance to self. In the case of a virus infection, however, the cross-presenting APC would capture tissue antigens and simultaneously receive a signal from viral products binding to pattern-recognition receptors. This process would convert the APC into a state ready for cross-priming, which leads to virus-specific CTL immunity. The main problem with this model is that it does not provide an obvious mechanism by which the cross-presenting APC can be activated to induce cross-priming to tumors or minor histocompatibility antigens.

The second model, proposed by Matzinger (93), is sometimes referred to as the "danger model" and relies on cell-derived signals to activate the APC. Instead of sensing pathogen products, the APC in the Matzinger model is designed to sense danger in the form of factors released from damaged cells. These factors could be as simple as heat shock proteins or mitochondrial products, factors that would normally be found only inside healthy cells. In this model, the immune system does not care about invasion by harmless parasites; instead, it focuses on generating immunity only when there is detectable harm being done to the body. In terms of cross-presentation, this approach to immunity means that the cross-presenting APC can constitutively capture tissue antigens and induce tolerance unless it is exposed to cellular signs of danger. In the presence of such danger, the cross-presenting APC will be converted into a cross-priming APC that will induce CTL immunity. The benefit of this model is that it can explain responses to tumors, which, due to uncontrolled growth, can become necrotic and release cellular signals of danger. The relationship between cross-priming and minor histocompatibility antigens is more difficult to explain, but preparation of the immunizing cells is likely to result in some level of damage, which may generate a source of danger.

At present, there are arguments for and against both the Janeway and Matzinger models. As far as cross-priming is concerned, however, Janeway's model does not easily explain cross-priming to tumors or minor antigens, where there are no apparent pathogen products. Thus, there is a tendency to favor the Matzinger model. However, rejection of Janeway's model should be approached with caution because it is difficult to rule out the presence of pathogen genes or gene products within cross-priming tissues such as tumors or transplanted material.

CONCLUSIONS

Though cross-priming was first described more than a quarter century ago, the field of cross-presentation still appears to be in its infancy. The relatively recent advent of transgenic technology, as well as the development of dendritic cell purification and culturing techniques, has provided us with several new insights into this process. However, we still have only a very basic understanding. In this review, we summarized our current knowledge of the mechanism of antigen capture, the phenotype of the APC, the molecular and cellular signals involved in cross-priming, and the factors that direct the immune system toward cross-tolerance or cross-priming. All of these areas need a great deal more investigation. When we consider the extensive role of cross-presentation in immunity to tumors, viruses, intracellular bacteria, and grafts, as well as cross-presentation's role in tolerance to self, we realize this is a field that certainly warrants future investment.

LITERATURE CITED

1. Bevan MJ. 1976. Cross-priming for a secondary cytotoxic response to minor H antigens with H-2 congenic cells which do not cross-react in the cytotoxic assay. *J. Exp. Med.* 143:1283–88

2. Heath WR, Kurts C, Miller JF, Carbone FR. 1998. Cross-tolerance: a pathway for inducing tolerance to peripheral tissue antigens. *J. Exp. Med.* 187:1549–53

3. Yewdell JW, Norbury CC, Bennink JR. 1999. Mechanisms of exogenous antigen presentation by MHC class I molecules in vitro and in vivo: implications for generating CD8+ T cell responses to infectious agents, tumors, transplants, and vaccines. *Adv. Immunol.* 73:1–77

4. Bennett SR, Carbone FR, Karamalis F, Miller JF, Heath WR. 1997. Induction of a CD8+ cytotoxic T lymphocyte response by cross-priming requires cognate CD4+ T cell help. *J. Exp. Med.* 186:65–70

5. Huang AY, Golumbek P, Ahmadzadeh M, Jaffee E, Pardoll D, Levitsky H. 1994. Role of bone marrow-derived cells in presenting MHC class I-restricted tumor antigens. *Science* 264:961–65

6. Sigal LJ, Crotty S, Andino R, Rock KL. 1999. Cytotoxic T-cell immunity to virus-infected non-haematopoietic cells requires presentation of exogenous antigen. *Nature* 398:77–80

7. Kurts C, Heath WR, Carbone FR, Allison J, Miller JF, Kosaka H. 1996. Constitutive class I-restricted exogenous presentation of self antigens in vivo. *J. Exp. Med.* 184:923–30

8. Morgan DJ, Kurts C, Kreuwel HT, Holst KL, Heath WR, Sherman LA. 1999. Ontogeny of T cell tolerance to peripherally expressed antigens. *Proc. Natl. Acad. Sci. USA* 96:3854–58

9. Huang AY, Bruce AT, Pardoll DM, Levitsky HI. 1996. In vivo cross-priming of

MHC class I-restricted antigens requires the TAP transporter. *Immunity* 4:349–55

10. Gooding LR, Edwards CB. 1980. H-2 antigen requirements in the in vitro induction of SV40-specific cytotoxic T lymphocytes. *J. Immunol.* 124:1258–62

11. Carbone FR, Bevan MJ. 1990. Class I-restricted processing and presentation of exogenous cell-associated antigen in vivo. *J. Exp. Med.* 171:377–87

12. Kundig TM, Bachmann MF, DiPaolo C, Simard JJ, Battegay M, Lother H, Gessner A, Kuhlcke K, Ohashi PS, Hengartner H, Zinkernagel R. 1995. Fibroblasts as efficient antigen-presenting cells in lymphoid organs. *Science* 268:1343–47

13. Ohashi PS, Oehen S, Buerki K, Pircher H, Ohashi CT, Odermatt B, Malissen B, Zinkernagel RM, Hengartner H. 1991. Ablation of "tolerance" and induction of diabetes by virus infection in viral antigen transgenic mice. *Cell* 65:305–17

14. Doe B, Selby M, Barnett S, Baenziger J, Walker CM. 1996. Induction of cytotoxic T lymphocytes by intramuscular immunization with plasmid DNA is facilitated by bone marrow-derived cells. *Proc. Natl. Acad. Sci. USA* 93:8578–83

15. Porgador A, Irvine KR, Iwasaki A, Barber BH, Restifo NP, Germain RN. 1998. Predominant role for directly transfected dendritic cells in antigen presentation to CD8+ T cells after gene gun immunization. *J. Exp. Med.* 188:1075–82

16. Kurts C, Kosaka H, Carbone FR, Miller JF, Heath WR. 1997. Class I-restricted cross-presentation of exogenous self-antigens leads to deletion of autoreactive CD8(+) T cells. *J. Exp. Med.* 186:239–45

17. Oldstone MB, Nerenberg M, Southern P, Price J, Lewicki H. 1991. Virus infection triggers insulin-dependent diabetes mellitus in a transgenic model: role

of anti-self (virus) immune response. *Cell* 65:319–31

18. Kurts C, Miller JF, Subramaniam RM, Carbone FR, Heath WR. 1998. Major histocompatibility complex class I-restricted cross-presentation is biased towards high dose antigens and those released during cellular destruction. *J. Exp. Med.* 188:409–14

19. Kurts C, Sutherland RM, Davey G, Li M, Lew AM, Blanas E, Carbone FR, Miller JF, Heath WR. 1999. CD8 T cell ignorance or tolerance to islet antigens depends on antigen dose. *Proc. Natl. Acad. Sci. USA* 96:12703–7

20. Deleted in proof

21. Pederson RA, Satkunarajah M, McIntosh CH, Scrocchi LA, Flamez D, Schuit F, Drucker DJ, Wheeler MB. 1998. Enhanced glucose-dependent insulinotropic polypeptide secretion and insulinotropic action in glucagon-like peptide 1 receptor -/- mice. *Diabetes* 47:1046–52

22. Kato K, Suzuki F, Nakajima T. 1983. Decrease in adipose S-100 protein levels by epinephrine in rat. *J. Biochem.* 93:311–13

23. Ansorge S, Wiederanders B, Riemann S, Brouwer A, Knook DL. 1984. Distribution of thiol-protein disulfide oxidoreductase, insulin-glucagon proteinase and cathepsin D in different cell types of the rat liver. *Biomed. Biochim. Acta* 43:1213–21

24. Chao J, Sostek M, Shimamoto K, Bank HL, Bigelow J, Margolius HS. 1980. Kallikrein content of rat pancreatic acinar cells or islets by direct radioimmunoassay. *Hoppe-Seylers Z. Physiol. Chem.* 361:1805–10

25. Benevolensky D, Belikova Y, Mohammadzadeh R, Trouve P, Marotte F, Russo-Marie F, Samuel JL, Charlemagne D. 2000. Expression and localization of the annexins II, V, and VI in myocardium from patients with end-stage heart failure. *Lab. Invest.* 80:123–33

26. Miceli MV, Tate DJ Jr, Alcock NW, Newsome DA. 1999. Zinc deficiency and

oxidative stress in the retina of pigmented rats. *Invest. Ophthalmol. Visual Sci.* 40:1238–44

27. Bellone M, Iezzi G, Rovere P, Galati G, Ronchetti A, Protti MP, Davoust J, Rugarli C, Manfredi AA. 1997. Processing of engulfed apoptotic bodies yields T cell epitopes. *J. Immunol.* 159:5391–99

28. Albert ML, Sauter B, Bhardwaj N. 1998. Dendritic cells acquire antigen from apoptotic cells and induce class I-restricted CTLs. *Nature* 392:86–89

29. Albert ML, Pearce SF, Francisco LM, Sauter B, Roy P, Silverstein RL, Bhardwaj N. 1998. Immature dendritic cells phagocytose apoptotic cells via alphavbeta5 and CD36, and cross-present antigens to cytotoxic T lymphocytes. *J. Exp. Med.* 188:1359–68

30. Ronchetti A, Rovere P, Iezzi G, Galati G, Heltai S, Protti MP, Garancini MP, Manfredi AA, Rugarli C, Bellone M. 1999. Immunogenicity of apoptotic cells in vivo: role of antigen load, antigen-presenting cells, and cytokines. *J. Immunol.* 163:130–36

31. Inaba K, Turley S, Yamaide F, Iyoda T, Mahnke K, Inaba M, Pack M, Subklewe M, Sauter B, Sheff D, Albert M, Bhardwaj N, Mellman I, Steinman RM. 1998. Efficient presentation of phagocytosed cellular fragments on the major histocompatibility complex class II products of dendritic cells. *J. Exp. Med.* 188:2163–73

32. Gallucci S, Lolkema M, Matzinger P. 1999. Natural adjuvants: endogenous activators of dendritic cells. *Nat. Med.* 5:1249–55

33. Arnold D, Faath S, Rammensee H, Schild H.1995. Cross-priming of minor histocompatibility antigen-specific cytotoxic T cells upon immunization with the heat shock protein gp96. *J. Exp. Med.* 182:885–89

34. Janetzki S, Blachere NE, Srivastava PK. 1998. Generation of tumor-specific cytotoxic T lymphocytes and memory T cells by immunization with tumor-derived

heat shock protein gp96. *J. Immunother.* 21:269–76

35. Udono H, Levey DL, Srivastava PK. 1994. Cellular requirements for tumor-specific immunity elicited by heat shock proteins: tumor rejection antigen gp96 primes CD8+ T cells in vivo. *Proc. Natl. Acad. Sci. USA* 91:3077–81

36. Lu Z, Yuan L, Zhou X, Sotomayor E, Levitsky HI, Pardoll DM. 2000. CD40–independent pathways of T cell help for priming of CD8(+) cytotoxic T lymphocytes. *J Exp Med.* 191:541–50

37. Savill J, Hogg N, Ren Y, Haslett C.1992. Thrombospondin cooperates with CD36 and the vitronectin receptor in macrophage recognition of neutrophils undergoing apoptosis. *J. Clin. Invest.* 90:1513–22

38. Rafii-Tabar E, Czitrom AA. 1986. Ontogeny of priming of cytotoxic T cells to minor alloantigens: the development of direct priming precedes that of cross-priming. *Eur. J. Immunol.* 16:1025–27

39. Hoglund P, Mintern J, Waltzinger C, Heath W, Benoist C, Mathis D. 1999. Initiation of autoimmune diabetes by developmentally regulated presentation of islet cell antigens in the pancreatic lymph nodes. *J. Exp. Med.* 189:331–39

40. Trudeau JD, Dutz JP, Arany E, Hill DJ, Fieldus WE, Finegood DT. 2000. Neonatal beta-cell apoptosis: a trigger for autoimmune diabetes? *Diabetes* 49:1–7

41. Petrik J, Arany E, McDonald TJ, Hill DJ. 1998. Apoptosis in the pancreatic islet cells of the neonatal rat is associated with a reduced expression of insulin-like growth factor II that may act as a survival factor. *Endocrinology* 139:2994–3004

42. Scaglia L, Cahill CJ, Finegood DT, Bonner-Weir S.1997. Apoptosis participates in the remodeling of the endocrine pancreas in the neonatal rat. *Endocrinology* 138:1736–41

43. Finegood DT, Scaglia L, Bonner-Weir S. 1995. Dynamics of beta-cell mass in the growing rat pancreas. Estimation with a simple mathematical model. *Diabetes* 44:249–56

44. Kovacsovics-Bankowski M, Clark K, Benacerraf B, Rock KL. 1993. Efficient major histocompatibility complex class I presentation of exogenous antigen upon phagocytosis by macrophages. *Proc. Natl. Acad. Sci. USA* 90:4942–46

45. Debrick JE, Campbell PA, Staerz UD. 1991. Macrophages as accessory cells for class I MHC-restricted immune responses. *J. Immunol.* 147:2846–51

46. Pulaski BA, Yeh KY, Shastri N, Maltby KM, Penney DP, Lord EM, Frelinger JG. 1996. Interleukin 3 enhances cytotoxic T lymphocyte development and class I major histocompatibility complex "re-presentation" of exogenous antigen by tumor-infiltrating antigen-presenting cells. *Proc. Natl. Acad. Sci. USA* 93:3669–74

47. Steinman RM, Cohn ZA. 1973. Identification of a novel cell type in peripheral lymphoid organs of mice. I. Morphology, quantitation, tissue distribution. *J. Exp. Med.* 137:1142–62

48. Witmer-Pack MD, Crowley MT, Inaba K, Steinman RM. 1993. Macrophages, but not dendritic cells, accumulate colloidal carbon following administration in situ. *J. Cell Sci.* 105:965–73

49. Sallusto F, Cella M, Danieli C, Lanzavecchia A. 1995. Dendritic cells use macropinocytosis and the mannose receptor to concentrate macromolecules in the major histocompatibility complex class II compartment: downregulation by cytokines and bacterial products. *J. Exp. Med.* 182:389–400

50. Norbury CC, Hewlett LJ, A.R. P, Shastri N Watts C. 1995. Class I MHC presentation of exogenous soluble antigen via macropinocytosis in bone marrow macrophages. *Immunity* 3:783–91

51. Norbury CC, Chambers BJ, Prescott AR, Ljunggren HG, Watts C. 1997. Constitutive macropinocytosis allows

TAP-dependent major histocompatibility complex class I presentation of exogenous soluble antigen by bone marrow-derived dendritic cells. *Eur. J. Immunol.* 27:280–88

52. Shen Z, Reznikoff G, Dranoff G, Rock KL. 1997. Cloned dendritic cells can present exogenous antigens on both MHC class I and class II molecules. *J. Immunol.* 158:2723–30

53. Mitchell DA, Nair SK, Gilboa E. 1998. Dendritic cell/macrophage precursors capture exogenous antigen for MHC class I presentation by dendritic cells. *Eur. J. Immunol.* 28:1923–33. Erratum. 1998. *Eur. J. Immunol.* 28(11):3891

54. Regnault A, Lankar D, Lacabanne V, Rodriguez A, Thery C, Rescigno M, Saito T, Verbeek S, Bonnerot C, Ricciardi-Castagnoli P, Amigorena S. 1999. Fc gamma receptor-mediated induction of dendritic cell maturation and major histocompatibility complex class I-restricted antigen presentation after immune complex internalization. *J. Exp. Med.* 189:371–80

55. Ke Y, Kapp JA. 1996. Exogenous antigens gain access to the major histocompatibility complex class I processing pathway in B cells by receptor-mediated uptake. *J. Exp. Med.* 184:1179–84

56. Reis E Sousa C, Germain RN. 1995. Major histocompatibility complex class I presentation of peptides derived from soluble exogenous antigen by a subset of cells engaged in phagocytosis. *J. Exp. Med.* 182:841–51

57. Harding CV, Song R. 1994. Phagocytic processing of exogenous particulate antigens by macrophages for presentation by class I MHC molecules. *J. Immunol.* 153:4925–33

58. Pfeifer JD, Wick MJ, Roberts RL, Findlay K, Normark SJ, Harding CV. 1993. Phagocytic processing of bacterial antigens for class I MHC presentation to T cells. *Nature* 361:359–62

59. Sauter B, Albert ML, Francisco L, Larson M, Somersan S, Bhardwaj N. 2000. Consequences of cell death: exposure to necrotic tumor cells, but not primary tissue cells or apoptotic cells, induces the maturation of immunostimulatory dendritic cells. *J. Exp. Med.* 191:423–34

60. Barnaba V, Franco A, Alberti A, Benvenuto R, Balsano F. 1990. Selective killing of hepatitis B envelope antigen-specific B cells by class I-restricted, exogenous antigen-specific T lymphocytes. *Nature* 345:258–60

61. Schoenberger SP, Toes RE, van der Voort EI, Offringa R, Melief CJ. 1998. T-cell help for cytotoxic T lymphocytes is mediated by CD40–CD40L interactions. *Nature* 393:480–83

62. Green EA, Wong FS, Eshima K, Mora C, Flavell RA. 2000. Neonatal tumor necrosis factor alpha promotes diabetes in nonobese diabetic mice by CD154–independent antigen presentation to CD8(+) T cells. *J. Exp. Med.* 191:225–38

63. Chiodoni C, Paglia P, Stoppacciaro A, Rodolfo M, Parenza M, Colombo MP. 1999. Dendritic cells infiltrating tumors cotransduced with granulocyte/macrophage colony-stimulating factor (GM-CSF) and CD40 ligand genes take up and present endogenous tumor-associated antigens, and prime naive mice for a cytotoxic T lymphocyte response. *J. Exp. Med.* 190:125–33

64. Banchereau J, Steinman RM. 1998. Dendritic cells and the control of immunity. *Nature* 392:245–52

65. Huang FP, Platt N, Wykes M, Major JR, Powell TJ, Jenkins CD, MacPherson GG. 2000. A discrete subpopulation of dendritic cells transports apoptotic intestinal epithelial cells to T cell areas of mesenteric lymph nodes. *J. Exp. Med.* 191:435–44

66. Josien R, Heslan M, Soulillou JP, Cuturi MC. 1997. Rat spleen dendritic cells express natural killer cell receptor protein 1 (NKR-P1) and have cytotoxic activity to select targets via a Ca2+-dependent mechanism. *J. Exp. Med.* 186:467–72

67. Clarke SR. 2000. The critical role of CD40/CD40L in the CD4-dependent generation of CD8+ T cell immunity. *J. Leukoc. Biol.* 67:607–14

68. Heath WR, Carbone FR. 1999. Cytotoxic T lymphocyte activation by cross-priming. *Curr. Opin. Immunol.* 11:314–18

69. Husmann LA, Bevan MJ. 1988. Cooperation between helper T cells and cytotoxic T lymphocyte precursors. *Ann. N.Y. Acad. Sci.* 532:158–69

70. Buller RM, Holmes KL, Hugin A, Frederickson TN, Morse HCd. 1987. Induction of cytotoxic T-cell responses in vivo in the absence of CD4 helper cells. *Nature* 328:77–79

71. Rahemtulla A, Fung-Leung WP, Schilham MW, Kundig TM, Sambhara SR, Narendran A Arabian A, Wakeham A, Paige CJ, Zinkernagel RM, Miller RG, Mak TW. 1991. Normal development and function of CD8+ cells but markedly decreased helper cell activity in mice lacking CD4. *Nature* 353:180–84

72. Liu Y, Mullbacher A. 1989. The generation and activation of memory class I MHC restricted cytotoxic T cell responses to influenza A virus in vivo do not require CD4+ T cells. *Immunol. Cell Biol.* 67:413–20

73. Cassell D, Forman J. 1988. Linked recognition of helper and cytotoxic antigenic determinants for the generation of cytotoxic T lymphocytes. *Ann. NY Acad. Sci.* 532:51–60

74. Keene JA, Forman J. 1982. Helper activity is required for the in vivo generation of cytotoxic T lymphocytes. *J. Exp. Med.* 155:768–82

75. Guerder S, Matzinger P. 1992. A fail-safe mechanism for maintaining self-tolerance. *J. Exp. Med.* 176:553–64

76. Ridge JP, Di Rosa F, Matzinger P. 1998. A conditioned dendritic cell can be a temporal bridge between a CD4+ T-helper and a T-killer cell. *Nature* 393:474–78

77. Bennett SR, Carbone FR, Karamalis F, Flavell RA, Miller JF, Heath WR. 1998. Help for cytotoxic-T-cell responses is mediated by CD40 signalling. *Nature* 393:478–80

78. Ruedl C, Kopf M, Bachmann MF. 1999. CD8(+) T cells mediate CD40-independent maturation of dendritic cells in vivo. *J. Exp. Med.* 189:1875–84

79. Grewal IS, Foellmer HG, Grewal KD, Xu J, Hardardottir F, Baron JL, Janeway C Jr, Flavell RA. 1996. Requirement for CD40 ligand in costimulation induction, T cell activation, and experimental allergic encephalomyelitis. *Science* 273:1864–67

80. Yang Y, Wilson JM. 1996. CD40 ligand-dependent T cell activation: requirement of B7–CD28 signaling through CD40. *Science* 273:1862–64

81. Cella M, Scheidegger D, Palmer-Lehmann K, Lane P, Lanzavecchia A, Alber G. 1996. Ligation of CD40 on dendritic cells triggers production of high levels of interleukin-12 and enhances T cell stimulatory capacity: T-T help via APC activation. *J. Exp. Med.* 184:747–52

82. Bianchi R, Grohmann U, Belladonna ML, Silla S, Fallarino F, Ayroldi E, Fioretti MC, Puccetti P. 1996. IL-12 is both required and sufficient for initiating T cell reactivity to a class I-restricted tumor peptide (P815AB) following transfer of P815AB-pulsed dendritic cells. *J. Immunol.* 157:1589–97

83. Wild J, Grusby MJ, Schirmbeck R, Reimann J. 1999. Priming MHC-I-restricted cytotoxic T lymphocyte responses to exogenous hepatitis B surface antigen is CD4+ T cell dependent. *J. Immunol.* 163:1880–87

84. Magram J, Connaughton SE, Warrier RR, Carvajal DM, Wu CY, Ferrante J, Stewart C, Sarmiento U, Faherty DA, Gately MK. 1996. IL-12–deficient mice are defective in IFN gamma production and type 1 cytokine responses. *Immunity* 4:471–81

85. Simmons CP, Mastroeni P, Fowler R, Ghaem-Maghami M, Lycke N, Pizza

M, Rappuoli R, Dougan G. 1999. MHC class I-restricted cytotoxic lymphocyte responses induced by enterotoxin-based mucosal adjuvants. *J. Immunol.* 163:6502–10

86. Forster I, Lieberam I. 1996. Peripheral tolerance of CD4 T cells following local activation in adolescent mice. *Eur. J. Immunol.* 26:3194–202

87. Adler AJ, Marsh DW, Yochum GS, Guzzo JL, Nigam A, Nelson WG, Pardoll DM. 1998. CD4+ T cell tolerance to parenchymal self antigens requires presentation by bone marrow derived antigen presenting cells. *J. Exp. Med.* 187:1555–64

88. Janeway CA Jr. 1992. The immune system evolved to discriminate infectious nonself from noninfectious self. *Immunol. Today.* 13:11–16

89. Medzhitov R, Preston-Hurlburt P, Janeway CA Jr. 1997. A human homologue of the Drosophila Toll protein signals activation of adaptive immunity. *Nature* 388:394–97

90. Medzhitov R, Janeway CA Jr. 1998. An ancient system of host defense. *Curr. Opin. Immunol.* 10:12–15

91. Medzhitov R, Janeway CA Jr. 1997. Innate immunity: the virtues of a nonclonal system of recognition. *Cell* 91:295–98

92. Poltorak A, He X, Smirnova I, Liu MY, Huffel CV, Du X, Birdwell D, Alejos E, Silva M, Galanos C, Freudenberg M, Ricciardi-Castagnoli P, Layton B, Beutler B. 1998. Defective LPS signaling in C3H/HeJ and C57BL/10ScCr mice: mutations in Tlr4 gene. *Science* 282:2085–88

93. Matzinger P. 1994. Tolerance, danger, and the extended family. *Annu. Rev. Immunol.* 12:991–1045

Annu. Rev. Immunol. 2001. 19:65–91

NONCYTOLYTIC CONTROL OF VIRAL INFECTIONS BY THE INNATE AND ADAPTIVE IMMUNE RESPONSE

Luca G. Guidotti and Francis V. Chisari

Department of Molecular and Experimental Medicine, Scripps Research Institute,
10550 North Torrey Pines Road, La Jolla, California 92037;
e-mail: guidotti@scripps.edu, fchisari@scripps.edu

Key Words noncytolytic antiviral mechanisms, viruses, cytokines, innate immunity, adaptive immunity

■ **Abstract** This review describes the contribution of noncytolytic mechanisms to the control of viral infections with a particular emphasis on the role of cytokines in these processes. It has long been known that most cell types in the body respond to an incoming viral infection by rapidly secreting antiviral cytokines such as interferon alpha/beta (IFN-α/β). After binding to specific receptors on the surface of infected cells, IFN-α/β has the potential to trigger the activation of multiple noncytolytic intracellular antiviral pathways that can target many steps in the viral life cycle, thereby limiting the amplification and spread of the virus and attenuating the infection. Clearance of established viral infections, however, requires additional functions of the immune response. The accepted dogma is that complete clearance of intracellular viruses by the immune response depends on the destruction of infected cells by the effector cells of the innate and adaptive immune system [natural killer (NK) cells and cytotoxic T cells (CTLs)]. This notion, however, has been recently challenged by experimental evidence showing that much of the antiviral potential of these cells reflects their ability to produce antiviral cytokines such as IFN-γ and tumor necrosis factor (TNF)-α at the site of the infection. Indeed, these cytokines can purge viruses from infected cells noncytopathically as long as the cell is able to activate antiviral mechanisms and the virus is sensitive to them. Importantly, the same cytokines also control viral infections indirectly, by modulating the induction, amplification, recruitment, and effector functions of the immune response and by upregulating antigen processing and display of viral epitopes at the surface of infected cells. In keeping with these concepts, it is not surprising that a number of viruses encode proteins that have the potential to inhibit the antiviral activity of cytokines.

0732-0582/01/0407-0065$14.00

INTRODUCTION AND OVERVIEW

The host-virus relationship is a dynamic process in which the virus attempts to minimize its visibility while the host attempts to prevent and eradicate infection with minimal collateral damage to itself. Initially, the virus must recognize, bind, and enter its target cells, and migrate to the appropriate cellular compartment. Here its genome is transcribed, translated, and replicated to permit the assembly and export of new virions so the infection can spread to additional susceptible cells and hosts. The host must be able to recognize the presence of the virus and eliminate it as quickly and efficiently as possible. This usually occurs as a stepwise series of events in which the infected cells and the immune system each play a critical role.

Depending on the nature of the infecting virus, the infected cells may be triggered by the virus to produce antiviral cytokines (e.g. IFN-α/β) that inhibit one or more steps in the viral life cycle, thereby limiting the extent of the infection. The same cytokines have the potential to recruit inflammatory cells into the infected tissue and to activate those cells to express effector functions, to upregulate MHC protein expression, and to enhance the processing and transport of viral peptides so they can be efficiently displayed by the MHC proteins at the surface of the infected cells.

The host must recognize the infecting virus and respond to it. Granulocytes, NK cells, and perhaps NKT cells constitute an early line of defense when they are attracted into the infected tissue by cytokines and chemokines produced by the infected cells and by secondarily activated resident macrophages. Although the target recognition element(s) of NK cells is not currently known, they have the potential to recognize the infected cells very early in the infection; e.g. before MHC class I expression is significantly induced. NK cells display at least two effector functions that can contribute to control of infection: First, they can kill infected cells; second, they are a rich source of inflammatory cytokines with antiviral activity, especially IFN-γ. NKT cells may also play a role in the early control of virus infections if they become activated in infected tissue during a viral infection, given their ability to produce IFN-γ. In addition, because they are unusually abundant in the liver (where they constitute one third of all resident lymphocytes under baseline conditions), they may play a special role in the control hepatic infections because they don't need to be recruited into that organ.

Host macrophages and dendritic cells also play a key role in the early control of infection by secreting chemokines as well as pro-inflammatory cytokines, such as interleukin (IL)-12 and IL-18 that can induce IFN-γ, and other cytokines, such as IL-1, IL-6, and TNF-α, that can have direct and indirect antiviral effects on their own. All of the foregoing events contribute to the development of the adaptive immune response to an infecting virus. When the infection occurs in nonlymphoid organs, the immune response likely occurs in regional lymph nodes to which apoptotic infected cells and debris are delivered by tissue-derived dendritic cells.

The derivative T cell populations can then home to the infected tissue, recognize viral antigen, and perform their effector functions, including the production of antiviral cytokines, especially IFN-γ and TNF-α.

IFN-γ and TNF-α can play a critical role in the control of viral infection at several different levels. First, they can recruit and activate macrophages, NK cells, and T cells to perform their effector functions, including the production of immunoregulatory and antiviral monokines and cytokines. Second, they can polarize the T cell response toward the development of antiviral effector functions needed for effective control of viral infections. Third, they can upregulate antigen processing, transport, and MHC expression locally in the infected cells. Finally, they can exert direct antiviral activity.

The antiviral effects of inflammatory cytokines are mediated by induced cellular pathways that interfere with one or more steps in the viral replication program resulting in complete or partial purging of the virus from the cell while maintaining its functional integrity. Only a few of these cellular pathways have been defined thus far. The best studied pathways to date are induced by interferon-alpha/beta, including $2'5'$ oligoadenylate synthetase–induced RNAse L (which degrades viral RNAs) and double-stranded RNA-activated protein kinase (PKR) (which inhibits viral protein synthesis). In recent studies, the molecular bases for posttranscriptional degradation of hepatitis B virus (HBV) RNA and posttranslational inhibition of HBV capsid formation/stability by inflammatory cytokines have been defined, and are discussed below. In view of the powerful direct and indirect antiviral activities of these products of the immune response, many viruses have developed ingenious evasion strategies to escape their effects, especially the large DNA viruses (e.g., poxviruses, herpesviruses) whose genome coding capacity is substantial enough to accommodate these functions, and these are discussed at the end of this review.

Finally, antiviral antibodies become detectable relatively late in most infections when they are thought to be primarily responsible for prevention of cell-to-cell spread and resistance to reinfection. However, in certain instances, antiviral antibodies may also control the production or release of virus from infected cells, and they may act synergistically with antiviral cytokines in this regard.

EARLY ANTIVIRAL EVENTS IN RESPONSE TO VIRUS INFECTION

Viral infection is a multiphase process that includes virus entry, genome replication, transcription, and translation of viral gene products, and the assembly and secretion of virions. One or more of these events may be detected by the infected cell, triggering it to secrete IFN-α/β or to activate other defense mechanisms such as apoptosis. Certain cell types can recognize an incoming infection even before the virus replicates. For example, neurons that are infected by Sindbis virus are capable of detecting an early step in viral entry (fusion of the viral envelope with the plasma membrane) and responding to it by undergoing apoptosis (1, 2, 3). Most cell types, however, recognize incoming viruses at a later stage by detecting double-stranded RNA (dsRNA) molecules that are produced during the replication process of many RNA and DNA viruses (4). Detection of dsRNA results in the induction of cytokines such as IFN type I (designated IFN-α/β herein), which is normally not synthesized by the uninfected cell (4). The induction of IFN-α/β occurs very rapidly (within a few hours) following viral infection (5). This early, virus-induced cytokine response is not limited to IFN-α/β. For example, certain viruses (such as HIV or lymphocytic choriomeningitis virus [LCMV]) have the potential to infect and rapidly activate macrophages to produce additional antiviral cytokines, such as TNF-α (6, 7), which can trigger independent antiviral activities. Nonetheless, the induction of IFN-α/β is widely accepted as the most immediate and important antiviral host response to many viral infections (5).

IFN-α/β has long been know to inhibit the replication of many viruses in vitro (5), including picornaviruses, retroviruses, influenza viruses, vesicular stomatitis virus (VSV), herpes simplex virus (HSV), vaccinia virus, adenovirus, reovirus (4), duck hepatitis B virus (DHBV) (8, 9), and others. Furthermore, many viruses (including vaccinia virus, VSV, LCMV, Semliki Forest virus, HSV, and HBV) are sensitive to the antiviral activity of IFN-α/β in vivo because they replicate uncontrollably in mice that either received neutralizing antibodies to IFN-α/β (10, 11) or that were genetically deficient for the IFN-α/β receptor (12–15) or IFN-γ (16). In most of these in vivo studies, however, it is difficult to determine whether IFN-α/β contributed to viral clearance by direct antiviral or indirect immunoregulatory mechanisms. Recently, however, IFN-α/β was shown to inhibit HBV replication noncytopathically in vivo, using HBV transgenic mice that are immunologically tolerant to the viral proteins (17, 18) and therefore do not respond to the immunoregulatory activity of the cytokine. Finally, it is important to note that different viruses can be differentially sensitive to IFN-α/β (4). Indeed, even different strains of the same virus can be differentially sensitive to IFN-α/β. For example, genetic variability in a region of the nonstructural protein 5A (NS5A) of hepatitis C virus (HCV) has been associated with different sensitivity of the different genotypes of HCV to IFN-α/β (19). In addition, several strains of LCMV (e.g. Armstrong, Aggressive, and WE) are very sensitive to IFN-α/β, whereas others (e.g. Traub, Cl 13-Armstrong, and Docile) are relatively resistant (11). Similarly, the relative antiviral activity of IFN-α/β against reovirus differs among various reovirus strains (20).

Besides its direct antiviral activities, IFN-α/β can inhibit cell division, stimulate effector functions of NK cells, CTLs, and macrophages, upregulate the expression of MHC class I and MHC class II molecules, induce Ig synthesis in B cells (5), and stimulate the proliferation of memory-phenotype T cells (21). All these functions suggest that IFN-α/β can control viral infections not only by its direct antiviral activities, but also by modulating the innate and adaptive immune response.

THE ROLE OF CELLS OF THE INNATE IMMUNE SYSTEM IN VIRAL CLEARANCE

Granulocytes, NK cells, NKT cells, macrophages, and dendritic cells are cellular components of the innate immune system. These cells are normally rapidly recruited and/or activated at the site of virus infection. They can participate in the antiviral response both directly (by killing infected cells and by producing antiviral cytokines and nitric oxide) and indirectly (by producing chemokines that recruit inflammatory cells into the infected tissue and by producing immunoregulatory cytokines that enable the adaptive immune response to recognize infected cells and perform antiviral effector functions).

Granulocytes

Granulocytes are short-lived phacocytic cells that contain neutrophilic, eosinophilic, and basophilic granules in their cytoplasm. Neutrophils, the most abundant leukocytes in the blood, are known to play a very important role against various bacterial infections (22). Their contribution to the antiviral response, however, remains unclear. Neutrophils are rapidly and abundantly recruited to the site of some viral infections, presumably being attracted by chemokines produced by virus-infected cells and by activated resident macrophages (22, 23). It has been proposed that antiviral molecules such as TNF-α and NO produced by neutrophils (and probably by other granulocytes as well) may contribute to the control of certain viral infections, e.g. HSV infection of the cornea (24) and respiratory syncytial virus (RSV) infection in the lung (25). The role of eosinophils and basophils in antiviral immunity is also poorly understood, although recent in vitro studies have shown that eosinophils can secrete granule ribonucleases (EDN/RNase 2 and ECP/RNase 3) that have antiviral activity against extracellular virions of RSV (26, 27). In addition it is likely that eosinophils and basophils contribute to the control of viral infections by their capacity to secrete a large variety of antiviral and immunoregulatory cytokines (including TNF-α, IL-1, IL-3, IL-4, IL-5, IL-6, IL-8, GM-CSF) (28–30) and chemokines (including eotaxin, RANTES, and IL-8) (31) upon virus infection [e.g. dengue virus (32) or influenza (33)] and after exposure to inflammatory cytokines (28, 34). Finally, granulocytes can play an indirect role in antiviral immunity by presenting viral antigen to antiviral T cells. For example, eosinophils have been recently shown to present rhinovirus (RV)- derived antigens to virus-specific T cells, resulting in T cell proliferation and T cell–dependent production of IFN-γ (35).

NK Cells

The role of NK cells in antiviral immunity has been extensively reviewed by Biron and colleagues in a recent issue of the *Annual Review of Immunology* (36). NK cells can be rapidly recruited into infected organs and tissues by chemoattractant factors produced by virally infected cells and activated resident macrophages (36), which are also a major source of IFN-α/β that induces NK cell proliferation and NK cell–mediated cytolysis of infected cells (36). Numerous NK cell receptors have been discovered, some of which (e.g. CD16, CD2, NKR-P1, CD28, Ly6, CD69, and others) positively regulate NK cell–dependent cytolysis and cytokine production, whereas others (e.g. Ly49, CD94/NKG2, KIRs) negatively regulate their activity when they recognize MHC class I at the infected cell surface (37). Thus, NK cells recognize virally infected cells before MHC class I expression is upregulated. This property is especially important for the control of infections of certain cell types (e.g. neurons and hepatocytes) that normally express little or no MHC class I, suggesting that NK cells may play a critical role in controlling neurotropic and hepatotropic infections. As discussed later in this review, several viruses downregulate MHC class I expression, apparently as a strategy to evade the adaptive immune response (38). This would make the NK cell response especially important for the control of these viral infections. Indeed, the importance of NK cells in the control of virus infection is also underscored by the ability of viruses to encode MHC class I homologues that have the potential to inhibit NK cell effector functions (38).

The relative importance of the cytolytic versus noncytolytic antiviral effector functions of NK cells is under investigation in many laboratories. While the cytolytic activity of these cells is clearly important, it is now well accepted that the production of IFN-γ and, perhaps, TNF-α by activated NK cells is critical for the control of several virus infections (36). Indeed, a large variety of DNA viruses, e.g. mouse cytomegalovirus (MCMV) (39–41), human cytomegalovirus (HCMV) (42), HSV (43), and adenovirus (44) as well as RNA viruses, e.g. influenza (45), vaccinia virus (46), ectromelia virus (47), and coxsackievirus (48), are sensitive to the cytokine-dependent antiviral activity of NK cells.

NKT Cells

NKT cells are a subset of T cells that express NK cell markers. They have an extremely limited TCR repertoire that recognizes glycolipid antigens restricted by the nonclassical MHC class I–like molecule CD1d, which is expressed on professional antigen presenting cells (49–51). Current evidence suggests that NKT cells are likely to play a role in immunity to intracellular bacteria and parasites, such as mycobacteria (52, 53), Toxoplasma gondii (54), malaria (55), and some tumors (56). Whether NKT cells play a role in the control of viral infections is currently undefined. Upon activation, however, NKT cells rapidly produce high levels of IFN-γ (and to a lesser extent IL-4) and increase their cytotoxic capacity (49); thus they have the potential to control viral infections. A recent study has shown that activation of the resident NKT cells of the liver by α-galactosylceramide inhibits HBV replication in the liver of transgenic mice (56a). This antiviral process is mediated by IFN-γ and IFN-α/β, which are produced in the liver of these animals by the NKT cells and also by other cells (NK cells, T cells, and macrophages) that they recruit. Since NKT cells account for 20–30% of intrahepatic lymphocytes in the normal liver, these results suggest that activation of NK T cells could play an important role in the control of viral replication during natural HBV nfection and perhaps other infections of the liver as well.

Macrophages

Macrophages are long-lived phagocytic cells that can circulate in the blood or reside in different organs and tissues. Macrophages phagocytose particulate and foreign material (microorganisms, red cells, immune complexes, endotoxin), and they also present antigens very efficiently to T lymphocytes (57). While the role of macrophages in the control of bacterial infections is well described (58), much less is known about the antiviral function of this cell type during viral infections. However, there is evidence that IL-1 and other products of the activated macrophages such as TNF-α and nitric oxide can control HSV (59), vaccinia virus (60), VSV (61), and mouse hepatitis virus (62) infections in vitro. Although the relevance of these observations remains to be confirmed in vivo, for several reasons, it is highly likely that macrophage activation represents a key step in the clearance of many virus infections. First, once activated by infecting viruses or NK-, NKT- or T cell–derived cytokines, macrophages produce cytokines (e.g. IFN-α/β, TNF-α, and nitric oxide) that have direct antiviral activity as well as other cytokines that have indirect immunoregulatory functions (e.g. IL-1, IL-6, IL-8, IL-10, IL-12, IL-18, GM-CSF) (57, 63).

The direct antiviral activity of macrophages in vivo was illustrated recently by studies performed in HBV transgenic mice. Following infection of newborn HBV transgenic mice with a strain of LCMV that replicates in the intrahepatic macrophages (Kupffer cells), HBV gene expression and replication in the hepatocytes were permanently abolished by the antiviral effects of IFN-α/β and TNF-α in the absence of inflammation or other antiviral cytokines because the mice were immunologically tolerant to LCMV. Furthermore, HBV replication is inhibited in the same HBV transgenic mice during the erythrocytic stage of malaria infection due to the activation of Kupffer cells that phacocytose malaria-infected erythrocytes (64). Other macrophage-derived cytokines (e.g. IL-12) inhibit in vivo the replication of a number of viruses, including HBV (65), HSV (66), and encephalomyocarditis virus (67). Similarly, IL-18 treatment of mice controls vaccinia virus (68) and HSV (69) infections. Most of these antiviral activities, however, are probably due to the ability of IL12 and IL-18 to induce IFN-γ, since they don't appear to display any direct antiviral potential themselves.

Macrophages also produce products such as nitric oxide shown to inhibit the replication of a number of viruses, including vaccinia virus, VSV, HSV, poliovirus, rhinovirus, MCMV, ectromelia (70), coxsackievirus (71), and HBV (72). Furthermore, activated macrophages produce chemokines (including IP-10, MIP1α, MIP1β, MCP-1, MCP-2, MCP-3, MCP-4, MCP-5, RANTES, gro-β, gro-α) (5) that not only recruit inflammatory cells and their antiviral products to the site of infection, but have direct antiviral activity themselves. Indeed, since chemokine receptors serve as membrane co-receptors for HIV, chemokines such as RANTES, and MIP1α and MIP1β, have been shown to be effective inhibitors of HIV-1 entry into susceptible cells by competing with the virus for receptor binding (73–75).

Dendritic Cells

Dendritic cells (DCs) are highly specialized in capturing and presenting antigens to T cells and stimulating the differentiation and proliferation of B cells (76, 77). Because of these functions, DCs are thought to be key modulators in the development of the adaptive immune response during viral infections. Although DCs have not yet been shown to exert direct antiviral activity themselves, they secrete a large variety of antiviral and immunoregulatory cytokines [including IFN-α/β (78), TNF-α, IL-1, IL-6, IL-12, and IL-18 (79)] following activation.

Based on the studies summarized thus far, it is clear that cytokines produced by virus-infected cells, phagocytic, and antigen presenting cells or by cells of the innate immune response can play a direct role in controlling the replication of many viruses during the initial phase of the infection and, due to their immunoregulatory activity, they can also contribute to the initiation of the adaptive immune response. The contribution of the latter to viral clearance relies upon the antiviral functions of CTLs, helper T cells (Th), and B cells.

THE ROLE OF CTLs IN VIRAL CLEARANCE

CTLs are primed by dendritic cells and other professional antigen presenting cells (APCs) in lymphoid organs (77). Whereas T helper cells can be primed by APCs that have internalized viral antigens secreted by other cells, priming of CTLs usually requires the processing of viral proteins that are either endogenously produced within or phagocytosed by professional APCs (77). For viruses that do not infect professional APCs, tissue-derived dendritic cells that have processed apoptotic virus-infected cells and debris are likely to migrate to the regional lymph nodes to allow CTL priming to occur (80). Primed CTLs clonally expand, leave the lymph nodes, home to the infected tissue, to recognize viral antigen and perform their effector functions. Depending upon the infection, virus-specific CTLs can be detected in the infected tissue as early as 5–7 days after exposure.

Contribution of CTL-Mediated Killing to Viral Clearance

It is widely assumed that clearance of intracellular viruses by the immune response requires the destruction of infected cells by virus-specific CTLs via perforin- or Fas-dependent pathways. This dogma has been challenged recently by experimental evidence showing that antiviral cytokines secreted by CTLs can purge susceptible viruses from living cells and that this process can be as efficient as or more efficient than the destructive potential of the CTLs (see below). Since the discovery of MHC-restriction (81), the antiviral function of the CTL response has been primarily studied by monitoring the cytolytic activity of CTLs in vitro. The cytolytic nature of the ^{51}Cr-release assay used in most studies, coupled with the exquisite specificity of the CTL-MHC interaction (virus A-specific CTLs kill virus A-infected MHC-matched cells but not virus A-infected MHC-mismatched or virus B-infected MHC-matched cells) (82), led to the conclusion that viral clearance by CTLs is due primarily to the destruction of infected cells. This notion was also supported by experimental evidence showing that mice deficient in perforin and/or Fas are unable to control certain viral infections, including LCMV (83, 84), Theiler's virus (85), influenza (86) and HSV (87). Based on these results, it is not surprising that the killing of infected cells has been viewed by many investigators as an absolute requirement for viral clearance to occur, especially for noncytopathic persistent viral infections.

While this may be correct for viruses that infect relatively few cells in an organ (88), CTLs are not likely to eradicate infections that affect large numbers of cells simply by killing them, especially in large vital organs such as the brain or liver, since the CTLs can be outnumbered by several orders of magnitude and because full functional recovery of the organ often occurs after complete viral clearance. This principle was clearly established in adoptive CTL transfer experiments using HBV transgenic mice (89–91) where it was shown that, upon antigen recognition, an HBV-specific CTL does not merely kill its target cell, but it also releases antiviral cytokines (especially IFN-γ and TNF-α) that can purge the virus from hundreds or thousands of additional infected cells noncytopathically. Thus, the antiviral power of the CTL response is many orders of magnitude greater than its destructive potential, explaining how an inherently inefficient process that requires direct physical contact between CTLs and target cells can control infections involving very large numbers of cells, and how it can do so without destroying the infected organs and killing the host.

Viral Clearance Requires Additional CTL Functions Besides Their Ability to Kill Infected Cells   The observation that the antiviral potential of the CTLs in the HBV transgenic mouse experiment was primarily mediated by noncytolytic cytokine-mediated mechanisms was not entirely surprising, since we had previously shown that TNF-α (92, 93) and IFN-α/β (93) inhibit HBV gene expression in the liver of transgenic mice. In addition, others had demonstrated reduced pathogenicity and accelerated viral clearance of vaccinia viruses expressing IFN-γ or TNF-α in normal and immunodeficient mice (94–97), and IFN-γ and TNF-α had been previously shown to contribute to viral clearance during murine cytomegalovirus (MCMV) infection in mice (98, 99). Furthermore, it was known that antibodies to IFN-γ could partially inhibit immune-mediated clearance of LCMV from infected tissues following the adoptive transfer of immune spleen cells (100) and that LCMV was not cleared when relatively high numbers of IFN-γ-deficient CTLs were passively transferred (101). In addition, LCMV replication was shown to be less efficiently controlled in mice that lack the IFN-γ receptor (12) or that have been treated with IFN-γ-specific antibodies (102).

While the infection models clearly demonstrated that IFN-γ and/or TNF-α contribute to the control of many viral infections, they didn't prove that the cytokines directly inhibited viral replication. Indeed, the antiviral effect could have been due to immunoregulatory activity of these cytokines or their ability to enhance antigen presentation or to stimulate the homing function or cytolytic function of innate or adaptive effector cells, thereby increasing their ability to kill the infected cells. Since the number of infected cells was not demonstrated in these models, the CTLs could have easily destroyed the infected cells without having a noticeable impact on the function of the infected tissues or the survival of the host, if they represented a small fraction of the total cells in vital organs or a high percentage of the cells in nonvital organs.

In contrast to these experiments, however, the direct antiviral potential of CTL-derived cytokines was clearly separated from their indirect immunoregulatory activity in the HBV transgenic mouse model. This could not be done in the natural infection models where viruses can reinfect potentially cured cells and where the immune response and other antiviral mechanisms can be activated, thereby obscuring the interpretation of the results. Unlike natural infections, HBV is not infectious for mice. In the transgenic mice, HBV is produced by each hepatocyte, but it cannot spread from cell to cell (17). Furthermore, the mice are profoundly immunologically tolerant to the virus (18, 103), so the immunoregulatory activities of the cytokines were not operative in these animals. Thus, it was possible to demonstrate that the intrahepatic induction of IFN-γ and TNF-α produced by adoptively transferred virus-specific CTLs in this model completely inhibited HBV replication in the liver in the absence of an immune response (15). Furthermore, the antiviral effect was observed less than 24 h after transfer of CTL clones (90) that were outnumbered 100-fold by HBV-expressing hepatocytes. Finally, HBV replication was abolished in the absence of liver disease following the transfer of HBV-specific CTLs from perforin-deficient (90) and Fas ligand–deficient mice (104).

This notion that cytokines produced by activated immune cells can play a direct role in viral clearance was subsequently confirmed in a number of infection models, including HBV. Indeed, a recent study in acutely HBV-infected chimpanzees showed that noncytopathic antiviral mechanisms contribute to HBV clearance since HBV DNA disappeared from the liver of acutely infected chimpanzees largely before the onset of liver disease, concomitant with the intrahepatic appearance of IFN-γ (105). Furthermore, the appearance of this cytokine in the chimp liver preceded the peak of T cell infiltration, suggesting that IFN-γ was produced initially by cells other than CTLs, perhaps NK and NKT cells. Along the same lines, duck hepatitis B virus (DHBV) infection has been recently shown to be susceptible to the noncytopathic antiviral activity of IFN-γ (106); and noncytopathic antiviral mechanisms mediated by T cell–derived cytokines (IFN-γ and/or TNF-α) have been shown to operate in other viral infections, including LCMV (107), adenovirus (15, 108, 109), mouse hepatitis virus (110, 111), and coxsackievirus (112, 113). Interestingly, expression of HIV RNA and viral replication is inhibited in vitro by currently undefined noncytolyic factors produced by HIV-specific CTLs upon antigen recognition (114, 115).

THE ROLE OF T HELPER CELLS IN VIRAL CLEARANCE

T helper (Th) cells play a key role in antiviral immunity. They participate in the antiviral response both directly (by producing antiviral cytokines) and indirectly (by providing help for B cells and CTLs). Th cells can be divided into two different subsets, Th1 and Th2 cells, based on their different cytokine profiles. Th1 cells produce IL-2, TNF-α, and IFN-γ, which possess antiviral activities and regulate the cellular immune response, whereas Th2 cells produce IL-4, IL-5, IL-10, and IL-13, which are known to stimulate antibody production (116). In spite of the fact that virus-specific Th2 cells can be detected following primary infection by viruses such as LCMV (117), virus-specific Th1 cells are usually much more abundant and reach very high numbers at the peak of the acute infection (118, 119); and their frequencies remain elevated following resolution of the infection (120). A role for Th1 cells in controlling viral infections is supported by experiments showing that they can clear influenza (121–123), VSV (124), and vaccinia virus infections (125, 126) in a CTL-independent manner. Both Th1-derived antiviral cytokines (e.g. IFN-γ and TNF-α) and Th cell–dependent antiviral antibodies have been thought to contribute to viral clearance in those experiments. A direct, cytokine-dependent antiviral role of Th1 cells has been shown in HBV transgenic mice. Passive transfer of HBV-specific Th1 cells into these immunologically tolerant animals resulted in recognition of viral antigens expressed by hepatic nonparenchymal cells, cytokine release, and suppression of viral replication in the liver (127).

The importance of Th cells in the induction of the antiviral CTL response can vary from virus to virus. For example whereas the CTL response to Sendai virus is virtually normal in the absence of Th cells, (128), lack of Th cells significantly impairs the CTL response to VSV, LCMV, and vaccinia virus (129, 130). Th cells can also play a critical role in maintaining the control of persisting viral infections. They can do so by sustaining CTL-dependent antiviral functions in persistent MHV infection (131), or by directly producing antiviral cytokines in persistent Friend virus (FV) infection (132). Finally, although Th cells have cytolytic activity in vitro, it is still unclear whether the destruction of infected cells by cytotoxic Th1 cells contributes to the control of viral infections in vivo (133, 134). If so, their antiviral potential should be limited to virally infected cells that express Fas on their surface.

THE ROLE OF ANTIVIRAL ANTIBODIES IN VIRAL CLEARANCE

Antiviral antibodies contribute to viral clearance mainly by blocking virus entry into susceptible cells and by removing infectious virions from the circulation, thereby preventing extracellular viral spread. This is a complex process that involves not only antiviral antibodies, but also the complement system and phagocytic cells. Coating of viruses with antibodies (neutralizing and non-neutralizing) can block the physical interaction of many viruses with their receptors, and it can also activate the complement system to lyse viruses (135, 136). The Fc portion of virus-bound antibodies can interact with Fc receptors present on the surface of phagocytic cells, thereby accelerating the removal of virions from the circulation (135–137).

Antibodies also perform antiviral functions that do not involve neutralization of extracellular virions. The deposition of antibodies on the surface of the infected cell may prevent the release of virions from the infected cell (2). In addition, the presence of antibodies on the cell surface could activate the complement to lyse the infected cell (135, 136). Other undefined antiviral mechanisms that are mediated by antibodies and do not require neutralization of extracellular virions play a role in the clearance of Sindbis virus from neurons. This notion is supported by two lines of evidence. First, antiviral antibodies are sufficient to clear Sindbis virus from infected neurons in vivo in the absence of T cells, complement (138), or interferons (139). Second, antiviral antibodies can clear Sindbis virus from infected neurons noncytopathically in vitro, initiating an antiviral effect that persists even after the antibodies are removed from the culture (138, 140). Antibodies can also contribute to the antiviral response in a more indirect way, e.g. by enhancing the presentation of viral antigens to T and B cells. Indeed, uptake of viral antigens by professional APCs in secondary lymphoid organs can be facilitated by the interaction of Fc receptors present on the surface of APCs with the Fc portion of virus-bound antibodies (141).

The relative contribution of antiviral antibodies to viral clearance can vary from virus to virus. Following primary infection, the IgM response is the first to appear (usually within few days of infection), and neutralizing IgM responses significantly lower the blood titer of several viruses, including VSV, LCMV, and Friend virus (FV) (142–144). As the IgM response fades, a T cell–dependent isotype switch occurs, and IgG (including neutralizing IgG) is generated. In the case of VSV, the appearance of neutralizing IgG can occur as early as one week after the infection (141), while neutralizing IgG usually peaks at later time points during other infections, including HBV or HCV (145, 146). The neutralizing IgG response further contributes to the removal of extracellular virus; it is also thought to be critical in controlling long-term infections that are not completely cleared, e.g. HBV (147, 148) or LCMV (149). Indeed, complete viral clearance following clinical recovery from HBV and LCMV infections may never occur because very small traces of these viruses can persist indefinitely. Neutralizing IgG probably inhibits the reemergence of these viruses, as has been recently shown for LCMV (150), presumably by blocking extracellular spread, although the precise mechanism for this antiviral function has been not yet defined. Finally, natural antibodies that represent the immunoglobulin repertoire of naive animals have been shown to contribute to the control of LCMV, VSV, and vaccinia virus by inhibiting extracellular spread and by enhancing immunogenicity through increased uptake of viral antigens in secondary lymphoid organs (151).

CYTOKINE-INDUCIBLE INTRACELLULAR MECHANISMS OF VIRAL INACTIVATION

IFN-α/β activates a variety of intracellular antiviral mechanisms and, often, more than one mechanism can be activated at the same time in an infected cell. Such mechanisms have the potential to target many steps in the viral life cycle (4, 152, 153). For example, viral entry of SV40, adenovirus, and retroviruses has been shown to be inhibited by IFN-α/β (4). Transcription, translation, assembly, and secretion of several DNA and RNA viruses can also be inhibited by IFN-α/β (4, 153). A large variety of IFN-inducible genes have been identified that are activated by the JAK-STAT signal transduction cascade (154). The recent advent of oligonucleotide arrays has facilitated identification of many IFN-inducible or repressed genes (155, 156). However, whether any of these genes have antiviral activity is not yet known, and the mechanism(s) they may trigger to control viral infections are not well understood.

Among the IFN-inducible genes, the 2'5' oligoadenylate synthetases, the Mx proteins, the double-stranded-RNA-activated protein kinase (PKR), and the double-stranded-RNA-specific adenosine deaminase systems are probably the best characterized. The 2'5'-oligoadenylate system mediates antiviral activities mainly by the induction of RNAse L, a cellular RNAse that degrades viral transcripts (157–159). This pathway has been shown to selectively reduce the intracellular RNA content of viruses such as HIV, encephalomyocardarditis virus, and vaccinia virus (160–162). The MxA protein is an interferon-induced GTPase that selectively inhibits influenza and bunyaviruses (163), probably via direct binding to viral ribonucleoprotein complexes (164) and blocking their import into the nucleus, as has been shown recently for Thoghoto virus infection (164).

Inhibition of viral protein synthesis initiation by the IFN-inducible PKR suppresses certain viral infections, including encephalomyocardarditis virus and reovirus (20, 154). The importance of the PKR system in HCV infection has been underlined by recent studies showing that HCV encodes proteins that may inhibit the antiviral activity of PKR. For instance, the interaction between the HCV E2 protein and PKR has been suggested to reduce the sensitivity of this virus to IFN-α/β (165). In addition, the nonstructural 5A protein of HCV inhibits PKR antiviral activity by blocking PKR dimerization (166, 167), a process that is required for the PKR-dependent phosphorylation of eIF-2alpha and the prevention of viral protein synthesis initiation.

IFN-α/β is also known to induce the double-stranded RNA-specific adenosine deaminase system that has the potential to inhibit viral protein synthesis by editing double-stranded viral RNA (168). This process can modulate the replication of different viruses, including reovirus, measles, and VSV (20). Recent experiments have shown that the antiviral effect of IFN-α/β on HBV replication in transgenic mice is due to inhibition of formation and/or destabilization of RNA-containing capsids, while transcription, translation, capsid maturation, and secretion seem not to be affected by this cytokine (169). Similarly, treatment of DHBV-infected hepatocyte cultures with duck IFN-α/β selectively depletes DHBV RNA-containing capsids (8). Additional, undefined intracellular antiviral pathways are also induced by IFN-α/β; and it has recently been shown that mice triply deficient for RNAse L, Mx1, and PKR are still partially resistant to VSV and encephalomyocardarditis virus (170). Identification of the nature of these antiviral pathways is an important area of investigation actively pursued in many laboratories at this time.

The known antiviral activities of IFN-γ and IFN-α/β are somewhat redundant because they activate an overlapping set of genes via related limbs of the JAK-STAT signal transduction cascade (154). Although TNF-α has antiviral activities that are often synergistic with IFN-γ (171), very little is known about the direct intracellular antiviral mechanisms activated by this cytokine (171). It is noteworthy that the intrahepatic induction of IFN-γ and TNF-α triggers the degradation of preformed HBV RNA in the nucleus of the hepatocyte (172). Recent studies have demonstrated that HBV mRNA stability is associated with the presence of a 45-kDa nuclear ribonucleoprotein (SSB/La) (173) that binds a predicted stem-loop structure in the viral RNA (174). IFN-γ and/or TNF-α trigger the cleavage of SSB/La, thereby exposing an endoribonuclease-sensitive site in the viral RNA; these events are associated with its degradation (T Heise, LG Guidotti, FV Chisari, unpublished results). Thus, the interaction between the SSB/La protein and the viral RNA stem-loop structure may contribute to HBV RNA stability under baseline conditions, and the cytokine-induced cleavage of SSB/La may facilitate the destabilization of viral RNA by exposing previously protected sequences to nuclear endoribonuclease activities that may themselves be induced by these cytokines.

INFECTED CELLS ARE ACTIVE PARTICIPANTS IN THE ANTIVIRAL RESPONSE

A fundamental requirement for cytokine-induced virus purging is that the intracellular antiviral mechanisms described above must be operative in the infected cell. Indeed, it is possible that such mechanisms may not operate in all cell types. If this is correct, one would expect that the same virus could be controlled by the immune system either by curative or cytodestructive mechanisms, depending upon the cell in which it replicates. Indeed, this is the case for LCMV as well as certain other viruses, including MCMV and vaccinia virus. For example, recent studies have shown that LCMV can be eliminated from the hepatocytes in a cytokine-dependent, noncytopathic bystander manner, whereas other events, presumably killing, are needed to eliminate LCMV from nonparenchymal cells of the liver and from the spleen, which do not purge the virus noncytopathically in response to the cytokines (107). Furthermore, the control of murine cytomegalovirus infection in the liver and vaccinia virus in the central nervous system primarily depend on IFN-dependent noncytopathic mechanisms, while cytopathic events probably contribute to the clearance of these viruses from other organs (175, 176). Clearly, much remains to be done to identify the intracellular responses that determine whether a cell will purge itself of a viral infection as far as exposure to antiviral cytokines.

VIRUS-INDUCED MECHANISMS THAT INTERFERE WITH THE ANTIVIRAL ACTIVITY OF THE INNATE AND ADAPTIVE IMMUNE RESPONSE

A number of viruses encode proteins that have the potential to inhibit the antiviral activity of the innate and adaptive immune response. Several comprehensive reviews have been written on this subject in the last few years (38, 171, 177–179). Briefly, both cytolytic and noncytolytic mechanisms of virus control can be inhibited by various viruses. For example, myxoma virus, adenovirus, HCMV, vaccinia virus, Epstein-Barr virus (EBV), and others have been shown to interfere with apoptosis by encoding products that either inhibit pro-apoptotic pathways or induce anti-apoptotic pathways (38). Since apoptosis of the infected cell (induced by the virus itself or by cytokines, NK cells, or T cells) is a component of the antiviral response, it is not surprising that several viruses have chosen to inhibit this process. Poxviruses and herpesviruses produce MHC class I homologues that have the potential to deliver negative regulatory signals to NK cells, thereby preventing them from expressing their effector functions (38). Conversely, MHC class I and MHC class II expression on the surface of the infected cell is inhibited by adenovirus (intracellular retention) (180), HCMV and MCMV (intracellular retention and degradation) (181–184), HIV (degradation) (185), Kaposi's sarcoma-associated herpesvirus (KSHV) (enhanced endocytosis) (186), and others (38). Inhibition of cell surface expression of MHC class I is also accomplished by herpesvirus-derived gene products that can target the function of the TAP (transporter associated with antigenic processing) proteins by direct interaction with both TAP1 and TAP2, thereby preventing their association (187, 188).

Obviously, virus-dependent mechanisms that diminish the recognition of infected cells by NK and T cells have the potential to inhibit both the direct cytolytic function of these cells and the production of antiviral cytokines. Given the importance of antiviral cytokines in the control of viral infections, it is not surprising that these molecules are also targeted specifically by different viruses. Two basic strategies are usually employed. The first reflects the ability of virus proteins to interfere with cytokine-induced signaling or with the antiviral activities of cytokine-induced genes intracellularly, e.g. the inhibition of the function of ISGF3 (a cellular transcription factor induced by IFN-α/β) by the E1A protein of adenovirus (189). The second is due to the ability of certain viral proteins to interfere with the antiviral activities of cytokines extracellularly, e.g. as cytokine antagonists or receptor analogues (189, 190), as is well known for viral proteins of various members of the poxvirus, herpesvirus, and retrovirus families (190).

Virus gene products interfere with the antibody response and the complement system. Herpesviruses produce Fc receptor-like molecules that can bind the Fc portion of virus-bound antibodies (38). This process may prevent recognition of virus-antibody complexes by the complement system and phagocytic cells. Finally, herpesviruses, vaccinia virus, EBV, and other viruses can produce proteins that inhibit complement activation by interfering with different molecules of the complement cascade (38).

CONCLUDING REMARKS

The tissue-sparing, noncytolytic antiviral mechanisms mediated by the innate and adaptive immune response described herein can be viewed as a host survival strategy to control infections of vital organs that would otherwise be destroyed if the only way to eliminate the infections was to kill all of the infected cells. Interestingly, by inhibiting viral replication and downregulating viral antigen expression, the same process could also function as a viral evasion strategy and contribute to viral persistence. Indeed, both scenarios may be correct, and they could even be operative at the same time in the same individual. If so, the noncytolytic process described in this review should be strongly favored during evolution because it provides a strong survival advantage for both the host and the virus. This notion is supported by the recent discovery that complete viral clearance probably never occurs after infection with viruses like HBV or LCMV, both of which are known to be susceptible to noncytopathic mechanisms of antiviral control. Identification of the cytokine-induced intracellular molecular events that control viral infections is an important area of investigation that will benefit by recent advances in functional genomics and proteomics. Future results from these studies will not only improve our understanding of the host-virus interactions that determine the outcome of infection, but they may also lead to the discovery of new approaches for the treatment of persistent viruses such as HBV, HCV, and HIV.

Visit the Annual Reviews home page at www.AnnualReviews.org

LITERATURE CITED

1. Jan JT, Griffin DE. 1999. Induction of apoptosis by Sindbis virus occurs at cell entry and does not require virus replication. *J. Virol.* 73:10296–10302
2. Griffin DE, Hardwick JM. 1999. Perspective: virus infections and the death of neurons. *Trends Microbiol.* 7:155–60

3. Koyama AH, Irie H, Fukumori T, Hata S, Iida S, Akari H, Adachi A. 1998. Role of virus-induced apoptosis in a host defense mechanism against virus infection. *J. Med. Invest.* 45:37–45
4. Vilcek J, Sen GC. 1996. Interferons and other cytokines. In *Virology*, ed. BN Fields,

DM Knipe, PM Howley, pp. 375-99. Philadelphia: Lippincott-Raven

5. Thomson A. 1998. *The Cytokine Handbook.* San Diego: Academic Press

6. Merrill JE, Chen IS. 1991. HIV-1, macrophages, glial cells, and cytokinesin AIDS nervous system disease. *Faseb J.* 5:2391–97

7. Guidotti LG, Borrow P, Hobbs MV, Matzke B, Gresser I, Oldstone MBA, Chisari FV. 1996. Viral cross talk: intracellular inactivation of the hepatitis B virus during an unrelated viral infection of the liver. *Proc. Natl. Acad. Sci. USA* 93:4589–94

8. Schultz U, Summers J, Staeheli P, Chisari FV. 1999. Elimination of duck hepatitis B virus RNA-containing capsids in duck interferon-alpha-treated hepatocytes. *J. Virol.* 73:5459–65

9. Protzer U, Nassal M, Chiang PW, Kirschfink M, Schaller H. 1999. Interferon gene transfer by a hepatitis B virus vector efficiently suppresses wild-type virus infection [see comments]. *Proc. Natl. Acad. Sci. USA* 96:10818–23

10. Gresser I. 1984. Role of interferon in resistance to viral infection in vivo. In *Interferons 2: Interferons and the Immune System,* ed. J. Vilcek, E De Mayer, pp. 221–47. Amsterdam: Elsevier Sci.

11. Moskophidis D, Battegay M, Bruendler M-A, Laine E, Gresser I, Zinkernagel R. 1994. Resistance of lymphocytic choriomeningitis virus to alpha/beta interferon and gamma interferon. *J. Virol.* 68:1951–55

12. Muller U, Steinhoff U, Reis LF, Hemmi S, Pavlovic J, Zinkernagel RM, Aguet M. 1994. Functional role of type I and type II interferons in antiviral defense. *Science* 264:1918–21

13. Kamijo R, Shapiro D, Gerecitano J, Le J, Bosland M, Vilcek J. 1994. Biological functions of IFN-gamma and IFN-alpha/beta: lessons from studies in gene knockout mice. *Hokkaido Igaku Zasshi* 69:1332–38

14. Leib DA, Harrison TE, Laslo KM, Machalek MA, Moorman NJ, Virgin HW. 1999. Interferons regulate the phenotype of wild-type and mutant herpes simplex viruses in vivo. *J. Exp. Med.* 189:663–72

15. McClary H, Koch R, Chisari FV, Guidotti LG. 2000. Relative sensitivity of hepatitis B virus and other hepatotropic viruses to the antiviral effects of cytokines. *J. Virol.* 74:2255–64

16. Deonarain R, Alcami A, Alexiou M, Dallman MJ, Gewert DR, Porter AC. 2000. Impaired antiviral response and alpha/beta interferon induction in mice lacking beta interferon. *J. Virol.* 74:3404–9

17. Guidotti LG, Matzke B, Schaller H, Chisari FV. 1995. High level hepatitis B virus replication in transgenic mice. *J. Virol.* 69:6158–69

18. Shimizu Y, Guidotti LG, Fowler P, Chisari FV. 1998. Dendritic cell immunization breaks cytotoxic T lymphocyte tolerance in hepatitis B virus transgenic mice. *J. Immunol.* 161:4520–29

19. Enomoto N, Sakuma I, Asahina Y, Kurosaki M, Murakami T, Yamamoto C, Ogura Y, Izumi N, Marumo F, Sato C. 1996. Mutations in the nonstructural protein 5A gene and response to interferon in patients with chronic hepatitis C virus 1b infection. *N. Engl. J. Med.* 334:77–81

20. Samuel CE. 1998. Reoviruses and the interferon system. *Curr. Top. Microbiol. Immunol.* 233:125–45

21. Tough DF, Sun S, Zhang X, Sprent J. 1999. Stimulation of naive and memory T cells by cytokines. *Immunol. Rev.* 170:39–47

22. Mollinedo F, Borregaard N, Boxer LA. 1999. Novel trends in neutrophil structure, function and development. *Immunol. Today* 20:535–37

23. Rossi D, Zlotnik A. 2000. The biology of chemokines and their receptors. *Annu. Rev. Immunol.* 18:217–42

24. Daheshia M, Kanangat S, Rouse BT. 1998. Production of key molecules by ocular

neutrophils early after herpetic infection of the cornea. *Exp. Eye Res.* 67:619–24

25. Wang SZ, Forsyth KD. 2000. The interaction of neutrophils with respiratory epithelial cells in viral infection. *Respirology* 5:1–10

26. Domachowske JB, Dyer KD, Adams AG, Leto TL, Rosenberg HF. 1998. Eosinophil cationic protein/RNase 3 is another RNase A-family ribonuclease with direct antiviral activity. *Nucleic Acids Res.* 26:3358–63

27. Rosenberg HF, Domachowske JB. 1999. Eosinophils, ribonucleases and host defense: solving the puzzle. *Immunol. Res.* 20:261–74

28. Sampson AP. 2000. The role of eosinophils and neutrophils in inflammation. *Clin. Exp. Allergy* 30(Suppl.) 1:22–27

29. Benyon RC, Bissonnette EY, Befus AD. 1991. Tumor necrosis factor-alpha dependent cytotoxicity of human skin mast cells is enhanced by anti-IgE antibodies. *J. Immunol.* 147:2253–58

30. Bradding P, Feather IH, Wilson S, Bardin PG, Heusser CH, Holgate ST, Howarth PH. 1993. Immunolocalization of cytokines in the nasal mucosa of normal and perennial rhinitic subjects. The mast cell as a source of IL-4, IL-5, and IL-6 in human allergic mucosal inflammation. *J. Immunol.* 151:3853–65

31. Kaplan AP, Kuna P, Reddigari SR. 1995. Chemokines and the allergic response. *Exp. Dermatol.* 4:260–65

32. King CA, Marshall JS, Alshurafa H, Anderson R. 2000. Release of vasoactive cytokines by antibody-enhanced dengue virus infection of a human mast cell/basophil line. *J. Virol.* 74:7146–50

33. Kawaguchi M, Kokubu F, Kuga H, Tomita T, Matsukura S, Kadokura M, Adachi M. 2000. Expression of eotaxin by normal airway epithelial cells after influenza virus A infection. *Int. Arch. Allergy Immunol.* 122(Suppl.) 1:44–49

34. Marshall JS, Bienenstock J. 1994. The role of mast cells in inflammatory reactions of

the airways, skin and intestine. *Curr. Opin. Immunol.* 6:853–59

35. Handzel ZT, Busse WW, Sedgwick JB, Vrtis R, Lee WM, Kelly EA, Gern JE. 1998. Eosinophils bind rhinovirus and activate virus-specific T cells. *J. Immunol.* 160:1279–84

36. Biron CA, Nguyen KB, Pien GC, Cousens LP, Salazar-Mather TP. 1999. Natural killer cells in antiviral defense: function and regulation by innate cytokines. *Annu. Rev. Immunol.* 17:189–220

37. Lanier LL. 1998. NK cell receptors. *Annu. Rev. Immunol.* 16:359–93

38. Tortorella D, Gewurz BE, Furman MH, Schust DJ, Ploegh HL. 2000. Viral subversion of the immune system. *Annu. Rev. Immunol.* 18:861–926

39. Bukowski JF, Woda BA, Welsh RM. 1984. Pathogenesis of murine cytomegalovirus infection in natural killer cell-depleted mice. *J. Virol.* 52:119–28

40. Orange JS, Wang B, Terhorst C, Biron CA. 1995. Requirement for natural killer cell-produced interferon g in defense against murine cytomegalovirus infection and enhancement of this defense pathway by interleukin 12 administration. *J. Exp. Med.* 182:1045–56

41. Orange JS, Biron CA. 1996. Characterization of early IL-12, IFN-α/β, and TNF effects on antiviral state and NK cell responses during murine cytomegalovirus infection. *J. Immunol.* 156:4746–56

42. Quinnan GV Jr, Kirmani N, Rook AH, Manischewitz JF, Jackson L, Moreschi G, Santos GW, Saral R, Burns WH. 1982. Cytotoxic T cells in cytomegalovirus infection: HLA-restricted T-lymphocyte and non-T-lymphocyte cytotoxic responses correlate with recovery from cytomegalovirus infection in bone-marrow-transplant recipients. *N. Engl. J. Med.* 307:7–13

43. Biron CA, Byron KS, Sullivan JL. 1989. Severe herpesvirus infections in an adolescent without natural killer cells [see comments]. *N. Engl. J. Med.* 320:1731–35

44. Sheil JM, Gallimore PH, Zimmer SG, Sopori ML. 1984. Susceptibility of adenovirus 2-transformed rat cell lines to natural killer (NK) cells: direct correlation between NK resistance and in vivo tumorigenesis. *J. Immunol.* 132:1578–82

45. Stein-Streilein J, Guffee J. 1986. In vivo treatment of mice and hamsters with antibodies to asialo GM1 increases morbidity and mortality to pulmonary influenza infection. *J. Immunol.* 136:1435–41

46. Bukowski JF, Woda BA, Habu S, Okumura K, Welsh RM. 1983. Natural killer cell depletion enhances virus synthesis and virus-induced hepatitis in vivo. *J. Immunol.* 131:1531–38

47. Delano ML, Brownstein DG. 1995. Innate resistance to lethal mousepox is genetically linked to the NK gene complex on chromosome 6 and correlates with early restriction of virus replication by cells with an NK phenotype. *J. Virol.* 69:5875–77

48. Godeny EK, Gauntt CJ. 1987. Murine natural killer cells limit coxsackievirus B3 replication. *J. Immunol.* 139:913–18

49. Bendelac A, Rivera MN, Park SH, Roark JH. 1997. Mouse CD1-specific NK1 T cells: development, specificity, and function. *Annu. Rev. Immunol.* 15:535–62

50. Brossay L, Jullien D, Cardell S, Sydora BC, Burdin N, Modlin RL, Kronenberg M. 1997. Mouse CD1 is mainly expressed on hemopoietic-derived cells. *J. Immunol.* 159:1216–24

51. Burdin N, Brossay L, Koezuka Y, Smiley ST, Grusby MJ, Gui M, Taniguchi M, Hayakawa K, Kronenberg M. 1998. Selective ability of mouse CD1 to present glycolipids: alpha- galactosylceramide specifically stimulates V alpha 14[+] NK T lymphocytes. *J. Immunol.* 161:3271–81

52. Sieling PA, Chatterjee D, Porcelli SA, Prigozy TI, Mazzaccaro RJ, Soriano T, Bloom BR, Brenner MB, Kronenberg M, Brennan PJ, et al. 1995. CD1-restricted T cell recognition of microbial lipoglycan antigens. *Science* 269:227–30

53. Apostolou I, Takahama Y, Belmant C, Kawano T, Huerre M, Marchal G, Cui J, Taniguchi M, Nakauchi H, Fournie JJ, Kourilsky P, Gachelin G. 1999. Murine natural killer T(NKT) cells contribute to the granulomatous reaction caused by mycobacterial cell walls. *Proc. Natl. Acad. Sci. USA* 96:5141–46

54. Denkers EY, Scharton-Kersten T, Barbieri S, Caspar P, Sher A. 1996. A role for CD4[+] NK1.1[+] T lymphocytes as major histocompatibility complex class II independent helper cells in the generation of CD8[+] effector function against intracellular infection. *J. Exp. Med.* 184:131–39

55. Schofield L, McConville MJ, Hansen D, Campbell AS, Fraser-Reid B, Grusby MJ, Tachado SD. 1999. CD1d-restricted immunoglobulin G formation to GPI-anchored antigens mediated by NKT cells. *Science* 283:225–29

56. Cui J, Shin T, Kawano T, Sato H, Kondo E, Toura I, Kaneko Y, Koseki H, Kanno M, Taniguchi M. 1997. Requirement for Valpha14 NKT cells in IL-12-mediated rejection of tumors. *Science* 278:1623–26

56a. Kakimi K, Guidotti LG, Koezuka Y, Chisari FV. 2000. Natural killer T cell activation inhibits HBV replication in vivo. *J. Exp. Med.* 192:921–30

57. Laskin DL, Pendino KJ. 1995. Macrophages and inflammatory mediators in tissue injury. *Annu. Rev. Pharmacol. Toxicol.* 35:655–77

58. Russell DG. 1995. Of microbes and macrophages: entry, survival and persistence. *Curr. Opin. Immunol.* 7:479–84

59. Wildy P, Gell PGH, Rhodes J, Newton A. 1982. Inhibition of herpes simplex virus multiplication by activated macrophages: a role of arginase. *Infect. Immun.* 37:40–45

60. Keller F, Wild MT, Kirn A. 1985. In vitro antiviral properties of endotoxin

activated rat Kupffer cells. *J. Leuk. Biol.*
38:293–303

61. Leblanc AP. 1989. Macrophage activation
for cytolysis of virally infected target cells.
J. Leuk. Biol. 45:345–50

62. Keller F, Schmitt C, Kirn A. 1988. Interaction of mouse hepatitis virus 3 with Kupffer cells explanted from susceptible and resistant mouse strains. Antiviral activity, interleukin-1 synthesis. *FEMS Microbiol. Immunol.* 1:87–95

63. Dinarello CA. 1999. Interleukin-18. *Methods* 19:121–32

64. Pasquetto V, Guidotti LG, Kakimi K, Tsuji M, Chisari FV. 2000. Host-virus interactions during malaria infection in hepatitis B virus transgenic mice. *J. Exp. Med.* 192:529–35

65. Cavanaugh VJ, Guidotti LG, Chisari FV. 1997. Interleukin-12 inhibits hepatitis B virus replication in HBV transgenic mice. *J. Virol.* 71:3236–43

66. Carr JA, Rogerson J, Mulqueen MJ, Roberts NA, Booth RF. 1997. Interleukin-12 exhibits potent antiviral activity in experimental herpesvirus infections. *J. Virol.* 71:7799–7803

67. Ozmen L, Aguet M, Trinchieri G, Garotta G. 1995. The in vivo antiviral activity of interleukin-12 is mediated by gamma interferon. *J. Virol.* 69:8147–50

68. Tanaka-Kataoka M, Kunikata T, Takayama S, Iwaki K, Ohashi K, Ikeda M, Kurimoto M. 1999. In vivo antiviral effect of interleukin 18 in a mouse model of vaccinia virus infection. *Cytokine* 11:593–99

69. Fujioka N, Akazawa R, Ohashi K, Fujii M, Ikeda M, Kurimoto M. 1999. Interleukin-18 protects mice against acute herpes simplex virus type 1 infection. *J. Virol.* 73:2401–9

70. Reiss CS, Komatsu T. 1998. Does nitric oxide play a critical role in viral infections? *J. Virol.* 72:4547–51

71. Saura M, Zaragoza C, McMillan A, Quick RA, Hohenadl C, Lowenstein JM, Lowenstein CJ. 1999. An antiviral mechanism of nitric oxide: inhibition of a viral protease. *Immunity* 10:21–28

72. Guidotti LG, McClary H, Moorhead Loudis J, Chisari FV. 2000. Nitric oxide inhibits hepatitis B virus replication in the liver of transgenic mice. *J. Exp. Med.* 191:1247–52

73. Cocchi F, DeVico AL, Garzino-Demo A, Arya SK, Gallo RC, Lusso P. 1995. Identification of RANTES, MIP-1$\alpha\beta$, and MIP-1β as the major HIV-suppressive factors produced by CD8$^+$ T cells. *Science* 270:1811–15

74. Lusso P. 1997. A chemokine trap for HIV co-receptors [news; comment] [see comments]. *Nat. Med.* 3:1074–75

75. Locati M, Murphy PM. 1999. Chemokines and chemokine receptors: biology and clinical relevance in inflammation and AIDS. *Annu. Rev. Med.* 50:425–40

76. Banchereau J, Steinman RM. 1998. Dendritic cells and the control of immunity. *Nature* 392:245–52

77. Steinman RM, Inaba K, Turley S, Pierre P, Mellman I. 1999. Antigen capture, processing, and presentation by dendritic cells: recent cell biological studies. *Hum. Immunol.* 60:562–67

78. Bender A, Albert M, Reddy A, Feldman M, Sauter B, Kaplan G, Hellman W, Bhardwa JN. 1998. The distinctive features of influenza virus infection of dendritic cells. *Immunobiology* 198:552–67

79. Stockwin LH, McGonagle D, Martin IG, Blair GE. 2000. Dendritic cells: immunological sentinels with a central role in health and disease. *Immunol. Cell Biol.* 78:91–102

80. Sallusto F, Lanzavecchia A. 1999. Mobilizing dendritic cells for tolerance, priming, and chronic inflammation [comment]. *J. Exp. Med.* 189:611–14

81. Zinkernagel RM, Doherty PC. 1974. Restriction of in vitro T cell–mediated cytotoxicity in lymphocytic choriomeningitis virus within a syngeneic or semiallogeneic system. *Nature* 248:701–3

82. Lukacher AE, Braciale VL, Braciale TJ. 1984. In vivo effector function of influenza virus-specific cytotoxic T lymphocyte clones is highly specific. *J. Exp. Med.* 160:814–26

83. Kagi D, Ledermann B, Burki K, Seiler P, Odermatt B, Olsen J, Podack ER, Zinkernagel R, Hengartner H. 1994. Cytotoxicity mediated by T cells and natural killer cells is greatly impaired in perforin-deficient mice. *Nature* 369:31–37

84. Walsh CM, Matloubian M, Liu C-C, Ueda R, Kurahara CG, Christensen JL, Huang MT, Young JD-E, Ahmed R, Clark WR. 1994. Immune function in mice lacking the perforin gene. *Proc. Natl. Acad. Sci. USA* 91:10854–58

85. Rossi CP, McAllister A, Tanguy M, Kagi D, Brahic M. 1998. Theiler's virus infection of perforin-deficient mice. *J. Virol.* 72:4515–19

86. Topham DJ, Tripp RA, Doherty PC. 1997. CD8+ T cells clear influenza virus by perforin or Fas-dependent processes. *J. Immunol.* 159:5197–5200

87. Holterman AX, Rogers K, Edelmann K, Koelle DM, Corey L, Wilson CB. 1999. An important role for major histocompatibility complex class I–restricted T cells, and a limited role for gamma interferon, in protection of mice against lethal herpes simplex virus infection. *J. Virol.* 73:2058–63

88. Harty JT, Tvinnereim AR, White DW. 2000. CD8+ T cell effector mechanisms in resistance to infection. *Annu. Rev. Immunol.* 18:275–308

89. Guidotti LG, Ando K, Hobbs MV, Ishikawa T, Runkel RD, Schreiber RD, Chisari FV. 1994. Cytotoxic T lymphocytes inhibit hepatitis B virus gene expression by a noncytolytic mechanism in transgenic mice. *Proc. Natl. Acad. Sci. USA* 91:3764–68

90. Guidotti LG, Ishikawa T, Hobbs MV, Matzke B, Schreiber R, Chisari FV. 1996. Intracellular inactivation of the hepatitis B

91. Guidotti LG, Chisari FV. 1999. Cytokine-induced viral purging–role in viral pathogenesis. *Curr. Opin. Microbiol.* 2:388–91

92. Gilles PN, Fey G, Chisari FV. 1992. Tumor necrosis factor-alpha negatively regulates hepatitis B virus gene expression in transgenic mice. *J. Virol.* 66:3955–60

93. Guidotti LG, Guilhot S, Chisari FV. 1994. Interleukin 2 and interferon alpha/beta downregulate hepatitis B virus gene expression in vivo by tumor necrosis factor dependent and independent pathways. *J. Virol.* 68:1265–70

94. Kohonen-Corish MRJ, King NJC, Woodhams CE, Ramshaw IA. 1990. Immunodeficient mice recover from infection with vaccinia virus expressing interferon-g. *Eur. J. Immunol.* 20:157–61

95. Karupiah G, Blanden RV, Ramshaw IA. 1990. Interferon gamma is involved in the recovery of athymic nude mice from recombinant vaccinia virus/interleukin 2 infection. *J. Exp. Med.* 172:1495–1503

96. Sambhi SK, Kohonen-Corish MRJ, Ramshaw IA. 1991. Local production of tumor necrosis factor encoded by recombinant vaccinia virus is effective in controlling viral replication *in vivo*. *Proc. Natl. Acad. Sci. USA* 88:4025–29

97. Ramshaw I, Ruby J, Ramsay A, Ada G, Karupiah G. 1992. Expression of cytokines by recombinant vaccinia viruses: a model for studying cytokines in virus infections in vivo. *Immunol. Rev.* 127:157–82

98. Lucin P, Pavic I, Polic B, Jonjic S, Koszinowski UH. 1992. Gamma interferon-dependent clearance of cytomegalovirus infection in salivary glands. *J. Virol.* 66:1977–84

99. Pavic I, Polic B, Crnkovic I, Lucin P, Jonjic S, Koszinowski UH. 1993. Participation of endogenous tumour necrosis factor {a} in host resistance to cytomegalovirus infection. *J. Gen. Virol.* 74:2215–23

100. Klavinskis LS, Geckeler R, Oldstone MBA. 1989. Cytotoxic T lymphocyte control of acute lymphocytic choriomeningitis virus infection: interferon gamma, but not tumour necrosis factor α, displays antiviral activity *in vivo. J. Gen. Virol.* 70:3317–25

101. Tishon A, Lewiski H, Rall G, VonHerrath M, Oldstone MBA. 1995. An essential role for type 1 interferon-gamma in terminating persistent viral infection. *Virology* 212:244–50

102. Leist TP, Eppler M, Zinkernagel RM. 1989. Enhanced virus replication and inhibition of lymphocytic choriomeningitis virus disease in anti-gamma interferon-treated mice. *J. Virol.* 63:2813–19

103. Wirth S, Guidotti LG, Ando K, Schlicht HJ, Chisari FV. 1995. Breaking tolerance leads to autoantibody production but not autoimmune liver disease in HBV envelope transgenic mice. *J. Immunol.* 154:2504–15

104. Nakamoto Y, Guidotti LG, Pasquetto V, Schreiber RD, Chisari FV. 1997. Differential target cell sensitivity to cytotoxic T lymphocyte-activated death pathways in vivo. *J. Immunol.* 158:5692–97

105. Guidotti LG, Rochford R, Chung L, Shapiro M, Purcell R, Chisari FV. 1999. Viral clearance without destruction of infected cells during acute HBV infection. *Science* 284:825–29

106. Schultz U, Chisari FV. 1999. Recombinant duck interferon gamma inhibits duck hepatitis B virus replication in primary hepatocytes. *J. Virol.* 73:3162–68

107. Guidotti LG, Borrow P, Brown A, McClary H, Koch R, Chisari FV. 1999. Noncytopathic clearance of lymphocytic choriomeningitis virus from the hepatocyte. *J. Exp. Med.* 189:1555–64

108. Benihoud K, Saggio I, Opolon P, Salone B, Amiot F, Connault E, Chianale C, Dautry F, Yeh P, Perricaudet M. 1998. Efficient, repeated adenovirus-mediated gene transfer in mice lacking both tumor necrosis factor alpha and lymphotoxin alpha. *J. Virol.* 72:9514–25

109. Zhang HG, Zhou T, Yang P, Edwards CK, 3rd Curiel DT, Mountz JD. 1998. Inhibition of tumor necrosis factor alpha decreases inflammation and prolongs adenovirus gene expression in lung and liver. *Hum. Gene Ther.* 9:1875–84

110. Lin MT, Hinton DR, Stohlman SA. 1998. Mechanisms of viral clearance in perforin-deficient mice. *Adv. Exp. Med. Biol.* 440:431–36

111. Parra B, Hinton DR, Marten NW, Bergmann CC, Lin MT, Yang CS, Stohlman SA. 1999. IFN-gamma is required for viral clearance from central nervous system oligodendroglia. *J. Immunol.* 162:1641–47

112. Horwitz MS, Krahl T, Fine C, Lee J, Sarvetnick N. 1999. Protection from lethal coxsackievirus-induced pancreatitis by expression of gamma interferon. *J. Virol.* 73:1756–66

113. Gebhard JR, Perry CM, Harkins S, Lane T, Mena I, Asensio VC, Campbell IL, Whitton JL. 1998. Coxsackievirus B3-induced myocarditis: perforin exacerbates disease, but plays no detectable role in virus clearance. *Am. J. Pathol.* 153:417–28

114. Levy JA, Mackewicz CE, Barker E. 1996. Controlling HIV pathogenesis: the role of the noncytotoxic anti-HIV response of CD8+ T cells. *Immunol. Today* 17:217–24

115. Mackewicz CE, Patterson BK, Lee SA, Levy JA. 2000. CD8(+) cell noncytotoxic anti-human immunodeficiency virus response inhibits expression of viral RNA but not reverse transcription or provirus integration. *J. Gen. Virol.* 81 Pt 5:1261–64

116. Mosmann TR, Coffman RL. 1989. Th-1 and Th-2 cells: different patterns of lymphokine secretion lead to different functional properties. *Annu. Rev. Immunol.* 7:145–73

117. Whitmire JK, Asano MS, Murali-Krishna K, Suresh M, Ahmed R. 1998. Long-term CD4 Th1 and Th2 memory following acute lymphocytic choriomeningitis virus infection. *J. Virol.* 72:8281–88

118. Varga SM, Welsh RM. 1998. Detection of a high frequency of virus-specific CD4$^+$ T cells during acute infection with lymphocytic choriomeningitis virus. *J. Immunol.* 161:3215–18

119. Varga SM, Welsh RM. 2000. High frequency of virus-specific interleukin-2-producing CD4$^{(+)}$ T cells and Th1 dominance during lymphocytic choriomeningitis virus infection. *J. Virol.* 74:4429–32

120. Varga SM, Welsh RM. 1998. Stability of virus-specific CD4$^+$ T cell frequencies from acute infection into long term memory. *J. Immunol.* 161:367–74

121. Eichelberger M, Allan W, Zijlstra M, Jaenisch R, Doherty PC. 1991. Clearance of influenza virus respiratory infection in mice lacking class I major histocompatibility complex-restricted CD8$^+$ T cells. *J. Exp. Med.* 174:875–80

122. Scherle PA, Palladino G, Gerhard W. 1992. Mice can recover from pulmonary influenza virus infection in the absence of class I–restricted cytotoxic T cells. *J. Immunol.* 148:212–17

123. Graham MB, Braciale VL, Braciale TJ. 1994. Influenza virus-specific CD4$^+$ T helper type 2 T lymphocytes do not promote recovery from experimental virus infection. *J. Exp. Med.* 180:1273–82

124. Maloy KJ, Burkhart C, Junt TM, Odermatt B, Oxenius A, Piali L, Zinkernagel RM, Hengartner H. 2000. CD4$^{(+)}$ T cell subsets during virus infection. Protective capacity depends on effector cytokine secretion and on migratory capability. *J. Exp. Med.* 191:2159–70

125. Spriggs MK, Koller BH, Sato T, Morrissey PJ, Fanslow WC, Smithies O, Voice RF, Widmer MB, Maliszewski CR. 1992. Beta 2-microglobulin-, CD8$^+$ T-cell-deficient mice survive inoculation with high doses of vaccinia virus and exhibit altered IgG responses. *Proc. Natl. Acad. Sci. USA* 89:6070–4

126. Kagi D, Seiler P, Pavlovic J, Ledermann B, Burki K, Zinkernagel RM, Hengartner H. 1995. The roles of perforin- and Fas-dependent cytotoxicity in protection against cytopathic and noncytopathic viruses. *Eur. J. Immunol.* 25:3256–62

127. Franco A, Guidotti LG, Hobbs MV, Pasquetto V, Chisari FV. 1997. Pathogenetic effector function of CD4-positive T-helper-1 cells in hepatitis B virus transgenic mice. *J. Immunol.* 159:2001–8

128. Hou S, Mo XY, Hyland L, Doherty PC. 1995. Host response to Sendai virus in mice lacking class II major histocompatibility complex glycoproteins. *J. Virol.* 69:1429–34

129. Leist TP, Kohler M, Zinkernagel RM. 1989. Impaired generation of anti-viral cytotoxicity against lymphocytic choriomeningitis and vaccinia virus in mice treated with CD4-specific monoclonal antibody. *Scand. J. Immunol.* 30:679–86

130. Battegay M, Bachmann MF, Burhkart C, Viville S, Benoist C, Mathis D, Hengartner H, Zinkernagel RM. 1996. Antiviral immune responses of mice lacking MHC class II or its associated invariant chain. *Cell Immunol.* 167:115–21

131. Doherty PC, Topham DJ, Tripp RA, Cardin RD, Brooks JW, Stevenson PG. 1997. Effector CD4$^+$ and CD8$^+$ T-cell mechanisms in the control of respiratory virus infections. *Immunol. Rev* 159:105–17

132. Hasenkrug KJ, Brooks DM, Dittmer U. 1998. Critical role for CD4$^{(+)}$ T cells in controlling retrovirus replication and spread in persistently infected mice. *J. Virol.* 72:6559–64

133. Hahn S, Erb P. 1999. The immunomodulatory role of CD4-positive cytotoxic T-lymphocytes in health and disease. *Int. Rev. Immunol.* 18:449–64

134. Hasenkrug KJ, Dittmer U. 2000. The role of CD4 and CD8 T cells in recovery and protection from retroviral infection: lessons from the friend virus model. *Virology* 272:244–49

135. Cooper NR, Nemerow GR. 1983. Complement, viruses, and virus-infected cells. *Springer Semin. Immunopathol.* 6:327–47

136. Cooper NR, Nemerow GR. 1984. The role of antibody and complement in the control of viral infections. *J. Invest. Dermatol.* 83:121s–27s

137. Burton DR, Williamson RA, Parren PW. 2000. Antibody and virus: binding and neutralization. *Virology* 270:1–3

138. Levine B, Hardwick JM, Trapp BD, Crawford TO, Bollinger RC, Griffin DE. 1991. Antibody-mediated clearance of alphavirus infection from neurons. *Science* 254:856–60

139. Byrnes AP, Durbin JE, Griffin DE. 2000. Control of Sindbis virus infection by antibody in interferon-deficient mice. *J. Virol.* 74:3905–8

140. Ubol S, Levine B, Lee SH, Greenspan NS, Griffin DE. 1995. Roles of immunoglobulin valency and the heavy-chain constant domain in antibody-mediated downregulation of Sindbis virus replication in persistently infected neurons. *J. Virol.* 69:1990–93

141. Bachmann MF, Zinkernagel RM. 1997. Neutralizing antiviral B cell responses. *Annu. Rev. Immunol.* 15:235–70

142. Brundler MA, Aichele P, Bachmann M, Kitamura D, Rajewsky K, Zinkernagel RM. 1996. Immunity to viruses in B cell–deficient mice: influence of antibodies on virus persistence and on T cell memory. *Eur. J. Immunol.* 26:2257–62

143. Seiler P, Kalinke U, Rulicke T, Bucher EM, Bose C, Zinkernagel RM, Hengartner H. 1998. Enhanced virus clearance by early inducible lymphocytic choriomeningitis virus-neutralizing antibodies in immunoglobulin-transgenic mice. *J. Virol.* 72:2253–58

144. Super HJ, Brooks D, Hasenkrug K, Chesebro B. 1998. Requirement for CD4(+) T cells in the Friend murine retrovirus neutralizing antibody response: evidence for functional T cells in genetic low-recovery mice. *J. Virol.* 72:9400–3

145. Chisari FV, Ferrari C. 1995. Hepatitis B virus immunopathogenesis. *Annu. Rev. Immunol.* 13:29–60

146. Koziel MJ. 1997. The role of immune responses in the pathogenesis of hepatitis C virus infection. *J. Viral. Hepat.* 4:31–41

147. Michalak TI, Pasquinelli C, Guilhot S, Chisari FV. 1994. Hepatitis B virus persistence after recovery from acute viral hepatitis. *J. Clin. Invest.* 93:230–39

148. Rehermann B, Ferrari C, Pasquinelli C, Chisari FV. 1996. The hepatitis B virus persists for decades after patients' recovery from acute viral hepatitis despite active maintenance of a cytotoxic T lymphocyte response. *Nat. Med.* 2:1104–8

149. Ciurea A, Klenerman P, Hunziker L, Horvath E, Odermatt B, Ochsenbein AF, Hengartner H, Zinkernagel RM. 1999. Persistence of lymphocytic choriomeningitis virus at very low levels in immune mice. *Proc. Natl. Acad. Sci. USA* 96:11964–69

150. Ciurea A, Klenerman P, Hunziker L, Horvath E, Senn BM, Ochsenbein AF, Hengartner H, Zinkernagel RM. 2000. Viral persistence in vivo through selection of neutralizing antibody-escape variants. *Proc. Natl. Acad. Sci. USA* 97:2749–54

151. Ochsenbein AF, Fehr T, Lutz C, Suter M, Brombacher F, Hengartner H, Zinkernagel RM. 1999. Control of early viral and bacterial distribution and disease by natural antibodies. *Science* 286:2156–59

152. Samuel CE. 1991. Antiviral actions of interferon. Interferon-regulated cellular proteins and their surprisingly selective antiviral activities. *Virology* 183:1–11

153. Stark GR, Kerr IM, Williams BR, Silverman RH, Schreiber RD. 1998. How

cells respond to interferons. *Annu. Rev. Biochem.* 67:227–64

154. Kalvakolanu DV, Borden EC. 1996. An overview of the interferon system: signal transduction and mechanisms of action. *Cancer Invest.* 14:25–53

155. Zhu H, Cong JP, Shenk T. 1997. Use of differential display analysis to assess the effect of human cytomegalovirus infection on the accumulation of cellular RNAs: induction of interferon-responsive RNAs. *Proc. Natl. Acad. Sci. USA* 94:13985–90

156. Der SD, Zhou A, Williams BR, Silverman RH. 1998. Identification of genes differentially regulated by interferon alpha, beta, or gamma using oligonucleotide arrays. *Proc. Natl. Acad. Sci. USA* 95:15623–28

157. Silverman RH. 1994. Fascination with 2-5A-dependent RNase: a unique enzyme that functions in interferon action. *J. Interferon Res.* 14:101–4

158. Terenzi F, deVeer MJ, Ying H, Restifo NP, Williams BR, Silverman RH. 1999. The antiviral enzymes PKR and RNase L suppress gene expression from viral and nonviral based vectors. *Nucleic Acids Res.* 27:4369–75

159. Dong B, Silverman RH. 1999. Alternative function of a protein kinase homology domain in 2′,5′-oligoadenylate dependent RNase L. *Nucleic Acids Res.* 27:439–45

160. Maitra RK, Silverman RH. 1998. Regulation of human immunodeficiency virus replication by 2′,5′-oligoadenylate-dependent RNase L. *J. Virol.* 72:1146–52

161. Li XL, Blackford JA, Hassel BA. 1998. RNase L mediates the antiviral effect of interferon through a selective reduction in viral RNA during encephalomyocarditis virus infection. *J. Virol.* 72:2752–59

162. Diaz-Guerra M, Rivas C, Esteban M. 1997. Inducible expression of the 2-5A synthetase/RNase L system results in in-

hibition of vaccinia virus replication. *Virology* 227:220–28

163. Haller O, Frese M, Kochs G. 1998. Mx proteins: mediators of innate resistance to RNA viruses. *Rev. Sci. Technol.* 17:220–30

164. Kochs G, Haller O. 1999. Interferon-induced human MxA GTPase blocks nuclear import of Thogoto virus nucleocapsids. *Proc. Natl. Acad. Sci. USA* 96:2082–86

165. Taylor DR, Shi ST, Romano PR, Barber GN, Lai MM. 1999. Inhibition of the interferon-inducible protein kinase PKR by HCV E2 protein [see comments]. *Science* 285:107–10

166. Gale MJ, Jr., Korth MJ, Tang NM, Tan SL, Hopkins DA, Dever TE, Polyak SJ, Gretch DR, Katze MG. 1997. Evidence that hepatitis C virus resistance to interferon is mediated through repression of the PKR protein kinase by the nonstructural 5A protein. *Virology* 230:217–27

167. Gale MJ, Jr., Korth MJ, Katze MG. 1998. Repression of the PKR protein kinase by the hepatitis C virus NS5A protein: a potential mechanism of interferon resistance. *Clin. Diagnos. Virol.* 10:157–62

168. Patterson JB, Thomis DC, Hans SL, Samuel CE. 1995. Mechanism of interferon action: double-stranded RNA-specific adenosine deaminase from human cells is inducible by alpha and gamma interferons. *Virology* 210:508–11

169. Wieland SF, Guidotti LG, Chisari FV. 2000. Intrahepatic induction of IFN-α/β eliminates viral RNA-containing capsids in HBV transgenic mice. *J. Virol.* 74:4165–73

170. Zhou A, Paranjape JM, Der SD, Williams BR, Silverman RH. 1999. Interferon action in triply deficient mice reveals the existence of alternative antiviral pathways. *Virology* 258:435–40

171. Herbein G, O'Brien WA. 2000. Tumor necrosis factor (TNF)-alpha and TNF receptors in viral pathogenesis. *Proc. Soc. Exp. Biol. Med.* 223:241–57

172. Tsui LV, Guidotti LG, Ishikawa T, Chisari FV. 1995. Post-transcriptional clearance of hepatitis B virus RNA by cytotoxic T lymphocyte-activated hepatocytes. *Proc. Natl. Acad. Sci. USA* 92:12398–12402

173. Heise T, Guidotti LG, Chisari FV. 1999. La autoantigen specifically recognizes a predicted stem-loop in hepatitis B virus RNA. *J. Virol.* 73:5767–76

174. Heise T, Guidotti LG, Cavanaugh VJ, Chisari FV. 1999. Hepatitis B virus RNA-binding proteins associated with cytokine-induced clearance of viral RNA from the liver of transgenic mice. *J. Virol.* 73:474–81

175. Kundig TM, Hengartner H, Zinkernagel RM. 1993. T cell–dependent IFN-gamma exerts an antiviral effect in the central nervous system but not in peripheral solid organs. *J. Immunol.* 150:2316–21

176. Tay CH, Welsh RM. 1997. Distinct organ-dependent mechanisms for the control of murine cytomegalovirus infection by natural killer cells. *J. Virol.* 71:267–75

177. Estcourt MJ, Ramshaw l A, Ramsay AJ. 1998. Cytokine responses in virus infections: effects on pathogenesis, recovery and persistence. *Curr. Opin. Microbiol.* 1:411–18

178. Kalvakolanu DV. 1999. Virus interception of cytokine-regulated pathways. *Trends Microbiol.* 7:166–71

179. Wall EM, Cao JX, Upton C. 1998. Subversion of cytokine networks by viruses. *Int. Rev. Immunol.* 17:121–55

180. Mahr JA, Gooding LR. 1999. Immune evasion by adenoviruses. *Immunol. Rev.* 168:121–30

181. Wiertz EJ, Tortorella D, Bogyo M, Yu J, Mothes W, Jones TR, Rapoport TA, Ploegh HL. 1996. Sec61-mediated transfer of a membrane protein from the endoplasmic reticulum to the proteasome for destruction [see comments]. *Nature* 384:432–38

182. Ahn K, Angulo A, Ghazal P, Peterson PA, Yang Y, Fruh K. 1996. Human cytomegalovirus inhibits antigen presentation by a sequential multistep process. *Proc. Natl. Acad. Sci. USA* 93:10990–5

183. Ziegler H, Thale R, Lucin P, Muranyi W, Flohr T, Hengel H, Farrell H, Rawlinson W, Koszinowski UH. 1997. A mouse cytomegalovirus glycoprotein retains MHC class I complexes in the ERGIC/cis-Golgi compartments. *Immunity* 6:57–66

184. Reusch U, Muranyi W, Lucin P, Burgert HG, Hengel H, Koszinowski UH. 1999. A cytomegalovirus glycoprotein reroutes MHC class I complexes to lysosomes for degradation. *Embo. J.* 18:1081–91

185. Kerkau T, Bacik I, Bennink JR, Yewdell JW, Hunig T, Schimpl A, Schubert U. 1997. The human immunodeficiency virus type 1 (HIV-1) Vpu protein interfeRes. with an early step in the biosynthesis of major histocompatibility complex (MHC) class I molecules. *J. Exp. Med.* 185:1295–1305

186. Coscoy L, Ganem D. 2000. Kaposi's sarcoma–associated herpesvirus encodes two proteins that block cell surface display of MHC class I chains by enhancing their endocytosis. *Proc. Natl. Acad. Sci. USA* 97:8051–56

187. Lacaille VG, Androlewicz MJ. 1998. Herpes simplex virus inhibitor ICP47 destabilizes the transporter associated with antigen processing (TAP) heterodimer. *J. Biol. Chem.* 273:17386–90

188. Galocha B, Hill A, Barnett BC, Dolan A, Raimondi A, Cook RF, Brunner J, McGeoch DJ, Ploegh HL. 1997. The active site of ICP47, a herpes simplex virus–encoded inhibitor of the major

histocompatibility complex (MHC)-encoded peptide transporter associated with antigen processing (TAP), maps to the NH2-terminal 35 residues. *J. Exp. Med.* 185:1565–72

189. Reich N, Pine R, Levy D, Darnell Jr. JE. 1988. Transcription of interferon-stimulated genes is induced by adenovirus particles but is suppressed by E1A products. *J. Virol.* 62:114–19

190. McFadden G, Lalani A, Everett H, Nash P, Xu X. 1998. Virus-encoded receptors for cytokines and chemokines. *Semin. Cell Dev. Biol.* 9:359–68

Annu. Rev. Immunol. 2001. 19:93–129

IMMUNOLOGY OF TUBERCULOSIS

Joanne L. Flynn[1] and John Chan[2]

[1]Department of Molecular Genetics and Biochemistry, University of Pittsburgh
School of Medicine, Pittsburgh, Pennsylvania 15261; e-mail: joanne@pitt.edu
[2]Departments of Medicine and Microbiology and Immunology, Albert Einstein
College of Medicine, Bronx, New York 10461; e-mail: jchan@aecom.yu.edu

Key Words T lymphocytes, macrophage, cytokine, chemokine,
Mycobacterium tuberculosis

■ **Abstract** The resurgence of tuberculosis worldwide has intensified research efforts directed at examining the host defense and pathogenic mechanisms operative
in *Mycobacterium tuberculosis* infection. This review summarizes our current understanding of the host immune response, with emphasis on the roles of macrophages,
T cells, and the cytokine/chemokine network in engendering protective immunity.
Specifically, we summarize studies addressing the ability of the organism to survive
within macrophages by controlling phagolysosome fusion. The recent studies on Toll-
like receptors and the impact on the innate response to *M. tuberculosis* are discussed.
We also focus on the induction, specificity, and effector functions of CD4$^+$ and CD8$^+$
T cells, and the roles of cytokines and chemokines in the induction and effector functions of the immune response. Presentation of mycobacterial antigens by MHC class
I, class II, and CD1 as well as the implications of these molecules sampling various
compartments of the cell for presentation to T cells are discussed. Increased attention
to this disease and the integration of animal models and human studies have afforded
us a greater understanding of tuberculosis and the steps necessary to combat this infection. The pace of this research must be maintained if we are to realize an effective
vaccine in the next decades.

INTRODUCTION

Mycobacterium tuberculosis is responsible for at least 1.5 million deaths per year,
worldwide. In most cases, tuberculosis is a curable disease, but restricted access
to health care is an impediment for many people in developing countries with this
disease. The organism is a slow-growing acid-fast bacillus transmitted primarily by
the respiratory route, and although it can cause disease in most organs, pulmonary
tuberculosis is most common. Estimates are that one third of the world's population
is infected with *M. tuberculosis*, but infection does not usually lead to active
disease. The immune response mounted to the infection is generally successful in
containing, although not eliminating, the pathogen. Acute active tuberculosis can
result in a small percentage of infections, probably due to the lack of initiation of

0732-0582/01/0407-0093$14.00

an appropriate immune response. In most cases of *M. tuberculosis* infection, the individual is asymptomatic and noninfectious. This clinical latency often extends for the lifetime of the individual. However, reactivation of the latent infection can occur in response to perturbations of the immune response, and active tuberculosis ensues. In many cases of active tuberculosis, an obvious immunodeficiency is not found. However, infection with human immunodeficiency virus, treatment with corticosteroids, aging, and alcohol or drug abuse increase the potential for reactivation of latent tuberculosis (1).

M. tuberculosis persists in macrophages within a granuloma in the organs of infected hosts. The granuloma consists of macrophages and giant cells, T cells, B cells, and fibroblasts. In latent infections, the state of the bacteria within the granuloma, or tubercle, is not known. The organism may be in a dormant non-replicating state, actively replicating but killed off by the immune response, or metabolically altered with limited or infrequent replicative cycles. Breakdown of immune responses designed to contain the infection can result in reactivation and replication of the bacilli, with necrosis and damage to lung tissue. Thus, a constant battle between the host and the mycobacterium is being waged, and the outcome depends on many factors. Why is the immune response mounted to *M. tuberculosis* sufficient to prevent most people from active disease but not capable of clearing the infection? A corollary to that question is how can we improve upon the natural immune response to *M. tuberculosis* with a vaccine? Clearly, the organism has developed mechanisms for evading elimination by a strong cell-mediated immune response. A more complete understanding of the roles each component of the immune system plays in protection or exacerbation of tuberculosis, as well as of the bacterium's weapons to evade those components, will enhance development of preventive and therapeutic strategies against this enormously successful pathogen.

MACROPHAGES

In Vitro Activation of Macrophage Antimycobacterial Functions

It is well established that murine macrophages possess antimycobacterial function in tissue culture systems (2–4). When activated by supernatants of immunologically stimulated lymphocytes, macrophages exhibited various degrees of antimycobacterial activity (5). Hydrogen peroxide (H_2O_2), one of the reactive oxygen intermediates (ROI) generated by macrophages via the oxidative burst, was the first identified effector molecule that mediated mycobacteriocidal effects of mononuclear phagocytes (6). The significance of ROI in host defense against *M. tuberculosis* remains controversial (see below). Later, gamma-interferon (IFN-γ) was found to be the key endogenous activating agent that triggers the antimycobacterial effects of murine macrophages (7, 8). Tumor necrosis factor-alpha (TNF-α), although ineffective when used alone, synergizes with IFN-γ to induce antimycobacterial effects of murine macrophages in vitro (9). A major effector mechanism responsible for the antimycobacterial activity of IFN-γ and TNF-α is induction of the production of nitric oxide and related reactive nitrogen intermediates (RNI) by macrophages via the action of the inducible form of nitric oxide synthase (NOS2): in fact, these two cytokines act synergistically to induce the expression of the RNI-generating pathway (10).

Compared to the murine system, much less is known about the activation of antimycobacterial activity in human macrophages. The enhanced susceptibility to mycobacterial infection of individuals functionally deficient in IFN-γ as a result of mutation in the IFN-γ receptor gene provides strong evidence that this cytokine plays a significant role in defense against *M. tuberculosis* in humans (11), although the infections afflicting IFN-γ-deficient individuals are mostly not caused by *M. tuberculosis*. In vitro evidence supporting a role for IFN-γ in defense against human tuberculosis has been scarce due to the lack of an experimental system in which the killing of *M. tuberculosis* by macrophages can be reproducibly demonstrated. Thus, reports of the effect of IFN-γ treated human macrophages on the replication of *M. tuberculosis* range from its being inhibitory (7) to enhancing (12). This inconsistency cast considerable doubt on the antimycobacterial capability of human mononuclear phagocytes until the demonstration that 1,25-dihydroxy vitamin D_3 [1,25-$(OH)_2D_3$], alone or in combination with IFN-γ and TNF-α, was able to activate macrophages to inhibit and/or kill *M. tuberculosis* in the human system (13–15). 1,25-$(OH)_2D_3$ is known to have an immunoregulatory role mediated through binding to the vitamin D receptor in immune cells including macrophages (16). Recently, 1,25-$(OH)_2D_3$ was reported to induce the expression of the NOS2 and *M. tuberculosis* inhibitory activity in the human HL-60 macrophage-like cell line (17). This observation thus identifies NO and related RNI as the putative antimycobacterial effectors produced by human macrophages. This controversial notion is further supported by recent evidence that IFN-γ-stimulated human macrophages cocultured with lymphocytes (obtained from *M. tuberculosis*-lysate/IFN-γ-primed peripheral mononuclear cells) exhibit mycobacteriocidal activity concomitant with the expression of NOS2 (18).

Antimycobacterial Effector Functions of Macrophages

The mononuclear phagocyte constitutes a potent antimicrobial component of cell-mediated immunity. The precise mechanisms by which these cells mediate killing or inhibition of bacterial pathogens, however, are not clearly understood. In this section, discussion of antimycobacterial effector functions of macrophages focuses on phagolysosome fusion, generation of ROI by the oxidative burst, production of RNI via the NOS2-dependent cytotoxic pathway as well as on the possible evasive mechanisms employed by the tubercle bacillus to escape killing by activated macrophages. Finally, the role of the recently discovered Toll-like receptors in innate immunity against *M. tuberculosis* is discussed.

Phagolysosome Fusion   The lysosome (19–21) is a complex vacuolar organelle of the late endocytic pathway. Within the lysosomal vacuoles are potent hydrolytic enzymes capable of degrading a whole range of macromolecules including microbes. These enzymes function optimally at acidic pH, a condition found within the intralysosomal milieu. The lysosome is, in fact, the most acidic organelle in animal cells: pH 4.5–5.0 (22); this acidic environment is maintained by membrane ATP-dependent proton pumps, the vacuolar H^+-ATPases (22, 23).

It is well established that phagosomes, the product of the endocytic pathway initiated by phagocytosis of large particles including microbes, can fuse with lysosomes. While phagocytic vacuoles can fuse with lysosomes in a single event, the formation of phagolysosomes is in general a dynamic process during which the phagosome matures, modified by transient fission and fusion with endocytic organelles (24, 25). Phagocytosed microorganisms are subject to degradation by intralysosomal acidic hydrolases upon phagolysosome fusion (26). This highly regulated event (24, 25) constitutes a significant antimicrobial mechanism of phagocytes. Examination of the interaction between isotopically labeled bacteria and macrophages revealed that certain organisms are degraded extensively within 2 h after phagocytosis (26). It appears that the antimicrobial activity of the phagolysosome is mediated, at least in part, by the degradative function of lysosomal hydrolases and/or direct and indirect effect of acidification. However, the precise mechanisms by which the hydrolases and acidification confer antimicrobial properties, as well as the process of acidification of the various endocytic compartments, are not completely understood (22, 27, 28). Elucidation of these mechanisms will facilitate our understanding of how *M. tuberculosis* evades the hostile environment of phagolysosomes.

Significant progress has been made in this area of mycobacterial research since D'Arcy Hart and colleagues hypothesized that prevention of phagolysosomal fusion is a mechanism by which *M. tuberculosis* survives inside macrophages (29, 30). This hypothesis was based on studies examining the interaction of *M. tuberculosis* and mouse macrophages by electron microscopy and labeling of lysosomes with electron-opaque ferritin (29). An important inference was that lack of fusion with lysosomes was observed only with phagosomes containing viable bacilli. This apparent relative inaccessibility of mycobacterial phagosomes to the endocytic pathway has been supported by subsequent studies, with the more recent ones employing techniques that exploit the progress made in identifying specific markers of various endocytic compartments (31, 32). Emerging evidence, however, suggests that the apparent nonfusigenic attribute of the mycobacterial phagosome may be restricted to specific endocytic compartments. In fact, the mycobacterial vacuole is a highly dynamic, fusion-competent structure that selectively fuses with specific endosomal vacuoles (33; and see below).

Early studies focused on *M. tuberculosis* products that might disrupt phagolysosome fusion. It has been reported that mycobacterial sulfatides (34), derivatives of multiacylated trehalose 2-sulfate, a lysosomotropic polyanionic glycolipid (35, 36), have the ability to inhibit phagolysosomal fusion. In vitro studies demonstrated that *M. tuberculosis* generates copious amounts of ammonia in cultures (concentrations of up to 20 mM have been detected) and is thought to be responsible for the inhibitory effect of culture supernates of virulent mycobacteria on phagolysosome fusion (37). This finding is in keeping with the observation that the weak base ammonium chloride affects saltatory movement of lysosomes as well as alkalinizes the intralysosomal compartment (37, 38). However, it is unlikely that the ability of ammonia to alkalinize intracellular vacuoles accounts for its inhibitory effect on phagolysosome fusion because other bases capable of raising intralysosomal pH actually promote phagolysosome fusion (37). Also unsettled is the absolute requirement of acidification of the phagosomes for fusion with lysosomes (22, 27, 28). Thus, the precise mechanisms by which ammonia prevents phagolysosome fusion remain to be determined. Nevertheless, by virtue of its ability to produce significant amounts of ammonia, the tubercle bacillus can evade the toxic environment within the lysosomal vacuole by inhibiting phagolysosome fusion and diminishing the potency of the intralysosomal enzymes via alkalinization.

Two mycobacterial enzyme systems related to ammonia metabolism have been the target of investigation in the context of the relationship of disruption of phagolysosomal fusion to intracellular survival. The mycobacterial urease, which catalyzes the conversion of urea to ammonia and carbon dioxide, has been cloned, purified, and characterized (39, 40). A BCG urease-negative mutant generated by allelic exchange was only slightly compromised in the ability to multiply and persist in the lungs of mice (41). The significance of mycobacterial urease in the survival of virulent *M. tuberculosis* remains to be tested. Another mycobacterial enzyme, glutamine synthetase, which has the potential to influence ammonia level via its participation in nitrogen metabolism, has also been studied with respect to its ability to affect intracellular survival of *M. tuberculosis* (42, 43). *M. tuberculosis* glutamine synthetase is released in abundance into culture supernatants; immunogold electron microscopy revealed its release into phagosomes in infected human monocytes. The release of this enzyme during in vitro growth is associated with the pathogenicity of the mycobacteria studied; it is released in large quantities by *M. tuberculosis* and *M. bovis*, but not by the relatively nonpathogenic *M. smegmatis* and *M. phlei* (39). A putative function of the released glutamine synthetase is to mediate the generation of poly(L-glutamic acid/glutamine), a cell wall structure found in pathogenic strains of mycobacteria (42, 43). Significantly, the glutamine synthetase inhibitor L-methionine-S-sulfoximine selectively blocks the growth of pathogenic mycobacteria, both in culture and in human monocytes (43). Although it is likely that the mechanism by which glutamine synthetase confers a growth advantage is through its role in cell wall synthesis, its potential role in influencing ammonia levels and affecting phagolysosomal fusion remains an intriguing possibility.

Recent work on the effect of the tubercle bacillus on the fusigenicity of phagosomes and lysosomes has focused on the mechanisms underlying the alteration of biochemical properties of vacuolar membrane components and intravacuolar contents. This endeavor has been greatly facilitated by advances in the biochemical

and molecular characterization of endocytosis, exocytosis, and particularly vesicle transport and protein sorting (44, 45), and has enhanced our understanding
of the interaction of mycobacteria-containing phagosomes with other compartments of the endocytic pathway. For example, the GTPases of the Ras family,
known to play a role in the interaction between various endocytic compartments
(24, 46, 47), have been a target of investigation aimed at understanding the inability of mycobacterial phagosomes to mature to phagolysosomes (48). Thus,
mycobacterial phagosomes retain Rab5, which plays a role in the interaction between early endocytic compartments and phagosomes (24, 25), and exclude Rab7
(49), a GTPase that regulates late endosomal membrane trafficking (48; and reviewed in 32). These results further define the point at which maturation of the
mycobacterial phagosome is arrested.

Vacuolar ATPase, normally present in maturing phagosomes, is thought to be acquired from endosomal compartments (22). The exclusion of vacuolar ATPase proton pumps from phagosomes containing live *M. tuberculosis* or *M. avium* (50–52)
provides a mechanism for the relative lack of acidification of mycobacterial phagosomes. While it remains to be proven whether alkalinization of mycobacterial vacuoles attenuates phagolysosomal fusion, increase in intralysosomal pH is likely to
help mycobacteria evade the adverse effect of an otherwise acidic environment. In
addition, results of these studies support an apparent inaccessibility of mycobacterial phagosomes to fusion with endocytic vacuoles. Thus, it was surprising that
phagosomes harboring live *M. avium* or *M. tuberculosis* acquire LAMP-1, the late
endosomal/lysosomal marker (39, 51, 52). Russell et al proposed that this apparent
paradox is attainable if mycobacterial phagosomes selectively block fusion with
specific subsets of a heterogeneous population of endosomal vacuoles (31). In a
study using GM1 ganglioside-bound cholera toxin B subunit as a probe to examine
the fusigenicity of mycobacterial phagosomes (31), it was observed that vacuoles
containing mycobacteria are a highly dynamic, fusion-competent organelle that
interact readily with certain plasmalemma constituents, behaving like recycling endosomes. The fusion characteristics of recycling endosomes as regulated by Rabs
are specific. Therefore mycobacterial vacuoles might possess similar selectivity
with respect to specific intracellular vesicles with which they fuse. Elucidation of
the biochemical and molecular mechanisms underlying this selectivity will likely
advance our understanding of the pathogenicity of *M. tuberculosis*.

The recent discovery of the TACO (*t*ryptophan *a*spartate-containing *co*at) protein provides the most succinct and direct mechanistic explanation for the inability
of mycobacteria-containing phagosomes to fuse with lysosomes (53). Analysis of
the biochemical composition of mycobacterial phagosomes obtained by organelle
electrophoresis of a microsomal fraction prepared from S-methionine/cysteine-
labeled, BCG-infected macrophages has identified a 50-kDa host cell polypeptide specific for phagosomes containing live bacilli. This polypeptide was not
detected in other subcellular fractions analyzed, including the phagosomes that
contain dead BCG, nor was it present in metabolically labeled bacteria. TACO contains 5 WD [Trp-Asp] repeats and exhibits homology to coronin, a *Dictyostelium*

discoidium WD repeat actin-binding protein involved in actin-based cytoskeletal rearrangements. TACO is present in lymphoid and myeloid cells, and it was associated with the cortical microtubule network in noninfected macrophages. By 2 h postinfection with BCG, TACO was almost completely relocalized (from the cortical distribution) to the BCG-containing phagosomal membrane, and it remained associated for a prolonged period of time. TACO was also detected in phagosomes containing dead BCG. However, the association was transient: Dissociation occurred within 2 h after phagocytosis. Thus, viability of phagocytosed bacilli is requisite to the retention of TACO. This process is not due to the lack of acidification of phagosomes containing live BCG because those containing dead bacilli, in the presence of NH_4Cl, a phagosome-alkalinizing agent, failed to retain TACO. By retaining TACO and thus intercepting the fusion of phagosome with lysosome, mycobacteria evade potent lysosomal antimicrobial functions of macrophages. Intriguingly, TACO is not expressed in Kupffer cells, the resident phagocytes of the liver, and may well account for the relative resistance of this organ to *M. tuberculosis* infection. Elucidation of the mechanisms by which *M. tuberculosis* contains phagosomes and retains TACO will provide insight into the pathogenesis of the tubercle bacillus.

Free Radical-Based Antimycobacterial Mechanisms: Reactive Oxygen Intermediates (ROI) and the Nitrogen Oxides High output nitric oxide (NO) production by immunologically activated macrophages is a major antimicrobial mechanism (54–56). These phagocytes, upon activation by appropriate agents such as IFN-γ and TNF-α, generate NO and related RNI via NOS2 using L-arginine as the substrate. The significance of these toxic nitrogen oxides in host defense against *M. tuberculosis* has been well documented, both in vitro and in vivo, particularly in the murine system (55–57). In the mouse, RNI play a protective role in both acute and chronic persistent infection (58, 59). More important, accumulating evidence strongly supports a role for RNI in host defense in human tuberculosis (60, 61). High-level expression of NOS2 has been detected immunohistochemically in macrophages obtained by pulmonary alveolar lavage from individuals with active pulmonary tuberculosis (60, 61). In addition, the level of exhaled NO increases in tuberculosis patients (61).

While the role of macrophage NOS2 in host defense against *M. tuberculosis* is well established, the significance of toxic oxygen species in the control of tuberculosis remains controversial. Despite the demonstration that H_2O_2 generated by cytokine-activated macrophages was mycobacteriocidal (6), the ability of ROI to kill *M. tuberculosis* remains to be confirmed (8, 62). Indeed, mycobacteria are capable of evading the toxic effect of ROI by various means (5). For example, mycobacterial components lipoarabinomannan (LAM) and phenolicglycolipid I (PGL-I) are potent oxygen radical scavengers (63, 64). In addition, mycobacterial sulfatides interfere with the oxygen radical–dependent antimicrobial mechanism of macrophages. Despite these findings, a role of ROI in defense against the tubercle bacillus cannot be entirely excluded. Mice deficient in the NADPH oxidase complex exhibit modestly enhanced susceptibility to *M. tuberculosis* infection (65, 66). More important, it has been reported that individuals with chronic granulomatous disease are more susceptible to tuberculosis (67).

The Toll-Like Receptors (TLR) and Innate Immunity in Tuberculosis   The recent discovery of the importance of the TLR protein family in immune responses in insects, plants, and vertebrates has provided new insight into the link between innate and adaptive immunity. The antimicrobial effects of the TLR family were discovered as a result of the convergence of two independent lines of research: the Toll-dependent control of embryonic dorsoventral patterning of *Drosophila melanogaster* (68) and the nuclear factor (NF)-κB-mediated cytokine activation signal transduction pathway in mammals (69). The proteins involved in directing Drosophila embryonic dorsal-ventral polarity (Toll/Cactus/Dorsal) bear striking functional and structural similarities with those responsible for the cytokine-induced activation cascade (IL-1 receptor/I-κ B/NF-κ B), the latter a critical pathway in infectious and inflammatory disease processes. Based on the Toll/IL-1 receptor, Cactus/I-κ B, and Dorsal/NF-κ B parallels, and exploiting the powerful genetic systems of Drosophila, Lemaitre et al (70, 81) hypothesized and demonstrated that Toll plays a critical role in conferring insect innate immunity against fungal infection. Soon thereafter, Medzhitov et al (71) showed that a human homolog of the Drosophila Toll protein signals activation of adaptive immunity. This human TLR is a transmembrane protein with a leucine-rich repeat in the extracellular domain. Its cytoplasmic domain is homologous to that of the human IL-1 receptor. Transfection of a constitutively active human mutant TLR results in the activation of NF-κB, as well as the expression of various NF-κB-controlled cytokines and the costimulatory molecule B7.1 (71). The TLR-dependent activation of the NF-κB pathway is mediated via the adapter protein MyD88 (72), which is also required for signal transduction through IL-1R (73). These studies provide strong evidence that human homologs of Drosophila Toll play a significant role in innate immunity. This notion is further supported by the demonstration that in the mouse, *lps*, the gene that mediates responsiveness to lipopolysaccharide and confers resistance to gram-negative bacilli, and the murine Tlr4 are allelic (74).

The number of members of the human and mouse TLR family has expanded considerably since the discovery of the participation of these molecules in innate immunity. More importantly, emerging evidence suggests that TLRs play an important role in the activation of immune cells by pathogens, including *M. tuberculosis*. Using a dominant negative TLR2 mutant and promoter reporter fusions, Brightbill et al (75) demonstrated that induction of IL-12 and NOS2 promoter activity in vitro by the 19-kDa mycobacterial lipoprotein is dependent on human TLR2. But the interactions between *M. tuberculosis* and TLRs soon proved to be more complex, and it appears that distinct mycobacterial components may interact with different members of the TLR family (76). In vitro studies using human TLR2– and/or TLR4–overexpressed in cell lines and murine macrophages in conjunction with an NF-κB activity reporter system have provided evidence that *M. tuberculosis* can immunologically activate cells via either TLR2 or TLR4 in a CD14-independent manner (76). Interestingly, while TLR2 expression confers responsiveness to LAM derived from rapidly growing mycobacteria (AraLAM), TLR4 does not. This ligand-receptor specificity is further demonstrated by the observations that (*a*) LAM prepared from *M. tuberculosis* or BCG (ManLAM), both slow-growing strains, does not induce TLR-dependent activation, and (*b*) cellular activation induced by the tubercle bacillus via TLR2 is mediated by a soluble heat-stable and protease resistant component, while that via TLR4 is dependent on a heat-sensitive cell-associated mycobacterial factor. Thus, it appears that *M. tuberculosis* can signal via both human TLR2 and TLR4 in a ligand-specific manner. The significance of TLR2 in *M. tuberculosis*-induced cellular signaling has been similarly observed in studies using a transfection system involving murine RAW macrophages and the dominant negative murine TLR2 and MyD88 mutants, in conjunction with measuring intracellular TNF-α as an index of activation (77). This latter study demonstrates that heat-killed *M. tuberculosis* elicits TLR2-dependent responsiveness. This responsiveness is completely inhibitable by dominant negative MyD88, while the inhibition with dominant negative TLR2 is incomplete, suggesting *M. tuberculosis* may signal through other TLRs (77); based on results of the above described studies conducted with human TLRs, TLR4 is a possibility. Indeed TLR4-deficient mice exhibit enhanced susceptibility to *M. tuberculosis* (M Fenton, personal communication). Finally, various mycobacterial components, including AraLAM, mycolylarabinogalactan-peptidoglycan complex, and total *M. tuberculosis* lipids can activate murine macrophages to produce TNF-α in a TLR2-dependent fashion (77). Thus, the ability of mycobacterial AraLAM to signal through both human and murine TLR2 is apparent in two different in vitro systems (76, 77). In sum, these results predict that the interaction between *M. tuberculosis* and the various TLRs is complex. This notion is in keeping with our current understanding of LPS signaling through TLRs. In the LPS studies, in vitro evidence indicates that while this microbial product can signal through human TLR2 (78, 79), it can interact only with murine TLR4, but not murine TLR2 (77). Functional analysis of TLR4-deficient mouse strains has provided evidence that there may be LPS signaling receptors in addition to TLR4; depending on the genetic background of mouse deletion mutants, genes that compensate for the lack of Tlr4 may exist (80).

In vitro studies have provided strong evidence that *M. tuberculosis* can signal through at least two TLRs: TLR2 and TLR4. However, much remains to be learned. For example, do TLRs other than TLR2 and TLR4 play a role in *M. tuberculosis*-induced macrophage activation? What is the fine specificity of mycobacterial components with respect to TLRs? Is the production of distinct sets of cytokines and chemokines induced by specific *M. tuberculosis* factors mediated via interaction with specific TLR? Is TLRs expressed in the tuberculous granuloma, and if so, are they differentially expressed during the various phases of infection: acute versus latent tuberculosis? With respect to the latter, specific intra-granulomatous TLRs may be expressed to sample mycobacterial components expressed during persistent infection in order to maintain an effective antimycobacterial response, as hypothesized by Underhill et al (77). Demonstrating the significance of the various TLRs in host defense against *M. tuberculosis* awaits rigorous in vivo experimentation.

CYTOKINES

The immune response to all pathogens is at least in part dependent on cytokines, which regulate all cells of the immune system. *M. tuberculosis* is no exception and in fact strongly induces cytokines during infection. The inflammatory response to this pathogen is crucial to the control of the infection but may also contribute to the chronic infection and associated pathology. In this section, the contributions of various cytokines to the response to *M. tuberculosis* are discussed.

Interleukin-12

Immunologic control of *M. tuberculosis* infection is based on a type 1 T cell response. IL-12 is induced following phagocytosis of *M. tuberculosis* bacilli by macrophages and dendritic cells (82, 83), which drives development of a TH1 response with production of IFN-γ. Mycobacteria are such strong IL-12 inducers that mycobacterial infection can skew the response to a secondary antigen toward a TH1 phenotype (84). IL-12 is a crucial cytokine in controlling *M. tuberculosis* infection. Early administration of IL-12 to *M. tuberculosis*-infected BALB/c mice resulted in significantly decreased bacterial numbers and increased mean survival time, although the mice still succumbed to the infection (85). In contrast, IL-12 had only marginal effects on the bacterial numbers in C57BL/6 mice (86), perhaps reflecting the more naturally resistant phenotype of this strain compared to BALB/c. The enhanced resistance of IL-12-treated BALB/c mice was not due to a clear TH2 to TH1 shift, as is seen in *Leishmania major* murine infections, since a measurable TH2 response was not observed in *M. tuberculosis*-infected BALB/c mice (85). Convincing evidence of the importance of IL-12 in resistance to tuberculosis was provided by IL-12p40–gene deficient mice. These mice were quite susceptible to infection and had a greatly increased bacterial burden, as well as decreased survival time, compared to control mice, probably due to the substantially reduced IFN-γ production in IL-12p40-/- mice (87). Humans with mutations in IL-12p40 or the IL-12 receptor genes present with reduced but not absent IFN-γ production from T cells and are more susceptible to disseminated BCG and *M. avium* infections, although *M. tuberculosis* infections were not reported (11; T. Ottenhof, personal communication). An intriguing study indicated that administration of IL-12 DNA could substantially reduce bacterial numbers in mice with a chronic *M. tuberculosis* infection (88), suggesting that induction of this cytokine is an important factor in the design of a tuberculosis vaccine.

Interferon γ

IFN-γ is a key cytokine in control of *M. tuberculosis* infection. This cytokine is produced by both CD4 and CD8 T cells in tuberculosis (89–94) as well as by NK cells. Recently there have been reports of IL-12-dependent IFN-γ production by alveolar macrophages infected with mycobacteria (95, 96). To date, IFN-γ knockout (GKO) mice are the most susceptible to virulent *M. tuberculosis* (97, 98). Individuals defective in genes for IFN-γ or the IFN-γ receptor are prone to serious mycobacterial infections, including *M. tuberculosis* (11). *M. tuberculosis* bacilli grew essentially unchecked in the organs of GKO mice, and although granulomas formed, they quickly became necrotic. Macrophage activation is defective in these mice, and NOS2 expression is low (98, 99), factors that likely contribute to the extreme susceptibility of the GKO mice. However, the mean survival time for *M. tuberculosis*-infected NOS2-/- mice is at least twice that of GKO mice (58, 98; JL Flynn & J Chan, unpublished data), suggesting that there are IFN-γ-dependent, NOS2-independent mechanisms of protection against tuberculosis.

Although IFN-γ production alone is insufficient to control *M. tuberculosis* infection, it is required for the protective response to this pathogen. However, IFN-γ is produced by healthy PPD$^+$ subjects as well as those with active tuberculosis. Although IFN-γ production may vary among subjects, and some studies suggest that IFN-γ levels are depressed in patients with active tuberculosis (100, 101), this cytokine may be unreliable as an immune correlate of protection. In fact, a recent study demonstrated that *M. tuberculosis* can prevent macrophages from responding adequately to IFN-γ (102). Mycobacterial components as well as live bacteria inhibited IFN-γ signaling in human macrophages by disrupting the association of the transcription activator STAT1 with the transcriptional coactivators CREB binding protein and p300. This ability of *M. tuberculosis* to limit activation of macrophages by IFN-γ suggests that the amount of IFN-γ produced by T cells may be less predictive of outcome than the ability of the cells to respond to this cytokine.

Interleukin-4

TH2 responses and IL-4 in tuberculosis are subjects of some controversy. *M. tuberculosis* is a potent inducer of IL-12, and thus IFN-γ responses are almost always detected in infected hosts. However, detection of IL-4 is variable, and although some reports have indicated that various TH2 responses exist in tuberculosis, it can be difficult to demonstrate. In human studies, a depressed TH1 response but not an enhanced TH2 response was observed in PBMC from tuberculosis patients (100, 101, 103). Elevated IFN-γ expression was detected in granulomas within lymph nodes of patients with tuberculous lymphadenitis, but little IL-4 mRNA was detected (100). These results and others indicated that in humans a strong TH2 response is not associated with tuberculosis. Certainly, the dominant TH2 response that accounts for susceptibility of certain mouse strains to

L. major is not observed with *M. tuberculosis*. BALB/c mice, while more susceptible than C57BL/6 mice to *M. tuberculosis*, do not exhibit a polarized or consistent TH2 response, even though their resistance can be augmented by exogenous IL-12 (85). A shift to a TH2 response was not observed in GKO (98) or IL-12p40-/- (87) mice infected with *M. tuberculosis*. These data suggest that the absence of a TH1 response to *M. tuberculosis* does not necessarily promote a TH2 response, and an IFN-γ deficiency, rather than the presence of IL-4 or other TH2 cytokines, prevents control of infection. Finally, IL-4-deficient mice on a C57BL/6 background were resistant to *M. tuberculosis* infection (104, 105), although a different result might arise if the IL-4 gene disruption was on a BALB/c (more susceptible) background. In a study of cytokine gene expression in the granulomas of patients with advanced tuberculosis by in situ hybridization, IL-4 was detected in 3/5 patients, but never in the absence of IFN-γ expression (106). The presence or absence of IL-4 did not correlate with improved clinical outcome or differences in granuloma stages or pathology. All the granulomas examined were from advanced tuberculosis cases and represent essentially a failure of the immune system to contain the infection. Extrapolation from these studies to speculate which cytokines might be expressed in granulomas that are functioning to prevent bacterial replication is difficult. Clearly, the presence or absence of IL-4 alone is not predictive of clinical outcome.

Tumor Necrosis Factor α

TNF-α is a cytokine with a long history in tuberculosis research and is believed to play multiple roles in immune and pathologic responses in tuberculosis. *M. tuberculosis* induces TNF-α secretion by macrophages, dendritic cells, and T cells (82, 83, 93, 94). This cytokine is required for control of acute *M. tuberculosis* infection. In mice deficient in TNF-α or the 55-kDa TNF receptor, *M. tuberculosis* infection resulted in rapid death of the mice, with substantially higher bacterial burdens compared to control mice (107, 108). The requirement for TNF-α in control of *M. tuberculosis* infection is complex, but in part this may be due to its role as a mediator of macrophage activation. TNF-α in synergy with IFN-γ induces NOS2 expression (9, 62, 109). In response to *M. tuberculosis* infection, NOS2 expression in the granulomas of TNFRp55-/- mice was delayed (107), although a similar delay was not observed in TNF-α-/- mice (108).

Convincing data on the importance of this cytokine in granuloma formation in tuberculosis and other mycobacterial diseases has been provided by a number of groups (107, 108, 110–112). In the absence of TNF-α or the 55-kDa TNF receptor, the granulomatous response is deficient following acute *M. tuberculosis* infection in murine models. The granulomas that do form are disorganized, with fewer activated or epithelioid macrophages (107); lymphocyte co-localization with macrophages is impaired (108). Clearly, TNF-α affects cell migration to and localization within tissues in *M. tuberculosis* infection. TNF-α influences expression of adhesion molecules as well as chemokines and chemokine receptors (see below), and this is certain to affect formation of functional granulomas in infected tissues. However, the multiple mechanisms by which TNF-α promotes effective granuloma formation, maintenance, and function remain to be determined.

TNF-α has also been implicated in the pathologic response of the host to *M. tuberculosis* infection and is often cited as a major factor in host-mediated destruction of lung tissue (113–115). Thalidomide treatment in *M. tuberculosis* infected mice, which downregulated the expression of inflammatory cytokines including TNF-α, IL-6, and IL-10, reduced the size of granulomas in the lungs without a change in bacterial numbers (115). Tipping the balance of TNF-α in the lungs may lead to increased pathology and necrosis. Recent experiments with recombinant BCG expressing TNF-α indicate that very high levels of TNF-α cause destructive inflammation (G Kaplan, personal communication). However, TNF-α is not a requirement for necrosis of lung tissue, as *M. tuberculosis* infection in TNF-α or TNF-receptor deficient mice resulted in necrosis associated with high bacterial numbers. Unexpected data from a murine model of chronic persistent tuberculosis suggested a role for TNF-α in limiting pathology of the lung (Mohan et al, submitted). Mice with a stable bacterial load 6 months after *M. tuberculosis* infection were treated with anti-TNF-α antibody. Neutralization of TNF-α resulted in 100% mortality. Bacterial numbers in the lungs of the anti-TNF antibody-treated mice increased, although not to levels predicted as lethal in this model, and then stabilized, suggesting that bacterial numbers alone may not account for the mortality of the mice. Histologic examination revealed that the lungs of the TNF-α-neutralized mice exhibited severe pathology, with disorganized granulomas, diffuse cellular infiltration, alveolar exudates, and in some cases, squamous metaplasia, which is a pathologic response to chronic inflammation. Such aberrant immunopathology in the absence of TNF-α suggests that this cytokine contributes to limiting the pathologic response in tuberculosis. Thus, TNF-α has an important role as a modulator of inflammation in this infection. An anti-inflammatory role for TNF-α has been suggested for *Corynebacterium parvum* infection, in which TNF-α-deficient mice responded to the infection with severe inflammation, resulting in death of the mice (116). Clearly the roles of TNF-α in protection and immunopathology in tuberculous infection are complex and multifaceted. Although limited data exist on the role of this cytokine in human tuberculosis, a recent report indicated that a patient undergoing treatment with anti-TNF-α antibody for rheumatoid arthritis developed fatal disseminated tuberculosis (117).

Interleukin-10

In contrast to TNF-α, IL-10 is generally considered to be primarily anti-inflammatory. This cytokine, produced by macrophages and T cells during *M. tuberculosis* infection, possesses macrophage deactivating properties, including downregulation of IL-12 production, which in turn decreases IFN-γ production by T cells. Macrophages from tuberculosis patients are suppressive for T cell proliferation in vitro, and inhibition of IL-10 partially reversed this suppression (118).

IL-10 directly inhibits CD4$^+$ T cell responses, as well as inhibiting APC function of cells infected with mycobacteria (119). Transgenic mice constitutively expressing IL-10 were less capable of clearing a BCG infection, although T cell responses including IFN-γ production were unimpaired (120). These results suggested that IL-10 may counter the macrophage activating properties of IFN-γ. However, IL-10-/- mice were not more resistant to acute *M. tuberculosis*, compared to wild-type mice (104). The role for IL-10 in modulating protection or pathology in tuberculosis awaits further experimentation.

Interleukin-6

IL-6 has also been implicated in the host response to *M. tuberculosis*. This cytokine has multiple roles in the immune response, including inflammation, hematopoiesis, and differentiation of T cells. A potential role for IL-6 in suppression of T cell responses was reported (121). In this study, BCG-infected macrophages were inefficient in stimulating T cell responses to an unrelated antigen, and this effect could be partially abrogated by neutralization of IL-6. Following low dose aerosol infection, early increases in lung burden, as well as decreased IFN-γ production, were observed in the IL-6-/- mice, compared to control mice, suggesting that IL-6 is important in the initial innate response to the pathogen (105). Once acquired immunity developed, the IL-6-/- mice controlled the infection and the mice survived. Memory responses to virulent aerosol challenge were also intact in IL-6-/- mice (105). The IL-6-/- mice did succumb to infection with a high i.v. dose of *M. tuberculosis* (122); in this case, the defective innate response may have been overwhelmed by the large number of bacteria introduced into the lungs.

Transforming Growth Factor-β

This classic anti-inflammatory cytokine has been implicated in suppression of T cell responses in tuberculosis patients (123). TGF-β is present in the granulomatous lesions of tuberculosis patients and is produced by human monocytes after stimulation with *M. tuberculosis* (124) or lipoarabinomannan (125). Reportedly it inhibits T cell responses to *M. tuberculosis* (123, 126) as well as participates in macrophage deactivation by inhibiting IFN-γ-induced NOS2 production (127). Regulation of this cytokine is very complex and occurs at various levels. The in vivo role of TGF-β in protection or pathology in tuberculosis has not been directly tested.

T CELLS

M. tuberculosis is a classic example of a pathogen for which the protective response relies on cell mediated immunity. This is primarily because the organism lives within cells, usually macrophages; thus T cell effector mechanisms, rather than antibody, are required to control or eliminate the bacteria. Historically, research was focused on the CD4$^+$ T cell response to tuberculosis, but recently there has been increased interest in the roles of CD8$^+$ T cells in the immune response to this pathogen. In the mouse model, within 1 week of infection with virulent *M. tuberculosis*, the number of activated CD4$^+$ and CD8$^+$ T cells in the lung-draining lymph nodes increases (128, 129). Between 2 and 4 weeks postinfection, both CD4$^+$ and CD8$^+$ T cells migrate to the lungs and demonstrate an effector/memory phenotype (CD44^{hi}CD45^{lo}CD62L$^-$); approximately 50% of these cells are CD69$^+$ (93, 128, 129). This indicates that activated T cells migrate to the site of infection and are interacting with APCs. The tuberculous granuloma contains both CD4 and CD8 T cells (130, 131) that likely participate in the continuous battle to contain the infection within the granuloma and prevent reactivation.

CD4 T Cells

M. tuberculosis resides primarily in a vacuole within the macrophage, and thus, MHC class II presentation of mycobacterial antigens to CD4$^+$ T cells is an obvious outcome of infection. It is not surprising that these cells are among the most important in the protective response against *M. tuberculosis*. Murine studies have shown by antibody depletion of CD4 T cells (132), adoptive transfer (133, 134), or the use of gene-disrupted mice (135, 136) that the CD4$^+$ T cell subset is required for control of infection. In humans, the tragedy of HIV has demonstrated that the loss of CD4$^+$ T cells greatly increases susceptibility to both acute and reactivation tuberculosis. In fact, HIV$^+$ PPD$^+$ subjects have 8–10% annual risk of developing active tuberculosis, compared to a 10% lifetime risk for PPD$^+$ HIV–patients (137).

Numerous studies indicate that CD4$^+$ T cells from infected subjects produce IFN-γ in response to a wide variety of mycobacterial antigens. The primary effector function of CD4$^+$ T cells is believed to be production of IFN-γ and possibly other cytokines, sufficient to activate macrophages, which can then control or eliminate intracellular organisms. Although IFN-γ production by CD4$^+$ T cells is undeniably a very important effector function of this subset, these cells most certainly have other, less obvious roles in controlling *M. tuberculosis* infection. In MHC class II-/- or CD4-/- mice, levels of IFN-γ were severely diminished very early in infection (135, 136). However, by 3 weeks postinfection, overall IFN-γ levels in the lungs appeared to be similar to wild type, with the CD8$^+$ T cell subset contributing substantially to this production (136). The mice were not rescued by this later IFN-γ production and succumbed to the infection. NOS2 expression by macrophages was also delayed in the CD4$^+$ T cell deficient mice but returned to wild-type levels in conjunction with IFN-γ expression (136).

These findings were extended in a murine model of chronic persistent *M. tuberculosis* infection (138). Mice infected with a low dose of *M. tuberculosis* were treated with anti-CD4 antibody beginning 6 months postinfection. The resulting CD4 T cell depletion caused rapid reactivation of the infection, and mice succumbed with high bacterial burdens in the lungs. IFN-γ levels overall were similar in the lungs of CD4$^+$ T cell–depleted and control (IgG-treated) mice, due to IFN-γ production by CD8$^+$ T cells. Most surprising, there was no apparent change in macrophage NOS2 production or activity in the CD4$^+$ T cell–depleted mice. This indicated that there are IFN-γ and NOS2-independent, CD4$^+$ T cell–dependent mechanisms for control of tuberculosis. Certainly IFN-γ production and subsequent induction of NOS2 are important effector functions for CD4$^+$ T cells, but clearly there are other roles for these cells. Most studies have focused on IFN-γ production by CD4$^+$ T cells in response to mycobacterial antigen, but other functions of CD4$^+$ T cells are likely to be important in the protective response and must be understood as correlates of immunity and as targets for vaccine design.

How might CD4$^+$ T cells contribute to the immune response against tuberculosis, apart from IFN-γ production? A role for CD4$^+$ T cells in activating or maturing APCs has been addressed in various systems. Interaction of CD40L on CD4$^+$ T cells with CD40 on macrophages or dendritic cells results in enhanced antigen presentation and costimulatory activity. This interaction may be important in *M. tuberculosis* infection, although CD40L-/- mice were not more susceptible to acute infection (139). It has also been reported that infection with *M. tuberculosis* matured dendritic cells in the absence of any T cells, and these cells were excellent APCs (83; K Bodnar, JL Flynn, submitted). However, the role for CD40-CD40L interaction, or the interaction of other molecules (i.e. OX40L-OX40), on the antimycobacterial functions of macrophages has not been addressed. The importance of CD4$^+$ T cells on priming and maintenance of CD8$^+$ T cell effector and memory functions has been demonstrated in viral models and may be dependent on CD40-CD40L interaction between CD4$^+$ T cells and APCs (140–142). Although many researchers have dismissed a role for B cells or antibody in protection against tuberculosis (143), recent studies suggest that these may contribute to the response to tuberculosis (144, 145). The importance of CD4$^+$ T cells for adequate B cell responses is known; understanding the effects of CD4$^+$ T cells on these cells in tuberculosis awaits a clearer picture of the role of B cells in this infection. CD4$^+$ T cells can also produce a multitude of cytokines in addition to IFN-γ including IL-2. It is likely that production of CD4$^+$ T cell cytokines at a certain time, or in close proximity to the macrophage or other cells, is important in controlling the infection. Finally, apoptosis or lysis of infected cells by CD4$^+$ T cells may also play a role in controlling infection (146, 147); human CD4$^+$ T cells can produce perforin and granulysin, although these molecules did not seem to participate in bacterial killing (D Canaday, WH Boom, personal communication). The effects of FasL- or TNF-α-induced apoptosis on *M. tuberculosis* viability in human and mouse macrophages is controversial; some studies report reduced bacterial numbers within macrophages after apoptosis (148), and others indicate this mechanism has little antimycobacterial effect (149, 150).

M. tuberculosis-infected macrophages appear to be diminished in their ability to present antigens to CD4$^+$ T cells, which would contribute to the inability of the host to eliminate a persistent infection. Presentation of soluble ovalbumin to a T cell hybridoma was reduced following *M. tuberculosis* infection of macrophages (151).

One mechanism by which *M. tuberculosis* infection might inhibit recognition of macrophages by CD4$^+$ T cells is by downregulation of cell surface expression of MHC class II molecules. The reports in the literature are somewhat contradictory on this point. Reiner and colleagues used virulent *M. tuberculosis* and human macrophages to clearly demonstrate that the greatest reduction in MHC class II expression occurred when the cells were also exposed to IFN-γ (152). The effect was dependent on multiplicity of infection (MOI) and dead bacilli were much less effective than live bacilli. However, IFN-γ mediated induction of MHC class II and class II transactivator (CIITA) gene expression was not inhibited by *M. tuberculosis* infection. Instead, post-Golgi transit of nascent MHC class II molecules into the endocytic pathway for antigen loading was impaired, resulting in intracellular sequestration and diminished cell surface expression. Although functional studies were not reported, the net effect of fewer MHC class II molecules at the cell surface would presumably be reduced antigen presentation. Other reports addressing a mechanism for reduced MHC class II presentation have used avirulent mycobacteria, such as *M. tuberculosis* H37Ra or BCG. Cell surface expression was decreased only slightly upon infection with H37Ra at high MOI ($\sim$40), but mRNA levels for I-A^k gene were decreased $\sim$75% (153). In this study, dead bacilli or lysates were as effective as live bacilli in reducing presentation of unrelated antigens by macrophages. BCG infection reduced IFN-γ-induced I-A^b and CIITA mRNA levels as well as cell surface levels of MHC class II in macrophages (154), in contrast to the *M. tuberculosis* experiments discussed above. Another APC, the dendritic cell has constitutively high levels of MHC class II. Infection of these cells with *M. tuberculosis* did not result in diminished MHC class II cell surface expression (83, 155). Thus, priming of CD4$^+$ T cells, a major function of dendritic cells in vivo, is less likely to be affected by *M. tuberculosis* infection. This is supported by the fact that a strong CD4$^+$ T cell response is mounted to *M. tuberculosis* infection. Another mechanism by which APCs contribute to defective T cell stimulation may be production of cytokines, including TGF-β (123, 126), IL-6 (121), or IL-10 (118, 126). Production of these cytokines by infected macrophages can directly and indirectly affect T cell proliferation and function. Clearly, substantial CD4$^+$ T cell responses are observed in patients infected with *M. tuberculosis*. The inadequacy of that response for elimination of bacteria may be partially at the level of recognition and activation of infected macrophages. *M. tuberculosis* is obviously equipped with numerous immune evasion strategies, including modulation of antigen presentation to avoid elimination by T cells.

CD8$^+$ T Cells

Although *M. tuberculosis* bacilli have been observed in the cytoplasm (156), most researchers believe that these organisms usually reside within a vacuole. Since MHC class I presentation is most efficient with cytoplasmic antigens, a possible role for CD8$^+$ T cells in the immune response to *M. tuberculosis* received little attention for many years. There were reports that CD8$^+$ T cells affected control of the infection, using antibody depletion or adoptive transfer in mice (132–134), although not all studies confirmed these data. Mice genetically disrupted in the genes for $\beta 2$ microglobulin or TAP, and thus deficient in MHC class I molecules and CD8 T cells, were quite susceptible to *M. tuberculosis* infection (130, 157, 158). An obstacle to the acceptance of CD8$^+$ T cells as an important component of the immune response was the difficulty in isolating *M. tuberculosis*-specific CD8$^+$ CTL from infected humans or mice. However, in recent years, CD8$^+$ T cells specific for mycobacterial antigens have been isolated from infected hosts or generated by immunization (90, 149, 159–165). Although recognition of the expected antigen by these cells has been demonstrated, recognition of cells infected with *M. tuberculosis*, the relevant in vivo target, has not always been reported. Since priming of CTL responses can occur by both infected cells and dendritic cells that take up apoptotic fragments of infected macrophages (166), the mere presence of CD8$^+$ T cells specific for an antigen in an infected host does not demonstrate that these cells can recognize infected cells in vivo. To be effective, CD8$^+$ T cells need to respond to infected macrophages, either by IFN-γ secretion or cytotoxic responses; therefore it is necessary to demonstrate this recognition by CD8$^+$ T cells specific for a defined mycobacterial antigen. Certain antigens may not be presented by infected cells, since little is known about MHC class I presentation of mycobacterial antigens. Recent studies in mice have demonstrated that CD8$^+$ T cells migrate to the lungs with kinetics similar to CD4$^+$ T cells following *M. tuberculosis* infection (93, 129). These cells are capable of producing IFN-γ and lysing infected macrophages (89, 93, 128, 129). CD8$^+$ T cells in mycobacterial infections are both classically and nonclassically restricted.

MHC Class I–Restricted CD8$^+$ T Cells   The reported MHC class I–restricted CD8$^+$ T cells from *M. tuberculosis*-infected or BCG-immunized mice and humans recognize several antigens, including 38-kDa (161), 65-kDa heat shock protein (150), and 19-kDa (163). Recently, MHC class I–restricted human CD8 T cell lines specific for three different antigens were demonstrated to recognize infected macrophages and in response produce IFN-γ and lyse the cells (S Cho, R Modlin, personal communication). Although one of the antigens identified was Ag85, a secreted protein, the other CD8$^+$ T cell lines recognized cytoplasmic antigens. In unpublished work, two classically restricted (HLA-B44 and HLA-B14) CD8 T cell clones from a PPD$^+$ subject present at high frequency in PBMC recognized the same protein, CFP10 (Mtb11) (D Lewinsohn, personal communication). Studies defining antigens recognized by CD8$^+$ T cells from infected hosts without active tuberculosis provide attractive vaccine candidates and support the notion that CD8$^+$ T cell responses as well as CD4$^+$ T cell responses must be stimulated to provide protective immunity.

The mechanism by which mycobacterial proteins gain access to the MHC class I molecules is not fully understood. In general, access of antigen to the cytoplasm for processing and transport to the lumen of the endoplasmic reticulum by TAP molecules is necessary for loading and presentation of epitopes by MHC class I molecules. Bacilli in macrophages have been found outside the phagosome 4-5 days after infection (156), but presentation of mycobacterial antigen by infected macrophages to CD8 T cells can occur as early as 12 h after infection, although recognition of the target improves over time (128). Two reports provide evidence for a mycobacteria-induced pore or break in the vesicular membrane surrounding the bacilli that might allow mycobacterial antigen to enter the cytoplasm of the infected cell. *M. tuberculosis* infection of macrophages facilitated MHC class I presentation of soluble ovalbumin in a TAP-dependent manner, indicating that ovalbumin taken up into phagosomes along with *M. tuberculosis* gained access to the cytoplasm (151). This effect was dependent on MOI as well as on the relative virulence of the organism used. Heat-killed or fixed *M. tuberculosis* did not facilitate presentation of ovalbumin, suggesting that *M. tuberculosis* actively generates the phagosome pore. In a model system using live cells and real time confocal microscopy, BCG infection of macrophages facilitated transport of molecules up to 70-kDa from the cytoplasm into the phagosomes containing the bacteria (168). This supports the presence of a presumably bidirectional pore induced by mycobacterial infection. The bacterium may use this pore to obtain nutrients or introduce toxic molecules into the cytoplasm. A consequence may be the introduction of a wide variety of mycobacterial antigens into the cytoplasm for processing and presentation by MHC class I molecules. There is also evidence for an alternative processing pathway for MHC class I–presented *M. tuberculosis* antigens that is insensitive to brefeldin A (169).

Nonclassically Restricted CD8 T Cells   CD1 molecules are nonpolymorphic antigen presenting molecules; Group I CD1 molecules include CD1a, b, and c, while Group II includes CD1d. An excellent review of the structure, distribution, and antigen-presenting capacity of these molecules was published recently (170). CD1 molecules have structural similarities to MHC class I molecules, with β2-microglobulin noncovalently bound to both molecules. However, the antigen binding groove of CD1 is much deeper and more hydrophobic than that of MHC class I or II molecules. In contrast to the peptide epitopes presented by MHC class Ia molecules, CD1 present lipids or glycolipids to T cells (for review, see 170). CD1-restricted T cells are often CD4$^-$8$^-$ or CD8$^+$, but a recent study indicated that CD1 could also present antigen to CD4$^+$ T cells (171). The first described nonprotein antigen presented by CD1b was mycolic acid (172), a mycobacterial cell wall component. Since then, additional mycobacterial lipid-containing antigens presented by CD1 have been reported, including LAM (173), phosphatidyl inositol mannoside (173), glucose monomycolate (174), and isoprenoid glycolipids (175). These discoveries provided evidence for a vastly increased antigenic repertoire that could be recognized by T cells.

Group 1 CD1 molecules appear to sample different compartments of the cell for antigen presentation. CD1a does not have an endosomal localization signal in its cytoplasmic tail, while CD1b and CD1c have a tyrosine-based endosomal targeting motif, YXXZ (176, 177). CD1a has been localized primarily at the plasma membrane and traffics in the recycling pathway of early endosomes (178, 179). CD1b was found primarily in late endosomal, phagolysosomal and MHC class II compartments (178–180). In contrast, although CD1c was observed in endosomal compartments, it was much more strongly expressed on the cell surface (180). Recent data indicate that lipids from mycobacteria within phagosomes can be transported in and exported from the cell in endocytic vesicles and can be taken up by bystander cells for presentation to T cells (181, SHE Kaufmann, personal communication). Differences in CD1 localization may be important in determining which lipid antigens are presented by each molecule, and this, together with MHC class I and class II molecule presentation, allows a full survey of mycobacterial antigens by T cells.

The actual role for CD1-restricted cells in the innate or adaptive immune response to *M. tuberculosis* remains to be elucidated. In early studies, CD1-restricted responses to mycobacterial lipids were generated in vitro from PBMC of both PPD$^+$ and PPD$^-$ subjects (172, 182). A recent study provided the first evidence of a recall T cell response to a CD1-restricted antigen in *M. tuberculosis*-exposed PPD$^+$ subjects. PBMC from these subjects proliferated to an isoprenoid glycolipid, in contrast to PBMC from PPD$^-$ subjects, and this proliferation was inhibited by anti-CD1c antibody (175). Effector functions of CD1-restricted CD8$^+$ T cells include IFN-γ production and cytotoxic activity, but the target of these cells in vivo may not be the macrophages. CD1 molecules are usually found on dendritic cells in vivo (183), although a low level expression on macrophages may be sufficient to allow recognition by CD1-restricted T cells in vivo. Dendritic cells present in the lungs may be stimulating CD1-restricted cells in the granuloma that can then have a bystander effect on infected macrophages. In vitro data indicate that dendritic cells can be infected with *M. tuberculosis* (83, 155), and perhaps the CD1-restricted cells serve to monitor this reservoir of infection. Clearly more research is necessary to elucidate the protective role that these cells might play in tuberculosis. This has been hampered by the fact that mice lack Group 1 CD1 molecules and have only CD1d. Mice deficient in CD1d are not more susceptible to *M. tuberculosis* than are wild-type mice (157, 158). The recent description of a full array of CD1 Group 1 molecules in the guinea pig (184) may provide a model for studying the direct role of T cells recognizing CD1-restricted antigens in the protective response to this infection.

MHC class Ib molecules are nonpolymorphic molecules encoded within the MHC locus and also present mycobacterial antigen to CD8$^+$ T cells. In one study, CD8 T cell clones isolated from two PPD-reactive donors recognized *M. tuberculosis*-infected dendritic cells and produced IFN-γ but were not restricted by HLA-A, B, C, DR, or DQ, nor by CD1 (164). To characterize the CD8 T cell response to this infection, an IFN-γ ELISPOT-based limiting dilution assay was used to estimate the frequency of classically restricted and nonclassically restricted CD8 T cells in *M. tuberculosis*-exposed but healthy subjects (165). In the two subjects, only 4% and 26% of the *M. tuberculosis*-reactive CD8 T cell clones were classically restricted, with the remainder nonclassically restricted (but not CD1 restricted). The data suggest that further investigation of the processing and presentation of mycobacterial antigens to CD8 T cells is necessary to understand the potential contribution of this subset to protection.

H2-M3 is a murine MHC class Ib molecule that presents N-formylated peptides to CD8$^+$ T cells. These peptides are produced primarily by bacteria or in the mitochondria. In *Listeria* infection, H2-M3 presentation of antigens is an early response, and H2-M3-restricted CD8$^+$ T cells do not appear to participate in a recall response (185). C-R Wang and colleagues have generated CD8$^+$ and CD4$^-$8$^-$ T cell lines specific for mycobacterial N-formylated peptides. These cell lines produce IFN-γ and specifically lyse *M. tuberculosis*–infected macrophages (T Chun, C-R Wang, personal communication). Immunization with two *M. tuberculosis*-derived H2-M3 binding peptides resulted in CTL responses and a reduction in bacterial numbers following *M. tuberculosis* aerosol challenge (217). The presence and role of H2-M3-restricted cells generated during *M. tuberculosis* infection of mice remains to be established.

Effector Functions of CD8$^+$ T Cells   There appear to be two primary effector functions for CD8$^+$ T cells in tuberculosis: lysis of infected cells and production of cytokines, namely IFN-γ. The relative contributions of these functions in the infection are unknown. The function of this subset in controlling or eliminating the infection is an important question with respect to design of effective vaccination or immunotherapeutic strategies.

CD8$^+$ T cells specific for mycobacterial antigens from both mouse and humans reported to date produce IFN-γ. The role of IFN-γ in mycobacterial infections is generally believed to be macrophage activation, and it is certainly likely that CD8$^+$ T cells can participate in this function. CD8$^+$ T cells from the lungs of infected mice are primed to produce IFN-γ, and secrete this cytokine upon TCR ligation or by interaction with *M. tuberculosis*–infected dendritic cells (93). However, unlike CD4$^+$ T cells, spontaneous ex vivo production of IFN-γ by CD8$^+$ T cells is very low, suggesting that production of this cytokine by CD8 T cells in the lungs is limited (93). This could be due to ineffective signals for IFN-γ production by infected APC in the lungs. One study indicated that the modest protection transferred to nude mice by CD8$^+$ T cells was at least partially dependent on IFN-γ production (135). However, the importance of IFN-γ production by CD8$^+$ T cells in an immunocompetent mouse remains to be tested.

Lysis of target cells by CD8$^+$ T cells can occur via perforin and granzymes or the Fas/FasL pathway. Perforin-mediated lysis is considered to be an important component of the CD8 T cell response in viral infections. However, lysing cells containing live bacteria capable of extracellular survival seems counterintuitive as a protective response. A hypothesis put forth by Stefan Kaufmann was that macrophages infected with *M. tuberculosis* that are incapable of eliminating the intracellular organisms, because of either defective activation or an overwhelming infection, would benefit from being lysed to allow release of the bacteria (186, 187).

The released bacteria could then be taken up by activated macrophages within the granuloma, and presumably contained or destroyed.

There is evidence for a more direct role for CD8$^+$ CTL in control of *M. tuberculosis* infection. Lysis of infected human dendritic cells and macrophages by CD1- and MHC class I–restricted CD8$^+$ T cells specific for *M. tuberculosis* antigens reduced intracellular bacterial numbers (149, 167). The killing of intracellular bacteria was dependent on perforin, and lysis through the Fas/FasL pathway did not reproduce this effect (149). Perforin was required to form a pore, but the molecule responsible for killing of intracellular organisms was granulysin, another cytotoxic granule protein (188). Incubation of *M. tuberculosis* with granulysin alone was sufficient for killing the organisms. Mice apparently do not have a gene or a homolog for granulysin (A Krensky, personal communication), so the contribution of this as a direct antimycobacterial function by CD8 T cells in murine tuberculosis is unknown. A recent paper indicates that a subset of murine CD8$^+$ clones specific for hsp60 that can transfer a degree of protection in vivo can lyse infected macrophages via a perforin-mediated mechanism. At high effector-to-target ratio (50:1), this lysis reduced bacterial numbers (150). The mycobacterial killing was dependent on perforin, and to a lesser extent on IFN-γ production. Skepticism about the relative importance of CD8$^+$ CTL function in mycobacterial infection arose from experiments indicating that mice deficient in perforin (P-/-) were capable of controlling acute *M. tuberculosis* infection (189, 190). However, recent data indicate that the CD8$^+$ T cells in P-/- mice are hyperactivated, suggesting a regulatory role for perforin in the immune system (191). Indeed, in P-/- mice infected with *M. tuberculosis*, a greater number of CD8 T cells were found in the lungs shortly after infection and expressed high levels of CD69 and CD25, compared to wild type (128). Most strikingly, IFN-γ production in the lungs by the CD8 T cell subset was increased at least fourfold in the P-/- mice, suggesting that a compensatory effect protects P-/- mice from acute infection. In a recent study, P-/- mice did succumb to infection, but at a late time point (158). Thus, because of compensatory effects, negative results in a knockout mouse may fail to reveal the importance of a particular effector mechanism.

CELL MIGRATION AND GRANULOMA FORMATION

A successful host inflammatory response to invading microbes requires precise coordination of myriad immunologic elements. An important first step is to recruit intravascular immune cells to the proximity of the infective focus and prepare them for extravasation. This is controlled by adhesion molecules and chemokines. Mice with a truncated intracellular adhesion molecule 1 (ICAM-1) were deficient in granuloma formation, although control of infection was not impaired (192). Chemokines contribute to cell migration and localization, as well as affect priming and differentiation of T cell responses (193, 194). Some of the difficulty in studying chemokine responses to infectious agents has been due to a lack of reagents, particularly in the murine system. In addition, it is important to recognize that the gene or protein expression levels of chemokines do not tell the whole story because chemokines work in a gradient and the "optimal" dose for attracting cells depends on a number of factors, including the receptors on the cells, other chemokine signals, and the strength of the signal over a specific area (195). Thus, judging responses by examining levels of expression of chemokines may not give an accurate picture of the contribution of an individual chemokine in response to the infection. Finally, each chemokine receptor has multiple ligands, and many chemokines can respond to more than one receptor on a wide variety of cells (196, 197). The functional consequences of this apparent redundancy are not yet understood, but it is clear that chemokine signaling and regulation are very complex.

Chemokines in *M. tuberculosis* infection have been investigated to a limited extent. In in vitro and in vivo murine models, *M. tuberculosis* induced production of a variety of chemokines, including RANTES, MIP1-α, MIP2, MCP-1, MCP-3, MCP-5, and IP10 (198, 199) (H Scott, JL Flynn, unpublished observations). Mice overexpressing MCP-1 (200), but not MCP1-/- mice (201), were more susceptible to *M. tuberculosis* infection than were wild-type mice. RANTES, MCP-1, MIP1α, and IL-8 were released by human alveolar macrophages upon infection with *M. tuberculosis* in vitro (202), and monocytes, lymph node cells, and bronchoalveolar lavage fluid from pulmonary TB patients had increased levels of a subset of these chemokines compared to healthy controls (202–204).

Chemokine receptors present on a variety of cells in the immune system can interact with a number of different ligands. In human studies, CCR5, the receptor for RANTES, MIP1-α, and MIP1-β, was increased on macrophages following in vitro *M. tuberculosis* infection and on alveolar macrophages in BAL from tuberculosis patients (205). CCR5 expression increased on T cells in nonhuman primates following inoculation with BCG (206). CCR2 is a receptor for MCP-1, 3, and 5 and is present on macrophages and activated T cells. CCR2-/- mice are extraordinarily susceptible to *M. tuberculosis* infection, and they exhibit a defect in macrophage recruitment to the lungs (J Ernst, personal communication). The relative resistance of MCP1-/- mice compared to CCR2-/- mice suggests that MCP-3 or MCP-5 may be important chemokines in the response to this infection. As more mice genetically deficient in chemokines and their receptors become available, the requirement for these molecules in the response to *M. tuberculosis* will be addressed.

Chemokine and chemokine receptor expression must contribute to the formation and maintenance of granulomas in chronic infections such as tuberculosis. Using instillation of PPD or schistosomal egg antigen beads, or injection of schistosomal eggs, to induce granulomas in lungs of mice, contributions of CCR1 and CCR2, as well as RANTES and MCP-1 to granuloma formation were reported (201, 207–211). The importance of TNF-α in granuloma formation and maintenance, as discussed above, is surely in part due to regulation of chemokines or chemokine receptors. The current literature indicates that TNF-α can upregulate expression of MIP1-α, MIP1-β, MIP2, MCP-1, CINC, and RANTES (212–215), and it can affect recruitment of neutrophils, lymphocytes, and monocytes/macrophages to certain sites. It has also been reported that TNF-α downregulates expression of CCR5 on human monocytes (212). LAM induction of IL-8, MCP-1, and MIP1 from human PBMC was partially inhibited by anti-TNF antibody (216). Any attempt to understand granuloma formation and maintenance, as well as immune responses in the lungs to *M. tuberculosis*, must include the study of chemokines and chemokine receptors.

SUMMARY

The protective and pathologic response to *M. tuberculosis* is complex and multifaceted, involving many components of the immune system. A clear picture of the network of immune responses to this pathogen, as well as an understanding of the effector functions of these components, is essential to the design and implementation of effective vaccines and treatments for tuberculosis. The combination of studies in animal models and human subjects, as well as technical advances in genetic manipulation of the organism, will be instrumental in enhancing our understanding of this immensely successful pathogen in the future.

ACKNOWLEDGMENTS

For sharing data and ideas before publication, we are grateful to Steve Porcelli, Stefan Kaufmann, Tom Ottenhof, Joel Ernst, David Lewinsohn, Matthew Fenton, Robert Modlin, Chyung-Ru Wang, Gilla Kaplan, David Canaday, W. Henry Boom, and Alan Krensky. We thank Natalya Serbina and Charles Scanga for critical reading of the manuscript and suggestions. This work was supported by NIH grants AIHL36990 (J.C. and J.L.F.), AI38411 (J.L.F.) and AI37859 (J.L.F.).

Visit the Annual Reviews home page at www.AnnualReviews.org

LITERATURE CITED

1. Chan J, Flynn JL. 2000. Latent and reactivation tuberculosis. *Einstein Q.* In press
2. Lurie M. 1942. Studies on the mechanism of immunity in tuberculosis. The fate of tubercle bacilli ingested by mononuclear phagocytes derived from normal and immunized animals. *J. Exp. Med.* 75:247
3. Suter E. 1952. The multiplication of tubercle bacilli within normal phagocytes in tissue cultures. *J. Exp. Med.* 96:137
4. Mackaness G. 1969. The influence of immunologically committed lymphoid cells on macrophage activation in vivo. *J. Exp. Med.* 129:973
5. Chan J, Kaufmann SHE. 1994. Immune mechanisms of protection. In *Tuberculosis: Pathogenesis, Protection and Control*, ed. BR Bloom, pp. 389–415. Washington, DC: Am. Soc. Microbiol.
6. Walker L, Lowrie DB. 1981. Killing of *Mycobacterium microti* by immunologically activated macrophages. *Nature* 293:69–70

7. Rook GAW, Steele J, Ainsworth M, Champion BR. 1986. Activation of macrophages to inhibit proliferation of *Mycobacterium tuberculosis*: comparison of the effects of recombinant gamma interferon on human monocytes and murine peritoneal macrophages. *Immunol.* 59:333–38

8. Flesch I, Kaufmann S. 1987. Mycobacterial growth inhibition by interferon-g activated bone marrow macrophages and differential susceptibility among strains of Mycobacterium tuberculosis. *J. Immunol.* 138:4408–13

9. Flesch I, Kaufmann SHE. 1990. Activation of tuberculostatic macrophage functions by gamma interferon, interleukin-4, and tumor necrosis factor. *Infect. Immun.* 58:2675–77

10. Ding AH, Nathan C, Stuehr D. 1988. Release of reactive nitrogen intermediates and reactive oxygen intermediates from mouse peritoneal macrophages. *J. Immunol.* 141:2407–12

11. Ottenhof TH, Kumararatne D, Casanova JL. 1998. Novel human immunodeficiencies reveal the essential role of type-1 cytokines in immunity to intracellular bacteria. *Immunol. Today* 19:491–94

12. Douvas G, Looker DL, Vatter AE, Crowle AJ. 1985. Gamma interferon activates human macrophages to become tumoricidal and leishmanicidal but enhances replication of macrophage-associated mycobacteria. *Infect. Immun.* 50:1–8

13. Crowle A, Ross EJ, May MH. 1987. Inhibition by 1,25(OH)2-vitamin D3 of the multiplication of virulent tubercle bacilli in cultured human macrophages. *Infect. Immun.* 55:2945–50

14. Rook GAW. 1988. The role of vitamin D in tuberculosis. *Am. Rev. Respir. Dis.* 138:768–70

15. Denis M. 1991. Killing of *Mycobacterium tuberculosis* within human monocytes: activation by cytokines and calcitriol. *Clin. Exp. Immunol.* 84:200–6

16. Rigby W. 1988. The immunobiology of vitamin D. *Immunol Today* 9:54–58

17. Rockett K, Brookes R, Udalova I, Vidal V, Hill AV, Kwiatkowski D. 1998. 1,25-Dihydroxyvitamin D3 induces nitric oxide synthase and suppresses growth of *Mycobacterium tuberculosis* in a human macrophage-like cell line. *Infect. Immun.* 66:5314–21

18. Bonecini-Almeida M, Chitale S, Boutsikakis I, Geng J, Doo H, He S, Ho JL. 1998. Induction of in vitro human macrophage anti-Mycobacterium tuberculosis activity: requirement for IFN-gamma and primed lymphocytes. *J. Immunol.* 160:4490–99

19. de Duve C, Wattiaux R. 1966. Functions of lysosomes. *Annu. Rev. Physiol.* 28:435–92

20. Bainton D. 1981. The discovery of lysosomes. *J. Cell Biol.* 91:66S–76S

21. Kornfeld S. 1987. Trafficking of lysosomal enzymes. *FASEB J.* 1:462–68

22. Mellman I, Fuchs R, Helenius A. 1986. Acidification of the endocytic and exocytic pathways. *Annu. Rev. Biochem.* 55:663–700

23. Ohkuma S, Poole B. 1978. Fluorescence probe measurement of the intralysosomal pH in living cells and the perturbation of pH by various agents. *Proc. Natl. Acad. Sci. USA* 75:3327–31

24. Desjardins M, Huber LA, Parton RG, Griffiths G. 1994. Biogenesis of phagolysosomes proceeds through a sequential series of interactions with the endocytic apparatus. *J. Cell Biol.* 124:677–88

25. Desjardins M. 1995. Biogenesis of phagolysosomes: the 'kiss and run' hypothesis. *Trends Cell Biol.* 5:183–86

26. Cohn Z. 1963. The fate of bacteria within phagocytic cells. I. The degradation of isotopically labeled bacteria by polymorphonuclear leucocytes and macrophages. *J. Exp. Med.* 117:27–42

27. Hackam D, Rotstein OD, Zhang WJ, Demaurex N, Woodside M, Tsai O, Grinstein S. 1997. Regulation of phagosomal acidification. Differential targeting of Na+/H+

exchangers, Na+/K+-ATPases, and vacuolar-type H+-atpases. *J. Biol. Chem.* 272:29810–20

28. Downey G, Botelho RJ, Butler JR, Moltyaner Y, Chien P, Schreiber AD, Grinstein S. 1999. Phagosomal maturation, acidification, and inhibition of bacterial growth in nonphagocytic cells transfected with FcgRIIA receptors. *J. Biol. Chem.* 274:28436–44

29. Armstrong J, D'Arcy Hart P. 1971. Response of cultured macrophages to *Mycobacterium tuberculosis*, with observations on fusion of lysosomes with phagosomes. *J. Exp. Med.* 134:713–40

30. D'Arcy Hart P, Armstrong J, Brown CA, Draper P. 1972. Ultrastructural study of the behavior of macrophages toward parasitic mycobacteria. *Infect. Immun.* 5:803–7

31. Russell D. 1995. Mycobacterium and Leishmania: stowaways in the endosomal network. *Trends Cell Biol.* 5:125–28

32. Deretic V, Fratti RA. 1999. Mycobacterium tuberculosis phagosome. *Mol. Microbiol.* 31:1603–9

33. Russell DG, Dant J, Sturgill-Koszycki S. 1996. *Mycobacterium avium-* and *Mycobacterium tuberculosis*-containing vacuoles are dynamic, fusion-competent vesicles that are accessible to glycosphingolipids from the host plasmalemma. *J. Immunol.* 156:4764–73

34. Goren M, D'Arcy Hart P, Young MR, Armstrong JA. 1976. Prevention of phagosome-lysosome fusion in cultured macrophages by sulfatides of *Mycobacterium tuberculosis*. *Proc. Nat. Acad. Sci. USA* 73:2510–14

35. Middlebrook G, Coleman CM, Schaeffer WB. 1959. Sulfolipid from virulent tubercle bacilli. *Proc. Natl. Acad. Sci. USA* 45:1801–4

36. Goren M, Brokl O, Roller P, Fales HM, Das BC. 1976. Sulfatides of *Mycobacterium tuberculosis*: the structure of the principal sulfatide (SL-1). *Biochemistry* 15:2728

37. Gordon A, D'Arcy Hart P, Young MR. 1980. Ammonia inhibits phagosome-lysosome fusion in macrophages. *Nature* 286:79–81

38. D'Arcy Hart P, Young MR, Jordan MM, Perkins WJ, Geisow MJ. 1983. Chemical inhibitors of phagosome-lysosome fusion in cultured macrophages also inhibit saltatory lysosomal movements. A combined microscopic and computer study. *J. Exp. Med.* 158:477–92

39. Clemens D, Horwitz MA. 1995. Characterization of the *Mycobacterium tuberculosis* phagosome and evidence that phagosomal maturation is inhibited. *J. Exp. Med.* 181:257–70

40. Reyrat J-M, Berthet F-X, Gicquel B. 1995. The urease locus of *Mycobacterium tuberculosis* and its utilization for the demonstration of allelic exchange in *Mycobacterium bovis* bacillus Calmette-Guerin. *Proc. Natl. Acad. Sci. USA* 92:8768–72

41. Reyrat J-M, Lopez-Ramirez G, Ofredo C, Gicquel B, Winter N. 1996. Urease activity does not contribute dramatically to persistence of *Mycobacterium bovis* bacillus Calmette-Guerin. *Infect. Immun.* 64:3934–36

42. Harth G, Clemens DL, Horwitz MA. 1994. Glutamine synthetase of *Mycobacterium tuberculosis*: extracellular release and characterization of its enzymatic activity. *Proc. Natl. Acad. Sci. USA* 91:9342–46

43. Harth G, Horwitz MA. 1999. An inhibitor of exported Mycobacterium tuberculosis glutamine synthetase selectively blocks the growth of pathogenic mycobacteria in axenic culture and in human monocytes: extracellular proteins as potential novel drug targets. *J. Exp. Med.* 189:1425–35

44. Schekman R, Orci L. 1996. Coat proteins and vesicle budding. *Science* 271:1526–33

45. Rothman J, Wieland FT. 1996. Protein sorting by transport vesicles. *Science* 272:227–34

46. Pfeffer S. 1992. GTP-binding proteins in

intracellular transport. *Trends Cell Biol.* 2:41–46

47. Zerial M, Stenmark H. 1993. Rab GT-Pases in vesicular transport. *Curr. Opin. Cell Biol.* 5:613–20

48. Via L, Deretic D, Ulmer RJ, Hibler NS, Huber LA, Deretic V. 1997. Arrest of mycobacterial phagosome maturation is caused by a block in vesicle fusion between stages controlled by rab5 and rab7. *J. Biol. Chem.* 272:13326–31

49. Press B, Feng Y, Hoflack B, Wandinger-Ness A. 1998. Mutant Rab7 causes the accumulation of cathepsin D and cation-independent mannose 6-phosphate receptor in an early endocytic compartment. *J. Cell Biol.* 140:1075–89

50. Crowle A, Dahl R, Ross E, May MH. 1991. Evidence that vesicles containing living, *virulent Mycobacterium tuberculosis* or *Mycobacterium avium* in cultured human macrophages are not acidic. *Infect. Immun.* 59:1823–31

51. Sturgill-Koszycki S, Schlesinger PH, Chakraborty P, Haddix PL, Collins HL, Fok AK, Allen D, Gluck SL, Heuser J, Russell DG. 1994. Lack of acidification in Mycobacterium phagosomes produced by exclusion of the vesicular proton-ATPase. *Science* 263:678–81

52. Xu S, Cooper A, Sturgill-Koszycki S, van Heyningen T, Chatterjee D, Orme I, Allen P, Russell DG. 1994. Intracellular trafficking in *Mycobacterium tuberculosis* and *Mycobacterium avium*-infected macrophages. *J. Immunol.* 153:2568–78

53. Ferrari G, Langen H, Naito M, Pieters JA. 1999. Coat protein on phagosomes involved in the intracellular survival of mycobacteria. *Cell* 97:435–47

54. Fang F. 1997. Mechanisms of nitric oxide-related antimicrobial activity. *J. Clin. Invest.* 99:2818–25

55. MacMicking J, Xie Q-W, Nathan C. 1997. Nitric oxide and macrophage function. *Annu. Rev. Immunol.* 15:323–50

56. Chan J, Flynn JL. 1999. Nitric oxide in *Mycobacterium tuberculosis* infection. In *Nitric Oxide and Infection*, ed. F Fang, pp. 281–310. New York: Plenum

57. Shiloh M, Nathan CF. 2000. Reactive nitrogen intermediates and the pathogenesis of Salmonella and mycobacteria. *Curr. Opin. Microbiol.* 3:35–42

58. MacMicking JD, North RJ, LaCourse R, Mudgett JS, Shah SK, Nathan CF. 1997. Identification of nitric oxide synthase as a protective locus against tuberculosis. *Proc. Natl. Acad. Sci. USA* 94:5243–48

59. Flynn JL, Scanga CA, Tanaka KE, Chan J. 1998. Effects of aminoguanidine on latent murine tuberculosis. *J. Immunol.* 160:1796–1803

60. Nicholson S, Bonecini-Almeida M, Silva JRL, Nathan C, Xie Q-W, Mumford R, Weidner JR, Calaycay J, Geng J, Boechat N, Linhares C, Rom W, Ho JL. 1996. Inducible nitric oxide synthase in pumonary alveolar macrophages from patients with tuberculosis. *J. Exp. Med.* 184:2293–2302

61. Wang C-H, Liu C-Y, Lin H-C, Yu C-T, Chung KF, Kuo HP. 1998. Increased exhaled nitric oxide in active pulmonary tuberculosis due to inducible NO synthase upregulation in alveolar macrophages. *Eur. Respir. J.* 11:809–15

62. Chan J, Xing Y, Magliozzo R, Bloom BR. 1992. Killing of virulent *Mycobacterium tuberculosis* by reactive nitrogen intermediates produced by activated murine macrophages. *J. Exp. Med.* 175:1111–22

63. Chan J, Fujiwara T, Brennen P, McNeil M, Turco SJ, Sibille JC, Snapper M, Aisen P, Bloom BR. 1989. Microbial glycolipids: possible virulence factors that scavenge oxygen radicals. *Proc. Natl. Acad. Sci. USA* 86:2453–57

64. Chan J, Fan X-D, Hunter SW, Brennan PJ, Bloom BR. 1991. Lipoarabinomannan, a possible virulence factor involved in persistence of Mycobacterium tuberculosis within macrophages. *Infect. Immun.* 59:1755–61

65. Adams L, Dinauer MC, Morgenstern DE,

Krahenbuhl JL. 1997. Comparison of the roles of reactive oxygen and nitrogen intermediates in the host response to Mycobacterium tuberculosis using transgenic mice. *Tuberculosis Lung Dis.* 78:237–56

66. Cooper A, Segal BH, Frank AA, Holland SM, Orme IM. 2000. Transient loss of resistance to pulmonary tuberculosis in p47phox-/- mice. *Infect. Immun.* 68:1231–34

67. Lau YL, Chan GC, Ha SY, Hui YF, Yuen KY. 1998. The role of the phagocytic respiratory burst in host defense agasint *Mycobacterium tuberculosis. Clin. Infect. Dis.* 26:226–27

68. Belvin M, Anderson KV. 1996. A conserved signaling pathway: the Drosophila toll-dorsal pathway. *Annu. Rev. Cell Dev. Biol.* 12:393–416

69. Baeuerle P, Henkel T. 1994. Function and activation of NF-kappa B in the immune system. *Annu. Rev. Immunol.* 12:141–79

70. Lemaitre B, Nicolas E, Michaut L, Reichhart JM, Hoffmann JA. 1996. The dorsoventral regulatory gene cassette spatzle/Toll/cactus controls the potent antifungal response in Drosophila adults. *Cell* 86:973–83

71. Medzhitov R, Preston-Hurlburt P, Janeway CA Jr. 1997. A human homologue of the Drosophila Toll protein signals activation of adaptive immunity. *Nature* 388:394–97

72. Medzhitov R, Preston-Hurlburt P, Kopp E, Stadlen A, Chen C, Ghosh S, Janeway CA Jr. 1998. MyD88 is an adaptor protein in the hToll/IL-1 receptor family signaling pathways. *Mol. Cell* 2:253–58

73. Hultmark D. 1994. Macrophage differentiation marker MyD88 is a member of the Toll/IL-1 receptor family. *Biochem. Biophys. Res. Commun.* 199:144–46

74. Poltorak A, He X, Smirnova I, Liu MY, Huffel CV, Du X, Birdwell D, Alejos E, Silva M, Galanos C, Freudenberg M, Ricciardi-Castagnoli P, Layton B, Beutler B. 1998. Defective LPS signaling in C3H/HeJ and C57BL/10ScCr mice: mutations in Tlr4 gene. *Science* 282:2085–88

75. Brightbill HD, Libraty DH, Krutzik SR, Yang RB, Belisle JT, Bleharski JR, Maitland M, Norgard MV, Plevy SE, Smale ST, Brennan PJ, Bloom BR, Godowski PJ, Modlin RL. 1999. Host defense mechanisms triggered by microbial lipoproteins through toll-like receptors. *Science* 285:732–36

76. Means TK, Wang S, Lien E, Yoshimura A, Golenbock DT, Fenton MJ. 1999. Human toll-like receptors mediate cellular activation by Mycobacterium tuberculosis. *J. Immunol.* 163:3920–27

77. Underhill DM, Ozinsky A, Smith KD, Aderem A. 1999. Toll-like receptor-2 mediates mycobacteria-induced proinflammatory signaling in macrophages. *Proc. Natl. Acad. Sci. USA* 96:14,459–63

78. Yang R, Mark MR, Gray A, Huang A, Xie MH, Zhang M, Goddard A, Wood WI, Gurney AL, Godowski PJ. 1998. Toll-like receptor-2 mediates lipopolysaccharide-induced cellular signalling. *Nature* 395:284–88

79. Schwandner R, Dziarski R, Wesche H, Rothe M, Kirschning CJ. 1999. Peptidoglycan- and lipoteichoic acid-induced cell activation is mediated by toll-like receptor 2. *J. Biol. Chem.* 274:17,406–9

80. Vogel S, Johnson D, Perera PY, Medvedev A, Lariviere L, Qureshi ST, Malo D. 1999. Functional characterization of the effect of the C3H/HeJ defect in mice that lack an Lps gene: in vivo evidence for a dominant negative mutation. *J. Immunol.* 162:5666–70

81. Lemaitre B, Reichhart JM, Hoffmann JA. 1997. Drosophila host defense: differential induction of antimicrobial peptide genes after infection by various classes of microorganisms. *Proc. Natl. Acad. Sci. USA* 94:14614–19

82. Ladel CH, Szalay G, Reidel D, Kaufmann SHE. 1997. Interleukin-12

secretion by *Mycobacterium tuberculosis*-infected macrophages. *Infect. Immun.* 65:1936–38

83. Henderson RA, Watkins SC, Flynn JL. 1997. Activation of human dendritic cells following infection with *Mycobacterium tuberculosis*. *J. Immunol.* 159:635–43

84. Sano K, Handea K, Tamura G, Shirato K. 1999. Ovalbumin (OVA) and Myocbacterium tuberculosis bacilli cooperatively polarize anti-OVA T-helper cells foward a Th1-dominant phenotype and ameliorate murine tracheal eosinophilia. *Am. J. Resp. Cell Molec. Biol.* 20:1260–67

85. Flynn JL, Goldstein MM, Triebold KJ, Sypek J, Wolf S, Bloom BR. 1995. IL-12 increases resistance of BALB/c mice to *Mycobacterium tuberculosis* infection. *J. Immunol.* 155:2515–24

86. Cooper AM, Roberts AD, Rhoades ER, Callahan JE, Getzy DM, Orme IM. 1995. The role of interleukin-12 in acquired immunity to *Mycobacterium tuberculosis* infection. *Immunology* 84:423–32

87. Cooper AM, Magram J, Ferrante J, Orme IM. 1997. Interleukin 12 (IL-12) is crucial to the development of protective immunity in mice intravenously infected with *Mycobacterium tuberculosis*. *J. Exp. Med.* 186:39–45

88. Lowrie DB, Tascon RE, Bonato VLD, Lima VMF, Faccioli LH, Stavropoulos E, Colston MJ, Hewinson RG, Moelling K, Silva CL. 1999. Therapy of tuberculosis in mice by DNA vaccination. *Nature* 400:269–71

89. Lyadova I, Yeremeev V, Majorov K, Nikonenko B, Khaidukov S, Kondratieva T, Kobets N, Apt A. 1998. An ex vivo study of T lymphocytes recovered from the lungs of I/St mice infected with and susceptible to *Mycobacterium tuberculosis*. *Infec. Immun.* 66:4981–88

90. Lalvani A, Brookes R, Wilkinson R, Malin A, Pathan A, Andersen P, Dockrell H, Pasvol G, Hill A. 1998. Human cytolytic and interferon gamma-secreting CD8+ T lymphocytes specific for *Mycobacterium tuberculosis*. *Proc. Natl. Acad. Sci. USA* 95:270–5

91. Orme I, Miller E, Roberts A, Furney S, Griffen J, Dobos K, Chi D, Rivoire B, Brennan P. 1992. T Lymphocytes mediating protection and cellular cytolysis during the course of *Mycobacterium tuberculosis* infection. *J. Immunol.* 148:189–96

92. Orme IM, Roberts AD, Griffen JP, Abrams JS. 1993. Cytokine secretion by CD4 T lymphocytes acquired in response to *Mycobacterium tuberculosis* infection. *J. Immunol.* 151:518–25

93. Serbina NV, Flynn JL. 1999. Early emergence of CD8+ T cells primed for production of Type 1 cytokines in the lungs of *Mycobacterium tuberculosis*-infected mice. *Infect. Immun.* 67:3980–88

94. Barnes PF, Abrams JS, Lu S, Sieling PA, Rea TH, Modlin RL. 1993. Patterns of cytokine production by *Mycobacterium*-reactive human T-cell clones. *Infect. Immun.* 61:197–203

95. Wang J, Wakeham J, Harkness R, Xing Z. 1999. Macrophages are a significant source of type 1 cytokines during mycobacterial infection. *J. Clin. Invest.* 103:1023–29

96. Fenton MJ, Vermeulen MW, Kim S, Burdick M, Strieter RM, Kornfeld H. 1997. Induction of gamma-interferon production in human alveolar macrophages by *Mycobacterium tuberculosis*. *Infect. Immun.* 65:5149–56

97. Cooper AM, Dalton DK, Stewart TA, Griffen JP, Russell DG, Orme IM. 1993. Disseminated tuberculosis in IFN-γ gene-disrupted mice. *J. Exp. Med.* 178:2243–48

98. Flynn JL, Chan J, Triebold KJ, Dalton DK, Stewart T, Bloom BR. 1993. An essential role for Interferon-γ in resistance to *Mycobacterium tuberculosis* infection. *J. Exp. Med.* 178:2249–54

99. Dalton DK, Pitts-Meek S, Keshav S, Figari IS, Bradley A, Stewart TA. 1993. Multiple defects of immune cell function

in mice with disrupted interferon-gamma genes. *Science* 259:1739–42

100. Lin Y, Zhang M, Hofman FM, Gong J, Barnes PF. 1996. Absence of a prominent TH2 cytokine response in human tuberculosis. *Infect. Immun.* 64:1351–56

101. Zhang M, Lin Y, Iyer DV, Gong J, Abrams JS, Barnes PF. 1995. T cell cytokine responses in human infection with *Mycobacterium tuberculosis*. *Infect. Immun.* 63:3231–34

102. Ting LM, Kim AC, Cattamanchi A, Ernst JD. 1999. *Mycobacterium tuberculosis* inhibits IFN-gamma transcriptional responses without inhibiting activation of STAT1. *J. Immunol* 163:3898–3906

103. Bhattacharyya S, Singla R, Dey AB, Prasad HK. 1999. Dichotomy of cytokine profiles in patients and high-risk healthy subjects exposed to tuberculosis. *Infect. Immun.* 67:5597–5603

104. North RJ. 1998. Mice incapable of making IL-4 and IL-10 display normal resistance in infection with *Mycobacterium tuberculosis*. *Clin. Exp. Immunol.* 113:55–58

105. Saunders BM, Frank AA, Orme IM, Cooper AM. 2000. Interleukin-6 induces early gamma interferon production in the infected lung but is not required for generation of specific immunity to *Mycobacterium tuberculosis* infection. *Infect. Immun.* 68:3322–26

106. Fenhalls G, Wong A, Bezuidenhout J, van Helden P, Bardin P, Lukey PT. 2000. In situ production of gamma interferon, interleukin-4, and tumor necrosis factor alpha mRNA in human lung tuberculous granuloma. *Infect. Immun.* 68:2827–36

107. Flynn JL, Goldstein MM, Chan J, Triebold KJ, Pfeffer K, Lowenstein CJ, Schreiber R, Mak TW, Bloom BR. 1995. Tumor necrosis factor-α is required in the protective immune response against *M. tuberculosis* in mice. *Immunity* 2:561–72

108. Bean AGD, Roach DR, Briscoe H, France MP, Korner H, Sedgwick JD,

Britton WJ. 1999. Structural deficiencies in granuloma formation in TNF gene-targeted mice underlie the heightened susceptibility to aerosol *Mycobacterium tuberculosis* infection, which is not compensated for by lymphotoxin. *J. Immunol.* 162:3504–11

109. Liew FY, Li Y, Millott S. 1990. Tumor necrosis factor-α synergizes with IFN-γ in mediating killing of *Leishmania major* through the induction of nitric oxide. *J. Immunol.* 145:4306–10

110. Ehlers S, Benin J, Kutschn S, Endres R, Rietschel ET, Pfeffer K. 1999. Fatal granuloma necrosis without exacerbated mycobacterial growth in tumor necrosis factor receptor p55 gene-deficient mice intravenously infected with *Mycobacterium avium*. *Infect. Immun.* 67:3571–79

111. Kindler V, Sappino A-P, Grau GE, Piguet P-F, Vassalli P. 1989. The inducing role of tumor necrosis factor in the development of bactericidal granulomas during BCG infection. *Cell* 56:731–40

112. Garcia I, Miyazaki Y, Marchal G, Lesslauer W, Vassalli P. 1997. High sensitivity of transgenic mice expressing soluble TNFR1 fusion protein to mycobacterial infections: synergistic action of TNF and IFN-gamma in the differentiation of protective granulomas. *Eur. J. Immunol.* 27:3182–90

113. Rook GAW, Taverne J, Leveton C, Steele J. 1987. The role of gamma-interferon, vitamin D3 metabolites and tumour necrosis factor in the pathogenesis of tuberculosis. *Immunology* 62:229–34

114. Rook GAW. 1990. Mycobacteria, cytokines and antibiotics. *Pathol. Biol. (Paris)* 38:276–80

115. Moreira AL, Tsenova-Berkova L, Wang J, Laochumroonvorapong P, Freeman S, Freedman GK. 1997. Effect of cytokine modulation by thalidomide on the granomatous response in murine tuberculosis. *Tubercle Lung Disease* 78:47–55

116. Hodge-Dufour J, Marino MW, Horton

MR, Jungbluth A, Durdick MD, Strieter RM, Noble PW, Hunter CA, Pure E. 1998. Inhibition of interferon γ induced interleukin 12 production: a potential mechanism for the anti-inflammatory activities of tumor necrosis factor. *Proc. Natl. Acad. Sci. USA* 95:13806–11

117. Maini R, St. Clair EW, Breedveld F, Furst D, Kalden J, Weisman M, Smolen J, Emery P, Harriman G, Feldman M, Lipsky P. 1999. Infliximab (chimeric anti-tumour necrosis factor a monoclonal antibody) versus placebo in rheumatoid arthritis patients receiving concomitant methotrexate: a randomized phase III trial. *Lancet* 354:1932–39

118. Gong J-H, Zhang M, Modlin RL, Linsley PS, Iyer D, Lin Y, Barnes PF. 1996. Interleukin-10 downregulates *Mycobacterium tuberculosis*-induced Th1 responses and CTLA4 expression. *Infect. Immun.* 64:913–18

119. Rojas M, Olivier M, Gros P, Barrera LF, Garcia LF. 1999. TNF-α and IL-10 modulate the induction of apoptosis by virulent *Mycobacterium tuberculosis* in murine macorphages. *J. Immunol.* 162:6122–31

120. Murray PJ, Yang L, Onufryk C, Tepper RI, Young RA. 1997. T cell-derived IL-10 antagonizes macrophage function in mycobacteria infection. *J. Immunol.* 158:315–21

121. VanHeyningen TK, Collins HL, Russell DG. 1997. IL-6 produced by macrophages infected with *Mycobacterium* species suppresses T cell responses. *J. Immunol.* 158:330–37

122. Ladel CH, Blum C, Dreher A, Reifenberg K, Kopf M, Kaufmann SHE. 1997. Lethal tuberculosis in Interleukin-6-deficient mutant mice. *Infect. Immun.* 65:4843–49

123. Hirsch CS, Ellner JJ, Blinkhorn R, Toossi Z. 1997. In vitro restoration of T cell responses in tuberculosis and augmentation of moncyte effector function against *Mycobacterium tuberculosis* by natural inhibitors of transforming growth factor beta. *Proc. Natl. Acad. Sci. USA* 94:3926–31

124. Toossi Z, Gogate P, Shiratsuchi H, Young T, Ellner J.J. 1995. Enhanced production of TGF-beta by blood monocytes from patients with active tuberculosis and presence of TGF-beta in tuberculosis granulomatous lung lesions. *J. Immunol.* 154:465

125. Dahl KE, Shiratsuchi H, Hamilton B, Ellner JJ, Toossi Z. 1996. Selective induction of transforming growth factor β in human monocytes by lipoarabinomannan of Mycobacterium tuberculosis. *Infect. Immun.* 64:399–405

126. Rojas RE, Balaji KN, Subramanian A, Boom WH. 1999. Regulation of human CD4+ αβ TCR+ and γδ TCR+ T cell responses to *Mycobacterium tuberculosis* by interleukin-10 and transforming growth factor β. *Infect. Immun.* 67:6461–72

127. Ding A, Nathan C, Srimal S. 1990. Macrophage deactivation factor and TFG-β inhibition of macrophage nitrogen oxide synthesis by IFN-γ. *J. Immunol.* 145:940–45

128. Serbina NV, Liu C-C, Scanga CA, Flynn JL. 2000. CD8+ cytotoxic T lymphocytes from lungs of *M. tuberculosis* infected mice express perforin in vivo and lyse infected macrophages. *J. Immunol.* 165:353–63

129. Feng CG, Bean AGD, Hooi H, Briscoe H, Britton WJ. 1999. Increase in gamma interferon-secreting CD8+, as well as CD4+ T cells in lungs following aerosol infection with *Mycobacterium tuberculosis*. *Infect. Immun.* 67:3242–47

130. Flynn JL, Goldstein MM, Triebold KJ, Koller B, Bloom BR. 1992. Major histocompatibility complex class I-restricted T cells are required for resistance to *Mycobacterium tuberculosis* infection. *Proc. Natl. Acad. Sci. USA* 89:12,013–17

131. Randhawa PS. 1990. Lymphocyte subsets in granulomas of human tuberculosis: an in situ immunofluorescence study using monoclonal antibodies. *Pathology* 22:153–55

132. Muller I, Cobbold S, Waldmann H, Kaufmann SHE. 1987. Impaired resistance to Mycobacterium tuberculosis infection after selective in vivo depletion of L3T4+ and Lyt2+ T cells. *Infect. Immunol.* 55:2037–41

133. Orme I, Collins F. 1984. Adoptive protection of the *Mycobacteria tuberculosis*-infected lung. *Cell. Immun.* 84:113–20

134. Orme I, Collins F. 1983. Protection against *Mycobacterium tuberculosis* infection by adoptive immunotherapy. *J. Exp. Med.* 158:74–83

135. Tascon RE, Stavropoulos E, Lukacs KV, Colston MJ. 1998. Protection against *Mycobacterium tuberculosis* infection by CD8 T cells requires production of gamma interferon. *Infect. Immun.* 66: 830–34

136. Caruso AM, Serbina N, Klein E, Triebold K, Bloom BR, Flynn JL. 1999. Mice deficient in CD4 T cells have only transiently diminished levels of IFN-γ, yet succumb to tuberculosis. *J. Immunol.* 162:5407–16

137. Selwyn PA, Hartel D, Lewis VA, Schoenbaum EE, Vermund SH, Klein RS, Walker AT, Freidland GH. 1989. A prospective study of the risk of tuberculosis among intravenous drug users with human immunodeficiency virus infection. *New Engl. J. Med.* 320:545–50

138. Scanga CA, Mohan VP, Yu K, Joseph H, Tanaka K, Chan J, Flynn JL. 2000. Depletion of CD4+ T cells causes reactivation of murine persistent tuberculosis despite continued expression of IFN-γ and NOS2. *J. Exp Med.* 192:347–58

139. Campos-Neto A, Ovendale P, Bement T, Koppi TA, Fanslow WC, Rossi MA, Alderson MR. 1998. CD40 ligand is not essential for the development of cell-mediated immunity and resistance to *Mycobacterium tuberculosis*. *J. Immunol.* 160:2037–41

140. Clarke SRM. 2000. The critical role of CD40/CD40L in the CD4-dependent generation of CD8+ T cell immunity. *J. Leuk. Biol.* 67:607–14

141. Andreasen SO, Christensen J, Marker O, Thomsen AR. 2000. Role of CD40 ligand and CD28 in induction and maintenance of antiviral CD8+ effector T cell responses. *J. Immunol.* 164:3689–97

142. Kalams SA, Walker BD. 1998. The critical need for CD4 help in maintaining effective cytotoxic T lymphocyte responses. *J. Exp. Med.* 188:2199–2204

143. Johnson CM, Cooper AM, Frank AA, Bonorino CB, Wysoki LJ, Orme IM. 1997. *Mycobacterium tuberculosis* aerogenic challenge infections in B cell-deficient mice. *Tubercle Lung Dis.* 78:257–61

144. Teitelbaum R, Glatman-Freedman A, Chen B, Robbins JB, Unanue E, Casadevall A, Bloom BR. 1998. A mAb recognizing a surface antigen of *Mycobacterium tuberculosis* enhances host survival. *Proc. Natl. Acad. Sci., U.S.A.* 95:15,688–93

145. Bosio CM, Gardner D, Elkins KL. 2000. Infection of B cell deficient mice with CDC1551, a clinical isolate of Mycobacterium tuberculosis: delay in dissemination and development of lung pathology. *J. Immunol.* 164:6417–25

146. Balcewicz-Sablinska MK, Keane J, Kornfeld H, Remold HG. 1998. Pathogenic *Mycobacterium tuberculosis* evades apoptosis of host macrophages by release of TNF-R2, resulting in inactivation of TNF-α. *J. Immunol.* 161:2636–41

147. Keane J, Balcewicz-Sablinska MK, Remold HG, Chupp GL, Meek BB, Fenton MJ, Kornfeld H. 1997. Infection by *Mycobacterium tuberculosis* promotes human alveolar macrophage apoptosis. *Infect. Immun.* 65:298–304

148. Oddo M, Renno T, Attainger A, Bakker T, MacDonald HR, Meylan PRA. 1998. Fas ligand-induced apoptosis of infected human macrophages reduces the viability of intracellular *Mycobacterium tuberculosis. J. Immunol.* 160:5448–54

149. Stenger S, Mazzaccaro R, Uyemura K, Cho S, Barnes P, Rosat J, Sette A, Brenner M, Porcelli S, Bloom B, Modlin R. 1997. Differential effects of cytolytic T cell subsets on intracellular infection. *Science* 276:1684–87

150. Silva CL, Lowrie DB. 2000. Identification and characterization of murine cytotoxic T cells that kill Mycobacterium tuberculosis. *Infect. Immun.* 68:3269–74

151. Mazzaccaro RJ, Gedde M, Jensen ER, van Santem HM, Ploegh HL, Rock KL, Bloom BR. 1996. Major histocompatibility class I presentation of soluble antigen facilitated by *Mycobacterium tuberculosis* infection. *Proc. Natl. Acad. Sci. USA* 93:11786–91

152. Hmama Z, Gabathuler R, Jefferies WA, Dejong G, Reiner NE. 1998. Attenuation of HLA-DR expression by mononuclear phagocytes infected with *Mycobacterium tuberculosis* is related to intracellular sequestration of immature class II heterodimers. *J. Immunol.* 161:4882–93

153. Noss EH, Harding CV, Boom WH. 2000. *Mycobacterium tuberculosis* inhibits MHC class II antigen processing in murine bone marrow macrophages. *Cell. Immunol.* 201:63–74

154. Wojciechowski W, DeSanctis J, Skamene E, Radzioch D. 1999. Attenuation of MHC class II expression in macrophages infected with Mycobacterium bovis BCG involves class II transactivator and depends on the Nramp1 gene. *J. Immunol.* 163:2688–96

155. Stenger S, Niazi KR, Modlin RL. 1998. Down-regulation of CD1 on antigen presenting cells by infection with *Mycobacterium tuberculosis. J. Immunol.* 161:3582–88

156. McDonough KA, Kress Y, Bloom BR. 1993. Pathogenesis of Tuberculosis: Interaction of *Mycobacterium tuberculosis* with macrophages. *Infect. Immun.* 61:2763–73

157. Behar SM, Dascher CC, Grusby MJ, Wang CR, Brenner MB. 1999. Susceptibility of mice deficient in CD1D or TAP1 to infection with *Mycobacterium tuberculosis. J. Exp. Med.* 189:1973–80

158. Sousa AO, Mazzaccaro R, Russell DG, Lee FK, Turner OC, Hong S, Van Kaer L, Bloom BR. 1999. Relative contributions of distinct MHC class I-dependent cell populations in protection to tuberculosis infection in mice. *Proc. Natl. Acad. Sci., USA* 97:4204–8

159. De Libero G, Flesch I, Kaufmann SHE. 1988. Mycobacteria-reactive Lyt-2+ T cell lines. *Eur. J. Immunol.* 18:59–66

160. Silva CL, Silva MF, Pietro R, Lowrie DB. 1994. Protection against tuberculosis by passive transfer with T-cell clones recognizing mycobacterial heat shock protein 65. *Immunology* 83:341–46

161. Zhu X, Stauss HJ, Ivanyi J, Vordermeier HM. 1997. Specificity of CD8+ T cells from subunit vaccinated or infected H-2b mice recognizing the 38 kDa antigen of Mycobacterium tuberculosis. *Int. Immunol.* 9:1669

162. Tan JS, Canady DH, Boom WH, Balaji KN, Schwander SK, Rich EA. 1997. Human alveolar T lymphocyte responses to *Mycobacterium tuberculosis* infection. *J. Immunol.* 159:290–97

163. Mohagheghpour N, Gammon D, Kawamura LM, van Vollenhoven A, Benike CJ, Engleman EG. 1998. CTL response to *Mycobacterium tuberculosis*: identification of an immunogenic epitope in the 19kDa lipoprotein. *J. Immunol.* 161:2400–

164. Lewinsohn D, Alderson M, Briden A, Riddell S, Reed S, Grabstein K.

1998. Characterization of human CD8+ T cells reactive with Mycobacterium tuberculosis-infected antigen presenting cells. *J. Exp. Med.* 187:1633–40

165. Lewinsohn DM, Briden AL, Reed SG, Grabstein KH, Alderson MR. 2000. Mycobacterium tuberculosis-reactive CD8+ T lymphocytes: the relative contribution of classical versus nonclassical HLA restriction. 165:925–30

166. Albert M, Sauter B, Bhardwaj N. 1998. Dendritic cells acquire antigen from apoptotic cells and induce class I-restricted CTLs. *Nature* 392:86–89

167. Cho S, Mehra V, Thoma-Uszynski S, Stenger S, Serbina N, Mazzaccaro R, Flynn JL, F. Barnes P, Southwood S, Celis E, Bloom BR, Modlin RL, Sette A. Antimicrobial activity of MHC class I restricted CD8+ T cells in human tuberculosis. *Proc. Natl. Acad. Sci. USA.* In press

168. Teitelbaum R, Cammer M, Maitland ML, Freitag NE, Condeelis J, Bloom BR. 1999. Mycobacterial infection of macrophages results in membrane-permeable phagosomes. *Proc. Natl. Acad. Sci. USA* 96:15190–95

169. Canaday DH, Ziebold C, Noss EH, Chervenak KA, Harding CV, Boom WH. 1999. Activation of human CD8+ $\alpha\beta$ TCR+ cells by *Mycobacterium tuberculosis* via an alternate class I MHC antigen processing pathway. *J. Immunol.* 162:372–79

170. Porcelli SA, Modlin RL. 1999. The CD1 system: antigen-presenting molecules for T cell recognition of lipids and glycolipids. *Annu. Rev. Immunol.* 17:297–329

171. Sieling PA, Ochoa M-T, Jullien D, Leslie DS, Sabet S, Rosat J-P, Burdick AE, Rea TH, Brenner MB, Porcelli SA, Modlin RL. 2000. Evidence for human CD4+ T cells in the CD1- restricted repertoire: derivation of mycobacteria-reactive T cells from leprosy lesions. *J. Immunol.* 164:4790–96

172. Beckman EM, Porcelli SA, Morita CT, Behar SM, Furlong ST, Brenner MB. 1994. Recognition of a lipid antigen by CD1-restricted $\alpha\beta$ + T cells. *Nature* 372:691–94

173. Sieling PA, Chatterjee D, Porcelli SA, Prigozy TI, Mazzaccaro RJ, Soriano T, Bloom BR, Brenner MB, Kronenberg M, Brennan PJ, Modlin RL. 1995. CD1-restricted T cell recognition of microbial lipoglycan antigens. *Science* 269:227–30

174. Moody DB, Reinhold BB, Guy MR, Beckman EM, Frederique DE, Furlong ST, Ye S, Reinhold VN, Sieling PA, Modlin RL, Besra GS, Porcelli SA. 1997. Structural requirements for glycolipid antigen recognition by CD1b-restricted T cells. *Science* 278:283–86

175. Moody DB, Ulrichs T, Muhlecker W, Young DC, Gurcha SS, Grant E, Rosaat J-P, Brenner MB, Costello CE, Besra GS, Porcelli SA. 2000. CD1c-mediated T-cell recognition of isoprenoid glycolipids in Mycobacterium tuberculosis infection. *Nature* 404:884–88

176. Jackman RM, Stenger S, Lee A, Moody DB, Rogers RA, Niazi KR, Peters PJ, Porcelli SA. 1998. The tyrosine containing cytoplasmic tail of CD1b is essential for its efficient presentation of bacterial lipid antigens. *Immunity* 8:341–51

177. Sugita M, Jackman RM, van Donselaar E, Behar SM, Rogers RA, Peters PJ, Brenner MB, Porcelli SA. 1996. Cytoplasmic tail-dependent localization of CD1b antigen-presenting molecules to MIICs. *Science* 273:349–52

178. Sugita M, Grant EP, van Donselaar E, Hsu VS, Rogers RA, Peters PJ, Brenner MB. 1999. Separate pathways for antigen presentation by CD1 molecules. *Immunity* 11:743–52

179. Schaible UE, Hagens K, Fischer K, Collins HL, Kaufmann SHE. 2000. Intersection of Group I CD1 molecules and mycobacteria in different intracellular

compartments of dendritic cells. *J. Immunol.* 164:4843–52

180. Briken V, Jackman RM, Watts GF, Rogers RA, Porcelli SA. 2000. Human CD1b and CD1c isoforms survey different intracellular compartments for the presentation of microbial lipid antigens. *J. Exp. Med.* 192:281–87

181. Beatty WL, Rhoades ER, Ullrich H-J, Chatterjee D, Heuser JE, Russell DG. 2000. Trafficking and release of mycobacterial lipids from infected macrophages. *Traffic* 1:235–47

182. Porcelli A, Morita CT, Brenner MB. 1992. CD1b restricts the response of human CD4-8- T lymphocytes to a microbial antigen. *Nature* 360:593–97

183. Sieling PA, Jullien D, Dahlem M, Rea TH, Modlin RL, Porcelli SA. 1999. CD1 expression by dendritic cells in human leprosy lesions: correlation with effective host immunity. *J. Immunol.* 162:1851–58

184. Dascher CC, Hiromatsu K, Naylor JW, Brauer PP, Brown KA, Storey JR, Behar SM, Kawasaki ES, Porcelli SA, Brenner MB, LeClair KP. 1999. Conservation of a CD1 multigene family in the guinea pig. *J. Immunol.* 163:5478–88

185. Kerksiek KM, Busch DH, Pilip IM, Allen SE, Pamer EG. 1999. H2-M3-restricted T cells in bacterial infection: rapid primary but diminished memory responses. *J. Exp. Med.* 190:195–204

186. Kaufmann S. 1988. CD8+ T lymphocytes in intracellular microbial infections. *Immunol. Today* 9:168–74

187. Kaufmann SHE. 1993. Immunity to intracellular bacteria. *Annu. Rev. Immunol.* 11:129–63

188. Stenger S, Hanson DA, Teitelbaum R, Dewan P, R NK, Froelich CS, Ganz T, Thomauszynski S, Melian A, Bogdan C, Porcelli SA, Bloom BR, Krensky AM, Modlin RL. 1998. An antimicrobial activity of cytotoxic T cells mediated by granulysin. *Science* 282:121–25

189. Cooper AM, D'Souza C, Frank AA, Orme IM. 1997. The course of *Mycobacterium tuberculosis* infection in the lungs of mice lacking expression of either perforin- or granzyme-mediated cytolytic mechanisms. *Infect. Immun.* 65:1317–20

190. Laochumroonvorapong P, Wang J, Liu CC, Ye W, Moreira AL, Elkon KB, Freedman VH, Kaplan G. 1997. Perforin, a cytotoxic molecule which mediates cell necrosis, is not required for the early control of mycobacterial infection in mice. *Infect. Immun.* 65:127–32

191. Matloubian M, Suresh M, Glass A, Galvan M, Chow K, Whitmire JK, Walsh GE, Clark WR, Ahmed R. 1999. A role for perforin in downregulating T-cell responses during chronic viral infection. *J. Virol.* 73:2527–36

192. Johnson C, Cooper AM, Frank AA, Orme IM. 1998. Adequate expression of protective immunity in the absence of granuloma formation in Myocbaterium tuberculosis-infected mice with a disruption in the intracellular adhesion molecule 1 gene. *Infect. Immun.* 66:1666–70

193. Bonecchi R, Bianchi G, Bordignon PP, D'Ambrosio D, Lang R, Borsatti A, Sozzani S, Allavena P, Gray PA, Mantovani A, Sinigaglia F. 1998. Differential expression of chemokine receptors and chemotactic responsiveness of type 1 T helper cells (Th1s) and Th2s. *J. Exp. Med.* 187:129–34

194. Sallusto F, Mackay CR, Lanzavecchia A. 2000. The role of chemokine receptors in primary, effector, and memory immune responses. *Annu. Rev. Immunol.* 18:593–620

195. Foxman EF, Campbell JJ, Butcher EC. 1997. Multistep navigation and combinatorial control of leukocyte chemotaxis. *J. Cell. Biol.* 139:1349–60

196. Luster AD. 1998. Chemokines: chemotactic cytokines that mediate inflammation. *N. Engl. J. Med.* 338:436–45

197. Baggiolini M, Dewald B, Moser B. 1997.

Human chemokines: an update. *Annu. Rev. Immunol.* 15:675–705

198. Orme IM, Cooper AM. 1999. Cytokine/chemokine cascades in immunity to tuberculosis. *Immunol. Today* 20:307–12

199. Rhoades ER, Cooper AM, Orme IM. 1995. Chemokine response in mice infected with *Mycobacterium tuberculosis*. *Infect. Immun.* 63:3871–77

200. Rutledge BJ, Rayburn H, Rosenberg R, North RJ, Gladue RP, Corless CL, Rollins BJ. 1995. High level monocyte chemoattractant protein-1 expression in transgenic mice increase their susceptibility to intracellular pathogens. *J. Immunol.* 155:4838–43

201. Lu B, Rutledge BJ, Gu L, Fiorillo J, Lukacs NW, Kunkel SL, North RJ, Gerard C, Rollins BJ. 1998. Abnormalities in monocyte recruitment and cytokine expression in monocyte chemoattractant protein 1-deficient mice. *J. Exp. Med.* 187:601–8

202. Sadek MI, Sada E, Toossi Z, Schwander SK, Rich EA. 1998. Chemokines induced by infection of mononuclear phagocytes with mycobacteria and present in lung alveoli during active pulmonary tuberculosis. *Am. J. Respir. Cell Mol. Biol.* 19:513–21

203. Kuarshima K, Mukaida N, Fujimura M, Yasui M, Nakazumi Y, Matsuda T, Matsushima K. 1997. Elevated chemokine levels in bronchoalveolar lavage fluid of tuberculosis patients. *Am. J. Resp. Crit. Care Med.* 155:1474–7

204. Lin YG, Gong J, Zhang M, Xue W, Barnes PF. 1998. Production of monocyte chemoattractant protein 1 in tuberculosis patients. *Infect. Immun.* 66:2319–22

205. Faziano M, Cappelli G, Santucci M, Mariani F, Amicosante M, Casarini M, Giosue S, Bisetti A, Colizzi V. 1999. Expression of CCR5 is increasedin human monocyte-derived macrophages and alveolar macrophages in the course of in vivo

and in vitro *Mycobacterium tuberculosis* infection. *AIDS Res. Human Retrovirus* 15:869

206. Croix DA, Capuano S III, Simpson L, Fallert BA, Fuller CL, Klein EC, Reinhart TA, Murphey-Corb M, Flynn JL. 2000. The effect of mycobacterial infection on virus load and disease progression in Simian Immunodeficiency Virus-infected rhesus monkeys. *AIDS Res. Human Retrovirus.* In press

207. Hogaboam CM, Bone-Larson CL, Lipinski S, Lukacs NW, Chensue SW, Strieter RM, Kunkel SL. 1999. Differential monocyte chemoattractant protein-1 and CCR2 expression by murine lung fibroblasts derived from Th1 and Th2 type pulmonary granuloma models. *J. Immunol.* 163:2193–201

208. Warmington KS, Boring L, Ruth JH, Sonstein J, Hogaboam CM, Curtis JL, Kunkel SL, Charo IR, Chensue SW. 1999. Effect of C-C chemokine receptor 2 (CCR2) knockout on type-2 (schistosomal antigen-elicited) pulmonary granuloma formation: analysis of cellular recruitment and cytokine responses. *Am. J. Pathol.* 154:1407–16

209. Boring L, Gosling J, Chensue SW, Kunkel SL, Farese GE Jr, Broxmeyer HE, Charo IF. 1997. Impaired monocyte migration and reduced type 1 (Th1) cytokine responses in C-C chemokine receptor 2 knockout mice. *J. Clin. Invest.* 100:2552–61

210. Gao JL, Wynn TA, Chang Y, Lee EJ, Broxmeyer HE, Cooper S, Tiffany HL, Westphal H, Kwon-Chung J, Murphy PM. 1997. Impaired host defense, hematopoiesis, granulomatous inflammation and type 1-type 2 cytokine balance in mice lacking CC chemokine receptor 1. *J. Exp. Med.* 185:1959–68

211. Chensue SW, Warmington KS, Allenspach EJ, Lu B, Gerard C, Kunkel SL, Lukacs NW. 1999. Differential expression and cross-regulatory function

of RANTES during mycobacterial (type 1) and schistosomal (type 2) antigen-elicited granulomatous inflammation. *J. Immunol.* 163:165–73

212. Lane BR, Markovitz DM, Woodford NL, Rochford R, Strieter RM, Coffey MJ. 1999. TNF-alpha inhibits HIV-1 replication in peripheral blood monocytes and alveolar macrophages by inducing the production of RANTES and decreasing C-C chemokine receptor 5 (CCR5) expression. *J. Immunol.* 163:3653–61

213. Czermak BJ, Sarma V, Bless NM, Schmal H, Friedl HP, Ward PA. 1999. In vitro and in vivo dependency of chemokine generation on C5a and TNF-*α*. *J. Immunol.* 162:2321–25

214. Crippen TL, Riches DW, Hyde DM. 1998. Differential regulation of the expression of cytokine-induced neutrophil chemoattractant by mouse macrophages. *Pathobiology* 66:24–32

215. Koyama S, Sato E, Nomura H, Kubo K, Miura M, Yamashita T, Nagai S, Izumi T. 1999. Monocyte chemotactic factors released from type II pneumocyte-like cells in respone to TNF-a and IL-1a. *Eur. Resp. J.* 13:820–28

216. Juffermans NP, Verbaon A, van Deventer SJ, van Deurekom H, Belisle JT, Ellis ME, Speelman P, van der Poll T. 1999. Elevated chemokine concentrations in sera of human immunodeficiency virus (HIV) seropositivie and HIV-seronegative patients with tuberculosis: a possible role for mycobacterial lipoarabinomannan. *Infect. Immun.* 67:4295–97

217. Dow SW, Roberts A, Vyas J, Rodgers J, Rich RR, Orme I, Potter TA. 2000. Immunization with f-Met peptides induces immune reactivity against Mycobacterium tuberculosis. *Tubercle Lund. Dis.* 80:5–13

Annu. Rev. Immunol. 2001. 19:131–61

TOLERANCE TO ISLET AUTOANTIGENS IN TYPE 1 DIABETES

Jean-François Bach and Lucienne Chatenoud

INSERM U 25, Hôpital Necker, 161 rue de Sèvres, 75743 Paris Cedex 15, France;
e-mail: bach@necker.fr

Key Words insulin, GAD, CD3, immunoregulation, Th2

■ **Abstract** Tolerance to β cell autoantigens represents a fragile equilibrium. Autoreactive T cells specific to these autoantigens are present in most normal individuals but are kept under control by a number of peripheral tolerance mechanisms, among which CD4$^+$ CD25$^+$ CD62L$^+$ T cell–mediated regulation probably plays a central role. The equilibrium may be disrupted by inappropriate activation of autoantigen-specific T cells, notably following to local inflammation that enhances the expression of the various molecules contributing to antigen recognition by T cells. Even when T cell activation finally overrides regulation, stimulation of regulatory cells by CD3 antibodies may reset the control of autoimmunity. Other procedures may also lead to disease prevention. These procedures are essentially focused on Th2 cytokines, whether used systemically or produced by Th2 cells after specific stimulation by autoantigens. Protection can also be obtained by NK T cell stimulation. Administration of β cell antigens or CD3 antibodies is now being tested in clinical trials in prediabetics and/or recently diagnosed diabetes.

INTRODUCTION

Insulin-dependent diabetes mellitus (IDDM) ensues from the selective aggression against insulin-secreting β cells of the islets of Langerhans by autoreactive T cells (1, 2). Both CD4 and CD8 T cells are involved in the pathogenesis of the spontaneous disease although monoclonal islet reactive CD4 or CD8 T cells may express diabetogenic properties on their own under particular experimental conditions. The nature of the triggering and/or of the target autoantigen(s) is elusive, and several candidates have been described, including insulin (or proinsulin), glutamic acid decarboxylase (GAD), IA-2, a tyrosine phosphatase, and heat shock protein 60 (hsp 60). A special case was made for GAD when it was shown that the β cell–directed transgenic expression of a GAD antisense oligonucleotide prevented diabetes in non-obese diabetic (NOD) mice (3). Although highly suggestive, these data require confirmation. It will be important to determine whether NOD mice genetically deficient in both GAD65 and GAD67 are protected from

0732-0582/01/0407-0131$14.00

131

diabetes at variance with NOD mice deficient only in GAD65 that do develop diabetes (4).

Islet-reactive T cells are present in the blood of healthy individuals as is illustrated by the possibility of raising GAD-specific T cell lines from normal peripheral blood lymphocytes (5). The peaceful coexistence of such "physiologic" autoreactive T cells with the organ expressing the target autoantigen suggests the possibility of ignorance or indifference. Indifference was initially described by Zinkernagel's group in double transgenic mice that express both a given antigen in their pancreatic β cells and the specific T cell receptor (TCR) on a large proportion of T cells, and which yet do not develop either insulitis or diabetes (6).

Which are the distinctive features of these physiologic autoreactive cells and of the pathogenic T cells incriminated in diabetes? What mechanisms drive the emergence of pathogenic T cells? What are the respective roles of activation of islet-reactive lymphocytes and of the decreased efficacy of peripheral tolerance mechanisms that maintain self-tolerance throughout life? How can one explain the rupture of this self-tolerance in diabetic subjects? Can one envision its restoration, which would represent the best approach in preventing the disease since it does not expose the subjects to the hazards of generalized immunosuppression? These are the main questions addressed in this review.

HOW IS TOLERANCE TO β CELL AUTOANTIGENS MAINTAINED IN NORMAL SUBJECTS?

Thymic or central deletion of β cell–reactive T cell clones is one major potential mechanism. Various autoantigens, including β cell autoantigens, are expressed in the thymus [as recently extensively demonstrated for insulin (7), I-A2, GAD, glucagon, somatostatin, pancreatic polypeptide, retinal-specific antigens, myelin basic protein (MBP), thyroglobulin, C reactive protein and serum amyloid protein] (for review, see 8).

It is plausible that T cells showing high affinity for these antigens are deleted through negative selection, which, however, is only partial since, as mentioned above, autoantigen reactive T cells, presumably of low affinity, are found in the peripheral blood of normal individuals.

It is interesting in this context that diabetes is prevented in both NOD mice and Bio Breeding (BB) rats upon intrathymic grafting of syngeneic or allogeneic islets (9–13).

Islets were implanted either at birth or within 4 weeks of age. Diabetes prevention was associated with absolute absence of insulitis in most animals. The specificity of the tolerance induced for the islet tissue was evidenced by the persistent infiltration of salivary glands (9, 10) and of the thyroid (13). The facts that spleen cells from tolerant islet-grafted NOD mice did not transfer diabetes into immunoincompetent hosts (10) and that cyclophosphamide did not break the tolerance in one study (9) are compatible with a preferential deletional mechanism. Such deletion could particularly involve CD8 cells as evidenced in intrathymic islet grafting experiments performed in the streptozotocin-induced diabetes model (14).

Similarly, transgenic expression in the thymus and the β cells of a viral antigen (which in this setting may be considered as an autoantigen) is associated with a delayed appearance of diabetes after infection with the virus, contrasting with the early onset disease observed when the viral antigen is expressed exclusively in β cells (15).

Self-reactive T cells escaping central deletion are kept under control by mechanisms of peripheral tolerance that include indifference, peripheral deletion, anergy, and/or immunoregulation.

The first three mechanisms have been investigated in TCR transgenic models (in which specific T cells present in high proportions) are easy to trace with specific anti-TCR or anti-clonotype antibodies. They are more difficult and almost impossible to address in less reductionist systems closer to the physiological polyclonal situation in normal individuals.

Deletion of self-reactive T cells taking place in the periphery is a major mechanism for maintaining self-tolerance as shown for anti-ovalbumin (OVA) transgenic mice expressing large amounts of OVA in pancreatic β cells (16). Different groups have analyzed other double transgenic mice expressing influenza hemagglutinin (HA) in β cells and different class II–restricted HA-specific TCRs. In none of these models was there any evidence for efficient peripheral T cell tolerance. Thus, in all cases, a spontaneous activation of HA-specific transgenic T cells was observed that led to variable disease patterns ranging from benign insulitis with no disease (17) to moderate (17, 18) or fulminant diabetes (19).

These differences have been ascribed to either the genetic non-MHC background where the transgene was expressed (17) or to the level of affinity of the TCR for the MHC-peptide complexes, a high-affinity TCR favoring a more aggressive disease independently of the overall frequency of TCR-specific T cells.

As previously mentioned, clear evidence for autoreactive T cell indifference came from double transgenic mice expressing lymphochoriomeningitis virus (LCMV) protein in β cells and a class I–restricted specific TCR (6).

Indifference differs as a mechanism from anergy in that it does not imply that T cells are in any way "paralyzed" but suggests rather that the autoantigen is not adequately presented to T cells. One may assume that presentation of the autoantigen by the target cell that produces it will generally not be immunogenic because of the lack of costimulation signals. Presentation by professional antigen-presenting cells (APCs) (cross-priming) is quantitatively insufficient to be operational.

This is not, however, a general feature transgenic mice since in similar HA double diabetes occurred very rapidly independently of the genetic background (20). Here again, it was proposed that, first, disease severity correlated with the TCR affinity for peptide-MHC complexes and, second, that costimulation may not be required for the activation of high-affinity TCR- bearing cells.

Thus, taken together, these data show that peripheral self-tolerance is not a common phenomenon in these models and that when it occurs indifference and peripheral deletion appear as the main mechanisms. Importantly, no data has been reported so far arguing for anergy as a mechanism in these spontaneous disease models. However, we shall see further that the situation may be significantly different after autoantigen administration.

Immunoregulation has long been considered controversial but is now established on a firm basis, even if the underlying mechanisms are still ill defined (21–23). The strongest evidence in favor of a control of self-reactivity by regulatory T cells mainly derives from experiments showing that selective cell depletion of normal T cells may lead to autoimmune disease. A very striking observation in this context is that of the polyautoimmune syndrome that follows post-natal (day 3) thymectomy in some mouse strains (24, 25). Similarly, PVG.RT1^u rats thymectomized as adults and sublethally irradiated develop thyroiditis and diabetes (26). In such cases, autoimmunity is prevented by administration of selected T cell subsets from nonthymectomized animals [CD25$^+$ T cells in the mouse (25), RT6$^+$ or CD62L$^+$ cells in the rat (27)]. Regulatory T cells may be demonstrated in the prediabetic stage in animal models of IDDM. Thus, in the NOD mouse, diabetes onset is accelerated by thymectomy at 3 weeks of age (28) or by cyclophosphamide (29). In the spleen or the thymus of prediabetic mice, one can demonstrate regulatory T cells that inhibit diabetes transfer into immunoincompetent hosts (30). Further studies of these regulatory T cells in this model have revealed that they are CD4$^+$ CD62L$^+$ and/or CD25$^+$ (30–32) and that their regulatory function does not rely on the production of T helper (Th) 2 cytokines (IL-4, IL-10) (33) even if Th2 cytokines can inhibit IDDM onset on their own (34–36). The antigen specificity of these regulatory T cells is an unanswered question. Experiments by P McCullagh in sheep and rats (37) and by D Mason in rats (38) favor such antigen specificity: in utero thyroid ablation induces the secondary appearance of a state of antithyroid autoreactivity that is specific to the thyroid, probably due to the absence of differentiation of thyroid-specific regulatory T cells. Similar experiments have been reported by O Taguchi in neonatally orchidectomized mice (39, 40).

LOSS OF SELF-TOLERANCE TO β CELL AUTOANTIGENS IN IDDM

T Cell Activation

Compelling evidence suggests that β cell autoantigen(s)-driven T cell activation is a mandatory step for the emergence of the aggressive "diabetogenic" lymphocyte response. This is well illustrated by the exhaustion of the pathogenic potential of T cells from the spleen of diabetic NOD mice when they are parked in β cell–deprived recipients, namely irradiated adult NOD recipients whose β cells have been destroyed by alloxan treatment (41). The tight major histocompatibility complex (MHC)-IDDM association may also be interpreted as the need for defined pathogenic β cell epitopes to be presented by selected MHC molecules. In the same vein, one may note that transgenic NOD mice overexpressing B7 (42) or tumor necrosis factor (TNF) (43) in β cells show enhanced activation of β–cell autoantigen-specific T cells and accelerated diabetes onset.

This activation essentially involves Th1 cells because it is accelerated by administration of IL-12 (44) and impaired by treatment with a monoclonal antibody to interferon (IFN) γ (45). Furthermore, IFNγ receptor–deficient NOD mice do not develop diabetes (46), whereas IL-4-deficient NOD mice do (47).

Much remains to be learned, though, on the primary events triggering this T cell activation. The privileged role of CD8 cells has been referred to on the basis that treatment of very young NOD mice (2–5 week old) with a depleting CD8 antibody prevented insulitis (48). Intra-islet inflammation may also play a key role independently of the nature of the initial insult. This inflammation, whether primary, induced by a non-immune assault (such as a viral infection), or secondary to the first wave of emerging pathogenic CD4$^+$ Th1 or CD8$^+$ cells, will promote antigen spreading of the anti-β cell response (49). Such spreading probably explains the large spectrum of β cell epitopes targeted by autoreactive T and B cells in overtly diabetic humans and NOD mice.

The nature of the APC, its location, and the repetition of the antigen stimulation may be crucial in determining the chronicity of the process. The modalities of autoantigen presentation leading to autoimmune diseases are still ill-defined, as illustrated by the surprising observation that nonprofessional APCs, namely fibroblasts transfected with a thyroid autoantigen gene and also MHC class-II genes, induce autoimmune thyroiditis that more closely resembles human thyroiditis than that observed after immunization with the soluble antigens in the presence of adjuvants (50, 51). One would also have to explain why NOD mice lacking B cells are protected from diabetes (52–54), which points to a major role of B cells in β cell autoantigen presentation.

Several mechanisms have been discussed to explain the onset of the activation of autoreactive T cells. Antigen mimicry has been proposed as an explanation for the overcoming of T cell tolerance to autoantigens (55). This hypothesis has received some support in the case of IDDM from observations of the sharing of T cell epitopes and/or sequence homology between GAD and a Coxsackie B3 virus protein (56). There is some epidemiological and serological evidence in favor of Coxsackie B virus infection in human IDDM, but it remains weak (1). Additionally, recent data showing the ability of Coxsackie virus to elicit IDDM in BDC2.5 TCR transgenic mice, which show a restricted repertoire of non-GAD specific transgenic CD4 pathogenic T cells, indicate that the diabetogenic effect of Coxsackie is not due to mimicry but to bystander damage and T cell activation (57).

An increased or aberrant β cell expression of MHC, costimulatory, or adhesion molecules is another possibility that elicited major interest when an abnormal expression of HLA class II antigens was first described on β cells from recently diagnosed diabetic patients (58). This observation, which was not consistently confirmed, is in any case difficult to interpret as a definite proof for a primary event since it could be secondary to the cytokine release induced by the initial immune response. In fact, the transgenic β cell–targeted IFN-γ expression in non-autoimmunity-prone BALB/c mice triggers autoimmune insulitis (59). Finally, the role of inflammation-induced abnormal expression of molecules involved in antigen recognition remains a strong possibility either by triggering the initial autoimmune reaction or by perpetuating it through antigen spreading (49). This is well illustrated by Theiler's disease, where antigen spreading elicited by the inflammation, secondary to the viral insult, is responsible for disease chronicity with its typical relapses (60).

Another hypothesis relates to non–antigen specific stimulation. A role for superantigens has been postulated on the basis of results showing that islet-infiltrating T cells isolated from the pancreas of two recently diagnosed IDDM patients expressed a Vβ7-biased T cell repertoire (61). This hypothesis was strengthened by the finding in IDDM patients of an endogenous retrovirus selectively expanding Vβ7-expressing T cells (62). Here again one may question the primary versus the exacerbating role of such stimulation.

The Protective Role of Immunoregulation

The development of diabetes that follows T cell activation by β cell autoantigens is under the control of immunoregulatory $CD4^+$ T cells. Diabetes onset is accelerated by thymectomy at weaning (28), disruption of costimulatory pathways (inactivation of the CD28 or B7 gene by homologous recombination, CTLA4-Ig treatment) (32, 63) or treatment of young prediabetic NOD mice with cyclophosphamide (29). Similarly, fulminant diabetes is observed in transgenic mice (between 4 and 6 weeks of age) expressing a TCR derived from a diabetogenic T cell clone in a monoclonal fashion, a model that excludes the presence of regulatory T cells using a distinct TCR (64—our unpublished results]. Such mice are obtained by backcrossing conventional TCR transgenic BDC2.5 NOD mice with TCR $C\alpha^{-/-}$ or scid NODs to avoid endogenous α chain recombination.

Conversely, disease onset may be significantly delayed or prevented by the transfer of immunoregulatory T cells (30). Thus, in conventional mixing experiments, the transfusion of purified $CD4^+$ $CD62L^+$ cells prevents diabetes transfer into immunoincompetent NOD recipients (i.e. adult irradiated NOD or NOD scid) by diabetogenic lymphocytes (30, 31, 33). In $CD28^{-/-}$ NOD mice, diabetes acceleration is abrogated by the transfer of purified $CD25^+$ cells (32).

An unsettled question concerns the role of Th2 cytokines in this immune regulation. Such cytokines can indeed prevent diabetes onset (34–36). Prevention of insulitis and diabetes is also observed in transgenic NOD mice overexpressing IL-4 in β cells (65). On the other hand, the protective effect of $CD4^+$ $CD62L^+$ T cells discussed above is not abrogated by treatment with antibodies to IL-4 and IL-10 (33), and $IL-4^{-/-}$ mice do not show accelerated diabetes onset (47).

Conclusions

The coexistence of β cell–driven autoimmunity and immunoregulation in prediabetic NOD mice raises the question of the nature of the events leading to diabetes onset. It is difficult to determine when the immune status shifts from indifference to benign autoreactivity since insulitis, which is the most reliable indicator, could initially be non-immune related (peri-insulitis is observed in non-autoimmunity-prone congenic NOD mice) (66). It is also difficult to determine whether the onset of disease is due to the mere overriding of immunoregulation by T cell activation or concomitantly involves a decline in immunoregulation. This decline could have more general consequences since diabetes onset is associated in NOD mice with other autoimmune manifestations such as sialitis, thyroiditis (67), autoimmune hemolytic anemia (68), and antinuclear antibodies (69).

GENETIC AND ENVIRONMENTAL INFLUENCES

As mentioned above, T cell activation by β cell antigens may be triggered by environmental factors such as β cell tropic viruses, superantigens, or other polyclonal T cell activators. Genetically, MHC genes are obviously central for the presentation of β cell autoantigen(s) to T cells of diabetes-prone individuals. Numerous diabetes non-MHC predisposing genes have been mapped, but most of them are yet unidentified. The association of the IDDM predisposing insulin gene promoter polymorphism with decreased level of thymic proinsulin expression is particularly interesting in the context of our discussion because it implies that high levels of thymic insulin expression would be protective (7, 70).

Immunoregulation is also influenced by environmental and genetic factors. A number of infections nonspecifically inhibit diabetes onset, probably through induction of regulatory T cells. This has notably been shown for mycobacteria (71), viruses (72) and parasites (73). The protection afforded by complete Freund's adjuvant (CFA) is transferable to non-CFA-treated NOD mice by CD4 T cells (71, 74) and is abrogated by cyclophosphamide treatment (75) or administration of antibodies to IL-4 and IL-10 (76). Genetic protection afforded by HLA DQB1*0602 could be explained by immunoregulation (there is no defect in GAD peptide binding by DQB1*0602 HLA molecules) (77). One may hypothesize that HLA DQB1*0602 DR15 alleles confer an active protection as indicated by the capacity of the corresponding HLA molecules to present efficiently GAD epitopes to T cells. It is interesting in this context to mention that transgenic NOD mice expressing H-2^b (78) or H-2^k (79) class II genes are actively protected from diabetes (protection is abrogated by cyclophosphamide treatment, and protected mice harbor effector cells). Non-MHC genes also seem important in the control of regulatory T cells. This is well exemplified by the very rapid diabetes onset (4 weeks of age) observed when a T cell receptor transgene from the diabetogenic CD4 T cell clone (BDC2.5) is expressed in the C57BL/6-IHa2^{g7} background as compared with the slow progressing disease seen in the NOD background (80). Recent data suggest that in the NOD mouse Idd9 affects immunoregulation because disease-resistant Idd9 congenic NOD mice show increased expression of IL-4 in islets (80a). A case was made for the CTLA4 gene in human IDDM (81), which could be in keeping with the presence of the CTLA4 gene in the Idd5 region (82). This is particularly interesting in view of disease acceleration by blockade of the CD28/B7 costimulatory pathway (63), but it remains to be proven that it is the CTLA4 gene itself that is incriminated.

RESTORATION OF SELF-TOLERANCE BY β CELL ANTIGEN ADMINISTRATION

Diabetes Can Be Prevented in NOD Mice by Early Administration of a Variety of Soluble β Cell Autoantigens

As just discussed, the propensity to develop diabetes in NOD mice is an obvious consequence of the loss of tolerance to β cell antigens. One might have expected in the first instance that it would be difficult to restore self-tolerance since NOD mice have been difficult to tolerize in several settings. Neonatal administration of allogeneic cells does not induce full long-term tolerance in conditions where this is achieved in other strains (83). Transgenic expression of a β cell antigen GAD (MHC class-I promoter driven) does not induce tolerance in NOD mice, whereas it does so in non-autoimmune prone BALB/c mice (84). Full protection from diabetes was obtained with transgenic expression of proinsulin (85), but here again without evidence for central tolerance. No clear explanation is available for such resistance to tolerance, although it has been related to Ia^{g7} instability (86). In this context, it is remarkable that the administration of a number of β cell autoantigens to prediabetic NOD mice prevents diabetes onset, particularly since these antigens, which are recognized as candidate diabetes antigens, have not been able to induce the disease after administration to non-autoimmunity prone mice in the presence of adjuvants. The only exception to this rule is the successful immunization of C57BL/6 mice against an hsp 60 peptide coupled to a bovine serum albumin carrier (87). However, in these experiments the disease observed was mild and transient.

The first data showing protection in NOD mice concerned GAD and were published concomitantly by D Kaufman, who used intravenous injection of the antigen (88), and R Tisch, who used intrathymic injection (without direct evidence that GAD acted in situ rather than by seeding to the periphery) (89). Similar results were subsequently reported by B Singh using GAD67 (90). Several investigators have characterized GAD epitopes in terms of their capacity to stimulate T cell proliferation in NOD mice and in human diabetics and to modify disease course after in vivo administration to NOD mice (protection, as just discussed for the entire molecule, and also acceleration). No clear consensus was obtained on the relative importance of the different GAD peptide tested as shown on Table 1.

Similar protection was reported with insulin following intravenous, subcutaneous, oral and nasal administration (91–100). The use in the initial experiments of the metabolically active hormone (91–93) precluded a clear interpretation of the data due to the "β cell rest" effect that has been associated with a decreased expression of some islet autoantigens (101). The fact that the same protective effect was later observed upon administration of the non–metabolically active purified insulin B chain strongly argued for a tolerogenic effect (97, 98).

Hsp60, and more particularly one of its constitutive peptides, p277, was also protective in NOD mice (102, 103). Hsp60 is not a β cell–specific autoantigen, but its expression on the membrane of β cell granules (104) may be assumed to be enhanced in inflamed islets.

Most of the data reported above deal with relatively early administration of the autoantigens (typically 3 weeks of age for the two initial reports using GAD). Later administration of the peptides, however, still acts preventively as demonstrated for GAD at 8 weeks of age (105) and up to 17 weeks of age for hsp p277 (103). It was even shown, and these data require confirmation, that administration of GAD to diabetic mice prevented disease recurrence on syngeneic islet grafts for 6 to 8 weeks, an effect not observed, in the same study, with insulin B chain and hsp p277 (105).

Diabetes Protection Is Associated with Immune Deviation

The fact that antigen-induced protection is transferable to naive recipients by $\alpha\beta$ CD4 T cells supports the notion of an active tolerance phenomenon. This was first demonstrated by H Weiner's group after oral insulin-induced tolerance using irradiated recipients (95). Several groups subsequently confirmed these initial experiments, using a cotransfer model, and extended them to other candidate tolerogens such as GAD (106) and hsp 60 (107) as well as insulin (97).

Administration of the various autoantigens in soluble form mostly leads to a Th2 immune deviation. This is well illustrated by the shift of autoantibody responses to GAD (105, 106) and hsp60 (108) toward the Th2-dependent IgG1 isotype and by the in vitro T cell response to the tolerogen that results in preferential IL-4, IL-5, and IL-10 production (108, 109). A GAD-reactive Th2 type T cell clone has been derived from GAD tolerized mice and shown to be protective in cotransfer experiments (R Tisch, personal communication). The role of Th2 cytokines is also supported by the fact that IL-4$^{-/-}$ NOD mice resist GAD-induced protection even though they do not exhibit any acceleration of the spontaneous disease (110).

Two interesting exceptions to this preferential CD4^{+} Th2 polarization have been reported. The first one deals with the identification of $\gamma\delta$ CD8 T cells as the mediators of protection elicited in NOD mice following nasal administration of aerosolized insulin (99, 100). Diabetes protection in this system was associated with production of IL-10 within pancreatic lymph nodes by the protective $\gamma\delta$ CD8 T cells. This role of $\gamma\delta$ CD8 T cells is at variance with data obtained with oral insulin where $\alpha\beta$ CD4 regulatory T cells have been incriminated (95, 96),

TABLE 1 Antigenic GAD 65 epitopes identified in NOD mice (adapted from Ref. 148 with permission of the authors)

GAD65 peptide[88]	Immunological relevance	Disease relevance
GADp6 (78–97) 35%/85%[a]	■ GAD-primed T-cell response[149, 150] ■ Spontaneous T-cell response in young mice or adjuvant-protected mice only[149, 150] ■ Predominant Th1-like response[149, 150]	■ Immunization results in some exacerbation of disease onset in spontaneous IDDM models in NOD mice[149, 150]
GADp14 (202–221) 95%/100%	■ GAD-primed T-cell response[149, 150] ■ Spontaneous T-cell response in mice of all ages[149, 150] ■ Substantially reduced response in adjuvant-protected mice[149, 150] ■ Dominant Th1-like response[149, 150]	■ Immunization results in >50% decrease in disease incidence in spontaneous IDDM model[149, 150] ■ Immunization results in substantial decrease in disease incidence in cyclophosphamide-accelerated IDDM[149, 150]
GADp15 (217–236) 75%/100%	■ GAD-primed T-cell response[149, 150] ■ Spontaneous T-cell response in mice of all ages[149, 150] ■ Enhanced response in adjuvant-protected mice[149, 150]	■ No significant effect on disease incidence[149, 150]

GADp17 (247–266) 80%/95%[a]	▪ Spontaneous response in older mice only[88] ▪ Nasal administration results in IgG1 antibodies, IL-5, reduced IFNγ[b] [88]	▪ Nasal administration reduced incidence of IDDM in spontaneous disease model[b] [88] ▪ T-cell clones have no effect on induction of disease[152] ▪ Subcutaneous administration has no effect on incidence of disease[153]
GADp34 (509–528) 60%/100%[a]	▪ Spontaneous response in mice of all ages[88] ▪ No spontaneous response in NOD mice[149, 150] ▪ Nasal administration results in IgG1 antibodies, IL-5, reduced IFNγ[b] [88]	▪ Nasal administration reduces incidence of IDDM in spontaneous disease model[b] [88] ▪ Clones could not be obtained with specificity to this peptide[152] ▪ Subcutaneous administration has no effect on incidence of disease[153]
GADp35 (524–543) 80%/100%[a]	▪ Spontaneous response in mice of all ages[88] ▪ No spontaneous response in NOD mice[149, 150, 151] ▪ Nasal administration results in IgG1 antibodies, IL-5, reduced IFNγ[b] [88]	▪ Nasal administration reduces incidence of IDDM in spontaneous disease model[b] [88] ▪ Clones have no effect on induction of disease[152] ▪ Subcutaneous administration has no effect on incidence of disease[153]

(a) Amino acid similarity to homologous peptide of mouse GAD67/mouse GAD65 respectively.
(b) Determined by administration of a "cocktail" of GADp17,34,35.

a difference perhaps due to the degradation of insulin in the digestive tract (99). The second exception deals with the possible involvement of TGFβ in oral insulin-induced tolerance. Tolerized mice expressed IL-4, IL-10, and TGFβ in their islets, whereas control mice essentially expressed IFNγ (111). It is important to determine whether these peculiarities are linked to the nature of the tolerogen or to its route of administration (i.e. preferentially involving the mucosal immune system).

Immune deviation also provides the most likely explanation of diabetes protection afforded by altered peptide ligands (APL). It was initially thought that APLs acted through blockade of the binding of diabetogenic peptides to MHC molecules. Data obtained with APLs in experimental allergic encephalomyelitis (EAE) (with abrogation of the protection by anti-IL-4 and anti-IL-10 antibodies) (112) rather suggest that APLs act through immune deviation. This is in keeping with the observation that diabetes prevention by MHC-blocking peptides requires the induction of an active immune response (113).

It has not proven possible to induce diabetes protection by early administration of GAD or insulin B chain to BB rats as described above for NOD mice (114, 115). It was even shown that oral insulin with adjuvant could accelerate disease onset in these animals (116). This difference might be explained by the absence of the regulatory RT6 cell type in BB rats, inasmuch as one assumes that the protection would have involved such regulatory cells.

Protection Is Associated with Bystander Suppression

NOD mice injected with GAD at an early age show decreased proliferation to this autoantigen as a reflection of the restoration of self-tolerance. Importantly, this unresponsiveness is not restricted to the tolerogen but spreads to other β cell autoantigens, notably insulin and hsp60 (88, 89). A similar spreading is also observed for Th2-type responses (IL-4 and IL-5 production and IgG1 autoantibodies) (109). These observations are reminiscent of those made in EAE where the protection afforded by oral administration of MBP spread to the response to proteolipid protein, the other major myelin autoantigen implicated in the disease (117). The general interpretation of these data is that the production of regulatory cytokines, discussed above, driven by the tolerogen within the target tissue affects the immune responses directed against the other locally expressed autoantigens. This interpretation is further illustrated by the prevention of diabetes observed after the oral administration of insulin in the lymphochoriomeningitis virus–induced diabetes model (118).

Anergy or Deletion as Alternative Mechanisms of β Cell Antigen-Induced Tolerance: Evidence in TCR Transgenic Models

It is difficult to demonstrate anergy or deletion of specific T cells in polyclonal models like conventional NOD mice since it has been impossible hitherto in these mice to incriminate a primary epitope at the origin of the pathogenic autoimmune response. The reduced proliferation to the tolerogenic antigens, which in any case is partial, is not very informative. Hence the interest of TCR transgenic models in which autoantigen-specific pathogenic T cells are overexpressed or even monoclonal (after backcrossing to TCR $C\alpha^{-/-}$, $Rag^{-/-}$ or scid mice).

Interesting data have been obtained in inducing tolerance to the target peptide in double transgenic mice that had not spontaneously developed tolerance due to insufficient central deletion, peripheral anergy, or indifference. Intravenous injection of the tolerogenic target peptide (HA) could induce tolerance inasmuch as the peptide administration was regularly repeated (119, 120). Interestingly, tolerance was associated with massive peptide-induced apoptosis of transgenic T cells in the thymus and also in the periphery (as demonstrated in thymectomized mice). Remnant transgenic T cells were shown to be unable to proliferate to the antigen and thus termed anergic (119, 120). One may, however, question this definition since this unresponsiveness was not reversible in the presence of exogenous IL-2 (119). Anergy was also incriminated in a similar model using HA peptide plus anti-CD4 antibody, but here again there was no reversal after IL-2 addition and anergic cells were shown to produce IL-10 (18).

Conclusions

All the evidence presented above tends to indicate that tolerization by β cell autoantigens essentially acts through immune deviation toward Th2 and/or perhaps Th3 responses leading to bystander suppression and eventually diabetes protection.

Anergy or deletion may occur in some models, but this does not exclude the role of immunoregulation, which could be more prevalent in nontransgenic mice with a full T cell repertoire.

RESTORATION OF SELF-TOLERANCE TO β CELL ANTIGENS BY CD3 ANTIBODY TREATMENT

Diabetes Remission Is Induced by CD3 Antibody

CD3 monoclonal antibodies are immunosuppressants like many antibodies to T cell receptors such as antibodies to CD4. They are also known to promote tolerance to allografts as shown in a rat model (121), a property again shared with CD4 antibodies. It could therefore be expected that CD3 antibodies would prevent diabetes onset in the NOD mouse. The surprise came from the very unexpected window of efficacy of the antibody with regard to disease course (122, 123). To have an effect the antibody has to be administered not more than 6 to 10 weeks before presumed diabetes onset, and even then this effect is transient, with a diabetes retardation of only 4 to 6 weeks. No diabetes retardation is seen if CD3 antibody is administered earlier, a finding at variance with experience gained with other immunointervention procedures, with the exception of neonatal injection of CD3 antibody itself, which provides a very long and complete protection (the reasons for which are still debated) (124). In fact, the antibody effect is the most spectacular in established disease, i.e. in already diabetic mice, inasmuch as mice are treated within one or two weeks following diabetes onset (before β cells are completely destroyed). The only other strategy for which such a major effect in overt disease was observed is the administration of anti-lymphocyte serum (125).

In CD3 antibody-treated mice insulitis is cleared rapidly within 2 or 3 days; glycemia normalizes after 2 to 3 weeks following a 5-day treatment. The remission is complete and definitive (follow-up of >6 months). The rate of remission depends on the disease severity, which is linked to breeding facilities. The milder the disease, the higher the remission rate (our unpublished results). The effect was initially described with the entire molecule (122), but it is also obtained with non-mitogenic F(ab′)2 fragments (123). It is even better with such F(ab′)2 fragments than with the entire molecule, probably due to the deleterious action on β cells of cytokines produced when the mitogenic antibody is used.

CD3-Induced Tolerance Is Best Explained by Activation of Regulatory T Cells

CD3 antibody, and even F(ab′)2 fragments although to a lesser degree, do induce some T cell depletion, but such depletion is incomplete and transient. Antigen modulation of the TCR CD3 complex is another major and more important mode of action but is also transient and vanishes as soon as the antibody disappears from serum (126). The same comment applies to antigen coating (blind folding). It is thus difficult to explain the very long duration of the effect of CD3 antibody in the NOD mouse by one of these three mechanisms.

Another more attractive hypothesis is immunoregulation. This hypothesis is indirectly suggested by the reappearance of insulitis in CD3-protected mice (at the periphery of the islets as is found in prediabetic mice after its initial clearance) (122). It is also indicated by the fact that the spleen cells from protected CD3 antibody–treated mice still transfer diabetes to immunoincompetent hosts (irradiated or scid NOD mice) (123).

Direct evidence for regulation comes from two sets of data. First, tolerance (defined here as operational tolerance) is broken down by one injection of cyclophosphamide (123). Second, CD4$^+$ CD62L$^+$ spleen cells from CD3 antibody-protected mice inhibit diabetes transfer afforded by diabetogenic cells (our unpublished results).

The active nature of tolerance and the possible role of cytokines are confirmed by inhibition of CD3 antibody-induced tolerance observed when cyclosporin A is administered concomitantly with CD3 antibody (123). There is no clear Th2 polarization though, except in the first few days following the antibody injection. Additionally, F(ab′)2 fragments that are fully active do not induce any detectable cytokine release even if they do elicit some cytokine transcription (as detected for IL-4 and IL-10 messages).

CD3 Antibody-Induced Tolerance Requires T Cell Preactivation

The preferential effect of the antibody in established disease suggests that CD3 antibodies are most active in inducing regulatory T cells when there is T cell preactivation. This is in keeping with JA Smith & JA Bluestone's observation that CD3 antibodies, and most notably their F(ab')2 fragments, preferentially induce the production of Th2 cytokines in cell lines presenting a marked state of activation (127). Although our data relate to non-Th2 regulatory T cells, one may assume that they are also a preferential target of CD3 antibody when activated, which would fit with the therapeutic effect on established diabetes (122). However, an explanation is still lacking for the molecular basis of the CD3 antibody-induced signaling in these activated cells and their relationship to immunoregulation.

Other Antibodies May Induce Tolerance Through a Similar Mechanism (CD4, CD40L, MHC Class II)

Prevention of diabetes onset has been reported for a number of other monoclonal antibodies administered in the early life of the NOD mouse. The most spectacular data concern MHC class II and CD4 antibodies. In the case of MHC class II antibodies (128), the effect was obtained only when they were administered before 6 weeks of age. As in the case of CD3 antibody, the therapeutic effect was associated with stimulation of CD4$^+$ regulatory cells (protection was transferable to non-antibody-treated mice). The effect was long lasting and was not reversed by cyclophosphamide.

Several CD4 antibodies protect NOD mice against diabetes. Dramatic results were obtained with GK1.5, a depleting CD4 antibody with long-term tolerance established when the antibody was administered at an early age for a sustained period of time [4 weeks (129) or 15 weeks (130)]. Nondepleting antibodies to CD4 were also protective when administered to recipients of diabetogenic T cells (131).

Interesting results were also reported with CD40L (132), CD8 (48, 125, 133), and TCR $\alpha\beta$ antibodies (134). In none of these cases, however, was long-term tolerance noted in already diabetic mice.

OTHER TOLERANCE-INDUCING PROTOCOLS

A very large number of immunotherapies have been shown to protect NOD mice against diabetes when administered early, at the prediabetic stage. We consider here only methods affording protection lasting for several months. All other procedures may be classified in the frame of nonspecific immunosuppression or immunoprotection but not tolerance, even as defined here in the broad sense of operational tolerance.

Intrathymic Islet Grafts

As mentioned above, grafting syngeneic islets within the thymus gland of NOD mice or BB rats protects them against subsequent development of diabetes (9, 10, 13). Importantly, this strategy has only been successfully applied in very young animals (less than 4 weeks of age). One may question its application at a more advanced age with regard to both its efficacy and the feasibility of performing the intrathymic transplantation in atrophic thymuses.

B Cell Depletion

B cell depletion may be obtained either by invalidating the Ig genes (Ig$^{-/-}$) (52, 53) or by treatment with anti-μ serum at birth (54). B cell depletion is associated with definitive diabetes protection (52–54) suggesting that B cells are involved in the loss of self-tolerance in NOD mice (perhaps through antigen presentation).

Allogeneic Bone Marrow Transplantation

NOD mice that have been irradiated as adults and grafted with allogeneic bone marrow cells do not develop diabetes when they survive the bone marrow transplantation (135), which suggests that reactivity to β cell antigens lies in the lymphoid stem cell. One cannot, however, exclude the possibility that diabetes prevention in these experiments is secondary to immunosuppression caused by the allogeneic reaction.

NK T Cell Stimulation

NK T cells represent a discrete T cell subset characterized by the use of an invariant TCR α chain (Vα14 Jα281) and by the coexistence of T cell and NK T cell markers (136). NK T cells produce large amounts of IL-4 (and IFNγ) in response to TCR cross-linking or to the glycolipid α-galactosyl ceramide (α-GalCer) presented by CD1d. The role of NK T cells in the control of autoimmunity is suggested by their numerical and functional deficiency in NOD (137) and SJL (138) mice, two autoimmunity-prone mice. The partial prevention of diabetes afforded by NK T cell overexpression in Vα14 Jα281 transgenic NOD mice (139) argues for the possible implication of NK T cells in the control of diabetes emergence in NOD mice. NK T cells may not act directly to downregulate diabetogenic T cells, as suggested by their absence in the thymus of 3-week-old NOD mice (137) where regulatory T cells of the CD4$^+$ CD62L$^+$ type are found (31). In fact, NK T cells are CD62L$^-$.

In any case, NK T cells could represent an interesting target for restoration or boosting of immunoregulation in NOD mice, since administration of α Gal-Cer protects against diabetes either when given early in the spontaneous disease (A Herbelin, L van Kaer, personal communication) or in cyclophosphamide-treated

NOD mice (T Delovitch, personal communication). In the latter case, protection is associated with Th2 polarization.

THREE TYPES OF REGULATORY CELLS

A link exists between spontaneous (physiologic) and inducible (restored) self-tolerance to β cell autoantigens (Figure 1, Table 2).

The data discussed in the preceding pages strongly suggest that distinct regulatory T cells play a major role in maintaining or restoring tolerance to β cell antigens. These various regulatory T cells can provisionally be classified in three major cell types:

— cytokine-dependent CD4 regulatory T cells, namely Th2 and Th3, to which one might add Tr1 cells, although as yet there is no data in diabetes on this cell type,

— CD4$^+$ CD25$^+$ CD62L$^+$ T cells that apparently do not depend on cytokine production and

— NK T cells.

This is not an exclusive list since in some settings other cell types might also be involved, notably $\gamma\delta$ CD8 T cells as reported in the case of nasally induced tolerance to insulin (99).

Th2 (and Th3) Cells in the Response to Soluble Autoantigens

It is now widely accepted that, under defined conditions of presentation, some antigens may give rise to immune responses essentially dependent on Th2 cytokines

TABLE 2   Subsets of lymphocytes mediating immunoregulation

	Autoimmune related regulatory T cells (ART cells)	NK T cells	Th2 cells
Experimental condition	Spontaneous (thymus) Anti-CD3	Spontaneous Boosted by α-GalCer	Peripheral (β-cell antigens) CFA
Cytokine production	Undetectable	IL-4, IFNγ	IL-4, IL-10
Inhibition by IL-4/IL-10 antibody	−	+	+
Phenotype	CD4$^+$ CD62L$^+$ CD25$^+$	CD4/DN CD62L$^-$ CD25$^-$ CD122$^+$	CD4$^+$

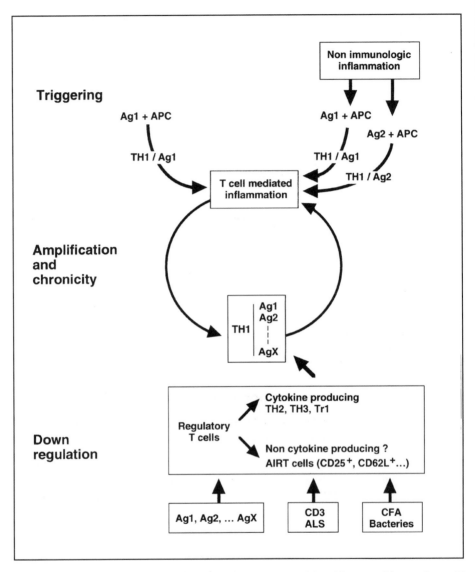

Figure 1 Activation of β cell antigen reactive T cells in IDDM and its control by regulatory T cells. Schematic representation of the immunopathological mechanisms in autoimmune diabetes.

(IL-4, IL-10, IL-13) or on TGFβ (Th3 cells). Th2 cells may also be induced by cell-associated antigens as in the case of allogeneic neonatal tolerance. But such examples are less common than those of stimulation by soluble antigens (allergens or soluble autoantigens in the absence of CFA as in experiments mentioned above using β cell autoantigens in the NOD mouse).

CD4$^+$ CD25$^+$ CD62L$^+$ in Response to Islet-Borne Autoantigens

Data derived from several models indicate the existence of regulatory T cells controlling the onset of pathologic autoimmunity. These models include (*a*) the post-thymectomy autoimmune syndromes described in the mouse (day 3 thymectomy) (24) and in the rat (adult thymectomy irradiation) (26), (*b*) the in utero thyroid ablation experiments in the sheep and in the rat (37, 38), (*c*) the orchectomy experiments in neonatal mice (39) and (*d*) the NOD mouse (prediabetic stage and CD3 antibody-treated diabetic mice) (28, 29, 31–33, 123).

Although it is far from established that the cells implicated in these four models represent a single cell type, there is a strong suggestion that these subsets at least grossly overlap.

Phenotypically, these cells, which we shall call autoimmune-related regulatory T cells or ART cells, are CD4$^+$ CD25$^+$ CD62L$^+$. It may be important to stress the fragility of these markers. Their stability is not established, and undoubtedly none of them is specific to the regulatory subset in question or related to their function. Twenty years after the initial mistakes on suppressor cells, we should not repeat the error of applying an overly specific label to ART cells.

There are no data indicating that ART cells produce cytokines or require them for their survival. IL-4$^{-/-}$ BALB/c mice still possess the CD25$^+$ cells defined on the basis of their capacity to inhibit the postnatal autoimmune syndrome (E Shevach, personal communication), and IL-4$^{-/-}$ NOD mice do not show accelerated disease progression (47) and possess regulatory T cells (assessed by co-transfer) at the prediabetic stage (33). Whether or not they act through membrane molecules such as CTLA4, as recently suggested in the post-thymectomy model (139a), or other molecules is still debatable.

ART cells appear early in ontogeny as suggested by P McCullagh & O Taguchi's experiments (37, 39). They are found in neonatal or 3-week-old mouse thymus as illustrated by the effects of early thymectomy in normal (24) and NOD (28) mice. Their differentiation requires the presence of the CD28-B7 costimulatory pathway, as demonstrated by diabetes acceleration in B7$^{-/-}$ or CD28$^{-/-}$ mice and diabetes protection in these mice after transfer of CD25$^+$ T cells derived from conventional NOD mice (32).

Lastly, ART cells are probably autoantigen-specific, as illustrated by thyroid and testis ablation experiments (37–39) that show organ-specific depletion of the regulatory cells. ART cells are activated by CD3 antibody treatment, and apparently not by soluble autoantigens, which induce Th2 or Th3 cells. As yet it is unclear whether their activation requires direct presentation by the target cells or presentation by professional APC present in the vicinity of the target cell. The question is still posed of the identity or difference in autoantigen presentation leading to either pathogenic autoimmunity or regulation of the ART cell type.

NK T Cell in the Control of the Differentiation of Regulatory T Cells

Intrathymic NK T cells produce IL-4 and IFNγ very early in development and could therefore play an important role in CD4 T cell subset differentiation. This is supported by the observation that $\beta 2m^{-/-}$ C57BL/6 mice that are NK T cell–deficient do not produce Th2-dependent IgE after polyclonal anti-IgD stimulation (140), and by the Th2 polarization (with high serum IgE levels) of transgenic mice overexpressing NK T cells (Vα14 Jα281 transgenics) (139, 141). The dependency is not absolute, however, since the NK T cell deficient CD1$^{-/-}$ mice (142) do mount Th2 responses. One possible explanation of the role of NK T cell deficiency in NOD or SJL mice is that NK T cells have an additional (but not mandatory) role in T cell–mediated regulation and that their effect is not necessarily direct but might derive from an indirect effect on the maintenance or survival of other regulatory T cell types (Th2 cells or ART cells).

TOLERANCE CLINICAL TRIALS

Autoantigens

Ongoing Trials   Several clinical trials of various autoantigens are under way in different clinical settings.

Parenteral or oral insulin has been used in a large-scale preventive protocol (DPT1) following encouraging Phase I studies (143, 144). The results of these trials are not yet available. Oral insulin has also been used in recently diagnosed diabetics with little or no effect. Insulin has been administered intranasally to prediabetics in a small-scale study (145).

GAD Phase I trials are being performed with the whole recombinant molecule.

The p277 peptide of hsp 60 is being used in Phase I/II trials in recently diagnosed diabetics, with promising data. In addition, the treatment appears safe since no acceleration of diabetes has been seen.

Comments   The strategy is very attractive since one may expect very limited toxicity of the autoantigen preparation. There is no risk of overimmunosuppression since in most protocols the autoantigen is used alone, without concomitant immunosuppressive treatment. It is also inexpensive, particularly when synthetic peptides are used in place of the whole recombinant molecules.

The risks differ in prediabetic and recently diagnosed subjects. In the first case (prediabetes) the main risk is that of acceleration of diabetes onset owing to undesirable idiosyncratic sensitization rather than tolerance. This risk is illustrated by the induction of diabetes observed in double transgenic mice expressing OVA in their β cells and anti-OVA TCR after oral administration of large doses of the antigen (146). However, the risk should not be exaggerated since these double transgenic mouse experiments were performed under extreme conditions and no disease aggravation was observed in any of the oral tolerance therapeutic trials performed so far. In the second case (recently diagnosed diabetes), efficacy may be insufficient because of the advanced stage of disease, except for hsp60 that has been shown to act late. Additionally, establishment of tolerance may take too long to be operational before most β cells are destroyed.

CD3 Antibodies

Ongoing Trials   Two clinical trials have been started to evaluate the effect of CD3 antibodies in recently diagnosed diabetics. In both trials, the antibody is administered for a short period of time (less than a month). The antibodies have been humanized by genetic engineering to ensure 1) that they are not mitogenic and thus do not lead to the massive cytokine release observed after the first injection of OKT3 (with severe clinical symptoms) (147), and 2) that they are not immunogenic. The endpoints are endogenous insulin production (C peptide) and to a lesser degree insulin requirement (U/kg).

Comments   The CD3 approach is also very attractive because its effects are both immediate (through the clearing of insulitis that follows the initiation of the treatment) and long lasting (through the stimulation of regulatory T cells). The treatment works at its best in already established disease even at a relatively advanced stage (122). The treatment is of short duration, which reduces the risk of overimmunosuppression and the cost.

The risk of a cytokine release syndrome is minimal, due to the antibody molecule modification, but cannot be formally excluded.

CONCLUSIONS

It appears that a number of therapeutic procedures can be proposed to restore self-tolerance to β cells in diabetes. It is remarkable that such perspectives of tolerance induction may be considered in a disease where the primary triggering autoantigen has not been formally identified. In the case of β cell antigen-induced diabetes protection, tolerance is mediated by bystander suppression induced by the tolerogen, whatever its role in the initiation of islet-specific autoimmunity. In the case of CD3 antibodies, which are by themselves non–antigen specific, tolerance specificity is afforded by the autoantigens expressed by the remnant β cells. The data and concepts discussed here for IDDM may also apply to most autoimmune diseases, particularly to those like IDDM that are mediated by Th1 T cells. In terms of basic understanding, they provide new insights into the cellular and molecular mechanisms of tolerance to self-antigens. From the therapeutic standpoint, they open new perspectives that are now being investigated clinically with the hope of proposing a specific and safe therapeutic approach to diseases that hitherto have essentially been tackled using relatively toxic and nonspecific chemicals, which involves the persistent risk of overimmunosuppression.

Visit the Annual Reviews home page at www.AnnualReviews.org

LITERATURE CITED

1. Bach JF. 1994. Insulin-dependent diabetes mellitus as an autoimmune disease. *Endocrine Rev.* 15(4):516–42
2. Delovitch TL, Singh B. 1997. The nonobese diabetic mouse as a model of autoimmune diabetes: immune dysregulation gets the NOD. *Immunity* 7(6):727–38
3. Yoon JW, Yoon CS, Lim HW, Huang QQ, Kang Y, Pyun KH, Hirasawa K, Sherwin RS, Jun HS. 1999. Control of autoimmune diabetes in NOD mice by GAD expression or suppression in beta cells. *Science* 284(5417):1183–87
4. Kash SF, Condie BG, Baekkeskov S. 1999. Glutamate decarboxylase and GABA in pancreatic islets: lessons from knock-out mice. *Hormone Metab. Res.* 31(5):340–44
5. Lohmann T, Leslie RDG, Londei M. 1996. T cell clones to epitopes of glutamic acid decarboxylase 65 raised from normal subjects and patients with insulin-dependent diabetes. *J. Autoimmun.* 9(3):385–89
6. Ohashi PS, Oehen S, Buerki K, Pircher H, Ohashi CT, Odermatt B, Malissen B, Zinkernagel RM, Hengartner H. 1991. Ablation of "tolerance" and induction of diabetes by virus infection in viral antigen transgenic mice. *Cell* 65(2):305–17
7. Vafiadis P, Bennett ST, Todd JA, Nadeau J, Grabs R, Goodyer CG, Wickramasinghe S, Colle E, Polychronakos C. 1997. Insulin expression in human thymus is modulated by INS VNTR alleles at the IDDM2 locus. *Nat. Genet.* 15(3):289–92
8. Hanahan D. 1998. Peripheral-antigen-expressing cells in thymic medulla: factors in self-tolerance and autoimmunity. *Curr. Opin. Immunol.* 10(6):656–62
9. Charlton B, Taylor-Edwards C, Tisch R, Fathman CG. 1994. Prevention of diabetes and insulitis by neonatal intrathymic islet administration in NOD mice. *J. Autoimmun.* 7(5):549–60
10. Gerling IC, Serreze DV, Christianson SW, Leiter EH. 1992. Intrathymic islet cell transplantation reduces beta-cell autoimmunity and prevents diabetes in NOD/Lt mice. *Diabetes* 41(12):1672–76
11. Nomura Y, Stein E, Mullen Y. 1993. Prevention of overt diabetes and insulitis by intrathymic injection of syngeneic islets in newborn nonobese diabetic (NOD) mice. *Transplantation* 56(3):638–42
12. Koevary SB, Blomberg M. 1992. Prevention of diabetes in BB/Wor rats by intrathymic islet injection. *J. Clin. Invest.* 89(2):512–16
13. Posselt AM, Barker CF, Friedman AL, Naji A. 1992. Prevention of autoimmune diabetes in the BB rat by intrathymic islet transplantation at birth. *Science* 256(5061):1321–24
14. Baumann EE, Buckingham F, Herold KC. 1995. Intrathymic transplantation of islet antigen affects CD8$^+$ diabetogenic T-cells resulting in tolerance to autoimmune IDDM. *Diabetes* 44(8):871–77
15. Von Herrath MG, Dockter J, Oldstone MB. 1994. How virus induces a rapid or slow onset insulin-dependent diabetes mellitus in a transgenic model. *Immunity* 1(3):231–42
16. Kurts C, Sutherland RM, Davey G, Li M, Lew AM, Blanas E, Carbone FR, Miller JF, Heath WR. 1999. CD8 T cell ignorance or tolerance to islet antigens depends on antigen dose. *Proc. Natl. Acad. Sci. USA* 96(22):12703–7
17. Scott B, Liblau R, Degermann S, Marconi LA, Ogata L, Caton AJ, McDevitt HO, Lo D. 1994. A role for non-MHC genetic

polymorphism in susceptibility to spontaneous autoimmunity. *Immunity* 1(1):73–82

18. Lanoue A, Bona C, Von Boehmer H, Sarukhan A. 1997. Conditions that induce tolerance in mature CD4$^+$ T cells. *J. Exp. Med.* 185(3):405–14

19. Radu DL, Brumeanu TD, McEvoy RC, Bona CA, Casares S. 1999. Escape from self-tolerance leads to neonatal insulin-dependent diabetes mellitus. *Autoimmunity* 30(4):199–207

20. Morgan DJ, Liblau R, Scott B, Fleck S, McDevitt HO, Sarvetnick N, Lo D, Sherman LA. 1996. CD8($^+$) T cell-mediated spontaneous diabetes in neonatal mice. *J. Immunol.* 157(3):978–83

21. Shevach EM. 2000. Regulatory T cells in autoimmunity. *Annu. Rev. Immunol.* 18(1):423–49

22. Sakaguchi S. 2000. Regulatory T cells: key controllers of immunologic self-tolerance. *Cell* 101(5):455–58

23. Mason D, Powrie F. 1998. Control of immune pathology by regulatory T cells. *Curr. Opin. Immunol.* 10(6):649–55

24. Nishizuka Y, Sakakura T. 1969. Thymus and reproduction: sex-linked dysgenesis of the gonad after neonatal thymectomy in mice. *Science* 166(906):753–55

25. Asano M, Toda M, Sakaguchi N, Sakaguchi S. 1996. Autoimmune disease as a consequence of developmental abnormality of a T cell subpopulation. *J. Exp. Med.* 184(2):387–96

26. Saoudi A, Seddon B, Fowell D, Mason D. 1996. The thymus contains a high frequency of cells that prevent autoimmune diabetes on transfer into prediabetic recipients. *J. Exp. Med.* 184(6):2393–98

27. Seddon B, Saoudi A, Nicholson M, Mason D. 1996. CD4$^+$CD8$^-$ thymocytes that express L-selectin protect rats from diabetes upon adoptive transfer. *Eur. J. Immunol.* 26(11):2702–8

28. Dardenne M, Lepault F, Bendelac A, Bach JF. 1989. Acceleration of the onset of diabetes in NOD mice by thymectomy

at weaning. *Eur. J. Immunol.* 19(5):889–95

29. Yasunami R, Bach JF. 1988. Antisuppressor effect of cyclophosphamide on the development of spontaneous diabetes in NOD mice. *Eur. J. Immunol.* 18(3):481–84

30. Boitard C, Yasunami R, Dardenne M, Bach JF. 1989. T cell-mediated inhibition of the transfer of autoimmune diabetes in NOD mice. *J. Exp. Med.* 169(5):1669–80

31. Herbelin A, Gombert JM, Lepault F, Bach JF, Chatenoud L. 1998. Mature mainstream TCR alpha beta($^+$)CD4($^+$) thymocytes expressing L-selectin mediate "active tolerance" in the nonobese diabetic mouse. *J. Immunol.* 161(5):2620–28

32. Salomon B, Lenschow DJ, Rhee L, Ashourian N, Singh B, Sharpe A, Bluestone JA. 2000. B7/CD28 costimulation is essential for the homeostasis of the CD4$^+$CD25$^+$ immunoregulatory T cells that control autoimmune diabetes. *Immunity* 12(4):431–40

33. Lepault F, Gagnerault MC. 2000. Characterization of peripheral regulatory CD4($^+$) T cells that prevent diabetes onset in nonobese diabetic mice. *J. Immunol.* 164(1):240–47

34. Rapoport MJ, Jaramillo A, Zipris D, Lazarus AH, Serreze DV, Leiter EH, Cyopick P, Danska JS, Delovitch TL. 1993. Interleukin 4 reverses T cell proliferative unresponsiveness and prevents the onset of diabetes in nonobese diabetic mice. *J. Exp. Med.* 178(1):87–99

35. Pennline KJ, Roque-Gaffney E, Monahan M. 1994. Recombinant human IL-10 prevents the onset of diabetes in the nonobese diabetic mouse. *Clin. Immunol. Immunopathol.* 71(2):169–75

36. Zaccone P, Phillips J, Conget I, Gomis R, Haskins K, Minty A, Bendtzen K, Cooke A, Nicoletti F. 1999. Interleukin-13 prevents autoimmune diabetes in NOD mice. *Diabetes* 48(8):1522–28

37. McCullagh P. 1996. The significance of

immune suppression in normal self tolerance. *Immunol. Rev.* 149:127–53

38. Seddon B, Mason D. 1999. Peripheral autoantigen induces regulatory T cells that prevent autoimmunity. *J. Exp. Med.* 189(5):877–82

39. Taguchi O, Nishizuka Y. 1987. Self tolerance and localized autoimmunity. Mouse models of autoimmune disease that suggest tissue-specific suppressor T cells are involved in self tolerance. *J. Exp. Med.* 165(1):146–56

40. Taguchi O, Kontani K, Ikeda H, Kezuka T, Takeuchi M, Takahashi T, Takahashi T. 1994. Tissue-specific suppressor T cells involved in self-tolerance are activated extrathymically by self-antigens. *Immunology* 82(3):365–69

41. Larger E, Becourt C, Bach JF, Boitard C. 1995. Pancreatic islet beta cells drive T cell-immune responses in the nonobese diabetic mouse model. *J. Exp. Med.* 181(5):1635–42

42. Wong S, Guerder S, Visintin I, Reich EP, Swenson KE, Flavell RA, Janeway CA. 1995. Expression of the co-stimulator molecule B7-1 in pancreatic beta-cells accelerates diabetes in the NOD mouse. *Diabetes* 44(3):326–29

43. Green EA, Flavell RA. 1999. Tumor necrosis factor-alpha and the progression of diabetes in non-obese diabetic mice. *Immunol. Rev.* 169():11–22

44. Trembleau S, Penna G, Bosi E, Mortara A, Gately MK, Adorini L. 1995. Interleukin 12 administration induces T helper type 1 cells and accelerates autoimmune diabetes in NOD mice. *J. Exp. Med.* 181(2):817–21

45. Debray-Sachs M, Carnaud C, Boitard C, Cohen H, Gresser I, Bedossa P, Bach JF. 1991. Prevention of diabetes in NOD mice treated with antibody to murine IFN gamma. *J. Autoimmun.* 4(2):237–48

46. Wang B, Andre I, Gonzalez A, Katz JD, Aguet M, Benoist C, Mathis D. 1997. Interferon-gamma impacts at multiple points during the progression of autoimmune diabetes. *Proc. Natl. Acad. Sci. USA* 94(25):13844–49

47. Wang B, Gonzalez A, Hoglund P, Katz JD, Benoist C, Mathis D. 1998. Interleukin-4 deficiency does not exacerbate disease in NOD mice. *Diabetes* 47(8):1207–11

48. Wang B, Gonzalez A, Benoist C, Mathis D. 1996. The role of CD8$^+$ T cells in the initiation of insulin-dependent diabetes mellitus. *Eur. J. Immunol.* 26(8):1762–69

49. Bach JF, Koutouzov S, Van Endert PM. 1998. Are there unique autoantigens triggering autoimmune diseases? *Immunol. Rev.* 164:139–55

50. Shimojo N, Kohno Y, Yamaguchi K, Kikuoka S, Hoshioka A, Niimi H, Hirai A, Tamura Y, Saito Y, Kohn LD, Tahara K. 1996. Induction of Graves-like disease in mice by immunization with fibroblasts transfected with the thyrotropin receptor and a class II molecule. *Proc. Natl. Acad. Sci. USA* 93(20):11074–79

51. Guo J, Wang Y, Rapoport B, McLachlan SM. 2000. Evidence for antigen presentation to sensitized T cells by thyroid peroxidase (TPO)-specific B cells in mice injected with fibroblasts co-expressing TPO and MHC class II. *Clin. Exp. Immunol.* 119(1):38–46

52. Serreze DV, Chapman HD, Varnum DS, Hanson MS, Reifsnyder PC, Richard SD, Fleming SA, Leiter EH, Shultz LD. 1996. B lymphocytes are essential for the initiation of T cell-mediated autoimmune diabetes: Analysis of a new "speed congenic" stock of NOD.Ig mu(null) mice. *J. Exp. Med.* 184(5):2049–53

53. Akashi T, Nagafuchi S, Anzai K, Kondo S, Kitamura D, Wakana S, Ono J, Kikuchi M, Niho Y, Watanabe T. 1997. Direct evidence for the contribution of B cells to the progression of insulitis and the development of diabetes in non-obese diabetic mice. *Int. Immunol.* 9(8):1159–64

54. Noorchashm H, Noorchashm N, Kern J, Rostami SY, Barker CF, Naji A. 1997. B-cells are required for the initiation of

insulitis and sialitis in nonobese diabetic mice. *Diabetes* 46(6):941–46

55. Albert LJ, Inman RD. 1999. Molecular mimicry and autoimmunity. *N. Engl. J. Med.* 341(27):2068–74

56. Atkinson MA, Bowman MA, Campbell L, Darrow BL, Kaufman DL, MacLaren NK. 1994. Cellular immunity to a determinant common to glutamate decarboxylase and Coxsackie virus in insulin-dependent diabetes. *J. Clin. Invest.* 94(5):2125–29

57. Horwitz MS, Bradley LM, Harbertson J, Krahl T, Lee J, Sarvetnick N. 1998. Diabetes induced by Coxsackie virus: initiation by bystander damage and not molecular mimicry. *Nature Med.* 4(7):781–85

58. Bottazzo GF, Dean BM, McNally JM, MacKay EH, Swift PG, Gamble DR. 1985. In situ characterization of autoimmune phenomena and expression of HLA molecules in the pancreas in diabetic insulitis. *N. Engl. J. Med.* 313(6):353–60

59. Sarvetnick N, Shizuru J, Liggitt D, Martin L, McIntyre B, Gregory A, Parslow T, Stewart T. 1990. Loss of pancreatic islet tolerance induced by beta-cell expression of interferon-gamma. *Nature* 346(6287):844–47

60. Miller SD, Vanderlugt CL, Begolka WS, Pao W, Yauch RL, Neville KL, Katz Levy Y, Carrizosa A, Kim BS. 1997. Persistent infection with Theiler's virus leads to CNS autoimmunity via epitope spreading. *Nat. Med.* 3(10):1133–36

61. Conrad B, Weidmann E, Trucco G, Rudert WA, Behboo R, Ricordi C, Rodriguez-Rilo H, Finegold D, Trucco M. 1994. Evidence for superantigen involvement in insulin-dependent diabetes mellitus aetiology. *Nature* 371(6495):351–55

62. Conrad B, Weissmahr RN, Boni J, Arcari R, Schupbach J, Mach B. 1997. A human endogenous retroviral superantigen as candidate autoimmune gene in type I diabetes. *Cell* 90(2):303–13

63. Green JM, Noel PJ, Sperling AI, Walunas TL, Gray GS, Bluestone JA, Thomp-

son CB. 1994. Absence of B7-dependent responses in CD28-deficient mice. *Immunity* 1(6):501–8

64. Kurrer MO, Pakala SV, Hanson HL, Katz JD. 1997. Beta cell apoptosis in T cell-mediated autoimmune diabetes. *Proc. Natl. Acad. Sci. USA* 94(1):213–18

65. Mueller R, Krahl T, Sarvetnick N. 1996. Pancreatic expression of interleukin-4 abrogates insulitis and autoimmune diabetes in nonobese diabetic (NOD) mice. *J. Exp. Med.* 184(3):1093–99

66. Wicker LS, Appel MC, Dotta F, Pressey A, Miller BJ, Delarato NH, Fischer PA, Boltz RC Jr, Peterson LB. 1992. Autoimmune syndromes in major histocompatibility complex (MHC) congenic strains of nonobese diabetic (NOD) mice. The NOD MHC is dominant for insulitis and cyclophosphamide-induced diabetes. *J. Exp. Med.* 176(1):67–77

67. Bernard NF, Ertug F, Margolese H. 1992. High incidence of thyroiditis and anti-thyroid autoantibodies in NOD mice. *Diabetes* 41(1):40–46

68. Baxter AG, Mandel TE. 1991. Hemolytic anemia in non-obese diabetic mice. *Eur. J. Immunol.* 21(9):2051–55

69. Humphreys-Beher MG, Brinkley L, Purushotham KR, Wang PL, Nakagawa Y, Dusek D, Kerr M, Chegini N, Chan EK. 1993. Characterization of antinuclear autoantibodies present in the serum from nonobese diabetic (NOD) mice. *Clin. Immunol. Immunopathol.* 68(3):350–56

70. Pugliese A, Zeller M, Fernandez A JR, Zalcberg LJ, Bartlett RJ, Ricordi C, Pietropaolo M, Eisenbarth GS, Bennett ST, Patel DD. 1997. The insulin gene is transcribed in the human thymus and transcription levels correlated with allelic variation at the INS VNTR-IDDM2 susceptibility locus for type 1 diabetes. *Nat. Genet.* 15(3):293–97

71. Qin HY, Sadelain MW, Hitchon C, Lauzon J, Singh B. 1993. Complete Freund's adjuvant-induced T cells prevent the

development and adoptive transfer of diabetes in nonobese diabetic mice. *J. Immunol.* 150(5):2072–80

72. Oldstone MB. 1990. Viruses as therapeutic agents. I. Treatment of nonobese insulin-dependent diabetes mice with virus prevents insulin-dependent diabetes mellitus while maintaining general immune competence. *J. Exp. Med.* 171(6):2077–89

73. Cooke A, Tonks P, Jones FM, O'Shea H, Hutchings P, Fulford AJ, Dunne DW. 1999. Infection with Schistosoma mansoni prevents insulin dependent diabetes mellitus in non-obese diabetic mice. *Parasite Immunol.* 21(4):169–76

74. McInerney MF, Pek SB, Thomas DW. 1991. Prevention of insulitis and diabetes onset by treatment with complete Freund's adjuvant in NOD mice. *Diabetes* 40(6):715–25

75. Shehadeh N, Calcinaro F, Bradley BJ, Bruchlim I, Vardi P, Lafferty KJ. 1994. Effect of adjuvant therapy on development of diabetes in mouse and man. *Lancet* 343(8899):706–7

76. Calcinaro F, Gambelunghe G, Lafferty KJ. 1997. Protection from autoimmune diabetes by adjuvant therapy in the non-obese diabetic mouse: the role of interleukin-4 and interleukin-10. *Immunol. Cell Biol.* 75(5):467–71

77. Bach JM, Otto H, Nepom GT, Jung G, Cohen H, Timsit J, Boitard C, Van Endert PM. 1997. High affinity presentation of an autoantigenic peptide in type I diabetes by an HLA class II protein encoded in a haplotype protecting from disease. *J. Autoimmun.* 10(4):375–86

78. Singer SM, Tisch R, Yang XD, McDevitt HO. 1993. An Abd transgene prevents diabetes in nonobese diabetic mice by inducing regulatory T cells. *Proc. Natl. Acad. Sci. USA* 90(20):9566–70

79. Slattery RM, Miller JF, Heath WR, Charlton B. 1993. Failure of a protective major histocompatibility complex class II molecule to delete autoreactive T cells in autoimmune diabetes. *Proc. Natl. Acad. Sci. USA* 90(22):10808–10

80. Gonzalez A, Katz JD, Mattei MG, Kikutani H, Benoist C, Mathis D. 1997. Genetic control of diabetes progression. *Immunity* 7(6):873–83

80a. Lyons PA, Hancock WW, Denny P, Lord CJ, Hill NJ, Siegmund T, Todd JA, Phillips MS, Hess JF, Chen SL, Fischer PA, Peterson LB, Wicker LS. 2000. The NOD Idd9 genetic intervcal influences the pathogenicity of insulitis and contains molecular variants of Cd30, Tnfr2, and Cd137. *Immunity* 13:107–15

81. Nistico L, Buzzetti R, Pritchard LE, Van Der Auwera B, Giovannini C, Bosi E, Larrad MT, Rios MS, Chow CC, Cockram CS, Jacobs K, Mijovic C, Bain SC, Barnett AH, Vandewalle CL, Schuit F, Gorus FK, Tosi R, Pozzilli P, Todd JA. 1996. The CTLA-4 gene region of chromosome 2q33 is linked to, and associated with, type 1 diabetes. *Hum. Mol. Genet.* 5(7):1075–80

82. Cornall RJ, Prins JB, Todd JA, Pressey A, Delarato NH, Wicker LS, Peterson LB. 1991. Type 1 diabetes in mice is linked to the interleukin-1 receptor and Lsh/Ity/Bcg genes on chromosome 1. *Nature* 353(6341):262–65

83. Bendelac A, Boitard C, Bach JF, Carnaud C. 1989. Neonatal induction of allogeneic tolerance prevents T cell-mediated autoimmunity in NOD mice. *Eur. J. Immunol.* 19(4):611–16

84. Geng LP, Solimena M, Flavell RA, Sherwin RS, Hayday AC. 1998. Widespread expression of an autoantigen-GAD65 transgene does not tolerize non-obese diabetic mice and can exacerbate disease. *Proc. Natl. Acad. Sci. USA* 95(17):10055–60

85. French MB, Allison J, Cram DS, Thomas HE, Dempsey-Collier M, Silva A, Georgiou HM, Kay TW, Harrison LC, Lew AM. 1997. Transgenic expression of mouse proinsulin II prevents

diabetes in nonobese diabetic mice. *Diabetes* 46(1):34–39

86. Carrasco-Marin E, Shimizu J, Kanagawa O, Unanue ER. 1996. The class II MHC I-Ag7 molecules from non-obese diabetic mice are poor peptide binders. *J. Immunol.* 156(2):450–58

87. Elias D, Marcus H, Reshef T, Ablamunits V, Cohen IR. 1995. Induction of diabetes in standard mice by immunization with the p277 peptide of a 60-kDa heat shock protein. *Eur. J. Immunol.* 25(10):2851–57

88. Kaufman DL, Clare-Salzler M, Tian J, Forsthuber T, Ting GSP, Robinson P, Atkinson MA, Sercarz EE, Tobin AJ, Lehmann PV. 1993. Spontaneous loss of T-cell tolerance to glutamic acid decarboxylase in murine insulin-dependent diabetes. *Nature* 366(6450):69–72

89. Tisch R, Yang XD, Singer SM, Liblau RS, Fugger L, McDevitt HO. 1993. Immune response to glutamic acid decarboxylase correlates with insulitis in non-obese diabetic mice. *Nature* 366(6450):72–75

90. Elliott JF, Qin HY, Bhatti S, Smith DK, Singh RK, Dillon T, Lauzon J, Singh B. 1994. Immunization with the larger isoform of mouse glutamic acid decarboxylase (GAD67) prevents autoimmune diabetes in NOD mice. *Diabetes* 43(12):1494–99

91. Gotfredsen CF, Buschard K, Frandsen EK. 1985. Reduction of diabetes incidence of BB Wistar rats by early prophylactic insulin treatment of diabetes-prone animals. *Diabetologia* 28(12):933–35

92. Bertrand S, de Paepe M, Vigeant C, Yale JF. 1992. Prevention of adoptive transfer in BB rats by prophylactic insulin treatment. *Diabetes* 41(10):1273–77

93. Atkinson MA, MacLaren NK, Luchetta R. 1990. Insulitis and diabetes in NOD mice reduced by prophylactic insulin therapy. *Diabetes* 39(8):933–37

94. Daniel D, Wegmann DR. 1996. Protection of nonobese diabetic mice from diabetes by intranasal or subcutaneous administration

of insulin peptide B-(9–23). *Proc. Natl. Acad. Sci. USA* 93(2):956–60

95. Zhang ZJ, Davidson L, Eisenbarth G, Weiner HL. 1991. Suppression of diabetes in nonobese diabetic mice by oral administration of porcine insulin. *Proc. Natl. Acad. Sci. USA* 88(22):10252–56

96. Bergerot I, Ploix C, Petersen J, Moulin V, Rask C, Fabien N, Lindblad M, Mayer A, Czerkinsky C, Holmgren J, Thivolet C. 1997. A cholera toxoid-insulin conjugate as an oral vaccine against spontaneous autoimmune diabetes. *Proc. Natl. Acad. Sci. USA* 94(9):4610–14

97. Muir A, Peck A, Clare-Salzler M, Song YH, Cornelius J, Luchetta R, Krischer J, MacLaren N. 1995. Insulin immunization of nonobese diabetic mice induces a protective insulitis characterized by diminished intraislet interferon-gamma transcription. *J. Clin. Invest.* 95(2):628–34

98. Karounos DG, Bryson JS, Cohen DA. 1997. Metabolically inactive insulin analog prevents type I diabetes in prediabetic NOD mice. *J. Clin. Invest.* 100(6):1344–48

99. Hanninen A, Harrison LC. 2000. Gamma delta T cells as mediators of mucosal tolerance: the autoimmune diabetes model. *Immunol. Rev.* 173:109–19

100. Harrison LC, Dempsey-Collier M, Kramer DR, Takahashi K. 1996. Aerosol insulin induces regulatory CD8 gamma delta T cells that prevent murine insulin-dependent diabetes. *J. Exp. Med.* 184(6):2167–74

101. Anastasi E, Dotta F, Tiberti C, Vecci E, Ponte E, Di Mario U. 1999. Insulin prophylaxis down-regulates islet antigen expression and islet autoimmunity in the low-dose Stz mouse model of diabetes. *Autoimmunity* 29(4):249–56

102. Elias D, Reshef T, Birk OS, Van Der Zee R, Walker MD, Cohen IR. 1991. Vaccination against autoimmune mouse diabetes with a T-cell epitope of the human 65-kDa

heat shock protein. *Proc. Natl. Acad. Sci. USA* 88(8):3088–91

103. Elias D, Cohen IR. 1994. Peptide therapy for diabetes in NOD mice. *Lancet* 343(8899):704–6

104. Brudzynski K, Martinez V, Gupta RS. 1992. Secretory granule autoantigen in insulin-dependent diabetes mellitus is related to 62 kDa heat-shock protein (hsp60). *J. Autoimmun.* 5(4):453–63

105. Tian JD, Clare-Salzler M, Herschenfeld A, Middleton B, Newman D, Mueller R, Arita S, Evans C, Atkinson MA, Mullen Y, Sarvetnick N, Tobin AJ, Lehmann PV, Kaufman DL. 1996. Modulating autoimmune responses to GAD inhibits disease progression and prolongs islet graft survival in diabetes-prone mice. *Nat. Med.* 2(12):1348–53

106. Tian J, Atkinson MA, Clare Salzler M, Herschenfeld A, Forsthuber T, Lehmann PV, Kaufman DL. 1996. Nasal administration of glutamate decarboxylase (GAD65) peptides induces Th2 responses and prevents murine insulin-dependent diabetes. *J. Exp. Med.* 183(4):1561–67

107. Elias D, Cohen IR. 1995. Treatment of autoimmune diabetes and insulitis in NOD mice with heat shock protein 60 peptide p277. *Diabetes* 44(9):1132–38

108. Elias D, Meilin A, Ablamunits V, Birk OS, Carmi P, Konen-Waisman S, Cohen IR. 1997. Hsp60 peptide therapy of NOD mouse diabetes induces a Th2 cytokine burst and downregulates autoimmunity to various beta-cell antigens. *Diabetes* 46(5):758–64

109. Tian J, Lehmann PV, Kaufman DL. 1997. Determinant spreading of T helper cell 2 (Th2) responses to pancreatic islet autoantigens. *J. Exp. Med.* 186(12):2039–43

110. Tisch R, Wang B, Serreze DV. 1999. Induction of glutamic acid decarboxylase 65- specific Th2 cells and suppression of autoimmune diabetes at late stages of disease is epitope dependent. *J. Immunol.* 163(3):1178–87

111. Hancock WW, Polanski M, Zhang J, Blogg N, Weiner HL. 1995. Suppression of insulitis in non-obese diabetic (NOD) mice by oral insulin administration is associated with selective expression of interleukin-4 and -10, transforming growth factor-beta, and prostaglandin-E. *Am. J. Pathol.* 147(5):1193–99

112. Gaur A, Boehme SA, Chalmers D, Crowe PD, Pahuja A, Ling N, Brocke S, Steinman L, Conlon PJ. 1997. Amelioration of relapsing experimental autoimmune encephalomyelitis with altered myelin basic protein peptides involves different cellular mechanisms. *J. Neuroimmunol.* 74 (1–2):149–58

113. Vaysburd M, Lock C, McDevitt H. 1995. Prevention of insulin-dependent diabetes mellitus in nonobese diabetic mice by immunogenic but not by tolerated peptides. *J. Exp. Med.* 182(3):897–902

114. Bieg S, Hanlon C, Hampe CS, Benjamin D, Mahoney CP. 1999. GAD65 and insulin B chain peptide (9–23) are not primary autoantigens in the type 1 diabetes syndrome of the BB rat. *Autoimmunity* 31(1):15–24

115. Petersen JS, MacKay P, Plesner A, Karlsen A, Gotfredsen C, Verland S, Michelsen B, Dyrberg T. 1997. Treatment with GAD65 or BSA does not protect against diabetes in BB rats. *Autoimmunity* 25(3):129–38

116. Bellmann K, Kolb H, Rastegar S, Jee P, Scott FW. 1998. Potential risk of oral insulin with adjuvant for the prevention of Type I diabetes: a protocol effective in NOD mice may exacerbate disease in BB rats. *Diabetologia* 41(7):844–47

117. Al-Sabbagh A, Miller A, Santos LM, Weiner HL. 1994. Antigen-driven tissue-specific suppression following oral tolerance: orally administered myelin basic protein suppresses proteolipid protein- induced experimental autoimmune encephalomyelitis in the SJL mouse. *Eur. J. Immunol.* 24(9):2104–9

118. Von Herrath MG, Dyrberg T, OldstoneMB. 1996. Oral insulin treatment suppresses virus-induced antigen-specific destruction of beta cells and prevents autoimmune diabetes in transgenic mice. *J. Clin. Invest.* 98(6):1324–31

119. Bercovici N, Delon J, Cambouris C, Escriou N, Debre P, Liblau RS. 1999. Chronic intravenous injections of antigen induce and maintain tolerance in T cell receptor- transgenic mice. *Eur. J. Immunol.* 29(1):345–54

120. Bercovici N, Heurtier A, Vizler C, Pardigon N, Cambouris C, Desreumaux P, Liblau R. 2000. Systemic administration of agonist peptide blocks the progression of spontaneous CD8-mediated autoimmune diabetes in transgenic mice without bystander damage. *J. Immunol.* 165(1):202–10

121. Nicolls MR, Aversa GG, Pearce NW, Spinelli A, Berger MF, Gurley KE, Hall BM. 1993. Induction of long-term specific tolerance to allografts in rats by therapy with an anti-CD3-like monoclonal antibody. *Transplantation* 55(3):459–68

122. Chatenoud L, Thervet E, Primo J, Bach JF. 1994. Anti-CD3 antibody induces long-term remission of overt autoimmunity in nonobese diabetic mice. *Proc. Natl. Acad. Sci. USA* 91(1):123–27

123. Chatenoud L, Primo J, Bach JF. 1997. CD3 antibody-induced dominant self tolerance in overtly diabetic NOD mice. *J. Immunol.* 158(6):2947–54

124. Hayward AR, Shreiber M. 1989. Neonatal injection of CD3 antibody into nonobese diabetic mice reduces the incidence of insulitis and diabetes. *J. Immunol.* 143(5):1555–59

125. Maki T, Ichikawa T, Blanco R, Porter J. 1992. Long-term abrogation of autoimmune diabetes in nonobese diabetic mice by immunotherapy with anti-lymphocyte serum. *Proc. Natl. Acad. Sci. USA* 89(8):3434–38

126. Chatenoud L, Baudrihaye MF, Kreis H, Goldstein G, Schindler J, Bach JF. 1982. Human in vivo antigenic modulation induced by the anti-T cell OKT3 monoclonal antibody. *Eur. J. Immunol.* 12(11):979–82

127. Smith JA, Tang QH, Bluestone JA. 1998. Partial TCR signals delivered by FcR-nonbinding anti-CD3 monoclonal antibodies differentially regulate individual Th subsets. *J. Immunol.* 160(10):4841–49

128. Boitard C, Bendelac A, Richard MF, Carnaud C, Bach JF. 1988. Prevention of diabetes in nonobese diabetic mice by anti-I-A monoclonal antibodies: transfer of protection by splenic T cells. *Proc. Natl. Acad. Sci. USA* 85(24):9719–23

129. Kurasawa K, Sakamoto A, Maeda T, Sumida T, Ito I, Tomioka H, Yoshida S, Koike T. 1993. Short-term administration of anti-L3T4 MoAb prevents diabetes in NOD mice. *Clin. Exp. Immunol.* 91(3):376–80

130. Shizuru JA, Taylor-Edwards C, Banks BA, Gregory AK, Fathman CG. 1988. Immunotherapy of the nonobese diabetic mouse: treatment with an antibody to T-helper lymphocytes. *Science* 240(4852):659–62

131. Hutchings P, O'Reilly L, Parish NM, Waldmann H, Cooke A. 1992. The use of a non-depleting anti-CD4 monoclonal antibody to reestablish tolerance to beta cells in NOD mice. *Eur. J. Immunol.* 22(7):1913–18

132. Balasa B, Krahl T, Patstone G, Lee J, Tisch R, McDevitt HO, Sarvetnick N. 1997. CD40 ligand-CD40 interactions are necessary for the initiation of insulitis and diabetes in nonobese diabetic mice. *J. Immunol.* 159(9):4620–27

133. Parish NM, Bowie L, Zusman Harach S, Phillips JM, Cooke A. 1998. Thymus-dependent monoclonal antibody-induced protection from transferred diabetes. *Eur. J. Immunol.* 28(12):4362–73

134. Sempe P, Bedossa P, Richard MF, Villa

MC, Bach JF, Boitard C. 1991. Anti-alpha/beta T cell receptor monoclonal antibody provides an efficient therapy for autoimmune diabetes in nonobese diabetic (NOD) mice. *Eur. J. Immunol.* 21(5):1163–69

135. Ikehara S, Ohtsuki H, Good RA, Asamoto H, Nakamura T, Sekita K, Muso E, Tochino Y, Ida T, Kuzuya H, Imura H, Hamashima Y. 1985. Prevention of type I diabetes in nonobese diabetic mice by allogenic bone marrow transplantation. *Proc. Natl. Acad. Sci. USA* 82(22):7743–47

136. Bendelac A, Rivera MN, Park SH, Roark JH. 1997. Mouse CD1-specific NK1 T cells: development, specificity, and function. *Annu. Rev. Immunol.* 15:535–62

137. Gombert JM, Herbelin A, Tancrede-Bohin E, Dy M, Carnaud C, Bach JF. 1996. Early quantitative and functional deficiency of NK1($^+$)-like thymocytes in the NOD mouse. *Eur. J. Immunol.* 26(12):2989–98

138. Yoshimoto T, Bendelac A, Hu-Li J, Paul WE. 1995. Defective IgE production by SJL mice is linked to the absence of CD4$^+$, NK1.1$^+$T cells that promptly produce interleukin 4. *Proc. Natl. Acad. Sci. USA* 92(25):11931–34

139. Lehuen A, Lantz O, Beaudoin L, Laloux V, Carnaud C, Bendelac A, Bach JF, Monteiro RC. 1998. Overexpression of natural killer T cells protects V alpha 14-J alpha 281 transgenic nonobese diabetic mice against diabetes. *J. Exp. Med.* 188(10):1831–39

139a. Takahashi T, Tagami T, Yamazaki S, Uede T, Shimizu J, Sakaguchi N, Mak TW, Sakaguchi S. 2000. Immunologic self-tolerance maintained by CD25+CD4+ regulatory T cells constitutively expressing cytotoxic T lymphocyte-associated antigen 4. *J. Exp. Med.* 192(2):303–9

140. Yoshimoto T, Bendelac A, Watson C, Hu-Li J, Paul WE. 1995. Role of NK1.1$^+$ T cells in a TH2 response and in immunoglobulin E production. *Science* 270(5243):1845–47

141. Bendelac A, Hunziker RD, Lantz O. 1996. Increased interleukin 4 and immunoglobulin E production in transgenic mice overexpressing NK1 T cells. *J. Exp. Med.* 184(4):1285–93

142. Smiley ST, Kaplan MH, Grusby MJ. 1997. Immunoglobulin E production in the absence of interleukin-4-secreting CD1-dependent cells. *Science* 275(5302):977–79

143. Keller RJ, Eisenbarth GS, Jackson RA. 1993. Insulin prophylaxis in individuals at high risk of type I diabetes. *Lancet* 341(8850):927–28

144. Kobayashi T, Nakanishi K, Murase T, Kosaka K. 1996. Small doses of subcutaneous insulin as a strategy for preventing slowly progressive beta-cell failure in islet cell antibody-positive patients with clinical features of NIDDM. *Diabetes* 45(5):622–26

145. Harrison LC, Honeyman MC, Steele C, Wright M, Gellert SA, Colman PG. 1999. Intranasal insulin trial (INIT) in preclinical type 1 diabetes. 10th Int. Congress of Mucosal Immunol., Amsterdam, Netherlands, June 27–July 1, 1999. *Immunol. Lett.* 69(1):72

146. Blanas E, Carbone FR, Allison J, Miller JF, Heath WR. 1996. Induction of autoimmune diabetes by oral administration of autoantigen. *Science* 274(5293):1707–9

147. Chatenoud L, Ferran C, Legendre C, Thouard I, Merite S, Reuter A, Gevaert Y, Kreis H, Franchimont P, Bach JF. 1990. In vivo cell activation following OKT3 administration. Systemic cytokine release and modulation by corticosteroids. *Transplantation* 49(4):697–702

148. Zechel MA, Chaturvedi P, Singh B. 1997. Characterization of immunodominant peptide determinants of IDDM-associated autoantigens in the NOD

mouse. *Res. Immunol.* 148(5):338–48

149. Zechel MA, Elliott JF, Atkinson MA, Singh B. 1998. Characterization of novel T-cell epitopes on 65 kDa and 67 kDa glutamic acid decarboxylase relevant in autoimmune responses in NOD mice. *J. Autoimmun.* 11(1):83–95

150. Zechel MA, Krawetz MD, Singh B. 1998. Epitope dominance: evidence for reciprocal determinant spreading to glutamic acid decarboxylase in non-obese diabetic mice. *Immunol. Rev.* 164:111–18

151. Chen SL, Whiteley PJ, Freed DC, Rothbard JB, Peterson LB, Wicker LS. 1994. Responses of NOD congenic mice to a glutamic acid decarboxylase-derived peptide. *J. Autoimmun.* 7(5):635–41

152. Schloot NC, Daniel D, Norbury-Glaser M, Wegmann DR. 1996. Peripheral T cell clones from NOD mice specific for GAD65 peptides: lack of islet responsiveness or diabetogenicity. *J. Autoimmun.* 9(3):357–63

153. Ramiya VK, Shang XZ, Pharis PG, Wasserfall CH, Stabler TV, Muir AB, Schatz DA, MacLaren NK. 1996. Antigen based therapies to prevent diabetes in NOD mice. *J. Autoimmun.* 9(3):349–56

Annu. Rev. Immunol. 2001. 19:163–96

ANTI-TNFα THERAPY OF RHEUMATOID ARTHRITIS: What Have We Learned?

Marc Feldmann and Ravinder N. Maini

Kennedy Institute of Rheumatology Division, Imperial College School of Medicine, 1 Aspenlea Road, London W6 8LH, United Kingdom; e-mail: m.feldmann@ic.ac.uk; r.maini@ic.ac.uk

Key Words   TNFα, cytokines, anti-TNFα antibodies and inhibitors, rheumatoid arthritis, immunotherapy

■ **Abstract**   Rheumatoid arthritis (RA), a systemic disease, is characterized by a chronic inflammatory reaction in the synovium of joints and is associated with degeneration of cartilage and erosion of juxta-articular bone. Many pro-inflammatory cytokines including TNFα, chemokines, and growth factors are expressed in diseased joints. The rationale that TNFα played a central role in regulating these molecules, and their pathophysiological potential, was initially provided by the demonstration that anti-TNFα antibodies added to in vitro cultures of a representative population of cells derived from diseased joints inhibited the spontaneous production of IL-1 and other pro-inflammatory cytokines. Systemic administration of anti-TNFα antibody or sTNFR fusion protein to mouse models of RA was shown to be anti-inflammatory and joint protective. Clinical investigations in which the activcity of TNFα in RA patients was blocked with intravenously administered infliximab, a chimeric anti-TNFα monoclonal antibody (mAB), has provided evidence that TNF regulates IL-6, IL-8, MCP-1, and VEGF production, recruitment of immune and inflammatory cells into joints, angiogenesis, and reduction of blood levels of matrix metalloproteinases-1 and -3. Randomized, placebo-controlled, multi-center clinical trials of human TNFα inhibitors have demonstrated their consistent and remarkable efficacy in controlling signs and symptoms, with a favorable safety profile, in approximately two thirds of patients for up to 2 years, and their ability to retard joint damage. Infliximab (a mAB), and etanercept (a sTNF-R-Fc fusion protein) have been approved by regulatory authorities in the United States and Europe for treating RA, and they represent a significant new addition to available therapeutic options.

INTRODUCTION

Rheumatoid arthritis is one of the commonest human autoimmune diseases, with a prevalence of 1%. There is a genetic predisposition, with the clearly defined involvement of HLA of DR4/DR1 (1). A shared epitope, a sequence between amino acid positions 70 and 74 of the DRB chain that is shared by DR4/DR1 susceptible haplotypes, has been identified (2). This implicates CD4$^+$ T cell recognition at some stage of the disease process (3). Concordance in twin studies is low, ranging from 35% (4) to 15% (5), indicating the role of nongenetic factors.

The clinical features are mostly due to inflammation and eventual damage to synovial joints of hands, feet, wrists, knees, hips, etc. In more severe cases, there is extra articular disease, and survival is impaired (6, 7).

The synovitis involves a massive leucocytic infiltrate chiefly consisting of macrophages, T lymphocytes, and plasma cells, and this is associated with augmented angiogenesis. Where the synovium abuts the cartilage and bone is the site of major joint damage. Details of the features of rheumatoid arthritis have been documented in detail elsewhere (8, 9).

Pathophysiology of TNFα

Despite the discovery of TNFα bioactivity in the 1970s by Old and colleagues (10, 11) and its cloning (12–14) under different names in the 1980s (such as cachectin by Cerami and colleagues), the pathophysiological effects of TNFα and its sister molecule lymphotoxin (15, 16) are still incompletely understood. It is clear that many of the in vitro experiments, performed with abundant recombinant TNFα (like many other cytokines) at supraphysiological doses, does not represent what happens in vivo at the much more limiting physiological doses, and in the presence of inhibitors and regulatory pathways. Based on in vitro analysis, it appears that TNFα, LTα, IL-1α and β have almost identical function, and GM-CSF exerts almost the same effects. Hence the concept of cytokine redundancy was conceived (17, 18), which suggested that many cytokines had almost the same properties, but the reasons for this cytokine redundancy were never clear. However, experiments in vivo using neutralizing antibodies and especially targeted mutations or gene knockouts have shown that cytokine redundancy is much less obvious in vivo.

The major source of TNFα is the cells of the monocyte/macrophage lineage, with T lymphocytes, neutrophils, mast cells, and endothelium also contributing under different circumstances. All potentially noxious stimuli, ranging from the physical (ultraviolet light, X-radiation, heat) to the chemical and immunological, can rapidly induce TNFα production and release (14, 19). In vivo TNFα is the most rapidly produced pro-inflammatory cytokine, with serum levels detectable in mice in 30 min (20). Probably the earliest TNFα comes from preformed stores by cleavage of membrane TNFα on macrophages, neutrophils, and activated T cells by TNFα converting enzyme (TACE/ADAM 17) (21), and release of cytoplasmic granules from mast cells and eosinophils. Subsequent release of TNFα is due to new synthesis, chiefly in macrophages and T lymphocytes.

If the rapid release of TNFα at times of stress is blocked, the expression of other pro-inflammatory cytokines, such as IL-1 and IL-6, is reduced (22). This and analogous in vitro data (23) suggest that TNFα in vivo coordinates the cytokine response to injury and acts as a fire alarm. The induction by TNFα of multiple chemokines and adhesion molecules (24, 25) is of major importance in rapidly attracting immune and inflammatory leukocytes to the site of injury and TNFα release. TNFα also acutely upregulates the function of the immune system (26, 27), but following prolonged exposure to an excess of TNFα, it is immunosuppressive (28).

More details of the multiple functions of TNFα can be found in the references (13, 14, 19).

Cytokine Network

The description of cytokines as chemical entities got off to a slow start. It seemed initially that many of the multiple biological activities, described for cell-free supernatants termed cytokines, were due to a small set of proteins. Thus interleukin (IL)-1 was independently discovered as lymphocyte activating factor, connective tissue degradative catabolin, and endogenous pyrogen (reviewed in 29). However, over 150 cytokines have been identified and cloned (30), and by genome sequencing many more cytokine-like molecules of unknown function have been uncovered. Many recently described cytokines are not secreted by cells but act by cell-to-cell contact, thus confounding the initial definition of cytokines as secreted proteins acting as short range intercellular messenger molecules. For an updated description of the current status of cytokines, see (30).

Cytokines are never expressed singly by a cell or tissue. Instead, an activated cell (e.g. a macrophage) produces a wide spectrum of cytokines. Similarly all cells express receptors for many, but not all, cytokines. Unlike hormones that are expressed constitutively, most cytokines are expressed transiently after an inducing stimulus. One of the most potent signals for inducing cytokines are other cytokines, and so the concept has arisen of a cytokine network in which cytokines induce or inhibit each other (17, 31, 32). This accounts, in part, for the complexity of cytokine expression found at any diseased tissue site such as the rheumatoid synovium. How this complex mixture of molecules, interacting with multiple cells, is regulated is currently only partly understood, but it is becoming evident that dysregulation of the cytokine network contributes in a major way to the pathogenesis and pathology of rheumatoid arthritis (31–37).

Key aspects of the cytokine network in health include the transient expression of cytokine genes in contrast to the constitutive but regulated expression of cytokine receptors. However, cytokine receptors also form part of the regulatory system as they are downregulated by ligand interaction and most importantly are cleaved by metalloproteinase enzymes (21, 38) to yield soluble cytokine receptors (39–41). Many, probably most of these soluble receptors [e.g. soluble IL-2 receptor (sIL-2R), soluble TNF-receptor (sTNF-R)] are still capable of binding the cytokine and hence act as inhibitors by competing with membrane-bound signaling receptors. Cleavage of receptors also reduces their cell surface density, and since cytokine receptors usually need to be aggregated by their ligand to generate a signal, the signaling capacity of the cell is inhibited.

Concomitantly, soon after the release of pro-inflammatory cytokines, other cytokines with chiefly anti-inflammatory properties are released that act to limit the duration and extent of the pro-inflammatory effect. These inhibitory cytokines include IL-10, TGFβ, IL-11, and IL-1 receptor antagonist (IL-1Ra) (35, 42–46).

The relatively easily accessible rheumatoid synovium has become the most extensively analyzed tissue site of a local immune and inflammatory reaction. Hence much is known about synovial cytokine expression. This has been studied in a variety of ways, for example, on fresh ex vivo tissue by immunohistology (47) or in situ hybridization (48), by examining its waste products found in the synovial fluid (49, 50), and also by short-term culture of synovial membrane cells in the absence of extrinsic stimulation (23). The latter technique permits the quantitative analysis of released proteins and their inhibitors, and it is the procedure we have studied most extensively. Using such cultures, we and others have documented expression of a great many cytokines in this tissue. The data has demonstrated that there is upregulation not only of pro-inflammatory cytokines but also of the anti-inflammatory cytokines and cytokine inhibitors, including soluble receptors (23, 47–57).

Our attempts to understand how this plethora of mediators was regulated in the absence of extrinsic stimulation (23) led us to use antibodies to cytokines as pharmacological antagonists. This revealed the profound effects of anti-TNFα antibody in reducing the production of IL-1 in rheumatoid synovial cultures and led us to the current understanding that TNFα was of major importance in regulating the activities of other cytokines (23, 33, 34). A grossly simplified summary of the cytokine network in RA is shown in Figure 1, which does not include the multiple cell interactions or the effects of cell recruitment and apoptosis that are most likely involved under physiological conditions at sites of inflammation.

Cytokine Expression and Regulation in RA

A summary of the many potentially important cytokines found in RA synovium is shown in Table 1. It shows that cytokines of essentially all classes are found with multiple activities, such as those with pro-inflammatory and anti-inflammatory

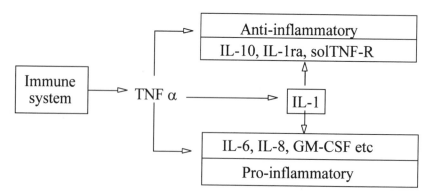

Figure 1   Cytokine cascade in rheumatoid arthritis. Modified from Feldmann, Elliott, Woody and Maini (1997) *Advances in Immunology* 64:283–350.

TABLE 1   Cytokine expression in rheumatoid arthritis

Cytokine	Expression	
	mRNA	**protein**
Pro-inflammatory		
IL-1α,β (interleukin 1)	+[a]	+
TNF (tumor necrosis factor alpha)	+	+
LT (lympotoxin)	+	±
IL-6 (interleukin 6)	+	+
GM-CSF (granulocyte macrophage colony stimulating factor)	+	+
M-CSF (macrophage colony stimulating factor)	+	+
LIF (leucocyte inhibitory factor)	+	+
Oncostatin M (oncostatin M)	+	+
IL-2 (interleukin 2)	+	±
IL-3 (interleukin 3)	−	−
IL-7 (interleukin 7)	?	?
IL-9 (interleukin 9)	?	?
IL-12 (interleukin 12)	+	+
IL-15 (interleukin 15)	+	+
IFN α,β (interferon alpha/beta)	+	+
IFN γ (interferon gamma)	+	±
IL-17 (interleukin 17)	+	+
IL-18 (interleukin 18)	+	+
Immunoregulatory		
IL-4 (interleukin 4)	±	−
IL-10 (interleukin 10)	+	+
IL-11 (interleukin 11)	+	+
IL-13 (interleukin 13)	+	+
TGF β (transforming growth factor beta)	+	+
Chemokines		
IL-8 (interleukin 8)	+	+
Gro α (melanoma growth stimulating activity)	+	+
MIP-1 (macrophage inflammatory protein)	+	+
MCP-1 (monocyte chemoattractant protein)	+	+
ENA-78 (epithelial neutrophil activating peptide 78)	+	+
RANTES (regulated upon activatioin T cell expressed & secreted)	+	+
Mitogens		
FGF (Fibroblast growth factor)	+	+
PDGF (Platelet-derived growth factor)	+	+
VEGF (vascular endothelial growth factor)	+	+

[a]Cytokines expressed in rheumatoid synovial tissue. + present, − absent
Modified after Feldmann, Brennan & Maini (1996), *Annual Review of Immunology* 14:397–440.

action, growth factors, interferons, etc. A major exception is IL-4 because the presence of this cytokine is very rarely reported in RA synovium. This could be of pathophysiological relevance, highlighting both the Th1 dominance of the immune-inflammatory process and the relative lack of its anti-inflammatory counter effect. In contrast other anti-inflammatory cytokines are upregulated and hence relatively abundant, including IL-10, IL-11, and TGFβ1. The latter are active in RA synovium, as neutralizing of IL-10 or IL-11, for example, markedly upregulates TNFα production (58, 59).

The complexity of cytokine expression in synovium obscures the role that any single cytokine might play in pathogenesis of disease. To this complexity, as noted by immunohistology, must be added microheterogeneity, in that cytokine expression varies from one region to another and is also different at the sites of cartilage and bone damage where the synovial membrane abuts on cartilage or bone, a tissue termed pannus (60, 61).

Despite this local heterogeneity, lost when the synovial tissue is dissociated, the regulation of rheumatoid cytokine expression studied in in vitro cultures was instrumental in providing the initial findings leading to a rationale for anti-TNFα therapy in rheumatoid arthritis. Many of the observations made in these rheumatoid synovial cultures have been verified to occur in vivo by analyses of clinical trials of anti-TNFα in rheumatoid patients (see below).

Cytokine expression in rheumatoid tissue has been extensively reviewed in recent years and hence is not documented in detail here. For comprehensive review see (33, 37).

Rationale for Anti-TNFα Therapy in RA

It is a misconception to think that TNFα was an obvious therapeutic target in the early 1990s since it is pro-inflammatory and present in synovium. The same could be said for IL-1, IL-6, GM-CSF, IL-8, and so on. The plethora of possible cytokine therapeutic targets and the concern about cytokine redundancy led some workers in the field to consider cytokines to be poor therapeutic targets. The prevailing view in the early 1990s was that blocking any one pro-inflammatory mediator in isolation would not be beneficial as those remaining would drive the biological processes.

The first clue that TNFα might be a good therapeutic target has already been alluded to, namely the effects of anti-TNFα antibody on cultures of dissociated rheumatoid synovial membranes (23). These cultures provide a good model of certain aspects of the disease as the cells in these suspensions, namely 30% T, 30%–40% macrophages, and fewer endothelial cells, fibroblasts, dendritic cells, plasma cells, B lymphocytes, etc, reaggregate in vitro and reproduce, in the absence of extrinsic stimulation, the molecules that are produced in vivo – e.g. TNFα, IL-1, GM-CSF, IL-6, VEGF, MMPs, PGE2, etc.

Addition of anti-TNFα antibody, but not the closely related anti-LTα antibody, inhibited production of IL-1 bioactivity (23). This prompted studies of other effects

TABLE 2   Rationale for anti-TNFα therapy

---

1. TNFα dependence of pro-inflammatory cytokines in rheumatoid synovial cultures
2. Anti TNFα ameliorates inflammation and joint destruction in murine collagen induced arthritis
3. Upregulated TNFα/TNF-R in joints in inflamed synovium and the destructive pannus-cartilage junction

---

of anti-TNFα in rheumatoid synovial cultures in vitro; downregulation of synovial GM-CSF (62), IL-6, IL-8 was noted (33). Hence blocking a single pro-inflammatory cytokine led to the diminution in production of other pro-inflammatory cytokines with closely related action in the diseased tissue (e.g. IL-1, GM-CSF, IL-6) and suggested that cytokine redundancy in this diseased tissue may not be a major problem.

As it is possible to artefactually induce pro-inflammatory cytokines rapidly in vitro, for example with LPS, which contaminates serum and glassware, the verification by immunohistologic approaches of upregulated TNF/TNF-receptor expression (not involving tissue culture) on freshly frozen tissue (47, 63) was a valuable confirmation that TNF/TNF-R interactions might be important in vivo. The findings also contributed to the emerging concept that TNFα might be a good therapeutic target in RA.

Whereas there are often significant differences between animal models of disease and the authentic human disease (64, 65), there are benefits of using animal models because physiological aspects of disease, e.g. cell trafficking, cannot be mimicked in vitro. Collagen-type II induced arthritis, which has many resemblances to RA but also some differences, was the model initially used to test whether TNFα blockade was beneficial in vivo. Several groups performed similar studies simultaneous with anti-TNFα agent and reported their results in 1992/1993 (66–69). All of them demonstrated a clear benefit of TNFα inhibition by antibodies or TNF-R Fc fusion proteins on collagen induced arthritis, most notably even if the treatment was begun after disease onset.

A summary of the rationale for anti-TNFα therapy of RA is presented in Table 2.

INHIBITORS OF TNFα IN CURRENT CLINICAL USE

At present (June 2000), the only drugs that are in clinical practice or in clinical trials to block TNFα are biologicals, protein-based drugs, either antibody to TNFα or based on TNFα receptors (e.g. linked to Fc dimers). These agents have the major advantage of specificity (70) but have significant disadvantages, including the need for repeated injection and their relative high cost compared to small organic chemical drugs (71).

Monoclonal Antibodies

Chimeric Monoclonal Anti-TNFα, Infliximab (Remicade^{TM})   This antibody was chimerized and is a mouse Fv, human IgG1, κ antibody of high affinity and neutralizing capacity with the potential for effector functions on human cells (72). This was the first anti-TNFα antibody used for therapy of RA (73) and is now approved for this indication and for Crohn's disease in the United States and more recently in Europe for both these indications.

Human Monoclonal Anti-TNFα Antibodies   Subsequent to the use of infliximab in clinical trials of RA, other anti-TNFα antibodies and fusion proteins, which had been developed for use in sepsis, were diverted for use in RA. The first of these was a humanized, complementarity determining region (CDR) grafted monoclonal antibody, CDP571, developed by Celltech (74). Subsequently, a human antibody, D2E7, produced by phage display by Cambridge Antibody Technology, has entered clinical development with BASF/Knoll (75). The newest entrant to the anti-TNFα antibody field is a PEG-linked Fab fragment, CDP870, from Celltech, which can be produced in E. coli (76).

TNF Receptor Based Biologicals

As the TNF receptors possess a high affinity for TNFα, these molecules in their soluble form are also potential TNFα inhibitors. The cleaved soluble p55 and p75 TNF receptors are present in body fluids at ng/ml concentrations (39–41), act as physiological inhibitors, and have been engineered as pharmaceutical inhibitors, as described below.

p75 TNF-R Fc Fusion Protein, Etanercept (Enbrel^{TM})   As TNFα is a trimer, a TNF-R dimer would more effectively compete with binding of TNFα to the membrane receptors than a mononomer and prevent cell signaling. Engineered p75 TNFR dimers linked to Fc portion of IgG were shown to be effective inhibitors, first in animal models (77) and subsequently in clinical trials.

p55 TNF-R Fc Fusion Protein, Lenercept   This is a similar dimer based on p55 TNF-R, but while it was effective in animal models (78), it was less successful in the clinic than etanercept or infliximal and has been abandoned.

Pegylated Truncated p55 TNF-R   A truncated p55 TNF-R was produced in order to overcome the immunogenicity of a dimeric pegylated full-length p55 TNF-R. It is PEG-linked to prolong its circulating half-life (79).

CLINICAL EFFICACY OF ANTI-TNFα BIOLOGICALS

Since clinical trials of anti-TNFα biologicals in RA began in 1992, the results have been very consistent, with all the TNFα inhibitors tested being efficacious

TABLE 3   Anti-TNF agents in clinical trials in rheumatoid arthritis

Name	Composition	Manufacturer
Monoclonal antibodies		
Infliximab, Remicade[TM]	Chimeric (mouse × human) mAb	Centocor, USA
CDP571	Humanized murine CDR3 engrafted mAb	Celltech, UK
D2E7	Human mAb	Cambridge Antibody Technology/BASF
Soluble TNFR:Fc (IgG) Fusion Proteins		
Etanercept, Enbrel[TM]	p75TNFR:Fc	Immunex/American Home Products
Lenercept	p55TNFR:Fc	Roche, Switzerland

(Table 3). In the absence of direct comparisons, it is not possible to conclude whether apparent differences in outcome measurement between these agents are due to pharmacological effects or clinical heterogeneity of patient populations. However, the concept of TNFα as a major therapeutic target in RA has been amply validated, and two of these agents, etanercept and infliximab, have been approved for treatment of rheumatoid arthritis by the FDA and the European agency. At the time of writing (June 2000), almost 100,000 rheumatoid patients have been treated with one or other of these agents.

Clinical Efficacy of Anti-TNFα, Infliximab

Infliximab was the first anti-TNFα agent to be used for the treatment of RA and is the most intensively investigated in clinical pharmacological studies. The first Phase I/II study was an open (nonplacebo controlled) trial of infliximab in long-standing active RA patients who had failed all prior therapy; it was initiated in May 1992. A high dose of anti-TNFα antibody was given (20 mg/kg over 2 weeks in either 2 or 4 infusions) (73) as animal model studies had demonstrated that efficacy required a dose in this range (67).

The clinical results were notable, with patients reporting alleviation of symptoms such as pain, morning stiffness, tiredness, and lethargy within hours; a reduction in the numbers of swollen joints and tender joints was observed by 2 to 4 weeks. While all 20 patients in this trial benefited to a variable degree, the response was temporary, lasting from 8 to 22 weeks (73). A subset of these patients was re-treated (with 10 mg/kg) for a further 3 cycles of infusions with infliximab; each followed with a renewed response of a similar magnitude and limited duration (80). These highly encouraging results laid the foundation for the concept that repeated long-term treatment with anti-TNFα was possible for chronic diseases such as RA.

A double-blind, randomized, placebo controlled clinical trial quickly followed and established efficacy of infliximab in controlling signs and symptoms of RA.

Seventy-three patients with active RA despite previous anti-rheumatic therapy were given a single intravenous infusion of infliximab at either high (10 mg/kg) or low (1 mg/kg) doses. The end point of this study was response to therapy evaluated at the end of four weeks by the Paulus criteria, a composite index requiring improvements in at least four out of six variables, including tender and swollen joint counts, duration of morning stiffness and reduction in ESR or C-reactive protein (CRP), and the patient's and physician's global assessment of disease activity.

The results of this intention-to-treat analysis were clear cut, in that 2/24 (8%) patients given placebo infusion met these criteria, compared with 11 out of 25 (44%) at the low dose and 19 of 24 (79%) at the high dose of infliximab. All patients were followed to relapse; the median duration of response at 1 mg/kg was found to last 3 weeks and at 10 mg/kg lasted 8 weeks (81). The degree of improvement was high, with a 60%–70% reduction in measures of disease activity such as tender or swollen joint counts and CRP. The results of this trial not only provided a formal proof of concept (73), they also stimulated initiation of clinical trials with other TNFα inhibitors, e.g. lenercept, etanercept, CDP571, which had been developed for use in sepsis.

As established RA is a chronic disease, the aim of the next most important clinical trial was to demonstrate that multiple doses of anti-TNFα could be administered safely over a prolonged period without any loss of efficacy. Thus, a longer term trial was initiated involving patients with active disease despite methotrexate (MTX) therapy. Five infusions of placebo or infliximab at three dose levels were administered, either with a continuing fixed low dose of methotrexate, or without methotrexate over a 14-week period, with a final assessment at 6 months (82). Since MTX in low doses once a week has become established as one of the more durable and effective therapies for RA, patients whose disease activity persisted despite this drug were recruited in this randomized placebo trial. The enhanced efficacy of anti-TNFα therapy by anti-CD4 antibody in collagen induced arthritis provided the rationale for the combination of infliximab and MTX which also has anti-T cell activity (83).

A total of 101 patients with longstanding active disease were stabilized on MTX 7.5 mg weekly and allocated to one of seven groups. A control group received placebo infusions (plus MTX), three groups received infliximab at 1, 3, or 10 mg/kg of body weight plus MTX, and another three groups at 1, 3, or 10 mg infliximab plus placebo tablets instead of MTX. The response was assessed by the Paulus criteria at baseline and over the next 6 months.

In the absence of MTX, there was a very clear dose response. Infliximab at a dose of 1 mg/kg yielded a 20% Paulus response in 60% of patients at 3 weeks, but this was not sustained despite repeated infusions. In contrast, 60% of patients receiving higher doses (3 mg/kg and 10 mg/kg) maintained benefit for about 16 weeks and diminished thereafter.

In the presence of MTX the results were different. All 3 doses (1, 3, 10 mg/kg) gave a sustained response, which at the higher two doses was sustained from the last treatment at 14 weeks to the 26th week and end of the trial. The reasons for the difference are discussed later.

A phase III randomized, placebo-controlled study, ATTRACT (anti-TNF therapy of rheumatoid arthritis with concomitant therapy), included patients with active disease despite their use of relatively high dose MTX–median dose, 15 mg/week. Some 428 patients from Europe and United States and Canada were enrolled and randomized into 5 groups. They were all maintained on MTX (last dose carried forward) and were given either 3 or 10 mg/kg infliximab at 0, 2, and 6 weeks and then continued at either 4 or 8 weekly intervals. The control group received MTX plus placebo infusions. The five groups were well matched for disease duration, severity, and disease activity at baseline (84).

This trial is continuing for two years, and the results have been decoded at 6 months (for signs and symptoms) and at 1 year (for X-ray assessment of joint damage) and at 2 years. There was a rapid onset of response, with a significant improvement in symptoms and signs by 2 weeks, and the great majority of patients achieved the American College of Rheumatology 20 criteria of response by 6 weeks, but with further increments in the number of responders up to 1 year (Figure 2). Over 60–70% change in individual parameters of disease activity was

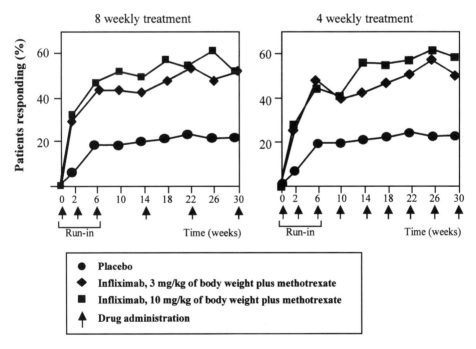

Figure 2 Efficacy of combination of infliximab and methotrexate versus methotrexate and placebo. Percentage of patients achieving a clinical response of 20% change from baseline as defined by the American College of Rheumatology criteria. Patients were treated with methotrexate (10–35 mg/week) and either placebo, 3 or 10 mg/kg inflixamab administered intravenously at time points indicated, in a DMARD unresponsive patient group with active disease despite methotrexate therapy (Maini et al; *Lancet* 1999–84).

achieved in the infliximab groups as compared to placebo. Between 50% and 60% of patients reached the 20% ACR criterion for improvement in all four active treatment groups. The sensitive biochemical marker of disease activity, CRP, reached normal limits within 2 weeks and remained at these concentrations throughout.

The 54-week end point of the ATTRACT trial was joint protection as judged by a change of deterioration in radiographs of the hands and feet, assessed by the Van der Heijde modification of the Sharp scoring system (85). This score attempts to assess cartilage and bone loss separately and has been shown to progress steadily during the disease, despite conventional (i.e. non anti-TNFα) therapy.

In the ATTRACT trial, the total Van der Heijde score (joint space narrowing and erosions in hands and feet) of the MTX alone group (placebo infusion) progressed as anticipated, with an increase in score of 4.0 (median) or 6.97 (mean). In contrast was a median score of 0.0 (mean 0.55) in the 340 patients treated with infliximab at various regimes. Zero change in the radiographic score from baseline in about 50% of the infliximab treated population was of interest as it occurred in patients who satisfied clinical responses assessed by the 20% ACR criteria as well as those who failed to do so. Moreover, the effect on halting of progression held true when the data were analyzed for a change in joint space narrowing and erosion counts separately (86) and subsequently at 2 years.

Results with CDP571, Humanized Anti-TNFα Monoclonal Antibody

The groups of Isenberg and of Panayi (87) reported that CDP571 was effective in RA patients at doses of 10 mg/kg, but not at 1 mg/kg. While this result was the first to confirm those obtained with infliximab, the CDP571 anti-TNFα appeared to be less effective than infliximab at equivalent doses. Its development seems to have been discontinued for RA, possibly because it appeared less effective; however, it is still in development for Crohn's disease (96).

D2E7 A Human Anti-TNFα Monoclonal Antibody

Whereas there are few publications with D2E7, a number of studies are published as abstracts. The overall picture is that D2E7 appears to be an effective anti-TNFα antibody, efficacious in RA by both subcutaneous and intravenous injection, over a range of doses. The clinical results so far appear to be comparable to those obtained with infliximab or etanercept (88–92). The mechanism of action studies so far indicate similar results to infliximab, for example, the reduction in IL-1 expression (93). Joint protection was described after long-term treatment (92).

TNFα Blockade with Etanercept (Enbrel™)

The efficacy of etanercept in RA has been demonstrated in a series of clinical trials that led to its approval by the FDA in November 1998. A dose ranging phase II study compared 0.25, 2, and 16 mg/m^2 etanercept subcutaneously twice a week for

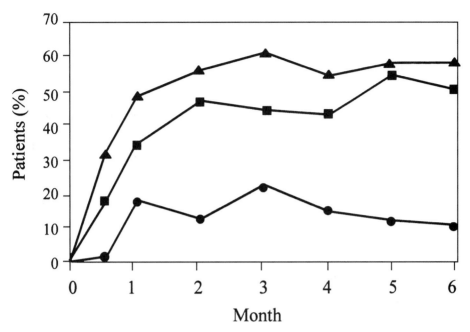

Figure 3 Efficacy of etanercept versus placebo. ACR 20% results in patients treated with two doses of etanercept or placebo injections administered subcutaneously twice weekly over a six-month period in DMARD unresponsive population. ▲ 25 mg etanercept, ■ 10 mg etanerce[t. ● placebo (Moreland et al, *Ann. Internal Med.* 1999).

three months. The highest dose yielded approximately a 60% reduction in swollen and tender joints, compared to 25% with placebo (94).

In a further trial, etanercept was administered at 10 or 25 mg subcutaneously twice per week for 6 months and compared to placebo. The 25 mg dose was efficacious at 3 and 6 months; 59% showed an ACR 20 response at 6 months, compared to 11% with placebo (95) (Figure 3).

Etanercept was added to treatment with MTX in another randomized trial involving 89 patients with active disease despite MTX therapy: 71% of the patients receiving MTX plus etanercept responded, versus 27% in the MTX plus placebo (96). In this trial there was no treatment group which received etanercept alone, hence it is not clear whether MTX plus etanercept is more efficacious than etanercept alone, as was demonstrated in infliximab trials in which treatment groups receiving infliximab alone could be compared with infliximab co-administered with MTX (82).

Other studies have investigated progression in joint damage using etanercept. The results were presented at the November 1999 American College of Rheumatology Meeting. Both 10 mg and 25 mg etanercept subcutaneously twice weekly for 1 year were compared to MTX in patients with active RA of less than 3 years' duration who had not previously been treated with methotrexate (97). Etanercept at 25 mg per week was at least as efficacious as MTX in controlling signs and symptoms and was better than MTX in retarding progression of erosions assessed by radiography of hands and feet in patients with erosions at base line, but not in patients without erosions on X-rays taken upon entry into the trial. No difference was noted in joint space narrowing. These data suggest that etanercept is more effective in controlling bone damage than cartilage damage in RA. Secondary end points were improved.

In a clinical trial on 69 children with juvenile severe poly-articular RA, treatment of patients with 0.4 mg/kg etanercept twice weekly for 90 days induced improvement in 74%. Over the next 9 months, half of the patients randomized to receive continuing etanercept had a disease relapse rate of 24%, in contrast to 77% of those receiving placebo (98). This result has led to the approval of etanercept for juvenile RA.

TNF-R p55 Fc (Lenercept)

This was the first TNF-R IgG Fc fusion protein to be extensively tested in the clinic in sepsis and then in RA. The results were positive, but were somewhat variable (99–102). The reasons for this inconsistency are not fully known, but two distinct hypotheses for this variation have been discussed. One is that there were batch-to-batch variations in the product, due to manufacturing problems. Another is that lenercept was more immunogenic in vivo than would have been predicted from its fully human derivation. Lesslauer and colleagues have reported that the extended peptide linker between the immunoglobulin Fc region and the TNF receptor was the immunogenic part of the molecule, and with time, antibodies generated extended to the TNF-R itself (103). If the latter hypothesis is correct, then agonistic effects due to crosslinking cell surface p55 receptors may have also contributed to variable results. It is noteworthy that Lesslauer reported agonistic antibodies in a small cohort (3 out of 7) of patients given subcutaneous lenercept, which would be more immunogenic. Changes in the half-life of lenercept were noted after the second injection compared to the first, which supports the concept that it was immunogenic. However in some clinical trials patients apparently showed sustained benefit over long periods of time.

PEG-ylated p55 TNF-R

This product has been shown to be active in rodent and primate models of arthritis and there is also preliminary evidence in rheumatoid arthritis phase I/II trials, which have been presented at meetings but not yet published in full (79, 104).

SAFETY OF ANTI-TNFα THERAPY

Overall, the available data both from clinical trials and less clearly from routine clinical practice suggest that the safety of TNFα inhibitors is at least as good as that of other anti-rheumatic drugs (34, 105, 106). In the clinical trial setting an increased incidence of upper respiratory tract infections has been reported in comparison to the placebo control groups for both infliximab and etanercept. However, the higher rates of discontinuations in the placebo treatment arms of the trials led to shorter periods of observation. When adjusted to equivalent periods of exposure to anti-TNFα therapy in 'patient-years' these differences became insignificant. It should be noted that patients used in the trials were generally those with longstanding and severe RA, and such patients have increased rates of co-morbidity, complications, and shortened life-spans. However, despite the reassuring early data the risk of developing tuberculosis and fungal infections will require continuing surveillance.

The conclusion from clinical trials is that the overall safety profile is good. There were initial scares about a possibly increased incidence of lymphoma in the early infliximab studies. However, the incidence of lymphomas is higher than expected in rheumatoid patients with severe disease and receiving other immunosuppressant drugs. These features describe the type of patient included in the infliximab trials. The risk observed to date in all clinical trials in which patients were exposed to infliximab is not higher than might be expected (84), but longer-term follow-up of a larger number of patients is required to definitively exclude or confirm an association. As regards other cancers, the data of anti-TNFα studies have revealed that the number of nonlymphoid malignancies is similar to the expected frequency by comparison with populations of this age, using the NIH Cancer databases.

One complication of interest is that there appears to be a small risk of drug-induced lupus. The mechanism is poorly understood and may be similar to that implicated in the worsening of disease following administration of anti-TNFα antibody and IL-10 therapy (which inhibits TNFα synthesis) in the murine NZB/W model of systemic lupus erythematosus (SLE) (107). NZB/W mice show a genetic deficiency of TNFα (108), which is corrected by administration of low doses of TNFα. TNFα knockouts also develop elevated levels of anti-double stranded (ds) DNA antibody (109), emphasizing the role of TNFα in regulating autoimmunity. Increase in anti-ds DNA antibodies occurs in up to 15% of patients given anti-TNFα antibody or fusion proteins (87, 110, 111), but only about 0.2% of patients treated with infliximab develop symptoms of SLE (111). The few patients reported to date have responded well to discontinuation of the antibody treatment, with complete reversal of the lupus syndrome. These results indicate that SLE is a cytokine-dependent disease but at a different end of the spectrum from RA. The risk of induced SLE by TNFα blocking therapy is therefore small, not dissimilar to that observed in the past in RA patients treated with D-penicillamine and sulphasalazine, so it is not a limitation in clinical practice.

With considerable evidence from TNFα knockout mice and other models that TNFα is important in the innate immune response and in the induction of adoptive immune responses, it is not surprising that there is a concern that bacterial, viral, or parasitic infections may be increased in prevalence or severity in anti-TNFα treated patients. Thus far there are no statistically augmented risks of serious infection during the trials, although in some increased antibiotic usage in anti-TNFα groups suggests that there may be a small difference. What will happen on a longer time scale of treatment is not clear, but as etanercept has already been on the market for over a year, the infectious risk does not appear to be a major issue. Whether different anti-TNFα agents have a different propensity to infection is not known. Safety is discussed in more detail in other reviews (32, 34).

MECHANISM OF ACTION OF ANTI-TNFα THERAPY

Overview

There are many reasons to study the mechanism of action of therapeutic agents, especially with biological agents, where the specificity of the drug is much easier to ascertain and verify than is the case for small organic chemicals. Study of the patients before and after therapy offers insights into the pathogenesis of the disease process.

This opportunity has been extensively seized with infliximab, and there are multiple papers published on mechanistic clinical studies using this antibody. It is not known whether the mechanism of action of a TNFα inhibitor like infliximab which is given at a high concentration and so yields a 'cytokine washout,' is the same as the effects of a TNFα inhibitor like etanercept, which is given repeatedly at lower doses leading to much lower blood levels. Thus infliximab blood levels reach to well over 100 μg/ml, whereas etanercept reaches steady state levels of 3 μg/ml.

Anti-TNFα Downregulates the Cytokine Cascade In Vivo

The effect of anti-TNFα on other 'downstream' cytokines in the RA synovial cultures such as IL-1 (23), GM-CSF and IL-6 (reviewed in 33) was a very important part of the rationale for anti-TNFα therapy, as it was based on studies of the diseased rheumatoid tissue, put into culture in the absence of extrinsic stimuli. It was thus of interest and importance to evaluate whether this inhibitory effect on other pro-inflammatory cytokines was also observed in vivo during clinical trials. The easiest cytokine to assay in vivo is IL-6, as there are elevated levels in RA patients, averaging about 100 pg/ml, and IL-6 is bioactive in serum.

Within a day of infliximab therapy, serum IL-6 concentrations fell to normal levels (112). This was not unexpected as it was already known that CRP, an inflammatory serum marker believed to be controlled chiefly by IL-6, normalized within a few days of treatment with anti-TNFα (73). The reduction of IL-6 is formal proof that TNFα regulates other pro-inflammatory cytokines. The speed and magnitude of the diminution of IL-6 within 24 h makes it likely to be a direct consequence of TNFα blockade on the cytokine network, rather than due to reduction in numbers of cells producing IL-6 in synovium, for example, which might be due to the indirect effects on leukocyte trafficking, or the killing of TNFα-producing cells that express surface TNF. These cells, chiefly macrophages, would also be the IL-6 producing cells.

Other evidence exists for downregulation of the other pro-inflammatory cytokines and chemokines by anti-TNF˙ in vivo. A reduction in IL-8, MCP-1 and

VEGF has been described (113, 114), and the group of Kalden has reported down-regulation of serum IL-1 (115).

A key question is how the reduction in multiple pro-inflammatory cytokines influences manifestations of disease. TNFα has been reported to reduce neuropathic pain (116), and reduction in TNFα may reduce pain by mechanisms involving the central nervous system. Joint swelling is due to fluid as well as cellular infiltration, and reduction in VEGF concentrations, a cytokine that was also cloned as vascular permeability factor, is likely to involve reduction in VEGF-induced permeability and contribute to the rapid reduction of joint swelling within two weeks of anti-TNFα therapy. The reduction in TNFα and the consequent reduction in IL-1 would be expected to reduce the synthesis of MMP and other degradative enzymes production. Support for this mechanism was obtained by serial studies of serum pro MMP levels, before and after anti-TNFα. There was a marked reduction in proMMP-3 and of proMMP-1 after infliximab, probably reflecting reduced joint synthesis (117). It would be expected that joint destruction would diminish as was subsequently established in longer term clinical trials (see Clinical Efficacy of Anti-TNFα Infliximab and 86).

Infliximab Diminishes Leukocyte Trafficking into Joints

The reduction in TNFα and the consequent reduction in IL-1 would have marked effects on endothelial activation (23). The diminution in endothelial adhesion molecules after anti-TNFα therapy has been monitored in the infliximab trials. Two approaches were used, the most quantitative of which was to measure the serum concentrations of soluble adhesion molecules, ICAM-1, E-selectin, and VCAM-1. Among these, the levels of E-selectin, which is an endothelial specific molecule, most probably reflects the adhesive properties of blood vessels more closely than those of ICAM-1 or VCAM-1, which are also expressed on many other cells in the synovium. Significant reductions in serum E-selectin and ICAM-1 were indeed detected (118). Less quantitative, but more relevant to the joint disease, was a semi-quantitative immunohistological analysis of synovial biopsies before and after anti-TNFα therapy. This had demonstrated, to 'blinded' observers, that the expression of the adhesion molecules E-selectin, ICAM-1, and VCAM-1 in the synovium was diminished after anti-TNFα antibody therapy (119).

It was discussed above that serum levels of many but not all chemokines are reduced after infliximab therapy. Together with the adhesion molecule data, this strongly suggests that leucocyte trafficking will be reduced as leucocyte trafficking critically involves both adhesion molecules and chemokines. It was possible to verify this directly in a small clinical trial using [111]indium labelled autologous granulocytes, reinfused into the patient before and 2 weeks after infliximab treatment (114). This trial showed reductions in granulocyte influx of 40%–50%.

While the [111]indium granulocyte joint cell uptake results strictly apply only to the granulocytes, it is very likely that other leucocytes are also entering joints more slowly after infliximab therapy because the requirements for chemokines and adhesion molecules for cell recruitment apply to all cells. Post-treatment synovial biopsies are much less cellular, with the numbers of T cells and macrophages reduced (119). Since T lymphocytes and macrophages also use the same spectrum of adhesion molecules as neutrophils, and relevant chemokines such as MCP-1 are downregulated, it is likely that there is reduced trafficking of all major leucocyte subsets into the joint. Cellularity is a balance between immigration and loss, and increased apoptosis, noted in the T lymphocytes areas (after infliximab therapy) may also contribute to the reduced cellularity found post treatment (P Taylor, unpublished data). It seems to do so in Crohn's disease after anti-TNFα therapy (Sander van Deventer, personal communication).

Infliximab Reduces VEGF and Angiogenesis in Inflamed Joints

Angiogenesis is a prominent feature of the chronic rheumatoid synovium, and so it was pertinent to investigate whether infliximab therapy was associated with re-duced angiogenesis in order to investigate the relationship between inflammation and angiogenesis. Initial studies focused on measurement of VEGF, a potent and endothelial specific growth factor that promotes angiogenesis. Following the pre-vious work of Fava and Koch, who had demonstrated high VEGF levels in rheuma-toid synovium (120, 121), we assayed longitudinal blood samples from patients in the infliximab trials on the assumption that raised serum levels of VEGF might reflect enhanced synovial synthesis of VEGF. Serial synovial biopsies would not be possible in a sufficient percentage of patients to permit accurate statistical anal-ysis. Pretreatment serum VEGF concentrations were indeed elevated; the degree of elevation correlated with a marker of disease activity, CRP, and was significantly reduced after infliximab therapy in two separate trials (113).

The partial reduction in serum VEGF levels led us to explore subsequently the possibility that angiogenesis was reduced in the synovium. Computerized image analysis of endothelium for multiple markers of endothelium (e.g. VWF, CD31) and neovasculature (αvβ3) has shown a reduced vascularity after infliximab ther-apy (122).

Infliximab Restores the Hematological Abnormalities in RA

There are multiple hematological abnormalities in active RA. For example the counts of neutrophils tend to be on the high side. A tendency to low hemoglobin (Hb) concentration is common in RA patients. In view of the profound effects of multiple cytokines upregulated in RA on hemopoiesis, it was of interest to investigate the effects of infliximab on the blood constituents of RA patients in the infliximab clinical trials.

In the first phase II trial, with an end point at 4 weeks, Hb levels fell over this 4-week period in the placebo-treated group, possibly due to blood loss for experimental analyses. With the 1 mg/kg infliximab treatment it stayed at the same level, but at 10 mg/kg, the Hb level was significantly elevated over the baseline. This result suggests that the anemia of RA, and by inference probably the anemia of other chronic inflammatory diseases, is cytokine dependent. Whether the anemia is an effect of TNFα or IL-6 or both is not clear, since both these cytokines are reported to diminish red cell production in certain in vitro systems (123).

Elevated platelet levels are a potentially dangerous consequence of RA, as elevated platelet levels may promote thrombotic and atherosclerotic complications. Infliximab diminished the elevated platelet levels to the normal range (81). The elevated fibrinogen levels commonly found in active RA patients are also likely to predispose to these diseases. However, there is as yet no evidence to support the hypothesis that infliximab is protective against coronary or cerebral thrombosis. The tendency of RA patients to have a moderate neutrophilia was normalized after infliximab therapy.

WHAT HAVE WE LEARNED?

Immunogenicity of Monoclonal Antibodies and Biologicals Is Variable and Can Be Contained

A real concern in the past has been the immunogenicity of antibodies. With murine monoclonals, this concern was borne out in clinical trials, for example of anti-IL-6, where initial efficacy rapidly waned (124). Subsequent antibodies were molecularly engineered to reduce the percentage of mouse sequences in an attempt to deal with this problem. Chimeric antibodies retain the mouse Fv antigen combining site, and thus they are three-quarters human (72). More complex techniques such as CDR grafting leading to humanized antibodies were designed to reduce potential immunogenicity further (125). With the phage display technique (126) it is possible to produce antibodies comprising only human sequences. This is also the case using transgenic mice that have had their Ig loci knocked out and replaced by human heavy and light chain loci (127, 128).

However, in all these cases it is possible to generate anti-idiotype antibodies directed against the binding site itself. This is well known, as the work of Oudin had demonstrated that autologous anti-idiotype antisera can be raised in rabbits (129). Hence the actual degree of immunogenicity of an antibody is difficult to predict. Fully human ones may still generate anti-idiotype or anti-allotype responses. Partly mouse ones, depending on which V regions are used, may not differ that much from the nearest human sequences.

The immunogenicity of antibodies may be reduced by a variety of procedures. First, there is evidence that aggregation of human antibodies augments their immunogenicity, just as was found previously in mice. Technical improvements in the preparation of the chimeric antibodies appear to have reduced the incidence of infusion reactions and diminished the incidence of antibody response to injected antibody (human anti-chimeric antibody—HACA) response.

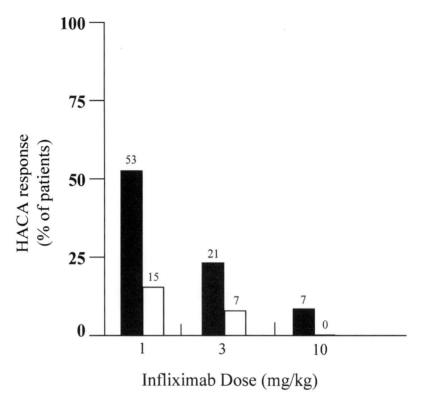

Figure 4 The incidence of human antichimeric antibodies (HACA) in patients treated with infliximab and methotrexate is inversely proportional to that of the dose of infleximab and is diminished in methotrexate. ■ infliximab alone; ❑ infliximab plus methotrexate (Maini et al, *Arthritis Rheum.* 1998).

Secondly, it is apparent that the frequency of the HACA response is inversely related to the amount of antibody infused (82). For example, 1 mg/kg of infliximab was much more frequently immunogenic than 3 mg/kg or 10 mg/kg (Figure 4). The mechanism for this inverse dose relationship appears to be high zone tolerance (HZT) extensively studied in the late 1960s, early 1970s. This was achieved by injection of high doses of soluble protein, and much of this old literature concerns deaggregated gamma globulin. HZT was described in many species (130–132), and whereas the inverse dose response is not formal proof of immunological tolerance, it is highly suggestive of HZT. The proof would require challenge with gamma globulin and adjuvant, which is clearly not possible.

Third, there is evidence that the frequency of the HACA response is diminished in the presence of methotrexate (MTX) (82, 133). This indicates that MTX has an immunosuppressive effect, as had been found by others (134).

With TNF-R fusion proteins, there have been variable results. Lenercept, the p55 TNF-R Fc fusion protein, was found to be highly immunogenic (103), and this contributed to its eventual abandonment. The first evidence for immunogenicity noted was a reduction in the half-life after the first dose, from 7 to 4 days. Subsequently the antibody response was measured, and epitopes recognized were mapped by Lesslauer and his colleagues. They found that the earliest epitopes recognized were in the hinge region, which is extended and differs in conformation from that of native Ig. The epitopes recognized then extended to the p55 TNF-R (103). As most monoclonal antibodies to the p55 TNF-R are agonistic (135), it is possible that agonistic antibodies were raised and that they contributed to the variable results obtained.

An analogous situation has been documented in mice with gene therapy with an adenovirus encoding for a human p55 TNF-R mouse Fc fusion protein. This was initially efficacious, but subsequently the benefit was lost and the disease activity rebounded to a level worse than that of the controls. The sera of these mice had antibodies to human p55 TNF-R, some of which cross-reacted with murine TNF-R (136).

In contrast, initial reports suggested that etanercept was non-immunogenic, but with more sensitive assays, antibodies to etanercept were detected in 16% of treated individuals (137). However, it is reported that these do not interfere with chronic therapy.

Chronic Treatment with Antibodies and Fusion Proteins Is Possible

When antibody therapy was first conceived, it was not known whether antibodies were going to be used for short term or whether they could also be used long term (i.e. several years). This question has been resolved, and it is possible to use some antibodies or fusion proteins long term. Patients have been treated with such agents for up to one year in open-label continuation studies (100) and with infliximab in a randomized controlled trial (86).

Hence, long-term therapy is possible provided the therapy is efficacious and of low immunogenicity. The current regimes for infliximab—3 or 10 mg/kg infusion in the presence of MTX, or of etanercept—25 mg s.c. twice per week—appear to fulfill these criteria. D2E7, a human antibody produced by phage display, has also been used for over a year (92).

Why Are There No Cures with Anti-TNFα Therapy?

Remission is rare in late active RA (138). Nevertheless our concept that there is a disregulated cytokine equilibrium, (31, 33) suggests that if the balance was normalized, the augmented anti-inflammatory pathways may restore homeostasis. One reason for the lack of sustained benefit when therapy is stopped emerged from monitoring the effect of anti-TNFα therapy on the endogenous cytokine inhibitors. Serum IL-1Ra and soluble TNF-R were found to diminish after infliximab (112). There is a suggestion in a small group of patients that serum IL-10 was augmented (139). However, serum IL-10 levels are low and may not reflect the situation in the synovium, since IL-10 production in in vitro rheumatoid synovial cultures is inhibited by anti-TNFα antibody (58).

These results suggest that additional therapeutic benefit may ensue by restoring cytokine inhibitor levels in anti-TNFα–treated patients. Whether it might be achieved by co-administration of IL-10 or IL-1Ra is not clear. We have shown in murine collagen–induced arthritis that anti-TNFα and IL-10 work additively (140); Feige et al (141) have shown that in rat arthritis models the therapeutic effect of TNF-inhibitor (TNF-R PEG) is augmented by IL-1Ra.

Our overall conclusion is that the TNFα overproduction, while a key pathogenic mechanism in the disease (in human and mouse), is certainly not the only pathogenic pathway implicated in maintaining disease chronicity. Other pathways likely to be involved in maintenance of chronicity include augmented angiogenesis (37, 122, 142), lack of synovial apoptosis (12, 143–145), and abnormalities of the immune system (146). It will be important to target these mechanisms of chronicity if a cure is to be achieved.

Combination Therapy Works

Studies in experimental systems, undertaken in the past, mainly in the mouse collagen–induced arthritis model of RA, have demonstrated that the benefit of anti-TNFα therapy may be augmented by a variety of forms of anti–T cell therapy. The first to be documented in detail was synergy with anti-CD4 antibodies (83), but synergy can also be documented with blockade of costimulatory molecules (CD80 and CD86), using CTLA-4Ig fusion protein or anti-CD3 antibodies (Williams, unpublished data).

The extrapolation of these data into human disease, requiring the application of unlicensed drugs in clinical trials, is unrealistic. The first combination therapy targeting the immune system as well as TNFα was performed using MTX, and was highly successful (82). This has led to the routine use of infliximab with MTX (82, 84, 86). Increased efficacy without increased toxicity has also subsequently been found using etanercept (96).

The optimum combination therapy has not yet been evaluated, and it is possible that in human RA, as in the mouse, additional anti–T cell therapy, for example with anti-CD4 or anti-CD3 or cyclosporin, may lead to benefit in the patients not responding to anti-TNFα therapy alone.

Pathogenesis of Joint Damage

It has been proposed that contrary to the conventional view, inflammation and joint destruction may not be causally related. Evidence that they are uncoupled and due to different processes, with joint destruction due to an 'autonomous' tumorlike mass of fibroblasts, has been put forward (147). This was established by transplanting human fibroblast-like synoviocytes derived from rheumatoid tissue into immunocompromised SCID mice and demonstrating invasion and destruction of co-implanted cartilage. However, the clinical joint protection studies with infliximab, etanercept, and D2E7 indicate that this process of joint destruction is also likely dependent on TNFα (86, 92, 97).

The control of joint destruction, and hence the preservation of function, has been viewed as the holy grail in the therapy of rheumatoid arthritis. Randomized controlled trials have provided evidence that drugs such as MTX, leflunomide, and sulphasalazine retard structural damage compared with placebo therapy. In the ATTRACT phase III trial, the 12-month radiological analysis demonstrated that cartilage and bone damage (assessed by a modified Sharp score) progressed relentlessly in the group with active disease resistant to MTX who continue to receive MTX and placebo infusions, but was arrested in the groups receiving both MTX and infliximab in about 50% of patients (86). Etanercept used alone also had bone protective effects (97). Follow-up studies with D2E7 over one year have shown radiological benefit, although this was not a randomized and fully blinded prospective study (92).

The rush of recent clinical trial results clearly suggests that the current biological anti-TNFα agents have major protective effects against joint destruction. These data in RA are reminiscent of the protection of cartilage and bone with anti-TNFα antibody therapy in collagen II–induced arthritis in mice (66, 67) especially when combined with anti-T cell therapy (83). Prior to these animal studies, in vitro experiments had shown that TNFα was able to induce cartilage damage (148, 149) and bone damage (150).

The relative contribution of IL-1 and TNFα in mediating tissue destruction continues to be debated. The view has been espoused that targeted IL-1 blockade is critical in regulating joint destruction (151). This claim is based on a combination of in vitro and in vivo studies, which demonstrate the superior potency of IL-1 over TNFα in the induction of cartilage and bone damage (152, 153).

Experimental data exist, however, that can reconcile the role of TNFα and IL-1 in this regard. The addition of anti-TNFα antibody to RA synovial cells in vitro reduced IL-1 synthesis (23), and subsequently evidence was obtained that this occurs in vivo following therapy with infliximab (115, 154). Downregulation of IL-1 production in RA patients has also been recently reported in patients treated with D2E7 by Van den Berg's group (93). The work of Dinarello and others has highlighted the synergy between TNFα and IL-1 in many systems (29). Hence, it is possible that depletion of TNFα not only reduces production of IL-1 in joints, but also diminishes the synergistic effect of TNFα and IL-1.

Since anti-TNFα therapy combined with MTX has proved to show an unexpected degree of joint protective effect, it seems likely that the added benefit from co-administration of other anti-cytokines may be small. However, anti-IL-1 therapy may prove beneficial in patients unresponsive to anti-TNFα therapy (30%–40% in some trials) and in conjunction with anti-TNFα therapy administered at suboptimal levels (141).

The mechanisms of bone damage in RA are not fully understood. Osteoclasts are believed to play an important role in erosions of bone. The strongest signal for the differentiation and activation of osteoclasts is provided by RANK ligand (RANKL, also known as ODF, TRANCE, or OPG ligand), which is expressed by mesenchymal cells (e.g. synoviocytes and osteoblasts) as well as T lymphocytes.

TNFα may itself be able to induce osteoclast differentiation, by-passing RANK, in vitro (155). This result is not surprising as RANK (receptor activated inducer of NFκB) signals chiefly by inducing NFκB, as does TNFα. Whether anti-TNFα therapy has any impact on RANKL expression, or on the levels of the soluble inhibitor of osteoclast activation, osteoprotegerin (OPG), which blocks RANKL, is not known at present. This is certainly possible as TNFα and IL-1 have been described to upregulate both RANKL and OPG (156, 157). The effect of anti-TNFα therapy on the critical RANKL/OPG balance remains to be established.

Perhaps the most important conclusion from the three recent studies of anti-TNFα blockade on protecting joints (86, 92, 97) is the awareness that targeting TNFα is effective even in late-stage disease. Whether blocking RANKL by raising OPG levels will have additional benefits to blocking TNFα alone is not known, but in the rat adjuvant arthritis model, the administration of OPG was associated with joint protection (158).

CONCLUSIONS

Anti-TNFα therapy is one of the current successes of the biotechnology industry, which has cloned cytokines and generated inhibitors to them. It is also one of the successes of research in the cytokine field aimed at understanding the key, rate-limiting cytokines involved in the pathogenesis of disease, which might be suitable therapeutic targets. The success of anti-TNFα therapy in RA has prompted clinical studies in related diseases, such as Crohn's disease, which have also been highly successful therapeutically (159, 160), and more recently in the treatment of psoriatic arthritis and ankylosing spondylitis. We anticipate that this is the beginning of a wave of new therapies based on a rational understanding of the molecular pathogenesis of complex diseases. Many of these therapies will be targeted at cytokines. For maximum impact on improving the quality of life and secondary prevention of morbidity and premature mortality, cytokine-regulating drugs will need to be used in early stages of the disease. Durability of benefit, safety, and pharmacoeconomic issues will determine whether the early promise of the success of this knowledge-based approach will prove to be a boon to sufferers of incurable and painful diseases.

Visit the Annual Reviews home page at www.AnnualReviews.org

LITERATURE CITED

1. Stasny P. 1978. Association of the B cell alloantigen DRW4 with rheumatoid arthritis. *N. Engl. J. Med.* 298:869–71
2. Gregersen PK, Silver J, Winchester RJ. 1987. The shared epitope hypothesis. An approach to understanding the molecular genetics of susceptibility to rheumatoid arthritis. *Arthritis Rheum.* 30:1205–13
3. Todd JA, Acha-Orbea H, Bell JI, Chao N, Fronek Z, Jacob CO, McDermott M, Sinha

AA, Timmerman L, Steinman L, McDevitt HO. 1988. A molecular basis for MHC class II-associated autoimmunity. *Science* 240:1003–9

4. Laurence JS. 1970. Rheumatoid arthritis: nature or nurture? *Ann. Rheum. Dis.* 29: 357–69

5. Silman AJ, MacGregor AJ, Thomson W, Holligan S, Carthy D, Farhan A, Ollier WER. 1993. Twin concordance rates for rheumatoid arthritis: results from a nationwide study. *Br. J. Rheumatol.* 32:903–7

6. Erhardt CC, Mumford PA, Venables PJW, Maini RN. 1989. Factors predicting a poor life prognosis in rheumatoid arthritis: an eight year prospective study. *Ann. Rheum. Dis.* 48:7–13

7. Pincus T, Callahan LF. 1993. What is the natural history of rheumatoid arthritis? *Rheum. Dis. Clin. North Am.* 19:123–51

8. Maini RN, Zvaifler NJSE. 1994. Rheumatoid arthritis. In *Rheumatology*, ed. JH Klippel, PA Dieppe, 3.1. - 3.14.8. London: Mosby Year Book Europe

9. Smolen JS, Kalden JR, Maini RN, eds. 1992. *Rheumatoid Arthritis*. Berlin: Springer-Verlag

10. Carswell EA, Old LJ, Kassel RL, Green S, Fiore N, Williamson B. 1975. An endotoxin-induced serum factor that causes necrosis of tumors. *Proc. Natl. Acad. Sci. USA* 72:3666–70

11. Old LJ. 1985. Tumor necrosis factor (TNF). *Science* 230:630–32

12. Pennica D, Nedwin GE, Hayflick JS, P.H.S, Derynck R, Palladino MA, Kohr WJ, Aggarwal BB, Goeddel DV. 1984. Human tumor necrosis factor: precursor structure expression and homology to lymphotoxin. *Nature* 312:724–29

13. Beutler B, Cerami A. 1988. Tumor necrosis, cachexia, shock, and inflammation: a common mediator. *Annu. Rev. Biochem.* 57:505–18

14. Vassalli P. 1992. The pathophysiology of tumor necrosis factors. *Annu. Rev. Immunol.* 10:411

15. Ruddle NH, Waksman BH. 1968. Cytotoxicity mediated by soluble antigen and lymphocytes in delayed hypersensitivity. I. Characterization of the phenomenon. *J. Exp. Med.* 128:1237–54

16. Gray PW, Aggarwal BB, Benton CV, Bringman TS, Henzel WJ, Jarrett JA, Leung DW, Moffat B, Ng P, Svedersky LP, Palladino MA, Nedwin GE. 1984. Cloning and expression of cDNA for human lymphotoxin, a lymphokine with tumor necrosis factor activity. *Nature* 312: 721–24

17. Vilcek J. 1998. The cytokines: an overview. In *The Cytokine Handbook*, ed. A. W. Thomson, pp. 1–20 Academic Press

18. Feldmann M, Dower S, Brennan FM. 1996. The role of cytokines in normal and pathological situations. In *Role of Cytokines in Autoimmunity*, ed. F. M. Brennan, M. Feldmann, pp. 1–23. Austin, TX: RG Landes Comp., Med. Intelligence Unit

19. Aggarwal BB, Samanta A, Feldmann M. 2000. TNFα. In *The Cytokine Reference*, ed. OJ, FM. New York: Academic Press.

20. Tracey KJ, Fong Y, Hesse DG, Manogue KR, Lee AT, Kuo GC, Lowry SF, Cerami A. 1987. Anti-cachectin/TNF monoclonal antibodies prevent septic shock during lethal bacteraemia. *Nature* 330:662–4

21. Black RA, Rauch CT, Kozlosky CJ, Peschon JJ, Slack JL, Wolfson MF, Castner BJ, Stocking KL, Reddy P, Srinivasan S, Nelson N, Boiani N, Schooley KA, Gerhart M, Davis R, Fitzner JN, Johnson RS, Paxton RJ, March CJ, Cerretti DP. 1997. A metalloproteinase disintegrin that releases tumour necrosis factor-alpha from cells. *Nature* 385:729–33

22. Fong Y, Tracey KJ, Moldawer LL, Hesse DG, Manogue KB, Kenney JS, Lee AT, Kuo GC, Allison AC, Lowry SF, Cerami A. 1989. Antibodies to cachectin/tumor necrosis factor reduce interleukin 1β and interleukin 6 appearance during lethal bacteremia. *J. Exp. Med.* 170:1627–33

23. Brennan FM, Chantry D, Jackson A, Maini R, Feldmann M. 1989. Inhibitory effect of TNF alpha antibodies on synovial cell interleukin-1 production in rheumatoid arthritis. *Lancet* 2:244–47

24. Doukas J, Pober JS. 1990. IFN-γ enhances endothelial activation induced by tumor necrosis factor but not IL-1. *J. Immunol.* 145:1727–33

25. Schroder JM, Sticherling M, Henneicke HH, Preissner WC, Christophers E. 1990. IL-1α or tumor necrosis factor-α stimulate release of three NAP-1/IL-8-related neutrophil chemotactic proteins in human dermal fibroblasts. *J. Immunol.* 144:2223–32

26. Yokota S, Geppert T, Lipsky P. 1988. Enhancement of antigen- and mitogen-induced human T lymphocyte proliferation by tumor necrosis factor-α. *J. Immunol.* 140:531–36

27. Gordon C, Wofsy D. 1990. Effects of recombinant murine tumor necrosis factor-α on immune function. *J. Immunol.* 144:1753–58

28. Cope AP, Londei M, Chu NR, Cohen SBA, Elliott MJ, Maini RN, Brennan FM, Feldmann M. 1994. Chronic exposure to tumor necrosis factor (TNF) in vitro impairs the activation of T cells through the T cell receptor/CD3 complex; reversal in vivo by anti-TNF antibodies in patients with rheumatoid arthritis. *J. Clin. Invest.* 94:749–60

29. Dinarello CA. 1994. The interleukin-1 family: 10 years of discovery. *FASEB J.* 8:1314–25

30. Oppenheim JJ, Feldmann M, eds. 2000. *The Cytokine Reference – A Comprehensive Guide to the Role of Cytokines in Health and Disease.* London: Academic Press.

31. Feldmann M, Brennan FM, Maini RN. 1996. Rheumatoid arthritis. *Cell.* 85:307–10

32. Maini RN, Feldmann M. 2000. *Pocket Reference to TNFα Antagonism and Rheumatoid Arthritis.* London: Science Press.

33. Feldmann M, Brennan FM, Maini RN. 1996. Role of cytokines in rheumatoid arthritis. *Annu. Rev. Immunol.* 14:397–440

34. Feldmann M, Elliott MJ, Woody JN, Maini RN. 1997. Anti TNFα therapy of rheumatoid arthritis. *Adv. Immunol.* 64:283–350

35. Arend WP, Dayer J-M. 1995. Inhibition of the production and effects of interleukin-1 and tumor necrosis factor α in rheumatoid arthritis. *Arthritis Rheum.* 38:151–60

36. Pisetsky DS. 2000. Tumor necrosis factor blockers in rheumatoid arthritis. *N. Engl. J. Med.* 342:810–11

37. Koch AE, Kunkel SL, Strieter RM. 1995. Cytokines in rheumatoid arthritis. *J. Invest. Med.* 43:28–38

38. Williams L, Gibbons DL, Gearing A, Feldmann M, Brennan FM. 1996. The synthetic metalloproteinase inhibitor BB-2275 blocks both p55 and p75 TNF receptor shedding, independent of its inhibitory effect on TNF processing. *J. Clin. Invest.* 97:2833–41

39. Seckinger P, Isaaz S, Dayer JM. 1988. A human inhibitor of tumor necrosis factor α. *J. Exp. Med.* 167:1511–16

40. Engelmann H, Aderka D, Rubinstein M, Rotman D, Wallach D. 1989. A tumor necrosis factor-binding protein purified to homogeneity from human urine protects cells from tumor necrosis factor toxicity. *J. Biol. Chem.* 264:11974–80

41. Olsson I, Lantz S, Nilsson E, Peetre C, Thysell H, Grubb A, Adolf G. 1989. Isolation and characterization of a tumor necrosis factor binding protein from urine. *Eur. J. Haematol.* 42:270–75

42. Moore KW, O'Garra A, de Waal Malefyt R, Vieira P, Mosmann TR. 1993. Interleukin-10. *Annu. Rev. Immunol.* 11:165–90

43. Roberts AB, Sporn MB. 1990. The transforming growth factors-beta. In *Handbook of Experimental Pharmacology*, ed. M. B. Sporn, A. B. Roberts, 95:419–72. Heidelberg: Springer Verlag

44. Trepicchio WL, Bozza M, Pedneault G, Dorner AJ. 1996. Recombinant human interleukin-11 attenuates the inflammatory response through down-regulation of pro-inflammatory cytokine release and nitric oxide production. *J. Immunol.* 157:3627–34

45. Keith JC Jr, Albert L, Sonis ST, Pfeiffer CJ, Schaub RG. 1994. IL-11, a pleiotropic cytokine: exciting new effects of IL-11 on gastrointestinal mucosal biology. *Stem Cells.* 1:79–89

46. Dayer JM, Burger D. 1994. Interleukin-1, tumor necrosis factor and their specific inhibitors. *Eur. Cytokine Netw.* 5:563–71

47. Chu CQ, Field M, Feldmann M, Maini RN. 1991. Localization of tumor necrosis factor α in synovial tissues and at the cartilage-pannus junction in patients with rheumatoid arthritis. *Arthritis Rheum.* 34:1125–32

48. Wood NC, Symons JA, Dickens E, Duff GW. 1992. In situ hybridization of IL-6 in rheumatoid arthritis. *Clin. Exp. Immunol.* 87:183–89

49. Saxne T, Palladino MA Jr, Heinegard D, Talal N, Wollheim FA. 1988. Detection of tumor necrosis factor α but not tumor necrosis factor β in rheumatoid arthritis synovial fluid and serum. *Arthritis Rheum.* 31:1041–45

50. Fontana A, Hentgartner H, Fehr K, Grob PJ, Cohen G. 1982. Interleukin-1 activity in the synovial fluid of patients with rheumatoid arthritis. *Rheumatol. Int.* 2: 49–56

51. Alvaro-Garcia JM, Zvaifler NJ, Brown CB, Kaushansky L, Firestein GS. 1991. Cytokines in chronic inflammatory arthritis. VI. Analysis of the synovial cells involved in granulocyte-macrophage colony stimulating factor production and gene expression in rheumatoid arthritis and its regulation by IL-1 and TNFα. *J. Immunol.* 146:3365–71

52. Hopkins SJ, Humphreys M, Jayson MI. 1988. Cytokines in synovial fluid. I. The presence of biologically active and im-munoreactive IL-1. *Clin. Exp. Immunol.* 72:422–27

53. Di Giovine FS, Nuki G, Duff GW. 1988. Tumour necrosis factor in synovial exudates. *Ann. Rheum. Dis.* 47:768–72

54. Alvaro-Garcia JM, Zvaifler NJ, Firestein GS. 1989. Cytokines in chronic inflammatory arthritis. IV. GM-CSF mediated induction of class II MHC antigen on human monocytes: a possible role in RA. *J. Exp. Med.* 146:865–75

55. Malyak M, Swaney RE, Arend WP. 1993. Levels of synovial fluid interleukin-1 receptor antagonist in rheumatoid arthritis and other arthropathies. *Arthritis Rheum.* 36:781–89

56. Miossec P, Naviliat M, D'Angeac AD, Sany J, Banchereau J. 1990. Low levels of interleukin-4 and high levels of transforming growth factor β in rheumatoid synovitis. *Arthritis Rheum.* 33:1180–87

57. Leech M, Metz C, Hall P, Hutchinson P, Gianis K, Smith M, Weedon H, Holdsworth SR, Bucala R, Morand EF. 1999. Macrophage migration inhibitory factor in rheumatoid arthritis: evidence of proinflammatory function and regulation by glucocorticoids. *Arthritis Rheum.* 42:1601–8

58. Katsikis PD, Chu CQ, Brennan FM, Maini RN, Feldmann M. 1994. Immunoregulatory role of interleukin 10 in rheumatoid arthritis. *J. Exp. Med.* 179:1517–27

59. Hermann JA, Hall MA, Maini RN, Feldmann M, Brennan FM. 1998. Important immunoregulatory role of interleukin-11 in the inflammatory process in rheumatoid arthritis. *Arthritis Rheum.* 41:1388–97

60. Allard SA, Muirden KD, Maini RN. 1991. Correlation of histopathological features of pannus with patterns of damage in different joints in rheumatoid arthritis. *Ann. Rheum. Dis.* 50:278–83

61. Zvaifler NJ, Firestein GS. 1994. Current comment: pannus and pannocytes: alternative models of joint destruction in rheumatoid arthritis. *Arthritis Rheum.* 37:783–89

62. Haworth C, Brennan FM, Chantry D, Turner M, Maini RN, Feldmann M. 1991. Expression of granulocyte-macrophage colony–stimulating factor in rheumatoid arthritis: regulation by tumor necrosis factor-alpha. *Eur. J. Immunol.* 21:2575–79

63. Deleuran BW, Chu CQ, Field M, Brennan FM, Mitchell T, Feldmann M, Maini RN. 1992. Localization of tumor necrosis factor receptors in the synovial tissue and cartilage-pannus junction in patients with rheumatoid arthritis. Implications for local actions of tumor necrosis factor alpha. *Arthritis Rheum.* 35:1170–78

64. Staines NA, Wooley PH. 1994. Collagen-induced arthritis—what can it teach us? *Br. J. Rheumatol.* 33:798–807

65. Korganow AS, Ji H, Mangialaio S, Duchatelle V, Pelanda R, Martin T, Degott C, Kikutani H, Rajewsky K, Pasquali JL, Benoist C, Mathis D. 1999. From systemic T cell self-reactivity to organ-specific autoimmune disease via immunoglobulins. *Immunity* 10:451–61

66. Thorbecke GJ, Shah R, Leu CH, Kuruvilla AP, Hardison AM, Palladino MA. 1992. Involvement of endogenous tumour necrosis factor α and transforming growth factor β during induction of collagen type II arthritis in mice. *Proc. Natl. Acad. Sci. USA* 89:7375–79

67. Williams RO, Feldmann M, Maini RN. 1992. Anti-tumor necrosis factor ameliorates joint disease in murine collagen-induced arthritis. *Proc. Natl. Acad. Sci. USA* 89:9784–88

68. Piguet PF, Grau GE, Vesin C, Loetscher H, Gentz R, Lesslauer W. 1992. Evolution of collagen arthritis in mice is arrested by treatment with anti-tumour necrosis factor (TNF) antibody or a recombinant soluble TNF receptor. *Immunology* 77:510–14

69. Wooley PH, Dutcher J, Widmer MB, Gillis S. 1993. Influence of a recombinant human soluble tumour necrosis factor receptor Fc fusion protein on type II collagen-induced arthritis in mice. *J. Immunol.* 151:6602–7

70. Breedveld FC. 2000. Therapeutic monoclonal antibodies. *Lancet* 355:735–40

71. Tugwell P. 2000. Pharmacoeconomics of drug therapy for rheumatoid arthritis. *Rheumatology* 39 (Suppl. 1):43–47

72. Knight DM, Trinh H, Le J, Siegel S, Shealy D, McDonough M, Scallon B, Moore AM, Vilcek J, Daddona P, Ghrayeb J. 1993. Construction and initial characterization of a mouse-human chimeric anti-TNF antibody. *Mol. Immunol.* 30:1443–53

73. Elliott MJ, Maini RN, Feldmann M, Long-Fox A, Charles P, Katsikis P, Brennan FM, Walker J, Bijl H, Ghrayeb J, Woody JN. 1993. Treatment of rheumatoid arthritis with chimeric monoclonal antibodies to tumor necrosis factor alpha. *Arthritis Rheum.* 36:1681–90

74. Sopwith M, Stephens S. 1999. An engineered human antibody for chronic therapy: CDP571. In *Biotechnology*, ed. H-J Rehn, G Reed, pp. 343–53. Weinham: Wiley-VCH. 2nd ed.

75. Jespers L, Roberts A, Mahler S, Winter G, Hoogenboom H. 1994. Guiding the selection of human antibodies from phage display repertoires to a single epitope of an antigen. *Biotechnology* 12:899–903

76. Hazleman B, Smith M, Moss K, Lisi L, Scott D, Sopwith M, Choy E, Isenberg D. 2000. Efficacy of a novel pegylated humanised anti-TNF fragment (CDP870) in patients with rheumatoid arthritis. *Rheumatology.* 39 (Suppl. 1):87

77. Mohler KM, Torrence DS, Smith CA. 1993. Soluble tumour necrosis factor (TNF) receptors are effective therapeutic agents in lethal endotoxemia and function simultaneously as both TNF carriers and TNF antagonists. *J. Immunol.* 151:1548–61

78. Lesslauer W, Tabuchi H, Gentz R, Brockhaus M, Schlaeger EJ, Grau G, Piguet PF, Pointaire P, Vassalli P, Loetscher H. 1991. Recombinant soluble TNF receptor proteins protect mice from LPS-induced lethality. *Eur. J. Immunol.* 21:2883–86

79. Edwards CKI. 1999. PEGylated recombinant human soluble tumour necrosis factor receptor type I (r-Hu-sTNF-RI): novel high affinity TNF receptor designed for chronic inflammatory diseases. *Ann. Rheum. Dis.* 58 (Suppl 1):173–81

80. Elliott MJ, Maini RN, Feldmann M, Long-Fox A, Charles P, Bijl H, Woody JN. 1994. Repeated therapy with monoclonal antibody to tumour necrosis factor α (cA2) in patients with rheumatoid arthritis. *Lancet* 344:1125–27

81. Elliott MJ, Maini RN, Feldmann M, Kalden JR, Antoni C, Smolen JS, Leeb B, Breedveld FC, Macfarlane JD, Bijl H, Woody JN. 1994. Randomised double-blind comparison of chimeric monoclonal antibody to tumour necrosis factor alpha (cA2) versus placebo in rheumatoid arthritis. *Lancet* 344:1105–10

82. Maini RN, Breedveld FC, Kalden JR, Smolen JS, Davis D, Macfarlane JD, Antoni C, Leeb B, Elliott MJ, Woody JN, Schaible TF, Feldmann M. 1998. Therapeutic efficacy of multiple intravenous infusions of anti-tumor necrosis factor alpha monoclonal antibody combined with low-dose weekly methotrexate in rheumatoid arthritis. *Arthritis Rheum.* 41:1552–63

83. Williams RO, Mason LJ, Feldmann M, Maini RN. 1994. Synergy between anti-CD4 and anti-TNF in the amelioration of established collagen-induced arthritis. *Proc. Natl. Acad. Sci. USA* 91:2762–66

84. Maini RN, St Clair EW, Breedveld F, Furst D, Kalden J, Weisman M, Smolen J, Emery P, Harriman G, Feldmann M, Lipsky P, Group AS. 1999. Infliximab (chimeric anti-tumour necrosis factor a monoclonal antibody) versus placebo in rheumatoid arthritis patients receiving concomitant methotrexate: a randomised phase III trial. *Lancet.* 354:1932–39

85. van der Heijde DM. 1996. Plain X-rays in rheumatoid arthritis: overview of scoring methods, their reliability and applicability. *Baillieres Clin. Rheumatol.* 10:435–53

86. Lipsky P, St. Clair W, Furst D, Breedveld F, Smolen J, Kalden JR, Weisman M, Emery P, Harriman G, an der Heijde D, Maini RN. 1999. 54 week clinical and radiographic results from the attract trial: a phase III study of infliximab (RemicadeTM) in patient with active RA despite methrotrexate (abstract). *Arthritis Rheum.* 42: S401

87. Rankin ECC, Choy EHS, Kassimos D, Kingsley GH, Sopwith SM, Isenberg DA, Panayi GS. 1995. The therapeutic effects of an engineered human anti-tumour necrosis factor alpha antibody (CD571) in rheumatoid arthritis. *Br. J. Rheumatol.* 34: 334–42

88. Kempeni J. 1999. Preliminary results of early clinical trials with the fully human anti-TNF monoclonal antibody D2E7. *Ann. Rheum. Dis.* 58 (Suppl. 1):I70–I2

89. van de Putte LBA, van Riel PLCM, den Broeder A, Sander O, Rau R, Binder C, Kruger K, Schattenkirchner M, Fenner H, Salfeld J, Bankmann Y, Kupper H, Kempeni J. 1998. A single dose placebo controlled phase I study of the fully human anti-TNF antibody D2E7 in patients with rheumatoid arthritis. *Arthritis Rheum.* 41: No. 9 (Suppl.), Ab.:148:S57

90. Schattenkirchner M, Kruger K, Sander O, Rau R, Kroot E-J, van Riel PLCM, van de Putte LBA, den Broeder A, Fenner H, Kempeni J, Kupper H. 1999. Efficacy and tolerability of weekly subcutaneous injections of the fully human anti-TNF antibody D2E7 in patients with rheumatoid arthritis—results of a phase I study. *Arthritis Rheum.* 41: No. 9 (Suppl.), Ab.:149:S57

91. Rau R, Herborn G, Sander O, van de Putte LBA, van Riel PLC, den Broeder A, Schattenkirchner M, Wastlhuber J, Rihl M, Fenner H, Kempeni J, Kupper H. 1999. Long-term efficacy and tolerability of multiple i.v. doses of the fully human anti-TNF antibody D2E7 in patients with rheumatoid arthritis. *Arthritis Rheum.* 41(9):(Suppl):S55

92. Rau R, Herborn G, Sander O, van de Putte LBA, van Riel PLC, den Broeder A, Schattenkirchner M, Wastlhuber J, Rihl M, Fenner H, Kempeni J, Kupper H. 1999. Long term treatment with the fully human anti TNF antibody D2E7 slows radiographic disease progression in rheumatoid arthritis. *Arthritis Rheum.* 42:(9)(Suppl.):S400

93. Barrera P, Joosten LAB, den Broeder AA, van de Putte LBA, van den Berg WB. 1999. Effect of a fully human anti TNFα monoclonal antibody on the local and systemic expression of TNFα and IL-1β. *Arthritis Rheum.* 42:(9)(Suppl.) (Abst.) 29:S75

94. Moreland LW, Baumgartner SW, Schiff MH, Tindall eA, Fleischmann RM, Weaver AL, Ettlinger RE, Cohen S, Koopman WJ, Mohler K, Widmer MB, Blosch CM. 1997. Treatment of rheumatoid arthritis with a recombinant human tumor necrosis factor receptor (p75)-Fc fusion protein. *N. Engl. J. Med.* 337:141–47

95. Moreland LW, Schiff MH, Baumgartner SW, Tindall EA, Fleischmann RM, Bulpitt KJ, Weaver AL, Keystone EC, Furst DE, Mease PJ, Ruderman EM, Hortwitz DA, Arkfield DG, Garrison L, D.J B, Blosch CM, Lange ML, McDonnell ND, Weinblatt ME. 1999. Etanercept therapy in rheumatoid arthritis. A randomized, controlled trial. *Ann. Intern. Med.* 130:478–86

96. Weinblatt ME, Kremer JM, Bankhurst AD, Bulpitt KJ, Fleischmann RM, Fox RI, Jackson CG, Lange M, Burge DJ. 1999. A trial of etanercept, a recombinant tumor necrosis factor receptor:Fc fusion protein, in patients with rheumatoid arthritis receiving methotrexate. *N. Engl. J. Med.* 340:253–59

97. Finck B, Martin R, Fleischmann R, Moreland L, Schiff M, Bathon J. 1999. A phase III trial of etanercept vs methotrexate (MTX) in early rheumatoid arthritis (Enbrel ERA trial). *Arthritis Rheum.* 42:S117

98. Lovell DJ, Giannini EH, Reiff PHA, Cawkwell GD, Silverman ED, Nocton JJ, Stein LD, Gedalia A, Ilowite NT, Wallace CA, Whitmore J, Finck BK. 2000. Etanercept in children with polyarticular juvenile rheumatoid arthritis. *N. Engl. J. Med.* 342:763–69

99. Sander O, Rau R, van Riel P, van de Putte L, Hasler F, Baudin M, Ludin E, McAuliffe T, Dickinson S, Kahny M-R, Lesslauer W, Van der Auwera P. 1996. Neutralization of TNF by Lenercept (TNFR55-IgG1, Ro 45-2081) in patients with rheumatoid arthritis treated for 3 months: results of a European phase II trial. *Arthritis Rheum.*, October 18–22, 1996, S242

100. Hasler F, van de Putte L, Baudin M, Lodin E, Durrwell L, McAuliffe T, van de Auwera P. 1996. Chronic TNF neutralization (up to 1 year) by lenercept (TNFR 55 IgG1, Ro 45-2081) in patients with rheumatoid arthitis: Results from open label extension of a double blind single-dose phase I study. *Arthritis Rheum.* 39(Suppl.):S243

101. Furst D, Weisman M, Paulus H, Bulpitt K, Weinblatt M, Polisson R, St. Clair P, Milnarik P, Baudin M, Ludin E, McAuliffe T, Kahry MR, Lesslauer W, Van de Auwera P. 1996. Neutralization of TNF by lenercept (TNFR 55 TgGt, Ro 45-2081) in patients with rheumatoid arthritis treated for 3 months: results of a phase II trial. *Arthritis Rheum.* S243

102. Cutolo M, Kirkham B, Bologna C, Sany J, Scott D, Books P, Forre O, Jain R, Kvien T, Markenson J, Seibold J, Sturrock R, Veys E, Edwards J, Zaug M, Durrwell L, Bisschops C, St Clair P, Milnarik P, Baudin M, Van der Auwera P. 1996. Loading/maintenance doses approach to neutralization of TNF by Lenercept (TNFR55-IgG1, Ro45-2081) inpatients with rheumatoid arthritis treated for 3 months: results of a double-blind placebo controlled phase II trial. *Arthritis Rheum.*, October 18–22, 1996, S243

103. Christen U, Thuerkauf R, Lesslauer W. 1998. Immunogenicity of a human

TNFR55-IgG1 fusion protein (Lenercept) in rheumnatoid arthritis (RA) and multiple sclerosis (MS) patients. *J. Interfer. Cytokine Res.* 18:A121

104. Moreland LW, McCabe D, Caldwell JR, Sach M, Weisman M, Henry G, Seely J, Martin SW, Yee C, Bendele AM, Frazier J, Kohno T, Cosenza ME, Lyons S, Dayer J-M, Cohen A, Edwards CKI. 1999. Recombinant methionyl human tumor necrosis factor binding protein PE-Gylated dimer (TNFbp Dimer) in patients with active refractory rheumatoid arthritis. *J. Rheumatol.* In press

105. Moreland LW, Heck LW Jr, Koopman WJ. 1997. Biologic agents for treating rheumatoid arthritis. Concepts and progress. *Arthritis Rheum.* 40:397–409

106. Kavanaugh AF. 1998. Anti-tumor necrosis factor-α monoclonal antibody therapy for rheumatoid arthritis. *Emerging Therapies Rheumatoid Arthritis* 24:593–614

107. Ishida H, Muchamuel T, Sakaguchi S, Andrade S, Menon S, Howard M. 1994. Continuous administration of anti-interleukin 10 antibodies delays onset of autoimmunity in NZB/W F1 mice. *J. Exp. Med.* 179:305–10

108. Jacob CO, McDevitt HO. 1988. Tumour necrosis factor-alpha in murine autoimmune 'lupus' nephritis. *Nature* 331:356–58

109. Ettinger R, Daniel N. 2000. TNF-deficient mice develop anti-nuclear autoantibodies (abs). *Scand. J. Immunol.* 51 (Suppl.):88

110. Maini RN, Elliott MJ, Charles PJ, Feldmann M. 1994. Immunological intervention reveals reciprocal roles for TNFα and IL-10 in rheumatoid arthritis and SLE. *Springer Semin. Immunopathol.* 16:327–36

111. Charles PJ, Smeenk RJT, DeJong J, Feldmann M, Maini RN. 2000. Assessment of antibodies to dsDNA induced in rheumatoid arthritis (RA) patients following treatment with infliximab, a monoclonal antibody to TNF alpha. *Arthritis Rheum.* In press

112. Charles P, Elliott MJ, Davis D, Potter A, Kalden JR, Antoni C, Breedveld FC, Smolen JS, Eberl G, deWoody K, Feldmann M, Maini RN. 1999. Regulation of cytokines, cytokine inhibitors, and acute-phase proteins following anti-TNF-alpha therapy in rheumatoid arthritis. *J. Immunol.* 163:1521–28

113. Paleolog EM, Young S, Stark AC, Mc-Closkey RV, Feldmann M, Maini RN. 1998. Modulation of angiogenic vascular endothelial growth factor by tumor necrosis factor alpha and interleukin-1 in rheumatoid arthritis. *Arthritis Rheum.* 41:1258–65

114. Taylor PC, Peters AM, Paleolog E, Chapman PT, Elliott MJ, McCloskey R, Feldmann M, Maini RN. 2000. Reduction of chemokine levels and leukocyte traffic to joints by tumor necrosis factor α blockade in patients with rheumatoid arthritis. *Arthritis Rheum.* 43:38–47

115. Lorenz HM, Antoni C, Valerius T, Repp R, Grunke M, Schwerdtner N, Nusslein H, Woody J, Kalden JR, Manger B. 1996. In vivo blockade of TNF-alpha by intravenous infusion of a chimeric monoclonal TNF-alpha antibody in patients with rheumatoid arthritis - Short term cellular and molecular effects. *J. Immunol.* 156:1646–53

116. Ignatowski TA, Covey WC, Knight PR, Severin CM, Nickola TJ, Spengler RN. 1999. Brain-derived TNF alpha mediates nueropathic pain. *Brain Res.* 841:70–77

117. Brennan FM, Browne KA, Green PA, Jaspar JM, Maini RN, Feldmann M. 1997. Reduction of serum matrix metalloproteinase 1 and matrix metalloproteinase 3 in rheumatoid arthritis patients following anti- tumour necrosis factor-alpha (cA2) therapy. *Br. J. Rheumatol.* 36:643–50

118. Paleolog EM, Hunt M, Elliott MJ, Feldmann M, Maini RN, Woody JN. 1996. Deactivation of vascular endothelium by

monoclonal anti-tumor necrosis factor α antibody in rheumatoid arthritis. *Arthritis Rheum.* 39:1082–91

119. Tak PP, Taylor PC, Breedveld FC, Smeets TJM, Daha MR, Kluin PM, Meinders AE, Maini RN. 1996. Decrease in cellularity and expression of adhesion molecules by anti-tumor necrosis factor α monoclonal antibody treatment in patients with rheumatoid arthritis. *Arthritis Rheum.* 39:1077–81

120. Fava RA, Olsen NJ, Spencer-Green G, Yeo KT, Yeo TK, Berse B, Jackman RW, Senger DR, Dvorak HF, Brown LF. 1994. Vascular permeability factor/endothelial growth factor (VPF/VEGF): accumulation and expression in human synovial fluids and rheumatoid synovial tissue. *J. Exp. Med.* 180:341–46

121. Koch AE, Harlow LA, Haines GK, Amento EP, Unemori EN, Wong WL, Pope RM, Ferrara N. 1994. Vascular endothelial growth factor. A cytokine modulating endothelial function in rheumatoid arthritis. *J. Immunol.* 152:4149–56

122. Maini RN, Taylor PC, Paleolog E, Charles P, Ballara S, Brennan FM, Feldmann M. 1999. Anti-tumour necrosis factor specific antibody (infliximab) treatment provides insights into the pathophysiology of rheumatoid arthritis. *Ann. Rheum. Dis.* 58(Suppl. 1):156–60

123. Davis D, Charles PJ, Potter A, Feldmann M, Maini RN, Elliott MJ. 1997. Anaemia of chronic disease in rheumatoid arthritis: in vivo effects of tumour necrosis factor a blockade. *Br. J. Rheumatol.* 36:950–56

124. Wijdenes J, Racadot E, Wendling D. 1994. Interleukin 6 antibodies in rheumatoid arthritis. *J. Interferon Res.* 14:297–98

125. Soderlind E, Ohlin M, Carlsson R. 1999. Complementarily-determining region (CDR) implantation: a theme of recombination. *Immunotechnology* 4:279–85

126. Winter G, Griffiths AD, Hawkins RE, Hoogenboom HR. 1994. Making antibodies by phage display technology. *Ann. Rev. Immunol.* 12:433–55

127. Fishwild DM, O'Donnell SL, Bengoechea T, Hudson DV, Harding F, Bernhard SL, Jones D, Kay RM, Higgins KM, Schramm SR, Lonberg N. 1996. High-avidity human IgG kappa monoclonal antibodies from a novel strain of minilocus transgenic mice. *Nat. Biotechnol.* 14:845–51

128. Green LL, Hardy MC, Maynard-Currie CE, Tsuda H, Louie DM, Mendez MJ, Abderrahim H, Noguchi M, Smith DH, Zeng Y, et al. 1994. Antigen-specific human monoclonal antibodies from mice engineered with human Ig heavy and light chain YACs. *Nat. Genet.* 7:13–21

129. Oudin J, J. M. 1963. A new form of allotype of rabbit gamma-globulins apparently correlated with antibody function and specificity C. *R. Acad. Sci.* 257:805–8

130. Dresser DW, Mitchison NA. 1968. The mechanism of immunological paralysis. *Adv. Immunol.* 8:129–81

131. Basten A, Miller JF, Sprent J, Cheers C. 1974. Cell-to-cell interaction in the immune response. X. T-cell-dependent suppression in tolerant mice. *J. Exp. Med.* 140:199–217

132. Chiller JM, Habicht GS, Weigle WO. 1970. Cellular sites of immunologic unresponsiveness. *Proc. Natl. Acad. Sci. USA* 65:551–56

133. Kavanaugh AF, Cush JJ, St Clair EW, McCune WJ, Braakman TAJ, Nichols LA, Lipsky PE. 1996. Anti-TNFα monoclonal antibody (mAb) treatment of rheumatoid arthritis (RA) patients with active disease on methotrexate (MTX): results of a double-blind, placebo controlled multicenter trial. *Arthritis Rheum.* 39:A575

134. Genestier L, Paillot R, Fournel S, Ferraro C, Miossec P, Revillard JP. 1998. Immunosuppressive properties of methotrexate: apoptosis and clonal deletion of activated peripheral T cells. *J. Clin. Invest.* 102:322–28

135. Espevik T, Brockhaus M, Loetscher H, Nonstad U, Shalaby R. 1990. Characterization of binding and biological effects of monoclonal antibodies against a human tumor necrosis factor receptor. *J. Exp. Med.* 171:415–26

136. Quattrocchi E, Dallman M, Feldmann M. 2000. Adenovirus mediated gene transfer of CTLA-4Ig fusion protein suppresses experimental autoimmune arthritis. *Arthritis Rheum.* 43:1688–97

137. Garrision L, McDonnell ND. 1999. Etanercept: theapeutic use in patients with rheumatoid arthritis. *Ann. Rheum. Dis* 58 (suppl 1):165–69

138. Pinals RS, Masi AT, Larsen RA. 1981. Preliminary criteria for clinical remission in rheumatoid arthritis. *Arthritis Rheum.* 24:1308–15

139. Ohshima S, Saeki Y, Mima T, Suemura M, Ishida H, Shimizu M, McClosky R, Kishimoto T. 1996. Possible mechanism for the long-term efficacy of anti-TNF alpha antibody (cA2) therapy in RA. *Arthritis Rheum.* 39, No. 9 (Suppl.):S242

140. Walmsley M, Katsikis PD, Abney E, Parry S, Williams RO, Maini RN, Feldmann M. 1996. Interleukin-10 inhibition of the progression of established collagen-induced arthritis. *Arthritis Rheum.* 39:495–503

141. Feige U, Hu YL, Julian E, Duryea D, Bolon B. 1999. Combining anti IL-1 and anti-TNF treatments provides better efficacy in rat adjuvant arthritis than does either agent alone. *Arthritis Rheum.* 42:S383:(A1875)

142. Paleolog E. 1996. Angiogenesis: a critical process in the pathogenesis of RA - a role for VEGF? *Br. J. Rheumatol.* 35:917–20

143. Hayashida K, Shimaoka Y, Ochi T, Lipsky PE. 2000. Rheumatoid arthritis synovial stromal cells inhibit apoptosis and upregulate Bcl-xL expression by B cells in a CD49/CD29-CD106-dependent mechanism. *J. Immunol.* 164:1110–16

144. Salmon M, Scheel-Toellner D, Huissoon AP, Pilling D, Shamsadeen N, Hyde H, D'Angeac AD, Bacon PA, Emery P, Akbar AN. 1997. Inhibition of T cell apoptosis in the rheumatoid synovium. *J. Clin. Invest.* 99 (3):439–46

145. Aupperle KR, Boyle DL, Hendrix M, Seftor EA, Zvaifler NJ, Barbosa M, Firestein GS. 1998. Regulation of synoviocyte proliferation, apoptosis, and invasion by the p53 tumor suppressor gene. *Am. J. Pathol.* 152:1091–98

146. Brennan FM, Hayes AL, Ciesielski CJ, Foxwell BMJ, Feldmann M. 2000. Cytokine activated T cells are important in TNFα synthesis in rheumatoid arthritis: P13 kinase and NF-κB pathways discriminate between cytokine and TCR activated T cells. Submitted

147. Muller-Ladner U, Gay RE, Gay S. 1998. Molecular biology of cartilage and bone destruction. *Curr. Opin. Rheumatol.* 10:212–19

148. Saklatvala J, Sarsfield SJ, Townsend Y. 1985. Pig interleukin -1. Purification of two immunologically different leukocyte proteins that cause cartilage resorption, lymphocyte activation and fever. *J. Exp. Med.* 162:1208–15

149. Saklatvala J. 1986. Tumour necrosis factor alpha stimulates resorption and inhibits synthesis of proteoglycan in cartilage. *Nature* 322:547–49

150. Gowen M, Mundy GG. 1986. Actions of recombinant interleukin 1, interleukin 2, and interferon gamma on bone resorption in vitro. *J. Immunol.* 136:2478–82

151. van den Berg WB. 1998. Joint inflammation and cartilage destruction may occur uncoupled. *Springer Semin. Immunopathol.* 20:149–64

152. Henderson B, Pettipher ER. 1989. Arthritogenic actions of recombinant IL-1 and tumour necrosis factor α in the rabbit: evidence for synergistic interactions between cytokines *in vivo*. *Clin. Exp. Immunol.* 75:306–10

153. Joosten LA, Helsen MM, Saxne T, van De Loo FA, Heinegard D, van Den Berg WB. 1999. IL-1 alpha beta blockade prevents cartilage and bone destruction in murine type II collagen-induced arthritis, whereas TNF-alpha blockade only ameliorates joint inflammation. *J. Immunol.* 163:5049–55

154. Ulfgren A-K, Andersson U, Engstrom M, Klareskog L, Maini RN, Taylor PC. 2000. Systemic anti-TNFα therapy in rheumatoid arthritis down-regulates synovial TNFα synthesis. Submitted

155. Kobayashi K, Takahashi N, Jimi E, Udagawa N, Takami M, Kotake S, Nakagawa N, Kinosaki M, Yamaguchi K, Shima N, Yasuda H, Morinaga T, Higashio K, Martin TJ, Suda T. 2000. Tumor necrosis factor alpha stimulates osteoclast differentiation by a mechanism independent of the ODF/RANKL-RANK interaction. *J. Exp. Med.* 191:275–86

156. Lacey DL, Timms E, Tan HL, Kelley MJ, Dunstan CR, Burgess T, Elliott R, Colombero A, Elliott G, Scully S, Hsu H, Sullivan J, Hawkins N, Davy E, Capparelli C, Eli A, Qian YX, Kaufman S, Sarosi I, Shalhoub V, Senaldi G, Guo J, Delaney J, Boyle WJ. 1998. Osteoprotegerin ligand is a cytokine that regulates osteoclast differentiation and activation. *Cell.* 93:165–76

157. Yasuda H, Shima N, Nakagawa N, Yamaguchi K, Kinosaki M, Mochizuki S, Tomoyasu a, Yano K, Goto M, Murakami A, Tsuda E, Morinaga T, Higashio K, Udagawa N, Takahashi N, Suda T. 1998. Osteoclast differentiation factor is a ligand for osteoprotegerin/osteoclastogenesis-inhibitory factor and is identical to TRANCE/RANKL. *Proc. Natl. Acad. Sci. USA* 95:3597–3602

158. Kong YY, Feige U, Sarosi I, Bolon B, Tafuri A, Morony S, Capparelli C, Li J, Elliott R, McCabe S, Wong T, Campagnuolo G, Moran E, Bogoch ER, Van G, Nguyen LT, Ohashi PS, Lacey DL, Fish E, Boyle WJ, Penninger JM. 1999. Activated T cells regulate bone loss and joint destruction in adjuvant arthritis through osteoprotegerin ligand. *Nature* 402:304–9

159. Present DHR, Targan P, Hanauer S, Mayer SB, van Hogezand L, Podolsky RA, Sands DK, Braakman TAJ, DeWoody KC, Schaible TF, van Deventer SJH. 1999. Infliximab for the treatment of fistulas in patients with Crohn's disease. *N. Engl. J. Med.* 340:1398–1405

160. van Dulleman HM, van Deventer SJ, W. HD, Bijl HA, Jansen J, Tytgat GN, Woody J. 1995. Treatment of Crohn's disease with anti-tumor necrosis factor chimeric monoclonal antibody (cA2). *Gastroenterology* 109:129–35

Annu. Rev. Immunol. 2001. 19:197–223

ACTIVATING RECEPTORS AND CORECEPTORS INVOLVED IN HUMAN NATURAL KILLER CELL-MEDIATED CYTOLYSIS

Alessandro Moretta,[1] Cristina Bottino,[2] Massimo Vitale,[2] Daniela Pende,[2] Claudia Cantoni,[1] Maria Cristina Mingari,[2,3] Roberto Biassoni,[2] Lorenzo Moretta[4]

[1]*Dipartimento di Medicina Sperimentale, Università degli Studi di Genova*
[2]*Istituto Nazionale per la Ricerca sul Cancro, Genova*
[3]*Dipartimento di Oncologia, Biologia e Genetica, Università degli Studi di Genova,
Italy; e-mail: alemoret@unige.it*
[4]*Instituto G-Geslini, Genova*

Key Words   natural cytotoxicity, NKG2D, 2B4, X-linked lymphoproliferative disease

■ **Abstract**   Natural killer cells can discriminate between normal cells and cells that do not express adequate amounts of major histocompatibility complex (MHC) class I molecules. The discovery, both in mouse and in human, of MHC-specific inhibitory receptors clarified the molecular basis of this important NK cell function. However, the triggering receptors responsible for positive NK cell stimulation remained elusive until recently. Some of these receptors have now been identified in humans, thus shedding some light on the molecular mechanisms involved in NK cell activation during the process of natural cytotoxicity. Three novel, NK-specific, triggering surface molecules (NKp46, NKp30, and NKp44) have been identified. They represent the first members of a novel emerging group of receptors collectively termed natural cytotoxicity receptors (NCR). Monoclonal antibodies (mAbs) to NCR block to differing extents the NK-mediated lysis of various tumors. Moreover, lysis of certain tumors can be virtually abrogated by the simultaneous masking of the three NCRs. There is a coordinated surface expression of the three NCRs, their surface density varying in different individuals and also in the NK cells isolated from a given individual. A direct correlation exists between the surface density of NCR and the ability of NK cells to kill various tumors. NKp46 is the only NCR involved in human NK-mediated killing of murine target cells. Accordingly, a homologue of NKp46 has been detected in mouse. Molecular cloning of NCR revealed novel members of the Ig superfamily displaying a low degree of similarity to each other and to known human molecules. NCRs are coupled to different signal transducing adaptor proteins, including CD3ζ, FcεRIγ, and KARAP/DAP12. Another triggering NK receptor is NKG2D. It appears to play either a complementary or a synergistic role with NCRs. Thus, the triggering of NK cells in the process of tumor cell lysis may often depend on the concerted action of NCR and

0732-0582/01/0407-0197$14.00   **197**

NKG2D. In some instances, however, it may uniquely depend upon the activity of NCR or NKG2D only. Strict NKG2D-dependency can be appreciated using clones that, in spite of their NCR[dull] phenotype, efficiently lyse certain epithelial tumors or leukemic cell lines. Other triggering surface molecules including 2B4 and the novel NKp80 appear to function as coreceptors rather than as true receptors. Indeed, they can induce natural cytotoxicity only when co-engaged with a triggering receptor. While an altered expression or function of NCR or NKG2D is being explored as a possible cause of immunological disorders, 2B4 dysfunction has already been associated with a severe form of immunodeficiency. Indeed, in patients with the X-linked lymphoproliferative disease, the inability to control Epstein-Barr virus infections may be consequent to a major dysfunction of 2B4 that exerts inhibitory instead of activating functions.

INTRODUCTION

The past ten years witnessed unpredictable advances in our knowledge of NK cells, their surface receptors, and the molecular mechanisms involved in their function. This favorable situation primarily stems from the discovery of inhibitory receptors specific for class I molecules (1–3). This allowed a better understanding of how NK cells can discriminate between normal major histocompatibility complex class I positive (MHC class I[+]) cells and cells that have lost the expression of MHC class I molecules as a consequence of tumor transformation or viral infection. It became apparent also that the effector function of NK cells is regulated by a balance between opposite signals delivered by the MHC class I–specific inhibitory receptors and by the activating receptors responsible for NK cell triggering. Upon ligation of activating receptors with membrane-bound molecules on surrounding tissues, NK cells would undergo blastogenesis, cytokine production, cytotoxicity, and migration. However, coligation of activating receptors with inhibitory receptors results in a dominant inhibitory effect that downregulates signals initiated via the activating pathways. These inhibitory signals are based on the involvement of tyrosine phosphatases that are required to terminate the activating signals dependent on the activity of tyrosine kinases. The common pathway generated by ligation of inhibitory receptors is characterized by tyrosine phosphorylation of immune tyrosine-based inhibitory motifs (ITIM) that recruit tyrosine phosphatases such as the Src homology 2 domain-containing phosphatase (SHP)-1 and SHP-2 (3–5), which are responsible for the inhibition of various NK cell–mediated effector functions.

In human NK cells both HLA-specific (1–3) and non HLA-specific (6–9) inhibitory receptors have been identified. The inhibitory receptors specific for HLA-class I consist of two structurally distinct families of molecules: the killer cell Ig-like receptors (KIR) and the killer cell lectin-like receptors (KLR). These receptors have also been detected in minor fractions of human CD8[+] T lymphocytes characterized by a memory phenotype (10–11). The inhibitory receptors prevent killing of normal cells and limit the production by NK cells of inflammatory cytokines including interferon-γ (IFN-γ), granulocyte macrophage-colony stimulating factor (GM-CSF), and tumor necrosis factor-α (TNF-α). Since surface expression of HLA-class I molecules is frequently altered as a consequence of tumor transformation (12–13) or viral infection (14–17), the main function of HLA-class I specific inhibitory receptors is to check the integrity of cells and to avoid damage to normal tissues. As originally proposed by Ljunggren & Kärre in the "missing self hypothesis" (18), the lack of expression, or simply the expression of inadequate amounts, of MHC class I molecules leads to NK-mediated killing of target cells. This would result in a number of receptor/MHC-class I interactions insufficient to inhibit NK cell triggering.

Although it is well established that, in the absence of efficient inhibition, both NK cell activation and expression of effector functions occur, the surface structures that provide the triggering signals leading to cytotoxicity have remained elusive until recently.

In this review we report on recently identified human activating NK receptors and coreceptors. Their discovery substantially helped to unfold the molecular mechanisms responsible for the induction of NK-mediated natural cytotoxicity in humans.

NK-MEDIATED NATURAL CYTOTOXICITY

That NK cells preferentially kill target cells that lack surface expression of MHC class I molecules (19–20) implies the existence of triggering receptors that recognize non-MHC ligands on these target cells. Unlike T lymphocytes that recognize MHC/peptide complexes using clonally distributed T cell receptors generated by gene rearrangement, NK cells appear to use triggering receptors that do not require this genetic process. Indeed, studies in mice with disrupted RAG-1 or RAG-2 genes indicated that NK cells could undergo normal development and express receptors capable of mediating natural cytotoxicity (21–22). These triggering receptors can initiate NK cell activation and target cell lysis, provided that NK cells are not turned off by ligation of MHC class I–specific inhibitory receptors, as it occurs when they interact with MHC class I-negative target cells. However target cell lysis could also be readily appreciated in the case of normal (MHC class I$^+$) target cells, provided that the interaction between MHC class I molecules and the inhibitory receptors was disrupted by the use of anti-MHC class I mAbs (23). This would mean that the activating receptors recognize ligands also on the surface of normal MHC class I$^+$ cells (for example, in humans, autologous PHA blasts). This may not be surprising in view of the strict requirement for a negative control exerted by the inhibitory receptors to prevent lysis of normal cells.

The link existing between NK cell triggering and inhibition is also emphasized by the fact that an efficient negative regulation of NK cell function requires the co-engagement of both activating and inhibitory receptors (24). Taken together, these data suggest that triggering NK receptors involved in natural cytotoxicity recognize non-MHC ligands expressed not only by abnormal but also by normal cells. This implies that at least some of these ligands are not confined to (or upregulated by) cells undergoing tumor transformation or viral infection. Several new experimental results support the notion that many different receptor-ligand interactions occur in NK/target cell triggering. Therefore, it is conceivable that some receptors recognize ligands primarily expressed by tumor cells, whereas others may bind ligands expressed by both normal and transformed cells. It is also likely that the putative triggering receptors may function in a synergistic fashion and that their contribution to NK cell activation may depend on the surface expression of their specific ligands on target cells (25). The existence of several molecules involved in NK cell triggering may also raise the question of whether a given molecule may function as a receptor, a coreceptor, or simply as an adhesion molecule. Some well-known surface molecules such as CD2 can actually be involved in NK cell killing (26, 27), at least against a few selected target cells. However, the expression of CD2 is not restricted to NK cells, and its function may rather be that of a coreceptor. Indeed, antibody-induced ligation of CD2 led to NK cell activation only in a fraction of CD2$^+$ NK cell clones (28). This suggests that NK-mediated cytolysis induced via CD2 may depend upon the simultaneous engagement of triggering receptor(s) expressed by a fraction of CD2$^+$ clones. Similar functional features may apply to other broadly expressed surface molecules such as DNAM-1 that have also been reported to trigger NK-mediated cytotoxicity upon ligation with specific mAbs (29).

A true NK receptor involved in natural cytotoxicity should mediate NK cell triggering independent of the engagement of other surface molecules. In addition, its surface expression may be expected to be mostly restricted to NK cells. The triggering surface molecules with both of these properties have recently been identified in humans and are referred to as natural cytotoxicity receptors (NCR)(25, 30).

NATURAL CYTOTOXICITY RECEPTORS

A useful strategy to search for triggering NK receptors has been based on the screening of mAbs capable of inducing NK-mediated killing of Fc receptor positive tumor target cells (in a redirected killing assay). This approach led to the identification of several molecules that, under these experimental conditions, were shown to mediate NK cell activation. However, several of these molecules were not restricted to NK cells, but in a way similar to CD2 and DNAM-1 were also expressed by T cells.

NKp46

Only in a few cases did mAbs inducing NK cell cytotoxicity in redirected killing assays display specific reactivity with NK cells. Although triggering molecules co-expressed by NK cells and other cell types may well be relevant, attention was focused primarily on those displaying NK specificity. The first mAb with this characteristic was obtained by immunizing mice with an NK clone displaying strong spontaneous cytotoxicity against a variety of NK-susceptible target cells. This mAb reacted with a novel 46-kDa cell surface molecule termed NKp46 (31). mAb-mediated cross-linking of NKp46 resulted in increases in cytotoxicity, Ca^{++} mobilization, and cytokine production. Analysis of cell distribution indicated that NKp46 was expressed by all NK cells (including the $CD56^{bright}$ $CD16^-$ subset) irrespective of their state of activation. Moreover, NKp46 was also found in immature NK cells undergoing in vitro maturation starting from $CD34^+$ cell precursors (A Moretta, unpublished results).

Molecular cloning of NKp46 (32) revealed a type I transmembrane glycoprotein belonging to the Ig superfamily. This glycoprotein is characterized by two C2-type Ig-like domains in the extracellular portion, followed by a stretch of amino acids, possibly forming a stem, which connects the ectodomain to the transmembrane region (Figure 1). The transmembrane region contains a positively charged amino acid (Arg), which may be involved in stabilizing the interaction(s) with associated molecules. The cytoplasmic portion does not contain tyrosine-based motifs typically involved in the activation of signal cascade(s). Biochemical analysis revealed that NKp46 molecules are coupled to intracytoplasmic transduction machinery by their association with CD3ζ and FcεRIγ adaptor proteins that contain immune tyrosine-based activating motifs (ITAM). These small polypeptides are

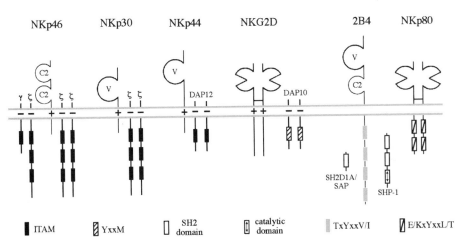

Figure 1   The surface receptors involved in natural cytotoxicity and their association with distinct signal transducing molecules. This simplified representation of the natural cytotoxicity receptors (NCR) NKp46, NKp30, and NKp44 as well as of NKG2D, 2B4, and NKp80 illustrates their molecular heterogeneity. NKp46, NKp30, NKp44, and 2B4 are type I glycoproteins belonging to the Ig-SF. NKG2D and NKp80 are dimeric type II glycoproteins belonging to the C-type lectin receptor family. Note that both NCR and NKG2D contain, in their transmembrane portion, positively charged amino acids involved in the association with signal-transducing molecules characterized by negatively charged residues. 2B4 and NKp80 do not contain charged residues in the transmembrane portion and are characterized by tyrosine-based motifs in their cytoplasmic tails.

characterized by short extracellular portions and by cytoplasmic tails containing three and one ITAM (33, 34), respectively, that become tyrosine phosphorylated upon receptor engagement. CD3ζ and FcεRIγ polypeptides are able to form disulfide-bonded homodimers or heterodimers (35). In NK cells, CD3ζ and FcεRIγ are also involved in intracellular signaling via CD16 (36–39) and are phosphorylated by tyrosine kinases of the Src family, such as p56lck (40, 41), followed by the recruitment of Syk (42, 43) and ZAP70 (44) tyrosine kinases.

The NKp46-encoding gene, similar to all the genes encoding KIR and ILT, maps on human chromosome 19 (32) within the leukocyte receptor complex (LRC) at 19q13.4 (45). Murine and rat homologues of human NKp46 have been cloned (46, 47) and found to display 58% and 59% amino acid identity, respectively, with the human protein. Remarkably, the murine NKp46-encoding gene maps on mouse chromosome 7, syntenic to human chromosome 19. Recent work by Tomasello et al (48) indicated that in double knockout mice lacking both CD3ζ and FcεRIγ chains the cytolytic activity against most target cells (including YAC, BW15.02, RMA, RMA-S, and C4.4.25) is profoundly reduced. This suggests that in mice NKp46 (or other, still undefined, murine receptors associated with ζ/γ polypeptides) may also play a prominent role in natural cytotoxicity mediated by murine NK cells.

NKp30

A second triggering surface molecule (termed NKp30) has been identified (49) that displays several features in common with NKp46. Thus, NKp30 is selectively expressed by all NK cells, including those expressing the CD56[bright] CD16$^-$ surface phenotype, as well as by immature NK cells derived in vitro from CD34$^+$ precursors (A Moretta, unpublished results). Moreover, mAb-mediated cross-linking of NKp30 resulted in cellular responses identical to those induced via NKp46 (i.e. Ca^{++} flux, cytotoxicity, and cytokine production). Biochemical analysis, however, revealed a molecular size of approximately 30 kDa, thus differing from NKp46. In addition, mAb-mediated surface modulation of NKp46 did not affect the expression of NKp30. Similar to NKp46 and CD16, NKp30 associated with CD3ζ chains that become tyrosine phosphorylated following cell treatment with pervanadate (49).

Molecular cloning of the cDNA encoding NKp30 revealed a member of the Ig superfamily. The extracellular portion is characterized by a single domain of the V-type and by a region rich in hydrophobic amino acids, potentially involved in protein/protein interactions, that connects the IgV-like domain with the transmembrane portion (Figure 1). The transmembrane region contains the positively charged amino acid Arg, probably involved in the association with CD3ζ chains, whereas the cytoplasmic portion lacks typical ITAM consensus sequences. The cDNA specific for NKp30 (49) was identical to an alternatively spliced form of the previously identified 1C7 gene (50). This gene maps to chromosome 6 in the TNF cluster of the MHC gene complex. Northern blot analysis, consistent with the reactivity of the anti-NKp30 mAb, revealed that NKp30 mRNA expression was essentially restricted to NK cells. On the other hand, in some non–NK cell lines that were negative for mRNA expression by Northern blot and by reactivity with anti-NKp30 mAb, transcripts could be identified by RT-PCR. This suggests that other cell types may express low levels of NKp30 transcripts that do not result in NKp30 expression on the cell surface.

NKp44

Another member of the NCR family displaying a molecular size of approximately 44 kDa has been termed NKp44 (51). Similar to NKp46 and NKp30, NKp44 could induce triggering of NK-mediated cytotoxicity upon cross-linking by specific mAbs. However, the expression of NKp44 was restricted to activated NK cells cultured in the presence of IL-2, whereas it was absent in fresh peripheral blood NK cells. Therefore, NKp44 represents the first marker specific for activated human NK cells. In this context, it is well known that following culture in the presence of IL-2, NK cells acquire increased cytolytic activity against NK susceptible targets. Moreover, they become cytolytic against targets that are resistant to fresh NK cells (52, 53). This may reflect, at least in part, the de novo expression of triggering receptors such as NKp44 that allow NK cells to recognize additional ligands on target cells.

NKp44 is a glycoprotein displaying a protein backbone of approximately 29 kDa that associates with the ITAM-bearing KARAP/DAP12 signal-transducing molecules that become tyrosine phosphorylated upon NKp44 cross-linking (51, 54). Molecular cloning of NKp44 (54) revealed a novel member of the Ig-SF characterized by a single extracellular V-type domain (Figure 1). The membrane-proximal portion of NKp44 contains a high proportion of Pro, Ser, and Thr that may confer an extended open conformation. The gene encoding NKp44, similar to that coding for NKp30, is located on human chromosome 6. NKp44 does not contain an ITAM in the cytoplasmic portion, while it is characterized by a trans-membrane region containing a charged amino acid (Lys) possibly involved in the association with KARAP/DAP12.

KARAP(55)/DAP12(56) are adaptor molecules that contain a single ITAM in the cytoplasmic portion and are expressed as disulfide-bonded homodimers. In NK cells, KARAP/DAP12 associate with other activating molecules including the HLA class I–specific receptors p50/KIR2DS (55–57) and NKG2C (58). A common feature of DAP12, CD3ζ, and FcεRIγ polypeptides is the presence in their transmembrane portions of negatively charged residues. The associated receptors in turn display positively charged amino acids. Although interactions between opposite charged amino acids are believed to be important for the receptor/adaptor association, other residues may play a crucial role. Indeed, a strict specificity exists in the association of a given receptor with a given adaptor molecule (53, 59). In this context, a recent study identified NK cell clones derived from a normal individual expressing p50.2/KIR2DS2 receptors that were unable to transduce activating signals. Sequence analysis revealed six mutations in the exon coding for the transmembrane portion. Notably one such mutation involved the charged lysine residue. Cotransfection experiments revealed that this naturally occurring p50.2/KIR2DS2 mutant displayed a dramatically reduced ability to associate with KARAP/DAP12 polypeptides (60).

THE SURFACE DENSITY OF NCR DICTATES THE ABILITY OF NK CELLS TO LYSE MOST TUMOR TARGET CELLS

It is well known that NK cell clones frequently display heterogeneity in their ability to kill a given HLA class I-negative target cell. In particular, in some of the individuals analyzed, two distinct groups of NK cell clones could be identified on the basis of the ability to kill a given NK susceptible target cell. Thus, some clones displayed strong cytolytic activity while others were poorly cytolytic. Since the target cells analyzed did not express either classical or nonclassical HLA-class I molecules, it seems unlikely that the functional heterogeneity of NK clones could result from the occurrence of inhibitory interactions between KIR or KLR and their ligands. On the other hand, clonal heterogeneity could reflect a differential expression of triggering receptors. Indeed, the surface density of NKp46 was markedly different in the two groups of clones. Thus, clones displaying strong cytolytic activity expressed high levels of NKp46, whereas the poorly cytolytic ones were characterized by low NKp46 surface density (61). Importantly, NKp46[bright] and NKp46[dull] clones were also characterized by a parallel high and low level of expression of NKp30 and NKp44 receptors (49). These findings indicate that it is possible to identify cells characterized by high or low natural cytotoxicity simply on the basis of NCR surface density.

NCR surface density did not correlate with the cytolytic potential of NK cells. Indeed, the magnitude of the cytolytic responses induced by anti-CD16 mAbs is comparable in NKp46[bright] and NCR[dull] NK clones. This indicates that the correlation between the NCR phenotype and the spontaneous cytotoxicity against NK susceptible target cells is likely to reflect different degrees of interactions between NCR and their ligands on target cells.

Although a correlation between the NCR[bright] phenotype and high levels of spontaneous cytotoxicity can be consistently detected when NK cells are tested against most target cells (including melanomas, EBV-LCL, lung carcinomas, PHA blasts, and xenogeneic target cells), exceptions to this rule do exist (25). Thus, target cells including T cell lymphomas (e.g. Jurkat and H9 cells), certain ovarian carcinomas (e.g. IGROV), and other epithelial tumor cell lines (e.g. HeLa) were efficiently killed by both NCR[bright] and NCR[dull] NK clones. This suggested that recognition and killing of these target cells could depend not only on NCR but also on additional triggering receptors expressed by NCR[dull] clones. These data suggested that analysis of NCR[dull] clones in cytolytic assays against susceptible target cells may be crucial in an attempt to identify novel, still undefined, triggering receptors.

The NCR density at the NK cell surface is remarkably stable. Indeed, it does not change under different culture conditions (including culture in the presence of different cytokines such as IL-2, IL-15, IL-12, and IL-18) (A Moretta, unpublished results). Thus, NK-cell clones derived from individuals characterized by high proportions of NCR^{bright} peripheral NK cells consistently display a NCR^{bright} phenotype. Likewise, in some individuals, both fresh and cultured cells, including NK clones, display a NCR^{dull} phenotype. Remarkably, fresh NK cells isolated from individuals with NCR^{bright} or NCR^{dull} phenotype also display major differences in their natural cytotoxicity (61). Finally, it is worth mentioning that some donors are characterized by a continuous rather than a bimodal distribution of the surface density of NCR. This reflects the presence of cells with intermediate levels of surface NCR. As expected, NK clones characterized by intermediate NCR surface expression also display intermediate levels of spontaneous cytotoxicity.

BLOCKING NCR RECOGNITION INHIBITS NATURAL CYTOTOXICITY

The finding that a given cell membrane molecule is able to initiate NK-mediated killing and that its surface density directly correlates with spontaneous killing is suggestive of a possible role as a receptor involved in target cell recognition and lysis. In order to demonstrate that NCR indeed had these properties, blocking experiments were performed in which NK clones were assessed for cytotoxicity against Fc receptor negative, NK-susceptible target cells, in the presence of anti-NCR mAb. In most instances, blocking of individual NCR resulted in partial inhibition of cytotoxicity (25, 32, 49, 51). This could be due to additional NCR interacting with their ligands on target cells. Indeed, only the combined use of mAbs directed to different NCR resulted in strong inhibition of cytolysis (25, 49). This would mean that the different NCR cooperate in target cell recognition and killing. The extent of this cooperation appears to be dictated by the type and/or the density of the ligands expressed on target cells. Thus, although no NCR ligands have been molecularly identified so far, the co-operation of the different NCR strongly suggests that most target cells express multiple ligands recognized by these receptors. Infrequently, lysis of a given target cell appears to be dependent upon the function of a single triggering receptor. One such example was provided by xenogeneic (murine) target cells. Indeed, lysis of murine cells by human NK cells only involved NKp46-mediated recognition. Thus, blocking experiments demonstrated that mAb-mediated masking of NKp46 prevented killing of murine target cells such as YAC, BW15.02, or P815 (25, 32). Therefore, the engagement of a single NCR may be sufficient to induce NK cell triggering and target cell lysis. However, the simultaneous engagement of different NCR, usually results in a more efficient target cell lysis. Hence, a given NK cell clone will kill human target cells more efficiently than murine target cells.

The fact that NKp46 recognizes ligands on murine cells, together with the identification of a murine (m) NKp46 homologue (46), suggested that this particular receptor/ligand interaction may be conserved during evolution. Accordingly, it is likely that the occurrence of such triggering interactions among species may cause difficulties in xenotransplantation. As reviewed recently by Auchincloss & Sachs (62), human NK cells are able to kill pig targets due to the failure of pig MHC class I molecules to interact with human HLA class I–specific inhibitory receptors (63, 64). In this context, different in vivo experiments revealed a high concentration of NK cells in cellular infiltrates associated with xenograft rejection (65). In addition, prolongation of xenograft survival has been achieved by combining the depletion of NK cells with other forms of immunosuppression (66). Thus, it is likely that the NK-mediated cytotoxicity in xenografts may be the result of the failure to engage HLA-specific inhibitory human receptors (due to inappropriate MHC ligands) together with the NK-mediated recognition of xenogeneic ligands (possibly via NKp46). It is also conceivable that additional receptor/ligand interactions may be involved in induction of NK cell triggering, depending upon the animal species used for xenotransplantation.

ROLE OF NKG2D IN NATURAL CYTOTOXICITY

NKG2D, a C-type lectin surface receptor, is a member of the NKG2 family encoded within the NK complex on human chromosome 12 (67). NKG2A, C, E, and F (68–71) show a high degree of identity with one another and form heterodimers with CD94 (68–71), some of which function as receptors for HLA-E (72–74). On the contrary, NKG2D is only distantly related to the other members of the family and does not couple with CD94 being expressed as a homodimer (75) (Figure 1). Unlike the other known triggering NK receptors, the surface expression of NKG2D requires association with a newly identified adaptor protein termed DAP10 (75) or KAP10 (76). DAP10 is characterized by the presence of a negatively charged residue in the transmembrane portion and by a YxxM motif in the cytoplasmic tail that, upon tyrosine phosphorylation, binds to PI 3-kinase. In contrast to NCR, the expression of which is confined to NK cells, NKG2D is also expressed by virtually all $TCR\gamma\delta^+$ and $CD8^+$ $TCR\alpha/\beta^+$ cells. NKG2D can mediate potent NK cell triggering in redirected killing assays. Moreover, blocking of NKG2D by specific mAbs leads to inhibition of NK cell–mediated cytotoxicity against certain target cells. Thus, NKG2D could represent an additional triggering receptor involved in target cell recognition and initiation of killing. It is important that the target cell ligands for NKG2D have been identified. These ligands are the closely related molecules MICA and MICB (77) that are encoded within the human MHC. MICA/B are stress-inducible molecules mostly expressed in epithelial tumors including breast, ovary, colon, kidney, and lung carcinomas (78, 79). The interaction between NKG2D and MICA/B leads to NK cell activation, while mAb-mediated disruption of this interaction inhibits cytotoxicity by both NK cell clones (80) and the NKL cell line (75). It is of note that ligation of NKG2D by specific mAb could induce triggering of cytotoxicity also in $TCR\gamma/\delta^+$ clones and in a fraction of $CD8^+TCR\alpha\beta^+$ $NKG2D^+$ clones. These data suggest that NKG2D may represent a triggering receptor responsible for the so-called NK-like activity mediated by some cytolytic T cells. Indeed a partial inhibition of the NK-like activity of some $CD8^+TCR\alpha/\beta^+$ cytolytic clones has been detected by the use of anti-NKG2D mAb (MC Mingari, unpublished results).

The role of NKG2D in NK-mediated natural cytotoxicity has recently been evaluated in human NK cell clones and compared to that of NCR (80). These studies have shown that in NCR^{bright} clones killing of various tumors was mostly NCR-dependent, whereas killing of other targets required triggering signals via both NCR and NKG2D. Further analysis of NCR^{dull} clones indicated that both the expression and the function of NKG2D did not correlate with the surface density of NCR. Indeed, comparable surface densities of NKG2D were detected in both NCR^{bright} and NCR^{dull} clones. Moreover, the magnitude of the cytolytic responses following NKG2D cross-linking was similar in the two groups of clones. Important information on the function of NKG2D has been obtained by the study of NCR^{dull} clones. In spite of the low expression of NCR, these clones could efficiently kill certain tumors. Indeed, the cytolytic activity of NCR^{dull} clones against $MICA^+$ target cells such as HeLa and IGROV was virtually abrogated by anti-NKG2D mAb. These data suggest that lysis of these tumors by NCR^{dull} clones is mostly NKG2D dependent. Thus, NKG2D plays an important role in NK cell activation, and its function is complementary to that of NCR (Figure 2).

A mouse (m) NKG2D has been identified (81) that displays a high degree of similarity with the human NKG2D. mNKG2D is expressed on resting and activated NK cells, LPS-activated macrophages, and activated $CD8^+$ T cells (82). While the existence of murine MIC homologues is still controversial, recent data show that mNKG2D interacts with two distinct ligands, H60 and Rae1 (82, 83) that are encoded on mouse chromosome 10. H60 (84) and Rae1 (85) contain an extracellular domain with similarity to the $\alpha1$ and $\alpha2$ domain of MHC-class I molecules and a serine-, threonine-, and proline (STP)-rich domain proximal to the cell membrane. While H60 has a cytoplasmic tail, Rae1 is a glycosyl-phosphatidyl-inositol (GPI)-linked protein. Experiments performed using H60 and Rae1-transfected cells show that their interaction with NKG2D induces both cytotoxicity (82, 83) and $IFN\gamma$ production by NK cells, and $TNF\alpha$ and nitric oxide by activated macrophages (82). Interestingly, genes encoding H60 and Rae1 homologues have been identified on human chromosome 6 on which also HLA genes are located. Moreover, the human ULBP genes (86, 87) are also located within this region. They encode for molecules that exhibit similarities to the $\alpha1$ and $\alpha2$ domains of MHC class I molecules that may interact with NKG2D.

2B4 FUNCTIONS AS A CORECEPTOR IN THE NK-MEDIATED NATURAL CYTOTOXICITY

2B4 was originally identified in mice (88) as a surface receptor expressed by NK, $CD8^+$, and $\gamma\delta$ T cells. Cross-linking of murine (m) 2B4 was shown to trigger NK

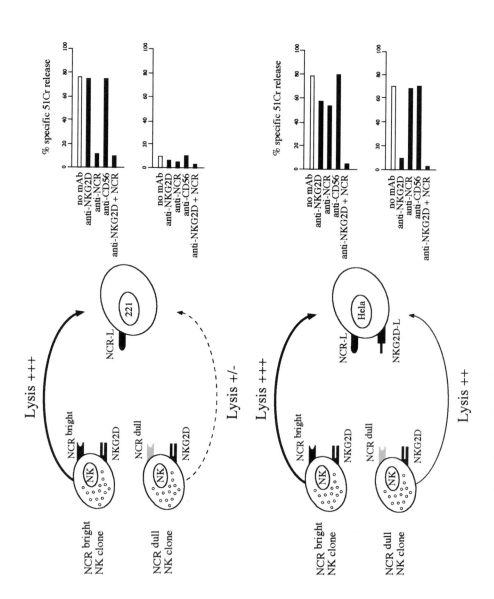

and T cell–mediated cytotoxicity, IFN-γ and IL-2 secretion, granule exocytosis (88), activation of $\gamma\delta$ T cells (89), and upregulation of egr-1 and c-fos mRNA expression (88). Molecular cloning (90) revealed a novel member of the CD2 subfamily (91) of the Ig-SF, which includes CD48, CD58, CD84, CDw150 (also termed SLAM), and Ly-9. Subsequently, molecular binding assays revealed that m2B4 bind with high affinity to CD48, a glycosyl-phosphatidyl-inositol (GPI)-anchored molecule, suggesting that CD48 may represent its physiological ligand (92, 93).

In humans, 2B4 was first described as a surface molecule recognized by the monoclonal antibodies PP35 (94) and C1.7 (95). These mAbs immunoprecipitated a 70-kDa glycoprotein expressed by all NK cells and by a $CD8^+$ T cell subset. mAb-mediated cross-linking could strongly enhance the NK-mediated cytotoxicity while, in contrast to the murine system, it had no effect on $CD8^+$ T cells (94, 95). Molecular cloning (96–99) revealed that the human (h) 2B4-encoding gene, similar to m2B4, is located on chromosome 1 in the CD2 subfamily cluster. h2B4 displays a 70% identity with m2B4 and is characterized by one membrane-distal IgV type domain and one membrane proximal Ig-C2 type domain (Figure 1). In accord with the lack of association of 2B4 with ITAM-containing polypeptides, the transmembrane portion does not contain charged amino acids. Interestingly, however, h2B4 is characterized by a long cytoplasmic tail containing four tyrosine-based motifs (TxYxxI/V). CD48 has been identified as the putative natural ligand of 2B4 also in humans (97, 98).

Figure 2   Role of NCRs or NKG2D in the NK-mediated target cell lysis. A correct understanding of the role played by NKp46, NKp30, and NKp44 (here collectively indicated as NCR, for sake of simplicity) or NKG2D in the NK-mediated natural cytotoxicity requires the analysis of different target cells as well as of NK cells characterized by either an NCR[bright] or an NCR[dull] surface phenotype. The upper part of the figure illustrates the NK-mediated cytolytic activity against the LCL 721.221. Lysis of these cells is fully dependent on the effect of NCR. Indeed, killing mediated by the NCR[bright] clone is blocked by mAb-mediated masking of NCR, whereas no effect is obtained by masking NKG2D. In addition, NCR[dull] clones fail to lyse 721.221 target cells. This reflects the expression of insufficient surface densities of NCRs by the effector cells and, most likely, the lack (or the expression of insufficient amounts) of NKG2D ligand(s) on target cells. The lower part of the figure shows the lysis of the epithelial tumor cell line HeLa by NCR[bright] or NCR[dull] clones. HeLa cells express the ligand for both NCRs and NKG2D. Note that the NCR[bright] clone-mediated lysis is partially inhibited by masking either NCRs or NKG2D, while a complete inhibition is achieved by the simultaneous addition of mAbs to NCRs and NKG2D. Remarkably, lysis of HeLa cells by NCR[dull] clones is uniquely dependent on the engagement of NKG2D. Indeed, cytolytic activity was abrogated by the addition of anti-NKG2D mAb. Taken together, these data indicate that, depending on the type of effector or target cells used, NCR and NKG2D may be differently involved in NK-mediated cytolysis. Namely, 1. Certain target cells are lysed in NCR-dependent fashion; 2. lysis of other targets may require both NCR and NKG2D when NCR[bright] effector cells are analyzed; and 3. lysis of the same targets uniquely involve NKG2D in the case of NCR[dull] effector NK cells.

Analysis of human NK cells revealed a sharp functional heterogeneity of 2B4 molecules. Thus, the ability of anti-2B4 mAb to induce NK cell activation in redirected killing assays was confined to a fraction of NK cell clones (94). These data have recently been clarified in studies showing that the apparent functional heterogeneity of 2B4 molecules actually reflects clonal differences in the co-engagement of triggering receptors (100). Thus, in a redirected killing assay against P815 murine target cells, only NCR^{bright} clones were triggered by anti-2B4 mAb. No triggering of NCR^{dull} clones occurred, although they expressed comparable surface densities of 2B4. Moreover, mAb-mediated modulation of NKp46 did not affect the surface expression of 2B4, but instead resulted in NK cells' unresponsiveness to anti-2B4 mAb. Since murine target cells (including P815) are known to express a ligand for NKp46 (see above), it is conceivable that the ability of 2B4 to mediate NK-cell triggering, in this experimental setting, may depend upon the extent of NKp46/NKp46-ligand interactions. Taken together, these data support the notion that in human NK cell–mediated natural cytotoxicity, NCRs function as triggering receptors, whereas 2B4 acts as a coreceptor (100). h2B4 has also been detected on a small subset of CD4$^+$ T cells, monocytes and basophils; however, its function in these cells, as well as in CD8$^+$ T cells, remains to be defined.

Consistent with the presence of tyrosine-based motifs in the cytoplasmic portion, tyrosine phosphorylation of 2B4 has been detected both in normal NK cells (98, 101) and in cell transfectants (99). However, controversial information exists on the molecular mechanisms involved in 2B4-mediated signaling. Thus, using cell transfectants (99), 2B4 has been shown to associate both with the Src homology 2 domain-containing protein (SH2D1A) (also termed SLAM-associated protein SAP)(102–104) and with the SHP-2 phosphatase. A recent study using normal NK cells confirmed that tyrosine-phosphorylation of 2B4 leads to association with SH2D1A/SAP (101). However, different from cell transfectants, 2B4 associated with SHP-1 rather than with SHP-2. Taken together these data suggest that, in normal NK cells, SH2D1A/SAP may sustain 2B4-mediated triggering responses by preventing the generation of inhibitory signals mediated by SHP-1. A recent study (105) showed that in normal human NK cells, 2B4 constitutively associates with the linker for activation of T cells (LAT) (106, 107). Importantly, specific engagement of 2B4, following cell triggering with an anti-2B4 mAb, resulted in tyrosine phosphorylation of both 2B4 and of the associated LAT molecules. Moreover, tyrosine phosphorylation of LAT led to the recruitment of intracytoplasmic signaling molecules including PLCγ and Grb2.

NKp80, A NOVEL SURFACE MOLECULE INVOLVED IN NK CELL TRIGGERING

Recently, a novel triggering surface molecule termed NKp80 has been identified by the generation of specific mAb (MA152 and LAP171) (108). NKp80 is expressed by virtually all fresh NK cells derived from peripheral blood as well as by a minor T cell subset characterized by the CD3$^+$ CD56$^+$ surface phenotype. In addition, the majority of the NK cell clones analyzed expressed NKp80. Cross-linking of NKp80 in a redirected killing assay could induce NK cell activation only in a fraction of NKp80$^+$ clones. This clonal heterogeneity correlated with the NCR^{bright} and the NCR^{dull} phenotype thus suggesting that, in a way similar to 2B4 (100), NKp80 may function as a coreceptor rather than as a classical receptor. Interestingly, NKp80 was involved in the process of NK-mediated cytolysis of allogeneic PHA blasts. Indeed, mAb-mediated blocking of NKp80 could partially inhibit killing of these target cells, although a complete inhibition was achieved only by the simultaneous blocking of NCR. Thus, NKp80 appears to function synergistically with NCR. Remarkably, NKp80-mediated recognition of target cells appears to be restricted to PHA blasts. Indeed, in experiments of mAb-mediated NKp80 blocking, no inhibitory effect could be detected on the lysis of various tumor cell lines. NKp80 is expressed at the cell surface as a dimer of approximately 80 kDa and, similar to 2B4, does not associate with classical ITAM-containing polypeptides. Molecular cloning revealed a type II transmembrane protein of 231 amino acids (aa) containing a C-type lectin domain (108). The transmembrane region is characterized by nonpolar amino acids, and the cytoplasmic tail contains two tyrosine-based motifs (Figure 1). The nucleotide alignment showed that the NKp80-encoding cDNA is identical to the recently described KLRF1 cDNA (109). KLRF1 transcripts were found in different cell types and, based on the sequence analysis, an inhibitory function was suggested for the predicted KLRF1-encoded molecule. Notably, however, the surface expression of NKp80 is mostly confined to NK cells, and it functions as an activating, rather than as an inhibitory, molecule (108).

POSSIBLE ROLE OF ACTIVATING HLA CLASS I-SPECIFIC RECEPTORS IN NK CELL–MEDIATED CYTOTOXICITY

The first receptors for HLA class I molecules (p58/KIR2DL) were identified by the generation of specific mAbs that, upon cross-linking, were shown to inhibit spontaneous NK-mediated cytotoxicity as well as the anti-CD16 mAb-induced redirected lysis (110–112). More recently, the activating forms of the HLA class I–specific receptors (p50/KIR2DS) have been identified (113, 114). As they react with the same mAb specific for their inhibitory counterpart, they could be disclosed on the basis of their triggering capability in redirected killing assays. The HLA class I–specific activating receptors are characterized by a short intracellular region that does not contain signaling motifs and by a transmembrane domain containing a positively charged amino acid possibly involved in the association with signal transducing adaptor molecules characterized by ITAM motifs (60, 114, 115). The adaptor molecule for both p50/KIR2DS (specific for HLA-C) and NKG2C (specific for HLA-E) activating receptors is represented by DAP12 (55–58). The actual role of HLA class I–specific triggering receptors in NK cell responses is still debated. The finding that p50/KIR2DS binds HLA-C with lower affinity as compared to its inhibitory counterpart (116) suggested the existence of a mechanism ensuring that inhibitory signals overrule triggering signals when both activating and inhibitory receptors are expressed on the same NK cell. This could be particularly relevant in the case of NK cells expressing triggering and inhibitory receptors specific for different HLA–class I molecules. In this case, the HLA–class I specific triggering receptors (similar to NCR or NKG2D) would be allowed to signal only when target cells have lost the expression of the HLA allele(s) recognized by the inhibitory receptor(s). This situation may occur in viral infections (17) or tumor transformation (13, 17, 117) that selectively downregulate a given HLA–class I allele.

The function of triggering NK receptors may be required during NK cell development from $CD34^+$ precursors for the selection of immature NK cells and for the expression of HLA class I–specific inhibitory receptors. However, it is now well established that the NK development is not affected in DAP12-knockout mice (DAP12−/−) (118) nor in DAP12 loss-of-function knockin mice (KΔY75/KΔY75)(98). Since these mice represent functional knockout models for all the activating forms of HLA class I–specific receptors, it is possible to conclude that shaping of the inhibitory receptor repertoire does not depend on the function of their activating counterparts. Consistent with these results, Ly49H and Ly49D activating receptors are expressed during NK cell development later than the inhibitory Ly49 receptors (119). Along this line, it is mandatory to analyze ζ/γ knockout mice (120) in order to define whether selection of immature NK cells and expression of HLA class I–specific inhibitory receptors is impaired under developmental conditions in which the function of NKp46 (or other ζ/γ-coupled receptors) is affected.

In conclusion, we would like to propose the following role for p50/KIR2DS and NKG2C activating receptors. They could initiate NK cell triggering in NK cells expressing a NCR^{dull} phenotype against (HLA-class I$^+$) target cells that do not express ligands for NKG2D. In support of this hypothesis, an inverse correlation has indeed been detected between the NCR^{bright} phenotype and the expression of NKG2C (61) or p50/KIR2DS (A. Moretta, unpublished observation).

SURFACE EXPRESSION AND FUNCTION OF TRIGGERING NK RECEPTORS IN HUMAN DISEASES

As the various triggering NK receptors have been identified only recently, little is yet known about their possible contribution to pathological conditions involving the immune system. For example, it is unknown whether individuals in whom most NK cells are characterized by low NCR surface density may be more susceptible to certain viral infections or even more prone to develop certain tumors. It is still unknown whether in TAP-deficient patients (121), characterized by low expression of HLA class I molecules, NCR cells display an NCR bright or dull phenotype. In these patients, the defect in KIR/HLA interactions (122, 123) could be counterbalanced by a reduced surface density of one or more triggering receptors in order to prevent NK-mediated autoreactivity.

The first evidence that an altered function of a triggering NK receptor may be responsible for a disease has recently been obtained in individuals affected by the X-linked lymphoproliferative disease (XLP). XLP is a severe inherited immune deficiency, characterized by abnormal immune responses to the Epstein-Barr virus (EBV) (124, 125). In most cases, prior to EBV infection, the immunological status of genotypically affected males is normal (126). After exposure to EBV, XLP males either succumb to fulminant infectious mononucleosis or develop lymphoma, hypo- or dys-gammaglobulinemia, and/or histiocytic infiltration leading to marrow aplasia. The gene defective in XLP has recently been identified (102–104). This gene is located at Xq25 and, in normal individuals, encodes for a 15-kDa intracytoplasmic protein characterized by a single SH2 domain, termed SH2D1A or SAP (see above).

SH2D1A/SAP is expressed in lymphoid tissues (thymus, spleen) and particularly in T and NK lymphocytes. Different mutations of the SH2D1A gene have been identified, the result of which is either the absence of SH2D1A/SAP molecule or the presence of truncated nonfunctional products. It has been proposed that the SH2D1A/SAP protein functions as a regulator of the signal transduction pathways initiated by at least two distinct human surface receptors belonging to the CD2 family, namely, the signaling lymphocytic activation molecule (SLAM), expressed on T and B cells (127), and 2B4.

This suggested that, in XLP patients, 2B4 molecules could be nonfunctional owing to the lack of SH2D1A/SAP. To explore this possibility, the function of 2B4 molecules in XLP patients has been analyzed in detail (101). Although different triggering receptors including CD16 and NCR displayed a normal function in XLP-NK cells, the signaling pathway initiated by 2B4 was dramatically altered. But there was not simply a lack of function of the 2B4; indeed, the engagement of 2B4 (by specific mAbs or its ligand CD48) resulted in the generation of inhibitory rather than activating signals. These signals blocked not only the spontaneous NK cytotoxicity, but also the target cell lysis induced via CD16 or NCR. As a consequence, XLP-NK cells could efficiently kill CD48$^-$ but not CD48$^+$ target cells.

Remarkably high densities of CD48 are expressed on EBV-infected LCL. Indeed, XLP-NK cells are unable to kill either HLA–class I$^-$ EBV$^+$ B cell lines (such as LCL 721.221 and Daudi) or HLA class I$^+$ autologous EBV$^+$ LCL (Figure 3). The cytolytic activity against HLA class I$^-$ LCL could be completely restored by mAb-mediated disruption of the 2B4/CD48 interactions, while disruption of both HLA/KIR and 2B4/CD48 interactions allowed XLP-NK cells to efficiently kill autologous EBV$^+$ LCL (101). Molecular analysis revealed that 2B4 molecules isolated from XLP patients were identical to those derived from normal NK cells. On the other hand (as expected) in XLP-NK cells, 2B4 did not associate with SH2D1A whereas, in a way similar to 2B4 molecules isolated from normal NK cells, it did associate with SHP-1 phosphatase. Whether SHP-1 is directly involved in the downregulation of the activating pathways initiated via CD16 and NCR has still to be investigated. Interestingly, preliminary data suggest that in XLP patients

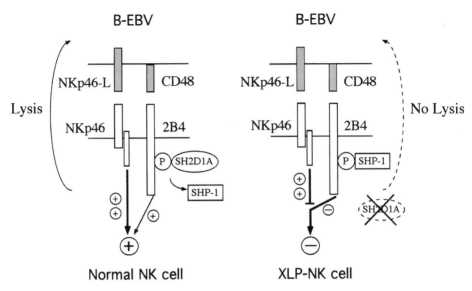

Figure 3 Function of 2B4 in normal individuals and in X-linked lymphoproliferative disease (XLP). In normal individuals, 2B4 functions as a coreceptor cooperating with triggering receptors (here the natural cytotoxicity receptor NKp46 is shown) to induce NK cell activation upon interaction with EBV-infected B cells. Note that B-EBV cells express the ligands for 2B4 (i.e. CD48) and the still undefined ligand for NKp46 (NKp46-L). The triggering function of 2B4 (upon engagement with CD48) appears to require the recruitment of the small intracytoplasmic molecule SH2D1A that likely prevents the generation of inhibitory signals mediated by SHP-1 phosphatase. The triggering signals delivered to NK cells via NKp46 and 2B4 lead to NK-cell activation and induction of cytolysis of B-EBV target cells. The molecular defect in XLP patients has recently been identified. The lack of a functional SH2D1A protein in these patients results in its lack of association to 2B4. This defect does not simply result in a nonfunctional 2B4 molecule. Indeed, in this case, 2B4 engagement extinguishes the triggering signals delivered via NKp46 or other activating receptors. As a consequence, NK cells (and most likely CD8[+] CTL) fail to lyse EBV-infected target cells (or to release relevant cytokines) and to control viral infection.

2B4 may also negatively regulate T cell–mediated responses (101). Therefore, it is conceivable also that specific CTL responses against EBV[+] B cells may also be impaired by a molecular mechanism similar to that responsible for NK cell dysfunction. Altogether, the altered function of 2B4 in XLP patients may account for a general inability of different cytolytic effector cells to control EBV infections.

CONCLUDING REMARKS

Over the past three years, important advances have been made toward a better definition of the molecular mechanisms by which NK cells function. Thus, thanks to the identification and the molecular characterization of NKp46, NKp30, NKp44, and NKG2D, the major players responsible for NK cell activation during natural cytotoxicity are mysterious no longer. Indeed, lysis of most tumors can now be explained on the ground of the interactions between NCR or NKG2D and their ligands on target cells. The strength of the "on" signals can be reinforced by the co-engagement of coreceptors. 2B4 and, in part, NKp80 may fulfill this role. In the case of HLA–class I$^+$ target cells, other players may go into action, namely, the activating counterparts of the HLA–class I-specific inhibitory receptors. The majority of the ligands for the activating receptors appear to be expressed also by normal cells. Therefore, in order to prevent serious cell damage, the activating receptors are usually under the control of HLA–class I-specific inhibitory receptors that provide the "off" signal. The activity of the inhibitory receptors strictly depends on the co-engagement of triggering receptors so that the inhibition will be induced only when necessary.

A remarkable finding is the complementary role played by the NCR and the NKG2D receptors. This function can be appreciated by the selection not only of particular tumors as target cells, but also of appropriate NK cell clones as effectors. For example, NK clones characterized by a NCR^{dull} phenotype fail to lyse many different tumor cells (that are efficiently killed by the NCR^{bright} clones in a NCR-dependent fashion). However, the same NCR^{dull} clones efficiently lyse certain tumors including HeLa, IGROV, and Jurkat cell lines: in this case, NKG2D is the major activating receptor responsible for target cell lysis.

While the ligands for NKG2D are represented by the MHC–class I-like MICA/B surface antigens and the natural ligand for 2B4 is CD48, the ligands for NCR are still undefined. It is evident that, since NCR are the major receptors responsible for the induction of natural cytotoxicity, the identification of their ligands may be relevant for tumor cell typing as well as for novel approaches of immunotherapy.

In view of their recent discovery, no information is available so far on possible defects of expression or function of NCRs or NKG2D in disease. It might be expected that such defects could lead to an impaired control of certain tumors or viral infections. On the other hand, a dysfunction of 2B4 has already been associated with X-linked lymphoproliferative disease.

In conclusion, the identification of various surface molecules regulating NK-cell function may help us to understand NK cell physiology and may also shed light on the pathogenesis of certain immune disorders. It may offer novel tools for therapeutic interventions in these diseases.

ACKNOWLEDGMENTS

This work was supported by grants awarded by Associazione Italiana per la Ricerca sul Cancro (A.I.R.C.), Istituto Superiore di Sanità (I.S.S.), Ministero della Sanità, and Ministero dell'Università e della Ricerca Scientifica e Tecnologica (M.U.R.S.T.), MURST 5%-CNR Biotechnology program 95/95 and Consiglio Nazionale delle Ricerche, Progetto Finalizzato Biotecnologie. Also the financial support of Telethon-Italy (grant no.E.0892) is gratefully acknowledged. We thank C Miriello for secretarial assistance.

Visit the Annual Reviews home page at www.AnnualReviews.org

LITERATURE CITED

1. Moretta A, Bottino C, Vitale M, Pende D, Biassoni R, Mingari MC, Moretta L. 1996. Receptors for HLA-class I molecules in human natural killer cells. *Annu. Rev. Immunol.* 14:619–48
2. Lanier LL. 1998. NK cell receptors. *Annu. Rev. Immunol.* 16:359–93
3. Long EO. 1999. Regulation of immune responses through inhibitory receptors. *Annu. Rev. Immunol.* 17:875–904
4. Bolland S, Ravetch JV. 1999. Inhibitory pathways triggered by ITIM-containing receptors. *Adv Immunol.* 72:149–77
5. Tomasello E, Blery M, Vely E, Vivier E. 2000. Signaling pathways engaged by NK cell receptors: double concerto for activating receptors, inhibitory receptors and NK cells. *Semin. Immunol. Apr;* 12(2):139–47
6. Poggi A, Pella N, Morelli L, Spada F, Ravello V, Sivori S, Augugliaro R, Moretta L, Moretta A. 1995. p40, a novel surface molecule involved in the regulation of the non-MHC restricted cytolytic activity in humans. *Eur. J. Immunol.* 25:369–76
7. Meyaard L, Adema GJ, Chang C, Woollatt E, Sutherland GR, Lanier LL, Phillips JH. 1997. LAIR-1, a novel inhibitory receptor expressed on human mononuclear leukocytes. *Immunity* 7:283–90
8. Cantoni C, Bottino C, Augugliaro R, Morelli L, Marcenaro E, Castriconi R, Vitale M, Pende D, Sivori S, Millo R, Biassoni R, Moretta L, Moretta A. 1999. Molecular and functional characterization of IRp60, a member of the immunoglobulin superfamily that functions as an inhibitory receptor in human natural killer cells. *Eur. J. Immunol.* 29:3148–59
9. Falco M, Biassoni R, Bottino C, Vitale M, Sivori S, Augugliaro R, Moretta L, Moretta A. 1999. Identification and molecular cloning of p75/AIRM1, a novel member of the sialoadhesin family which functions as an inhibitory receptor in human natural killer cells. *J. Exp. Med.* 190:793–802
10. Mingari MC, Schiavetti F, Ponte M, Vitale C, Maggi E, Romagnani S, Demarest J, Pantaleo G, Fauci AS, Moretta L. 1996. Human CD8$^+$ T lymphocyte subsets that express HLA class I-specific inhibitory receptors represent oligoclonally or monoclonally expanded cell populations. *Proc. Natl. Acad. Sci. USA.* 93:12433–38
11. Mingari MC, Moretta A, Moretta L. 1998. Regulation of KIR expression in human T lymphocytes. A safety mechanism which may impair protective T cell responses. *Immunol. Today* 19:153–57
12. Garrido F, Ruiz-Cabello F, Cabrera T, Pérez-Villar JJ, Lòpez-Botet M, Duggan-Keen M, Stern PL. 1997. Implications for immunosurveillance of altered HLA-class I phenotypes in human tumours. *Immunol. Today* 18:89–95
13. Garrido F. 1996. MHC molecules in normal and neoplastic cells. *Int. J. Cancer* 6:1–10
14. Ploegh HL. 1998. Viral strategies of immune evasion. *Science* 280:248–53
15. Biron CA. 1997. Activation and function of natural killer cell responses during viral infections. *Curr. Opin. Immunol.* 9:24–34
16. Zeidler R, Eissner G, Meissner P, Uebel S, Tampe R, Lazis S, Hammerschmidt W. 1997. Downregulation of TAP1 in B lymphocytes by cellular and Epstein-Barr virus-encoded interleukin-10. *Blood* 90:2390–97
17. Cohen GB, Gandhi RT, Davis DM, Mandelboim O, Chen BK, Strominger JL, Baltimore D. 1999. The selective downregulation of class I major histocompatibility complex proteins by HIV-1 protects HIV-infected cells from NK cells. *Immunity* 10:661–71
18. Ljunggren HG, Karre K. 1990. In search of the "missing self". MHC molecules

and NK cell recognition. *Immunol. Today* 11:237–44

19. Moretta A, Biassoni R, Bottino C, Pende D, Vitale M, Poggi A, Mingari MC, Moretta L. 1997. Major histocompability complex class I-specific receptors on human natural killer and T lymphocytes. *Immunol. Rev.* 155:105–17

20. Moretta L, Ciccone E, Moretta A, Hoglund P, Ohlén C, Karre K. 1992. Allorecognition by NK cells: nonself or no self? *Immunol. Today* 13:300–06

21. Shinkai Y, Rathbun G, Lam KP, Oltz EM, Stewart V, Mendelsohn M, Charron J, Datta M, Young F, Stall AM, Alt FW. 1992. RAG-2-deficient mice lack mature lymphocytes owing to inability to initiate V(D)J rearrangement. *Cell* 68:855–67

22. Mombaerts P, Iacomini J, Johnson RS, Herrup K, Tonegawa S, Papaioannou VE. 1992. RAG-1-deficient mice have no mature B and T lymphocytes. *Cell* 68:869–77

23. Ciccone E, Pende D, Vitale M, Nanni L, Di Donato C, Bottino C, Morelli L, Viale O, Amoroso A, Moretta and Moretta L. 1994. Self Class I molecules protect normal cells from lysis mediated by autologous natural killer cells. *Eur. J. Immunol.* 24:1003–6

24. Bléry M, Delon J, Trautman A, Cambiaggi A, Olcese L, Biassoni R, Moretta L, Moretta A, Daeron M, Vivier E. 1997. Reconstituted killer-cell-inhibitory receptors for MHC class I molecules control mast cell activation induced via immunoreceptor tyrosine-based activation motifs. *J. Biol. Chem.* 272:8989–96

25. Moretta A, Biassoni R, Bottino C, Mingari MC, Moretta L. 2000. Natural cytotoxicity receptors that trigger human NK-mediated cytolysis. *Immunol. Today* 21:228–34

26. Siliciano RF, Pratt JC, Schmidt RE, Ritz J, Reinherz EL. 1985. Activation of cytolytic T lymphocyte and natural killer cell function through the T11 sheep erythrocyte binding protein. *Nature* 317:428–30

27. Bolhuis RL, Roozemond RC, Van de Griend RJ. 1986. Induction and blocking of cytolysis in CD2+, CD3– NK and CD2+, CD3+ cytotoxic T lymphocytes via CD2 50 kD sheep erythrocyte receptor. *J. Immunol.* 136:3939–44

28. Lanier LL, Corliss B, Phillips JH. 1997. Arousal and inhibition of human NK cells. *Immunol. Rev.* 155:145–54

29. Shibuya A, Campbell D, Hannum C, Yssel H, Franz-Bacon K, McClanahan T, Kitamura T, Nicholl J, Sutherland GR, Lanier LL, Phillips JH. 1996. DNAM-1, a novel adhesion molecule involved in the cytolytic function of T lymphocytes. *Immunity* 4:573–81

30. Bottino C, Biassoni R, Millo R, Moretta L, Moretta A. 2000. The human natural cytotoxicity receptors (NCR) that induce HLA class I-independent NK cell triggering. *Human Immunol.* 61:1–6

31. Sivori S, Vitale M, Morelli L, Sanseverino L, Augugliaro R, Bottino C, Moretta L, Moretta A. 1997. p46, a novel natural killer cell-specific surface molecule which mediates cell activation. *J. Exp. Med.* 186: 1129–36

32. Pessino A, Sivori S, Bottino C, Malaspina A, Morelli L, Moretta L, Biassoni R, Moretta A. 1998. Molecular cloning of NKp46: a novel member of the immunoglobulin superfamily involved in triggering of natural cytotoxicity. *J. Exp. Med.* 188:953–60

33. Reth M. 1989. Antigen receptor tail clue. *Nature* 338:383–84

34. Cambier JC. 1995. New nomenclature for the Reth motif. *Immunol. Today* 16:110

35. Orloff DG, Ra CS, Frank SJ, Klausner RD, Kinet JP. 1990. Family of disulphide-linked dimers containing the zeta and eta chains of the T-cell receptor and the gamma chain of Fc receptors. *Nature* 347:189–91

36. Lanier LL, Yu G, Phillips JH. 1989. Co-association of CD3 zeta with a receptor (CD16) for IgG Fc on human natural killer cells. *Nature* 342:803–5

37. Wirthmueller U, Kurosaki T, Murakami MS, Ravetch JV. 1992. Signal transduction

by Fc gamma RIII (CD16) is mediated through the gamma chain. *J. Exp. Med.* 175:1381–90

38. Daeron M. 1997. Fc receptor biology. *Annu. Rev. Immunol.* 15:203–34

39. Ravetch JV, Kinet JP. 1991. Fc receptors. *Annu. Rev. Immunol.* 9:457–92

40. Ting AT, Dick CJ, Schoon RA, Karnitz LM, Abraham RT, Leibson PJ. 1995. Interaction between lck and syk family tyrosine kinases in Fc gamma receptor-initiated activation of natural killer cells. *J. Biol. Chem.* 270:16415–21

41. Salcedo TW, Kurosaki T, Kanakaraj P, Ravetch JV, Perussia B. 1993. Physical and functional association of p56^{lck} with Fc gamma RIIIA (CD16) in natural killer cells. *J. Exp. Med.* 177:1475–80

42. Brumbaugh KM, Binstadt BA, Billadeau DD, Schoon RA, Dick CJ, Ten RM, Leibson PJ. 1997. Functional role for Syk tyrosine kinase in natural killer cell-mediated natural cytotoxicity. *J. Exp. Med.* 186:1965–74

43. Stahls A, Liwszyc GE, Couture C, Mustelin T, Andersson LC. 1994. Triggering of human natural killer cells through CD16 induces tyrosine phosphorylation of the p72syk kinase. *Eur. J. Immunol.* 24:2491–96

44. Cone JC, Lu Y, Trevillyan JM, Bjorndahl JM, Phillips CA. 1993. Association of the p56^{lck} protein tyrosine kinase with the Fc gamma RIIIA/CD16 complex in human natural killer cells. *Eur. J. Immunol.* 23:2488–97

45. Wilson MJ, Torkar M, Haude A, Milne S, Jones T, Sheer D, Beck S, Trowsdale J. 2000. Plasticity in the organization and sequences of human KIR/ILT gene families. *Proc. Natl. Acad. Sci. USA* 97:4778–83

46. Biassoni R, Pessino A, Bottino C, Pende D, Moretta L, Moretta A. 1999. The murine homologue of the human NKp46, a triggering receptor involved in the induction of natural cytotoxicity. *Eur. J. Immunol.* 29:1014–20

47. Falco M, Cantoni C, Bottino C, Moretta A, Biassoni R. 1999. Identification of the rat homologue of the human NKp46 triggering receptor. *Immunol. Lett.* 68:411–14

48. Tomasello E, Desmoulins PO, Chemin K, Guia S, Cremer H, Ortaldo J, Love P, Kaiserlian D, Vivier E. 2000. Combined natural killer cell and dendritic cell functional deficiency in KARAP/DAP12 loss-of-function mutant mice. *Immunity* 13:355–64

49. Pende D, Parolini S, Pessino A, Sivori S, Augugliaro R, Morelli L, Marcenaro E, Accame L, Malaspina A, Biassoni R, Bottino C, Moretta L, Moretta A. 1999. Identification and molecular characterization of NKp30, a novel triggering receptor involved in natural cytotoxicity mediated by human natural killer cells. *J. Exp. Med.* 190:1505–16

50. Neville MJ, Campbell RD. 1999. A new member of the Ig superfamily and a V-ATPase G subunit are among the predicted products of novel genes close to the TNF locus in the human MHC. *J. Immunol.* 162:4745–54

51. Vitale M, Bottino C, Sivori S, Sanseverino L, Castriconi R, Marcenaro R, Augugliaro R, Moretta L, Moretta A. 1998. NKp44, a novel triggering surface molecule specifically expressed by activated Natural Killer cells is involved in non-MHC restricted tumor cell lysis. *J. Exp. Med.* 187:2065–72

52. Ferrini S, Miescher S, Zocchi MR, Von Fliedner V, Moretta A. 1987. Phenotypic and functional characterization of recombinant interleukin-2 (rIL-2)-induced killer cells: analysis at the population and the clonal level. *J. Immunol.* 138:1297–1302

53. Rosenberg A, Lotze MT. 1986. Cancer immunotherapy-2 and interleukin-2-activated lymphocytes. *Annu. Rev. Immunol.* 4:681–09

54. Cantoni C, Bottino C, Vitale M, Pessino A, Augugliaro R, Malaspina A, Parolini S, Moretta L, Moretta A, Biassoni R. 1999.

NKp44, a triggering receptor involved in tumor cell lysis by activated human Natural Killer cells, is a novel member of the immunoglobulin superfamily. *J. Exp. Med.* 189:787–96

55. Olcese L, Cambiaggi A, Semenzato G, Bottino C, Moretta A, Vivier E. 1997. Human killer cell activatory receptors for MHC class I molecules are included in a multimeric complex expressed by natural killer cells. *J. Immunol.* 158:5083–86

56. Lanier LL, Corliss BC, Jun W, Leong C, Phillips JH. 1998. Immunoreceptor DAP12 bearing a tyrosine-based activation motifs is involved in activating NK cells. *Nature* 391:703–7

57. Campbell KS, Cella M, Carretero M, Lopez-Botet M, Colonna M. 1998. Signaling through human killer cell activating receptors triggers tyrosine phosphorylation of an associated protein complex. *Eur. J. Immunol.* 28:599–609

58. Lanier LL, Corliss B, Wu J, Phillips JH. 1998. Association of DAP12 with activating CD94/NKG2C NK cell receptors. *Immunity* 8:693–1

59. Lanier LL. 2000. Turning on natural killer cells. *J. Exp. Med.* 191:1259–62

60. Bottino C, Falco M, Sivori S, Moretta L, Moretta A, Biassoni R. 2000. Identification and molecular characterization of a natural mutant of the p50.2/KIR2DS activating NK receptor that fails to mediate NK cell triggering. *Eur. J. Immunol.* In press

61. Sivori S, Pende D, Bottino C, Marcenaro E, Pessino A, Biassoni R, Moretta L, Moretta A. 1999. NKp46 is the major triggering receptor involved in the natural cytotoxicity of fresh or cultured human natural killer cells. Correlation between surface density of NKp46 and natural cytotoxicity against autologous, allogeneic or xenogeneic target cells. *Eur. J. Immunol.* 29:1656–66

62. Auchincloss H Jr, Sachs DH. 1998. Xenogeneic transplantation. *Annu. Rev. Immunol.* 16:433–70

63. Chan DV, Auchincloss H Jr. 1996. Human anti-pig cell-mediated cytotoxicity in vitro involves non-T as well as T cell components. *Xenotransplantation* 3:158–65

64. Seebach JD, Yamada K, McMorrow IM, Sachs DH, DerSimonian H. 1996. Xenogeneic human anti-pig cytotoxicity mediated by activated natural killer cells. *Xenotransplantation* 3:188–97

65. Inverardi L, Samaja M, Motterlini R, Mangili F, Bender JR, Pardi R. 1992. Early recognition of a discordant xenogeneic organ by human circulating lymphocytes. *J. Immunol.* 149:1416–23

66. Umesue M., Mayumi H., Nishimura Y, Kong Y-Y, Omoto K, Murakami Y, Nomoto K. 1996. Donor-specific prolongation of rat skin graft survival induced by rat-donor cells and cyclophosphamide under coadminstration of monoclonal antibodies against T cell receptor and natural killer cells in mice. *Transplantation* 61: 116–24

67. Houchins JP, Yabe T, McSherry C, Bach FH. 1991. DNA sequence analysis of NKG2, a family of related cDNA clones encoding type II integral membrane proteins on human natural killer cells. *J. Exp. Med.* 173:1017–20

68. Carretero M, Cantoni C, Bellón T, Bottino C, Biassoni R, Rodríguez A, Pérez-Villar JJ, Moretta L, Moretta A, López-Botet M. 1997. The CD94 and NKG2-A C-type lectins covalently assamble to form a a NK cell inhibitory receptor for HLA class I molecules. *Eur. J. Immunol.* 27:563–67

69. Lazetic S, Chang C, Houchins JP, Lanier LL, Phillips JH. 1996. Human natural killer cell receptors involved in MHC class I recognition are disulphide-linked heterodimers of CD94 and NKG2 subunits. *J. Immunol.* 157:4741–45

70. Cantoni C, Biassoni R, Pende D, Sivori S, Accame L, Pareti L, Semenzato G, Moretta L, Moretta A, Bottino C. 1998. The activating form of CD94 receptor complex. CD94 covalently associates with the Kp39 protein

that represents the product of the NKG2-C gene. *Eur. J. Immunol.* 28:327–38

71. Plougastel B, Trowsdale J. 1997. Cloning of NKG2-F, a new member of the NKG2 family of human natural killer cell receptor genes. *Eur. J. Immunol.* 27:2835–39

72. Braud VM, Allan DSJ, O'Callaghan CA, Soderstrom K, D'Andrea A, Ogg GS, Lazetic S, Young NT, Bell JI, Phillips JH, Lanier LL, McMichael AJ. 1998. HLA-E binds to natural killer cell receptors CD94/ NKG2A, B and C. *Nature* 391:795–99

73. Borrego F, Ulbrecht M, Weiss EH, Coligan JE, Brooks AG. 1998. Recognition of human histocompatibility leukocyte antigen (HLA)-E complexed with HLA class I signal sequence-derived peptides by CD94/NKG2 confers protection from natural killer cell-mediated lysis. *J. Exp. Med.* 187:813–18

74. Lee N, Llano M, Carretero M, Ishitani A, Navarro F, Lòpez-Botet M, Gheraty D. 1998. HLA-E is a major ligand for the natural killer inhibitory receptor CD94/ NKG2A. *Proc. Natl. Acad. Sci. USA* 95: 5199–5204

75. Wu J, Song Y, Bakker AB, Bauer S, Spies T, Lanier LL, Phillips JH. 1999. An activating immunoreceptor complex formed by NKG2D and DAP10. *Science* 285:730–32

76. Chang C, Dietrich J, Harpur AG, Lindquist JA, Haude A, Loke YW, King A, Colonna M, Trowsdale J, Wilson MJ. 1999. KAP10, a novel transmembrane adapter protein genetically linked to DAP12 but with unique signaling properties. *J. Immunol.* 163:4651–54

77. Bauer S, Groh V, Wu J, Steinle A, Phillips JH, Lanier LL, Spies T. 1999. Activation of NK cells and T cells by NKG2D, a receptor for stress-inducible MICA. *Science* 285:727–29

78. Groh V, Bahram S, Bauer S, Herman A, Beauchamp M, Spies T. 1996. Cell stress-regulated human major histocompatibility complex class I gene expressed in gastroin-testinal epithelium. *Proc. Natl. Acad. Sci. USA* 93:12445–50

79. Groh V, Rhinehart R, Secrist H, Bauer S, Grabstein KH, Spies T. 1999. Broad tumor-associated expression and recognition by tumor-derived gamma delta T cells of MICA and MICB. *Proc. Natl. Acad. Sci. USA* 96:6879–84

80. Pende D, Cantoni C, Vitale M, Rivera P, Castriconi R, Marcenaro S, Nahni M, Biassoni R, Bottino C, Moretta A, Moretta L. 2000. Involvement of NKG2D in the tumor cell by normal NK cells: complementary role with NKp46, NKp44 and NKp30 natural cytotoxicity receptors. Submitted

81. Ho EL, Heusel JW, Brown MG, Matsumoto K, Scalzo AA, Yokoyama WM. 1998. Murine NKG2D and CD94 are clustered within the natural killer complex and are expressed independently in natural killer cells. *Proc. Natl. Acad. Sci. USA* 95:6320–25

82. Diefenbach A, Jamieson AM, Liu SD, Shastri N, Raulet DH. 2000. Ligands for the murine NKG2D receptor: expression by tumor cells and activation of NK cells and macrophages. *Nat. Immunol.* 1:119–26

83. Cerwenka A, Bakker ABH, McClanahan T, Wagner J, Wu J, Phillips JH, Lanier LL. 2000. Retinoic acid early inducible genes define a ligand family for the activating NKG2D receptor in mice. *Immunity* 12:721–27

84. Malarkannan S, Shih PP, Eden PA, Horng T, Zuberi AR, Christianson G, Roopenian D, Shastri N. 1998. The molecular and functional characterization of a dominant minor H antigen, H60. *J. Immunol.* 161:3501–9

85. Nomura M, Zou Z, Joh T, Takihara Y, Matsuda Y, Shimada K. 1996. Genomic structures and characterization of Rae1 family members encoding GPI-anchored cell surface proteins and expressed predominantly in embryonic mouse brain. *J. Biochem.* (Tokyo). 120:987–95

86. Cosman D, Mullberg J, Fanslow W,

Armitage R, Chin W, et al. 2000. The human cytomegalovirus (HCMV) glycoprotein, UL16, binds to the MHC class I-related protein, MICB/PERB11, and to two novel, MHC class I-related molecules, ULBP1 and ULBP2. *Faseb J.* 14:A1018

87. Chalupny J, Cosman D, Mullberg J, Chin W, Cassiano I, et al. 2000. Soluble forms of the novel MHC class I-related molecules, ULBP1 and ULBP2, bind to, and functionally activate NK cells. *Faseb J.* 14:A1018

88. Garni-Wagner BA, Purohit A, Mathew PA, Bennett M, Kumar V 1993. A novel function-associated molecule related to non-MHC-restricted cytotoxicity mediated by activated natural killer cells and T cells. *J. Immunol.* 151:60–70

89. Schuhmachers G, Ariizumi K, Mathew PA, Bennett M, Kumar V, Takashima A. 1995. Activation of murine epidermal gamma delta T cells through surface 2B4. *Eur. J. Immunol.* 25:1117–20

90. Mathew PA, Garni-Wagner BA, Land K, Takashima A, Stoneman E, Bennett M, Kumar V. 1993. Cloning and characterization of the 2B4 gene encoding a molecule associated with non-MHC-restricted killing mediated by activated natural killer cells and T cells. *J. Immunol.* 151:5328–37

91. Davis SJ, van der Merwe PA. 1996. The structure and ligand interactions of CD2: implications for T-cell function. *Immunol Today* 17:177–87

92. Brown MH, Boles K, van der Merwe PA, Kumar V, Mathew PA, Barclay AN. 1998. 2B4, the natural killer and T cell immunoglobulin superfamily surface protein, is a ligand for CD48. *J. Exp. Med.* 188:2083–90

93. Latchman Y, McKay PF, Reiser H. 1998. Identification of the 2B4 molecule as a counter-receptor for CD48. *J. Immunol.* 161:5809–12

94. Moretta A., Bottino C, Tripodi G, Vitale M, Pende D, Morelli L, Augugliaro R, Barbaresi M, Ciccone E, Millo R, Moretta L. 1992. Novel surface molecules involved

in human NK cell activation and triggering of the lytic machinery. *Int. J. Cancer.* (Suppl.) 7:6–10

95. Valiante NM, Trinchieri G. 1993. Identification of a novel signal transduction surface molecule on human cytotoxic lymphocytes. *J. Exp. Med.* 178:1397–406

96. Boles KS, Nakajima H, Colonna M, Chuang SS, Stepp SE, Bennett M, Kumar V, Mathew PA. 1999. Molecular characterization of a novel human natural killer cell receptor homologous to mouse 2B4. *Tissue Antigens* 54:27–34

97. Kubin MZ, Parsley DL, Din W, Waugh JY, Davis-Smith T, Smith CA, Macduff BM, Armitage RJ, Chin W, Cassiano L, Borges L, Petersen M, Trinchieri G, Goodwing RG. 1999. Molecular cloning and biological characterization of NK cell activation-inducing ligand, a counterstructure for CD48. *Eur. J. Immunol.* 29:3466–77

98. Nakajima H, Cella M, Langen H, Friedlein A, Colonna M. 1999. Activating interactions in human NK cell recognition: the role of 2B4-CD48. *Eur. J. Immunol.* 29:1676–83

99. Tangye SG, Lazetic S, Woollatt E, Sutherland GR, Lanier LL, Phillips JH. 1999. Human 2B4, an activating NK cell receptor, recruits the protein tyrosine phosphatase SHP-2 and the adaptor signaling protein SAP. *J. Immunol.* 162:6981–85

100. Sivori S, Parolini S, Falco M, Marcenaro E, Biassoni R, Bottino C, Moretta L and Moretta A. 2000. 2B4 functions as a coreceptor in human natural killer cell activation. *Eur. J. Immunol.* 30:787–93

101. Parolini S, Bottino C, Falco M, Augugliaro R, Silvia Giliani S, Franceschini R, Ochs H.D, Wolf H, Bonnefoy J-Y, Biassoni R, Moretta L, Notarangelo LD, Moretta A. 2000. X-linked lymphoproliferative disease: 2B4 molecules displaying inhibitory rather than activating function are responsible for the inability of NK cells to kill EBV-infected cells. *J. Exp. Med.* 192:337–46

102. Nichols KE, Harkin DP, Levitz S, Krainer M, Kolquist KA, Genovese C, Bernard A, Ferguson M, Zuo L, Snyder E, Buckler AJ, Wise C, Ashley J, Lovett M, Valentine MB, Look AT, Gerald W, Housman DE, Haber DA. 1998. Inactivating mutations in an SH2 domain-encoding gene in X-linked lymphoproliferative syndrome. *Proc. Natl. Acad. Sci. USA* 95:13765–770

103. Coffey A.J., Brooksbank RA, Brandau O, Oohashi T, Howell GR, Bye JM, Cahn AP, Durham J, Heath P, Wray P, Pavitt R, Wilkinson J, Leversha M, Huckle E, Shaw-Smith CJ, Dunham A, Rhodes S, Schuster V, Porta G, Yin L, Serafini P, Sylla B, Zollo M, Franco B, Bolino A, Seri M, Lanyi A, Davis JR, Webster DW, Harris A, Lenoir G, de St Basile G, Jones A, Behloradsky BH, Achatz H, Murken HJ, Fassler R, Sumegi J, Romeo G, Vaudin M, Ross MT, Meindl A, Bentley DR. 1998. Host response to EBV infection in X-linked lymphoproliferative disease results from mutations in an SH2-domain encoding gene. *Nat. Genet.* 20:129–35

104. Sayos J, Wu C, Morra M, Wang N, Zhang X, Allen D, van Schaik S, Notarangelo L, Geha R, Roncarolo MG, Oettgen H, De Vries JE, Aversa G, Terhorst C. 1998. The X-linked lymphoproliferative-disease gene product SAP regulates signals induced through the co-receptor SLAM. *Nature* 395:462–69

105. Bottino C, Augugliaro R, Castriconi R, Nanni M, Biassoni R, Moretta L, Moretta A. 2000. Analysis of the molecular mechanism involved in 2B4-mediated NK cell activation: evidence that human 2B4 is physically and functionally associated with the linker for activation of T cells (LAT). *Eur. J. Immunol.* In press

106. Zhang W, Sloan-Lancaster J, Kitchen J, Trible R-P, Samelson L-E. 1998. LAT: the ZAP-70 tyrosine kinase substrate that links T cell receptor to cellular activation. *Cell* 92:83–92

107. Jevremovic D, Billadeau D-D, Schoon R-A, Dick C-J, Irvin B-J, Zhang W, Samelson L-E, Abraham R-T and Leibson P-J. 1999. A role for the adaptor protein LAT in human NK cell-mediated cytotoxicity. *J. Immunol.* 162:2453–56

108. Vitale M, Falco M, Castriconi R, Parolini S, Zambello R, Semenzato G, Biassoni R, Bottino C, Moretta L, Moretta A. 2000. Identification of NKp80 a novel triggering molecule expressed by human natural killer cells. *Eur. J. Immunol.* In press

109. Roda-Navarro P, Arce I, Renedo M, Montgomery K, Kucherlapati R, Fernandez-Ruiz E. 2000. Human KLRF1, a novel member of the killer cell lectin-like receptor gene family: molecular characterization, genomic structure, physical mapping to the NK gene complex and expression analysis. *Eur. J. Immunol.* 30:568–76

110. Moretta A, Tambussi G, Bottino C, Tripodi G, Merli A, Ciccone E, Pantaleo G, Moretta L. 1990. A novel surface antigen expressed by a subset of human CD3⁻CD16⁺ natural killer cells. Role in cell activation and regulation of cytolytic function. *J. Exp. Med.* 171:695–14

111. Moretta A, Bottino C, Pende D, Tripodi G, Tambussi G, Viale O, Orengo AM, Barbaresi M, Merli A, Ciccone E, Moretta L. 1990. Identification of four subset of human CD3⁻CD16⁺ NK cells by the expression of clonally distributed functional surface molecules. Correlation between subset assignment of NK clones and ability to mediate specific alloantigen recognition. *J. Exp. Med.* 172:1589–98

112. Moretta A, Vitale M, Bottino C, Orengo AM, Morelli L, Augugliaro R, Barbaresi M, Ciccone E, Moretta L. 1993. P58 molecules as putative receptors for MHC class I molecules in human natural killer (NK) cells. Anti-p58 antibodies reconstitute lysis of MHC class I-protected cells in NK clones displaying different specificities. *J. Exp. Med.* 178:597–604

113. Moretta A, Sivori S, Vitale M, Pende D, Morelli L, Augugliaro R, Bottino C Moretta L. 1995. Existence of both inhibitory (p58) and activatory (p50) receptors for HLA.C molecules in human natural killer cells. *J. Exp. Med.* 182:875–84

114. Bottino C, Sivori S, Vitale M, Cantoni C, Falco M, Pende D, Morelli L, Augugliaro R, Semenzato G, Biassoni R, Moretta L, Moretta A. 1996. A novel surface molecule homologous to the p58/p50 family of receptors is selectively expressed on a subset of human natural killer cells and induces both triggering of cell functions and proliferation. *Eur. J. Immunol.* 26:1816–24

115. Biassoni R, Cantoni C, Falco M, Verdiani S, Bottino C, Vitale M, Conte R, Poggi A, Moretta A, Moretta L. 1996. The HLA-C specific "activatory" and "inhibitory" natural killer cell receptors display highly homologous extracellular domains but differ in their transmembrane and intracytoplasmic portions. *J. Exp. Med.* 183:645–50

116. Biassoni R, Pessino A, Malaspina A, Cantoni C, Bottino C, Sivori S, Moretta L, Moretta A. 1997. Role of amino acid position 70 in the binding affinity of p50.1 and p58.1 receptors for CW4 molecules. *Eur. J. Immunol.* 27:3095–99

117. Ikeda H, Lethé B, Lehmann F, Van Baren N, Baurain JF, De Smet C, Chambost H, Vitale M, Moretta A, Boon T, Coulie PG. 1997. Characterization of an antigen that is recognized on a melanoma showing partial HLA-loss by CTL expressing an inhibitory receptor. *Immunity* 6:199–8

118. Bakker ABH, Hoek RM, Cerwenka A, Blom B, Lucian L, McNeil T, Murray R, Phillips JH, Sedgwick JD, Lanier LL. 2000. DAP12-deficient mice fail to develop autoimmunity due to impaired antigen priming. *Immunity* 13:345–53

119. Smith HR, Chuang HH, Wang LL, Salcedo M, Heusel JW, Yokoyama WM. 2000. Nonstochastic coexpression of activation receptors on murine natural killer cells. *J. Exp. Med.* 191:1341–54

120. Shores EW, Ono M, Kawabe T, Sommers CL, Tran T, Lui K, Udey MC, Ravetch J, Love PE. 1998. T cell development in mice lacking all T cell receptor zeta family members (Zeta, eta, and Fc epsilon RI gamma). *J. Exp. Med.* 187:1093–101

121. De la Salle H, Hanau D, Fricker D, Urlacher A, Kelly A, Salamero J, Powis SH, Donato L, Bausinger H, Laforet M, Jeras M, Spehner D, Bieber T, Falkenrodt A, Cazenave JP, Trowsdale J, Tongio MM. 1994. Homozygous human TAP peptide transporter mutation in HLA class I deficiency. *Science* 265:237–41

122. Zimmer J, Donato L, Hanau D, Cazenave JP, Tongio MM, Moretta A, de la Salle H. 1998. Activity and phenotype of natural killer cells in peptide transporter (TAP)-deficient patients (type I bare lymphocyte syndrome). *J. Exp. Med.* 187:117–22

123. Teisserenc H, Schmitt W, Blake N, Dunbar R, Gadola S, Gross WL, Exley A, Cerundolo V. 1997. A case of primary immunodeficiency due to a defect of the major histocompatibility gene complex class I processing and presentation pathway. *Immunol Lett.* 57:183–87

124. Purtilo DT, Cassel CK, Yang JPS. 1974. Fatal infectious mononucleosis in familial lymphohistiocytosis. *N. Engl. J. Med.* 201:736 (Letter)

125. Seemayer TA, Gross CK, Egeler RM, Pirruccello SJ, Davi JR, Kelly CM, Okano M, Lanyi A. Sumeegi J. 1995. X-linked lymphoproliferative disease: twenty five years after discovery. *Pediatr. Res.* 38:471–78

126. Sullivan Jl, Woda BA. 1989. X-linked proliferative syndrome. *Immunodef. Rev.* 1:325–47

127. Cocks BG, Change CC, Garballido J, Yssel H, de Vries JE, Aversa G. 1995. A novel receptor involved in T-cell activation. *Nature* 376:260–63

Annu. Rev. Immunol. 2001. 19:225–52

Complexities of CD28/B7: CTLA-4 Costimulatory Pathways in Autoimmunity and Transplantation

Benoît Salomon[1] and Jeffrey A. Bluestone[2]

[1]The Committee on Immunology, Ben May Institute for Cancer Research and Department of Pathology, University of Chicago, Chicago, Illinois 60637
[2]UCSF Diabetes Center, University of California, San Francisco, California 94143-0540; e-mail: jbluest@diabetes.ucsf.edu

Key Words   T cell costimulation, CD28, B7, tolerance

■ **Abstract**   Recent advances in the understanding of T cell activation have led to new therapeutic approaches in the treatment of immunological disorders. One attractive target of intervention has been the blockade of T cell costimulatory pathways, which result in more selective effects on only those T cells that have encountered specific antigen. In fact, in some instances, costimulatory pathway antagonists can induce antigen-specific tolerance that prevents the progression of autoimmune diseases and organ graft rejection. In this review, we summarize the current understanding of these complex costimulatory pathways including the individual roles of the CD28, CTLA-4, B7-1 (CD80), and B7-2 (CD86) molecules. We present evidence that suggests that multiple mechanisms contribute to CD28/B7-mediated T cell costimulation in disease settings that include expansion of activated pathogenic T cells, differentiation of Th1/Th2 cells, and the migration of T cells into target tissues. Additionally, the negative regulatory role of CTLA-4 in autoimmune diseases and graft rejection supports a dynamic but complex process of immune regulation that is prominent in the control of self-reactivity. This is most apparent in regulation of the $CD4^+CD25^+CTLA-4^+$ immunoregulatory T cells that control multiple autoimmune diseases. The implications of these complexities and the potential for use of these therapies in clinical immune intervention are discussed.

INTRODUCTION

The ability to discriminate between self and nonself is perhaps the most fundamentally important aspect of immune regulation. This property translates into the immune recognition and destruction of infectious invaders while normal host tissues are left untouched. This highly selective response is characterized by a complicated set of T cell regulatory mechanisms that have been described over the past decades. One such mechanism designed to maintain the fidelity of the

0732-0582/01/0407-0225$14.00

immune response is the requirement of two distinct signals for effective activation of antigen-specific T cells: an antigen-specific signal via the T cell receptor (Signal 1) and a noncognate costimulatory signal (Signal 2) that is provided by soluble factors or cell-surface molecules on the antigen presenting cell (APC). The integration of these two signals triggers cell division and differentiation to effectors and regulators of the immune response. Aside from the critical biological implications of costimulation, the identification of a costimulatory signal has important implications for clinical intervention as the effects of costimulation blockade would be restricted to only those T cells whose antigen-specific receptors have been engaged, i.e. T cells already receiving signal 1. Thus, in principal, the selective blockade of T cell costimulation offers an antigen-specific mode of targeting immune responses without actual knowledge of the specific antigen involved.

Although investigators have studied the T cell receptor and its fundamental function for decades, they only recently discovered the existence and characterization of the second costimulatory signal. Experiments in the late 1980s showed that T cell clones failed to proliferate in the absence of costimulatory signals and became refractory to further activation (1). The finding that T cell inactivation, termed T cell anergy, was a direct consequence of regulated IL-2 production (2) led to the search for a master costimulatory signal that targeted the IL-2 pathway. This search resulted in the identification of the CD28/B7 pathway as a prominent costimulatory pathway for T cells (3, 4). Although additional costimulatory pathways have since been identified, including CD40 ligand (CD154)/CD40, CD2/CD58, LFA-1 (CD18)/ICAM-1 (CD54), and others, the CD28/B7 pathway remains one of the most potent and well-characterized costimulatory interactions. As discussed below, there is increasing evidence that CD28 engagement leads to multiple effects on immune responses in addition to the regulation of IL-2 production. The pleiotropic activitiees of CD28 support the potential clinical usefulness of CD28/B7 blockade in immune intervention.

The effectiveness of costimulatory blockade was first demonstrated in the early 1990s using CTLA-4Ig, an engineered fusion protein that binds with high affinity the two ligands of CD28, B7-1 (CD80) and B7-2 (CD86) (5). This antagonist inhibited islet xenograft rejection and induced long-lasting immune tolerance (6). Subsequently, a number of preclinical studies have demonstrated the primary importance of the CD28/B7 pathway in the prevention of graft rejection in rodents and primates. In fact, antagonists of this pathway, alone or in combination with CD40L/CD40 blockade, have been especially effective in treating autoimmune diseases in preclinical models of these diseases (7–12). Thus, these agents remain among the most promising for the induction of long-term, stable tolerance.

However, the complexity of regulation of these diseases by T cell costimulation blockade has now become apparent. The relative importance of the various costimulation pathways is highly dependent on the tissue expression, the nature of the inflammatory response, and the state of the reactive T cell subset. Apparent contradictions in the in vivo effects of costimulatory blockade abound in the literature. For example, in experimental autoimmune encephalitis [(EAE), a rodent model of multiple sclerosis] the effects of blocking B7 costimulation vary significantly depending on the dosing and the timing of antagonist administration, the strain of mouse or rat used, and the protocol used to induce the disease in EAE (for reviews, see 13–16). In some instances, blocking B7 costimulation reduces the severity of EAE; whereas in different disease settings, similar treatments actually led to an exacerbation of autoimmune symptoms.

This review attempts to clarify the current state of knowledge regarding the various mechanisms by which the CD28/B7 T costimulatory pathway impacts autoimmune diseases and transplantation. The pleiotropic effects of this regulatory system are highlighted by the diversity of its functions in immune regulation, including (*a*) T cell activation and differentiation, (*b*) tissue migration, and (*c*) its role in peripheral tolerance induction. The role of the CD40/CD154 pathway is also discussed because of the inherent similarities between it and the CD28/B7 pathway as well as the growing interest in CD40/CD154 blockade clinically in the treatment of autoimmune diseases and transplantation. Finally, we summarize recent data on the utility of these T cell costimulation pathways blockade in autoimmune diseases and transplantation in nonhuman primates and humans.

THE CD28:CTLA-4/B7 COSTIMULATORY PATHWAY REGULATES IMMUNITY BY MULTIPLE MECHANISMS

The CD28/B7 Costimulatory Pathway Regulates T Cell Activation by Inhibiting Cell Expansion

The differential importance of the CD28/B7 pathway in T cell activation of naïve and differentiated T cells has been studied extensively over the past decade. In vitro studies have shown that antigen-specific proliferation of naïve T cells isolated from TCR transgenic mice is exquisitely dependent on CD28/B7 costimulation (17–20). Most prominent are the findings that the disruption of the CD28/B7 interaction dramatically reduces the frequency of proliferating cells and the number of cell divisions of previously activated cells (21, 22). The dependence of cell proliferation on CD28 is due to several mechanisms. CD28 costimulation increases transcription and mRNA stability of IL-2, a critical T cell growth factor (4, 23–25). CD28 costimulation induces increased expression of the anti-apoptotic protein Bcl-X$_L$ that promotes cell survival in vitro (18, 26) and in vivo (27–30). Thus, CD28 ligation is essential for sustained proliferation of T cells. Finally, in addition to its distal effects on T cell activation, CD28 costimulation decreases the threshold of T cell activation (31). In naïve T cells, this occurs by promoting the formation of an immunological synapse (32, 33).

Although a potent stimulator of T cell activation, CD28 costimulation is not always required, especially under circumstances where a strong or sustained Ag-specific signal is available (34–36). This finding is most readily apparent in models that use different antigenic peptides. T cell activation by weak peptide agonists or low concentrations of peptides is generally dependent on CD28 costimulation, whereas CD28 dependency decreases under conditions of high antigenic load or strong peptide agonists (19, 22, 35–37). It is significant to note that in contrast to the study of naïve T cells, studies on proliferation and cytokine production (IFN-γ, IL-4) by recently activated T cells and memory T cells demonstrate that these cells are less dependent on CD28 costimulation (38–41). This could be due to constitutive expression of activated lck, which localizes to the TCR complex and thus decreases the threshold for T cell activation (42).

The critical importance of CD28/B7 costimulation in T cell activation has led to multiple studies that examine the role of costimulation in experimental models of autoimmune diseases. Several tissue-specific autoimmune disease models have been developed in rodents by breaking tolerance through immunization with self-proteins and peptides. Early studies showed that disruption of CD28/B7 costimulation at the time of immunization was associated invariably with the reduction of the severity of the pathology and, in some cases, with complete disease prevention. For instance, CD28/B7 blockade by CTLA-4Ig or, in some cases, anti-B7 mAbs reduced disease severity in mouse models of multiple sclerosis (for review, see 13–15), myocarditis (43), arthritis (44), thyroiditis (45), and myasthenia gravis (46).

Much of the research into the clinical effects of CD28/B7 costimulation blockade has focused on EAE as a model for the human disease multiple sclerosis (MS) (47, 48). EAE is a demyelinating disease of the central nervous system (CNS) that is mediated by CD4$^+$ T helper-type 1 (Th1) cells. It can be induced in several strains of animals by immunization with various myelin proteins or their immunodominant peptide epitopes [derived from myelin basic protein, proteolipoprotein, (MOG)] (47, 48). Initial studies were performed at the onset of the disease. In these studies, the complete blockade of CD28/B7 interactions resulted in the reduction of EAE. This effect correlated with a decrease in proliferation of CNS-reactive T cells in the draining lymph nodes 10–15 days after immunization, a time when the first clinical symptoms appear (37, 49). The investigators suggested that CD28/B7 blockade in this system limited T cell expansion in vivo. The decreased severity of EAE following CD28/B7 disruption was not associated with a reduction of T cell proliferation to the immunizing antigen in other experimental systems (50, 51). In these settings, alternative mechanisms, such as regulation of the Th1/Th2 balance, alteration in T cell migration, the induction of T cell unresponsiveness, or the emergence of a suppressive mechanism due to the lack of CD28 costimulation, were more likely to be involved as discussed below.

Important to note, and more clinically relevant, have been the studies of CD28/B7 costimulation after disease onset. These studies have relied on a murine relapsing-remitting EAE (R-EAE) that is induced by immunization with the immunodominant proteolipid protein epitope (PLP139–151) (52, 53). Following active immunization, the mice exhibit a paralytic acute phase followed by spontaneous remission and subsequent clinical relapses, an evolution comparable to that of MS. Several studies have shown that blockade of the CD28/B7 pathway during the acute or remission phases of EAE prevents further relapses (54, 55). Moreover, targeted administration of CTLA-4Ig to the brain, which is the site of ongoing pathogenic immune responses, by gene therapy (56) increased the efficiency of the drug as compared to systemic injection (57–59). The therapeutic effects of blocking CD28/B7 after disease onset might not have been predicted based on the previous observations that the stimulation of recently activated T cells and memory T cells was CD28-independent (20, 38, 39). However, two important features of the disease provide an explanation for this unanticipated result. Unlike T cells that respond to conventional foreign antigens, the T cell receptors of autoreactive T cells often have weak affinities to their ligands. Thus, the activation of autoreactive T cells may be more dependent on CD28/B7 costimulation than the activation of T cells to foreign Ag. Indeed, ex vivo proliferation of myelin-autoreactive T cells purified from mice that were developing acute EAE were shown to remain dependent on CD28/B7 costimulation (58, 60). Equally important were the observations by several groups that showed that the clinical relapses did not result from memory T cell reactivation but were a consequence of activation of naïve autoreactive T cells triggered by endogenously presented non-cross-reactive myelin epitopes elicited as a result of autoimmune tissue destruction. Several groups have demonstrated the critical role of this phenomenon, termed epitope spreading, in the progression of ongoing disease (61, 62). Indeed, we have shown that relapses of disease in SJL mice can be prevented by blocking CD28 costimulation during disease remission. In this setting, the therapy had minimal effects on the reactivity of the primary PLP139-specific T cell responses but totally blocked epitope spreading (54).

Thus, the effects of costimulatory blockade on an ongoing autoimmune disease may be limited to the inhibition of naïve T cell activation and expansion, and they may not be sufficient to block ongoing autoimmunity. In this regard, we have explored the role of the CD28/B7 pathway in the pathogenesis of diabetes using the NOD mouse, a spontaneous model of autoimmune disease. In these studies, we demonstrated that treatment of NOD mice early in the disease process (between 2 to 7 weeks of age) with anti-B7-2 mAb prevented the development of diabetes. However, late therapy had no effect on disease progression. In fact, although CTLA-4Ig was quite effective in blocking islet graft rejection in normal mice (63), it was ineffective in prolonging graft survival following graft rejection in diabetic NOD animals (CG Park, GL Szot, JA Bluestone, unpublished observations).

In summary, the findings support a primary role for CD28/B7 activation in the initiation but not reactivation of any immune response. The mechanistic basis for this difference is not known but most likely reflects functional and biochemical differences between naïve and memory T cells. First, naïve T cells are exquisitely dependent on IL-2 as their primary growth factor. Second, the threshold of signal transduction required for memory T cell reactivation is substantially reduced such that the biochemical signals that promote T cell activation in naïve T cells become less critical. Therefore, the potential for bypassing CD28 costimulation is likely to be problematic in settings where chronic antigen exposure exists. Moreover, the existence of epitope spreading and, thus, the presence of autoreactive T cells at different stages of differentiation will complicate the outcome of costimulation blockade in the clinical setting where intervention, by necessity, will be after disease onset.

The CD28/B7 Costimulatory Pathway Regulates Th1/Th2 Differentiation

T cells can be divided into distinct subsets based on their cytokine production profile. Th1 T cells produce inflammatory cytokines such as IFN-γ and TNF-α that mediate pathogenic responses in infectious disease, autoimmunity, and transplantation. In contrast, Th2 T cells produce IL-4, IL-5, and IL-10. These cytokines are critical for the development of humoral responses and increasingly have been shown to modulate the Th1 response through a bystander suppressive effect on Th1 cell differentiation. Inflammatory cytokines play a pathogenic role in many tissue-specific autoimmune diseases (for review, see 64). In contrast, Th2 cells have been reported to regulate these same diseases (65) or, in some instances, to promote pathogenic antibody-mediated autoimmunity.

CD28/B7 costimulation regulates the Th1/Th2 balance. Differentiation of naïve CD4$^+$ T cells toward Th2 is strictly dependant on CD28/B7 costimulation. In vitro experiments showed that in the absence of CD28 costimulation IL-4, IL-5, and IL-10 cytokines are not produced, whereas IFN-γ production is not severely affected (20, 66–68). The critical role of CD28 in Th2 differentiation has been implicated in a number of experimental autoimmune disease settings. Several groups demonstrated that the decreased severity of EAE following CD28 antagonism is not associated with changes in T cell expansion (50, 51). In studies by Kuchroo and others, prevention of EAE by B7 costimulation blockade during disease induction is associated with a shift of CNS-autoreactive T cells in draining lymph nodes (50) and in the CNS (69) toward a Th2 phenotype.

Similar findings have been observed in NOD mice. Exogenous injection of IL-4 or other Th2 cytokines or overexpression in the Th2 cytokines in islets protects mice from the disease (70). Thus, in contrast to R-EAE, NOD diabetes is exquisitely Th2 dependent. Thus, perhaps it was not surprising that blockade of the CD28/B7 pathway via disruption of the CD28 gene expression led to an earlier onset, increased incidence, and increased severity of autoimmunity in NOD mice as compared to their littermate controls. The absence of a requirement for CD28 in the initial activation of naïve islet autoreactive T cells likely resulted from the repeated activation of these cells due to the chronicity of antigen exposure in this autoimmune strain of mice. Indeed, sustained activation of naïve T cell overcomes the requirement for CD28 costimulation (35). However, the islet autoreactive T cells that develop produced Th1 cytokines but not immunoregulatory Th2 cytokines. This change in cytokine balance led to decreased levels of Th2-type anti-GAD antibodies and a more severe insulitis, which suggests one reason for the exacerbation of diabetes (71). Similar and predictable results were obtained following treatment of young NOD mice with a stimulating anti-CD28 mAb. The islet infiltrating NOD T cells that were produced increased levels of IL-4 and prevented the development of autoimmune diabetes (72). The critical role of CD28-dependent Th2 development and the subsequent inhibition of disease were not observed when treating older NOD mice. In fact, under certain conditions, CD28 antagonist therapies blocked the development of late stage disease. These results emphasize the paradox of CD28/B7 costimulation. Effective blockade of the pathway preferentially blocks Th2 versus Th1 differentiation; however, once an established effector T cell population has developed, proliferation of Th1 cells but not of Th2 cells is dependent on CD28/B7 costimulation (20, 38, 39).

The role of CD28/B7 costimulation has been analyzed in models of autoimmunity mediated by pathogenic Th2 responses. As an example, in the NZB/NZW mouse strain, which develops an antibody-dependent lupus-like autoimmune syndrome, treatment with CTLA-4Ig or a combination of anti-B7-1 and anti-B7-2 Abs prevented the development and progression of the disease (73, 74). In this setting, the blockade of CD28/B7 interactions had a most dramatic effect on Th2 differentiation and subsequent production of antibodies (5, 75). Thus, the therapeutic effects of blocking CD28/B7 in this autoimmune model were likely due to the critical role of this pathway in the CD4-dependent humoral response (73, 74). However, it should be emphasized that these lupus-like diseases also exhibit a Th1 component, thus therapies directed at both arms of the T cell response are likely to be the most effective therapies. In this regard, Wofsy and colleagues have shown recently that a combination of CTLA-4Ig and cyclophosphomide was most effective in preventing the autoimmune disease in the NZB/NZW strain of mice (D Wofsy, personal communication).

In summary, these results emphasize the delicate balance of the immune response and highlight the uncertain outcome of immune manipulation in complex autoimmune diseases. The blockade of the CD28/B7 pathway can affect this cytokine balance to protect or to exacerbate disease depending on the nature of disease pathogenesis and the ability of the autoreactive T cells to expand in the absence of adequate costimulation. Although inhibition of Th2 differentiation following CD28/B7 blockade has the potential to prevent antibody-mediated diseases such as lupus, it can also lead to exacerbation of Th1-mediated diseases such as autoimmune diabetes. For instance, disease progression in NZB/NZW F1 (lupus) mice can be blocked by a short course of CTLA4-Ig combined with anti-CD40L mAb administered at the onset of disease (76). There was long-lasting inhibition of autoantibody production and renal disease. Thus, it is likely that a combination of therapies will be essential to abrogate disease in these settings. In this regard, we have recently bred the CD40LKO to the highly disease-prone CD28KO NOD mice. The combined disruption of both costimulatory pathways protected the mice from developing diabetes (BS Salomon, L Rhee, JA Bluestone, unpublished observations).

The CD28/B7 Costimulatory Pathway Regulates Cell Migration

In addition to its role in regulating T cell activation and Th1/Th2 differentiation, the CD28/B7 costimulatory pathway has been implicated in cell migration and inflammation. CD28 costimulation is required for the production of chemokines such as MIP-1α and MIP-1β (77) as well as CXCR4, a chemokine receptor that is upregulated following CD28/B7 engagement (78). In contrast, the CCR5 chemokine receptor is downregulated following CD28 signaling. These results may explain recent studies in CD28 and B7 genetically disrupted animals. B7-1/B7-2KO and CD28KO mice develop a potent T cell proliferative response to the immunizing myelin-derived proteins as evidenced by the presence of autoreactive T cells in the lymphoid tissue that produce high levels of the pathogenic TNF-α and IFN-γ cytokines. However, these mice do not develop EAE (51, 79). Further studies showed that the CD28KO mice exhibited a significantly decreased delayed-type hypersensitivity response to the myelin-derived Ag, which suggests that there was decreased or altered T cell trafficking of the pathogenic T cells into the inflammatory sites of the CNS (51). It is important to note that chemokines are essential in the migration of mononuclear cells into the CNS and in the pathogenesis of EAE (80). In fact, active immunization of B6 CD28KO mice with the neural peptide led not to EAE but rather to an autoimmune meningitis with a mononuclear inflammation in the leptomeninges, but not in the parenchyma of the CNS as normally observed in EAE (81). Thus, one underappreciated function of the CD28/B7 costimulatory pathway in tissue-specific autoimmune diseases is its control of inflammatory cell migration and thus the target tissue of autoimmune attack.

CD28/B7 Costimulation is Essential for the Homeostasis of the CD25$^+$CD4$^+$ Immunoregulatory T Cells

Recently, a unique population of peripheral CD4$^+$ T cells has been shown to be essential for the maintenance of tolerance to tissue-specific self-antigens. These regulatory T cells express CD25 as well as a constellation of other cell surface markers including low levels of CD45RB and high levels of Mel-14 and CD38. Removal of the CD25$^+$CD4$^+$ T cells in the nonautoimmune-prone BALB/c mice results in the spontaneous development of various T cell-mediated autoimmune diseases (e.g. thyroiditis, gastritis, and insulin-dependent diabetes mellitus), and reconstitution of this subset prevents development of autoimmunity (for review, see 82). As discussed previously, CD28KO and B7-1/B7-2KO NOD mice develop severe diabetes. In both the CD28- and B7-deficient mice, the population of CD25$^+$CD4$^+$ T cells, which regulate diabetes in NOD mice, was severely depleted. The absence of these cells was responsible for the increased diabetes due to CD28/B7 disruption (83). Thus, CD28/B7 interaction is essential for the homeostasis of the immunoregulatory CD25$^+$CD4$^+$ T cells.

THE ROLE OF CTLA-4/B7 INTERACTIONS IN THE REGULATION OF IMMUNITY AND TOLERANCE

Autoimmune diseases result from the failure of the immune system to develop tolerance to self-proteins. For many years, investigators considered the negative selection of autoreactive T cells in the thymus as the major mechanism of tolerance to self-tissues. However, increasing evidence collected during the last decade has demonstrated the importance of peripheral tolerance and active regulation in autoimmunity. For example, researchers have found autoreactive T cells in the circulation in normal humans and rodents not prone to develop autoimmune diseases (40, 41, 84). These cells reside in lymphoid tissues in a nonpathogenic naïve state. Expression of B7 molecules in target tissues breaks this tolerance and generates an autoimmune disease (85, 86). Over the past few years, the CTLA-4/B7 pathway has emerged as a major regulator of peripheral tolerance.

CTLA-4 (CD152) is a member of a class of cell surface molecules capable of terminating early events in the receptor-mediated signaling cascade (87). Expression of CTLA-4 is dependent on CD28/B7 engagement (88, 89). In contrast to CD28, CTLA-4 negatively regulates T cell function. For example, in vitro blockade of CTLA-4 by mAbs enhances mouse T cell proliferation, whereas CTLA-4 cross-linking inhibits IL-2 production, cell cycle progression, and anti-CD3-induced cyclins (89–91). Thus, the engagement of CD28 not only enhances immunity as described above but also positions the system for self-regulation later in the course of an immune response. Additional support for a regulatory role of CTLA-4 has been shown in vivo. CTLA-4-deficient mice develop a lymphoproliferative disorder that results from uncontrolled polyclonal CD4$^+$ T cell expansion, apparently a result of dysregulated tolerance to peripheral auto-antigens. This disease results in the death of the CTLA-4–deficient mice within three to four weeks of age (92–94). The lymphoproliferative disorder of CTLA-4–deficient mice is due, at least in part, to the role of CTLA-4 in downregulating T cell activation. However, bone marrow chimeric mice with mixed populations of CTLA-4–deficient and CTLA-4–expressing T cells do not develop this disease (95). This finding suggests that CTLA-4 expressed by a T cell subpopulation exerts a dominant control on the proliferation of other T cells, which limits autoreactivity. Finally, CTLA-4 engagement is critical for tolerance induced following the intravenous injection of a soluble antigen (96) or membrane bound tolerogens (TN Eager, SD Miller, and JA Bluestone, unpublished results). The administration of anti-CTLA-4 mAb to mice concurrently or even after antigen-specific tolerance induction reverses clonal inactivation of the antigen-reactive T cells.

CTLA-4 regulates peripheral tolerance by a number of different mechanisms. First, CTLA-4 regulates the activation of pathogenic T cells by directly modulating T cell receptor signaling (i.e. TCRζ chain phosphorylation) (87) as well as downstream biochemical signals (i.e. ERK activation) (97). The mechanistic basis for these effects remains controversial as some investigators failed to find a role for the intracytoplasmic tail of CTLA-4, which prompted investigators to question what the precise role of its PI-3 kinase and SHP-2 phosphatase binding activity is. Thus, some researchers have suggested that one consequence of CTLA-4 expression is simply to competitively block CD28/B7 interactions (98, 99). In this regard, it is important to note that CTLA-4 function only in *cis* in association with TCR engagement, and unlike CD28 will not function in *trans* when B7 is expressed on a antigen-deficient APC (100). This restricted activity differs from CD28 function. Second, recent studies have shown that the $CD4^+CD25^+$ immunoregulatory T cells constitutively express CTLA-4 (83). In fact, signaling via CTLA-4 is essential for the function of these cells (101, 102). Thus, CTLA-4 may regulate signal transduction in the cells, which leads to differentiation into regulatory T cells; or alternatively, CTLA-4 engagement on the effector cells may alter signal transduction and subsequent cytokine production. Cross-linking of CTLA-4 induces secretion of the immunoregulatory TGF-β cytokine (103), which provides one possible mechanism of action for the $CD4^+CTLA-4^+CD25^+$ regulatory T cells. Third, CTLA-4 signaling affects T helper cell differentiation. Blocking CTLA-4/B7 interactions during an immune response promotes Th2 differentiation (104). Furthermore, T cells from CTLA-4 KO mice are skewed toward a Th2 phenotype (105, 106).

Although the findings appear to suggest multiple functional effects of CTLA-4 in altering immune function, we propose that these apparently different activities are all related. Our model stems from an assumption that the major effect of CTLA-4 is to alter the threshold of T cell activation by altering early events in TCR signaling. Previous studies have shown that slight differences in the proximal biochemical signals in T cells can lead to alterations in Th1/Th2 balance, cell survival, and expansion and functional activities. In fact, studies by Suthanthiran and colleagues (107) demonstrated that treatment of T cells with cyclosporine A, a calcineurin inhibitor that modulates calcium mobilization, leads to the generation of a TGFβ-producing T cells that are similar to the $CD4^+CTLA-4^+CD25^+$ regulatory T cells. Thus, the effects of CTLA-4 engagement whether directed at the inhibition of CD28 signaling, modulation of proximal TCR signals, or downstream effector pathways of T cell activation result in altered T cell differentiation and downregulation of immune responses. These findings not only support the potential therapeutic effects of treatments that block the CD28:CTLA-4/B7 pathway but also emphasize the potential of these treatments to inadvertently exacerbate the disease process by blocking the incorrect (i.e. CTLA-4 versus CD28) pathway. In an effort to develop more selective therapeutics, we have developed specific cell-surface-bound single chain monoclonal antibodies to selectively target the individual pathways (100).

CTLA-4 is involved in the maintenance of tolerance in autoimmune diseases. Several investigators have shown that treatment of mice with an anti-CTLA-4 mAb leads to exacerbation of autoimmune disease. In vivo blockade of CTLA-4/B7 interactions by monoclonal anti-CTLA-4 mAbs exacerbates EAE induced by PLP139-151 (108–110). In our studies, both intact Ig and F(ab) fragments of anti-CTLA-4 mAb were used with similar effects, which suggests that these reagents were blocking CTLA-4–mediated events (108). Similar results were observed following adoptive transfer of primed EAE-specific T cells, wherein in vivo blockade of CTLA-4 in recipient mice resulted in exacerbation of disease (108). These findings support an essential role in the initial triggering of the pathogenic PLP139-151-specific responses. Treatment of mice during the first remission after the acute phase of R-EAE resulted in greater incidence and severity of relapses. In fact, CTLA-4 blockade resulted in the enhancement of responses to the inducing epitope (PLP139-151) as well as the acceleration of the spreading responses to other epitopes, such as PLP178-191 and MBP84-104 (111). Thus, blockade of CTLA-4/B7 engagement prevents disease remission and exacerbates relapses with the acceleration of epitope spreading. Similar effects have been observed in NOD mice that express TCR transgenes specific for an islet Ag. However, in this model, CTLA-4 blockade exacerbated the development of diabetes only when administrated early before the onset of insulitis (112) and only in BDC2.5 NOD mice, which are populated by both transgenic and endogenous T cells; this finding suggests that the CTLA-4 blockade may be affecting the regulatory T cell subset. In this scenario, the $CD4^+CTLA-4^+CD25^+$ regulatory T cells function via CTLA-4 either to alter the APCs or to lead to the production of regulatory cytokines such as TGF-β or IL-10.

Finally, the CTLA-4/B7 pathway has been implicated in the genetic predisposition of certain humans to autoimmune diseases. Investigators have identified polymorphisms of the CTLA-4 gene that are associated with a susceptibility to autoimmune diseases such as diabetes and thyroiditis (113, 114) as well as a predisposition toward spontaneous abortion (115). In addition, soluble CTLA-4 and natural Abs to CTLA-4, which could antagonize CD28/B7 or CTLA-4/B7 interactions, have been observed in several autoimmune diseases in humans (116, 117). Together these findings demonstrate a vital role for CTLA-4 in modulating autoimmune T cell responses.

THE DIFFERENTIAL ROLES OF B7-1 AND B7-2 IN AUTOIMMUNITY

Both B7-1 and B7-2 Interactions with CD28 Influence Autoimmune Disease

Blocking B7 costimulation depends on interrupting both B7-1 and B7-2 interactions with CD28. CTLA-4Ig is effective in binding and disrupting both pathways. However, multiple studies have suggested that the individual CD28/CTLA-4 ligands may have different functions in the course of disease. Thus, efforts that utilize B7-deficient mice and specific monoclonal antibodies have been made to dissect these pathways. Initial studies that used anti-B7-1 and anti-B7-2 mAbs identified distinct therapeutic effects in models of autoimmune diseases and transplantation. For example, treatment of R-EAE with anti-B7-1 mAb reduced disease severity, whereas anti-B7-2 mAb exacerbated the disease (50, 60). In contrast, treatment of NOD mice with anti-B7-1 mAb worsened the spontaneous diabetes, whereas anti-B7-2 mAb had protective effects (118). Investigators have suggested that B7-2 and B7-1 selectively interact with CD28 versus CTLA-4 during the autoimmune response. This selective interaction leads to opposite outcomes (i.e. peripheral tolerance versus in T cell activation). However, other differences including inherent structural differences, unique signaling functions of the B7 molecules when expressed on APCs, and differences in the temporal kinetics or tissue-specific expression of the CD28 ligands are likely to also be involved as summarized below.

The kinetics of expression of B7-1 and B7-2 are different. B7-2 is constitutively expressed on dendritic cells and rapidly upregulated on activated T and B cells. In most primary immunization models, B7-2 provides the dominant costimulatory signal (20, 119). In contrast, B7-1 is not expressed on resting lymphocytes and only weakly expressed on DC. B7-1 is also upregulated following immune activation, but its expression peaks significantly later on these cells (120). Moreover, though B7-2 expression is largely restricted to hematopoietic cells, B7-1 is upregulated on a variety of other nonhematopoietic cell types including parenchymal cells of the pancreas, nervous tissue, heart, and liver. Different cytokines are responsible for upregulating the different B7 molecules, depending on their cell type and tissue location (120). In fact, we demonstrated recently that exposure of cells to agents damaging to DNA results in rapid upregulation of B7-1 but not B7-2 on tumor cells (121). The molecular basis for this difference appears to be the activation of NFκB, which leads to selective activation of the B7-1 locus. These observations have led to the notion that the dominance of the individual molecules is very much dependent on the location of the pathogenic immune response. In situations where B7-2 is preferentially expressed over B7-1, such as the early immune responses to soluble nominal Ag within the draining lymphoid tissue, B7-2 is the major ligand of CD28; thus it provides the dominant costimulatory signals in early T cell activation (75, 122). In contract, B7-1 plays a more significant role in sustaining T cell costimulation at distal inflammatory sites. This is especially true in autoimmune inflammation where type 1 interferons, nitrous oxide, or NFκB-inducing cytokines induce upregulation of B7-1. In humans, the expression of B7-1 is especially critical because endothelial cells present in allograft tissue or target organs will likely express both B7-1 and MHC class II in response to inflammatory responses. This finding may explain why B7-1 blockade is more effective in large animal preclinical settings than in many rodent models.

Investigators have made efforts to model the individual roles of B7-1 and B7-2 in both experimentally induced and spontaneous autoimmune diseases in mice. In most instances, B7-2 is the dominant costimulatory ligand. Collagen-induced arthritis, experimental myasthenia gravis, EAE, and autoimmune uveitis were all inhibited by anti-B7-2 mAbs. B7-2 KO NOD mice do not develop spontaneous diabetes. Similarly, anti-B7-2 mAb treatment inhibited the development of the diabetes in NOD as well as disease progression in another model of autoimmune diabetes (83, 123). The dominance of B7-2 in these models is similar to its role as the dominant costimulatory signal in T cell responses to exogenous antigens such as viruses and vaccinations as well as in T cell responses to foreign antigens. These results could be explained by a selective expression of B7-2 in the target tissues. Stephens & Kay demonstrated that B7-2 is predominantly expressed over B7-1 in islets during the late pathogenic phase of the disease (124). Similar findings have been documented in murine models of lupus and other autoimmune diseases of exocrine tissues where anti-B7-2 treatment, but not anti-B7-1 treatment, prevented disease progression (45, 74, 125). However, anti-B7-2 therapy is not effective during the late phase of the NOD disease progression. Treatment of NOD mice after 10 weeks of age had no effect on disease progression. These results suggest that either the major role of B7-2 is in the primary lymphoid tissues as described above or the autoimmune response evolves into a CD28-independent T cell response. This latter possibility is supported by studies performed in the CD28KO mice, which develop devastating autoimmune diabetes. The CD28 costimulation independent response is a consequence of the repeated activation of the autoimmune T cells due to the chronic nature of the disease. These results parallel those of certain virus infections in the CD28KO animals, wherein the immune responses to most pathogenic viruses are CD28-independent and can be mimicked by continuous antigen exposure (35).

Although B7-2 is a predominant costimulatory molecule, several studies have shown that the combination of B7-1 and B7-2 blockade is most effective in blocking animal models of autoimmunity and transplant rejection. This is most evident in the mouse lupus model as either CTLA-4Ig or a combination of anti-B7-1 and anti-B7-2 mAbs are most effective in blocking the development of the disease (73, 126). Researchers have observed similar results in asthma, allergy, and other autoimmune models. In fact, the most significant effect of B7-1 blockade occurs in EAE. Blocking B7-1, but not B7-2, with mAb during the initiation phase of EAE in mice decreased severity of the disease (50, 60). Moreover, relapses of disease in SJL mice can be prevented by treatment with F(ab) fragments of anti-B7-1 mAbs during disease remission. Several reports have noted that B7-1 is preferentially expressed during activation of the inflammatory process in EAE and MS. Indeed, B7-1 was upregulated, relative to B7-2, on CNS-infiltrating cells during the course of relapsing EAE (127). Similarly, the number of B7-1–expressing cells was increased during active paralytic phases in plaques in the brain and in the cerebrospinal fluid in MS (128–131). Thus, there is a strong correlation between B7-1 and active phase of the disease. Therefore, under these conditions, B7-1 becomes the dominant costimulatory molecule for activation of naïve T cells that are reactive with the additional pathogenic epitopes uncovered during the primary disease (127). In summary, both B7-1 and B7-2 can play an active role in promoting CD28-mediated T cell costimulation. B7-2 acts early and does so predominately within the primary lymphoid tissue, whereas B7-1 acts later during an immune/autoimmune response at the site of inflammation.

Selective Expression of B7-1 and B7-2 Molecules Can Influence the Tissue-Specificity of Autoimmunity

The previous discussion emphasized the relative importance of B7-1 and B7-2 in the development and progression of individual autoimmune diseases. However, recent data from our laboratory suggest that these molecules can actually influence the target tissues for autoimmune destruction in mice with a predisposition for autoimmunity. As stated above, breeding the B7-2-deficiency into the NOD background prevents the development of autoimmune diabetes in these animals. In fact, the B7-2KO NOD mice were free of insulitis even at 30 weeks of age. We also observed decreased inflammation in the salivary glands, another affected tissue in NOD mice (83). However, the B7-2KO NOD mice still maintained an autoimmune repertoire as islet antigen-specific autoreactive T cells were detected in the spleen. Thus, the elimination of B7-2 seemed to have prevented the migration and localization of pathogenic T cells in target organs. Surprisingly, B7-2KO NOD mice developed a peripheral neuropathy that started after 20 weeks of age with severe inflammation of the peripheral nerves that was composed of T cells and dendritic cells (BS Salomon, JA Bluestone, unpublished results). Pathogenic $CD4^+$ T cells mediated this spontaneous autoimmune disease. Because CD28/B7 costimulation regulates migration of inflammatory cells in target tissues, tissue-specific expression of B7-1 and B7-2 may influence the type of autoimmunity in an autoimmune disease–prone individual. The decision between severe autoimmune diabetes and emergence of a cryptic autoimmune neuropathy would depend on the relative expression of the B7-1 and B7-2 molecules, with B7-1 preferentially expressed in neural tissues versus preferential expression of B7-2 in the endocrine system as discussed above.

B7-1 Interacts Selectively with CTLA-4 to Downregulate Autoimmune Disease

Unlike B7-2 blockade, the consequence of B7-1 blockade is not always predictable. In some cases, the expression of B7-1 downregulates responses mediated by CTLA-4–expressing activated T cells. Certain inflammatory conditions create a potential for an efficient interaction between CTLA-4 and locally expressed B7-1 that may lead to the termination of T cell activation at the inflammatory site (132). In fact, under some circumstances, blockade of B7-1 leads to exacerbation of disease progression. For instance, treatment of NOD mice with anti-B7-1 mAb resulted in the exacerbation of diabetes. Similar results were observed in B7-1KO NOD mice. Anti-B7-1 mAb therapy can exacerbate R-EAE in a temporal pattern that is identical to the one observed following anti-CTLA-4 mAb treatment. The reason for the selective interaction between CTLA-4 and B7-1 may go beyond the similar temporal and tissue-specific expression of the two molecules. Recent structural studies by Davis and colleagues, who solved the crystal structure of human B7-1, determined that there exists within the B7-1 but not the B7-2 molecule a highly hydrophobic face without glycosylation sites that could promote homod-imer formation. The potential for homodimerization, coupled with the localization of the B7-1 binding site to the outside face of CTLA-4, would promote a multi-meric lattice on the surface of the T cell/APC interaction that would considerably increase the avidity of this interaction as compared to interactions of either B7-1/CD28 or B7-2/CTLA-4 (133).

In summary, blocking B7-1 and B7-2 costimulation is usually most effective in preventing or treating autoimmune diseases. However, under some circumstances, B7-1 provides a critical interaction with CTLA-4 to block pathogenic T cell re-sponses and thereby protects the individual from autoimmune diseases. Thus, the application of these therapeutics may have different outcomes depending on the disease setting and stage of the disease.

T CELL COSTIMULATION BLOCKADE PROLONGS GRAFT SURVIVAL AND INDUCES TOLERANCE

Although the results of costimulation blockade in the treatment of autoimmune diseases have been complicated, the potential for these therapies within transplant models has been more straightforward. It has long been assumed that the ultimate goal in transplantation is to induce immune tolerance of the graft. This would allow for long-term graft survival without the need to treat with hazardous non-specific immunosuppressive drugs. Experiments performed during the last decade indicated that blocking T cell costimulation could help to achieve such a goal. Based on our accumulated findings, both CD28/B7 costimulation and the costim-ulatory pathway that involves interaction between the CD40 ligand expressed by activated T cells and the CD40 ligand expressed by APC are critical for allograft rejection. First, long-term graft survival can be efficiently induced by blocking CD28/B7 or CD40/CD40L pathways with similar features. Second, the combina-tion of the two treatments has synergistic effects and is a promising strategy in transplantation.

Initial experiments showed that short term treatment with CTLA-4Ig at the time of graft implantation induced long-term acceptance of human islets in mice (6) and cardiac allografts in rats (134). Blocking B7 costimulation increased ro-dent allograft survival of kidney, liver, and lung transplants (16). In some cases, the therapy inhibited the rejection of a second donor, but not of a third party transplant, without the use of any additional immunosuppressive drugs. In addition, the ther-apy also eliminated chronic rejection (135–137). The relative importance of host versus donor B7 expression in allograft rejection has been examined in a murine heart model. In this setting, vascularized heart allografts survived long-term in B7-1/B7-2-deficient recipients. However, hearts from wild-type and B7-1/B7-2-deficient animals were rejected with the same kinetics after allograft transplanta-tion. These findings suggest that B7-expressing host APCs play a critical role in the rejection of heart allografts in mice (138, 139). A recent study in a mouse xenograft model (140) demonstrated that immunization of mice with peptides derived from pig B7 molecules led to the induction of an anti-pig B7 antibody response that blocked graft rejection, which suggests an important role for the direct pathway of donor graft recognition in this transplant setting.

The use of CD28 antagonists has been adopted with modest effects in non-human primates. Cynomologus monkeys treated with either CTLA-4Ig (7, 9) or a combination of anti-B7 mAbs (141) retained their allogeneic islet or kidney transplants significantly longer than untreated animals. However, all animals rejected their grafts within 100 days or so. CTLA4-Ig therapy abrogated the humoral response in all of the recipients. Similar inhibition of the alloantibody response has been obtained in the renal allograft model (T Pearson, L Larsen, unpublished observations). More recently, Alan Kirk has presented data demonstrating that an anti-human B7-1 monoclonal antibody can significantly prolong renal allograft survival alone or with anti-human B7-2 (unpublished observations). Thus, these results raised the possibility that CD28/B7 blockade could be an important but insufficient weapon in the treatment of transplant rejection and the induction of graft tolerance. In this regard, the blockade of B7 costimulation increased allogeneic skin graft survival but did not induce tolerance; thus it provided an excellent model in the attempt to complement CD28 blockade in tolerance-inducing protocols. Blocking CD40/CD40L interaction by using anti-CD40L mAbs in experimental rodent and primate transplant models represents a powerful adjunct strategy to prevent graft rejection. In rodents, this treatment prevented acute cardiac allograft rejection (142, 143); and even more relevant to human medicine, it markedly prolonged allograft survival of kidney and islets in nonhuman primates long after discontinuation of therapy (9, 144, 145). A loss of donor-specific alloreactivity, with maintenance of anti-third party responsiveness, has been demonstrated in both models. The combination of CD40/CD40L and CD28/B7 blockade therapies has synergistic effects in preventing both acute and chronic rejection (9–12, 143, 146); although some conflicting data resulted in models that used highly immunogenic skin allografts (10, 143). Finally, in cardiac, islet, and skin allograft transplantation, the therapeutic benefits of blocking B7 or CD40 costimulation was significantly enhanced if the treatment was simultaneously associated with injection of donor cells (16, 147–156). This latter treatment, termed donor-specific transfusion (DST), likely increased stimulation of host alloreactive T cells (157) and, in a context of a tolerogenic setting, enhanced tolerance induction.

CD40/CD40L or CD28/B7 blockade during transplantation induced a decrease of proliferation of alloreactive T cells and an increase of their death by apoptosis (143, 151, 158). Blocking this death suppressed tolerance to the allografts (158, 159). CTLA-4 engagement and the production of both IFN-γ and IL-2 were required during tolerance induction because of their anti-proliferative and pro-apoptotic properties for activated T cells (151, 158, 160, 161).There is strong evidence that calcineurin inhibitors may antagonize the therapeutic effects of costimulation blockade, which suggests that intact T cell receptor signaling may be required for tolerance induction to allografts. Thus, blocking CD28/B7 and CD40/CD40L pathways individually or in combination is now a reproducible strategy to induce long-term survival and tolerance of cardiac, islet, or kidney allografts in rodents.

CLINICAL EXPERIENCE

CD28/B7 blockade has been used in clinical trials. First, the in vitro principle that TCR stimulation during CD28/B7 blockade results in T cell anergy has been applied in a pilot clinical trial involving bone marrow allograft transplantation in an attempt at reducing graft-vs-host disease (GVHD) (162). GVHD is a complication that arises when donor T cells recognize recipient cells as allogeneic and foreign. Recipient peripheral blood leukocytes were collected from 12 patients before myeloablation. In order to induce anergy of donor T cells specific for recipient allo-MHC, donor bone marrow cells were cultured in vitro with irradiated host leukocytes in the presence of CTLA-4Ig. Restimulation in vitro showed reduced responses of donor T cells against recipient, but not third party cells, which suggests that donor-specific anergy had occurred. The incidence of GVHD following transfusion of these cells into patients was relatively low, which suggests the potential efficacy of this type of treatment. However, further studies are warranted that prospectively compare the incidence of GVHD when donor cells are injected without preincubation with CTLA-4Ig.

Human CTLA-4Ig has been used in vivo as well. Forty-three patients with stable psoriasis vulgaris received four infusions of the soluble chimeric protein CTLA-4Ig (163). Forty-six percent of the patients achieved a 50% or greater sustained improvement in clinical disease activity, with greater effects observed in the highest-dosing cohorts. Improvement in these patients was associated with quantitative reduction in epidermal hyperplasia and correlated with quantitative reduction in skin-infiltrating T cells. No marked increase in the rate of intra-lesional T cell apoptosis was identified, which suggests that the decreased number of T cells in the lesions was probably attributable to an inhibition of T cell proliferation, T cell recruitment, and/or apoptosis of antigen-specific T cells at extra-lesional sites. It is important to note that, although altered antibody responses to T cell–dependent neoantigens were observed, immunologic tolerance to these antigens was not demonstrated. This study illustrates the importance of the CD28 pathway in the pathogenesis of psoriasis and suggests a potential therapeutic use for this novel immunomodulatory approach in an array of T cell–mediated diseases. However, the data also emphasizes that tolerance induction, as defined by experiments in vitro and in small animals in vivo, may not reflect functional mechanisms in humans in vivo.

Finally, industry-sponsored Phase I/II clinical renal transplant and autoimmunity trials using long-term anti-CD154 maintenance therapy protocols are now underway. The results of these trials will be extremely helpful in the design of studies that use anti-CD154 in combination with other agents (e.g. anti-B7s, CTLA-4Ig, rapamycin) for tolerance induction.

PERSPECTIVES

Throughout the 1990s, most immune therapies in transplantation and autoimmunity have employed a standard nonspecific immunosuppressive regimen after transplantation. Although new immunosuppressive agents are continuously under development, the ultimate goal of the treatment of transplant rejection and the cure of autoimmune diseases is immunologic tolerance. Drugs and protocols aimed at "tricking" the immune system to recognize nonself as self or to retrain autoimmune cells will provide true cures for these diseases. Over the past eight years, multiple studies in rodents and nonhuman primates demonstrated the extraordinary therapeutic potential of blocking T cell costimulation in various models, autoimmune diseases, and transplantation. Although the initial experiences with agents blocking these pathways in nonhuman primates have been somewhat disappointing, new second-generation reagents and optimized protocols are being developed. These agents are targeted to specific antigen-reactive T cells and offer more selective effects on the immune response. However, we must remember that in our small animal studies similar therapies can exacerbate autoimmune diseases by depleting important immunoregulatory T cells or inhibiting the negative immunoregulation by CTLA-4. Thus, to be successful, the approaches will have to take into account the multiple effects of costimulation blockade as well as the timing and duration of the therapies.

Visit the Annual Reviews home page at www.AnnualReviews.org

LITERATURE CITED

1. Jenkins MK, Schwartz RH. 1987. Antigen presentation by chemically modified splenocytes induces antigen-specific T cell unresponsiveness in vitro and in vivo. *J. Exp. Med.* 165:302–19
2. DeSilva DR, Urdahl KB, Jenkins MK. 1991. Clonal anergy is induced in vitro by T cell receptor occupancy in the absence of proliferation. *J. Immunol.* 147:3261–67
3. Harding FA, McArthur JG, Gross JA, Raulet DH, Allison JP. 1992. CD28-mediated signaling co-stimulates murine T cells and prevents induction of anergy in T cell clones. *Nature* 356:607–9
4. Jenkins MK, Taylor PS, Norton SD, Urdahl KB. 1991. CD28 delivers a costimulatory signal involved in antigen-specific IL-2 production by human T cells. *J. Immunol.* 147:2461–66
5. Linsley PS, Wallace PM, Johnson J, Gibson MG, Greene JL, Ledbetter JA, Singh C, Tepper MA. 1992. Immunosuppression in vivo by a soluble form of the CTLA-4 T cell activation molecule. *Science* 257:792–95
6. Lenschow DJ, Zeng Y, Thistlethwaite JR, Montag A, Brady W, Gibson MG, Linsley PS, Bluestone JA. 1992. Long-term survival of xenogeneic pancreatic islet grafts induced by CTLA4Ig. *Science* 257:789–92
7. Levisetti MG, Padrid PA, Szot GL, Mittal N, Meehan SM, Wardrip CL, Gray GS, Bruce DS, Thistlethwaite JR, Jr., Bluestone JA. 1997. Immunosuppressive effects of human CTLA4-Ig in a non-human primate model of allogeneic pancreatic islet transplantation. *J. Immunol.* 159:5187–91
8. Pearson TC, Alexander DZ, Winn KJ, Linsley PS, Lowry RP, Larsen CP. 1994.

Transplantation tolerance induced by CTLA4-Ig. *Transplantation* 57:1701–6

9. Kirk AD, Harlan DM, Armstrong NN, Davis TA, Dong Y, Gray GS, Hong X, Thomas D, Fechner JH Jr, Knechtle SJ. 1997. CTLA4-Ig and anti-CD40 ligand prevent renal allograft rejection in primates. *Proc. Natl. Acad. Sci. USA* 94:8789–94

10. Larsen CP, Elwood ET, Alexander DZ, Ritchie SC, Hendrix R, Tucker-Burden C, Cho HR, Aruffo A, Hollenbaugh D, Linsley PS, Winn KJ, Pearson TC. 1996. Long-term acceptance of skin and cardiac allografts after blocking CD40 and CD28 pathways. *Nature* 381:434–38

11. Sun H, Subbotin V, Chen C, Aitouche A, Valdivia LA, Sayegh MH, Linsley PS, Fung JJ, Starzl TE, Rao AS. 1997. Prevention of chronic rejection in mouse aortic allografts by combined treatment with CTLA4-Ig and anti-CD40 ligand monoclonal antibody. *Transplantation* 64:1838–43

12. Elwood ET, Larsen CP, Cho HR, Corbascio M, Ritchie SC, Alexander DZ, Tucker-Burden C, Linsley PS, Aruffo A, Hollenbaugh D, Winn KJ, Pearson TC. 1998. Prolonged acceptance of concordant and discordant xenografts with combined CD40 and CD28 pathway blockade. *Transplantation* 65:1422–28

13. Karandikar NJ, Vanderlugt CL, Bluestone JA, Miller SD. 1998. Targeting the B7/CD28:CTLA-4 costimulatory system in CNS autoimmune disease. *J. Neuroimmunol.* 89:10–18

14. Racke MK, Ratts RB, Arredondo L, Perrin PJ, Lovet T Racke A. 2000. The role of costimulation in autoimmune demyelination. *J. Neuroimmunol.* 107:205–15

15. Anderson DE, Sharpe AH, Hafler DA. 1999. The B7-CD28/CTLA-4 costimulatory pathways in autoimmune disease of the central nervous system. *Curr. Opin. Immunol.* 11:677–83

16. Sayegh MH, Turka LA. 1998. The role of T cell costimulatory activation pathways in transplant rejection. *N. Engl. J. Med.* 338:1813–21

17. Lucas PJ, Negishi I, Nakayama K, Fields LE, Loh DY. 1995. Naive CD28-deficient T cells can initiate but not sustain an in vitro antigen-specific immune response. *J. Immunol.* 154:5757–68

18. Sperling AI, Auger JA, Ehst BD, Rulifson IC, Thompson CB, Bluestone JA. 1996. CD28/B7 interactions deliver a unique signal to naive T cells that regulates cell survival but not early proliferation. *J. Immunol.* 157:3909–17

19. Bachmann MF, McKall-Faienza K, Schmits R, Bouchard D, Beach J, Speiser DE, Mak TW, Ohashi PS. 1997. Distinct roles for LFA-1 and CD28 during activation of naive T cells: adhesion versus costimulation. *Immunity* 7:549–57

20. Schweitzer AN, Sharpe AH. 1998. Studies using antigen-presenting cells lacking expression of both B7-1 (CD80) and B7-2 (CD86) show distinct requirements for B7 molecules during priming versus restimulation of Th2 but not Th1 cytokine production. *J. Immunol.* 161:2762–71

21. Wells AD, Gudmundsdottir H, Turka LA. 1997. Following the fate of individual T cells throughout activation and clonal expansion. Signals from T cell receptor and CD28 differentially regulate the induction and duration of a proliferative response. *J. Clin. Invest.* 100:3173–83

22. Gudmundsdottir H, Wells AD, Turka LA. 1999. Dynamics and requirements of T cell clonal expansion in vivo at the single-cell level: Effector function is linked to proliferative capacity. *J. Immunol.* 162:5212–23

23. Lindsten T, June CH, Ledbetter JA, Stella G, Thompson CB. 1989. Regulation of lymphokine messenger RNA stability by a surface-mediated T cell activation pathway. *Science* 244:339–43

24. Fraser JD, Irving BA, Crabtree GR, Weiss A. 1991. Regulation of interleukin-2 gene

enhancer activity by the T cell accessory molecule CD28. *Science* 251:313–16

25. Norton SD, Zuckerman L, Urdahl KB, Shefner R, Miller J, Jenkins MK. 1992. The CD28 ligand, B7, enhances IL-2 production by providing a costimulatory signal to T cells. *J. Immunol.* 149:1556–61

26. Boise LH, Minn AJ, Noel PJ, June CH, Accavitti MA, Lindsten T, Thompson CB. 1995. CD28 costimulation can promote T cell survival by enhancing the expression of Bcl-XL. *Immunity* 3:87–98

27. Kearney ER, Walunas TL, Karr RW, Morton PA, Loh DY, Bluestone JA, Jenkins MK. 1995. Antigen-dependent clonal expansion of a trace population of antigen-specific CD4$^+$ T cells in vivo is dependent on CD28 costimulation and inhibited by CTLA-4. *J. Immunol.* 155:1032–36

28. Vella AT, Mitchell T, Groth B, Linsley PS, Green JM, Thompson CB, Kappler JW, Marrack P. 1997. CD28 engagement and proinflammatory cytokines contribute to T cell expansion and long-term survival in vivo. *J. Immunol.* 158:4714–20

29. Judge TA, Wu Z, Zheng XG, Sharpe AH, Sayegh MH, Turka LA. 1999. The role of CD80, CD86, and CTLA4 in alloimmune responses and the induction of long-term allograft survival. *J. Immunol.* 162:1947–51

30. Howland KC, Ausubel LJ, London CA, Abbas AK. 2000. The roles of CD28 and CD40 ligand in T cell activation and tolerance. *J. Immunol.* 164:4465–70

31. Viola A, Lanzavecchia A. 1996. T cell activation determined by T cell receptor number and tunable thresholds. *Science* 273:104–6

32. Viola A, Schroeder S, Sakakibara Y, Lanzavecchia A. 1999. T lymphocyte costimulation mediated by reorganization of membrane microdomains. *Science* 283:680–82

33. Wulfing C, Davis MM. 1998. A receptor/cytoskeletal movement triggered by costimulation during T cell activation. *Science* 282:2266–69

34. Green JM, Noel PJ, Sperling AI, Walunas TL, Gray GS, Bluestone JA, Thompson CB. 1994. Absence of B7-dependent responses in CD28-deficient mice. *Immunity* 1:501–8

35. Kundig TM, Shahinian A, Kawai K, Mittrucker HW, Sebzda E, Bachmann MF, Mak TW, Ohashi PS. 1996. Duration of TCR stimulation determines costimulatory requirement of T cells. *Immunity* 5:41–52

36. Teh HS, Teh SJ. 1997. High concentrations of antigenic ligand activate and do not tolerize naive CD4 T cells in the absence of CD28/B7 costimulation. *Cell. Immunol.* 179:74–83

37. Oliveira-dos-Santos AJ, Ho A, Tada Y, Lafaille JJ, Tonegawa S, Mak TW, Penninger JM. 1999. CD28 costimulation is crucial for the development of spontaneous autoimmune encephalomyelitis. *J. Immunol.* 162:4490–95

38. Croft M, Bradley LM, Swain SL. 1994. Naive versus memory CD4 T cell response to antigen. Memory cells are less dependent on accessory cell costimulation and can respond to many antigen-presenting cell types including resting B cells. *J. Immunol.* 152:2675–85

39. London CA, Lodge MP, Abbas AK. 2000. Functional responses and costimulator dependence of memory CD4$^+$ T cells. *J. Immunol.* 164:265–72

40. Lovet T Racke AE, Trotter JL, Lauber J, Perrin PJ, June CH, Racke MK. 1998. Decreased dependence of myelin basic protein-reactive T cells on CD28-mediated costimulation in multiple sclerosis patients. A marker of activated/memory T cells. *J. Clin. Invest.* 101:725–30

41. Scholz C, Patton KT, Anderson DE, Freeman GJ, Hafler DA. 1998. Expansion of autoreactive T cells in multiple sclerosis is independent of exogenous B7 costimulation. *J. Immunol.* 160:1532–38

42. Bachmann MF, Gallimore A, Linkert S, Cerundolo V, Lanzavecchia A, Kopf M, Viola A. 1999. Developmental regulation of

Lck targeting to the CD8 coreceptor controls signaling in naive and memory T cells. *J. Exp. Med.* 189:1521–30

43. Bachmaier K, Pummerer C, Shahinian A, Ionescu J, Neu N, Mak TW, Penninger JM. 1996. Induction of autoimmunity in the absence of CD28 costimulation. *J. Immunol.* 157:1752–57

44. Tada Y, Nagasawa K, Ho A, Morito F, Ushiyama O, Suzuki N, Ohta H, Mak TW. 1999. CD28-deficient mice are highly resistant to collagen-induced arthritis. *J. Immunol.* 162:203–8

45. Peterson KE, Sharp GC, Tang H, Braley-Mullen H. 1999. B7.2 has opposing roles during the activation versus effector stages of experimental autoimmune thyroiditis. *J. Immunol.* 162:1859–67

46. Shi FD, He B, Li H, Matusevicius D, Link H, Ljunggren HG. 1998. Differential requirements for CD28 and CD40 ligand in the induction of experimental autoimmune myasthenia gravis. *Eur. J. Immunol.* 28:3587–93

47. Gonatas NK, Greene MI, Waksman BH. 1986. Genetic and molecular aspects of demyelination. *Immunol. Today* 7:121–26

48. Wekerle H. 1991. Immunopathogenesis of multiple sclerosis. *Acta Neurol.* 13:197–204

49. Cross AH, Girard TJ, Giacoletto KS, Evans RJ, Keeling RM, Lin RF, Trotter JL, Karr RW. 1995. Long-term inhibition of murine experimental autoimmune encephalomyelitis using CTLA-4–Fc supports a key role for CD28 costimulation. *J. Clin. Invest.* 95:2783–89

50. Kuchroo VK, Das MP, Brown JA, Ranger AM, Zamvil SS, Sobel RA, Weiner HL, Nabavi N, Glimcher LH. 1995. B7-1 and B7-2 costimulatory molecules activate differentially the Th1/Th2 developmental pathways: application to autoimmune disease therapy. *Cell* 80:707–18

51. Girvin AM, Dal Canto MC, Rhee L, Salomon B, Sharpe A, Bluestone JA, Miller SD. 2000. A critical role for B7/CD28 costimulation in experimental autoimmune encephalomyelitis: a comparative study using costimulatory molecule–deficient mice and monoclonal antibody blockade. *J. Immunol.* 164:136–43

52. Tuohy VK, Lu Z, Sobel RA, Laursen RA, Lees MB. 1989. Identification of an encephalitogenic determinant of myelin proteolipid protein for SJL mice. *J. Immunol.* 142:1523–27

53. McRae BL, Kennedy MK, Tan LJ, Dal Canto MC, Picha KS, Miller SD. 1992. Induction of active and adoptive relapsing experimental autoimmune encephalomyelitis (EAE) using an encephalitogenic epitope of proteolipid protein. *J. Neuroimmunol.* 38:229–40

54. Miller SD, Vanderlugt CL, Lenschow DJ, Pope JG, Karandikar NJ, Dal Canto MC, Bluestone JA. 1995. Blockade of CD28/B7-1 interaction prevents epitope spreading and clinical relapses of murine EAE. *Immunity* 3:739–45

55. Perrin PJ, June CH, Maldonado JH, Ratts RB, Racke MK. 1999. Blockade of CD28 during in vitro activation of encephalitogenic T cells or after disease onset ameliorates experimental autoimmune encephalomyelitis. *J. Immunol.* 163:1704–10

56. Croxford JL, O'Neill JK, Ali RR, Browne K, Byrnes AP, Dallman MJ, Wood MJ, Feldmann M, Baker D. 1998. Local gene therapy with CTLA4-immunoglobulin fusion protein in experimental allergic encephalomyelitis. *Eur. J. Immunol.* 28:3904–16

57. Khoury SJ, Akalin E, Chandraker A, Turka LA, Linsley PS, Sayegh MH, Hancock WW. 1995. CD28-B7 costimulatory blockade by CTLA4Ig prevents actively induced experimental autoimmune encephalomyelitis and inhibits Th1 but spares Th2 cytokines in the central nervous system. *J. Immunol.* 155:4521–24

58. Arima T, Rehman A, Hickey WF, Flye MW. 1996. Inhibition by CTLA4Ig of

experimental allergic encephalomyelitis. *J. Immunol.* 156:4916–24

59. Cross AH, San M, Keeling RM, Karr RW. 1999. CTLA-4-Fc treatment of ongoing EAE improves recovery but has no effect upon relapse rate. Implications for the mechanisms involved in disease perpetuation. *J. Neuroimmunol.* 96:144–47

60. Racke MK, Scott DE, Quigley L, Gray GS, Abe R, June CH, Perrin PJ. 1995. Distinct roles for B7-1 (CD-80) and B7-2 (CD-86) in the initiation of experimental allergic encephalomyelitis. *J. Clin. Invest.* 96:2195–203

61. Lehmann PV, Forsthuber T, Miller A, Sercarz EE. 1992. Spreading of T cell autoimmunity to cryptic determinants of an autoantigen. *Nature* 358:155–57

62. McRae BL, Vanderlugt CL, Dal Canto MC, Miller SD. 1995. Functional evidence for epitope spreading in the relapsing pathology of experimental autoimmune encephalomyelitis. *J. Exp. Med.* 182:75–85

63. Tran HM, Nickerson PW, Restifo AC, Ivis-Woodward MA, Patel A, Allen RD, Strom TB, O'Connell PJ. 1997. Distinct mechanisms for the induction and maintenance of allograft tolerance with CTLA4-Fc treatment. *J. Immunol.* 159:2232–39

64. Liblau RS, Singer SM, McDevitt HO. 1995. Th1 and Th2 CD4$^+$ T cells in the pathogenesis of organ-specific autoimmune diseases. *Immunol. Today* 16:34–38

65. Homann D, Holz A, Bot A, Coon B, Wolfe T, Petersen J, Dyrberg TP, Grusby MJ, von Herrath MG. 1999. Autoreactive CD4$^+$ T cells protect from autoimmune diabetes via bystander suppression using the IL-4/Stat6 pathway. *Immunity* 11:463–72

66. Rulifson IC, Sperling AI, Fields PE, Fitch FW, Bluestone JA. 1997. CD28 costimulation promotes the production of Th2 cytokines. *J. Immunol.* 158:658–65

67. Salomon B, Bluestone JA. 1998. LFA-1 interaction with ICAM-1 and ICAM-2 regulates Th2 cytokine production. *J. Immunol.* 161:5138–42

68. Rogers PR, Croft M. 2000. CD28, Ox-40, LFA-1, and CD4 modulation of Th1/Th2 differentiation is directly dependent on the dose of antigen. *J. Immunol.* 164:2955–63

69. Khoury SJ, Gallon L, Verburg RR, Chandraker A, Peach R, Linsley PS, Turka LA, Hancock WW, Sayegh MH. 1996. Ex vivo treatment of antigen-presenting cells with CTLA4Ig and encephalitogenic peptide prevents experimental autoimmune encephalomyelitis in the Lewis rat. *J. Immunol.* 157:3700–5

70. Falcone M, Sarvetnick N. 1999. Cytokines that regulate autoimmune responses. *Curr. Opin. Immunol.* 11:670–76

71. Lenschow DJ, Herold KC, Rhee L, Patel B, Koons A, Qin HY, Fuchs E, Singh B, Thompson CB, Bluestone JA. 1996. CD28/B7 regulation of Th1 and Th2 subsets in the development of autoimmune diabetes. *Immunity* 5:285–93

72. Arreaza GA, Cameron MJ, Jaramillo A, Gill BM, Hardy D, Laupland KB, Rapoport MJ, Zucker P, Chakrabarti S, Chensue SW, Qin HY, Singh B, Delovitch TL. 1997. Neonatal activation of CD28 signaling overcomes T cell anergy and prevents autoimmune diabetes by an IL-4–dependent mechanism. *J. Clin. Invest.* 100:2243–53

73. Finck BK, Linsley PS, Wofsy D. 1994. Treatment of murine lupus with CTLA4Ig. *Science* 265:1225–27

74. Nakajima A, Azuma M, Kodera S, Nuriya S, Terashi A, Abe M, Hirose S, Shirai T, Yagita H, Okumura K. 1995. Preferential dependence of autoantibody production in murine lupus on CD86 costimulatory molecule. *Eur. J. Immunol.* 25:3060–69

75. Borriello F, Sethna MP, Boyd SD, Schweitzer AN, Tivol EA, Jacoby D, Strom TB, Simpson EM, Freeman GJ, Sharpe AH. 1997. B7-1 and B7-2 have overlapping, critical roles in immunoglobulin class switching and germinal center formation. *Immunity* 6:303–13

76. Daikh DI, Finck BK, Linsley PS, Hollenbaugh D, Wofsy D. 1997. Long-term inhibition of murine lupus by brief simultaneous blockade of the B7/CD28 and CD40/gp39 costimulation pathways. *J. Immunol.* 159:3104–8

77. Herold KC, Lu J, Rulifson I, Vezys V, Taub D, Grusby MJ, Bluestone JA. 1997. Regulation of C-C chemokine production by murine T cells by CD28/B7 costimulation. *J. Immunol.* 159:4150–53

78. Carroll RG, Riley JL, Levine BL, Feng Y, Kaushal S, Ritchey DW, Bernstein W, Weislow OS, Brown CR, Berger EA, June CH, St. Louis DC. 1997. Differential regulation of HIV-1 fusion cofactor expression by CD28 costimulation of CD4⁺ T cells. *Science* 276:273–76

79. Chang TT, Jabs C, Sobel RA, Kuchroo VK, Sharpe AH. 1999. Studies in B7-deficient mice reveal a critical role for B7 costimulation in both induction and effector phases of experimental autoimmune encephalomyelitis. *J. Exp. Med.* 190:733–40

80. Karpus WJ, Lukacs NW, McRae BL, Strieter RM, Kunkel SL, Miller SD. 1995. An important role for the chemokine macrophage inflammatory protein-1 alpha in the pathogenesis of the T cell-mediated autoimmune disease, experimental autoimmune encephalomyelitis. *J. Immunol.* 155:5003–10

81. Perrin PJ, Lavi E, Rumbley CA, Zekavat SA, Phillips SM. 1999. Experimental autoimmune meningitis: a novel neurological disease in CD28–deficient mice. *Clin. Immunol.* 91:41–49

82. Sakaguchi S. 2000. Regulatory T cells: key controllers of immunologic self-tolerance. *Cell* 101:455–58

83. Salomon B, Lenschow DJ, Rhee L, Ashourian N, Singh B, Sharpe A, Bluestone JA. 2000. B7/CD28 costimulation is essential for the homeostasis of the CD4⁺CD25⁺ immunoregulatory T cells that control autoimmune diabetes. *Immunity* 12:431–40

84. Lohmann T, Leslie RD, Londei M. 1996. T cell clones to epitopes of glutamic acid decarboxylase 65 raised from normal subjects and patients with insulin-dependent diabetes. *J. Autoimmun.* 9:385–89

85. Guerder S, Meyerhoff J, Flavell R. 1994. The role of the T cell costimulator B7-1 in autoimmunity and the induction and maintenance of tolerance to peripheral antigen. *Immunity* 1:155–66

86. von Herrath MG, Guerder S, Lewicki H, Flavell RA, Oldstone MB. 1995. Coexpression of B7-1 and viral ("self") transgenes in pancreatic beta cells can break peripheral ignorance and lead to spontaneous autoimmune diabetes. *Immunity* 3:727–38

87. Lee KM, Chuang E, Griffin M, Khattri R, Hong DK, Zhang W, Straus D, Samelson LE, Thompson CB, Bluestone JA. 1998. Molecular basis of T cell inactivation by CTLA-4. *Science* 282:2263–66

88. Alegre ML, Noel PJ, Eisfelder BJ, Chuang E, Clark MR, Reiner SL, Thompson CB. 1996. Regulation of surface and intracellular expression of CTLA4 on mouse T cells. *J. Immunol.* 157:4762–70

89. Walunas TL, Bakker CY, Bluestone JA. 1996. CTLA-4 ligation blocks CD28-dependent T cell activation. *J. Exp. Med.* 183:2541–50

90. Walunas TL, Lenschow DJ, Bakker CY, Linsley PS, Freeman GJ, Green JM, Thompson CB, Bluestone JA. 1994. CTLA-4 can function as a negative regulator of T cell activation. *Immunity* 1:405–13

91. Krummel MF, Allison JP. 1996. CTLA-4 engagement inhibits IL-2 accumulation and cell cycle progression upon activation of resting T cells. *J. Exp. Med.* 183:2533–40

92. Tivol EA, Borriello F, Schweitzer AN, Lynch WP, Bluestone JA, Sharpe AH. 1995. Loss of CTLA-4 leads to massive lymphoproliferation and fatal multiorgan tissue destruction, revealing a critical negative regulatory role of CTLA-4. *Immunity* 3:541–47

93. Waterhouse P, Penninger JM, Timms E, Wakeham A, Shahinian A, Lee KP, Thompson CB, Griesser H, Mak TW. 1995. Lymphoproliferative disorders with early lethality in mice deficient in CTLA-4. *Science* 270:985–88

94. Chambers CA, Sullivan TJ, Allison JP. 1997. Lymphoproliferation in CTLA-4–deficient mice is mediated by costimulation-dependent activation of CD4+ T cells. *Immunity* 7:885–95

95. Bachmann MF, Kohler G, Ecabert B, Mak TW, Kopf M. 1999. Cutting edge: lymphoproliferative disease in the absence of CTLA-4 is not T cell autonomous. *J. Immunol.* 163:1128–31

96. Perez VL, Van Parijs L, Biuckians A, Zheng XX, Strom TB, Abbas AK. 1997. Induction of peripheral T cell tolerance in vivo requires CTLA-4 engagement. *Immunity* 6:411–17

97. Calvo CR, Amsen D, Kruisbeek AM. 1997. Cytotoxic T lymphocyte antigen 4 (CTLA-4) interferes with extracellular signal-regulated kinase (ERK) and Jun NH2-terminal kinase (JNK) activation, but does not affect phosphorylation of T cell receptor zeta and ZAP70. *J. Exp. Med.* 186:1645–53

98. Thompson CB, Allison JP. 1997. The emerging role of CTLA-4 as an immune attenuator. *Immunity* 7:445–50

99. Masteller EL, Chuang E, Mullen AC, Reiner SL, Thompson CB. 2000. Structural analysis of CTLA-4 function in vivo. *J. Immunol.* 164:5319–27

100. Griffin MD, Hong DK, Holman PO, Lee KM, Whitters MJ, O'Herrin SM, Fallarino F, Collins M, Segal DM, Gajewski TF, Kranz DM, Bluestone JA. 2000. Blockade of T cell activation using a surface-linked single-chain antibody to CTLA-4 (CD152). *J. Immunol.* 164:4433–42

101. Read S, Malmstrom V, Powrie F. 2000. Cytotoxic T lymphocyte-associated antigen 4 plays an essential role in the function of CD25+CD4+ regulatory cells that control intestinal inflammation. *J. Exp. Med.* 192:295–302

102. Takahashi T, Tagami T, Yamazaki S, Uede T, Shimizu J, Sakaguchi N, Mak TW, Sakaguchi S. 2000. Immunologic self-tolerance maintained by CD25+CD4+ regulatory T cells constitutively expressing cytotoxic T lymphocyte-associated antigen 4. *J. Exp. Med.* 192:303–10

103. Chen W, Jin W, Wahl SM. 1998. Engagement of cytotoxic T lymphocyte-associated antigen 4 (CTLA-4) induces transforming growth factor beta (TGF-beta) production by murine CD4+ T cells. *J. Exp. Med.* 188:1849–57

104. Walunas TL, Bluestone JA. 1998. CTLA-4 regulates tolerance induction and T cell differentiation in vivo. *J. Immunol.* 160:3855–60

105. Khattri R, Auger JA, Griffin MD, Sharpe AH, Bluestone JA. 1999. Lymphoproliferative disorder in CTLA-4 knockout mice is characterized by CD28-regulated activation of Th2 responses. *J. Immunol.* 162:5784–91

106. Oosterwegel MA, Mandelbrot DA, Boyd SD, Lorsbach RB, Jarrett DY, Abbas AK, Sharpe AH. 1999. The role of CTLA-4 in regulating Th2 differentiation. *J. Immunol.* 163:2634–39

107. Prashar Y, Khanna A, Sehajpal P, Sharma VK, Suthanthiran M. 1995. Stimulation of transforming growth factor-beta 1 transcription by cyclosporine. *FEBS Lett.* 358:109–12

108. Karandikar NJ, Vanderlugt CL, Walunas TL, Miller SD, Bluestone JA. 1996. CTLA-4: a negative regulator of autoimmune disease. *J. Exp. Med.* 184:783–88

109. Perrin PJ, Maldonado JH, Davis TA, June CH, Racke MK. 1996. CTLA-4 blockade enhances clinical disease and cytokine production during experimental allergic encephalomyelitis. *J. Immunol.* 157:1333–36

110. Hurwitz AA, Sullivan TJ, Krummel MF, Sobel RA, Allison JP. 1997.

Specific blockade of CTLA-4/B7 interactions results in exacerbated clinical and histologic disease in an actively-induced model of experimental allergic encephalomyelitis. *J. Neuroimmunol.* 73:57–62

111. Karandikar NT, Eagar TN, Vanderlugt CL, Bluestone JA, Miller SD. 2000. CTLA-4 downregulates epitope spreading and mediates remission in relapsing experimental autoimmune encephalomyelitis. *J. Neuroimmunol.* In press

112. Luhder F, Hoglund P, Allison JP, Benoist C, Mathis D. 1998. Cytotoxic T lymphocyte-associated antigen 4 (CTLA-4) regulates the unfolding of autoimmune diabetes. *J. Exp. Med.* 187:427–32

113. Awata T, Kurihara S, Iitaka M, Takei S, Inoue I, Ishii C, Negishi K, Izumida T, Yoshida Y, Hagura R, Kuzuya N, Kanazawa Y, Katayama S. 1998. Association of CTLA-4 gene A-G polymorphism (IDDM12 locus) with acute-onset and insulin-depleted IDDM as well as autoimmune thyroid disease (Graves' disease and Hashimoto's thyroiditis) in the Japanese population. *Diabetes* 47:128–29

114. Marron MP, Zeidler A, Raffel LJ, Eckenrode SE, Yang JJ, Hopkins DI, Garchon HJ, Jacob CO, Serrano-Rios M, Martinez Larrad MT, Park Y, Bach JF, Rotter JI, Yang MC, She JX. 2000. Genetic and physical mapping of a type 1 diabetes susceptibility gene (IDDM12) to a 100-kb phagemid artificial chromosome clone containing D2S72-CTLA4-D2S105 on chromosome 2q33. *Diabetes* 49:492–99

115. Kaufman KA, Bowen JA, Tsai AF, Bluestone JA, Hunt JS, Ober C. 1999. The CTLA-4 gene is expressed in placental fibroblasts. *Mol. Hum. Reprod.* 5:84–87

116. Matsui T, Kurokawa M, Kobata T, Oki S, Azuma M, Tohma S, Inoue T, Yamamoto K, Nishioka K, Kato T. 1999. Autoantibodies to T cell costimulatory molecules

in systemic autoimmune diseases. *J. Immunol.* 162:4328–35

117. Oaks MK, Hallett KM. 2000. Cutting edge: a soluble form of CTLA-4 in patients with autoimmune thyroid disease. *J. Immunol.* 164:5015–18

118. Lenschow DJ, Ho SC, Sattar H, Rhee L, Gray G, Nabavi N, Herold KC, Bluestone JA. 1995. Differential effects of anti-B7-1 and anti-B7-2 monoclonal antibody treatment on the development of diabetes in the nonobese diabetic mouse. *J. Exp. Med.* 181:1145–55

119. Lenschow DJ, Zeng Y, Hathcock KS, Zuckerman LA, Freeman G, Thistlethwaite JR, Gray GS, Hodes RJ, Bluestone JA. 1995. Inhibition of transplant rejection following treatment with anti–B7-2 and anti–B7-1 antibodies. *Transplantation* 60:1171–78

120. Lenschow DJ, Walunas TL, Bluestone JA. 1996. CD28/B7 system of T cell costimulation. *Annu. Rev. Immunol.* 14:233–58

121. Sojka DK, Donepudi M, Bluestone JA, Mokyr MB. 2000. Melphalan and other anticancer modalities up-regulate B7-1 gene expression in tumor cells. *J. Immunol.* 164:6230–36

122. Sperling AI, Bluestone JA. 1996. The complexities of T cell co-stimulation: CD28 and beyond. *Immunol. Rev.* 153:155–82

123. Chakrabarti D, Hultgren B, Stewart TA. 1996. IFN-alpha induces autoimmune T cells through the induction of intracellular adhesion molecule-1 and B7.2. *J. Immunol.* 157:522–28

124. Stephens LA, Kay TW. 1995. Pancreatic expression of B7 co-stimulatory molecules in the nonobese diabetic mouse. *Int. Immunol.* 7:1885–95

125. Saegusa K, Ishimaru N, Yanagi K, Haneji N, Nishino M, Azuma M, Saito I, Hayashi Y. 2000. Treatment with anti-CD86 costimulatory molecule prevents the autoimmune lesions in murine Sjogren's syndrome (SS) through up-regulated Th2

response. *Clin. Exp. Immunol.* 119:354–60

126. Kinoshita K, Tesch G, Schwarting A, Maron R, Sharpe AH, Kelley VR. 2000. Costimulation by B7-1 and B7-2 is required for autoimmune disease in MRL-Fas lpr mice. *J. Immunol.* 164:6046–56

127. Karandikar NJ, Vanderlugt CL, Eagar T, Tan L, Bluestone JA, Miller SD. 1998. Tissue-specific up-regulation of B7-1 expression and function during the course of murine relapsing experimental autoimmune encephalomyelitis. *J. Immunol.* 161:192–99

128. Windhagen A, Newcombe J, Dangond F, Strand C, Woodroofe MN, Cuzner ML, Hafler DA. 1995. Expression of costimulatory molecules B7-1 (CD80), B7-2 (CD86), and interleukin 12 cytokine in multiple sclerosis lesions. *J. Exp. Med.* 182:1985–96

129. Windhagen A, Maniak S, Gebert A, Ferger I, Heidenreich F. 1999. Costimulatory molecules B7-1 and B7-2 on CSF cells in multiple sclerosis and optic neuritis. *J. Neuroimmunol.* 96:112–20

130. Genc K, Dona DL, Reder AT. 1997. Increased CD80+ B cells in active multiple sclerosis and reversal by interferon beta-1b therapy. *J. Clin. Invest.* 99:2664–71

131. Monteyne P, Guillaume B, Sindic CJ. 1998. B7-1 (CD80), B7-2 (CD86), interleukin-12 and transforming growth factor- beta mRNA expression in CSF and peripheral blood mononuclear cells from multiple sclerosis patients. *J. Neuroimmunol.* 91:198–203

132. Bluestone JA. 1995. New perspectives of CD28-B7-mediated T cell costimulation. *Immunity* 2:555–59

133. Ikemizu S, Gilbert RJ, Fennelly JA, Collins AV, Harlos K, Jones EY, Stuart DI, Davis SJ. 2000. Structure and dimerization of a soluble form of B7-1. *Immunity* 12:51–60

134. Turka LA, Linsley PS, Lin H, Brady W, Leiden JM, Wei RQ, Gibson ML, Zheng XG, Myrdal S, Gordon D, Thompson C. 1992. T cell activation by the CD28 ligand B7 is required for cardiac allograft rejection in vivo. *Proc. Natl. Acad. Sci. USA* 89:11102–105

135. Russell ME, Hancock WW, Akalin E, Wallace AF, Glysing-Jensen T, Willett TA, Sayegh MH. 1996. Chronic cardiac rejection in the LEW to F344 rat model. Blockade of CD28-B7 costimulation by CTLA4Ig modulates T cell and macrophage activation and attenuates arteriosclerosis. *J. Clin. Invest.* 97:833–38

136. Azuma H, Chandraker A, Nadeau K, Hancock WW, Carpenter CB, Tilney NL, Sayegh MH. 1996. Blockade of T cell costimulation prevents development of experimental chronic renal allograft rejection. *Proc. Natl. Acad. Sci. USA* 93:12439–44

137. Onodera K, Chandraker A, Volk HD, Ritter T, Lehmann M, Kato H, Sayegh MH, Kupiec-Weglinski JW. 1999. Distinct tolerance pathways in sensitized allograft recipients after selective blockade of activation signal 1 or signal 2. *Transplantation* 68:288–93

138. Mandelbrot DA, Furukawa Y, McAdam AJ, Alexander SI, Libby P, Mitchell RN, Sharpe AH. 1999. Expression of B7 molecules in recipient, not donor, mice determines the survival of cardiac allografts. *J. Immunol.* 163:3753–57

139. Szot GL, Zhou P, Sharpe AH, He G, Kim O, Newell KA, Bluestone JA, Thistlethwaite JR Jr. 2000. Absence of host B7 expression is sufficient for long-term murine vascularized heart allograft survival. *Transplantation* 69:904–9

140. Rogers NJ, Mirenda V, Jackson I, Dorling A, Lechler RI. 2000. Costimulatory blockade by the induction of an endogenous xenospecific antibody response. *Nature Immunol.* 2:163–68

141. Ossevoort MA, Ringers J, Kuhn EM, Boon L, Lorre K, van den Hout Y, Bruijn JA, de Boer M, Jonker M, de Waele P.

1999. Prevention of renal allograft rejection in primates by blocking the B7/CD28 pathway. *Transplantation* 68:1010–18

142. Larsen CP, Alexander DZ, Hollenbaugh D, Elwood ET, Ritchie SC, Aruffo A, Hendrix R, Pearson TC. 1996. CD40-gp39 interactions play a critical role during allograft rejection. Suppression of allograft rejection by blockade of the CD40-gp39 pathway. *Transplantation* 61:4–9

143. Li Y, Li XC, Zheng XX, Wells AD, Turka LA, Strom TB. 1999. Blocking both signal 1 and signal 2 of T cell activation prevents apoptosis of alloreactive T cells and induction of peripheral allograft tolerance. *Nat. Med.* 5:1298–302

144. Kenyon NS, Chatzipetrou M, Masetti M, Ranuncoli A, Oliveira M, Wagner JL, Kirk AD, Harlan DM, Burkly LC, Ricordi C. 1999. Long-term survival and function of intrahepatic islet allografts in rhesus monkeys treated with humanized anti-CD154. *Proc. Natl. Acad. Sci. USA* 96:8132–37

145. Kenyon NS, Fernandez LA, Lehmann R, Masetti M, Ranuncoli A, Chatzipetrou M, Iaria G, Han D, Wagner JL, Ruiz P, Berho M, Inverardi L, Alejandro R, Mintz DH, Kirk AD, Harlan DM, Burkly LC, Ricordi C. 1999. Long-term survival and function of intrahepatic islet allografts in baboons treated with humanized anti-CD154. *Diabetes* 48:1473–81

146. Lehnert AM, Yi S, Burgess JS, O'Connell PJ. 2000. Pancreatic islet xenograft tolerance after shorT term costimulation blockade is associated with increased CD4+ T cell apoptosis but not immune deviation. *Transplantation* 69:1176–85

147. Lin H, Bolling SF, Linsley PS, Wei RQ, Gordon D, Thompson CB, Turka LA. 1993. Long-term acceptance of major histocompatibility complex mismatched cardiac allografts induced by CTLA4Ig plus donor-specific transfusion. *J. Exp. Med.* 178:1801–6

148. Sayegh MH, Zheng XG, Magee C, Hancock WW, Turka LA. 1997. Donor antigen is necessary for the prevention of chronic rejection in CTLA4Ig-treated murine cardiac allograft recipients. *Transplantation* 64:1646–50

149. Pearson TC, Alexander DZ, Hendrix R, Elwood ET, Linsley PS, Winn KJ, Larsen CP. 1996. CTLA4-Ig plus bone marrow induces long-term allograft survival and donor specific unresponsiveness in the murine model. Evidence for hematopoietic chimerism. *Transplantation* 61:997–1004

150. Niimi M, Pearson TC, Larsen CP, Alexander DZ, Hollenbaugh D, Aruffo A, Linsley PS, Thomas E, Campbell K, Fanslow WC, Geha RS, Morris PJ, Wood KJ. 1998. The role of the CD40 pathway in alloantigen-induced hyporesponsiveness in vivo. *J. Immunol.* 161:5331–37

151. Iwakoshi NN, Mordes JP, Markees TG, Phillips NE, Rossini AA, Greiner DL. 2000. Treatment of allograft recipients with donor-specific transfusion and anti-CD154 antibody leads to deletion of alloreactive CD8+ T cells and prolonged graft survival in a CTLA4-dependent manner. *J. Immunol.* 164:512–21

152. Hancock WW, Sayegh MH, Zheng XG, Peach R, Linsley PS, Turka LA. 1996. Costimulatory function and expression of CD40 ligand, CD80, and CD86 in vascularized murine cardiac allograft rejection. *Proc. Natl. Acad. Sci. USA* 93:13967–72

153. Rossini AA, Mordes JP, Markees TG, Phillips NE, Gordon EJ, Greiner DL. 1999. Induction of islet transplantation tolerance using donor specific transfusion and anti-CD154 monoclonal antibody. *Transplant Proc.* 31:629–32

154. Markees TG, Phillips NE, Noelle RJ, Shultz LD, Mordes JP, Greiner DL, Rossini AA. 1997. Prolonged survival of mouse skin allografts in recipients treated with donor splenocytes and antibody to CD40 ligand. *Transplantation* 64:329–35

155. Markees TG, Phillips NE, Gordon EJ, Noelle RJ, Shultz LD, Mordes JP, Greiner DL, Rossini AA. 1998. Long-term survival of skin allografts induced by donor splenocytes and anti-CD154 antibody in thymectomized mice requires CD4$^+$ T cells, interferon-gamma, and CTLA4. *J. Clin. Invest.* 101:2446–55

156. Parker DC, Greiner DL, Phillips NE, Appel MC, Steele AW, Durie FH, Noelle RJ, Mordes JP, Rossini AA. 1995. Survival of mouse pancreatic islet allografts in recipients treated with allogeneic small lymphocytes and antibody to CD40 ligand. *Proc. Natl. Acad. Sci. USA* 92:9560–64

157. Hamano K, Rawsthorne MA, Bushell AR, Morris PJ, Wood KJ. 1996. Evidence that the continued presence of the organ graft and not peripheral donor microchimerism is essential for maintenance of tolerance to alloantigen in vivo in anti-CD4 treated recipients. *Transplantation* 62:856–60

158. Dai Z, Konieczny BT, Baddoura FK, Lakkis FG. 1998. Impaired alloantigen-mediated T cell apoptosis and failure to induce long-term allograft survival in IL-2–deficient mice. *J. Immunol.* 161:1659–63

159. Wells AD, Li XC, Li Y, Walsh MC, Zheng XX, Wu Z, Nunez G, Tang A, Sayegh M, Hancock WW, Strom TB, Turka LA. 1999. Requirement for T-cell apoptosis in the induction of peripheral transplantation tolerance. *Nat. Med.* 5:1303–7

160. Konieczny BT, Dai Z, Elwood ET, Saleem S, Linsley PS, Baddoura FK, Larsen CP, Pearson TC, Lakkis FG. 1998. IFN-gamma is critical for long-term allograft survival induced by blocking the CD28 and CD40 ligand T cell costimulation pathways. *J. Immunol.* 160:2059–64

161. Judge TA, Tang A, Spain LM, Deans-Gratiot J, Sayegh MH, Turka LA. 1996. The in vivo mechanism of action of CTLA4Ig. *J. Immunol.* 156:2294–99

162. Guinan EC, Boussiotis VA, Neuberg D, Brennan LL, Hirano N, Nadler LM, Gribben JG. 1999. Transplantation of anergic histoincompatible bone marrow allografts. *N. Engl. J. Med.* 340:1704–14

163. Abrams JR, Lebwohl MG, Guzzo CA, Jegasothy BV, Goldfarb MT, Goffe BS, Menter A, Lowe NJ, Krueger G, Brown MJ, Weiner RS, Birkhofer MJ, Warner GL, Berry KK, Linsley PS, Krueger JG, Ochs HD, Kelley SL, Kang S. 1999. CTLA4Ig-mediated blockade of T cell costimulation in patients with psoriasis vulgaris. *J. Clin. Invest.* 103:1243–52

Annu. Rev. Immunol. 2001. 19:253–74

GP120: Biologic Aspects of Structural Features

Pascal Poignard, Erica Ollmann Saphire, Paul WHI Parren, and Dennis R. Burton

Departments of Immunology and Molecular Biology, The Scripps Research Institute, 10550 North Torrey Pines Road, La Jolla, California 92037; e-mail: poignard@scripps.edu, burton@scripps.edu

Key Words HIV-1, HIV envelope protein gp120, HIV antibodies, neutralization, AIDS vaccines

■ **Abstract** HIV-1 particles are decorated with a network of densely arranged envelope spikes on their surface. Each spike is formed of a trimer of heterodimers of the gp120 surface and the gp41 transmembrane glycoproteins. These molecules mediate HIV-1 entry into target cells, initiating the HIV-1 replication cycle. They are a target for entry-blocking drugs and for neutralizing Abs that could contribute to vaccine protection. The crystal structure of the core of gp120 has been recently solved. It reveals the structure of the conserved HIV-1 receptor binding sites and some of the mechanisms evolved by HIV-1 to escape Ab responses. The gp120 consists of three faces. One is largely inaccessible on the native trimer, and two faces are exposed but apparently have low immunogenicity, particularly on primary viruses. We have modeled HIV-1 neutralization by a CD4 binding site monoclonal Ab, and we propose that neutralization takes place by inhibition of the interaction between gp120 and the target cell membrane receptors as a result of steric hindrance. Knowledge of gp120 structure and function should assist in the design of new drugs as well as of an effective vaccine. In the latter case, circumventing the low immunogenicity of the HIV-1 envelope spike is a major challenge.

INTRODUCTION

To combat the spread of HIV-1 infection, new treatments and an effective vaccine are greatly needed. The HIV-1 envelope glycoproteins, gp120 and gp41, are important molecules for both therapeutic and prophylactic approaches. First, they mediate HIV entry and therefore are a potential target for drugs aimed at blocking the first step of the viral replication cycle. Second, the envelope glycoproteins are the target of neutralizing Abs and could be the basis of the humoral component of a vaccine. Recently, great progress has been made in understanding HIV-1 entry and structure/function relationships in viral envelope glycoproteins. A compound that blocks HIV-1 entry has demonstrated convincing efficacy at controlling HIV-1

0732-0582/01/0407-0253$14.00

replication in patients, providing a proof of principle for this class of therapeutics. Furthermore HIV-1 envelope glycoproteins have been crystallized, bringing new insights for drug and vaccine design. This review summarizes the recent progress in the understanding of the gp120 structure and function, and focuses on our view of the area since a number of more general reviews have been published previously (1–3).

HIV-1 ENVELOPE GLYCOPROTEINS

HIV is an enveloped virus decorated with spikes on its surface that are essential for viral entry into target cells. These envelope spikes consist of a protein complex that comprises a cell-surface attachment glycoprotein, gp120, and a membrane spanning protein, gp41. Virus binding to the target cell takes place via a sequential interaction between gp120 and HIV cellular receptors: the CD4 molecule and members of the chemokine family receptors, termed HIV coreceptors. The CD4 molecule is a member of the immunoglobulin superfamily, mainly expressed on T lymphocytes, macrophages, and dendritic cells. Binding of gp120 to CD4 is not sufficient to permit HIV entry, which, in addition, requires the interaction of the gp120 envelope glycoprotein with a member of the chemokine receptor family (4). Chemokine receptors are seven transmembrane domain proteins that contain four extracellular domains: an amino-terminal domain and three extracellular loops. The two major coreceptors used by HIV-1 to enter target cells are CCR5 (5–8) and CXCR4 (9). CCR5 functions as the principal coreceptor for macrophage tropic strains (R5 strains), whereas CXCR4 is used by T tropic strains (X4 strains). Dual tropic HIV-1 strains (R5X4 strains) can use both coreceptors. Other coreceptors of less well understood importance in vivo have been reported (4). The tropism of envelope glycoproteins for either coreceptors depends on the ability of gp120 to interact directly with these receptors. The importance of CCR5 has been demonstrated by the discovery that a homozygous 32 bp deletion in the CCR5 gene confers resistance to HIV infection (10, 11). Failure of most individuals homozygous for the CCR5Δ32 deletion to become infected suggests that X4 viruses are inefficient at establishing an infection in a naïve host (8). Indeed R5 viruses are prevalent during the early phase of infection (12). Furthermore, heterozygosity for the CCR5Δ32 deletion delays progression to disease, probably because of a decrease of coreceptor expression (13–16). This observation suggests that interference with the viral entry process could be beneficial to infected individuals.

GP120 STRUCTURE

The HIV-1 envelope glycoprotein complex is initially produced as a single chain glycoprotein precursor, gp160, which is cleaved by a cellular protease. Gp160 cleavage yields the cell-surface attachment glycoprotein, gp120, and the membrane spanning protein, gp41. The two HIV envelope glycoproteins are noncovalently

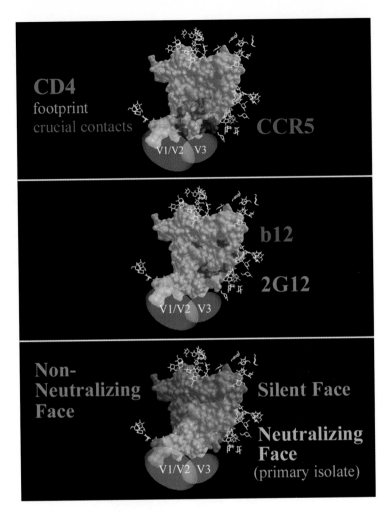

Figure 1 The structure of the gp120 core.

Top panel: The CD4-gp120 interface is shown in yellow. Proposed crucial residues for the binding of CD4 and CCR5 are highlighted in orange and blue, respectively.

Middle panel: Proposed crucial residues for the binding of monoclonal Abs b12 and 2G12 are highlighted in red and green, respectively.

Bottom panel: The faces of the gp120 core. The neutralizing face of primary viruses is highlighted in yellow. The neutralizing face of TCLA viruses corresponds to the grey and yellow surface.

Gp120 surfaces were generated using coordinates from Kwong et al. (22). Graphics were produced using MSMS (98) and visualized in PMV (99). Modeling of carbohydrates was based on preferred structures and torsion angles as in (100, 101) and done using TOM/FRODO (102).

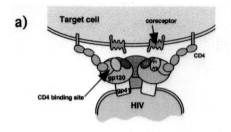

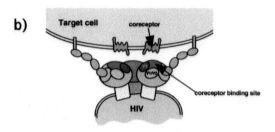

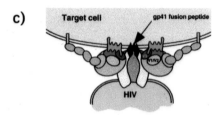

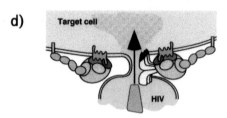

Figure 2 Schematic model of HIV-1 entry.

a) The first step of HIV-1 entry is the binding of the gp120 surface molecule to its receptor, the CD4 molecule, at the surface of the target cell.

b) Ligation of CD4 to gp120 leads to conformational changes in the envelope complex that permit exposure of the coreceptor binding site.

c) The gp41 fusion peptide inserts into the target cell membrane leading to the formation of the prehairpin intermediate.

d) The formation of the coiled-coil leads to membrane fusion and to the penetration of HIV-1 genetic information into the target cell.

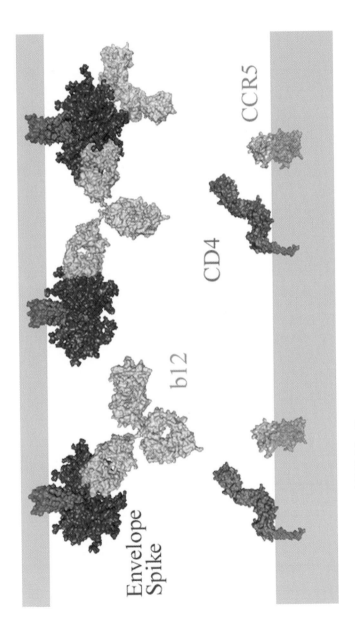

Figure 3 Model of neutralization of HIV-1 by Abs.
The Ab b12 binds to envelope spikes on the viral membrane (top) and prevents interaction with cell membrane viral receptors (bottom).

Envelope trimer assembly was done as in (31) using TOM/FRODO (102), and carbohydrates were added. Coordinates for gp120, gp41, CD4 and CCR5 are from (22), (54), (103) and (104), respectively. Coordinates for b12 are from E. Ollman Saphire et al. (manuscript in preparation).

linked and assemble into an oligomer, most likely a trimer (see below), of gp120-gp41 heterodimers that is expressed at the cell surface and then, following viral budding, at the virion surface (17, 18).

The surface envelope glycoprotein gp120 is a heavily glycosylated protein with carbohydrates accounting for about 40% to 50% of the molecular weight. It is composed of five constant regions (C1–C5) interspersed with five variable regions (V1–V5) (19, 20). Until recently, little information on gp120 structure was available. The only clues came from functional analysis of variant viruses, topographical mapping based on monoclonal Ab binding analysis, crystallographic and NMR studies of small portions of gp120, and molecular modeling with reference to homologous viral proteins of known structure. These studies suggested that the conserved regions of gp120 form a central core, whereas the variable regions, with the exception of V5, are bracketed with cysteine disulfide bonds and form four loops that emanate from the surface of the protein (for review, see 21).

The understanding of gp120 structure advanced remarkably with the resolution, by the groups of W Hendrickson and J Sodroski of the crystal structure of a complex formed between the gp120 core, the membrane distal 2 domains of the CD4 molecule and an antibody Fab fragment (22). We summarize below the main features of the gp120 crystal structure, but for an exhaustive description the reader is referred to the excellent original papers and accompanying reviews (22–24). To obtain crystals that diffracted with sufficient resolution, a gp120 core molecule was used that lacks the variable loops V1-V2 and V3 and amino- and carboxy-terminal sequences and that had been enzymatically stripped of over 90% of its carbohydrates. The loops were replaced with the tripeptide linker Gly-Ala-Gly. The final deglycosylated ΔV3, ΔV1-V2 gp120 core retains 67% of the envelope amino acid content of the full-length molecule and has a molecular weight of 35 kDa. Despite the modifications, the core retains structural integrity as shown by its ability to bind CD4 and to interact with a number of antibodies at levels comparable to the full-length molecule (25). Although the variable regions V3, V1-V2 are deleted, the core still contains some variable fragments—the V4 and V5 loops as well as surface loops termed LD and LE. The crystal structure at 2.5 Å resolution revealed that the gp120 core is composed of 25 β-strands, 5 α-helices, and 10 loop segments and that it folds into an heart-shaped globular structure with dimensions of $5 \times 5 \times 2.5$ nm. It is interesting that the gp120 structure is unrelated to any previous protein structure described. The core is formed of an inner domain and an outer domain that are linked by a four-stranded sheet termed the bridging sheet. Among different clades of HIV-1, the inner domain is more conserved than the outer domain. The crystal structure reveals that all three domains of the gp120 core are important for CD4 and coreceptor binding.

The Receptor Binding Sites on gp120

The receptor binding sites are potential targets for therapeutic intervention as they are likely to be conserved among different strains of HIV and need to be exposed on the gp120 surface at least transiently for the virus to enter the target cell.

The CD4 Binding Site   On gp120, the CD4 binding site is located in a depression formed at the interface of the outer and inner domains with the bridging sheet (22). Surprisingly, half of the residues of gp120 that contact CD4 do so only through main-chain atoms, which might help in escape from Abs as discussed below. Figure 1 (see color insert) shows the footprint of CD4 binding on the gp120 core, with proposed crucial contact residues highlighted in orange. The surface of interaction between gp120 and CD4 is large, covering 800 Å^2 on gp120 and 740 Å^2 on CD4. On gp120, the contact surface includes two unusually large cavities. The larger cavity (about 280 Å^3) is shallow and filled with water molecules. It is lined with gp120 residues that do not form many direct contacts with CD4. This allows variability to occur within the otherwise conserved CD4 binding site. The second cavity (about 150 Å^3) is hydrophobic, approximately spherical, and is deeply buried within gp120. It is located at the interface between the three domains and is lined by highly conserved residues. Upon CD4 ligation, the entrance of this cavity is plugged by Phe43 of CD4, which is crucial for the gp120-CD4 interaction.

The Coreceptor Binding Sites   The gp120 residues involved in the coreceptor CCR5 binding site were characterized by analysis of the binding of a panel of gp120 mutants to CCR5 (26). Site-directed mutagenesis of gp120 was carried out using structural information from the crystal structure of gp120 and in particular from knowledge of the contact residues of gp120 and the CD4-induced (CD4i) Ab 17b. The epitope recognized by this Ab (see below) overlaps the CCR5 binding site as suggested by the greater exposure of both the CCR5 binding site and the 17b epitope upon CD4 binding to gp120 and by the competition of CD4i Abs for the binding of gp120 to CCR5 (27). The results of the mutagenic analysis suggest that the CCR5 binding site is one of the most highly conserved surfaces on the gp120 core, even more conserved than the CD4 binding site (26). The CCR5 binding site is located on the gp120 core in relatively close proximity to the CD4 binding site (Figure 1, see color insert). The residues involved in CCR5 binding are found near or within the bridging sheet on the gp120 core. Some of these residues likely contact the coreceptor molecule directly. Residues of the V3 loop are probably involved in CCR5 binding, potentially forming a discontinuous binding site with the conserved core elements, but these residues are absent from the crystal structure. The surface of the CCR5 binding site on the gp120 core is highly basic. This should favor interaction with the acidic N-terminal portion of the coreceptor (28–30).

Importantly, exposure of the highly conserved coreceptor binding site requires that gp120 first binds CD4 (22, 26). Models of the gp120 oligomer suggest that, after CD4 ligation, the bridging sheet is oriented toward the target cell (24, 31). Experimental data suggest that binding to CD4 leads to the repositioning of the V1-V2 loop and to the exposure or the formation of the coreceptor binding site (32). However, other gp120 conformational changes must also be involved as coreceptor binding of a V1-V2 loop-deleted gp120 is still CD4 dependent (27).

As described earlier, there are two principal HIV-1 coreceptors CCR5 and CXCR4. The binding sites of these two coreceptors share characteristics such as increased exposure upon CD4 binding and competition with CD4i Abs and anti-V3 loop Abs for binding to gp120. Furthermore, a simple V3 substitution can convert a CXCR4-using virus into one using CCR5 (33, 34). It is then likely that both coreceptors interact with a similar region of gp120, but they may not share contact residues. Some reports suggest that the affinity of gp120 for CXCR4 and for CCR5 may be different. Monomeric gp120 from R5 viruses binds poorly in the absence of soluble CD4, whereas monomeric gp120 from X4 viruses can bind CXCR4 with detectable affinity (27, 35). CD4-independent viruses that possess a constitutively exposed coreceptor binding site on the gp120 surface have been described (34–37). However, all HIV primary isolates described to date are CD4 dependent, and the relevance of such CD4-independent viruses in vivo is unknown. Of note, multiple regions of the coreceptor, including the N terminus and the extracellular loops are involved in the gp120-coreceptor interaction (48). Furthermore diverse virus strains differ in their relative dependence on receptor domains, showing that the virus is flexible in its interaction with the coreceptor (38).

Other Potentially Conserved Exposed Sites on gp120   It has recently been demonstrated that heparan sulfate can influence the binding of HIV to some cells. Mondor et al have shown that binding to HeLa cells is CD4 independent but depends on an interaction with heparan sulfate at the cell surface (39). The role of heparan sulfate in vivo is unclear especially as the main target cells for HIV-1, CD4 T cells, and macrophages express little heparan sulfate on their surface. The ability to interact with heparan sulfate has been reported to be specific for X4 viruses. Moulard et al have shown that gp120 binding to heparan sulfate is dependent on coreceptor usage (40). Gp120 molecules from X4 and R5X4 viruses bind polyanions strongly, whereas R5 gp120 do not. The interaction with polyanions is mainly mediated by the V3 loop, and this interaction is followed by a second weaker interaction probably with the coreceptor binding region. This interaction resembles the gp120-coreceptor interaction, involving the V3 loop and the coreceptor binding site, but is limited to X4 and X4R5 gp120 molecules. The relevance of this observation in vivo is unclear. HIV-1 may use binding to polyanion as an initial means of attachment to the cell surface before forming a specific stronger interaction with CD4 and coreceptor.

Another interaction of gp120 with a cell surface molecule has been described recently and may be of greater relevance for HIV-1 pathogenesis. Previously gp120 had been shown to bind with high affinity to a C-type lectin isolated from a placental cDNA library (41). This molecule is now known to be a dendritic cell-specific lectin (DC-SIGN) (42). Geijtenbeek et al reported recently that this molecule is not used by HIV-1 as an entry receptor but may facilitate the capture and transport of HIV from mucosal surfaces to secondary lymphoid organs rich in T cells (43). Surprisingly, DC-SIGN can enhance infection of T cells in *trans*. The interaction of DC-SIGN with gp120 is independent of binding to CD4 and CCR5. Further, as mannan blocks the binding of DC-SIGN to gp120, it is probable that it interacts with carbohydrate moieties on gp120. However, that the lectin domain interacts with the polypeptide backbone of gp120 cannot be ruled out.

THE ENVELOPE SPIKE

The gp120-gp41 heterodimers associate in a trimer to form spikes at the virus surface that we term the native trimer. As discussed below, the oligomerization of the envelope glycoproteins has important consequences for their antigenicity and immunogenicity. The structure of the envelope spike is unknown. Modeling of the entire oligomer, including gp41, is not possible as the structure of gp41 in its gp120-associated state is not known. By analogy with the HA_2 protein of influenza virus, gp41 is currently thought to exist in a metastable non-coiled-coil conformation when associated with gp120 (44). A model of gp120 trimer has been proposed (24, 31). This model suggests that the surface of the gp120 trimer is roughly hemispherical. The inner domain of gp120 faces the trimer axis, whereas the outer domain is mostly exposed on the surface of the oligomer. The coreceptor binding site is close to the trimer axis and faces the target cell surface after CD4 ligation to gp120. The surface that faces the target cell is highly basic and includes the V3 loop. The model suggests that three CD4 molecules can bind obliquely to a gp120 trimer without steric interference.

The envelope spikes have been studied by electronic microscopy. These studies show that on the viral particle the envelope spikes form densely arranged knobs (45, 46). The diameter of each knob is about 14 nm and its height is 9 to 10 nm. The knobs are organized on the virion according to a skew class of icosahedral symmetry (45, 46). The ultrastructural studies suggest that mature HIV particles are icosahedral, comprising 20 faces and 12 vertices, and possess about 72 spikes (45–47). This symmetry follows the organization of the underlaying matrix protein p17 Gag. Trimers of the matrix protein associate in a hexagonal network of icosahedral symmetry that forms a hole into which gp41 can insert, determining the position of each spike on the viral surface (48–51). Measurement of electronic microscopy images of the viral particle show that the distance from the center of one spike to the next is about 21 to 22 nm (45, 46, 51).

HIV-1 ENTRY

The HIV entry process is complex. The first step is the binding of the CD4 molecule to gp120 at the surface of the viral particle as shown in Figure 2 (see color insert). Experimental evidence and the recently published gp120 structure suggest that CD4 binding induces conformational changes within the bridging sheet as well as between this sheet and the inner and outer domains of gp120 (22, 52, 53). These conformational changes lead to the exposure or the formation of the high-affinity coreceptor binding site (26). These rearrangements in gp120 involve a movement of the V1-V2 stem away from the underlying coreceptor binding site while the V3 loop may move toward this binding site (32). Binding of the coreceptor to gp120 results in further conformational changes that lead to gp41 activation into its fusion-active state.

It is currently thought that, as discussed above, gp41 exists in a metastable non-coiled-coil conformation when associated with gp120 and that, similarly to influenza virus HA_2, gp41 uses the coiled-coil formation as a spring-loaded mechanism to bring the viral and cell membranes closer (44, 54, 55). It has been proposed that following coreceptor binding the envelope glycoprotein complex undergoes conformational changes that lead to the insertion of gp41 fusion peptide into the membrane of the target cell and to the formation of a prehairpin intermediate where gp41 is both a viral and a cell membrane protein. One study suggests that the prehairpin intermediate is induced rapidly after binding of gp120 to its receptors and has a lifetime of minutes (56). The prehairpin intermediate is followed by the formation of a gp41 coiled-coil structure, leading to the apposition of membranes and ultimately to fusion. The formation of the coiled-coil may lead to the dissociation of gp120 from gp41, the gp120 molecule possibly remaining anchored to the target cell membrane through CD4 and coreceptor binding. The fusion events are poorly understood, and how many gp41 trimers are required in order to form a fusion pore is not yet known.

Of note, the mechanism of promotion of HIV-1 entry by DC-SIGN is not known. DC-SIGN might induce conformational rearrangements that enhance the interaction between gp120 and CD4 or the coreceptor or facilitate other entry steps (43).

GP120 ANTIGENICITY AND IMMUNOGENICITY

It has been long recognized that Abs can inhibit HIV-1 infectivity. Such Abs, termed neutralizing Abs, are directed against the envelope glycoproteins of HIV. Studies in animal models suggest that neutralizing Abs may be an important component of an efficient HIV vaccine (105–108). However, it is proving extremely difficult to generate HIV-1 envelope molecules that elicit such neutralizing Abs. Knowledge of the HIV-1 envelope glycoproteins structure may help understanding of how HIV-1 has evolved to escape humoral immunity and may permit the design of more efficient vaccines. A number of reviews have recently discussed HIV-1 neutralization in a general way (1, 57); here we focus on structural aspects of the interaction of neutralizing Abs with HIV-1 envelope glycoproteins.

Studies of the binding of monoclonal Abs to gp120 and of Ab cross-competition suggested the existence on gp120 of two faces (58, 59). These studies showed that neutralizing epitopes cluster on gp120 to form a surface that was termed the neutralizing face. By contrast, non-neutralizing epitopes cluster on another face on the gp120 core, forming a non-neutralizing face. Analysis of Ab binding to the envelope trimer expressed at the surface of HIV-infected cells suggested that the non-neutralizing epitopes are not exposed on the oligomeric form of gp120, being hidden within the trimer (58, 60). Structural studies of gp120 have then confirmed the existence of a neutralizing and a non-neutralizing face predicted by Ab cross-competition analysis (24, 59) and have revealed the presence of a third face, termed by Wyatt et al. the silent face (23).

The Silent Face of gp120

The heavy glycosylation of gp120 has long been thought to contribute to reduction of protein epitope exposure and to enhance viral evasion from Ab (61). Indeed carbohydrate side chains scarcely induce Ab responses, as they appear to the immune system as "self." It is interesting that the crystal structure of gp120 showed that most carbohydrates locate on a single face on the outer domain of the gp120 core (24). Models of gp120 trimerization suggest that this face is well exposed at the surface of the envelope oligomer (24, 31). The poor immunogenicity of this face has led to its designation as the "silent face." The face also contains the variable loops V4, V5, LA, LC, LD, and LE.

The Non-Neutralizing Face of gp120

This face induces a strong Ab response in infected individuals. However, Abs that bind epitopes belonging to this surface do not neutralize HIV-1. The non-neutralizing face corresponds to the inner domain of gp120 core and is relatively conserved (22). Analysis of Ab binding to gp120 trimer complexes expressed at the surface of infected cells as well as models of gp120 trimer suggest that this surface is buried within the gp120 trimer and is not exposed at the surface of the envelope oligomeric complex on the viral particle (24, 31, 60). Therefore, Abs that bind to epitopes on the non-neutralizing face cannot bind to virions and have no neutralizing activity. This view has been disputed by reports suggesting that some non-neutralizing epitopes could be exposed at the surface of the oligomeric gp120 on the virion surface (62–65). As explained below, in view of the probable mechanism of neutralization, we favor the hypothesis that non-neutralizing epitopes correspond to epitopes that are not exposed on the gp120 trimer and that all exposed epitopes are neutralizing. As the non-neutralizing face is well exposed at the surface of soluble monomeric gp120, it has been proposed that such Abs are elicited by gp120 shed from the viral particles and/or infected cells. However, as the gp160 precursor and monomeric gp120 share similar antigenicity, an alternative is that non-neutralizing Abs are elicited in response to gp160 found in quantities in debris of dying HIV-infected cells (66). Indeed the affinity of a number of human Abs is greater for gp160 than for gp120, suggesting that the former may be the eliciting Ag in vivo. It could also be hypothesized that such Abs are raised against viruses that bear partially shed spikes, exposing monomeric gp120 on their surface. Such particles would indeed be stronger immunogens than free monomeric gp120 (67).

The Neutralizing Face of gp120

To replicate, HIV-1 must interact with its receptors on target cells. As a consequence, part of the surface of gp120 has to be both exposed and conserved. The neutralizing face corresponds to this surface. However, HIV has evolved astute mechanisms to escape the Ab response, and the gp120 structure shows that this face is still relatively occluded (22, 24). In particular, the two most conserved regions, the receptor binding sites, are poorly accessible to Abs. Furthermore, the neutralizing epitopes are mainly accessible on viruses that have been adapted to immortalized T cell lines (T cell line adapted or TCLA isolates). These viruses are very sensitive to neutralization. By contrast, primary isolates, i.e. viruses that have been passaged only a limited number of times on activated primary lymphocytes, are much less sensitive to Ab neutralization (68). Differences in the quaternary structure of the envelope complex can presumably explain the differences between TCLA viruses and primary isolates to neutralization. The gp120 trimer of TCLA adopts a relatively open conformation, allowing the exposure in particular of the CD4 binding site, the coreceptor binding site, and the V3 loop. In contrast, it has been proposed that the primary isolate trimeric complex has a more closed conformation, reducing acceessibility of the receptor binding sites and preventing the binding of neutralizing Abs (57, 69–71). Primary isolates are significantly more representative of patient isolates than TCLA viruses. An ideal vaccine should essentially induce Abs that can neutralize a broad range of primary isolates. Only two broadly neutralizing anti-gp120 monoclonal Abs, both of human origin, have been described to date (72). The first Ab, b12, binds to an epitope overlapping the CD4 binding site (73–75). The second Ab, 2G12, recognizes a unique epitope located on the outer domain of gp120 (76). Below is a description of the neutralizing epitopes on gp120. The b12 and 2G12 epitopes are important for the neutralization of primary and TCLA viruses. The CD4 binding site in general, the variable loops, and the coreceptor binding site are more significant for TCLA viruses.

CD4 Binding Site; The b12 Epitope   The CD4 binding site revealed by the crystal structure of CD4 bound-gp120 has been described above. However, it should be stressed that the CD4 binding site conformation in this structure may not correspond to the one recognized by Abs. Indeed, as explained above, binding of CD4 to gp120 induces important conformational changes in the envelope glycoprotein. The CD4 binding site, as seen by Abs and by the immune system, is unliganded and might adopt a different conformation than the one described in the crystal structure of CD4-liganded gp120. Nevertheless, the structure of an unliganded gp120 would then be more informative in understanding more thoroughly immunogenicity from the perspective of vaccine design. The gp120 crystal structure that has been determined gives useful information on the epitopes of CD4 binding site Abs (22). As expected, residues critical for Abs that compete with CD4 binding locate within the CD4 binding domain. The location, close to the coreceptor binding site, of residues Asp 368 and Glu 370, known to be important for the binding of most CD4 binding site Abs (24, 77), shows that these epitopes also overlap the coreceptor binding site. This explains why anti-CD4 binding site Abs tend to compete with CD4i Abs (59, 78). Interestingly, the structure of CD4-bound gp120 reveals some of the features that HIV has evolved to escape anti-CD4 binding site Abs despite the need to keep this region conserved and exposed enough for receptor ligation. The first difficulty for Abs is to access the CD4 binding site recessed within the gp120 core. Indeed, the Fab of an Ab molecule is "wider" than CD4 (two Ig domains compared to one). In addition the binding site is flanked by variable and glycosylated regions that will likely diminish its effective immunogenicity. The large hydrophilic cavity of the CD4 binding site tolerates gp120 mutations, and this may facilitate viral escape from anti-CD4 binding site Abs. Some of the residues of gp120 that contact CD4 do so through their main-chain atoms. As Abs mostly contact residues via their side chains, this may permit the variation of residues involved in receptor binding and the escape from neutralizing Ab without detrimental effects on CD4 binding. Finally, the CD4 binding site is partially masked by the V1-V2 loop (22, 32).

Despite all these considerations, a number of Abs directed against the CD4 binding site neutralize TCLA viruses, suggesting that their epitopes are relatively well exposed on the virion surface (68). However, only the anti-CD4 binding site Ab b12 neutralizes a broad range of primary isolates (72). This Ab differs from all the other anti-CD4 binding site Abs described to date by its sensitivity to V1-V2 loop deletion (75). It is not known whether the Ab contacts the V1-V2 loop or if the sensitivity is only due to an indirect effect of conformational rearrangements following V1-V2 deletion. Analysis of Ab competition studies showed that b12 is the anti-CD4 binding site Ab that is most sensitive to anti-V2 competition, which might suggest that b12 contacts the V1-V2 loop (59). The proposed b12 contact residues, as determined by mutagenesis (75), are shown in Figure 1 (see color insert). It should be restated that this structure corresponds to the CD4-liganded gp120 and that gp120 may adopt another conformation prior to ligation.

The 2G12 Epitope   The 2G12 epitope is a unique neutralization site located on the outer domain of gp120 (Figure 1, see color insert). 2G12 binding is sensitive to deglycosylation (76). It is impaired by mutations that alter N-linked carbohydrate sites localized in the C2, C3, V4, and C4 regions (76). This Ab can neutralize a broad range of TCLA and primary isolates (72, 79), and it is therefore likely that 2G12 binds, at least to some extent, to carbohydrate structures that are well conserved between isolates. Interestingly, although it is potently neutralizing, 2G12 does not interfere with CD4 and coreceptor binding. This Ab specificity is uncommon in sera from HIV-1-infected individuals (76).

Variable Loops   The V3 loop is a good TCLA isolate neutralizing epitope (1). Some anti-V3 loop Abs have a limited activity against particular primary isolates. However, primary isolates are in general poorly neutralized by anti-V3 loop Abs (72). The V3 loop is probably located close to the coreceptor binding site.

Consistently anti-V3 Abs block coreceptor binding to gp120 (80). The V3 loop is absent from the published gp120 crystal structure. The structure of V3 loop peptides conjugated with monoclonal Abs suggest that the V3 loop can adopt at least two different conformations (81). One of these two conformations was found three times for three different monoclonal Abs, suggesting that this conformation might be conserved (R Stanfield, personal communication). As one of these Abs can neutralize some primary isolates, this V3 loop conformation may be conserved among some primary isolates. Overall, however, the variability of the V3 loop conformation on gp120 or envelope trimer remains unclear.

The importance of V1-V2 loop epitopes for neutralization, in particular of primary isolates, remains uncertain. The neutralizing potency of the V1-V2 Abs described to date is quite limited (82) (J Moore, personal communication), and the variability of the V1-V2 loop remains an important obstacle for broad neutralization.

CD4 Induced Epitope   CD4 induced (CD4i) Abs bind to gp120 with greater affinity when gp120 is complexed to CD4 (78). As discussed before, these Abs recognize an epitope that overlaps the coreceptor binding site. The published gp120 crystal structure reveals the interaction of the Fab fragment of the CD4i Ab 17b with CD4 bound-gp120 (22). The Fab fragment covers a surprisingly small surface of 455 Å of gp120, centered on residues of the bridging sheet and the stem of the V1-V2 loop and oriented toward the target cell membrane. The coreceptor binding site is the most conserved surface of gp120 and could be a promising target for neutralization (26). However, mAb 17b neutralizes TCLA viruses very poorly and primary isolates not at all. It appears that the 17b epitope is largely masked prior to CD4 binding by the V1-V2 loop. Furthermore, in contrast to binding of soluble CD4, the binding of cell surface CD4 to virus does not appear to make available the epitope to binding by 17b to allow neutralization. Presumably the binding of gp120 to cell surface CD4 brings the viral envelope complex so close to the target cell that although this region is accessible to coreceptor, it is not accessible to Ab. It may be that HIV-1 has evolved to use CD4 to provide a means to hide the conserved coreceptor binding site in order to prevent Ab neutralization (34).

Gp120 Structure and Ab Neutralization

The recent determination of the crystal structures of the neutralizing Ab b12 (E Ollmann Saphire, manuscript in preparation) and of gp120 (22) gives us the opportunity to model the interaction of gp120 with this neutralizing Ab. As shown in Figure 3 (see color insert), we modeled the binding of b12 to the gp120 oligomer at the surface of a viral particle about to encounter a target cell. The crystal structure of the b12 Ab shows that, consistent with previous knowledge, the Ab could extend about 18 nm from the tip of one Fab to the other and about 16 nm from the tip of a Fab to the tip of the Fc; the individual Fab and Fc fragments have dimensions of about $7 \times 4.5 \times 4$ nm and $7 \times 6 \times 3.5$ nm, respectively. Furthermore the hinge region gives a high flexibility to the Ab molecule. Gp120 on the other hand adopts a more compact conformation; the core has dimensions of $5 \times 5 \times 2.5$ nm (22). As discussed above, the gp120 trimer at the surface of the virus forms a knob of 14nm diameter and about 9 to 10 nm height above the viral membrane. The space occupied by an Ab molecule thus compares to or even surpasses the space occupied by a gp120 trimer. In addition, the spikes are equally distributed on the viral surface every 21 nm, which means that the outer edge of a spike approaches within 7 nm of its neighbors (45, 51). Therefore, considering the space occupied by the Ab and the close proximity of the spikes, when an Ab molecule is bound to gp120, the Fc (and possibly the free Fab) is likely to project from the virus surface as a result of steric hindrance and geometric constraints (Figure 3, see color insert). The structure solved for CD4 suggests that the membrane distal domains are parallel to the cell surface and that the first domain probably extends no further than 7 nm from the cell surface. Then, taking into account the respective sizes of the envelope trimer, the Ab and the CD4 molecule, it becomes unlikely that, when b12 Ab molecules are bound to an array of gp120 spikes, the viral and cellular membranes can approach close enough for the binding of gp120 to CD4 to take place, even though free CD4 binding sites may still be available on the spikes in question (Figure 3, see color insert).

We have previously shown that neutralization of HIV-1 by Abs against gp120 is determined primarily by occupancy of sites on the virion, irrespective of the epitope recognized (83). The molecular model shown in Figure 3 (see color insert) is in agreement with these results and refines the model that we have previously proposed (83). It is apparent that steric constraints will be roughly similar wherever an Ab molecule is attached to the gp120 trimer and will probably hinder further interaction with cellular receptors. This view is consistent with the inhibition of virus attachment to target cells observed for different anti-gp120 Abs against distinct epitopes (84, 85). The orientation of gp120 within the trimer suggests that the bivalent binding of an Ab to two gp120 molecules within the same trimer would require an extreme flexibility of the molecule, and this is unlikely (31). However, the short distance separating the viral spikes certainly permits bivalent binding of Abs to gp120 molecules belonging to different spikes, which would lead to increased avidity of the Ab.

In a recent review we calculated the stoichiometry of HIV neutralization, based on a comparison of the neutralization behavior of HIV-1 with a number of other viruses and on the work of Schönning et al (2, 86). It was determined that the attachment of approximately 70 IgG molecules per virion is required for neutralization, which is equivalent to about one IgG molecule per spike (2). Neutralization of HIV-1 is therefore suggested to be the result of coating of the viral surface with Ab molecules to a critical density. In the model that we propose, any epitope exposed on the envelope spike can mediate neutralization as long as the critical coating density can be achieved. On the gp120 moiety of primary isolate envelope spikes, only two neutralizing epitopes are known to be exposed, forming the small neutralizing face shown in Figure 1 (see color insert). It should be noted that the term "neutralizing face" can be misunderstood. It simply defines the area to which neutralizing Abs have been isolated to date and does not imply that Abs against the "silent face" cannot be neutralizing. However, under normal circumstances Abs against the latter region are not induced because of tolerance to carbohydrates. Ab 2G12 appears to be an exception and, in a sense, it could equally well be viewed to recognize the silent face as the neutralizing face.

VACCINE DESIGN

How can structural information help us design a vaccine that induces a strongly neutralizing Ab response? The structure of gp120 suggests that the virus escapes the Ab response first by burying much of the envelope glycoprotein surface (the non-neutralizing face), and second by decreasing the immunogenicity of the exposed surfaces (the neutralizing face and the silent face) on the envelope spike. Immunization with monomeric gp120, where the non-neutralizing face and the N- and C-terminal parts that interact with gp41 are exposed, has yielded Abs that bind to monomeric gp120 but not to the native oligomer and in particular not to the native oligomer of primary isolates (68). These Abs are consequently non-neutralizing.

Immunization with the native envelope trimer may force the immune system to focus on the neutralizing epitopes exposed on the surface of the trimer, leading to the production of neutralizing Abs. Different approaches are possible. Virions chemically inactivated by modification of the nucleocapsid zinc finger motifs conserve a native conformation of the envelope oligomers and could be used for immunization (87). Attempts to produce stable soluble envelope glycoprotein trimers that conserve a native conformation are currently in progress, and some approaches may be promising. Yang et al have introduced GCN4 trimeric helices at the C-terminus of a soluble form of the envelope glycoprotein in order to stabilize the trimerization (88, 89). Binley et al have proposed the addition of cysteines into the envelope glycoproteins in order to permit the creation of disulfide bridges between gp120 and gp41 and the stabilization of the gp120-gp41 interaction (90).

These approaches may be impaired by the low immunogenicity of the envelope trimer; modifications of gp120 might be required in order to increase immunogenicity. Removal of carbohydrates has been proposed to lead to greater immunogenicity and to the production of a better neutralizing Ab response (91). Removal of variable loops may also permit the exposure of otherwise hidden conserved surfaces. The difficulty with these approaches will be to increase immunogenicity without altering the antigenicity of the oligomeric gp120. This might prove difficult to achieve.

Other approaches may be required. According to the model of neutralization we have championed, any exposed surface on the trimer is a potential neutralizing epitope. The silent face is a well-exposed surface, with very low immunogenicity in part because of its heavy glycosylation. However, gp120 possesses carbohydrate moieties that are conserved among isolates as shown by the broad neutralization obtained with the 2G12 Ab (24, 72). A better understanding of gp120 carbohydrates and circumvention of their low immunogenicity could in principle make the HIV silent face a target for neutralizing Abs.

If the spike immunogenicity problem cannot be solved, we may have to look beyond HIV-1 surface envelope proteins and to envisage the use of mimotopes (92). Approaches based on available potent neutralizing Abs can be proposed. Complementary molecules could be selected from protein fragment libraries or retroviral libraries or designed from the knowledge of Ab structure. Finally, approaches that aim at increasing the Ab response in general, such as dendritic cell-targeted immunization, may have to be coupled to the approaches described above in order to raise strong neutralizing Ab responses.

SMALL MOLECULE DESIGN

The inhibition of HIV-1 entry as a therapeutic strategy has been recently validated by a clinical study that demonstrated that a compound, T20, which targets gp41 and blocks HIV-1 entry, is highly efficient at controlling viral replication in patients (93). This raised the hope that entry-blocking agents will be the next generation of anti-HIV drugs (94). Small molecules that bind to gp120 with high affinity and block crucial steps of viral entry would be desirable. The complex strategies that HIV has evolved to evade Abs may not be as efficient against small compounds. The resolution of the structure of gp120 might help the design of such agents. In particular the two conserved binding sites are potential targets for therapeutic intervention (95). However, as explained before, the unliganded gp120 molecule may adopt a different conformation than the CD4-liganded crystal structure that has been solved. The Phe43 cavity of the CD4 binding site might thus not be preserved in the absence of CD4 (22). The coreceptor binding site is an attractive target as it is very conserved, but its access is difficult because it is mostly hidden before CD4 ligation. However, in contrast to Abs, small compounds may be able to access the coreceptor binding site after CD4 binding despite steric constraints due to the proximity of the cell membrane. Molecules that mimic CD4 could trigger conformational changes and expose the coreceptor binding site, permitting the binding of small coreceptor binding inhibitors. Of note, the resolution of the crystal structure of a fragment of gp41 has permitted an elegant series of studies resulting in the identification of a pocket on gp41 as a potential drug target (55, 96). Small peptides have been designed that block this cavity and inhibit HIV-1 entry (97).

CONCLUDING REMARKS

Despite the hundreds of monoclonal Abs of rodent and human origin that have been generated against gp120, only two Abs that potently neutralize a broad range of primary isolates are available to date: the Abs b12 and 2G12. This illustrates the success of the strategies evolved by HIV to avoid Ab inactivation. Recent progress in the knowledge of HIV envelope glycoprotein structure further elucidates some of the viral strategies of Ab evasion. Although the targets of neutralizing Abs are now better understood, we still do not have immunogens that will elicit these Abs at useful levels. This remains a major challenge for vaccine design. The success of the T20 peptide, which targets gp41, will certainly intensify the search for small molecules that interfere with the viral entry process. This class of drug will, one hopes, be in common use in future years. The search for such small molecules and for improved immunogens would benefit from increased structural knowledge of gp120, especially from a crystal structure of an unliganded gp120 and of the gp120-gp41 trimeric complex.

ACKNOWLEDGMENTS

We thank J Sodroski and Z Huang for gp120 and CCR5 coordinates, respectively. We are grateful to J Sodroski and R Wyatt for critical review of the manuscript. EOS wishes to acknowledge Ian A Wilson for generous support. This work was supported by grants from the National Institute of Health AI45357(to PP), AI40377 (to PWHI), GM46192-05 (to IAW), AI33292 and HL59727 (to DRB).

Visit the Annual Reviews home page at www.AnnualReviews.org

LITERATURE CITED

1. Parren PWHI, Moore JP, Burton DR, Sattentau QJ. 1999. The neutralizing antibody response to HIV-1: viral evasion and escape from humoral immunity. *Aids* 13:S137–62

2. Parren PWHI, Burton DR. 2000. The antiviral activity of antibodies in vitro and in vivo. *Adv. Immunol.* In press

3. Sattentau QJ, Moulard M, Brivet B, Botto F, Guillemot JC, Mondor I, Poignard P, Ugolini S. 1999. Antibody neutralization of HIV-1 and the potential for vaccine design. *Immunol. Lett.* 66:143–49

4. Berger EA, Murphy PM, Farber JM. 1999. Chemokine receptors as HIV-1 coreceptors: roles in viral entry, tropism, and disease. *Annu. Rev. Immunol.* 17:657–700

5. Alkhatib G, Combadiere C, Broder C, Feng Y, Kennedy P, Murphy P, Berger E. 1996. CC CKR5: a RANTES, MIP-1alpha, MIP-1beta receptor as a fusion cofactor for macrophage-tropic HIV-1. *Science* 272:1955–58

6. Deng H, Liu R, Ellmeier W, Choe S, Unutmaz D, Burkhart M, Di Marzio P, Marmon S, Sutton R, Hill C, Davis C, Peiper S, Schall T, Littman D, Landau N. 1996. Identification of a major co-receptor for primary isolates of HIV-1. *Nature* 381:661–66

7. Doranz B, Rucker J, Yi Y, Smyth R, Samson M, Peiper S, Parmentier M, Collman R, Doms R. 1996. A dual-tropic primary HIV-1 isolate that uses fusin and the beta-chemokine receptors CKR-5, CKR-3, and CKR-2b as fusion cofactors. *Cell* 85:1149–58

8. Dragic T, Litwin V, Allaway G, Martin S, Huang Y, Nagashima K, Cayanan C, Maddon P, Koup R, Moore JP, Paxton W. 1996. HIV-1 entry into CD4+ cells is mediated by the chemokine receptor CC-CKR-5. *Nature* 381:667–73

9. Feng Y, Broder CC, Kennedy PE, Berger EA. 1996. HIV-1 entry cofactor: functional cDNA cloning of a seven-transmembrane,

G protein-coupled receptor. *Science* 272: 872–77

10. Liu R, Paxton WA, Choe S, Ceradini D, Martin SR, Horuk R, MacDonald ME, Stuhlmann H, Koup RA, Landau NR. 1996. Homozygous defect in HIV-1 coreceptor accounts for resistance of some multiply-exposed individuals to HIV-1 infection. *Cell* 86:367–77

11. Samson M, Libert F, Doranz B, Rucker J, Liesnard C, Farber C, Saragosti S, Lapoumeroulie C, Cognaux J, Forceille C, Muyldermans G, Verhofstede C, Burton-boy G, Georges M, Imai T, Rana S, Yi Y, Smyth R, Collman R, Doms R, Vassart G, Parmentier M. 1996. Resistance to HIV-1 infection in caucasian individuals bearing mutant alleles of the CCR-5 chemokine receptor gene. *Nature* 382:722–25

12. Connor R, Sheridan K, Ceradini D, Choe S, Landau N. 1997. Change in coreceptor use correlates with disease progression in HIV-1-infected individuals. *J. Exp. Med.* 185:621–28

13. Dean M, Carrington M, Winkler C, Huttley G, Smith M, Allikmets R, Goedert J, Buchbinder S, Vittinghoff E, Gomperts E, Donfield S, Vlahov D, Kaslow R, Saah A, Rinaldo C, Detels R, O'Brien S. 1996. Genetic restriction of HIV-1 infection and progression to AIDS by a deletion allele of the CKR5 structural gene. Hemophilia Growth and Development Study, Multicenter AIDS Cohort Study, Multicenter Hemophilia Cohort Study, San Francisco City Cohort, ALIVE Study. *Science* 273:1856–62

14. Smith M, Dean M, Carrington M, Winkler C, Huttley G, Lomb D, Goedert J, O'Brien T, Jacobson L, Kaslow R, Buchbinder S, Vittinghoff E, Vlahov D, Hoots K, Hilgartner M, O'Brien S. 1997. Contrasting genetic influence of CCR2 and CCR5 variants on HIV-1 infection and disease progression. Hemophilia Growth and Development Study (HGDS), Multicenter AIDS Cohort Study (MACS), Multicenter Hemophilia Cohort Study (MHCS), San Francisco City Cohort (SFCC), ALIVE Study. *Science* 277:959–65

15. Zimmerman P, Buckler-White A, Alkhatib G, Spalding T, Kubofcik J, Combadiere C, Weissman D, Cohen O, Rubbert A, Lam G, Vaccarezza M, Kennedy P, Kumaraswami V, Giorgi J, Detels R, Hunter J, Chopek M, Berger E, Fauci A, Nutman T, Murphy P. 1997. Inherited resistance to HIV-1 conferred by an inactivating mutation in CC chemokine receptor 5: studies in populations with contrasting clinical phenotypes, defined racial background, and quantified risk. *Mol. Med.* 3:23–36

16. Michael NL, Chang G, Louie LG, Mascola JR, Dondero D, Birx DL, Sheppard HW. 1997. The role of viral phenotype and CCR-5 gene defects in HIV-1 transmission and disease progression. *Nat. Med.* 3:338–40

17. Lu M, Blacklow SC, Kim PS. 1995. A trimeric structural domain of the HIV-1 transmembrane glycoprotein. *Nat. Struct. Biol.* 2:1075–82

18. Kowalski M, Potz J, Basiripour L, Dorfman T, Goh WC, Terwilliger E, Dayton A, Rosen C, Haseltine W, Sodroski J. 1987. Functional regions of the envelope glycoprotein of human immunodeficiency virus type 1. *Science* 237:1351–55

19. Leonard CK, Spellman NW, Riddle L, Harris RJ, Thomas JN, Gregory TJ. 1990. Assignment of intrachain disulphide bonds and characterization of potential glycosylation sites of the type 1 recombinant human immunodeficiency virus envelope glycoprotein (gp120) expressed in Chinese hamster ovary cells. *J. Biol. Chem.* 265:10373–82

20. Starlich BR, Hahn BH, Shaw GM, McNeely PD, Modrow S, Wolf H, Parks ES, Parks WP, Josephs SF, Gallo RC. 1986. Identification and characterisation of conserved and variable regions in the envelope gene of HTLV-III/LAV, the retrovirus of AIDS. *Cell* 45:637–48

21. Burton DR, Montefiori D. 1997. The antibody response in HIV-1 infection. *AIDS* 11(Suppl A):S87–S98

22. Kwong PD, Wyatt R, Robinson J, Sweet RW, Sodroski J, Hendrickson WA. 1998. Structure of an HIV gp120 envelope glycoprotein in complex with the CD4 receptor and a neutralizing human antibody. *Nature* 393:648–59

23. Wyatt R, Sodroski J. 1998. The HIV-1 envelope glycoproteins: fusogens, antigens, and immunogens. *Science* 280:1884–88

24. Wyatt R, Kwong PD, Desjardins E, Sweet RW, Robinson J, Hendrickson WA, Sodroski JG. 1998. The antigenic structure of the HIV gp120 envelope glycoprotein. *Nature* 393:705–11

25. Binley JM, Wyatt R, Desjardins E, Kwong PD, Hendrickson W, Moore JP, Sodroski J. 1998. Analysis of the interaction of antibodies with a conserved enzymatically deglycosylated core of the HIV type 1 envelope glycoprotein 120. *AIDS Res. Hum. Retroviruses* 14:191–98

26. Rizzuto CD, Wyatt R, Hernandez-Ramos N, Sun Y, Kwong PD, Hendrickson WA, Sodroski J. 1998. A conserved HIV gp120 glycoprotein structure involved in chemokine receptor binding. *Science* 280:1949–53

27. Wu L, Gerard NP, Wyatt R, Choe H, Parolin C, Ruffing N, Borsetti A, Cardoso AA, Desjardin E, Newman W, Gerard C, Sodroski J. 1996. CD4-induced interaction of primary HIV-1 gp120 glycoproteins with the chemokine receptor CCR-5. *Nature* 384:179–83

28. Farzan M, Choe H, Vaca L, Martin K, Sun Y, Desjardins E, Ruffing N, Wu L, Wyatt R, Gerard N, Gerard C, Sodroski J. 1998. A tyrosine-rich region in the N terminus of CCR5 is important for human immunodeficiency virus type 1 entry and mediates an association between gp120 and CCR5. *J. Virol.* 72:1160–64

29. Dragic T, Trkola A, Lin SW, Nagashima KA, Kajumo F, Zhao L, Olson WC, Wu L, Mackay CR, Allaway GP, Sakmar TP, Moore JP, Maddon PJ. 1998. Amino-terminal substitutions in the CCR5 coreceptor impair gp120 binding and human immunodeficiency virus type 1 entry. *J. Virol.* 72:279–85

30. Rabut GE, Konner JA, Kajumo F, Moore JP, Dragic T. 1998. Alanine substitutions of polar and nonpolar residues in the amino-terminal domain of CCR5 differently impair entry of macrophage- and dualtropic isolates of human immunodeficiency virus type 1. *J. Virol.* 72:3464–68

31. Kwong PD, Wyatt R, Sattentau QJ, Sodroski J, Hendrickson WA. 2000. Oligomeric modeling and electrostatic analysis of the gp120 envelope glycoprotein of human immunodeficiency virus. *J. Virol.* 74:1961–72

32. Wyatt R, Moore JP, Accola M, Desjardin E, Robinson J, Sodroski J. 1995. Involvement of the V1/V2 variable loop structure in the exposure of human immunodeficiency virus type 1 gp120 epitopes induced by receptor binding. *J. Virol.* 69:5723–33

33. Choe H, Farzan M, Sun Y, Sullivan N, Rollins B, Ponath P, Wu L, Mackay C, LaRosa G, Newman W, Gerard N, Gerard C, Sodroski J. 1996. The beta-chemokine receptors CCR3 and CCR5 facilitate infection by primary HIV-1 isolates. *Cell* 85:1135–48

34. Hoffman TL, LaBranche CC, Zhang W, Canziani G, Robinson J, Chaiken I, Hoxie JA, Doms RW. 1999. Stable exposure of the coreceptor-binding site in a CD4-independent HIV-1 envelope protein. *Proc. Natl. Acad. Sci. USA* 96:6359–64

35. Hesselgesser J, Halks-Miller M, DelVecchio V, Peiper SC, Hoxie J, Kolson DL, Taub D, Horuk R. 1997. CD4-independent association between HIV-1 gp120 and CXCR4: functional chemokine receptors are expressed in human neurons. *Curr. Biol.* 7:112–21

36. Bandres JC, Wang QF, O'Leary J, Baleaux F, Amara A, Hoxie JA, Zolla-Pazner S,

Gorny MK. 1998. Human immunodeficiency virus (HIV) envelope binds to CXCR4 independently of CD4, and binding can be enhanced by interaction with soluble CD4 or by HIV envelope deglycosylation. *J. Virol.* 72:2500–4

37. Dumonceaux J, Nisole S, Chanel C, Quivet L, Amara A, Baleux F, Briand P, Hazan U. 1998. Spontaneous mutations in the env gene of the human immunodeficiency virus type 1 NDK isolate are associated with a CD4-independent entry phenotype. *J. Virol.* 72:512–19

38. Bieniasz PD, Cullen BR. 1998. Chemokine receptors and human immunodeficiency virus infection. *Front. Biosci.* 3:D44–58

39. Mondor I, Ugolini S, Sattentau QJ. 1998. Human immunodeficiency virus type 1 attachment to HeLa CD4 cells is CD4 independent and gp120 dependent and requires cell surface heparans. *J. Virol.* 72: 3623–34

40. Moulard M, Lortat-Jacob H, Mondor I, Roca G, Wyatt R, Sodroski J, Zhao L, Olson W, Kwong PD, Sattentau QJ. 2000. Selective interactions of polyanions with basic surfaces on human immunodeficiency virus type 1 gp120. *J. Virol.* 74:1948–60

41. Curtis BM, Scharnowske S, Watson AJ. 1992. Sequence and expression of a membrane-associated C-type lectin that exhibits CD4-independent binding of human immunodeficiency virus envelope glycoprotein gp120. *Proc. Natl. Acad. Sci. USA* 89:8356–60

42. Geijtenbeek TB, Torensma R, van Vliet SJ, van Duijnhoven GC, Adema GJ, van Kooyk Y, Figdor CG. 2000. Identification of DC-SIGN, a novel dendritic cell-specific ICAM-3 receptor that supports primary immune responses. *Cell* 100:575–85

43. Geijtenbeek TB, Kwon DS, Torensma R, van Vliet SJ, van Duijnhoven GC, Middel J, Cornelissen IL, Nottet HS, KewalRamani VN, Littman DR, Figdor CG, van Kooyk Y. 2000. DC-SIGN, a dendritic cell-specific HIV-1-binding protein that enhances trans-infection of T cells. *Cell* 100:587–97

44. Chan DC, Kim PS. 1998. HIV entry and its inhibition. *Cell* 93:681–84

45. Gelderblom HR, Hausmann EH, Ozel M, Pauli G, Koch MA. 1987. Fine structure of human immunodeficiency virus (HIV) and immunolocalization of structural proteins. *Virology* 156:171–76

46. Ozel M, Pauli G, Gelderblom HR. 1988. The organization of the envelope projections on the surface of HIV. *Arch. Virol.* 100:255–66

47. Nermut MV, Grief C, Hashmi S, Hockley DJ. 1993. Further evidence of icosahedral symmetry in human and simian immunodeficiency virus. *AIDS Res. Hum. Retroviruses* 9:929–38

48. Rao Z, Belyaev AS, Fry E, Roy P, Jones IM, Stuart DI. 1995. Crystal structure of SIV matrix antigen and implications for virus assembly. *Nature* 378:743–47

49. Nermut MV, Hockley DJ, Bron P, Thomas D, Zhang WH, Jones IM. 1998. Further evidence for hexagonal organization of HIV gag protein in prebudding assemblies and immature virus-like particles. *J. Struct. Biol.* 123:143–49

50. Nermut MV, Hockley DJ, Jowett JB, Jones IM, Garreau M, Thomas D. 1994. Fullerene-like organization of HIV gag-protein shell in virus-like particles produced by recombinant baculovirus. *Virology* 198:288–96

51. Forster MJ, Mulloy B, Nermut MV. 2000. Molecular modelling study of HIV p17gag (MA) protein shell utilising data from electron microscopy and X-ray crystallography. *J. Mol. Biol.* 298:841–57

52. Sattentau QJ, Moore JP. 1991. Conformational changes induced in the human immunodeficiency virus envelope glycoprotein by soluble CD4 binding. *J. Exp. Med.* 174:407–15

53. Sattentau QJ, Moore JP, Vignaux F, Traincard F, Poignard P. 1993. Conformational changes induced in the envelope

glycoproteins of the human and simian immunodeficiency viruses by soluble receptor binding. *J. Virol.* 67:7383–93

54. Weissenhorn W, Dessen A, Harrison SC, Skehel JJ, Wiley DC. 1997. Atomic structure of the ectodomain from HIV-1 gp41. *Nature* 387:426–30

55. Chan DC, Fass D, Berger JM, Kim PS. 1997. Core structure of gp41 from the HIV envelope glycoprotein. *Cell* 89:263–73

56. Jones PL, Korte T, Blumenthal R. 1998. Conformational changes in cell surface HIV-1 envelope glycoproteins are triggered by cooperation between cell surface CD4 and co-receptors. *J. Biol. Chem.* 273:404–9

57. Burton DR. 1997. A vaccine for HIV type 1: the antibody perspective. *Proc. Natl. Acad. Sci. USA* 94:10018–23

58. Moore JP, Sattentau QJ, Wyatt R, Sodroski J. 1994. Probing the structure of the human immunodeficiency virus surface glycoprotein gp120 with a panel of monoclonal antibodies. *J. Virol.* 68:469–84

59. Moore JP, Sodroski J. 1996. Antibody cross-competition analysis of the human immunodeficiency virus type 1 gp120 exterior envelope glycoprotein. *J. Virol.* 70:1863–72

60. Sattentau QJ, Moore JP. 1995. Human immunodeficiency virus type 1 neutralization is determined by epitope exposure on the gp120 oligomer. *J. Exp. Med.* 182:185–96

61. Alexander S, Elder JH. 1984. Carbohydrate dramatically influences immune reactivity of antisera to viral glycoprotein antigens. *Science* 226:1328–30

62. Stamatatos L, Zolla-Pazner S, Gorny MK, Cheng-Mayer C. 1997. Binding of antibodies to virion-associated gp120 molecules of primary-like human immunodeficiency virus type 1 (HIV-1) isolates: effect on HIV-1 infection of macrophages and peripheral blood mononuclear cells. *Virology* 229:360–69

63. Fouts TR, Trkola A, Fung MS, Moore JP. 1998. Interactions of polyclonal and

monoclonal anti-glycoprotein 120 antibodies with oligomeric glycoprotein 120-glycoprotein 41 complexes of a primary HIV type 1 isolate: relationship to neutralization. *AIDS Res. Hum. Retroviruses* 14:591–97

64. Nyambi PN, Gorny MK, Bastiani L, van der Groen G, Williams C, Zolla-Pazner S. 1998. Mapping of epitopes exposed on intact human immunodeficiency virus type 1 (HIV-1) virions: a new strategy for studying the immunologic relatedness of HIV-1. *J. Virol.* 72:9384–91

65. Nyambi PN, Mbah HA, Burda S, Williams C, Gorny MK, Nadas A, Zolla-Pazner S. 2000. Conserved and exposed epitopes on intact, native, primary human immunodeficiency virus type 1 virions of group M. *J. Virol.* 74:7096–7107

66. Parren PWHI, Burton DR, Sattentau QJ. 1997. HIV-1 antibody–debris or virion? *Nat. Med.* 3:366–67

67. Bachmann MF, Zinkernagel RM. 1997. Neutralizing antiviral B cell responses. *Annu. Rev. Immunol.* 15:235–70

68. Poignard P, Klasse PJ, Sattentau QJ. 1996. Antibody neutralization of HIV-1. *Immunol. Today* 17:239–46

69. Moore JP, Cao Y, Qing L, Sattentau QJ, Pyati J, Koduri R, Robinson J, Barbas CF 3rd, Burton DR, Ho DD. 1995. Primary isolates of human immunodeficiency virus type 1 are relatively resistant to neutralization by monoclonal antibodies to gp120, and their neutralization is not predicted by studies with monomeric gp120. *J. Virol.* 69:101–9

70. Fouts TR, Binley JM, Trkola A, Robinson JE, Moore JP. 1997. Neutralization of the human immunodeficiency virus type 1 primary isolate JR-FL by human monoclonal antibodies correlates with antibody binding to the oligomeric form of the envelope glycoprotein complex. *J. Virol.* 71:2779–85

71. Bou-Habib DC, Roderiquez G, Oravecz T, Berman PW, Lusso P, Norcross MA. 1994.

Cryptic nature of envelope V3 region epitopes protects primary monocytotropic human immunodeficiency virus type 1 from antibody neutralization. *J. Virol.* 68:6006–13

72. D'Souza MP, Livnat D, Bradac JA, Bridges SH. 1997. Evaluation of monoclonal antibodies to human immunodeficiency virus type 1 primary isolates by neutralization assays: performance criteria for selecting candidate antibodies for clinical trials. AIDS Clinical Trials Group Antibody Selection Working Group. *J. Infect. Dis.* 175:1056–62

73. Burton DR, Barbas CF 3d, Persson M, Koenig S, Chanock R, Lerner R. 1991. A large array of human monoclonal antibodies to type 1 human immunodeficiency virus from combinatorial libraries of asymptomatic seropositive individuals. *Proc. Natl. Acad. Sci. USA* 88:10134–37

74. Burton DR, Pyati J, Koduri R, Sharp SJ, Thornton GB, Parren PWHI, Sawyer LS, Hendry RM, Dunlop N, Nara PL, et al. 1994. Efficient neutralization of primary isolates of HIV-1 by a recombinant human monoclonal antibody. *Science* 266:1024–27

75. Roben P, Moore JP, Thali M, Sodroski J, Barbas CF 3rd, Burton DR. 1994. Recognition properties of a panel of human recombinant Fab fragments to the CD4 binding site of gp120 that show differing abilities to neutralize human immunodeficiency virus type 1. *J. Virol.* 68:4821–28

76. Trkola A, Purtscher M, Muster T, Ballaun C, Buchacher A, Sullivan N, Srinivasan K, Sodroski J, Moore JP, Katinger H. 1996. Human monoclonal antibody 2G12 defines a distinctive neutralization epitope on the gp120 glycoprotein of human immunodeficiency virus type 1. *J. Virol.* 70:1100–8

77. Thali M, Furman C, Ho DD, Robinson J, Tilley S, Pinter A, Sodroski J. 1992. Discontinuous, conserved neutralization epitopes overlapping the CD4-binding region of human immunodeficiency virus type 1 gp120 envelope glycoprotein. *J. Virol.* 66:5635–41

78. Thali M, Moore JP, Furman C, Charles M, Ho DD, Robinson J, Sodroski J. 1993. Characterization of conserved human immunodeficiency virus type 1 gp120 neutralization epitopes exposed upon gp120-CD4 binding. *J. Virol.* 67:3978–88

79. Trkola A, Pomales AB, Yuan H, Korber B, Maddon PJ, Allaway GP, Katinger H, Barbas CF 3rd, Burton DR, Ho DD, et al. 1995. Cross-clade neutralization of primary isolates of human immunodeficiency virus type 1 by human monoclonal antibodies and tetrameric CD4-IgG. *J. Virol.* 69:6609–17

80. Trkola A, Dragic T, Arthos J, Binley JM, Olson WC, Allaway GP, Cheng-Mayer C, Robinson J, Maddon PJ, Moore JP. 1996. CD4-dependent, antibody-sensitive interactions between HIV-1 and its co-receptor CCR-5. *Nature* 384:184–87

81. Stanfield R, Cabezas E, Satterthwait A, Stura E, Profy A, Wilson I. 1999. Dual conformations for the HIV-1 gp120 V3 loop in complexes with different neutralizing fabs. *Structure Fold. Des.* 7:131–42

82. Pinter A, Honnen WJ, Kayman SC, Trochev O, Wu Z. 1998. Potent neutralization of primary HIV-1 isolates by antibodies directed against epitopes present in the V1/V2 domain of HIV-1 gp120. *Vaccine* 16:1803–11

83. Parren PWHI, Mondor I, Naniche D, Ditzel HJ, Klasse PJ, Burton DR, Sattentau QJ. 1998. Neutralization of human immunodeficiency virus type 1 by antibody to gp120 is determined primarily by occupancy of sites on the virion irrespective of epitope specificity. *J. Virol.* 72:3512–19

84. Ugolini S, Mondor I, Parren PWHI, Burton DR, Tilley SA, Klasse PJ, Sattentau QJ. 1997. Inhibition of virus attachment to CD4+ target cells is a major mechanism of T cell line-adapted HIV-1 neutralization. *J. Exp. Med.* 186:1287–98

85. Valenzuela A, Blanco J, Krust B, Franco R, Hovanessian AG. 1997. Neutralizing antibodies against the V3 loop of human immunodeficiency virus type 1 gp120 block the CD4-dependent and -independent binding of virus to cells. *J. Virol.* 71:8289–98

86. Schönning K, Lund O, Lund OS, Hansen JE. 1999. Stoichiometry of monoclonal antibody neutralization of T-cell line-adapted human immunodeficiency virus type 1. *J. Virol.* 73:8364–70

87. Rossio JL, Esser MT, Suryanarayana K, Schneider DK, Bess JW Jr, Vasquez GM, Wiltrout TA, Chertova E, Grimes MK, Sattentau Q, Arthur LO, Henderson LE, Lifson JD. 1998. Inactivation of human immunodeficiency virus type 1 infectivity with preservation of conformational and functional integrity of virion surface proteins. *J. Virol.* 72:7992–8001

88. Yang X, Florin L, Farzan M, Kolchinsky P, Kwong PD, Sodroski J, Wyatt R. 2000. Modifications that stabilize human immunodeficiency virus envelope glycoprotein trimers in solution. *J. Virol.* 74:4746–54

89. Yang X, Farzan M, Wyatt R, Sodroski J. 2000. Characterization of stable, soluble trimers containing complete ectodomains of human immunodeficiency virus type 1 envelope glycoproteins. *J. Virol.* 74:5716–25

90. Binley JM, Sanders RW, Clas B, Schuelke N, Master A, Guo Y, Kajumo F, Anselma DJ, Maddon PJ, Olson WC, Moore JP. 2000. A recombinant human immunodeficiency virus type 1 envelope glycoprotein complex stabilized by an intermolecular disulfide bond between the gp120 and gp41 subunits is an antigenic mimic of the trimeric virion-associated structure. *J. Virol.* 74:627–43

91. Reitter JN, Means RE, Desrosiers RC. 1998. A role for carbohydrates in immune evasion in AIDS. *Nat. Med.* 4:679–84

92. Burton DR, Parren PWHI. 2000. Vaccines and the induction of functional antibodies: time to look beyond the molecules of natural infection? *Nat. Med.* 6:123–25

93. Kilby JM, Hopkins S, Venetta TM, DiMassimo B, Cloud GA, Lee JY, Alldredge L, Hunter E, Lambert D, Bolognesi D, Matthews T, Johnson MR, Nowak MA, Shaw GM, Saag MS. 1998. Potent suppression of HIV-1 replication in humans by T-20, a peptide inhibitor of gp41-mediated virus entry. *Nat. Med.* 4:1302–7

94. Blair WS, Lin PF, Meanwell NA, Wallace OB. 2000. HIV-1 entry—an expanding portal for drug discovery. *Drug Discov. Today.* 5:183–94

95. Vita C, Drakopoulou E, Vizzavona J, Rochette S, Martin L, Menez A, Roumestand C, Yang YS, Ylisastigui L, Benjouad A, Gluckman JC. 1999. Rational engineering of a miniprotein that reproduces the core of the CD4 site interacting with HIV-1 envelope glycoprotein. *Proc. Natl. Acad. Sci. USA* 96:13091–96

96. Chan DC, Chutkowski CT, Kim PS. 1998. Evidence that a prominent cavity in the coiled coil of HIV type 1 gp41 is an attractive drug target. *Proc. Natl. Acad. Sci. USA* 95:15613–17

97. Eckert DM, Malashkevich VN, Hong LH, Carr PA, Kim PS. 1999. Inhibiting HIV-1 entry: discovery of D-peptide inhibitors that target the gp41 coiled-coil pocket. *Cell* 99:103–15

98. Sanner MF, Olson AJ, Spehner JC. 1996. Reduced surface: an efficient way to compute molecular surfaces. *Biopolymers* 38:305–20

99. Sanner MF. 1999. Python: a programming language for software integration and development. *J. Mol. Graph. Model.* 17:57–61

100. Wormald MR, Wooten EW, Bazzo R, Edge CJ, Feinstein A, Rademacher TW, Dwek RA. 1991. The conformational effects of N-glycosylation on the tailpiece from serum IgM. *Eur. J. Biochem.* 198:131–39

101. Imberty A, Perez S. 1995. Stereochemistry of the N-glycosylation sites in glycoproteins. *Protein Eng.* 8:699–709

102. Jones TA. 1985. Diffraction methods for biological macromolecules. Interactive computer graphics: FRODO. *Methods Enzymol.* 115:157–71

103. Wu H, Kwong PD, Hendrickson WA. 1997. Dimeric association and segmental variability in the structure of human CD4. *Nature* 387:527–30

104. Zhou N, Luo Z, Hall JW, Luo J, Han X, Huang Z. 2000. Molecular modeling and site-directed mutagenesis of CCR5 reveal residues critical for chemokine binding and signal transduction. *Eur. J. Immunol.* 30:164–73

105. Gauduin MC, Parren PW, Weir R, Barbas CF, Burton DR, Koup RA. 1997. Passive immunization with a human monoclonal antibody protects hu-PBL-SCID mice against challenge by primary isolates of HIV-1. *Nat. Med.* 3:1389–93

106. Shibata R, Igarashi T, Haigwood N, Buckler-White A, Ogert R, Ross W, Willey R, Cho MW, Martin MA. 1999. Neutralizing antibody directed against the HIV-1 envelope glycoprotein can completely block HIV-1/SIV chimeric virus infections of macaque monkeys. *Nat. Med.* 5:204–10

107. Baba TW, Liska V, Hofmann-Lehmann R, Vlasak J, Xu W, Ayehunie S, Cavacini LA, Posner MR, Katinger H, Stiegler G, Bernacky BJ, Rizvi TA, Schmidt R, Hill LR, Keeling ME, Lu Y, Wright JE, Chou TC, Ruprecht RM. 2000. Human neutralizing monoclonal antibodies of the IgG1 subtype protect against mucosal simian-human immunodeficiency virus infection. *Nat. Med.* 6:200–6

108. Mascola JR, Stiegler G, VanCott TC, Katinger H, Carpenter CB, Hanson CE, Beary H, Hayes D, Frankel SS, Birx DL, Lewis MG. 2000. Protection of macaques against vaginal transmission of a pathogenic HIV-1/SIV chimeric virus by passive infusion of neutralizing antibodies. *Nat. Med.* 6:207–10

Annu. Rev. Immunol. 2001. 19:275–90

IGG FC RECEPTORS

Jeffrey V. Ravetch and Silvia Bolland

Laboratory of Molecular Genetics and Immunology, Rockefeller University,
1230 York Ave, New York, NY 10021; e-mail: ravetch@rockefeller.edu

Key Words   FcR, immune complex, inflammation, hypersensitivity, autoimmune

■ **Abstract**   Since the description of the first mouse knockout for an IgG Fc receptor seven years ago, considerable progress has been made in defining the in vivo functions of these receptors in diverse biological systems. The role of activating $Fc\gamma Rs$ in providing a critical link between ligands and effector cells in type II and type III inflammation is now well established and has led to a fundamental revision of the significance of these receptors in initiating cellular responses in host defense, in determining the efficacy of therapeutic antibodies, and in pathological autoimmune conditions. Considerable progress has been made in the last two years on the in vivo regulation of these responses, through the appreciation of the importance of balancing activation responses with inhibitory signaling. The inhibitory FcR functions in the maintenance of peripheral tolerance, in regulating the threshold of activation responses, and ultimately in terminating IgG mediated effector stimulation. The consequences of deleting the inhibitory arm of this system are thus manifested in both the afferent and efferent immune responses. The hyperresponsive state that results leads to greatly magnified effector responses by cytotoxic antibodies and immune complexes and can culminate in autoimmunity and autoimmune disease when modified by environmental or genetic factors. $Fc\gamma Rs$ offer a paradigm for the biological significance of balancing activation and inhibitory signaling in the expanding family of activation/inhibitory receptor pairs found in the immune system.

INTRODUCTION

Fc receptors for IgG were identified over 35 years ago with the observation that IgG antibodies could be directly cytophilic for macrophages when presented as opsonized RBCs (1). This binding property of IgG antibodies was independent of the F(ab) region of the antibody and required only Fc interactions. Subsequent in vitro studies established the role of these receptors in triggering effector responses such as macrophage phagocytosis, NK cell ADCC, neutrophil activation, and the paradoxical inhibition of B cell activation by IgG immune complexes (2–6). Our current understanding of IgG FcRs has been greatly enhanced by the molecular cloning of the murine genes 15 years ago, followed soon after by their human counterparts and the recently described crystal structures for both the receptors and ligand complexes defined in the last year (7–16). Two general classes of IgG FcRs are now recognized—the activation receptors, characterized by the presence of a cytoplasmic ITAM sequence associated with the receptor, and the inhibitory receptor, characterized by the presence of an ITIM sequence (Figure 1, see color insert) (17–19). These two classes of receptors function in concert and are usually found coexpressed on the cell surface. Because activation and inhibitory receptors bind IgG with comparable affinity and specificity (17, 20), coengagement of both signaling pathways is thus the rule, setting thresholds for and ultimately determining the magnitude of effector cell responses. This appreciation of the balanced function of these receptors has been primarily developed through the analysis of mice deficient in either receptor or signaling pathway. This review focuses on these in vivo studies and the implications of those studies for the role of these receptors in maintaining tolerance, shaping the antibody repertoire, and determining the cellular outcome of engagement of FcRs by IgGs. The gene structures, cellular expression, binding affinities, polymorphisms, and subclass specificities of these receptors have been extensively reviewed in the past, and the reader is directed to those studies for further details (17, 18, 20, 21).

ACTIVATION FcγRs

These molecules are characterized by the presence of an ITAM motif either intrinsic to the receptor, as in the case of the human FcγRIIA (a receptor not found in the mouse), or more commonly, as part of an associated subunit, the γ or ζ chain, as in FcγRI and FcγRIIIA, receptors conserved between mouse and human (17, 18, 20). (A neutrophil specific decoy receptor, FcγRIIIB, is additionally found in humans that binds IgG immune complexes without triggering activation.) Activation receptors bind IgG either with relatively high affinity (10^{-9}) for the case of FcγRI or with low affinity (10^{-6}), as is the case for FcγRIIA and IIIA (17, 20). Cross-linking of the ligand binding extracellular domain results in tyrosine phosphorylation of the ITAM by members of the src kinase family, with subsequent recruitment of SH2 containing signaling molecules that bind the phosphorylated ITAM, most notably the syk kinase family of molecules. Depending on the particular cell type activated by the Fc receptor, different kinases are involved in these signaling pathways. For instance, FcγRIIIA aggregation activates lck in NK cells, while FcγRIIA or FcγRIIIA activate lyn and hck in monocytic and mast cells (22, 23). Likewise, syk is activated in mast cells and macrophages, whereas the related kinase ZAP70 is activated in NK cells (24–26). Subsequent signaling pathways associated with cellular activation by FcγRs are similar to that observed for other ITAM-containing receptors such as the BCR and TCR (27, 28). Early events include the activation of PI3 kinase, the enzymatic activity of which leads to production of PIP$_3$ and recruitment of PH domain containing molecules, such as PLCγ and Tec kinases, through a PIP$_3$-PH domain interaction (29–31). Myeloid cells contain several Tec kinases, named Btk, Itk, and Emt (32), that can all be activated upon Fc receptor aggregation. The newly discovered adaptor molecules

SLP-76 and BLNK link Syk activation with Btk and PLCγ responses in FcR-dependent macrophage activation (33). Ultimately, activation of PLCγ leads to generation of IP3, DAG, and sustained calcium mobilization. The significance of this activity for FcR function has been appreciated by the analysis of PLCγ2-deficient mice, which are defective for FcγRIII-dependent NK cell function (34). An example of some of the possible signaling pathways activated by FcγRIII aggregation is shown in Figure 2 (see color insert). Cellular phenotypes associated with FcγR activation receptors include degranulation, phagocytosis, ADCC, transcription of cytokine genes, and release of inflammatory mediators (2–4). In general, these phenotypes are indicative of the central role of these receptors in mediating inflammatory responses to cytotoxic IgGs or IgG immune complexes.

Activation FcγRs are found on most effector cells of the immune system, notably monocytes, macrophages, NK cells, mast cells, eosinophils, neutrophils, and platelets, while absent from lymphoid cells. In general, activation and inhibitory FcγRs are coexpressed on the same cell, a physiologically important means of setting thresholds for activating stimuli, because the IgG ligand will coengage both receptors. The ratio of expression of these two opposing signaling systems will determine the cellular response. It is, therefore, not surprising that these receptors are modulated in their expression during the differentiation and development of effector cells and by cytokine activation of these cells (17, 35, 36).

INHIBITORY FcγR

In both mouse and human, a single gene for an inhibitory FcγR, FcγRIIB, encodes a single chain glycoprotein characterized by a ligand-binding extracellular domain highly homologous to its activation counterparts, but containing the distinctive inhibitory or ITIM sequence in its cytoplasmic domain. The inhibitory FcR binds IgG with low affinity (10^{-6}), interacting with immune complexes only at physiological concentration of antibody (17, 20). The prototype six amino acid ITIM cytoplasmic sequence, I/V/L/SxYxxL/V, in which x denotes any amino acid, has been found in a growing number of receptors, most notably the NK inhibitory molecules that bind MHC class I (19, 37–40). The inhibitory activity of FcγRIIB, embedded in the cytoplasmic domain of the single chain FcγRIIB molecule, was defined as a 13 amino acid sequence AENTITYSLLKHP, shown to be both necessary and sufficient to mediate the inhibition of BCR-generated calcium mobilization and cellular proliferation (41, 42). Significantly, phosphorylation of the tyrosine of this motif was shown to occur upon BCR coligation and was required for its inhibitory activity (42). This modification generated an SH2 recognition domain that is the binding site for the inhibitory signaling molecule SHIP that leads to the abrogation of ITAM activation signaling by hydrolyzing the membrane inositol phosphate PIP3, itself the product of receptor activation (Figure 3, see color insert) (43). In the absence of PIP3, binding proteins of the PH domain class (e.g. Btk and PLCγ) are released from the membrane and a sustained calcium signal is blocked by preventing influx of extracellular calcium through the capacitance-coupled channel (44, 45). FcγRIIB phosphorylation also leads to an arrest of BCR triggered proliferation by potentially perturbing the activation of MAP kinases and preventing the recruitment of the anti-apoptotic protein kinase, Akt (46–49).

In addition to its expression on B cells, where it is the only IgG Fc receptor, FcγRIIB is widely expressed on effector cells such as macrophages, neutrophils, and mast cells, missing only from T and NK cells (17, 20). FcγRIIB displays three separable inhibitory activities, two of which are dependent on the ITIM motif and one independent of this motif. Coengagement of FcγRIIB to an ITAM-containing receptor leads to tyrosine phosphorylation of the ITIM by the lyn kinase, recruitment of SHIP, and the inhibition of ITAM-triggered calcium mobilization and cellular proliferation (43, 50, 51). However, inhibition of calcium mobilization and arrest of cellular proliferation, while both ITIM-dependent processes, are the result of different signaling pathways. Calcium inhibition requires the phosphatase activity of SHIP to hydrolyse PIP_3 and the ensuing dissociation of PH domain containing proteins like Btk and PLCγ (Figure 3) (44, 45, 52). The net effect is to block calcium influx and prevent sustained calcium signaling. Calcium-dependent processes such as degranulation, phagocytosis, ADCC, cytokine release, and proinflammatory activation are all blocked. Arrest of proliferation in B cells is also dependent upon the ITIM pathway, through the activation of the adaptor protein dok and subsequent inactivation of MAP kinases (47, 48). The role of SHIP in this process has not been fully delineated, although it can affect proliferation in several ways. SHIP, through its catalytic phosphatase domain, can prevent recruitment of the PH domain survival factor Akt by hydrolysis of PIP_3 (46, 49). SHIP also contains PTB domains that could act to recruit dok to the membrane and provide access to the lyn kinase that is involved in its activation. Dok-deficient B cells are unable to mediate FcγRIIB triggered arrest of BCR-induced proliferation, while retaining their ability to inhibit a calcium influx, demonstrating the dissociation of these two ITIM-dependent pathways (48).

The third inhibitory activity displayed by FcγRIIB is independent of the ITIM sequence and is displayed upon homo-aggregation of the receptor. Under these conditions of FcγRIIB clustering, a proapoptotic signal is generated through the transmembrane sequence (Figure 4, see color insert). This proapoptotic signal is blocked by recruitment of SHIP, which occurs upon coligation of FcγRIIB to the BCR, due to the Btk requirement for this apoptotic pathway. This novel activity has been reported only in B cells and has been proposed to act as a means of maintaining peripheral tolerance for B cells that have undergone somatic hypermutation (Figure 4) (53).

Fcγ Rs IN THE AFFERENT RESPONSE

The ability of IgG immune complexes to influence the afferent response has been known for over 50 years and can be either enhancing or suppressive, depending on the precise combination of antibody and antigen and the mode of

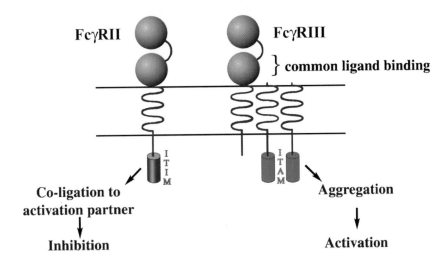

Figure 1 Schematic representation of an activation/inhibitory Fc receptor pair.

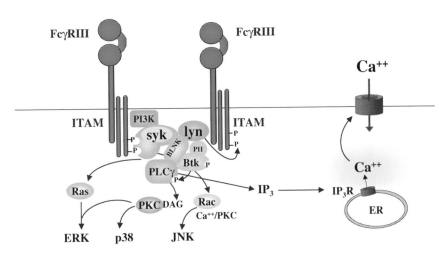

Figure 2 Cellular activation by FcgRIII aggregation. This figure shows an example of the possible signaling pathways initiated upon FcR ITAM phosphorylation.

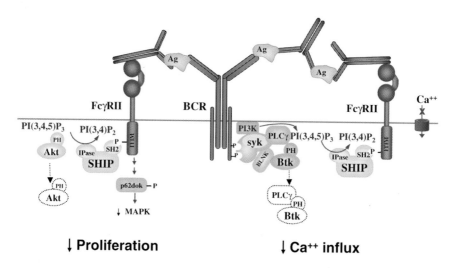

Figure 3 Signaling pathways triggered by BCR-FcγRII co-ligation. Cellular activation is inhibited by recruitment of the inositol phosphatase SHIP to the FcγR phosphorylated ITIM.

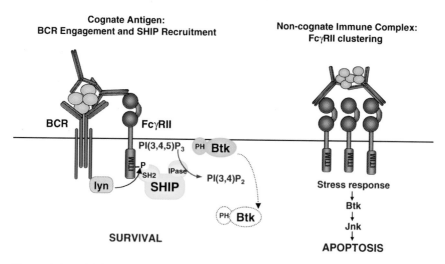

Figure 4 A model for the role of FcγRIIB in affinity maturation of germinal center B cells.

administration (54). Recent studies have attempted to define the molecular mechanisms behind these activities using defined mouse strains with mutations in activation or inhibitory FcRs. Direct effects on B cells stem from the ability of the inhibitory $Fc\gamma RIIB$ molecule to influence the state of B cell activation and survival by providing a means to discriminate between those rare somatically hypermutated germinal center B cells that have high-affinity cognate antigen binding from the predominant population with low-affinity and potentially cross-reactive specificities. Because antigen is retained in the form of immune complexes on follicular dendritic cells (FDC), it can interact with B cells either through $Fc\gamma RIIB$ alone, resulting in apoptosis, or by coengaging $Fc\gamma RIIB$ with BCR, favoring survival, as summarized in Figure 4. Support for a role of $Fc\gamma RIIB$ in the maintenance of peripheral tolerance comes from the observation that $Fc\gamma RIIB$-knockout mice on the C57Bl/6 background develop autoimmune disease in a B cell–autonomous manner (55). Those animals develop anti-DNA and antichromatin antibodies and then succumb to a fatal, autoimmune glomerulonephritis at 8 months of age. The phenotype is strain-dependent and is not seen in Balb/c or 129 strains of mice. $Fc\gamma RIIB$ thus acts as a genetic susceptibility factor for autoimmune disease, under the control of epistatic modifiers, to suppress the emergence of autoreactivity and maintain peripheral tolerance. Further support for this conclusion is provided by the observations that autoimmune strains of mice, like B/W F1, have reduced surface expression of $Fc\gamma RIIB$ attributed to DNA polymorphisms in the promoter region of the gene encoding this receptor (56, 57). This reduced expression of $Fc\gamma RIIB$ is thus suggested to contribute to the increased susceptibility of these animals to the development of autoantibodies and autoimmune disease.

If $Fc\gamma RIIB$ indeed functions in vivo to maintain peripheral tolerance, then its loss should allow for the emergence of autoantibodies when otherwise resistant animals are challenged with potentially cross-reactive antigens. This hypothesis has been validated in models of collagen-induced arthritis and Goodpasture's syndrome. $Fc\gamma RIIB$-deficient mice, on the nonpermissive $H-2^b$ haplotype, develop arthritis when immunized with bovine type II collagen (58). The loss of $Fc\gamma RIIB$ thus bypasses the requirement for the specific $H-2^{q,r}$ alleles previously demonstrated to be required in this model by allowing $Fc\gamma RIIB$-deficient autoreactive B cell clones to expand and produce pathogenic autoantibodies. When the permissive DBA/1 strain ($H-2^q$) is made deficient in $Fc\gamma RIIB$, autoantibody development is augmented and disease is greatly enhanced. In a similar manner, immunization of $H-2^b$ mice deficient in $Fc\gamma RIIB$ with bovine type IV collagen results in cross-reactive autoantibodies to murine type IV collagen, with dramatic pathogenic effects (59). These mice develop hemorrhagic lung disease and glomerulonephritis with a "ribbon deposition" pattern of immune complexes in the glomuli of affected animals. These characteristics are indicative of Goodpasture's syndrome, a human disease not previously modeled in an animal species.

Immune complexes can either enhance or suppress the humoral response depending on the kind of Fc receptor engaged and the cell type involved. Expression of the inhibitory FcγRIIB on B cells provides a mechanism for the suppressive effects of immune complexes on antibody production, particularly during the germinal center reaction when immune complexes retained on FDCs interact with somatically hypermutated B cells. The enhancing property of immune complexes on the afferent response is likely to arise from the expression of FcRs on antigen presenting cells, like dendritic cells (60–62). DCs express all three classes of IgG FcR. While in vitro studies have suggested that triggering of activation FcRs can induce DC maturation, the in vivo significance of this pathway has not been established (63). The ability of FcRs, particularly FcγRI, to internalize ICs could provide a mechanism for enhanced presentation and augmented antibody responses, while the presence of the inhibitory FcγRIIB molecule appears to reduce the enhancing effect (64, 65). Mice deficient in RIIB display enhanced antibody responses to soluble antibody-antigen complexes, in some cases dramatically so (66), which is likely to result from enhanced presentation. In addition, in vitro studies suggest that internalization through specific FcRs on APCs may influence the epitopes presented and T cell response generated as a result (63). At the present time there is a growing body of data to suggest that FcRs are indeed involved in enhancing the afferent response, by influencing antigen presentation and cognate T cell interactions. It is also possible that FcRs function on APCs in the establishment of tolerance by influencing the differentiation of DCs and their capacity to induce either anergy or T cell activation. The precise role of each Fc receptor expressed on APCs will require conditional knockouts of these molecules on specific DC populations to resolve the contribution of these systems to the generation of an appropriate antibody response.

FcRs IN THE EFFERENT RESPONSE

The first FcR knockout to be described was for the common activation subunit, the γ chain, required for surface assembly and signaling of FcγRI and FcγRIII as well as FcεRI (67). Mice deficient in the γ chain were systematically studied in diverse models of inflammation and found to be unable to mediate IgG-triggered inflammatory responses, attributed to the loss of the low-affinity activation receptor FcγRIII (67–73). This was further confirmed by the analysis of FcγRIII-deficient mice constructed by deletion of the receptor α-chain (74, 75). Subsequent studies on mice deficient in the inhibitory FcγRIIB molecule established the opposing action of this receptor, such that mice deficient in that receptor displayed enhanced B cell responses, autoimmunity, and augmented IgG-mediated inflammation (55, 58, 59, 71, 76–78). The general finding, discussed in detail below, illustrates that IgGs initiate their effector responses in vivo through coengagement of activating and inhibitory FcRs. The physiological response is thus the net of the opposing activation and inhibitory signaling pathways each receptor triggers and is determined by the level of expression of each receptor and the selective avidity of the IgG ligand.

TYPE I—IMMEDIATE HYPERSENSITIVITY

Both cutaneous and systemic models of passive anaphylaxis, induced by IgE, were studied in FcRγ chain–deficient mice and were found to be absent, fully consistent with the observations obtained in FcεRI–α chain deficient mice, confirming the role of the high-affinity IgE receptor in mediating IgE-induced anaphylactic responses (67, 79). FcγRIIB deficient mice, challenged in this model, displayed an unexpected enhancement of IgE-mediated anaphylaxis, suggesting a physiological interaction between this inhibitory receptor and FcεRI (80). The molecular basis for this modulation of FcεRI signaling by FcγRIIB has not been determined, although previous studies have indicated that IgE can bind with low affinity to FcγRII/III, suggesting a mechanism for coengagement of these receptors (81, 82). In addition to FcεRI, mast cells also express the IgG FcRs RIIB and RIII (82). Passive systemic anaphylaxis induced by IgG was attenuated in FcRγ chain–deficient and FcγRIII-deficient mice, indicating the capacity of IgG and FcγRIII to mediate mast cell activation in vivo (80, 83). FcγRIIB deficient mice were enhanced in IgG-induced anaphylaxis (76, 80). Surprisingly, active anaphylaxis, induced by immunization with antigen in alum, was enhanced in FcεRI-deficient mice and FcγRIIB-deficient mice and attenuated in FcRγ– and FcγRIII-deficient mice (83, 84). These animals all displayed antigen specific antibodies of both the IgE and IgG classes, indicating that the active anaphylaxis seen, which was FcγRIII dependent and FcεRI independent, was primarily attributed to IgG antibodies. The enhancement of anaphylactic responses in FcεRI animals resulted from the increased expression of FcγRIII on mast cells in these mice, normally limited by the availability of the common γ chain. In the absence of FcεRI α chain, FcRγ chain is available to associate with FcγRIII–α chain and assemble on the cell surface as a functional signaling receptor (84). These studies indicated the importance of the γ chain in regulating the level of surface expression of FcεRI and FcγRIII. Since γ chain is also associated with other members of the activation/inhibition paired receptors expressed on mast cells, such as PIRA/PIRB (85, 86), the intracellular competition between these diverse α subunits and the common γ chain will determine the level of surface expression of individual receptors and thus their ability to respond to specific biological stimuli. The absolute level of surface expression of FcRs on mast cells is clearly of therapeutic significance in both IgE- and IgG-mediated inflammatory responses; modulation of γ chain expression could thus represent a new therapeutic avenue for intervention in diseases like anaphylaxis and asthma.

TYPE II INFLAMMATION—CYTOTOXIC IgG

Cytotoxic IgGs are found in a variety of autoimmune disorders and have been developed for therapeutic indications in the treatment of infectious and neoplastic diseases. The mechanisms by which these antibodies trigger cytotoxicity in vivo have been investigated in FcR knockout mice. Anti-RBC antibodies trigger erythrophagocytosis of IgG opsonized RBCs in an FcR-dependent manner; γ chain–deficient mice were protected from the pathogenic effect of these antibodies, while complement C3 deficient mice were indistinguishable from wild-type animals in their ability to clear the targeted RBCs (69, 87, 88). FcγRIII plays the dominant role in this process for IgG1, 2a and 2b isotypes of antibodies; IgG3 antibodies were not pathogenic, consistent with its minimal engagement by FcRs. Experimental models of ITP, using mouse IgG2a antiplatelet antibodies to trigger thrombocytopenia, yielded similar results; FcRγ-deficient or FcγRIII-deficient mice were protected from the pathogenic activity of these antibodies, while C3-deficient mice were fully susceptible to antibody induced thrombocytopenia (87, 88). FcγRIIB-deficient mice were indistinguishable from wild-type animals in their ability to mediate anti-RBC or antiplatelet clearance, indicating that the specific effector cells involved in clearance were not expressing significant levels of this inhibitory receptor constitutively (89) (A Samuelsson, JV Ravetch, unpublished results). In other models of cytotoxic antibody responses, the dependence of activation FcRs was similar to the cases cited above. In a model of *Cryptococcus neoformans*-induced disease, passive immunization with mouse IgG1, 2a and 2b antibodies resulted in protection in wild-type, but not FcRγ chain– or FcγRIII-deficient animals; IgG3 antibodies enhanced disease in wild-type and FcR-deficient strains, again indicating that a distinct pathway, not requiring known FcγRs, is involved in IgG3 antibody–mediated internalization of this pathogen (90). While IgG3 antibodies have been reported to bind to FcγRI in vitro (91), the studies cited above indicate that different receptors are involved in vivo for IgG3 activity in this type of experimental system.

IgG antibodies raised to mouse glomerular basement membrane preparations induce acute glomerulonepthritis in wild-type, but not FcRγ– or FcγRIII-deficient animals (78, 92). FcγRIIB-deficient animals displayed enhanced disease in this model, indicating that the effector cells involved were constitutively expressing significant levels of FcγRIIB (78). Similar results were obtained when DBA/1 animals were immunized with bovine type II collagen to induce arthritis. Deficiency of FcRγ chain protected the mice from the pathogenic effects of the anticollagen antibodies generated in these mice (93). As mentioned above, deficiency of FcγRIIB in the DBA/1 CIA model resulted in enhanced disease, through increased autoantibody production and elevated effector responses (58).

A dramatic example of the importance of these pathways in determining the in vivo activity of cytotoxic antibodies was obtained in models of antitumor antibody response. In a syngenic murine model of metastatic melanoma, an IgG2a antimelanocyte antibody was able to reduce tumor metastasis in wild-type animals but was ineffective in FcRγ-deficient mice (94). In the absence of FcγRIIB, the activity of the antibody was enhanced 50-fold, indicating that the in vivo cytotoxic activity of the antibody was the net of activation and inhibitory receptor engagement (77). Identical results were obtained in xenograft models in nude mice, using human breast carcinoma or lymphoma lines and either murine IgG1 or humanized

IgG1 antibodies. A point mutation that eliminated FcR binding abolished the in vivo cytotoxic activity of the antibodies, while not affecting the in vitro growth inhibitory activity, again illustrating the difference between in vivo and in vitro mechanisms (77). The conclusions that can be drawn from these studies support a dominant role for FcγRIII in mediating cytotoxicity by IgG antibodies. FcγRIIB restricts the effector response in those situations where the effector cell expresses this inhibitory molecule. Through manipulation of IgG-Fc receptor interactions at either the receptor or antibody interface, cytotoxic antibodies can either be enhanced in their activity for therapeutic benefit in infectious and neoplastic disease or blocked in their ability to trigger effector responses as a means of treating IgG antibody mediated, organ-specific autoimmune diseases, or attenuating adverse side effects observed with some therapeutic antibodies. The availability of crystallographic data on these interactions will clearly guide the design of antibodies to optimize specific Fc-FcR interactions.

TYPE III RESPONSES—IMMUNE COMPLEX–MEDIATED INFLAMMATION

The classic example of this reaction, the Arthus reaction, has been studied in a variety of FcR and complement-deficient animals. The initial studies were performed using the cutaneous reverse passive Arthus reaction, in which antibody was injected intradermally and antigen given intravenously. An inflammatory response developed within 2 h, characterized by edema, hemorrhage, and neutrophil infiltration. This reaction was performed in a variety of complement-deficient and FcR-deficient animals (68, 87). The results from several independent studies confirmed the initial observations, that IgG immune complexes triggered cutaneous inflammatory reactions even in the absence of complement but displayed an absolute requirement for FcγRIII activation (75). FcγRIIB modulated the magnitude of the response, with enhanced Arthus reactions observed in FcγRIIB-deficient strains (76). The effector cell in the cutaneous reaction was determined to be the mast cell, as demonstrated by the use of mast cell–deficient strains and by mast cell reconstitution studies (95). The generality of this result was demonstrated in similar reactions performed in the lung, illustrating the FcR dependence and relative complement independence of this response (71). Thus, all studies have observed an absolute dependence on FcR expression in the Arthus reaction. However, some studies have reported partial attenuation of the Arthus reaction in mouse strains deficient in C3 and have suggested a synergistic involvement of both FcRs and early components of the complement cascade (96–98). It is more likely that the partial attenuation of the Arthus reaction reported in those studies is the result of IgM contamination in commercial IgG preparations of antibodies used or the effects of traumatic insult, two conditions in which complement has been demonstrated to be involved in effector cell activation. Deficiency in C5a or its receptor has also been reported to result in a partial reduction in the magnitude of the response in IC-induced lung inflammation (98). The conclusions consistent with these data on the Arthus reaction in the mouse is the strict requirement for the activation FcγRIII in initiating IgG immune complex inflammation, once again limited in its response by the expression of the inhibitory FcγRIIB. C5a activation may be a distal response to FcγRIII engagement in some specific models as one of downstream effector molecules involved in the later stages of the inflammatory response.

The significance of the FcR pathway in initiating immune complex inflammation in autoimmune disease was established by investigating a spontaneous murine model of lupus, the B/W F1 mouse. The Arthus reaction results predicted the absolute requirement of activation FcγR in initiating inflammation and tissue damage in immune complex diseases like lupus. The FcRγ chain deletion was backcrossed onto the NZB and NZW strains for eight generations and the intercrossed progeny were segregated into B/W FcR$\gamma^{-/-}$ and FcR$\gamma^{+/-}$. Anti-DNA antibodies and circulating immune complexes developed in all animals; immune complex and complement C3 deposition was similarly observed in all animals. However, mice deficient in the common γ chain showed no evidence of glomerulonephritis and had normal life expectancy, while mice heterozygous for the γ chain mutation developed glomerulonephritis and had reduced viability as has been described for B/W F1 animals (70). Reconstitution studies have confirmed that disease segregates with bone marrow derived cells expressing FcRγ, suggesting a model in which the IgG immune complexes deposited in the kidney triggered inflammation by FcR activation of bone marrow derived, circulating effector cells, most likely monocytes (RA Clynes, JV Ravetch, unpublished results). These results indicate that intervention in the effector stage of immune complex diseases, like lupus, would be accomplished by blocking FcγRIII activation to prevent initiation of effector cell responses. Early components of complement seem not to be required for initiating the inflammatory reponses, whereas later components like C5a may be downstream of FcR activation. Whether species selectivity exists favoring one pathway in rodents (FcRs) and another in humans (complement) remains to be determined, but such selectivity is unlikely given the conservation of both systems in a wide variety of species.

CONCLUSIONS

Receptors for the Fc portion of IgG play a significant role in vivo in maintaining peripheral tolerance by deleting autoreactive B cells, which can arise during somatic hypermutation in germinal centers, in augmenting T cell responses by enhancing antigen presentation by dendritic cells, and in mediating the coupling of antigen recognition to effector cell activation. Central to the correct functioning of these responses is the balance that is maintained through the pairing of activation and inhibitory receptors that coengage the IgG ligand; perturbations in either component result in pathological responses. Studies in mice deficient in individual

FcRs have provided the necessary insights for defining comparable activities in human autoimmune diseases and suggest ways in which manipulation of the Igg-FcR interaction may lead to new classes of therapeutics for the treatment of these diseases. Conversely, engineering of therapeutic antibodies targeted to eliminate infectious or neoplastic disease will likely benefit from optimization of their Fc domains for interaction with specific Fc receptors.

ACKNOWLEDGMENTS

The authors wish to acknowledge the support of the National Institutes of Health and the Nalitt Foundation.

Visit the Annual Reviews home page at www.annualReviews.org

LITERATURE CITED

1. Berken A, Benacerraf B. 1966. Properties of antibodies cytophilic for macrophages. *J. Exp. Med.* 123:119–44

2. Young JD, Ko SS, Cohn ZA. 1984. The increase in intracellular free calcium associated with IgG gamma 2b/gamma 1 Fc receptor-ligand interactions: role in phagocytosis. *Proc. Natl. Acad. Sci. USA* 81:5430–34

3. Anderson CL, Shen L, Eicher DM, Wewers MD, Gill JK. 1990. Phagocytosis mediated by three distinct Fc gamma receptor classes on human leukocytes. *J. Exp. Med.* 171:1333–45

4. Titus JA, Perez P, Kaubisch A, Garrido MA, Segal DM. 1987. Human K/natural killer cells targeted with hetero-cross-linked antibodies specifically lyse tumor cells in vitro and prevent tumor growth in vivo. *J. Immunol.* 139:3153–58

5. Chan PL, Sinclair NRSC. 1971. Regulation of the immune response: V. An analysis of the function of the Fc portion of antibody in suppression of an immune response with respect to interaction with components of the lymphoid system. *Immunology* 21:967–87

6. Phillips NE, Parker DC. 1983. Fc-dependent inhibition of mouse B cell activation by whole anti-mu antibodies. *J. Immunol.* 130:602–6

7. Ravetch JV, Luster AD, Weinshank R, Kochan J, Pavlovec A, Portnoy DA, Hulmes J, Pan YC, Unkeless JC. 1986. Structural heterogeneity and functional domains of murine immunoglobulin G Fc receptors. *Science* 234:718–25

8. Lewis VA, Koch T, Plutner H, Mellman I. 1986. A complementary DNA clone for a macrophage lymphocyte Fc receptor. *Nature* 324:372–75

9. Hogarth PM, Hibbs ML, Bonadonna L, Scott BM, Witort E, Pietersz GA, McKenzie IF. 1987. The mouse Fc receptor for IgG (Ly-17): molecular cloning and specificity. *Immunogenetics* 26:161–68

10. Brooks DG, Qiu WQ, Luster AD, Ravetch JV. 1989. Structure and expression of human IgG FcRII(CD32). Functional heterogeneity is encoded by the alternatively spliced products of multiple genes. *J. Exp. Med.* 170:1369–85

11. Hibbs ML, Bonadonna L, Scott BM, McKenzie IF, Hogarth PM. 1988. Molecular cloning of a human immunoglobulin G Fc receptor. *Proc. Natl. Acad. Sci. USA* 85:2240–44

12. Stengelin S, Stamenkovic I, Seed B. 1988. Isolation of cDNAs for two distinct human Fc receptors by ligand affinity cloning. *Embo J.* 7:1053–59

13. Stuart SG, Trounstine ML, Vaux DJ, Koch

T, Martens CL, Mellman I, Moore KW. 1987. Isolation and expression of cDNA clones encoding a human receptor for IgG (Fc gamma RII). *J. Exp. Med.* 166:1668–84

14. Perussia B, Tutt MM, Qiu WQ, Kuziel WA, Tucker PW, Trinchieri G, Bennett M, Ravetch JV, Kumar V. 1989. Murine natural killer cells express functional Fc gamma receptor II encoded by the Fc gamma R alpha gene. *J. Exp. Med.* 170:73–86

15. Maxwell KF, Powell MS, Hulett MD, Barton PA, McKenzie IF, Garrett TP, Hogarth PM. 1999. Crystal structure of the human leukocyte Fc receptor, Fc gammaRIIa. *Nat. Struct. Biol.* 6:437–42

16. Sondermann P, Huber R, Oosthuizen V, Jacob U. 2000. The 3.2-A crystal structure of the human IgG1 Fc fragment-Fc gammaRIII complex. *Nature* 406:267–73

17. Ravetch JV, Kinet JP. 1991. Fc receptors. *Annu. Rev. Immunol.* 9:457–92

18. Daeron M. 1997. Fc receptor biology. *Annu. Rev. Immunol.* 15:203–34

19. Bolland S, Ravetch JV. 1999. Inhibitory pathways triggered by ITIM-containing receptors. *Adv. Immunol.* 72:149–77

20. Hulett MD, Hogarth PM. 1994. Molecular basis of Fc receptor function. *Adv. Immunol.* 57:1–127

21. Jefferis R, Lund J, Pound JD. 1998. IgG-Fc-mediated effector functions: molecular definition of interaction sites for effector ligands and the role of glycosylation. *Immunol. Rev.* 163:59–76

22. Ghazizadeh S, Bolen JB, Fleit HB. 1994. Physical and functional association of Src-related protein tyrosine kinases with Fc gamma RII in monocytic THP-1 cells. *J. Biol. Chem.* 269:8878–84

23. Salcedo TW, Kurosaki T, Kanakaraj P, Ravetch JV, Perussia B. 1993. Physical and functional association of p56lck with Fc gamma RIIIA (CD16) in natural killer cells. *J. Exp. Med.* 177:1475–80

24. Agarwal A, Salem P, Robbins KC. 1993. Involvement of p72syk, a protein-tyrosine kinase, in Fc gamma receptor signaling. *J. Biol. Chem.* 268:15900–5

25. Cone JC, Lu Y, Trevillyan JM, Bjorndahl JM, Phillips CA. 1993. Association of the p56lck protein tyrosine kinase with the Fc gamma RIIIA/CD16 complex in human natural killer cells. *Eur. J. Immunol.* 23:2488–97

26. Crowley MT, Costello PS, Fitzer-Attas CJ, Turner M, Meng F, Lowell C, Tybulewicz VL, DeFranco AL. 1997. A critical role for Syk in signal transduction and phagocytosis mediated by Fcgamma receptors on macrophages. *J. Exp. Med.* 186:1027–39

27. Weiss A, Littman DR. 1994. Signal transduction by lymphocyte antigen receptors. *Cell* 76:263–74

28. Kurosaki T. 1999. Genetic analysis of B cell antigen receptor signaling. *Annu. Rev. Immunol.* 17:555–92

29. Salim K, Bottomley MJ, Querfurth E, Zvelebil MJ, Gout I, Scaife R, Margolis RL, Gigg R, Smith CI, Driscoll PC, Waterfield MD, Panayotou G. 1996. Distinct specificity in the recognition of phosphoinositides by the pleckstrin homology domains of dynamin and Bruton's tyrosine kinase. *Embo J.* 15:6241–50

30. Ferguson KM, Lemmon MA, Schlessinger J, Sigler PB. 1995. Structure of the high affinity complex of inositol trisphosphate with a phospholipase C pleckstrin homology domain. *Cell* 83:1037–46

31. Falasca M, Logan SK, Lehto VP, Baccante G, Lemmon MA, Schlessinger J. 1998. Activation of phospholipase C gamma by PI 3-kinase-induced PH domain-mediated membrane targeting. *Embo J.* 17:414–22

32. Kawakami Y, Yao L, Han W, Kawakami T. 1996. Tec family protein-tyrosine kinases and pleckstrin homology domains in mast cells. *Immunol. Lett.* 54:113–17

33. Bonilla FA, Fujita RM, Pivniouk VI, Chan AC, Geha RS. 2000. Adapter proteins SLP-76 and BLNK both are expressed

by murine macrophages and are linked to signaling via Fcgamma receptors I and II/III. *Proc. Natl. Acad. Sci. USA* 97:1725–30

34. Wang D, Feng J, Wen R, Marine JC, Sangster MY, Parganas E, Hoffmeyer A, Jackson CW, Cleveland JL, Murray PJ, Ihle JN. 2000. Phospholipase Cgamma2 is essential in the functions of B cell and several Fc receptors. *Immunity* 13:25–35

35. Weinshank RL, Luster AD, Ravetch JV. 1988. Function and regulation of a murine macrophage-specific IgG Fc receptor, Fc gamma R-alpha. *J. Exp. Med.* 167:1909–25

36. van de Winkel JG, Capel PJ. 1993. Human IgG Fc receptor heterogeneity: molecular aspects and clinical implications. *Immunol. Today.* 14:215–21

37. Unkeless JC, Jin J. 1997. Inhibitory receptors, ITIM sequences and phosphatases. *Curr. Opin. Immunol.* 9:338–43

38. Vivier E, Daeron M. 1997. Immunoreceptor tyrosine-based inhibition motifs. *Immunol. Today* 18:286–91

39. Lanier LL. 1998. NK cell receptors. *Annu. Rev. Immunol.* 16:359–93

40. Long EO. 1999. Regulation of immune responses through inhibitory receptors. *Annu. Rev. Immunol.* 17:875–904

41. Amigorena S, Bonnerot C, Drake JR, Choquet D, Hunziker W, Guillet JG, Webster P, Sautes C, Mellman I, Fridman WH. 1992. Cytoplasmic domain heterogeneity and functions of IgG Fc receptors in B lymphocytes. *Science* 256:1808–12

42. Muta T, Kurosaki T, Misulovin Z, Sanchez M, Nussenzweig MC, Ravetch JV. 1994. A 13-amino-acid motif in the cytoplasmic domain of Fc gamma RIIB modulates B-cell receptor signalling. *Nature* 368:70–73

43. Ono M, Bolland S, Tempst P, Ravetch JV. 1996. Role of the inositol phosphatase SHIP in negative regulation of the immune system by the receptor Fc-gamma-RIIB. *Nature* 383:263–66

44. Bolland S, Pearse RN, Kurosaki T, Ravetch JV. 1998. SHIP modulates immune receptor responses by regulating membrane association of Btk. *Immunity* 8:509–16

45. Scharenberg AM, El-Hillal O, Fruman DA, Beitz LO, Li Z, Lin S, Gout Cantley LC, Rawlings DJ, Kinet JP. 1998. Phosphatidylinositol-3,4,5-trisphosphate (PtdIns-3,4,5-P3)/Tec kinase-dependent calcium signaling pathway: a target for SHIP-mediated inhibitory signals. *EMBO J.* 17:1961–72

46. Liu Q, Sasaki T, Kozieradzki I, Wakeham A, Itie A, Dumont DJ, Penninger JM. 1999. SHIP is a negative regulator of growth factor receptor-mediated PKB/Akt activation and myeloid cell survival. *Genes Dev.* 13:786–91

47. Tamir I, Stolpa JC, Helgason CD, Nakamura K, Bruhns P, Daeron M, Cambier JC. 2000. The RasGAP-binding protein p62dok is a mediator of inhibitory FcgammaRIIB signals in B cells. *Immunity* 12:347–58

48. Yamanashi Y, Tamura T, Kanamori T, Yamane H, Nariuchi H, Yamamoto T, Baltimore D. 2000. Role of the rasGAP-associated docking protein p62(dok) in negative regulation of B cell receptor-mediated signaling. *Genes Dev.* 14:11–16

49. Aman MJ, Lamkin TD, Okada H, Kurosaki T, Ravichandran KS. 1998. The inositol phosphatase SHIP inhibits Akt/PKB activation in B cells. *J. Biol. Chem.* 273:33922–28

50. Daeron M, Latour S, Malbec O, Espinosa E, Pina P, Pasmans S, Fridman WH. 1995. The same tyrosine-based inhibition motif, in the intracytoplasmic domain of Fc gamma RIIB, regulates negatively BCR-, TCR-, and FcR-dependent cell activation. *Immunity* 3:635–46

51. Malbec O, Fong DC, Turner M, Tybulewicz VL, Cambier JC, Fridman WH, Daeron M. 1998. Fc epsilon receptor I-associated lyn-dependent phosphorylation of Fc gamma receptor IIB during

negative regulation of mast cell activation. *J. Immunol.* 160:1647–58

52. Ono M, Okada H, Bolland S, Yanagi S, Kurosaki T, Ravetch JV. 1997. Deletion of SHIP or SHP-1 reveals two distinct pathways for inhibitory signaling. *Cell* 90:293–301

53. Pearse RN, Kawabe T, Bolland S, Guinamard R, Kurosaki T, 1999. SHIP recruitment attenuates Fc gamma RIIB-induced B cell apoptosis. *Immunity* 10:753–60

54. Heyman B. 2000. Regulation of antibody responses via antibodies, complement, and Fc receptors. *Annu. Rev. Immunol.* 18:709–37

55. Bolland S, Ravetch JV. 2000. Spontaneous autoimmune disease in FcγRII deficient mice results from strain-specific epistasis. *Immunity* 13:277–85

56. Jiang Y, Hirose S, Abe M, Sanokawa-Akakura R, Ohtsuji M, Mi X, Li N, Xiu Y, Zhang D, Shirai J, Hamano Y, Fujii H, Shirai T. 2000. Polymorphisms in IgG Fc receptor IIB regulatory regions associated with autoimmune susceptibility. *Immunogenetics* 51:429–35

57. Pritchard NR, Cutler AJ, Uribe S, Chadban SJ, Morley BJ, Smith KG. 2000. Autoimmune-prone mice share a promoter haplotype associated with reduced expression and function of the Fc receptor FcgammaRII. *Curr. Biol.* 10:227–30

58. Yuasa T, Kubo S, Yoshino T, Ujike A, Matsumura K, Ono M, Ravetch JV, Takai T. 1999. Deletion of Fcgamma receptor IIB renders H-2(b) mice susceptible to collagen-induced arthritis. *J. Exp. Med.* 189:187–94

59. Nakamura A, Yuasa T, Ujike A, Ono M, Nukiwa T, Ravetch JV, Takai T. 2000. Fcgamma receptor IIB-deficient mice develop Goodpasture's syndrome upon immunization with type IV collagen: a novel murine model for autoimmune glomerular basement membrane disease. *J. Exp. Med.* 191:899–906

60. Banchereau J, Steinman RM. 1998. Dendritic cells and the control of immunity. *Nature* 392:245–52

61. Amigorena S, Bonnerot C. 1999. Fc receptor signaling and trafficking: a connection for antigen processing. *Immunol. Rev.* 172:279–84

62. Hamano Y, Arase H, Saisho H, Saito T. 2000. Immune complex and Fc receptor-mediated augmentation of antigen presentation for in vivo Th cell responses. *J. Immunol.* 164:6113–19

63. Regnault A, Lankar D, Lacabanne V, Rodriguez A, Thery C, Rescigno M, Saito T, Verbeek S, Bonnerot C, Ricciardi-Castagnoli P, Amigorena S. 1999. Fcgamma receptor-mediated induction of dendritic cell maturation and major histocompatibility complex class I-restricted antigen presentation after immune complex internalization. *J. Exp. Med.* 189:371–80

64. Minskoff SA, Matter K, Mellman I. 1998. Fc gamma RII-B1 regulates the presentation of B cell receptor-bound antigens. *J. Immunol.* 161:2079–83

65. Baiu DC, Prechl J, Tchorbanov A, Molina HD, Erdei A, Sulica A, Capel PJ, Hazenbos WL. 1999. Modulation of the humoral immune response by antibody-mediated antigen targeting to complement receptors and Fc receptors. *J. Immunol.* 162:3125–30

66. Wernersson S, Karlsson MC, Dahlstrom J, Mattsson R, Verbeek JS, Heyman B. 1999. IgG-mediated enhancement of antibody responses is low in Fc receptor gamma chain-deficient mice and increased in Fc gamma RII-deficient mice. *J. Immunol.* 163:618–22

67. Takai T, Li M, Sylvestre D, Clynes R, Ravetch JV. 1994. FcR gamma chain deletion results in pleiotrophic effector cell defects. *Cell* 76:519–29

68. Sylvestre DL, Ravetch JV. 1994. Fc receptors initiate the Arthus reaction: redefining the inflammatory cascade. *Science* 265:1095–98

69. Clynes R, Ravetch JV. 1995. Cytotoxic antibodies trigger inflammation through Fc receptors. *Immunity* 3:21–26

70. Clynes R, Dumitru C, Ravetch JV. 1998. Uncoupling of immune complex formation and kidney damage in autoimmune glomerulonephritis. *Science* 279:1052–54

71. Clynes R, Maizes JS, Guinamard R, Ono M, Takai T, Ravetch JV. 1999. Modulation of immune complex-induced inflammation in vivo by the coordinate expression of activation and inhibitory Fc receptors. *J. Exp. Med.* 189:179–85

72. Ravetch JV, Clynes RA. 1998. Divergent roles for Fc receptors and complement in vivo. *Annu. Rev. Immunol.* 16:421–32

73. Wakayama H, Hasegawa Y, Kawabe T, Hara T, Matsuo S, Mizuno M, Takai T, Kikutani H, Shimokata K. 2000. Abolition of anti-glomerular basement membrane antibody-mediated glomerulonephritis in FcRgamma-deficient mice. *Eur. J. Immunol.* 30:1182–90

74. Hazenbos WL, Heijnen IA, Meyer D, Hofhuis FM, Renardel de Lavalette CR, Schmidt RE, Capel PJ, van de Winkel JG, Gessner JE, van den Berg TK, Verbeek JS. 1998. Murine IgG1 complexes trigger immune effector functions predominantly via Fc gamma RIII (CD16). *J. Immunol.* 161:3026–32

75. Hazenbos WL, Gessner JE, Hofhuis FM, Kuipers H, Meyer D, Heijnen IA, Schmidt RE, Sandor M, Capel PJ, Daeron M, van de Winkel JG, Verbeek JS. 1996. Impaired IgG-dependent anaphylaxis and Arthus reaction in Fc gamma RIII (CD16) deficient mice. *Immunity* 5:181–88

76. Takai T, Ono M, Hikida M, Ohmori H, Ravetch JV. 1996. Augmented humoral and anaphylactic responses in Fc gamma RII-deficient mice. *Nature* 379:346–49

77. Clynes RA, Towers TL, Presta LG, Ravetch JV. 2000. Inhibitory Fc receptors modulate in vivo cytotoxicity against tumor targets. *Nat. Med.* 6:443–46

78. Suzuki Y, Shirato I, Okumura K, Ravetch JV, Takai T, Tomino Y, Ra C. 1998. Distinct contribution of Fc receptors and angiotensin II-dependent pathways in anti-GBM glomerulonephritis. *Kidney Int.* 54:1166–74

79. Dombrowicz D, Flamand V, Brigman KK, Koller BH, Kinet JP. 1993. Abolition of anaphylaxis by targeted disruption of the high affinity immunoglobulin E receptor alpha chain gene. *Cell* 75:969–76

80. Ujike A, Ishikawa Y, Ono M, Yuasa T, Yoshino T, Fukumoto M, Ravetch JV, Takai T. 1999. Modulation of immunoglobulin (Ig)E-mediated systemic anaphylaxis by low-affinity Fc receptors for IgG. *J. Exp. Med.* 189:1573–79

81. Bocek P Jr, Draberova L, Draber P, Pecht I. 1995. Characterization of Fc gamma receptors on rat mucosal mast cells using a mutant Fc epsilon RI-deficient rat basophilic leukemia line. *Eur. J. Immunol.* 25:2948–55

82. Takizawa F, Adamczewski M, Kinet JP. 1992. Identification of the low affinity receptor for immunoglobulin E on mouse mast cells and macrophages as Fc gamma RII and Fc gamma RIII. *J. Exp. Med.* 176:469–75

83. Miyajima I, Dombrowicz D, Martin TR, Ravetch JV, Kinet JP, Galli SJ. 1997. Systemic anaphylaxis in the mouse can be mediated largely through IgG1 and Fc gammaRIII. Assessment of the cardiopulmonary changes, mast cell degranulation, and death associated with active or IgE- or IgG1-dependent passive anaphylaxis. *J. Clin. Invest.* 99:901–14

84. Dombrowicz D, Flamand V, Miyajima I, Ravetch JV, Galli SJ, Kinet JP. 1997. Absence of Fc epsilonRI alpha chain results in upregulation of Fc gammaRIII-dependent mast cell degranulation and anaphylaxis. Evidence of competition between Fc epsilonRI and Fc gammaRIII for limiting amounts of FcR beta and gamma chains. *J. Clin. Invest.* 99:915–25

85. Kubagawa H, Chen CC, Ho LH, Shimada TS, Gartland L, Mashburn C, Uehara T, Ravetch JV, Cooper MD. 1999. Biochemical nature and cellular distribution of the paired immunoglobulin-like receptors, PIR-A and PIR-B. *J. Exp. Med.* 189:309–18

86. Maeda A, Kurosaki M, Kurosaki T. 1998. Paired immunoglobulin-like receptor (PIR)-A is involved in activating mast cells through its association with Fc receptor gamma chain. *J. Exp. Med.* 188:991–95

87. Sylvestre D, Clynes R, Ma M, Warren H, Carroll MC, Ravetch JV. 1996. Immunoglobulin G-mediated inflammatory responses develop normally in complement-deficient mice. *J. Exp. Med.* 184:2385–92

88. Fossati-Jimack L, Reininger L, Chicheportiche Y, Clynes R, Ravetch JV, Honjo T, Izui S. 1999. High pathogenic potential of low-affinity autoantibodies in experimental autoimmune hemolytic anemia. *J. Exp. Med.* 190:1689–96

89. Schiller C, Janssen-Graalfs I, Baumann U, Schwerter-Strumpf K, Izui S, Takai T, Schmidt RE, Gessner JE. 2000. Mouse FcgammaRII is a negative regulator of FcgammaRIII in IgG immune complex-triggered inflammation but not in autoantibody-induced hemolysis. *Eur. J. Immunol.* 30:481–90

90. Yuan R, Clynes R, Oh J, Ravetch JV, Scharff MD. 1998. Antibody-mediated modulation of Cryptococcus neoformans infection is dependent on distinct Fc receptor functions and IgG subclasses. *J. Exp. Med.* 187:641–48

91. Gavin AL, Barnes N, Dijstelbloem HM, Hogarth PM. 1998. Identification of the mouse IgG3 receptor: implications for antibody effector function at the interface between innate and adaptive immunity. *J. Immunol.* 160:20–23

92. Park SY, Ueda S, Ohno H, Hamano Y, Tanaka M, Shiratori T, Yamazaki T, Arase H, Arase N, Karasawa A, Sato S, Ledermann B, Kondo Y, Okumura K, Ra C, Saito T. 1998. Resistance of Fc receptor-deficient mice to fatal glomerulonephritis. *J. Clin. Invest.* 102:1229–38

93. Kleinau S, Martinsson P, Heyman B. 2000. Induction and suppression of collagen-induced arthritis is dependent on distinct fcgamma receptors. *J. Exp. Med.* 191:1611–16

94. Clynes R, Takechi Y, Moroi Y, Houghton A, Ravetch JV. 1998. Fc receptors are required in passive and active immunity to melanoma. *Proc. Natl. Acad. Sci. USA* 95:652–56

95. Sylvestre DL, Ravetch JV. 1996. A dominant role for mast cell Fc receptors in the Arthus reaction. *Immunity* 5:387–90

96. Hopken UE, Lu B, Gerard NP, Gerard C. 1997. Impaired inflammatory responses in the reverse arthus reaction through genetic deletion of the C5a receptor. *J. Exp. Med.* 186:749–56

97. Strachan AJ, Woodruff TM, Haaima G, Fairlie DP, Taylor SM. 2000. A new small molecule C5a receptor antagonist inhibits the reverse-passive Arthus reaction and endotoxic shock in rats. *J. Immunol.* 164:6560–65

98. Baumann U, Kohl J, Tschernig T, Schwerter-Strumpf K, Verbeek JS, Schmidt RE, Gessner JE. 2000. A codominant role of Fc gamma RI/III and C5aR in the reverse Arthus reaction. *J. Immunol.* 164:1065–70

Annu. Rev. Immunol. 2001. 19:291–330

REGULATION OF THE NATURAL KILLER CELL RECEPTOR REPERTOIRE

David H. Raulet, Russell E. Vance
and Christopher W. McMahon
*Department of Molecular and Cell Biology and Cancer Research Laboratory, University
of California, Berkeley, California 94720-3200; e-mail: raulet@uclink4.berkeley.edu*

Key Words inhibitory receptor, Ly49, KIR, CD94/NKG2, MHC

■ **Abstract** Natural killer cells express inhibitory receptors specific for MHC class I proteins and stimulatory receptors with diverse specificities. The MHC-specific receptors discriminate among different MHC class I alleles and are expressed in a variegated, overlapping fashion, such that each NK cell expresses several inhibitory and stimulatory receptors. Evidence suggests that individual developing NK cells initiate expression of inhibitory receptor genes in a sequential, cumulative, and stochastic fashion. Superimposed on the receptor acquisition process are multiple education mechanisms, which act to coordinate the stimulatory and inhibitory specificities of developing NK cells. One process influences the complement of receptors expressed by individual NK cells. Other mechanisms may prevent NK cell autoaggression even when the developing NK cell fails to express self-MHC-specific inhibitory receptors. Together, these mechanisms ensure a self-tolerant and maximally discriminating NK cell population. Like NK cells, a fraction of memory phenotype CD8[+] T cells, as well as other T cell subsets, express inhibitory class I–specific receptors in a variegated, overlapping fashion. The characteristics of these cells suggest that inhibitory receptor expression may be a response to prior antigenic stimulation as well as to poorly defined additional signals. A unifying hypothesis is that both NK cells and certain T cell subsets initiate expression of inhibitory receptors in response to stimulation.

INTRODUCTION

Natural killer (NK) cells are bone marrow–derived lymphocytes that were originally categorized by their large, granular morphology and their ability to lyse a variety of tumor targets and infected cells (1). In addition, NK cells can secrete potent levels of cytokines (especially IFN-γ and TNF-α) and chemokines (MIP-1 family members and RANTES) (for a review, see 2). In contrast to T and B cell responses to antigen, which typically require a proliferation phase, the innate NK cell response is immediate, implying that NK cells are involved in curbing pathogens during the initial several days of infection. Indeed, there is strong evidence that

0732-0582/01/0407-0291$14.00

NK cells contribute to the defense against intracellular bacteria (3) and parasites (4) and that they are critical for controlling several types of viral infection (2, 5). Despite the well-described antitumor activity of NK cells in vitro (6, 7) and in certain in vivo models (8), their role in the defense against spontaneous neoplastic transformation remains less well established.

NK cells do not require the specialized gene rearrangement machinery that assembles T and B cell antigen receptor genes (9). Nevertheless, NK cells exhibit a clear capacity to discriminate target cells. In the case of tumor cell targets, sensitivity to NK cells was correlated in many instances with decreased levels of MHC expression (10). NK cells are also able to reject MHC-different bone marrow grafts, especially in scenarios where the donor graft lacks MHC molecules of the host (for example, an MHC$^{a/b}$ host often rejects MHC$^{a/a}$ grafts) (11). These observations led to the formulation of the "missing self" hypothesis by Kärre and colleagues (12), which states that NK cells ignore potential targets expressing normal levels of autologous class I molecules and attack cells that do not. This view received strong support from studies with genetically engineered mice (13–16), which demonstrated that NK cells attack otherwise normal cells that lack some or all self-MHC class I molecules. The missing self hypothesis provided a satisfying rationale for NK cell function in vivo, since transformed and infected cells often downregulate or lose class I surface expression (17, 18). A molecular mechanism for missing self-recognition was established when several MHC class I–specific receptors were discovered that inhibit NK cell function (reviewed below).

Missing self-recognition is only one of several modes of NK cell–target cell discrimination. Under some conditions, NK cells attack even class I$^+$ tumor cells. As reviewed below, many stimulatory receptors on NK cells have been identified, some specific for ligands that are upregulated on tumor cells and stressed cells, and others apparently specific for ligands on normal cells. These disparate recognition systems can be understood in a model in which NK cells are regulated by the balance of signaling via stimulatory receptors, specific for diverse ligands, and inhibitory receptors, specific for MHC class I molecules.

Inhibitory Receptor Overview

The first inhibitory MHC-specific receptors to be discovered were the Ly49 receptors in rodents (19, 20), which bind directly to classical MHC class I (i.e. class Ia) molecules (21–26). More than 10 different Ly49 receptors have been identified in B6 mice, though just 8 of these are of the inhibitory type (27–29). Only a single nonfunctional Ly49-like gene has been identified in humans (30, 31). The second family discovered was the killer cell immunoglobulin-like receptors (KIR) family, which appears to be functional in primates but not rodents, and which also bind directly to class Ia molecules (32–37). Most people are estimated to have on the order of 10 different KIR genes, though not all of these are inhibitory (38–41). The third family is functional in both primates and rodents, and it consists of CD94/NKG2 heterodimers (42–45). Several NKG2 isoforms can pair with the CD94 "common"

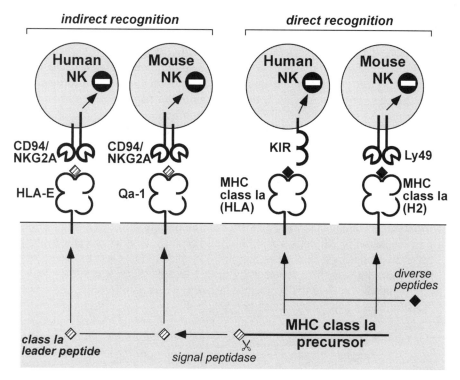

Figure 1 NK cells can detect self-MHC class Ia molecules directly or indirectly. In direct recognition (depicted on the right), MHC class I (class Ia) molecules are bound directly by NK receptors. In humans, these receptors are members of the killer cell immunoglobulin-like receptor (KIR) family, whereas Ly49 receptors fulfill a comparable role in mice. In indirect recognition (depicted on the left), NK cells recognize class Ia–derived leader peptides rather than mature MHC class Ia molecules themselves. The leader peptides are presented on the cell surface by a specialized nonclassical class I (class Ib) molecule called HLA-E (in humans) and Qa-1 (in mice), and the class Ib/leader peptide complex is bound by the heterodimeric CD94/NKG2A inhibitory receptor (present on human and murine NK cells). It should be noted that not all class Ia molecules contain a leader peptide that can be bound by HLA-E/Qa-1; moreover, not all class Ia molecules are directly recognized by KIR/Ly49 receptors.

chain; only CD94/NKG2A is known to be inhibitory. CD94/NKG2 receptors perceive class Ia molecules indirectly by specifically recognizing peptides processed from the leader sequences of class Ia molecules, bound into the groove of a nonclassical class Ib molecule, Qa-1 in mice (46) or HLA-E in humans (47–49) (see Figure 1). Direct and indirect recognition of class Ia molecules may serve complementary roles in inhibiting NK cells.

The two receptor families that recognize class Ia molecules directly, Ly49 receptors and KIR, are likely functionally analogous, even though the former are disulfide-linked homodimers bearing homology to type II C-type lectins, and the latter are type I monomeric Ig-like receptors. Significantly, all three receptor families exhibit the capacity to discriminate between different allelic class Ia isoforms. Individual Ly49 receptors (19, 24, 50) and KIR (51, 52) exhibit varying degrees of discrimination in reactivity to different class Ia molecules. The CD94/NKG2 receptors also effectively discriminate between different class Ia isoforms because some class Ia molecules do not contain the leader peptide recognized by these receptors (53, 54).

An important feature of all the inhibitory receptors is that each is expressed on a subset of NK cells that overlaps partially with the expression of other class I–specific inhibitory receptors. Thus, multiple receptors are usually expressed on each cell, and a complex combinatorial repertoire of NK specificities is generated. The *variegated* pattern of receptor expression allows individual NK cells to discriminate among cells expressing different class I molecules. For example, a host cell that downregulates only one MHC class I molecule will elicit a strong response by the subset of NK cells whose only self-specific inhibitory receptor recognizes that particular molecule. Cells that have completely lost class I expression will be even more sensitive to attack by most NK cells. Studies of tumor cells and virus-infected cells have documented instances where both selective and complete loss of class I expression occurs (17, 55).

The variegated pattern of receptor expression suggests a stochastic mechanism in the choice of which receptor genes are expressed by each NK cell. The stochastic pattern of expression applies to Ly49 receptors in mice (56) and KIR in humans (57, 58), despite their structural dissimilarities, as well as to the NKG2 subunits of the shared CD94/NKG2 receptors (46, 58, 59). The expression, or not, of the various receptor subunits in NK cell subpopulations is evident at the level of mRNA as well (60, 61), suggesting differential transcriptional control of receptor gene expression. Receptor variegation poses interesting questions as to how expression of receptor genes is initiated and maintained in individual NK cells.

All three of the families of inhibitory receptors signal through motifs in their cytoplasmic domains, called immunoreceptor tyrosine-based inhibitory motifs (ITIM) (62). Upon receptor engagement, ITIM are tyrosine-phosphorylated and recruit protein tyrosine phosphatases such as SHP-1 and possibly SHP-2 (63–67). Since inhibition is apparent at early activation steps such as calcium mobilization (68), the phosphatases probably interfere in an early step of NK cell stimulation pathways.

Stimulatory Receptor Overview

For many years, the characterization of stimulatory receptors on NK cells lagged behind that of inhibitory NK receptors, and during this time it was widely thought that generic adhesion or costimulatory molecules, such as LFA-1, might be responsible for most NK activation (69). However, accumulating evidence reviewed in this volume of *Annual Review of Immunology* by Moretta et al implicates numerous stimulatory receptors in various NK-target interactions.

Stimulatory receptors on NK cells can be broadly divided into those that recognize MHC class I–like ligands and those that do not. Ligands for many receptors in the latter class remain unknown, but some examples of stimulatory ligands for NK cells are MICA/B, Rae1, and H60 (which bind to NKG2D) (70–72), cell bound IgG (which binds to the $Fc\gamma R$), and CD48 (which binds to 2B4 and CD2) (73). Interestingly, if interactions between MHC molecules and receptors on NK cells are prevented, NK cells will attack normal autologous lymphoblasts (15, 16, 74), a fact suggesting that some stimulatory receptors on NK cells react with non-MHC ligands expressed by normal cells. Candidate receptors for such reactions include NKp30, NKp44, and NKp46 receptors (75), as well as the NK1.1 antigen (NKR-P1C) (76). Where tested, most of the non-MHC-specific stimulatory receptors are expressed by most if not all NK cells (72, 75, 77–79), presumably allowing individual NK cells to respond to numerous insults.

Strikingly, MHC class I–specific stimulatory receptors are found within each of the three families of class I–specific receptors. The KIR contain the stimulatory KIR2DS and KIR3DS, the NKG2 family contains the stimulatory NKG2C and E receptors (42, 80), and the Ly49 family contains stimulatory Ly49D and Ly49H receptors (though a class I specificity for Ly49H has yet to be assigned) (81–84).

The MHC class I–specific stimulatory receptors, unlike most non-MHC-specific stimulatory receptors, are expressed in a variegated and possibly stochastic fashion on subsets of NK cells (58, 81, 84). Expression of these stimulatory receptors overlaps with expression of class I–specific inhibitory receptors such that stimulatory and inhibitory receptors of the same class I–specificity are often not expressed by the same NK cell. A beneficial consequence of this expression pattern is that a target cell that has lost an inhibitory class I allele while retaining a stimulatory class I allele would become highly sensitive to attack. In general, class I–specific stimulatory receptors tend to recognize their class I ligands with lower affinity than do their inhibitory counterparts (85, 86). Although the significance of this observation remains uncertain, an intriguing speculation is that class I–specific stimulatory receptors may function preferentially when class I levels are high, as may occur in some viral infections due to the local release of interferons. Alternatively, it is possible that the stimulatory isoforms are in some sense pathogen-specific. For example, their purpose may be (or may have been) to detect (and therefore counter) decoy class I homologs (18) that viruses produce for the purpose of inhibiting NK cells. Or, class I–specific stimulatory receptors may recognize specific complexes of self-MHC bound to viral or tumor antigen-derived epitopes.

NK stimulatory receptors generally associate with small transmembrane adapter proteins that transmit activation signals, including KARAP/DAP12 (87, 88), $CD3\zeta$, $FcR\gamma$ (89), and DAP10/KAP10 (90, 91). It is thought that each of these adapters is expressed by all NK cells but associates only with a distinct subset of the stimulatory receptors. NK cells from mice or humans with mutations in one of these genes, KARAP/DAP12, exhibit only a subtle phenotype and can still attack most NK target cells (92, 93). These data confirm the idea that NK cell activation is multifactorial and does not rely on a single signaling adapter.

NK Cell Education

Although a stochastic mechanism appears to underlie the initial expression of inhibitory receptor genes, the final functional repertoire of NK receptor expression is shaped by education processes based on the MHC class I alleles that happen to be expressed by the host. The education processes are still poorly understood, but their ultimate effects are to ensure a repertoire of NK cells that is both self-tolerant and useful. The education process must take into account both the inhibitory and stimulatory receptors that individual NK cells express.

Here we review the present understanding of the NK repertoire, including, (a) the mechanisms that initiate and maintain expression of inhibitory NK cell receptors, generating a diverse repertoire of specificities; (b) the self-tolerant state of NK cells and the evidence for the involvement of various mechanisms in imposing self-tolerance; (c) the evidence that education mechanisms maximize the discriminatory properties of the repertoire; and (d) the similarities and differences between the repertoires of NK cell inhibitory receptors expressed by NK cells versus T cells.

INITIATION AND MAINTENANCE OF RECEPTOR EXPRESSION

Stochastic Expression of Receptor Genes

All three MHC-specific NK receptor families are expressed in a variegated, overlapping fashion. The frequency of NK cells co-expressing a given combination of receptors can usually be well estimated as the product of the frequencies of NK cells expressing each receptor (the "product rule") (56, 58), suggesting that different receptor genes are expressed with a substantial degree of independence. Independent receptor gene expression is consistent with stochastic initiation of receptor gene expression in individual developing NK cells.

While the product rule provides a good estimate for most combinations of Ly49 genes or KIR genes (56, 58, 61), deviations have been noted (84), especially in the co-expression of inhibitory with stimulatory Ly49 receptors. Some combinations of inhibitory Ly49 genes also show minor deviations (T Hanke and DH Raulet, unpublished data). In addition, NK cells co-expressing CD94/NKG2A with certain KIR were underrepresented in panels of human NK clones (58). Similarly, murine NK cells co-expressing CD94/NKG2A and certain Ly49 receptors were marginally underrepresented among murine NK cells (46, 84, 94).

Deviations from the product rule are expected, since education mechanisms exist to adjust the repertoire based on the available MHC molecules, which would be expected to skew the repertoire from a random pattern (95). Moreover, certain receptor genes may exhibit commonalities in regulation, which could also result in preferential co-expression. For example, recent data indicate that the transcription factor TCF-1 may control expression of Ly49A and Ly49D but have little or no role in the expression of other Ly49 genes (96).

To the extent that it has been examined in mice and humans, it appears that the NK repertoire contains cells expressing virtually every possible set of receptors. With estimates that each NK cell can express anywhere from three to seven class I–specific receptors (58, 61), the maximum number of receptor combinations in the repertoire, or its complexity, can be approximated. Humans and mice, each with approximately 10 different inhibitory MHC-specific receptors, possess approximately 1000 different types of NK cells expressing different receptor combinations[1]. It is possible, of course, that many of these combinations would not be found in a given individual, depending on the outcome of the education processes.

Monoallelic Expression of NK Receptor Genes

Ly49 genes exhibit sequence polymorphisms that have made it possible to discriminate expression of two Ly49 alleles at the same locus in Ly49 heterozygous mice. Such analyses have revealed the striking fact that Ly49 genes are expressed in a largely monoallelic fashion (60, 97, 98). That is, most NK cells in a Ly49 heterozygote that express a given Ly49 receptor express either the maternal or the paternal allele of the gene, but not both. This applies to all Ly49 genes examined, including Ly49A, Ly49G2, and Ly49C. Where examined, a smaller, but significant, population of NK cells co-expresses both alleles. Preliminary evidence indicates that the NKG2A inhibitory NK receptor gene is also expressed in a predominantly monoallelic fashion (94). It has not yet been tested whether the KIR genes are expressed in a monoallelic fashion. Monoallelic gene expression had been previously demonstrated in the case of olfactory receptor genes (99) and was subsequently reported for several cytokine genes (100–103). In the case of the cytokine genes, co-expression of both alleles occurs in a fraction of cells, similar to the pattern observed for the Ly49 genes. It is attractive to speculate that monoallelic expression is characteristic of genes encoding molecules that must be expressed in a variegated fashion in order to generate a repertoire of specificities or functions within a given class of cells.

Why are Ly49 genes expressed in a monoallelic fashion? One possibility is that allelic versions of Ly49 receptors typically differ in specificity. Monoallelic expression would then ensure that many NK cells express only one of the specificities. Although some allelic versions of Ly49 receptors may differ in specificity, no such difference was observed for Ly49C alleles, the only case yet examined comprehensively (24). An alternative perspective is that monoallelic expression of NK receptors serves no function per se but is rather the outcome of the specialized

---

[1]There are 120 ways that an NK cell could express 3 different inhibitory receptors from a pool of 10 receptors. In addition, there are 210 ways that an NK cell could express four of 10 receptors. Similarly, there are 252, 210, and 120 ways that an NK cell could express 5, 6, or 7 receptors from the pool of 10. Thus, there are total of $120 + 210 + 252 + 210 + 120 = 912$ possible cell types in a repertoire of NK cells expressing 3 to 7 receptors from a pool of 10 receptors.

mechanism for selecting a random subset of NK receptor genes for expression in individual NK cells (56, 60). Indeed, data suggest that this mechanism acts locally to stably regulate *cis*-acting control sequences associated with each Ly49 allele, independent of neighboring Ly49 genes or of the Ly49 allele on the opposite chromosome. For example, the fraction of NK cells that co-expresses both Ly49 alleles of a given Ly49 gene roughly approximates (albeit in some cases exceeds) the product rule estimates derived by multiplying the frequencies of NK cells expressing each allele (97, 98) (DM Tanamachi, T Hanke, DH Raulet, unpublished results). These findings suggest that the two Ly49A alleles in a cell are expressed with some independence, presumably because they are chosen for expression by the same stochastic mechanism that selects different Ly49 loci for expression. Furthermore, the choice of a given receptor allele for expression does not influence which allele is expressed at a second Ly49 locus nearby (60). For example, in the case of NK cells that co-express Ly49A and Ly49G2, there is an approximately equal likelihood that the two expressed Ly49 genes will be on the same or different chromosomes (98) (DM Tanamachi, T Hanke, DH Raulet, unpublished results).

The mechanisms that underlie random allelic expression of Ly49 genes are not known. One possibility is that *trans*-acting factors necessary to stably initiate (or possibly repress) Ly49 gene expression are limiting during a stage or stages when the gene expression pattern is established. The factors might be limiting in the sense that only a few are available per cell. Or, they may be limiting in a kinetic sense, such that there is only a modest probability that the factors will succeed in binding the regulatory elements of a given Ly49 allele within a limited time period. One candidate for such a factor is the transcription factor TCF-1. In heterozygous TCF-1$^{+/-}$ mice, only half as many NK cells expressed Ly49A as in wild-type TCF-1$^{+/+}$ mice (96). Since halving the TCF-1 gene dosage lowered the frequency of Ly49A$^+$ NK cells, it was plausibly suggested that TCF-1 represents a limiting factor for Ly49A gene expression.

Maintenance of Receptor Gene Expression

The preponderance of evidence suggests that once an NK receptor gene is successfully activated, its expression is stably maintained in the cell, even as it undergoes multiple rounds of proliferation. In the human system, long-term NK clones sustain expression of specific KIR and CD94/NKG2 receptors for many cell generations (57). In mice, sorted populations expressing specific Ly49 receptors maintain receptor expression for at least 10 days after transfer to irradiated recipient mice in vivo (104), and for at least 1–2 weeks of in vitro expansion in IL-2 (19). NK cells expressing CD94/NKG2 receptors maintained expression after transfer in vivo (105). In addition, NK cells from Ly49A heterozygous mice, sorted for expression of one of the two Ly49A alleles, maintained expression of that allele after expansion in culture (97) (DM Tanamachi, T Hanke, DH Raulet, unpublished results). These data argue for stable receptor expression, although they cannot rule out the possibility that NK cells extinguish receptor expression under certain circumstances in vivo.

Ontogeny of Receptor Gene Expression

Little is known concerning the ontogeny of NK receptor expression in humans. Some data indicate that CD94 and KIR are already expressed by NK cells in the human fetal liver (106) (L Lanier, personal communication).

With one possible exception (107), Ly49 receptors are initially expressed after birth in mice (104, 108), and the proportion of NK cells expressing each Ly49 receptor increases gradually over the first several weeks of life. In contrast, most murine NK cells express CD94/NKG2A at birth (61, 105, 108). Since the CD94/NKG2A receptor is reactive with all known MHC haplotypes, it has been proposed that this receptor prevents most neonatal and prenatal NK cells from attacking self-cells (105, 108). After birth, the proportion of CD94/NKG2A$^+$ NK cells gradually decreases to approximately 50% in the adult. Evidence suggested that the decrease in CD94/NKG2A$^+$ NK cells is not due to loss of the receptor from cells that already expressed it (105). One possibility is that progenitor cells in the adult initiate expression of the NKG2A gene in a variegated fashion, while neonatal and prenatal progenitor cells initiate expression in all cells.

Conditions Inducing Receptor Expression

Several studies have investigated the stimuli that promote receptor expression using in vitro models of NK cell development. Human progenitor cells cultured in vitro with cytokines, particularly IL-15, developed into NK cells, many of which expressed CD94/NKG2A receptors (106, 109, 110). Little or no KIR expression was induced in these cultures, suggesting that additional signals are required for initiation of KIR expression.

Similarly, CD94/NKG2A receptors were expressed by murine NK cells differentiating in vitro under the influence of cytokines (111; see also 112). No initiation of Ly49 gene expression occurred in these cultures. The initiation of Ly49 expression required additional undefined signals from stromal cells, since efficient Ly49 receptor expression occurred when NK cells developed in cultures containing both cytokines and bone marrow stromal cells or the OP9 stromal cell line (113, 114).

Developmentally Ordered Expression of Ly49 Receptor Genes

Evidence suggests that Ly49 receptors are expressed sequentially in a cumulative fashion during development. For example, cells with the NK phenotype (NK1.1$^+$CD3$^-$), but lacking expression of most Ly49 receptors, can initiate expression of Ly49 receptors on a fraction of cells after transfer to host mice (104, 105) or after culture in vitro on bone marrow stromal cells in the presence of cytokines (114). Furthermore, a fraction of NK cells expressing Ly49A or Ly49G2 can initiate expression of additional Ly49 receptors after transfer in vivo (104) or culture in vitro (114), while maintaining expression of Ly49A or Ly49G2, respectively.

Several studies suggest that there are restraints on the order in which different Ly49 receptors can be expressed during development. The first indication was that transferred Ly49A$^-$NK1.1$^+$ cells never initiate expression of Ly49A, either in vitro or in vivo, but do initiate expression of Ly49G2, Ly49C/I, and Ly49F on a fraction of cells (104, 114). Since Ly49A$^+$ NK cells arose in these experiments when NK1.1$^-$ lymphoid-restricted progenitor cells were employed, it was proposed that commitment to express Ly49A precedes acquisition of the NK1.1 marker, while commitment to express the other receptors can occur after NK1.1 expression. Moreover, Ly49G2$^+$NK1.1$^+$ cells were able to initiate expression of Ly49C/I genes, but not Ly49A, while Ly49A$^+$ NK cells were able to initiate expression of both Ly49G2 and Ly49C/I genes. These data are consistent with at least two models. In one, the capacity to activate Ly49 genes progresses in a sequence, e.g. Ly49A only → Ly49G2 only → Ly49C/I, etc. In the other model, all Ly49 genes are initially available for activation, and the capacity to activate some genes is lost before others, e.g. Ly49A/G2/C/I → Ly49G2/C/I → Ly49C/I. In both models, only a fraction of cells at each stage actually succeed in activating a relevant gene.

Another study was in accord that Ly49 gene expression occurs in an ordered fashion but differed as to the order (115). In this study, early NK-committed progenitors were precultured in cytokines and subsequently cloned at limiting dilution on stromal layers in the presence of cytokines. As determined by RT-PCR of RNA from clones at various days thereafter, Ly49G2 was expressed first, followed by Ly49C/I, and finally by Ly49A. The two studies are in fact not necessarily contradictory because the former study addresses the timing of commitment to express different Ly49 genes, while the latter study addresses the order in which the genes are actually expressed. The relative timing of commitment versus actual expression may vary for different Ly49 genes. Alternatively, the discrepant results may reflect differences in the experimental protocols used or the precursor cells tested.

NK CELL SELF-TOLERANCE

Tolerance to MHC-Identical Cells

That NK cells can mediate alloreactivity was first recognized in studies of bone marrow graft rejection by irradiated mice (11, 116). Many instances of bone marrow graft rejection by NK cells can be attributed to the absence on the graft of MHC molecules present in the host. For example, D8 mice, which are B6 (H-2^b) mice that transgenically express D^d as a self-antigen, reject B6 bone marrow grafts that lack D^d (13). This type of missing self recognition can also account, at least in part, for the rejection of fully MHC-different cells by NK cells. NK cells in H-2^d mice reject H-2^b bone marrow cells, H-2^d NK cells lyse H-2^b target cells in vitro, and human peripheral blood NK cells can often lyse allogeneic PHA blasts in vitro. It should also be noted that NK cells in B6 mice reject D8 bone marrow (13), indicating that in some instances NK cells can also positively recognize the presence of allogeneic MHC molecules. The latter reaction was recently attributed to an interaction between the stimulatory Ly49D receptor and the D^d class I molecule (117).

While NK cells often attack MHC-different target cells, they exhibit tolerance to MHC-identical target cells. The self-tolerance of NK cells is clearly a property that is acquired in the host, as opposed to being directly inherited. This is implicit in the fact that there is no obvious genetic mechanism to coordinate the inheritance of receptor genes that confer MHC specificity and the MHC genes themselves, which are on a different chromosome. In fact, the alloreactivity of NK cells cannot be attributed to inheritance of specific sets of receptor genes per se, since MHC congenic mice such as B10 and B10.D2 have the same NK receptor genes (20), yet exhibit mutual NK alloreactivity in vivo (118).

NK Cell Tolerance in Class I–Deficient Mice

The control of NK cell self-tolerance by MHC molecules is also evident in studies of MHC class I–deficient mice. In perhaps the clearest example of missing-self recognition, NK cells from normal mice attack bone marrow cells or lymphoblasts from class I–deficient mice (14–16). Interestingly, however, class I–deficient $\beta2m^{-/-}$ gene targeted mice exhibit no evidence of autoimmunity and do not reject class I–deficient cells (14). An identical phenotype is observed in other class I–deficient mouse models including $TAP^{-/-}$ (119), double mutant $TAP^{-/-}\beta2m^{-/-}$ (120), and double mutant $K^{b-/-}D^{b-/-}$ (121, 122) mice. Similarly, NK cells from TAP-deficient humans also exhibit reduced activity against class I–deficient target cells (123). The results as a whole indicate that self-tolerance can occur in the complete absence of ligands for any of the known MHC class I–specific receptors. Class I–deficient mice contain normal (15) or even elevated (122) numbers of NK cells, indicating that self-tolerance in these mice does not result from wholesale NK cell deletion, nor does it reflect the failure of NK cells to develop.

Cell Types Mediating Self-Tolerance of NK Cells

Developing NK cells are exposed to neighboring hematopoietic cells as well as various nonhematopoietic stromal cells during development in the bone marrow. Experiments utilizing bone marrow or fetal liver chimeras suggest that encounters with both types of cells contribute to self-tolerance. The presence of class I$^-$ hematopoietic cells in the chimeras, even when the host was class I$^+$, was sufficient to dominantly induce at least a partial state of tolerance as tested by subsequently challenging the mice with class I$^-$ bone marrow grafts (16, 124). The presence of nonhematopoietic class I$^-$ host cells had an even more substantial effect, inducing nearly complete tolerance (124). These data indicate that encounters with either hematopoietic or nonhematopoietic class I$^-$ cells can induce tolerance, with the latter cells playing a possibly larger role. Similar results were seen in other experimental systems (125, 126). In one set of experiments using mosaic mice that express D^d as a transgene on only a fraction of cells, as few as 10% D^d-negative H-2^b cells dominantly induced tolerance to H-2^b cells, despite the presence of neighboring D^{d+} cells (126).

The dominant activity of ligand-negative cells in inducing tolerance is significant because it rules out a simple positive selection model of NK cell education. In this model, encounters of NK cells expressing self-reactive inhibitory receptors with ligand-positive cells promote the survival or functional maturation of NK cells, whereas encounters with ligand-negative cells have no effect. The data do not rule out positive selection per se but do indicate that this cannot be the sole mechanism of tolerance induction.

Reversal of Self-Tolerance

A variety of data indicate that self-tolerance of NK cells can be broken in some instances by culturing the cells in high doses of IL-2 (125–127). In one study, NK cells from the D^d-transgenic mosaic mice described above were separated into those that expressed D^d and those that did not, and both populations were cultured in IL-2 for a short period. Within one day of separation, the D^{d+} fraction rapidly acquired the capacity to lyse B6 (H-2^b) target cells, suggesting that tolerance in this system is rapidly reversible (126). An earlier study showed that NK cells from F1 into parent bone marrow chimeras establish tolerance to grafts from the parental host, but that this tolerance was broken after culturing chimeric cells in IL-2 (125). Finally, a recent study showed that culture for four days in IL-2 reverses the self-tolerant state of NK cells from class I–deficient mice (127). The physiological significance of data obtained by culturing cells in abnormally high doses of IL-2 is open to question. The results are significant, however, because they raise a question as to the nature of a tolerant state that can be so rapidly reversed. Significantly, while IL-2 reversed tolerance in each of the experimental models discussed above, it had less (128, 129) or no (126, 130) effect in reversing self-tolerance of NK cells from normal mice. As is discussed below, one possible explanation is that culture in IL-2 reverses self-tolerance of only a fraction of NK cells in normal mice.

The "At Least One" Hypothesis

While there is general agreement that the self-tolerance of NK cells is imposed by a developmental process, the mechanisms involved are still poorly understood. One attractive hypothesis that has been discussed widely in the literature is that the formation of the NK cell repertoire is regulated such that every NK cell in a given individual expresses "at least one" inhibitory receptor specific for one or another self-MHC class I molecule. A process that equips every NK cell with a self-specific receptor would not only account for self-tolerance, it would also maximize the number of useful NK cells, i.e. those that can attack autologous cells that have downregulated class I molecules.

Evidence in favor of the at-least-one theory came from an analysis of panels of human NK clones from two individuals. Each NK clone derived from a given donor expressed at least one known inhibitory receptor specific for one of the donor's class I MHC molecules, and each clone was inhibited from lysing self-target cells (58). One caveat of the study was that it did not conclusively demonstrate that all of the NK cells originally resident in the donors expressed self-specific receptors. If NK cells exist that do not express self-specific receptors, they may be difficult to grow continuously in culture and so cannot be cloned.

The at-least-one hypothesis suggests that MHC genes should impact the frequencies of freshly isolated NK cells expressing different inhibitory receptors. Such alterations are well documented in mice, where MHC-congenic and MHC-deficient strains can be examined (131, 132), though it has not been shown that all murine NK cells express a self-specific receptor. In contrast, MHC-dependent alterations in KIR expression by freshly isolated human NK cell populations have not been detected (133). While considerable differences in repertoire between individuals were observed, no obvious correlation with MHC allotypes was discerned. Nor was there evidence that the levels of KIR or CD94/NKG2 receptors at the cell surface are affected by the MHC allotype of the host. The failure to observe such correlations in humans is difficult to interpret, since the effects of MHC allotypic differences may be obscured by variability in non-MHC genes and possibly by environmental factors.

In the murine system, some evidence suggests that NK cells with self-MHC-specific inhibitory receptors contribute preferentially to the NK cell pool, a prediction of the at-least-one hypothesis. This evidence was obtained with a transgene that directs expression of Ly49A (specific for $H-2^d$) in all developing NK cells. Bone marrow cells from transgenic and wild-type mice, both $H-2^d$, were mixed and inoculated in irradiated $H-2^d$ recipients. The resulting transgenic lymphocytes contained a marginally higher ratio of NK cells to B cells compared to nontransgenic lymphocytes in the same chimeras, or compared to transgenic or nontransgenic lymphocytes in similar mixed chimeras prepared in the $H-2^b$ background (134). The authors concluded that engagement of Ly49A on NK cells enhanced the survival of the cells, their proliferation, or the pace of their development. Another report indicated that NK cells expressing a self-MHC-specific stimulatory receptor (Ly49D in $H-2^d$ mice) usually co-expressed an $H-2^d$-specific inhibitory receptor (135). A caveat of this finding is that since most Ly49 receptors are $H-2^d$-specific, most Ly49D$^+$ NK cells co-express $H-2^d$-specific inhibitory receptors even in $H-2^b$ mice.

Intriguing though these data are, other evidence in the murine system suggests that not all NK cells express self-specific inhibitory receptors. For example, the only known receptors with a clearly defined specificity for $H-2^b$ class Ia molecules are Ly49C, Ly49I, and CD94/NKG2A. Analyses performed by single cell RT-PCR (61) or by staining NK cells with antibodies and/or tetramers against all of these receptors (59, 94) suggest that approximately 25% of NK cells in B6 (H-2^b) mice do not express any of the known H-2^b-specific receptors. The important caveat remains that other as-yet-undiscovered H-2^b-specific inhibitory receptors may exist. There is no evidence, however, that NK cells lacking Ly49C, I, and NKG2A in H-2^b mice are inhibited by self-MHC class I molecules, suggesting that they do not express novel H-2^b-specific inhibitory receptors (RE Vance, DH Raulet, unpublished data). In conclusion, attractive as the "at least one" hypothesis is, some new data raise doubts about its validity, at least in mice.

Modulation of Cell Surface Ly49 Receptors: Role in Self-Tolerance

It is well established that the cell surface levels of Ly49 receptors are downmodulated by interactions with self-class I molecules. Ly49A, Ly49C, and Ly49G2 are all expressed at lower levels (two to tenfold) in mice that express cognate MHC ligands (130, 131,136–138). It has been proposed that the downmodulation of Ly49 receptors in the presence of the ligand is part of a process that calibrates the reactivity of NK cells with self-MHC ligands (139). The term "calibration" was initially coined to refer to receptor downmodulation but is sometimes broadened to include MHC-dependent changes in the sizes of different Ly49-expressing subsets (see below for discussion of this phenomenon). As is discussed below, however, the two phenomena are mechanistically unrelated and are probably unrelated in their functional role. Here, use of the term calibration refers solely to changes in receptor cell surface levels.

In a common representation of the calibration model, it is proposed that receptor cell surface levels vary so as to create an optimal balance between inhibition and stimulation, such that the resulting NK cell is poised at the brink of reactivity. This would have the related effects of contributing to the establishment of self-tolerance and ensuring the maximal sensitivity of each NK cell to even minor alterations in target cell MHC levels. The idea that alterations in cell surface Ly49 levels calibrate NK cell specificity assumes that such changes demonstrably alter NK cell specificity, and it implies that such changes should tend toward an optimal level. Since the KIR (133) and CD94/NKG2 receptors (RE Vance, DH Raulet, unpublished data) have not been generally observed to undergo downmodulation in the presence of MHC ligands, this form of receptor calibration presumably does not apply to these receptors.

To address whether changes in Ly49 cell surface levels alter NK cell sensitivity to class I ligands, NK cells from MHC-different mice were compared. These NK cells express different levels of Ly49 receptors. NK cells expressing high Ly49 levels were more readily inhibited by target cell class I molecules (121, 140). It is plausible that the functional differences in these studies were due to altered cell surface levels of Ly49 receptors, but other causes were not ruled out. For example, the NK cells compared are expected to differ in the number of different Ly49 receptors expressed (see below), which could also alter the sensitivity of the cell to class I–mediated inhibition. Another possibility is that the differences in sensitivity reflect stable alterations in stimulatory receptor pathways.

While receptor levels may impact the sensitivity of NK cells to class I inhibition, some evidence suggests that Ly49 cell surface levels do not tend toward an optimum level. Using Ly49A transgenic mice, it was observed that the cell surface expression of a Ly49A transgene, like that of the endogenous Ly49A gene, was downmodulated in H-2^d mice, which (unlike H-2^b mice) contain a ligand for Ly49A (141, 142). A Ly49A transgenic mouse that expressed "normal" levels of Ly49A in the H-2^b background was compared to a Ly49A transgenic that expressed threefold lower levels of Ly49A. When the transgenes were crossed into an H-2^d background, both the high- and low-expressing lines exhibited a threefold reduction in levels of cell-surface Ly49A, due to the presence of H-2^d (141). These data suggested that Ly49 downmodulation is a generic response to ligand engagement and does not tend toward an optimal setpoint. Moreover, Ly49 receptor levels are not a stable property of mature NK cells. Thus, transfer of mature NK cells from mice lacking a Ly49A ligand to mice expressing the D^d ligand resulted in a very rapid downmodulation of Ly49A (143).

A likely possibility is that Ly49 downmodulation reflects the rapid internalization of receptor after ligand-engagement, as occurs with many other receptors. Consistent with this hypothesis, receptor downmodulation is independent of transcription (141). Moreover, MHC-dependent downmodulation of transgenically expressed Ly49A was clearly apparent in cells that normally do not express the receptor, such as B cells (DM Tanamachi, DH Raulet, unpublished data). These findings suggest that modulation of receptor levels can occur independently of NK cell development and is not a consequence of it. Of course, tolerance-inducing mechanisms would need to take into account any alteration in the sensitivity of NK cells to MHC ligands that resulted from receptor modulation.

Self-Tolerance of NK Cells Lacking Self-MHC-Specific Inhibitory Receptors

As already discussed, class I–deficient mice contain normal numbers of NK cells that are not autoaggressive, arguing that NK cells need not express self-MHC-specific receptors to achieve self-tolerance (15). As mentioned, evidence suggests that normal mice may also contain a class of NK cells that do not express self-MHC-specific receptors. An important finding is that several effector functions are impaired in NK cells from class I–deficient mice, compared to those of normal mice. Equally significant is that the impairment is not absolute. For example, NK cells from class I–deficient mice exhibited reduced but not absent antibody-dependent cellular cytotoxicity (ADCC) (120) and reverse-ADCC (redirected lysis) (M-F Wu, DH Raulet, unpublished data) activities. In addition, NK cells from class I–deficient mice usually exhibited a reduced capacity to attack YAC-1 tumor target cells, though this phenotype is variable and was not observed in all experiments (15, 16, 121). The picture that emerges is that NK cells from class I–deficient mice are essentially devoid of activity against class I–deficient normal cells, and they exhibit reduced functional activity in several other assays. NK cells with defects in components of the inhibitory signaling pathway, such as the SHP-1 tyrosine phosphatase, may also acquire a hyporesponsive phenotype (144). Thus, hyporesponsiveness may result either from the absence of class I ligands or from impaired signaling by class I–specific inhibitory receptors.

As discussed above, NK cells from class I–deficient mice cultured in high doses of IL-2 attain the capacity to lyse autologous lymphoblasts, indicating that these conditions reverse the hyporesponsive state (127). In contrast, similar cultures of unseparated NK cells from class I^+ mice are less affected (126, 128–130), and cultures of sorted NK cells expressing known self-specific inhibitory receptors retain the self-tolerant state (129, 130, 145). These findings are consistent with the notion that NK cells in normal mice are a mixture of two types of cells, those that express self-MHC-specific inhibitory receptors and those that lack self-MHC-specific receptors and are hyporesponsive. Presumably, culture in IL-2 reverses self-tolerance of only the latter set.

At least three general models can be considered for the self-tolerance of NK cells from class I–deficient mice. One model proposes that stimulatory signal transduction pathways, or even the stimulatory receptors themselves, may be downregulated or dampened in NK cells that have never encountered cognate class I ligands (120, 121). While at least some stimulatory receptors such as NKR-P1C (NK1.1 antigen, (15)) and Ly49D (T Hanke, DH Raulet, unpublished data) are expressed at normal levels on NK cells in class I–deficient mice, this may not be true for other stimulatory receptors or for relevant signaling molecules. A second related model is that the inhibitory signal transduction pathway may exhibit a basal level of activity even in the absence of ligands; stable elevation of this basal activity in the NK cells that develop in class I–deficient mice could swing the balance in favor of nonresponsiveness. A third model is that NK cells can express undiscovered inhibitory receptors specific for unidentified non-MHC ligands (120). Such receptors may be preferentially expressed by NK cells that have never encountered class I ligands, accounting for the failure of these cells to attack normal class I–deficient target cells.

MECHANISMS TO MINIMIZE RECEPTOR CO-EXPRESSION MAXIMIZE NK CELL FUNCTIONALITY

Several lines of evidence indicate that the receptor repertoire of NK cells, in terms of the frequencies of NK cells expressing different receptors, is impacted by MHC class I molecules expressed by the host. For example, in $\beta 2m^{-/-}$, $TAP^{-/-}$, or $\beta 2m^{-/-}TAP^{-/-}$ mice, the frequencies of NK cells expressing each of several Ly49 receptors were marginally higher, and the frequencies of NK cells co-expressing various receptor pairs or trios were substantially higher (120, 131, 132) as compared to class I$^+$ mice. Thus, the most pronounced effect of MHC class I expression is in limiting the extent of Ly49 receptor overlap.

It is important to emphasize that the alterations in frequencies of Ly49-defined NK cell subsets discussed here are accomplished by a completely different mechanism than the previously discussed alterations in cell surface Ly49 levels. Receptor cell surface levels adapt very rapidly to the presence of cognate ligands and are controlled by a posttranscriptional process. In contrast, receptor expression per se is controlled at the level of mRNA (97, 98, 141), presumably transcription, and appears to be a stable developmentally regulated property of NK cells.

Studies with Ly49 transgenic mice suggested that the effect of MHC molecules on the Ly49 repertoire is to limit the number of NK cells co-expressing multiple Ly49 receptors specific for self-MHC. A transgene encoding the Ly49A receptor was expressed early in the developmental pathway in all NK cells. The transgene had no effect on the endogenous repertoire in mice that lacks ligands for Ly49A. In H-2^d mice, which express the D^d Ly49A ligand, the transgene caused a substantial reduction in the frequency of NK cells expressing Ly49G2, endogenous Ly49A (141), and some other Ly49 receptors (T Hanke, DH Raulet, unpublished data). Recent experiments demonstrate that a Ly49G2 transgene exerts a similar effect on the expression of endogenous Ly49 receptors (T Hanke, DH Raulet, unpublished data). Thus, expression of one receptor specific for self-MHC reduces the probability that other self-specific receptors will be expressed.

Similar conclusions were obtained in in vitro experiments using a clonogenic system for NK cell development. When Ly49A transgenic NK precursors differentiated on class I–deficient bone marrow stromal cell layers, most of the resulting clones contained Ly49G2$^+$ NK cells. When the same precursors differentiated on H-2^d stromal cells (displaying a Ly49A ligand), many fewer clones contained Ly49G2$^+$ NK cells (114). These data suggest that during NK cell development, Ly49 interactions with MHC molecules on stromal cells act to minimize co-expression of self-specific Ly49 receptors.

Why should the co-expression of multiple self-MHC-specific receptors by NK cells be disfavored? An attractive possibility is based on the finding that MHC class I loss events are often selective, in that cells may lose one class Ia molecule and not another. For example, HIV-infected cells reportedly downregulate HLA-A and HLA-B molecules, but not HLA-C molecules (55). Rather than downregulating all class I expression, tumor cells often extinguish expression of just one or another class Ia gene, or even one or another class Ia allele in the case of MHC heterozygotes (17). NK cells that co-express receptors specific for different self–class I molecules may be unable to attack self-cells that have lost just one. Minimizing co-expression of self-specific receptors could also maximize the sensitivity of NK cells to small changes in the cell surface levels of host cell class I molecules.

At least two mechanistic models can account for the restricted co-expression of self-MHC-specific receptors by NK cells. In a selection model, NK cells that express "too many" self-MHC-specific receptors would die or fail to proliferate.

An alternative, adaptive model was suggested by the finding that NK cells acquire expression of Ly49 receptors in a sequential and cumulative fashion. It was proposed that this process is regulated by Ly49–class I interactions (56). If an NK cell expresses only nonself class I–specific receptors, it is free to activate additional receptor genes. If it expresses a sufficient number of self-MHC-specific receptors, however, subsequent rounds of receptor gene initiation would be inhibited. For example, in the Ly49A transgenic mice, engagement of the transgenic receptor inhibits subsequent initiation of other NK receptor genes, such as Ly49G2. This "regulated-sequential" model predicts that early engagement of Ly49 receptors, as in the Ly49A transgenic H-2^d mice, will inhibit expression of both self-specific and nonself-specific Ly49 receptors. The selection model predicts that only cells expressing self-specific endogenous receptors will be affected (95). Consistent with the regulated-sequential model, data indicate that utilization of both self-specific and nonself-specific receptors is diminished in the Ly49A transgenic mice (T Hanke and DH Raulet, unpublished data).

INTEGRATION OF STIMULATORY AND INHIBITORY SIGNALING IN NK CELL DEVELOPMENT

Since class I–deficient but otherwise normal cells are sensitive to NK cells, some stimulatory ligands must be constitutively expressed by at least some normal cells. Furthermore, certain class I–specific stimulatory receptors (e.g. KIR2DS, KIR3DS, Ly49D, CD94/NKG2C) are expressed in a variegated fashion by different NK cell subsets. Thus, depending on which stimulatory receptors are expressed, and whether the host animal happens to express ligands for MHC-specific receptors, the summed autostimulation received by individual NK cells is expected to vary. These considerations lead to the question: How are the stimulatory and inhibitory signals that emanate from self-cells integrated to ensure self-tolerance of individual NK cells?

Coordination of stimulatory and inhibitory signals can be easily accounted for in a selection model of NK cell tolerance, assuming that selection is delayed until after the cell has initiated expression of all relevant receptors. When the NK cell eventually interacts with self "selecting cells," the outcome of selection (i.e. cell death, survival, and/or proliferation) would be determined by the balance of stimulatory and inhibitory signaling that the NK cell receives. However, as discussed above, several lines of evidence suggest that NK cell tolerance is, at least in part, an adaptive process.

How could stimulatory and inhibitory signaling be balanced in an adaptive process? Several mechanisms can be envisaged: (a) One possibility is that the first receptors expressed by developing NK cells are stimulatory receptors. At this stage, the cells would presumably be immature and nonlytic. The engagement of self-ligands by these stimulatory receptors would then transmit signals that induce the de novo expression of inhibitory receptors, which are expressed in a sequential and cumulative fashion. When the cell eventually expresses one or more self-MHC-specific inhibitory receptors of sufficient strength to overcome the stimulatory signal, induction of additional receptors would be inhibited. At this point, the NK cell could mature fully by upregulating its sensitivity to stimulatory ligands. In encounters with self-cells, however, inhibition would just counteract stimulation, preventing autoaggression. (*b*) A converse mechanism is that NK cells express inhibitory receptors before they express stimulatory receptors. NK cells would then be permitted to initiate expression of stimulatory receptor genes to match the level of inhibition provided by the inhibitory receptors. (*c*) In a third model, these mechanisms may be combined. NK cells would ratchet up their stimulatory and inhibitory receptors in concert, such that the expression of an inhibitory receptor stimulates the expression of a stimulatory receptor, which in turn stimulates the expression of another inhibitory receptor. (*d*) A fourth model balances not the number or strength of each type of expressed receptor, but the efficiency of the relevant signal transduction pathway. Depending on the number and strength of inhibitory and stimulatory receptors expressed by each NK cell, the efficiency of the stimulatory and/or inhibitory signal transducing pathways could be stably adjusted to come into balance. Only then would the NK cell mature.

The available data does not allow these possibilities to be readily discriminated. It is unclear, for example, whether stimulatory or inhibitory receptors are generally expressed in a specific order relative to each other in NK cell development. A recent ontogenic analysis shows that the stimulatory Ly49D and Ly49H receptors are expressed on NK cells at about the same time after birth, or just slightly delayed, compared to the inhibitory receptors (84). Since new precursors are continuously differentiating, however, the ontogenic pattern does not necessarily reflect the order in which receptors are expressed on individual developing NK cells. It also remains possible that some stimulatory receptors, for example those specific for non-MHC ligands, are expressed early in the differentiation process, whereas the MHC-specific stimulatory receptors are expressed later. Consistent with the idea that some stimulatory receptors are expressed early in ontogeny, if not in development, fetal NK cells exhibit lytic activity against tumor targets (107, 146). Moreover, Fc receptors and the NKR-P1C stimulatory receptor are both expressed early in NK cell ontogeny (147, 148).

Some evidence supports the conclusion that stimulatory signals induce the expression of inhibitory receptors on developing NK cells. Mice deficient in the *src*-family tyrosine kinase *fyn* tend to express fewer inhibitory Ly49 receptors than do *fyn*-positive mice (W Held, personal communication). Since the *fyn* kinase is involved in lymphocyte activation, as opposed to inhibition, one interpretation of the data is that stimulatory signals promote de novo expression of inhibitory receptors. The data are also consistent with a selection model, in which developing NK cells that receive excess stimulation are selected against. If stimulatory signaling is partly impaired, more NK cells with fewer inhibitory receptors would survive the selection process.

THE INHIBITORY RECEPTOR REPERTOIRE EXPRESSED BY T CELLS

Although the inhibitory MHC class I-specific receptors are often described as NK receptors, each type is also expressed by fractions of various T cell subsets. Unlike NK cells, relatively few human and mouse T cells express these receptors. The role of the inhibitory receptors in the immune response of T cells has not been clearly established. A comparison of NK cells and T cells in terms of their repertoire of inhibitory receptors is nevertheless worthwhile, as it may hint at the underlying shared mechanisms in repertoire formation and function.

Phenotype of T Cells Expressing Inhibitory Class I–Specific Receptors

Individual KIR and CD94 receptors are normally expressed by up to 5% of peripheral blood T cells (149–154). Although CD4 T cells with KIR could be detected and cloned (150), the vast majority of KIR$^+$ T cells are CD8$^+$CD4$^-$ cytotoxic T lymphocytes (CTL). A corresponding population has been described in mice. Approximately 10% of murine CD8$^+$TCR$\alpha\beta^+$ T cells express at least one of the inhibitory Ly49 receptors, while expression of these receptors on conventional CD4 T cells is very rare (155, 156). A significant proportion of the CD8$^+$ Ly49$^+$ T cells also express other NK markers, including CD94/NKG2A, NKR-P1C, and the DX5 antigen (155, 156) (CW McMahon, RE Vance, DH Raulet, unpublished data).

NK receptor expression is also prominent in several nonconventional T cell populations: TCR$\gamma\delta$ T cells, intraepithelial lymphocytes, and the CD1d-restricted T cells often called NK T cells. In adult humans, the majority of peripheral $\gamma\delta$ T cells bear Vγ9Vδ2 TCR that recognize nonpeptide phosphoantigens in an MHC-independent manner. The various KIR are expressed by 1%–20% of circulating Vγ9Vδ2 T cells, and the CD94/NKG2A receptor is expressed by about 80% of Vγ9Vδ2 cells (157–161). CD1d-restricted T cells are a unique population of CD4$^-$CD8$^-$ or CD4$^+$CD8$^-$ TCR$\alpha\beta^+$ T cells in mice and humans that recognize lipid antigens presented by the nonclassical class I molecule CD1d (162). In mice, these cells usually express NKR-P1C and often express Ly49 family members. Notably, however, KIR was rarely expressed in a panel of human CD1d-restricted T cell lines, although NKR-P1A was expressed on essentially all such cells (163). It remains to be established whether human CD1d-restricted T cells in vivo express KIR.

In general, T cells that express inhibitory class I–specific receptors exhibit the phenotypic markers of memory T cells. In humans, KIR$^+$ CTL bear surface markers indicative of previous activation (CD45RO, CD29, CD44, CD18, CD57), and they lack markers for naïve T cells (CD45RA) (152). Likewise, murine Ly49$^+$ CTL express Ly6C and CD122 (IL-2Rβ) and are CD44^{hi} (156). Many of these memory markers are also expressed on KIR$^+$ $\gamma\delta$ T cells, CD1d-restricted T cells, and NK cells, suggesting that prior and/or chronic activation may underlie inhibitory receptor expression by these cells.

Specificity of T Cells Expressing Inhibitory Receptors

Inhibitory receptors cannot be detected on the majority of human CTL clones, but KIR$^+$ and CD94/NKG2A$^+$ CTL specific for HIV or melanoma antigens have been documented (164–169). Interestingly, many of the KIR$^+$ T cells in humans are present as expanded oligoclonal populations (152). Oligoclonal CD8$^+$ T cell populations have been proposed to represent T cells responsive to persistent antigens or self-antigens (170). In mice, by contrast, the CD8$^+$Ly49$^+$ population is apparently not oligoclonal, since it exhibits a near normal TCR Vβ distribution and is fairly consistent in size in individual animals of a given strain (156, 171). The mice studied, however, were somewhat younger than the age when oligoclonal CD8$^+$ T cell populations typically become detectable in mice (172). Whether oligoclonal murine CD8$^+$ T cell expansions express Ly49 receptors has not been reported, and it remains unclear whether the CD8$^+$Ly49$^+$ and CD8$^+$KIR$^+$ populations are strictly analogous.

It is perhaps significant that the nonconventional T cell subsets that express inhibitory receptors are thought to be specific for self-antigens. These include the Vγ9Vδ2 population, specific for self-phospho-antigens, and the TCR$\alpha\beta^+$ CD1d-restricted T cells, specific for lipid antigens presented by CD1d. Notably, only some Vγ9Vδ2 T cell clones were found to be overtly self-reactive, as defined by the capacity to lyse class I–deficient Daudi cells; the Daudi-reactive clones were much more likely to express CD94/NKG2A receptors than were clones that didn't lyse Daudi targets (158). These findings raise the possibility that inhibitory receptors on T cells may function in some cases to prevent uncontrolled autoreactivity, which is consistent with the proposal that inhibitory receptor expression by T cells is generally a response to persistent antigenic stimulation.

Function of Inhibitory Receptors on T Cells

Several methods have been used to demonstrate that class I–specific inhibitory receptors can functionally inhibit both cytolysis and cytokine secretion by human TCR$\alpha\beta^+$ and TCR$\gamma\delta^+$ CTL clones (149, 150, 158, 159, 165, 166, 168, 173–177). For more detailed reviews, see (178, 179). All of these studies utilized CTL clones (or in some cases, cultured lines), and whether freshly isolated cells behave in a similar manner remains to be determined.

In mice, studies with Ly49-transgenic mice indicate that these NK receptors can inhibit alloantigen-induced and antiviral responses by conventional T cells (24, 180, 181). However, CTL that naturally express Ly49 receptors appear to be less sensitive to inhibition, as Ly49 expressed on CTL isolated from normal mice was found to inhibit only early activation events, but not target cell killing or cytokine release (156). Likewise, TCR-mediated stimulation of Jurkat T cells transfected with Ly49G2 (182) and primed CTL from mice expressing a KIR transgene (183) did not appear to be attenuated by inhibitory receptor cross-linking. It is not clear whether the failure to observe strong inhibition in the latter experiments reflects the relatively low cell surface level of Ly49 receptors on T cells, the use of nonphysiological T cell triggering assays, or a difference in the relevant signal transduction pathways between naïve T cells and memory T cells. There is evidence that murine CD1d-restricted T cells can be inhibited via Ly49 engagement, as antigen-independent target lysis by NK1.1$^+$ Ly49$^+$ T cells cultured from the liver is reduced by Ly49 cross-linking (155).

Stage at Which Inhibitory Receptors Are Expressed by T Cells

Much evidence suggests that expression of inhibitory receptors by T cells typically occurs during or after activation of fully mature T cells. One indication, as previously noted, is that T cells that express inhibitory class I–specific receptors bear surface markers indicative of previous activation. In addition, recently matured conventional CD4$^+$ and CD8$^+$ T cells in the thymus do not express inhibitory receptors, nor do cord blood T lymphocytes from newborn humans (152, 153) or T cells with a naïve phenotype in the periphery of adult mice or humans (156). Additional evidence with fetal liver chimeric mice demonstrated that Ly49 receptor expression by CD8$^+$ T cells is dependent on expression of class I molecules by hematopoietic cells, suggesting that inhibitory receptor expression requires class I antigen presentation (156). Furthermore, in TCR transgenic mice raised in the absence of antigen, T cells expressing the TCR transgene were notably devoid of Ly49 receptors (156). It is more difficult to establish the stage at which inhibitory receptor expression occurs on CD1d-restricted T cells or Vγ9Vδ2 T cells, but it is perhaps telling that both types of cells are responsive to self-antigens and exhibit a memory or activated phenotype. Together, the data suggest that upregulation of inhibitory receptors occurs only after encounter with antigen, at least with respect to CD8$^+$ T cells, and possibly more generally.

In the case of the CD94/NKG2A receptor, upregulation on mature T cells has been demonstrated directly. Both IL-15 and TGF-β induce CD94/NKG2A expression on a large fraction of human CD8 T cells undergoing antigenic stimulation in vitro (109, 184). Interestingly, KIR are upregulated very poorly under the same conditions. In mice the CD94/NKG2A receptor is expressed on essentially all in vitro–stimulated CD8$^+$ T cells, T cell clones, and LCMV-specific CTL isolated from mice at the peak of infection (AJ Zajac, CW McMahon, R Ahmed, DH Raulet, unpublished data). Little Ly49 expression is observed under any of these conditions. These data suggest that CD94/NKG2A receptors can be expressed rapidly by mature CD8$^+$ T cells of any specificity, whereas expression of Ly49 and KIR is limited to special conditions or antigen specificities.

Stability and Overlap of Inhibitory Receptor Expression by T Cells

Little direct analysis has been done of the stability of KIR or Ly49 expression by T cells, though KIR$^+$ clones and sorted cells reportedly maintain receptor expression in culture (57, 185). In one study, it was observed that fewer

TABLE 1   Overlapping expression of Ly49 family members on murine CD8$^+$ CTL[a]

	Ly49G2 [7.2, 61.0][b]		Ly49C/I [3.2, 27.1]		Ly49F [8.7, 73.7]	
	% of CD8$^+$	% of Ly49$^+$CD8$^+$	% of CD8$^+$	% of Ly49$^+$CD8$^+$	% of CD8$^+$	% of Ly49$^+$CD8$^+$
LY49A [3.7, 31.3]	2.4[c] (0.27)[d]	20.3 (19.1)	0.7 (0.12)	5.9 (8.5)	2.6[c] (0.32)[d]	22.0 (23.1)
LY49G2 [7.2, 61.0]			1.3 (0.23)	11.0 (16.5)	4.9 (0.63)	41.5 (45.0)
LY49C,I [3.2, 27.1]					1.8 (0.28)	15.3 (20.1)

[a]Analysis by three color staining of nylon wool passed splenocytes pooled from three B6 mice, using JR9-318 (Ly49A), 4D11 (Ly49G2), SW5E6 (Ly49C and I), and HBF-719 (Ly49F) mAbs. Unpublished data of CW McMahon and DH Raulet.

[b]The numbers in brackets refer to cells expressing the indicated Ly49 as a percentage of CD8$^+$ T cells (first number) or of Ly49$^+$ CD8$^+$ T cells (second number). Ly49$^+$ CD8$^+$ cells are defined as the CD8$^+$ population that stains with a mixture of all the Ly49 mAbs listed (and therefore expresses one or more Ly49 receptors).

[c]Percentage of cells that co-express the two indicated Ly49 family members.

[d]Percentage of cells predicted by the product rule to co-express the two indicated Ly49 receptors.

CD1d-restricted NK1.1$^+$ T cells in the liver express Ly49 receptors compared to those in the thymus (186). The authors proposed that Ly49 expression is extinguished on many of the thymic CD1d-restricted T cells before or shortly after they migrate to the liver. It has not been ruled out, however, that the liver is populated by a selected set of thymic CD1d-restricted T cells, which is relatively deficient in Ly49$^+$ cells. The stability of CD94/NKG2A expression was investigated in mice that had cleared an LCMV infection months earlier. Although most of the cells still expressed detectable CD94/NKG2, the cell surface levels were substantially lower than at the peak of the response (AJ Zajac, CW McMahon, R Ahmed, DH Raulet, unpublished data). Whether activated CD8$^+$ T cells ever completely extinguish CD94/NKG2A expression is uncertain.

T cells, like NK cells, express inhibitory receptors in a variegated fashion, with extensive overlap in the expression of different receptors. The frequencies of human T cells expressing each KIR varies, and individual KIR$^+$ T cells often co-express additional KIR, ILT2/LIR-1, or CD94/NKG2 receptors (151–153, 169). Similar variegated overlapping expression of Ly49 receptors can also be observed on murine CD8$^+$ T cells (Table 1). On the other hand, some intriguing differences were noted between the pattern of receptor expression in NK cells and T cells. First, some receptors are expressed at different relative frequencies in the two populations. For example, Ly49F is one of the least frequently expressed inhibitory receptors among murine NK cells, but it is the most commonly expressed receptor among CD8$^+$ T cells (156) (Table 1). Furthermore, in mice, the stimulatory Ly49 isoforms (Ly49D and Ly49H) cannot be detected on CTL (84, 155, 156); however, human T cells reportedly do express stimulatory KIR (149, 154, 187). Second, as a fraction of all CD8$^+$ T cells, or even of memory (CD44^{hi}) CD8$^+$ T cells, the frequencies of cells co-expressing pairs of Ly49 receptors are higher than predicted by the product rule (Table 1). The product rule assumes that all cells in the studied population have the potential to express each receptor. A higher than expected overlap can be explained if stochastic Ly49 expression is allowed in only a subset of the population examined. Indeed, if one assumes that this subset can be defined as the population that expresses at least one of the five receptors tested in Table 1, the product rule predicts the overlap of different receptors with reasonable accuracy (Table 1).

Influence of MHC on the Receptor Repertoire

A key issue regarding the expression of inhibitory receptors by T cells is whether MHC molecules shape the repertoire, as has been observed for NK cells. Thus far, it has been difficult to observe alterations in the inhibitory receptor repertoire among T cells in normal mice that can be attributed to MHC molecules. The data on this point are sparse, however, and further investigation is warranted. Interestingly, it is reported that mice that express transgenes for both a human inhibitory KIR and its HLA ligand accumulate an abnormally large number of memory phenotype CD8 T cells (S Ugolini, E Vivier, personal communication). This observation has led to the hypothesis that class I binding by inhibitory NK receptors on CTL may encourage the formation or maintenance of memory cells. If so, it might be predicted that memory CD8$^+$ T cells would be selectively enriched for expression of self-MHC-specific inhibitory receptors. This possibility has not been rigorously tested. Also untested is whether mechanisms operate in T cells to minimize co-expression of self-MHC-specific inhibitory receptors, as observed in the case of NK cells.

SUMMARY: How to Generate a Functional and Self-Tolerant NK Repertoire

Although many fundamental questions remain, many features of the NK repertoire are beginning to emerge. In principle, the mechanisms that regulate the NK repertoire should ensure that NK cells are self-tolerant (nonresponsive to normal self cells) and maximally useful (responsive to abnormal or missing self). The following is a summary of some of the key findings from the disparate material discussed in the body of the review. At the same time, it is useful to put the results in the context of a model. Therefore, while there is currently little consensus on the broad underlying mechanisms, one speculative view of some of the key processes is presented below.

In adult animals, NK precursors are believed to arise in the bone marrow. Once committing to the NK lineage, these early precursors undergo a process of NK receptor acquisition, which is promoted by cytokines such as IL-15 and undefined signals from stromal cells. It appears that many inhibitory receptors are specific for MHC class I, whereas stimulatory receptors recognize a broader range of ligands including MHC molecules, non-MHC ligands that are upregulated on transformed or stressed cells, and constitutively expressed non-MHC self-ligands.

Importantly, both inhibitory and stimulatory receptors specific for MHC class I are distributed among NK cells by a stochastic mechanism that operates independently on each receptor gene allele. Consequently, the genes are expressed in variegated fashion and are predominantly monoallelically expressed, at least in the case of Ly49 and NKG2A genes. The pattern of inhibitory receptor expression by T cells is also consistent with a stochastic process, though clear qualitative differences have been noted between the inhibitory receptor repertoires of T cells and NK cells. In contrast to the MHC-specific receptors, several of the non-MHC-specific stimulatory receptors (e.g. NKRP1C, NKG2D, NKp46) appear to be expressed by all or nearly all NK cells. Some data suggest that expression of non-MHC-specific stimulatory receptors is an early event in NK cell development. On the other hand, MHC-specific stimulatory receptors in mice, such as Ly49D, appear at a similar or even delayed time in ontogeny as inhibitory Ly49 receptors.

Repertoire Formation as a Zero-Sum Game

An interesting possibility is that acquisition of inhibitory receptors occurs in NK cells that are receiving a net stimulatory signal from interactions with self-cells (Figure 2). Studies of mice harboring a mutation in a stimulatory signaling pathway ($fyn^{-/-}$) are consistent with this possibility. In addition, it would parallel the situation for $CD8^+$ T cells, where several lines of evidence suggest that stimulation through the T cell receptor promotes the acquisition of inhibitory receptors. In the case of NK cells, stimulation at the early stages of development might be mediated by receptors specific for non-MHC self-ligands. Subsequent expression of other stimulatory receptors reactive with self-ligands, such as self-MHC-specific stimulatory receptors, might provoke additional rounds of inhibitory receptor expression (see Figure 2). This mechanism would tend to counteract the expression of stimulatory receptors, pushing the cell toward a "zero-sum" balance between stimulation and inhibition (depicted as the diagonal line in Figure 2). Conversely, it is also possible that an excess of self-specific inhibitory receptors promotes expression of stimulatory receptors, but there are no data on this possibility.

Evidence indicates that acquisition of inhibitory MHC-specific receptors occurs in a sequential fashion. Acquisition of the CD94/NKG2A inhibitory receptor may be an early event, but only approximately 50% of NK cells in the adult express this receptor. In mice, Ly49 receptor expression is apparently a relatively late event, and there appears to be an order in which different Ly49 family members have the potential to be expressed. Expression of a given receptor gene allele is quite stable once initiated. Over time, these processes establish the complex combinatorial repertoire of NK cells, with each cell expressing multiple inhibitory (and stimulatory) specificities.

Evidence indicates that co-expression of multiple self-MHC-specific inhibitory receptors by NK cells is minimized. This finding is readily explained by the proposal that initiation of inhibitory receptor gene expression occurs only when NK

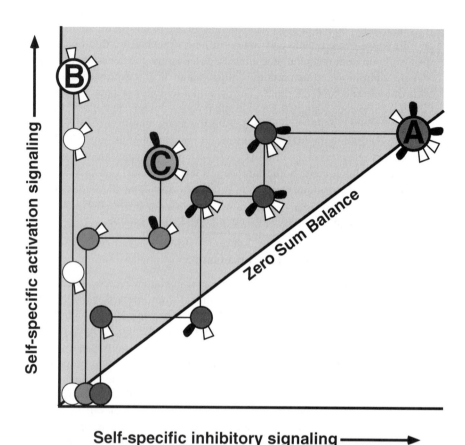

Figure 2   Model for how stimulatory and inhibitory interactions are integrated during the receptor acquisition phase of NK cell development. In this model, the expression and subsequent signaling by stimulatory receptors (white) drives the expression of inhibitory receptors (black). The shaded section indicates a net stimulatory signal, which provokes de novo expression of inhibitory receptors. Receptors are acquired stochastically until the process is terminated by unknown factors. Cell "A" has achieved balance in the amplitudes of positive and negative signals (influenced by the number of receptors, ligand affinities, and other factors) and is therefore self-tolerant and maximally sensitive to changes in host cell class I MHC expression. Cell "B" lacks self-specific inhibitory receptors (it may express non-self-specific inhibitory receptors); these cells are rendered hyporesponsive by an unknown mechanism. Cell "C" has both stimulatory and inhibitory self-specific receptors but has not attained a zero sum balance of signaling; subsequent fine tuning mechanisms may conceivably bring the cell into balance. Not depicted in the Figure is the possibility that some cells may express inhibitory receptors before stimulatory receptors.

cells receive a net stimulatory signal (Figure 2). Expression of one self-MHC-specific inhibitory receptor would at least partially counteract stimulatory signals, decreasing the likelihood of subsequent rounds of de novo expression of inhibitory receptors. A benefit of this proposed mechanism is that it imparts to NK cells a greater capacity to attack self-cells that have extinguished expression of only one of the several class Ia molecules normally expressed in an individual. In addition, since the process would tend toward an approximate balance of stimulation vs inhibition in many NK cells, the population as a whole would be more sensitive to changes in MHC class I levels.

Importantly, there appears to be an upper limit to the average number of inhibitory receptors that NK cells can express. Even in class I–deficient mice, where Ly49 and CD94/NKG2A receptors cannot engage ligands and counteract stimulatory signals, only a subset of all the receptor genes are expressed in each NK cell (albeit a greater average number than in normal mice). The basis for this limit remains uncertain. One possibility is that NK cells are only permitted to acquire receptors for a limited period of time during their development. Alternatively, the factors required to initiate expression of these receptor genes may be present in limiting quantities within the developing NK cell.

NK cells are clearly alloreactive but self-tolerant, and a major current challenge is to understand how self-tolerance is achieved. The zero-sum model proposed above, if allowed to continue to completion, would ultimately result in each NK cell expressing at least one self-MHC-specific inhibitory receptor to counteract stimulatory signals. The resulting NK cells would presumably be self-tolerant because stimulation and inhibition by self-ligands would be balanced. However, although the data are not definitive, some evidence suggests that a significant number of NK cells in normal mice do not express self-MHC-specific receptors. Furthermore, in the complete absence of MHC class I–mediated inhibition, as in class I–deficient mice, NK cells clearly achieve self-tolerance. It can be proposed that some NK cells in normal mice never succeed in expressing self–class I specific receptors, possibly because of the stochastic nature of the receptor acquisition process and the upper limit in the number of receptors that individual NK cells can express. These uninhibited cells may achieve self-tolerance by downregulating either the stimulatory receptors specific for self-ligands or components of the corresponding stimulatory signal transduction pathways. The adoption of this hyporesponsive state may occur either during the receptor acquisition process itself or, alternatively, during a later phase of NK development. In fact, it is plausible that the developing NK cells start out in a hyporesponsive state, only acquiring a heightened level of stimulatory sensitivity when inhibitory receptors are subsequently expressed and engaged. Regardless of the specific mechanism, it is important to emphasize that these cells are not predicted to be useless, as the NK cells in class I–deficient mice retain some capacity to attack tumor cells and certain other NK target cells. Perhaps the hyporesponsive state applies preferentially to stimulatory receptors that are self specific as opposed to tumor cell specific.

Together, the receptor acquisition and education processes would establish different sets of useful NK cells. Figure 3 summarizes the discriminatory properties

NK subsets in an MHC^{a+b} host

subset with inhibitory receptors specific for:

		MHC^a	MHC^b	MHC^{a+b}	none
	MHC^a	not useful self-tolerant	most useful vs MHC^{b-} targets self-tolerant	useful vs MHC^{b-} targets? self-tolerant	autoreactive? therefore: deleted? hyporesponsive?
constitutive self ligand		useful vs MHC^{a-} targets self-tolerant	useful vs MHC^{b-} targets self-tolerant	useful vs MHC^o targets self-tolerant	autoreactive? therefore: deleted? hyporesponsive?
stress-inducible self ligand		most useful vs stressed MHC^{a-} targets self-tolerant	most useful vs stressed MHC^{b-} targets self-tolerant	most useful vs stressed MHC^o targets self-tolerant	most useful vs stressed MHC^{a+b} targets self-tolerant

subset with stimulatory receptors specific for:

Figure 3 The mechanisms that distribute stimulatory and inhibitory receptors to NK cells have the potential to generate NK subsets with distinct functional characteristics. The figure depicts 12 potential subsets in a host expressing MHC^a and MHC^b molecules. The NK cells in this host could potentially express inhibitory receptors that are: (*a*) specific for MHC^a only (but not MHC^b); (*b*) specific for MHC^b only (but not MHC^a); (*c*) specific for MHC^a and MHC^b. A fourth category of NK cells is also considered: that is, those failing to express any self-specific MHC receptors ("none"). Three categories of stimulatory receptors are considered: (*a*) stimulatory receptors specific for MHC^a; (*b*) stimulatory receptors specific for constitutively expressed self-ligands; and (*c*) stimulatory receptors specific for self-ligands that are only induced on stressed or infected cells. The expected functional specificities of each NK subset is indicated within the relevant box. The fate of NK cells failing to express self-specific inhibitory receptors remains uncertain. Some of these cells may be deleted or rendered hyporesponsive by an as-yet-undetermined mechanism. It should be emphasized, however, that these cells are not necessarily useless, particularly if they express stimulatory receptors specific for inducible self-ligands (lower right box).

of different types of NK cells that would be expected to arise in the mature NK repertoire. This picture is consistent with recent research suggesting that NK cells employ multiple recognition systems so as to be responsive to diverse abnormalities arising from various infections and tumorigenesis.

ACKNOWLEDGMENTS

We thank James Carlyle, Andreas Diefenbach, and Amanda Jamieson for constructive comments, and Werner Held, Lewis Lanier, Alessandro Moretta, Lorenzo Moretta, and Eric Vivier for unpublished manuscripts. Work cited from our laboratory was supported by grants from the National Institutes of Health to DHR. REV is a Howard Hughes Predoctoral Fellow and CWM is a recipient of a postdoctoral fellowship from the Cancer Research Institute/Chase Manhattan Bank.

Visit the Annual Reviews home page at www.AnnualReviews.org

LITERATURE CITED

1. Trinchieri G. 1989. Biology of natural killer cells. *Adv. Immunol.* 47:187–376
2. Biron CA, Nguyen KB, Pien GC, Cousens LP, Salazar-Mather TP. 1999. Natural killer cells in antiviral defense: function and regulation by innate cytokines. *Annu. Rev. Immunol.* 17:189–220
3. Unanue ER. 1997. Studies in listeriosis show the strong symbiosis between the innate cellular system and the T-cell response. *Immunol. Rev.* 158:11–25
4. Scharton-Kersten TM, Sher A. 1997. Role of natural killer cells in innate resistance to protozoan infections. *Curr. Opin. Immunol.* 9:44–51
5. Biron CA, Byron KS, Sullivan JL. 1989. Severe herpes virus infections in an adolescent without natural killer cells. *N. Engl. J. Med.* 320:1731–35
6. Herberman RB, Nunn ME, Lavrin DH. 1975. Natural cytotoxic reactivity of mouse lymphoid cells against syngeneic and allogeneic tumors. I. Distribution of reactivity and specificity. *Int. J. Cancer* 16:216–29
7. Kiessling R, Klein E, Wigzell H. 1975. "Natural" killer cells in the mouse. I. Cytotoxic cells with specificity for mouse Moloney

leukemia cells. Specificity and distribution according to genotype. *Eur. J. Immunol.* 5:112–17
8. Seaman W, Sleisenger M, Eriksson E, Koo G. 1987. Depletion of natural killer cells in mice by monoclonal antibody to NK-1.1. Reduction in host defense against malignancy without loss of cellular or humoral immunity. *J. Immunol.* 138:4539–44
9. Murphy W, Kumar V, Bennett M. 1987. Rejection of bone marrow allografts by mice with severe combined immunodeficiency (SCID). *J. Exp. Med.* 165:1212–17
10. Ljunggren H-G, Karre K. 1985. Host resistance directed selectively against H-2-deficient lymphoma variants. *J. Exp. Med.* 162:1745–59
11. Bennett M. 1987. Biology and genetics of hybrid resistance. *Adv. Immunol.* 41:333–443
12. Karre K, Ljunggren HG, Piontek G, Kiessling R. 1986. Selective rejection of H-2-deficient lymphoma variants suggests alternative immune defense strategy. *Nature* 319:675–78
13. Ohlen C, Kling G, Höglund P, Hansson M, Scangos G, Bieberich C, Jay G, Karre K. 1989. Prevention of allogeneic bone

marrow graft rejection by H-2 transgene in donor mice. *Science* 246:666–68

14. Bix M, Liao N-S, Zijlstra M, Loring J, Jaenisch R, Raulet D. 1991. Rejection of class I MHC-deficient hemopoietic cells by irradiated MHC-matched mice. *Nature* 349:329–31

15. Liao N, Bix M, Zijlstra M, Jaenisch R, Raulet D. 1991. MHC class I deficiency: susceptibility to natural killer (NK) cells and impaired NK activity. *Science* 253: 199–202

16. Hoglund P, Ohlen C, Carbone E, Franksson L, Ljunggren H, Latour A, Koller B, Karre K. 1991. Recognition of β2-microglobulin-negative (β2m⁻) T-cell blasts by natural killer cells from normal but not from β2m⁻ mice: nonresponsiveness controlled by β2m⁻ bone marrow in chimeric mice. *Proc. Natl. Acad. Sci. USA* 88:10332–36

17. Garrido F, Ruiz-Cabello F, Cabrera T, Perez-Villar JJ, Lopez-Botet M, Duggan-Keen M, Stern PL. 1997. Implications for immunosurveillance of altered HLA class I phenotypes in human tumours. *Immunol. Today* 18:89–95

18. Tortorella D, Gewurz BE, Furman MH, Schust DJ, Ploegh HL. 2000. Viral subversion of the immune system. *Annu. Rev. Immunol.* 18:861–926

19. Karlhofer FM, Ribaudo RK, Yokoyama WM. 1992. MHC class I alloantigen specificity of Ly-49⁺ IL-2 activated natural killer cells. *Nature* 358:66–70

20. Yokoyama WM, Seaman WE. 1993. The Ly-49 and NKR-P1 gene families encoding lectin-like receptors on natural killer cells: the NK gene complex. *Annu. Rev. Immunol.* 11:613–35

21. Kane K. 1994. Ly-49 mediates EL4 lymphoma adhesion to isolated class I major histocompatibility complex molecules. *J. Exp. Med.* 179:1011–15

22. Daniels BF, Karlhofer FM, Seaman WE, Yokoyama WM. 1994. A natural killer cell receptor specific for a major histocompat-ibility complex class I molecule. *J. Exp. Med.* 180:687–92

23. Brennan J, Mager D, Jefferies W, Takei F. 1994. Expression of different members of the Ly-49 gene family defines distinct natural killer cell subsets and cell adhesion properties. *J. Exp. Med.* 180:2287–95

24. Hanke T, Takizawa H, McMahon CW, Busch DH, Pamer EG, Miller JD, Altman JD, Liu Y, Cado D, Lemonnier FA, Bjorkman PJ, Raulet DH. 1999. Direct assessment of MHC class I binding by seven Ly49 inhibitory NK cell receptors. *Immunity* 11:67–77

25. Michaelsson J, Achour A, Salcedo M, Kase-Sjostrom A, Sundback J, Harris RA, Karre K. 2000. Visualization of inhibitory Ly49 receptor specificity with soluble major histocompatibility complex class I tetramers. *Eur. J. Immunol.* 30:300–7

26. Tormo J, Natarajan K, Margulies DH, Mariuzza RA. 1999. Crystal structure of a lectin-like natural killer cell receptor bound to its MHC class I ligand. *Nature* 402:623–31

27. Smith HRC, Karlhofer FM, Yokoyama WM. 1994. Ly-49 multigene family expressed by IL-2-activated NK cells. *J. Immunol.* 153:1068–79

28. Wong S, Freeman JD, Kelleher C, Mager D, Takei F. 1991. Ly-49 multigene family. New members of a superfamily of type II membrane proteins with lectin-like domains. *J. Immunol.* 147:1417–23

29. McQueen KL, Lohwasser S, Takei F, Mager DL. 1999. Expression analysis of new Ly49 genes: most transcripts of Ly49j lack the transmembrane domain. *Immunogenetics* 49:685–91

30. Westgaard IH, Berg SF, Orstavik S, Fossum S, Dissen E. 1998. Identification of a human member of the Ly-49 multigene family. *Eur. J. Immunol.* 28:1839–46

31. Barten R, Trowsdale J. 1999. The human Ly-49L gene. *Immunogenetics* 49:731–34

32. Moretta A, Vitale M, Borrino C, Orengo A, Morelli L, Augugliaro R, Barbaresi M, Ciccone E, Moretta L. 1993. P58 molecules as putative receptors for major histocompatibility complex (MHC) class I molecules in human natural killer (NK) cells. Anti-p58 antibodies reconstitute lysis of MHC class I-protected cells in NK clones displaying different specifities. *J. Exp. Med.* 178:597–604

33. Wagtmann N, Biassoni R, Cantoni C, Verdiani S, Malnati M, Vitale M, Bottino C, Moretta L, Moretta A, Long E. 1995. Molecular clones of the p58 natural killer cell receptor reveal Ig-related molecules with diversity in both the extra- and intra-cellular domains. *Immunity* 2:439–49

34. Colonna M, Samaridis J. 1995. Cloning of immunoglobulin-superfamily members associated with HLA-C and HLA-B recognition by human natural killer cells. *Science* 268:405–8

35. D'Andrea A, Chang C, Bacon K, McClanahan T, Phillips J, Lanier LL. 1995. Molecular cloning of NKB1: a natural killer cell receptor for HLA-B allotypyes. *J. Immunol.* 155:2306–10

36. Long EO, Burshtyn DN, Clark WP, Peruzzi M, Rajagopalan S, Rojo S, Wagtmann N, Winter CC. 1997. Killer cell inhibitory receptors: diversity, specificity and function. *Immunol. Rev.* 155:135–44

37. Boyington JC, Motyka SA, Schuck P, Brooks AG, Sun PD. 2000. Crystal structure of an NK cell immunoglobulin-like receptor in complex with its class I MHC ligand. *Nature* 405:537–43

38. Uhrberg M, Valiente N, Shum B, Shilling H, Lienert-Weidenbach K, Corliss B, Tyan D, Lanier L, Parham P. 1997. Human diversity in killer cell inhibitory receptor genes. *Immunity* 7:753–63

39. Suto Y, Ishikawa Y, Kasahara M, Kasai F, Yabe T, Akaza T, Juji T. 1998. Gene arrangement of the killer cell inhibitory receptor family on human chromosome 19q13.4 detected by fiber-FISH. *Immunogenetics* 48:235–41

40. Martin AM, Freitas EM, Witt CS, Christiansen FT. 2000. The genomic organization and evolution of the natural killer immunoglobulin-like receptor (KIR) gene cluster. *Immunogenetics* 51:268–80

41. Wilson MJ, Torkar M, Haude A, Milne S, Jones T, Sheer D, Beck S, Trowsdale J. 2000. Plasticity in the organization and sequences of human KIR/ILT gene families. *Proc. Natl. Acad. Sci. USA* 97:4778–83

42. Houchins JP, Yabe T, McSherry C, Bach FH. 1991. DNA sequence analysis of NKG2, a family of related cDNA clones encoding type II integral membrane proteins on human natural killer cells. *J. Exp. Med.* 173:1017–20

43. Lazetic S, Chang C, Houchins JP, Lanier LL, Phillips JH. 1996. Human natural killer cell receptors involved in MHC class I recognition are disulfide-linked heterodimers of CD94 and NKG2 subunits. *J. Immunol.* 157:4741–45

44. Carretero M, Cantoni C, Bellon T, Bottino C, Biassoni R, Rodriguez A, Perez-Villar JJ, Moretta L, Moretta A, Lopez-Botet M. 1997. The CD94 and NKG2-A C-type lectins covalently assemble to form a natural killer cell inhibitory receptor for HLA class I molecules. *Eur. J. Immunol.* 27:563–67

45. Brooks AG, Posch PE, Scorzelli CJ, Borrego F, Coligan JE. 1997. NKG2A complexed with CD94 defines a novel inhibitory natural killer cell receptor. *J. Exp. Med.* 185:795–800

46. Vance RE, Kraft JR, Altman JD, Jensen PE, Raulet DH. 1998. Mouse CD94/NKG2A is a natural killer cell receptor for the nonclassical MHC class I molecule Qa-1^b. *J. Exp. Med.* 188:1841–48

47. Braud VM, Allan DSJ, O'Callaghan CA, Soderstrom K, D'Andrea A, Ogg GS, Lazetic S, Young NT, Bell JI, Phillips JH, Lanier LL, McMichael AJ. 1998. HLA-E binds to natural killer cell receptors

CD94/NKG2A, B, and C. *Nature* 391:795–99

48. Borrego F, Ulbrecht M, Weiss EH, Coligan JE, Brooks AG. 1998. Recognition of human histocompatibility leukocyte antigen (HLA)-E complexed with HLA class I signal sequence-derived peptides by CD94/NKG2 confers protection from natural killer cell-mediated lysis. *J. Exp. Med.* 187:813–18

49. Lee N, Llano M, Carretero M, Ishitani A, Navarro F, Lopez-Botet M, Geraghty DE. 1998. HLA-E is a major ligand for the natural killer inhibitory receptor CD94/NKG2A. *Proc. Natl. Acad. Sci. USA* 95:5199–204

50. Takei F, Brennan J, Mager DL. 1997. The Ly49 family: genes proteins and recognition of class I MHC. *Immunol. Rev.* 155:67–77

51. Moretta A, Bottino C, Vitale M, Pende D, Biassoni R, Mingari MC, Moretta L. 1996. Receptors for HLA class-I molecules in human natural killer cells. *Annu. Rev. Immunol.* 14:619–48

52. Litwin V, Gumperz J, Parham P, Phillips J, Lanier LL. 1994. NKB1: a natural killer cell receptor involved in the recognition of polymorphic HLA-B molecules. *J. Exp. Med.* 180:537–43

53. Braud VM, Allan DS, McMichael AJ. 1999. Functions of nonclassical MHC and non-MHC-encoded class I molecules. *Curr. Opin. Immunol.* 11:100–8

54. Aldrich CJ, DeCloux A, Woods AS, Cotter RJ, Soloski MJ, Forman J. 1994. Identification of a Tap-dependent leader peptide recognized by alloreactive T cells specific for a class Ib antigen. *Cell* 79:649–58

55. Cohen GB, Gandhi RT, Davis DM, Mandelboim O, Chen BK, Strominger JL, Baltimore D. 1999. The selective downregulation of class I major histocompatibility complex proteins by HIV-1 protects HIV-infected cells from NK cells. *Immunity* 10:661–71

56. Raulet DH, Held W, Correa I, Dorfman J, Wu M-F, Corral L. 1997. Specificity, tolerance and developmental regulation of natural killer cells defined by expression of class I-specific Ly49 receptors. *Immunol. Rev.* 155:41–52

57. Moretta A, Bottino C, Pende D, Tripodi G, Tambussi G, Viale O, Orengo A, Barbaresi M, Merli A, Ciccone E, Moretta L. 1990. Identification of four subsets of human CD3-CD16+ natural killer (NK) cells by the expression of clonally distributed functional surface molecules: correlation between subset assignment of NK clones and ability to mediate specific alloantigen recognition. *J. Exp. Med.* 172:1589–98

58. Valiante N, Uhberg M, Shilling H, Lienert-Weidenbach K, Arnett K, D'Andrea A, Phillips J, Lanier L, Parham P. 1997. Functionally and structurally distinct NK cell receptor repertoires in the peripheral blood of two human donors. *Immunity* 7:739–51

59. Salcedo M, Bousso P, Ljunggren HG, Kourilsky P, Abastado JP. 1998. The Qa-1b molecule binds to a large subpopulation of murine NK cells. *Eur. J. Immunol.* 28:4356–61

60. Held W, Roland J, Raulet DH. 1995. Allelic exclusion of Ly49 family genes encoding class I-MHC-specific receptors on NK cells. *Nature* 376:355–58

61. Kubota A, Kubota S, Lohwasser S, Mager DL, Takei F. 1999. Diversity of NK cell receptor repertoire in adult and neonatal mice. *J. Immunol.* 163:212–16

62. Burshtyn DN, Yang W, Yi T, Long EO. 1997. A novel phosphotyrosine motif with a critical amino acid at position −2 for the SH2 domain-mediated activation of the tyrosine phosphatase SHP-1. *J. Biol. Chem.* 272:13066–72

63. Burshtyn D, Scharenberg A, Wagtmann N, Rajagopalan S, Peruzzi M, Kinet J-P, Long EO. 1996. Recruitment of tyrosine phosphatase HCP by the NK cell inhibitory receptor. *Immunity* 4:77–85

64. Olcese L, Lang P, Vely F, Cambiaggi A, Marguet D, Blery M, Hippen KL, Biassono R, Moretta A, Moretta L, Cambier J, Vivier E. 1996. Human and mouse killer-cell inhibitory receptors recruit Ptp1c and Ptp1d protein tyrosine phosphatases. *J. Immunol.* 156:4531–34

65. Campbell KS, Dessing M, Lopez-Botet M, Cella M, Colonna M. 1996. Tyrosine phosphorylation of a human killer inhibitory receptor recruits protein tyrosine phosphatase 1C. *J. Exp. Med.* 184:93–100

66. Binstadt BA, Brumbaugh KM, Dick CJ, Scharenberg AM, Williams BL, Colonna M, Lanier LL, Kinet JP, Abraham RT, Leibson PJ. 1996. Sequential involvement of Lck and SHP-1 with MHC-recognizing receptors on NK cells inhibits FcR-initiated tyrosine kinase activation. *Immunity* 5:629–38

67. Vély F, Olivero S, Olcese L, Moretta A, Damen JE, Liu L, Krystal G, Cambier JC, Daëron M, Vivier E. 1997. Differential association of phosphatases with hematopoietic co-receptors bearing immunoreceptor tyrosine-based inhibition motifs. *Eur. J. Immunol.* 27:1994–2000

68. Leibson PJ. 1997. Signal transduction during natural killer cell activation: inside the mind of a killer. *Immunity* 6:655–61

69. Lanier LL, Corliss B, Phillips JH. 1997. Arousal and inhibition of human NK cells. *Immunol. Rev.* 155:145–54

70. Bauer S, Groh V, Wu J, Steinle A, Phillips JH, Lanier LL, Spies T. 1999. Activation of NK cells and T cells by NKG2D, a receptor for stress-inducible MICA. *Science* 285:727–29

71. Cerwenka A, Bakker ABH, McClanahan T, Wagner J, Wu J, Phillips JH, Lanier LL. 2000. Retinoic acid early inducible genes define a ligand family for the activating NKG2D receptor in mice. *Immunity* 12:721–27

72. Diefenbach A, Jamieson AM, Liu SD, Shastri N, Raulet DH. 2000. Novel ligands for the murine NKG2D receptor: expression by tumor cells and activation of NK cells and macrophages. *Nature Immunol.* 1:119–26

73. Tangye SG, Phillips JH, Lanier LL. 2000. The CD2-subset of the Ig superfamily of cell surface molecules: receptor-ligand pairs expressed by NK cells and other immune cells. *Semin. Immunol.* 12:149–57

74. Ciccone E, Pende D, Vitale M, Nanni L, Di Donato C, Bottino C, Morelli L, Viale O, Amoroso A, Moretta A, et al. 1994. Self class I molecules protect normal cells from lysis mediated by autologous natural killer cells. *Eur. J. Immunol.* 24:1003–6

75. Pende D, Parolini S, Pessino A, Sivori S, Augugliaro R, Morelli L, Marcenaro E, Accame L, Malaspina A, Biassoni R, Bottino C, Moretta L, Moretta A. 1999. Identification and molecular characterization of NKp30, a novel triggering receptor involved in natural cytotoxicity mediated by human natural killer cells. *J. Exp. Med.* 190:1505–16

76. Kung SK, Miller RG. 1995. The NK1.1 antigen in NK-mediated F1 antiparent killing in vitro. *J. Immunol.* 154:1624–33

77. Koo GC, Peppard JR. 1984. Establishment of monoclonal anti-NK-1.1 antibody. *Hybridoma* 3:301–3

78. Sivori S, Vitale M, Morelli L, Sanseverino L, Augugliaro R, Bottino C, Moretta L, Moretta A. 1997. p46, a novel natural killer cell-specific surface molecule that mediates cell activation. *J. Exp. Med.* 186:1129–36

79. Sentman CL, Hackett JJ, Moore TA, Tutt MM, Bennett M, Kumar V. 1989. Pan natural killer cell monoclonal antibodies and their relationship to the NK1.1 antigen. *Hybridoma* 8:605–14

80. Vance RE, Jamieson AM, Raulet DH. 1999. Recognition of the class Ib molecule Qa-1(b) by putative activating receptors CD94/NKG2C and CD94/NKG2E on mouse natural killer cells. *J. Exp. Med.* 190:1801–12

81. Mason LH, Anderson SK, Yokoyama WM, Smith HRC, Winkler-Pickett R, Ortaldo JR. 1996. The Ly49D receptor activates murine natural killer cells. *J. Exp. Med.* 184:2119–28

82. Smith KM, Wu J, Bakker AB, Phillips JH, Lanier LL. 1998. Ly-49D and Ly-49H associate with mouse DAP12 and form activating receptors. *J. Immunol.* 161:7–10

83. Nakamura MC, Linnemeyer PA, Niemi EC, Mason LH, Ortaldo JR, Ryan JC, Seaman WE. 1999. Mouse Ly-49D recognizes H-2D(d) and activates natural killer cell cytotoxicity. *J. Exp. Med.* 189:493–500

84. Smith HRC, Chuang HH, Wang LL, Salcedo M, Heusel JW, Yokoyama WM. 2000. Nonstochastic coexpression of activation receptors on murine natural killer cells. *J. Exp. Med.* 191:1341–54

85. Valés-Gómez M, Reyburn HT, Erskine RA, Lopez-Botet M, Strominger JL. 1999. Kinetics and peptide dependency of the binding of the inhibitory NK receptor CD94/NKG2-A and the activating receptor CD94/NKG2-C to HLA-E. *EMBO J.* 18:4250–60

86. Vales-Gomez M, Reyburn HT, Erskine RA, Strominger J. 1998. Differential binding to HLA-C of p50-activating and p58-inhibitory natural killer cell receptors. *Proc. Natl. Acad. Sci. USA* 95:14326–31

87. Olcese L, Cambiaggi A, Semenzato G, Bottino C, Moretta A, Vivier E. 1997. Human killer cell activatory receptors for MHC class I molecules are included in a multimeric complex expressed by natural killer cells. *J. Immunol.* 158:5083–86

88. Lanier LL, Corliss BC, Wu J, Leong C, Phillips JH. 1998. Immunoreceptor DAP12 bearing a tyrosine-based activation motif is involved in activating NK cells. *Nature* 391:703–7

89. Wirthmueller U, Kurosaki T, Murakami MS, Ravetch JV. 1992. Signal transduction by Fc gamma RIII (CD16) is mediated through the gamma chain. *J. Exp. Med.* 175:1381–90

90. Chang C, Dietrich J, Harpur AG, Lindquist JA, Haude A, Lake YW, King A, Colonna M, Trowsdale J, Wilson MJ. 1999. KAP10, a novel transmembrane adapter protein genetically linked to DAP12 but with unique signaling properties. *J. Immunol.* 163:4652–54

91. Wu J, Song Y, Bakker AB, Bauer S, Spies T, Lanier LL, Phillips JH. 1999. An activating immunoreceptor complex formed by NKG2D and DAP10. *Science* 285:730–32

92. Tomasello E, Desmoulins PO, Chemin K, Guia S, Cremer H, Ortaldo J, Love P, Kaiserlian D, Vivier E. 2000. Combined natural killer cell and dendritic cell functional deficiency in KARAP/DAP12 loss-of-function mutant mice. *Immunity* 13:355–64

93. Bakker ABH, Hoek RM, Cerwenka A, Blom B, Lucian L, McNeil T, Murray R, Phillips JH, Sedgwick JD, Lanier LL. 2000. AP12-deficient mice fail to develop autoimmunity due to impaired antigen priming. *Immunity* 13:345–53

94. Vance RE. 2000. *Natural killer cell receptors for nonclassical major histocompatibility complex class I molecules of the mouse.* PhD dissertation, Univ. Calif., Berkeley

95. Vance RE, Raulet DH. 1998. Toward a quantitative analysis of the repertoire of class I MHC-specific inhibitory receptors on natural killer cells. *Curr. Top. Microbiol. Immunol.* 230:135–60

96. Held W, Kunz B, Lowin-Kropf B, van de Wetering M, Clevers H. 1999. Clonal acquisition of the Ly49A NK cell receptor is dependent on the trans-acting factor TCF-1. *Immunity* 11:433–42

97. Held W, Raulet DH. 1997. Expression of the *Ly49A* gene in murine natural killer cell clones is predominantly but not exclusively mono-allelic. *Eur. J. Immunol.* 27:2876–84

98. Held W, Kunz B. 1998. An allele-specific, stochastic gene expression process controls

the expression of multiple Ly49 family genes and generates a diverse, MHC-specific NK cell receptor repertoire. *Eur. J. Immunol.* 28:2407–16

99. Chess A, Simon I, Cedar H, Axel R. 1994. Allelic inactivation regulates olfactory receptor gene expression. *Cell* 78:823–34

100. Bix M, Locksley RM. 1998. Independent and epigenetic regulation of the interleukin-4 alleles in CD4+ T cells. *Science* 281:1352–54

101. Hollander GA, Zuklys S, Morel C, Mizoguchi E, Mobisson K, Simpson S, Terhorst C, Wishart W, Golan DE, Ghan A, Burakoff S. 1998. Monoallelic expression of the interleukin-2 locus. *Science* 279:2118–21

102. Rivière I, Sunshine MJ, Littman DR. 1998. Regulation of IL-4 expression by activation of individual alleles. *Immunity* 9:217–28

103. Rhoades KL, Singh N, Simon I, Glidden B, Cedar H, Chess A. 2000. Allele-specific expression patterns of interleukin-2 and pax-5 revealed by a sensitive single-cell RT-PCR analysis. *Curr. Biol.* 10:789–92

104. Dorfman JR, Raulet DH. 1998. Acquisition of Ly49 receptor expression by developing natural killer cells. *J. Exp. Med.* 187:609–18

105. Salcedo M, Colucci F, Dyson PJ, Cotterill LA, Lemonnier FA, Kourilsky P, Di Santo JP, Ljunggren HG, Abastado JP. 2000. Role of Qa-1(b)-binding receptors in the specificity of developing NK cells. *Eur. J. Immunol.* 30:1094–1101

106. Jaleco AC, Blom B, Res P, Weijer K, Lanier LL, Phillips JH, Spits H. 1997. Fetal liver contains committed NK progenitors, but is not a site for development of CD34+ cells into T cells. *J. Immunol.* 159:694–702

107. Van Beneden K, De Creus A, Debacker V, De Boever J, Plum J, Leclercq G. 1999. Murine fetal natural killer cells are functionally and structurally distinct from adult natural killer cells. *J. Leukocyte Biol.* 66:625–33

108. Sivakumar PV, Gunturi A, Salcedo M, Schatzle JD, Lai WC, Kurepa Z, Pitcher L, Seaman MS, Lemonnier FA, Bennett M, Forman J, Kumar V. 1999. Cutting edge: expression of functional CD94/NKG2A inhibitory receptors on fetal NK1.1+Ly-49-cells: a possible mechanism of tolerance during NK cell development. *J. Immunol.* 162:6976–80

109. Mingari MC, Ponte M, Bertone S, Schiavetti F, Vitale C, Bellomo R, Moretta A, Moretta L. 1998. HLA class I-specific inhibitory receptors in human T lymphocytes: interleukin 15-induced expression of CD94/NKG2A in superantigen- or alloantigen-activated CD8+ T cells. *Proc. Natl. Acad. Sci. USA* 95:1172–77

110. Yu H, Fehniger TA, Fuchshuber P, Thiel KS, Vivier E, Carson WE, Caligiuri MA. 1998. Flt3 ligand promotes the generation of a distinct CD34(+) human natural killer cell progenitor that responds to interleukin-15. *Blood* 92:3647–57

111. Toomey JA, Salcedo M, Cotterill LA, Millrain MM, Chrzanowska-Lightowlers Z, Lawry J, Fraser K, Gays F, Robinson JH, Shrestha S, Dyson PJ, Brooks CG. 1999. Stochastic acquisition of Qa1 receptors during the development of fetal NK cells in vitro accounts in part but not in whole for the ability of these cells to distinguish between class I-sufficient and class I-deficient targets. *J. Immunol.* 163:3176–84

112. Sivakumar PV, Bennett M, Kumar V. 1997. Fetal and neonatal NK1.1+ Ly-49- cells can distinguish between major histocompatibility complex class I(hi) and class I(lo) target cells: evidence for a Ly-49-independent negative signaling receptor. *Eur. J. Immunol.* 27:3100–4

113. Williams NS, Klem J, Puzanov IJ, Sivakumar PV, Bennett M, Kumar V. 1999.

Differentiation of NK1.1+, Ly49+ NK cells from flt3+ multipotent marrow progenitor cells. *J. Immunol.* 163:2648–56

114. Roth C, Carlyle JR, Takizawa H, Raulet DH. 2000. Clonal acquisition of inhibitory Ly49 receptors on differentiating NK cell precursors is successively restricted and regulated by stromal cell class I MHC. *Immunity* 13:143–53

115. Williams NS, Kubota A, Bennett M, Kumar V, Takei F. 2000. Clonal analysis of NK cell development from bone marrow progenitors in vitro: orderly acquisition of receptor gene expression. *Eur. J. Immunol.* 30:2074–82

116. Kiessling R, Hochman PS, Haller O, Shearer GM, Wigzell H, Cudkowicz G. 1977. Evidence for a similar or common mechanisms for natural killer cell activity and resistance to hemopoietic grafts. *Eur. J. Immunol.* 7:655–63

117. Raziuddin A, Longo DL, Mason L, Ortaldo JR, Bennett M, Murphy WJ. 1998. Differential effects of the rejection of bone marrow allografts by the depletion of activating versus inhibiting Ly-49 natural killer cell subsets. *J. Immunol.* 160:87–94

118. Cudkowicz G, Bennett M. 1971. Peculiar immunobiology of bone marrow allografts. I. Graft rejection by irradiated responder mice. *J. Exp. Med.* 134:83–102

119. Ljunggren H-G, Van Kaer L, Ploegh HL, Tonegawa S. 1994. Altered natural killer cell repertoire in *Tap-1* mutant mice. *Proc. Natl. Acad. Sci. USA* 91:6520–24

120. Dorfman JR, Zerrahn J, Coles MC, Raulet DH. 1997. The basis for self-tolerance of natural killer cells in β2m⁻ and TAP-1⁻ mice. *J. Immunol.* 159:5219–25

121. Hoglund P, Glas R, Menard C, Kase A, Johansson MH, Franksson L, Lemmonier F, Karre K. 1998. Beta2-microglobulin-deficient NK cells show increased sensitivity to MHC class I-mediated inhibition, but self tolerance does not depend upon

target cell expression of H-2Kᵇ and Dᵇ heavy chains. *Eur. J. Immunol.* 28:370–78

122. Grigoriadou K, Menard C, Perarnau B, Lemonnier FA. 1999. MHC class Ia molecules alone control NK-mediated bone marrow graft rejection. *Eur. J. Immunol.* 29:3683–90

123. Zimmer J, Donato L, Hanau D, Cazenave JP, Tongio MM, Moretta A, de la Salle H. 1998. Activity and phenotype of natural killer cells in peptide transporter (TAP)-deficient patients (type I bare lymphocyte syndrome). *J. Exp. Med.* 187:117–22

124. Wu M-F, Raulet DH. 1997. Class I-deficient hematopoietic cells and non-hematopoietic cells dominantly induce unresponsiveness of NK cells to class I-deficient bone marrow grafts. *J. Immunol.* 158:1628–33

125. Kung SK, Miller RG. 1997. Mouse natural killer subsets defined by their target specificity and their ability to be separately rendered unresponsive in vivo. *J. Immunol.* 158:2616–26

126. Johansson MH, Bieberich C, Jay G, Karre K, Hoglund P. 1997. Natural killer cell tolerance in mice with mosaic expression of major histocompatibility complex class I transgene. *J. Exp. Med.* 186:353–64

127. Salcedo M, Andersson M, Lemieux S, Van Kaer L, Chambers BJ, Ljunggren H-G. 1998. Fine tuning of natural killer cell specificity and maintenance of self tolerance in MHC class I-deficient mice. *Eur. J. Immunol.* 28:1315–21

128. Chadwick BS, Miller RG. 1992. Hybrid resistance in vitro. Possible role of both class I MHC and self peptides in determining the level of target cell sensitivity. *J. Immunol.* 148:2307–13

129. Dorfman JR, Raulet DH. 1996. Major histocompatibility complex genes determine natural killer cell tolerance. *Eur. J. Immunol.* 26:151–55

130. Olsson MY, Karre K, Sentman CL. 1995. Altered phenotype and function of

natural killer cells expressing the major histocompatibility complex receptor Ly-49 in mice transgenic for its ligand. *Proc. Natl. Acad. Sci. USA* 92:1649–53

131. Held W, Dorfman JR, Wu M-F, Raulet DH. 1996. Major histocompatibility complex class I-dependent skewing of the natural killer cell Ly49 receptor repertoire. *Eur. J. Immunol.* 26:2286–92

132. Salcedo M, Diehl AD, Olsson-Alheim MY, Sundbäck J, Van Kaer L, Karre K, Ljunggren H-G. 1997. Altered expression of Ly49 inhibitory receptors on natural killer cells from MHC class I deficient mice. *J. Immunol.* 158:3174–80

133. Gumperz JE, Valiante NM, Parham P, Lanier LL, Tyan D. 1996. Heterogeneous phenotypes of expression of the NKB1 natural killer cell class I receptor among individuals of different human histocompatibility leukocyte antigens types appear genetically regulated, but not linked to major histocompatibililty complex haplotype. *J. Exp. Med.* 183:1817–27

134. Lowin-Kropf B, Held W. 2000. Positive impact of inhibitory Ly49 receptor-MHC class I interaction on NK cell development. *J. Immunol.* 165:91–95

135. George TC, Ortaldo JR, Lemieux S, Kumar V, Bennett M. 1999. Tolerance and alloreactivity of the Ly49D subset of murine NK cells. *J. Immunol.* 163:1859–67

136. Sykes M, Harty MW, Karlhofer FM, Pearson DA, Szot G, Yokoyama W. 1993. Hematopoietic cells and radioresistant host elements influence natural killer cell differentiation. *J. Exp. Med.* 178:223–29

137. Karlhofer FM, Hunziker R, Reichlin A, Margulies DH, Yokoyama WM. 1994. Host MHC class I molecules modulate in vivo expression of a NK cell receptor. *J. Immunol.* 153:2407–16

138. Gosselin P, Lusigan Y, Brennan J, Takei F, Lemieux S. 1997. The NK2.1 receptor is encoded by Ly-49C and its expression is regulated by MHC class I alleles. *Int. Immunol.* 9:533–40

139. Sentman CL, Olsson MY, Karre K. 1995. Missing self recognition by natural killer cells in MHC class I transgenic mice. A 'receptor calibration' model for how effector cells adapt to self. *Semin. Immunol.* 7:109–19

140. Olsson-Alheim MY, Salcedo M, Ljunggren HG, Karre K, Sentman CL. 1997. NK cell receptor calibration: effects of MHC class I induction on killing by Ly49Ahigh and Ly49Alow NK cells. *J. Immunol.* 159:3189–94

141. Held W, Raulet DH. 1997. Ly49A transgenic mice provide evidence for a major histocompatibility complex-dependent education process in NK cell development. *J. Exp. Med.* 185:2079–88

142. Fahlen L, Khoo NKS, Daws MR, Sentman CL. 1997. Location-specific regulation of transgenic Ly49A receptors by major histocompatibility complex class I molecules. *Eur. J. Immunol.* 27:2057–65

143. Kase A, Johansson MH, Olsson-Alheim MY, Karre K, Hoglund P. 1998. External and internal calibration of the MHC class I-specific receptor Ly49A on murine natural killer cells. *J. Immunol.* 161:6133–38

144. Lowin-Kropf B, Kunz B, Beermann F, Held W. 2000. Impaired natural killing of MHC class I-deficient targets by NK cells expressing a catalytically inactive form of SHP-1. *J. Immunol.* 165:1314–21

145. Yu YY, George T, Dorfman J, Roland J, Kumar V, Bennett M. 1996. The role of Ly49A and 5E6 (Ly49C) molecules in hybrid resistance mediated by murine natural killer cells against normal T cell blasts. *Immunity* 4:67–76

146. Carlyle JR, Michie AM, Cho SK, Zúñiga-Pflücker JC. 1998. Natural killer cell development and function precede alpha beta T cell differentiation in mouse fetal thymic ontogeny. *J. Immunol.* 160:744–53

147. Rodewald HR, Moingeon P, Lucich JL, Dosiou C, Lopez P, Reinherz EL. 1992. A population of early fetal thymocytes

expressing Fc gamma RII/III contains precursors of T lymphocytes and natural killer cells. *Cell* 69:139–50

148. Carlyle JR, Michie AM, Furlonger C, Nakano T, Lenardo MJ, Paige CJ, Zúniga-Pflücker JC. 1997. Identification of a novel developmental stage marking lineage commitment of progenitor thymocytes. *J. Exp. Med.* 186:173–82

149. Ferrini S, Cambiaggi A, Meazza R, Sforzini S, Marciano S, Mingari MC, Moretta L. 1994. T cell clones expressing the natural killer cell-related p58 receptor molecule display heterogeneity in phenotypic properties and p58 function. *Eur. J. Immunol.* 24:2294–98

150. Phillips JH, Gumperz JE, Parham P, Lanier LL. 1995. Superantigen-dependent, cell-mediated cytotoxicity inhibited by MHC class I receptors on T lymphocytes. *Science* 268:403–5

151. Mingari MC, Ponte M, Cantoni C, Vitale C, Schiavetti F, Bertone S, Bellomo R, Cappai AT, Biassoni R. 1997. HLA-class I-specific inhibitory receptors in human cytolytic T lymphocytes: molecular characterization, distribution in lymphoid tissues and co-expression by individual T cells. *Int. Immunol.* 9:485–91

152. Mingari MC, Schiavetti F, Ponte M, Vitale C, Maggi E, Romagnani S, Demarest J, Pantaleo G, Fauci AS, Moretta L. 1996. Human CD8+ T lymphocyte subsets that express HLA class I-specific inhibitory receptors represent oligoclonally or monoclonally expanded cell populations. *Proc. Natl. Acad. Sci. USA* 93:12433–38

153. Speiser DE, Valmori D, Rimoldi D, Pittet MJ, Liénard D, Cerundolo V, MacDonald HR, Cerottini JC, Romero P. 1999. CD28-negative cytolytic effector T cells frequently express NK receptors and are present at variable proportions in circulating lymphocytes from healthy donors and melanoma patients. *Eur. J. Immunol.* 29:1990–99

154. André P, Brunet C, Guia S, Gallais H, Sampol J, Vivier E, Dignat-George F. 1999. Differential regulation of killer cell Ig-like receptors and CD94 lectin-like dimers on NK and T lymphocytes from HIV-1-infected individuals. *Eur. J. Immunol.* 29:1076–85

155. Ortaldo JR, Winkler-Pickett R, Mason AT, Mason LH. 1998. The Ly-49 family: regulation of cytotoxicity and cytokine production in murine CD3+ cells. *J. Immunol.* 160:1158–65

156. Coles MC, McMahon CW, Takizawa H, Raulet DH. 2000. Memory CD8 T lymphocytes express inhibitory MHC-specific Ly49 receptors. *Eur. J. Immunol.* 30:236–44

157. Battistini L, Borsellino G, Sawicki G, Poccia F, Salvetti M, Ristori G, Brosnan CF. 1997. Phenotypic and cytokine analysis of human peripheral blood gamma delta T cells expressing NK cell receptors. *J. Immunol.* 159:3723–30

158. Halary F, Peyrat MA, Champagne E, Lopez-Botet M, Moretta A, Moretta L, Vie H, Fournie JJ, Bonneville M. 1997. Control of self-reactive cytotoxic T lymphocytes expressing gamma delta T cell receptors by natural killer inhibitory receptors. *Eur. J. Immunol.* 27:2812–21

159. Fisch P, Meuer E, Pende D, Rothenfusser S, Viale O, Kock S, Ferrone S, Fradelizi D, Klein G, Moretta L, Rammensee HG, Boon T, Coulie P, van der Bruggen P. 1997. Control of B cell lymphoma recognition via natural killer inhibitory receptors implies a role for human Vgamma9/Vdelta2 T cells in tumor immunity. *Eur. J. Immunol.* 27:3368–79

160. Aramburu J, Balboa MA, Ramirez A, Silva A, Acevedo A, Sanchez-Madrid F, De Landazuri MO, López-Botet M. 1990. A novel functional cell surface dimer (Kp43) expressed by natural killer cells and T cell receptor-gamma/delta+ T lymphocytes. I. Inhibition of the

IL-2-dependent proliferation by anti-Kp43 monoclonal antibody. *J. Immunol.* 144:3238–47

161. Rubio G, Aramburu J, Ontanon J, Lopez-Botet M, Aparicio P. 1993. A novel functional cell surface dimer (kp43) serves as accessory molecule for the activation of a subset of human gamma delta T cells. *J. Immunol.* 151:1312–21

162. Bendelac A, Rivera MN, Park S-H, Roark JH. 1997. Mouse CD1-specific NK1 T cells: development, specificity, and function. *Annu. Rev. Immunol.* 15:535–62

163. Davodeau F, Peyrat MA, Necker A, Dominici R, Blanchard F, Leget C, Gaschet J, Costa P, Jacques Y, Godard A, Vie H, Poggi A, Romagné F, Bonneville M. 1997. Close phenotypic and functional similarities between human and murine alphabeta T cells expressing invariant TCR alpha-chains. *J. Immunol.* 158: 5603–11

164. De Maria A, Ferraris A, Guastella M, Pilia S, Cantoni C, Polero L, Mingari MC, Bassetti D, Fauci AS, Moretta L. 1997. Expression of HLA class I-specific inhibitory natural killer cell receptors in HIV-specific cytolytic T lymphocytes: impairment of specific cytolytic functions. *Proc. Natl. Acad. Sci. USA* 94:10285–88

165. Ikeda H, Lethe B, Lehmann F, Va Baren N, Baurain J-F, De Smet C, Chambost H, Vitlae M, Moretta A, Boon T, Coulie P. 1997. Characterization of an antigen that is recognized on a melanoma showing partial HLA loss by CTL expressing an NK inhibitory receptor. *Immunity* 6:199–208

166. Noppen C, Schaefer C, Zajac P, Schütz A, Kocher T, Kloth J, Heberer M, Colonna M, De Libero G, Spagnoli GC. 1998. C-type lectin-like receptors in peptide-specific HLA class I-restricted cytotoxic T lymphocytes: differential expression and modulation of effector functions in clones sharing identical TCR structure

and epitope specificity. *Eur. J. Immunol.* 28:1134–42

167. Huard B, Karlsson L. 2000. KIR expression on self-reactive CD8+ T cells is controlled by T-cell receptor engagement. *Nature* 403:325–28

168. Speiser DE, Pittet MJ, Valmori D, Dunbar R, Rimoldi D, Liénard D, MacDonald HR, Cerottini JC, Cerundolo V, Romero P. 1999. In vivo expression of natural killer cell inhibitory receptors by human melanoma-specific cytolytic T lymphocytes. *J. Exp. Med.* 190:775–82

169. Deleted in proof

170. Posnett DN, Sinha R, Kabak S, Russo C. 1994. Clonal populations of T cells in normal elderly humans: the T cell equivalent to "benign monoclonal gammapathy". *J. Exp. Med.* 179:609–18

171. Eberl G, Lees R, Smiley ST, Taniguchi M, Grusby MJ, MacDonald HR. 1999. Tissue-specific segregation of CD1d-dependent and CD1d-independent NK T cells. *J. Immunol.* 162:6410–19

172. Callahan JE, Kappler JW, Marrack P. 1993. Unexpected expansions of CD8-bearing cells in old mice. *J. Immunol.* 151:6657–69

173. Mingari M, Vitale C, Cambiaggi A, Schiavetti F, Melioli G, Ferrini S, Poggi A. 1995. Cytolytic T lymphocytes displaying natural killer (NK)-like activity: expression of NK related functional receptors for HLA class I moleules (p58 and CD94) and inhibitory effect on the TCR-mediated target cell lysis or lymphokine production. *Int. Immunol.* 7:697–703

174. Nakajima H, Tomiyama H, Takiguchi M. 1995. Inhibition of gamma delta T cell recognition by receptors for MHC class I molecules. *J. Immunol.* 155:4139–42

175. D'Andrea A, Chang C, Phillips JH, Lanier LL. 1996. Regulation of T cell lymphokine production by killer cell inhibitory receptor recognition of self HLA class I alleles. *J. Exp. Med.* 184: 789–94

176. Poccia F, Cipriani B, Vendetti S, Colizzi V, Poquet Y, Battistini L, López-Botet M, Fournié JJ, Gougeon ML. 1997. CD94/NKG2 inhibitory receptor complex modulates both anti-viral and anti-tumoral responses of polyclonal phosphoantigen-reactive V gamma 9V delta 2 T lymphocytes. *J. Immunol.* 159:6009–17

177. Le Dréan E, Vély F, Olcese L, Cambiaggi A, Guia S, Krystal G, Gervois N, Moretta A, Jotereau F, Vivier E. 1998. Inhibition of antigen-induced T cell response and antibody-induced NK cell cytotoxicity by NKG2A: association of NKG2A with SHP-1 and SHP-2 protein-tyrosine phosphatases. *Eur. J. Immunol.* 28:264–76

178. Mingari MC, Ponte M, Vitale C, Bellomo R, Moretta L. 2000. Expression of HLA class I-specific inhibitory receptors in human cytolytic T lymphocytes: a regulated mechanism that controls T-cell activation and function. *Hum. Immunol.* 61:44–50

179. Ugolini S, Vivier E. 2000. Regulation of T cell function by NK cell receptors for classical MHC class I molecules. *Curr. Opin. Immunol.* 12:295–300

180. Held W, Cado D, Raulet DH. 1996. Transgenic expression of the Ly49A natural killer cell receptor confers class I major histocompatibility complex (MHC)-specific inhibition and prevents bone marrow allograft rejection. *J. Exp. Med.* 184:2037–41

181. Zajac AJ, Vance RE, Held W, Sourdive DJD, Altman JD, Raulet DH, Ahmed R. 1999. Impaired anti-viral T cell responses due to expression of the Ly49A inhibitory receptor. *J. Immunol.* 163:5526–34

182. Ortaldo JR, Winkler-Pickett R, Willette-Brown J, Wange RL, Anderson SK, Palumbo GJ, Mason LH, McVicar DW. 1999. Structure/function relationship of activating Ly-49D and inhibitory Ly-49G2 NK receptors. *J. Immunol.* 163:5269–77

183. Cambiaggi A, Darche S, Guia S, Kourilsky P, Abastado JP, Vivier E. 1999. Modulation of T-cell functions in KIR2DL3 (CD158b) transgenic mice. *Blood* 94:2396–2402

184. Bertone S, Schiavetti F, Bellomo R, Vitale C, Ponte M, Moretta L, Mingari MC. 1999. Transforming growth factor-beta-induced expression of CD94/NKG2A inhibitory receptors in human T lymphocytes. *Eur. J. Immunol.* 29:23–29

185. Moretta A, Tambussi G, Bottino C, Tripodi G, Merli A, Ciccone E, Pantaleo G, Moretta L. 1990. A novel surface antigen expressed by a subset of human CD3− CD16+ natural killer cells. Role in cell activation and regulation of cytolytic function. *J. Exp. Med.* 171:695–714

186. MacDonald HR, Lees RK, Held W. 1998. Developmentally regulated extinction of Ly-49 receptor expression permits maturation and selection of NK1.1$^+$ T cells. *J. Exp. Med.* 187:2109–14

187. Mandleboim O, Davis DM, Reyburn HT, Valés-Gómez M, Sheu EG, Pazmany L, Strominger JL. 1996. Enhancement of class II-restricted T cell responses by costimulatory NK receptors for class I MHC proteins. *Science* 274:2097–3100

Annu. Rev. Immunol. 2001. 19:331–73

The Bare Lymphocyte Syndrome and the Regulation of MHC Expression

Walter Reith and Bernard Mach

Jeantet Laboratory of Molecular Genetics, Department of Genetics and Microbiology, University of Geneva Medical School, 1 rue Michel-Servet, 1211 Geneva 4, Switzerland; e-mail: Walter.Reith@medecine.unige.ch, Bernard.Mach@medecine.unige.ch

Key Words MHC class II deficiency, primary immunodeficiency disease, transcription regulation, CIITA, RFX

■ **Abstract** The bare lymphocyte syndrome (BLS) is a hereditary immunodeficiency resulting from the absence of major histocompatibility complex class II (MHCII) expression. Considering the central role of MHCII molecules in the development and activation of CD4$^+$ T cells, it is not surprising that the immune system of the patients is severely impaired. BLS is the prototype of a "disease of gene regulation." The affected genes encode RFXANK, RFX5, RFXAP, and CIITA, four regulatory factors that are highly specific and essential for MHCII genes. The first three are subunits of RFX, a trimeric complex that binds to all MHCII promoters. CIITA is a non-DNA-binding coactivator that functions as the master control factor for MHCII expression. The study of RFX and CIITA has made major contributions to our comprehension of the molecular mechanisms controlling MHCII genes and has made this system into a textbook model for the regulation of gene expression.

PREAMBLE: BLS as a Unique Model System

Major histocompatibility complex class II (MHCII) deficiency (official WHO nomenclature) is frequently also referred to as the bare lymphocyte syndrome (BLS). It is a rare form of inherited immunodeficiency having an autosomal recessive mode of inheritance. The disease is characterized by the lack of expression of MHCII molecules, which leads to severe immunodeficiency, recurrent infections, and frequently to death in early childhood (1–5). BLS exhibits several remarkable and unique features that have fascinated geneticists, immunologists, and specialists in the regulation of gene expression.

From the point of view of medical genetics, BLS is of special interest for at least three reasons. First, the genes implicated in the phenotypic manifestation of the disease, namely the family of MHCII genes on chromosome 6, are in fact intact. The genes that are mutated in BLS are distinct from the MHCII genes themselves and are located on different chromosomes (Figure 1). Mutations in

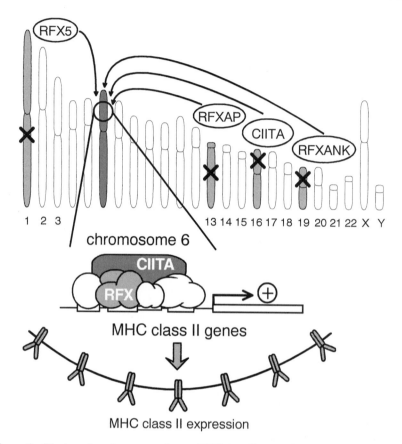

Figure 1   The bare lymphocyte syndrome (BLS) is a disease of MHCII gene regulation. BLS is characterized by a dissociation between the genes that are mutated in the disease (*top: RFX5, RFXAP, CIITA* and *RFXANK* on chromosomes 1, 13, 16 and 19, respectively) and the genes whose lack of expression accounts for the observed phenotype (*bottom*, MHCII genes on chromosome 6).

any one of these non-MHC genes are responsible for the lack of MHCII expression. This dissociation between the genes that are defective in the disease and those that are implicated in the observed phenotype is highly unusual (Figure 1). Second, although BLS is a monogenic disease in which a single defective gene is responsible for the entire clinical picture, and although the disease is clinically homogeneous, it can result from mutations in any one of four distinct genes (Figure 1). Curiously, a genetic defect in each of these four genes leads to the same clinical syndrome. This genetic heterogeneity associated with clinical homogeneity is also unusual. Thirdly, BLS represents the prototype of a "disease of gene regulation." The affected genes encode four *trans*-acting regulatory factors that are essential and highly specific for the control of MHCII gene expression (Figure 1).

It is evident that the last point explains the aforementioned distinction between the genetic defects and their phenotypic manifestations.

From the point of view of the control of the immune response, as well as of the regulation of gene expression in general, elucidation of BLS at the molecular level has led to numerous seminal findings. First, it is fair to say that the discovery of the four regulatory genes implicated in BLS has represented a major contribution to what we know today about the molecular basis of the regulation of MHCII gene expression. Given the tight and complex nature of this regulation, and its central role in the control of the immune response, the contribution of BLS to immunology has been remarkable. Second, identification of the four regulatory genes affected in BLS has provided us with a unique example of four transcription factors that are both essential and specific for the control of MHCII expression. This also represents a rather unusual situation because most transcription factors exhibit functional redundancy with other factors and/or exert pleiotropic effects via their control over numerous unrelated target genes. Finally, dissection of the mechanisms by which the four regulatory factors affected in BLS exert their control over MHCII genes has provided us with a textbook model for the regulation of gene expression. In particular, it has emphasized the essential role of protein-protein interactions in transcriptional control and the importance of cooperativity as a means for generating specificity.

The first part of this review covers BLS as a disease, discusses its molecular basis, and summarizes the discovery, between 1993 and 1998, of the four affected regulatory genes and the transacting factors that they encode. The second part deals with the contribution that the discovery of these four transactivators has made to our current understanding of the mechanisms regulating the expression of MHCII genes.

INTRODUCTION: Function and Regulation of MHCII Expression

MHCII molecules are heterodimeric (α/β) transmembrane glycoproteins. In humans there are three MHCII isotypes—HLA-DR, HLA-DQ, and HLA-DP—each of which is composed of a distinct pair of α and β chains. The genes encoding the α and β chains of HLA-DR, HLA-DQ, and HLA-DP are clustered in the D region of the MHC on the short arm of chromosome 6 (6). MHCII molecules are specialized for the presentation of peptides to the antigen receptor (TCR) of CD4$^+$ T helper cells. Engagement of MHCII–peptide complexes by the TCR of CD4$^+$ T cells is a key event in the development, activation, and regulation of the adaptive immune system. First, the recognition of MHCII–peptide complexes on epithelial cells and bone marrow–derived cells in the thymus is central to the positive and negative selection processes that sculpt the TCR repertoire of the CD4$^+$ T cell population (7). Second, the priming, propagation, and regulation of antigen-specific immune responses by CD4$^+$ T cells requires the interaction of their TCR with MHCII–peptide complexes displayed on antigen presenting cells (APC) (8). These APC are specialized for the MHCII-mediated presentation of peptides derived from the internalization and processing of exogenous protein antigens. Finally, the life span of CD4$^+$ T cells in the periphery is influenced by interactions with cells expressing MHCII molecules (7). Given these key functions of MHCII molecules, it is not surprising that defects in their expression have severe immunopathological consequences. The inability to express MHCII molecules leads to a severely crippled immune system that is incapable of responding adequately to foreign antigens (1–5). In contrast, aberrant or inappropriate MHCII expression has been incriminated in certain CD4$^+$ T cell–mediated autoimmune diseases (9). These two points emphasize the importance of correctly regulated MHCII expression for the control of the immune response in health and disease. For nearly two decades, a detailed elucidation of the molecular mechanisms that regulate MHCII expression has therefore represented a major challenge in molecular immunology.

Constitutive MHCII expression is generally restricted to a small number of cells of the immune system (4, 10–13). These include primarily bone marrow–derived APCs, namely dendritic cells (DCs), B cells, and cells of the monocyte/macrophage lineage. MHCII expression is also characteristic of epithelial cells in the thymus. Finally, in humans, activated T cells express MHCII. Constitutive expression in all three APC lineages is regulated as a function of developmental stage. Maturation of DCs is accompanied by an increase in cell surface MHCII expression. Activation of macrophages by stimuli such as interferon gamma (IFNγ) also leads to enhanced MHCII expression. In contrast, MHCII expression is extinguished upon differentiation of B cells into plasma cells.

The majority of non–bone marrow–derived cell types generally do not express MHCII molecules. However, MHCII expression can be induced in these cells by a variety of stimuli, of which IFNγ is most potent and well known. IFNγ–induced MHCII expression can be further modulated by a diverse array of other influences. For example, TGFβ, IFNβ, TNFα, IL-1, infection by a variety of pathogens, and certain drugs can attenuate or block the induction of MHCII expression by IFNγ.

Both constitutive and IFNγ–induced MHCII expression are controlled primarily at the level of transcription by a highly conserved regulatory region situated within the first 150 base pairs upstream of the transcription initiation site (4, 10–13). This promoter proximal regulatory region consists of four cis-acting elements referred to as the S (also called W or Z), X, X2, and Y boxes. These four elements are highly conserved in their sequence, orientation, order, and spacing relative to each other, and they function together as a single composite MHCII regulatory module (4, 11–13). The same architecture is evident in the promoters of all MHCII genes from every species that has been examined. A similar arrangement has also been conserved in the promoter regions of the MHCII-related *Ii, HLA-DM*, and *HLA-DO* genes (14–19), which code for proteins implicated in the intracellular traffic and peptide loading of MHCII molecules (20–22). Finally, it has recently also been appreciated that a region resembling the MHCII regulatory module contributes, albeit to a lesser extent, to expression of the MHC class I (MHCI) and $\beta2$ microglobulin (*B2M*) genes (23–27).

With the aim of dissecting the molecular mechanisms regulating transcription of MHCII genes, a considerable amount of effort has been devoted to the identification of transcription factors that bind to the MHCII regulatory module. Over 20 different nuclear factors capable of binding in vitro to the S, X, X2, and Y boxes were identified and/or cloned (4, 10–13). This complexity led to considerable confusion and controversy regarding the functional relevance and importance of all these MHCII promoter-binding factors. Distinguishing the factors that control transcription of MHCII genes from those that are functionally irrelevant represented a formidable task. This problem was solved to a large extent by a genetic approach. This genetic approach relied on the elucidation of the molecular defects underlying the absence of MHCII expression in the bare lymphocyte syndrome (BLS). Isolation of the genes that are defective in BLS has led to the unequivocal identification of CIITA and the multiprotein RFX complex, two key regulatory factors that activate transcription of the genes encoding the MHCII, HLA-DM, HLA-DO, Ii, and MHCI molecules (28–34).

PART 1: MHCII Deficiency or the Bare Lymphocyte Syndrome

Clinical Manifestations and Pathology

Patients suffering from a primary immunodeficiency syndrome characterized by a defect in MHC expression were first reported in the late 1970s and early 1980s (35–40). Curiously, the term BLS (41) was initially used to describe a reduced level of MHCI molecules in patients in which MHCII expression was not examined. Since then, a constant and profound defect in MHCII expression has been recognized as the major cause of the syndrome, and the disease was thus formally named MHCII deficiency by the World Health Organization (42). However, the term BLS is still widely used as a synonym for MHCII deficiency. The disease has been assigned the MIM (Mendelian Inheritance in Man) number 209920.

BLS is a rare autosomal recessive disease. Fewer than 80 patients coming from about 60 unrelated families have been formally reported worldwide. As expected for a rare inherited disease, there is a high incidence of consanguinity in the affected families (43). A majority of the affected families are from North Africa, but Turkey and Spain are also well represented (1, 3, 43).

The lack of expression of MHCII antigens results in a severe defect in both cellular and humoral immunity, and the patients thus exhibit an extreme vulnerability to infections (1–3, 5). This includes viral, bacterial, and fungal as well as protozoal infections. Clinical manifestations typical of BLS include mainly recurrent infections of the gastrointestinal tract, pneumonitis, and bronchitis. Severe septicemia is also common. Multiple infectious agents are responsible for the infections.

Pseudomonas and Salmonella, as well as cytomegalovirus, are found frequently. Major clinical findings resulting from bacterial infections of the gastrointestinal tract are protracted diarrhea, malabsorption, and failure to thrive. Infections start within the first year of life, and there is a dramatic progression of various types of infectious complications, generally leading to death before the age of 10. All of the clinical manifestations of the disease are related to infections and presumably result from the lack of MHCII expression. From a clinical point of view, no distinction has been made between BLS patients belonging to the four genetic complementation groups (see below). The most common clinical manifestations of BLS are summarized in Table 1. A more detailed presentation of the clinical picture of BLS can be found elsewhere (1–3, 5).

Laboratory Findings and Immunological Features

The most striking and constant immunological feature of BLS is the absence of cellular and humoral immune responses to foreign antigens (1–3, 5). Interestingly, all of the immunological features and anomalies recognized in BLS patients can be accounted for by the lack of MHCII expression and by its consequences in terms of antigen presentation. Surprisingly, the immunological anomalies exhibited by BLS patients, including their laboratory parameters, are notoriously variable from patient to patient. However, as observed for the clinical manifestations, no correlation has been recognized with the four distinct genetic groups of patients defined by the individual regulatory genes that are affected (see below).

Detailed accounts of the immunological features and laboratory findings typical of BLS have been published previously (1–3, 5). Patients are unable to mount T cell–mediated immune responses in vivo, and their T cells are not activated in vitro by antigens to which the patients have been exposed. Humoral immune responses are also severely affected: Hypogammaglobulinemia is characteristic, and antibody responses to immunizations and infections are reduced or absent (Table 1). The total numbers of circulating T and B lymphocytes is normal, but the number of $CD4^+$ T lymphocytes is reduced (Table 1). The severity of this reduction varies from patient to patient. The remaining $CD4^+$ T lymphocytes do not exhibit major abnormalities in their TCR repertoire, and they seem to be functionally normal as judged by alloreactivity and responses to mitogens. Their physiological responses to MHCII mediated antigen presentation have however not been studied thoroughly. The presence of a significant number of residual $CD4^+$ T lymphocytes in patients that fail to express MHCII molecules remains an interesting paradox. Residual expression of MHCII molecules in the thymus, although not clearly documented, or alternative pathways for positive selection of $CD4^+$ T cells, have been mentioned as possible explanations (see below).

Abnormal Expression of MHCII Genes

Since the initial descriptions of the disease, understanding the cause of BLS has represented a challenge for immunologists interested in the crucial role of MHCII and of its remarkably tight regulation in the control of the immune response.

TABLE 1   Clinical manifestations and immunological features of BLS

Clinical manifestations	Fraction of patients[1]
Repeated severe infections	47/47
Protracted diarrhea	45/47
Lower respiratory tract infections	40/47
Failure to thrive	34/47
Severe viral infections	27/47
Upper respiratory infections	24/47
Mucocutaneous candidiasis	16/47
Progressive liver disease	8/47
Cryptosporidiosis	8/47
Autoimmune cytopenia	4/47
Sclerosing cholangitis	5/47
Immunological findings	**Fraction of patients[1]**
Complete absence of MHCII expression:	
B cells	36/37
monocytes	31/37
PHA activated T cells	32/37
Residual MHCII expression:	
monocytes	6/37
PHA activated T cells	5/37
Reduction of MHCI expression:	
mononuclear cells	23/30
CD4+ lymphopenia	28/31
Serum immunoglobulins:	
decreased IgG	18/22
decreased IgM	23/32
decreased IgA	25/32
Decreased or absent antibody response to:	
immunizations	15/16
microbial antigens	26/26

[1]data adapted from Reith et al., 1999 (2).

Numerous research groups therefore turned to the study of the molecular basis of BLS as a way to learn more about the regulation of MHCII expression. Here we describe the progress that was made toward this goal in a chronological order, as a succession of logical experimental milestones. We are very grateful for the long-term collaborations between our laboratory and those who provided the BLS cell lines that made our studies possible, particularly the laboratories of C Griscelli (Paris) and M Hadam (Hanover).

As described in the Introduction, two distinct modes of MHCII expression are normally observed in healthy individuals: constitutive expression in a restricted number of highly specialized cells, and inducible expression in response to specific stimuli, particularly IFNγ. In BLS, both constitutive and inducible expression of MHCII antigens abolished (1–3, 5). The lack of cell surface MHCII molecules is evident on all professional antigen-presenting cells, including B cells, macrophages such as Kupfer cells in the liver, and dendritic cells such as Langerhans cells in the skin. Activated T cells remain MHCII negative. Moreover, cells that are not of bone marrow origin, such as thymic epithelial cells and endothelial cells, also lack MHCII molecules. Finally, cells from the patients do not express MHCII molecules following stimulation with IFNγ.

This general lack of cell surface MHCII expression was confirmed at the level of intracellular MHCII proteins (44). The next step was to show that no MHCII mRNA could be detected in any of the cell types and conditions studied (3, 44–46). It was further shown that the deficiency in expression concerned the α- and β-chain genes coding for the HLA-DR, HLA-DQ, and HLA-DP molecules, implying a general block in the expression of all MHCII genes (3, 44–46). More recently, a partial block in the expression of the MHCII-related genes encoding HLA-DM, HLA-DO, and the Ii chain was also described (15, 47, 48).

Occasional weak residual expression of MHCII antigens and mRNA has been reported in certain BLS patients (Table 1). This residual expression has been described both for constitutive expression in certain cell types and for inducible expression in response to IFNγ (1–3, 5). We have not observed such a leaky phenotype in most of the EBV-transformed BLS B cell lines that we have studied. In addition to the complete extinction of MHCII expression, a relatively minor reduction in the level of MHCI molecules has been observed in BLS (Table 1) (1–3, 5). Again, this reduction in MHCI is not evident, at least at the level of cell surface expression, in most of the typical BLS B cell lines that we have studied.

BLS Is a Disease of Gene Regulation Involving Defects in "Transacting" Factors

The demonstration that BLS is a disease of gene regulation represented a key step in the elucidation of BLS. The fact that all MHCII genes were found to be silent first suggested that there was a general defect acting in *trans* on the entire gene family. To test this hypothesis we studied the affected families for transmission of both the disease phenotype and the MHC locus on chromosome 6 (3, 45). The two clearly did not cosegregate, indicating that the genetic defect(s) responsible for BLS reside outside of the MHC. It was the merit of the late Claude de Préval to publish these findings in a 1985 *Nature* paper entitled "A trans-acting class II regulatory gene, unlinked to the MHC, controls the regulation of HLA class II expression" (45). This statement was formally confirmed 8 years later when we identified and cloned the first *trans*-acting gene affected in BLS (29 see below). Another important confirmation of the regulatory nature of the BLS defect came from cell fusion experiments demonstrating that MHCII expression can be reactivated upon fusion of MHCII negative cells affected in two different genes (see below) (43, 49–51). Finally, it was subsequently shown that MHCII promoters remain silent in functional studies performed in BLS cells (52, 53) and that nuclear extracts from BLS cells cannot support in vitro transcription from MHCII promoters (54). The realization that BLS is due to defects in regulatory factors specific for MHCII genes suggested that elucidation of the genetic basis of BLS was likely to lead, beyond the scope of the disease itself, to the discovery of genes and factors directly involved in the important but elusive molecular mechanisms controlling MHCII expression.

Genetic Heterogeneity in BLS

The search for the genetic defects underlying BLS became even more exciting and challenging when it was found that the disease is genetically heterogeneous and that patients could be classified into four distinct complementation groups (Table 2, groups A to D). The conclusion that the disease is genetically heterogeneous was drawn from somatic cell fusion experiments performed with MHCII-negative cell lines derived from BLS patients (43, 49–51, 55). In certain combinations MHCII expression was clearly restored, indicating that the two cell lines belong to distinct genetic complementation groups. These studies revealed the existence of four

TABLE 2   Genetic, biochemical and molecular heterogeneity in BLS

BLS complementation group	A	B	C	D
Prototypical patients	BLS-2, BCH	BLS-1, Ra	SJO, Ro	DA, ABI
Number of unrelated families	5	26	5	6
Prototypical in vitro mutant	RJ2.2.5	None	G1B	6.1.6
Number of in vitro mutants	3	None	1	1
MHCII expression	Absent	Absent	Absent	Absent
MHCII promoter activity	Absent	Absent	Absent	Absent
Binding of RFX	Yes	No	No	No
Promoter occupancy in vivo	Occupied	Bare	Bare	Bare
Affected gene	*MHC2TA*	*RFXANK*	*RFX5*	*RFXAP*
MIM number	600005	603200	601863	601861
mRNA sequence entry	X74301	AF094760	X85786	Y12812
Chromosomal localization	16p13	19p12	1q21.1–21.3	13q14
Protein	CIITA	RFXANK	RFX5	RFXAP
Length (amino acids)	1'130	269	616	272
Apparent molecular weight	130 kD	33 kD	75 kD	36 kD
No. distinct mutations in BLS	5	7	5	3

complementation groups (43, 49–51,55). It is now known that the majority of patients (26 out of 42 families) belong to group B, while groups A, C, and D correspond respectively to 5, 5, and 6 unrelated families (Table 2) (56). In addition to cells from BLS patients, several in vitro–generated mutant MHCII-negative cell lines have also been allocated to the complementation groups. These include RJ2.2.5 (group A), G1B (group C), and 6.1.6 (group D) (Table 2) (49–51, 57–59). The identification of four genetic complementation groups strongly suggested the existence of genetic loci corresponding to four key MHCII regulatory genes. This greatly strengthened the interest in the genetic and molecular basis of BLS because it implied that elucidation of this rare disease should lead to the discovery of four distinct regulatory genes that are all essential and specific for the control of MHCII expression.

As mentioned earlier, none of the clinical, pathological, or immunological features observed in BLS patients is typical of or unique to one of the four genetic groups. The syndrome is therefore genetically heterogeneous but clinically and phenotypically homogeneous. There is, however, an interesting correlation between individual BLS groups and the ethnic origin of the patients: Patients from group B are predominantly of North African origin while those from group A are mainly Hispanic (43).

Atypical Form of Deficiency in MHCII Expression

A family affected by an atypical and much less severe form of deficiency in MHCII expression has been described (60–62). Defective expression in the two patients from this family does not concern all MHCII genes equally. In B cell lines derived from these two patients, the *HLA-DRB*, *HLA-DQB*, and *HLA-DPA* genes are silent while the *HLA-DRA*, *HLA-DQA*, and *HLA-DPB* genes are expressed (62). Interestingly, the silent genes are present in one transcriptional orientation within the MHCII locus, whereas the active ones are found in the opposite orientation (62). This intriguing discordant pattern of expression remains unexplained. Impairment of the immune response is considerably less severe in the two atypical patients than in classical BLS (60, 61). This has been suggested to be due to the fact that the deficiency in MHCII expression does not affect all cell types to the same extent. Indeed, investigations of MHCII-dependent immune functions in these patients indicate the presence of competent MHCII positive APCs (60, 61). As expected from their unusual phenotype, the atypical patients represent a distinct medical and genetic entity compared to the classical BLS groups A to D (62). The molecular defect underlying this atypical form of immunodeficiency has not yet been elucidated.

DNA-Binding of RFX Distinguishes Between
Two Types of Molecular Defect in BLS

RFX (Regulatory Factor X) is a DNA-binding protein complex first identified in MHCII positive B cells on the basis of its ability to bind in vitro to the X box of MHCII promoters (30). Binding activity of the RFX complex was studied extensively with nuclear extracts prepared from various wild-type and BLS cell lines (30, 54, 63). It was recognized rather early that two types of BLS defects could be defined on the basis of the presence of the RFX complex (Table 2). Binding of RFX was found to be normal in wild-type cells as well as in cells from BLS patients in group A. On the other hand, cells from patients in groups B, C, and D were specifically devoid of RFX binding activity. This observation indicated that the genetic defects in groups B–D affect the integrity or binding activity of the RFX complex, while the defect in group A is independent of RFX.

Interestingly, there is a tight correlation between the status of RFX binding activity in vitro and the state of occupancy of MHCII promoters in vivo (Table 2). This was analyzed either by mapping of DNAseI hypersensitive sites (64) or by in vivo footprint experiments (65, 66). BLS cells lacking a functional RFX, complex (groups B, C and D) exhibit a "bare" promoter phenotype in which the X, X2, and Y sequences of MHCII promoters are not bound by their cognate DNA-binding proteins (65, 66). In contrast, wild-type cells as well as cells from BLS patients in group A exhibit both normal RFX binding activity in vitro and normal MHCII promoter occupancy in vivo (65, 66). The fact that not only the X box, but also the X2 and Y boxes are unoccupied in vivo in the absence of RFX, points to a crucial role of RFX in facilitating overall promoter occupation. It is now clear that this is explained by the fact that RFX entertains strong cooperative binding interactions with other MHCII promoter binding factors (67–71), including the Y box binding factor NF-Y (72) and the X2 box binding factor X2BP (67). The importance of these cooperative protein-protein interactions in the specificity of gene activation is discussed further below.

CIITA: The Regulatory Gene and Factor
Affected BLS Group A

Paradoxically, although the deficiency in RFX offered an experimental approach toward the identification and cloning of the genes affected in BLS groups B–D, the first BLS gene and factor to be discovered was the one affected in group A (29). The strategy employed relied on the genetic complementation of RJ2.2.5, one of the in vitro generated cell lines classified in group A. Following transfection of RJ2.2.5 with a B cell cDNA library prepared in an episomal expression vector, plasmids capable of correcting the genetic defect were rescued from cells in which MHCII expression was restored. This approach led to the isolation of cDNA clones encoding the MHC class II transactivator CIITA (Figure 2) (29). The human gene (*MHC2TA*) encoding CIITA is localized on chromosome 16 (16p13) (Figure 1). The mouse gene (*Mhc2ta*) is situated in a syntenic region of mouse chromosome 16 (V Steimle, B Mach, unpublished data). This localization is consistent with previous experiments demonstrating that regulatory genes present on the human and mouse chromosomes 16 (the *AIR-1* locus) are required for expression of MHCII genes (73, 74). The entire intron-exon structure of the mouse *Mhc2ta* gene has been determined. It consists of 19 exons spanning 42 kb of genomic DNA

The non-DNA-binding coactivator CIITA (BLS complementation group A)

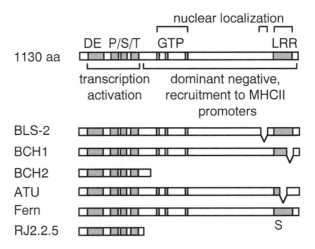

Figure 2 Structure, function, and mutation of CIITA, the regulatory factor that is affected in BLS complementation group A. A schematic map of the CIITA protein is shown at the top. The three sequences constituting a GTP binding domain, the leucine-rich repeat domain (LRR), the acidic region (DE), and 3 segments rich in proline, serine, and threonine (P/S/T) are represented by grey boxes. Regions that function in activation of transcription, in recruitment to MHCII promoters, in nuclear localization, and as a dominant negative mutant are indicated. Mutations affecting the *MHC2TA* gene have been determined in four BLS patients (BLS-2, BCH, ATU, and Fern) and in the in vitro generated cell line RJ2.2.5. The effects of the mutations at the level of the CIITA protein are represented schematically.

(W Reith, B Mach, unpublished data). Defects in the *MHC2TA* gene account for patients in complementation group A (Figure 2). Expression vectors encoding CIITA can reactivate expression of all three MHCII isotypes when transfected into cell lines from complementation group A (29). Wild-type levels of *Ii, HLA-DMA*, and *HLA-DMB* expression are also restored (47, 75). Five different mutations of the *MHC2TA* gene have been characterized in BLS patients from group A (29, 56, 76–78). Both alleles of the *MHC2TA* gene are also mutated in RJ2.2.5 (29, 79).

The Genes Encoding RFX, the DNA-Binding Complex Affected in BLS Groups B to D

Purification of RFX demonstrated that it consists of three subunits having apparent molecular weights of 75, 36, and 33 kDa (33, 54, 80). This suggested that defects in the genes encoding these three subunits were likely to account for the absence of RFX binding activity in cells from BLS groups B, C, and D. Isolation of the genes encoding the three subunits of RFX confirmed this interpretation (31–34).

We called these genes *RFXANK, RFX5*, and *RFXAP* and demonstrated that they are indeed mutated in BLS complementation groups B, C, and D, respectively (Table 2, Figure 3) (31–33).

RFX5: The Regulatory Gene and Factor Affected in BLS Group C   *RFX5*, the gene encoding the largest (75 kDa) subunit of the RFX complex, was isolated by the same genetic complementation approach that led to the cloning of CIITA (32). Briefly, *RFX5* cDNA clones were isolated by virtue of their ability to restore MHCII expression upon transfection into SJO, a cell line derived from a BLS patient in complementation group C (32). RFX5 derives its name from the fact that it is the fifth isolated member of a family of DNA-binding proteins capable of recognizing the MHCII X box (81). All members of this RFX family share a common motif called the RFX DNA-binding domain (Figure 3) (81, 82). The human *RFX5* gene is situated in a subcentromeric region of the long arm of chromosome 1 (1q21.1–21.3) (83). The corresponding mouse gene maps to a syntenic region of chromosome 3 (W Reith, unpublished data). The entire intron-exon structure of the mouse *Rfx5* gene has been determined and shown to consist of 10 exons (W Reith, unpublished data). Defects in *RFX5* account for the existence of complementation group C (Figure 3). Mutations in *RFX5* have been characterized in five patients from group C (32, 56, 83–85). A missense mutation has also been identified in G1B, an in vitro generated MHCII regulatory mutant (59).

RFXAP: The Regulatory Gene and Factor Affected in BLS Group D   *RFXAP*, the gene encoding the second subunit of the RFX complex was identified using a biochemical approach (31). To isolate *RFXAP*, we purified the RFX complex, isolated its 36 kDa subunit, derived peptide sequences from this polypeptide, and then cloned the corresponding gene. The gene was called *RFXAP* (RFX Associated Protein) because it encodes a protein that interacts directly with RFX5 (31). The human *RFXAP* gene is situated on the long arm of chromosome 13 (55). The genomic structure of the mouse *Rfxap* gene has been determined and shown to consist of only 3 exons (W Reith, unpublished data). Defects in the *RFXAP* gene account for complementation group D (Figure 3). Three different mutations have been identified in six unrelated families (31, 55, 56, 86). An in vitro generated mutant (6.1.6) has also been shown to contain mutations in *RFXAP* (31).

RFXANK: The Regulatory Gene and Factor Affected in BLS Group B   *RFXANK* (also called *RFXB*), the gene encoding the last subunit of RFX, was also discovered thanks to biochemical approaches relying on purification of the RFX complex. It was identified on the basis of peptide sequences derived from the smallest 33 kDa subunit of RFX. We named the gene *RFXANK* because it encodes a factor containing a protein-protein interaction domain consisting of ankyrin repeats (Figure 3) (33). Subsequently, another group independently isolated the same gene and proposed the name RFXB (34). The human *RFXANK* gene consists of 10 exons spanning 9 kb of genomic DNA and is situated on the short arm of

Subunits of the RFX complex

1) RFXANK (BLS complementation group B)

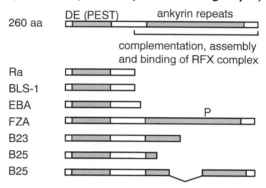

2) RFX5 (BLS complementation group C)

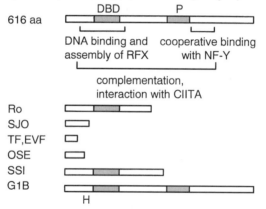

3) RFXAP (BLS complementation group D)

chromosome 19 (19p12) (33, 34). Defects in the *RFXANK* gene account for patients in complementation group B (33, 34, 87), which contains over 70% of all known BLS patients (Figure 3). Transfection of the *RFXANK* cDNA into cell lines from group B restores expression of all MHCII isotypes (33, 34). The *RFXANK* gene was found to be mutated in 26 unrelated patients (33, 34, 56, 87, 88). Only seven different mutations were identified in these patients (Figure 3). One of the mutations was found in 19 unrelated patients, indicating the existence of a founder effect (87).

Therapeutic Perspectives

Carrier Detection and Prenatal Diagnosis for BLS   Prenatal diagnosis or carrier detection on a population-wide scale is not justified because BLS is a very rare disease. However, these procedures could be valuable for families in which patients have already been identified, or when a consanguineous union is envisaged in a high-risk population. Thanks to the identification of the molecular defects underlying BLS, mutated alleles of the *MHC2TA*, *RFXANK*, *RFX5*, and *RFXAP* genes can now be screened for directly. This will permit healthy carriers to be identified unambiguously and should allow the development of accurate and reliable procedures for prenatal diagnosis.

Gene Therapy for BLS   Bone marrow transplantation (BMT) is currently the only curative treatment for BLS (89). Compared to other immunodeficiency syndromes, the success rate of BMT for BLS has been rather poor (89). This does not appear to be a peculiar characteristic of the BLS disease. Instead, it is likely to be due mainly to other criteria, such as diagnosis at a late age (89, 90). Identification of the affected genes has raised the hope that gene therapy will represent a potential alternative to BMT. Introduction of the wild-type MHC2TA, RFXANK, RFX5, or RFXAP genes into hematopoietic stem cells of BLS patients in complementation groups A, B, C, or D, respectively, would represent a logical therapeutic strategy. The *Mhc2ta* and *Rfx5* knockout mice (see below) will be invaluable for

---

Figure 3 Structure, function, and mutation of the RFX subunits that are affected in BLS complementation groups B, C, and D. Schematic maps of the RFXANK, RFX5, and RFXAP subunits are shown. The acidic region (DE) and ankyrin repeat domain of RFXANK, the DNA binding domain and proline rich segment of RFX5, and the acidic (DE), basic and glutamine-rich (Q) regions of RFXAP are represented as gray boxes. The regions that are required for complementation of BLS cells, for assembly and binding of the RFX complex, for cooperative binding between RFX and NF-Y, and for interaction with CIITA are indicated. Mutations in RFXANK, RFX5, and RFXAP have been characterized in BLS patients (Ra, BLS-1, EBA, FZA, B23, and B25 for RFXANK; Ro, SJO, TF/EVF, OSE, and SSI for RFX5; ABI, DA, ZM, and Sha/ShG for RFXAP) and in two in vitro generated cell lines (G1B and 6.1.6). The effects of the mutations at the level of the RFXANK, RFX5, and RFXAP proteins are represented schematically.

developing gene therapy procedures for BLS. Defective selection of CD4$^+$ T cells, resulting from the lack of MHCII expression on thymic epithelial cells, might be anticipated to represent an obstacle to gene therapy for BLS. However, the fact that classical BMT can cure BLS suggests that restoring MHCII expression on non–bone marrow–derived cells, such as thymic epithelial cells, is not absolutely essential. Another potential concern is that the therapeutic transgene could induce ectopic or abnormal levels of MHCII expression, which could have deleterious consequences and compromise the success of gene therapy. This will probably not be a major problem for RFX5, RFXANK (the largest group of patients), and RFXAP, which are expressed ubiquitously at nonlimiting levels in all cell types. On the other hand, this may represent a major dilemma in the case of CIITA because expression of the MHC2TA gene is tightly regulated.

Therapeutic Modulation of MHCII Expression   MHCII expression is severely impaired in BLS patients. The same is true for most cell types in the mouse models of the disease (see below). This implies that no bypass or alternative pathway can compensate efficiently for a deficiency in RFX or CIITA. Moreover, although there are indications that the specificity of RFX and CIITA is not as strict as previously believed (see below), the expression of MHCII genes remains the major system in which these transcription factors are essential. Because of these features, inhibitors of CIITA, RFXANK, RFXAP, and RFX5 would be anticipated to have an efficient and selective effect on MHCII expression. CIITA, RFXANK, RFXAP, and RFX5 may thus represent prime targets for novel immunomodulatory drugs having wide applications in situations in which inhibition of MHCII expression might be desirable or beneficial, such as organ transplantation, autoimmune diseases, and inflammation in general.

The immunogenicity and rejection of tumors can be enhanced by activating MHCII expression, alone or in combination with costimulatory molecules (91–94). This has raised hopes that the introduction of CIITA into tumor cells to activate MHCII expression might enhance tumor immunogenicity and contribute to the success of tumor immunotherapy. Experiments designed to address the validity of this approach have been initiated (95).

Lessons from Mouse Models for BLS

Knockout mice that reproduce the molecular defects of BLS patients in groups A and C have been constructed by targeting of the *Mhc2ta* and *Rfx5* genes (96–99). Both of these models reproduce the major immunopathological characteristics of the human disease. There is a strong reduction of constitutive MHCII expression on professional APCs (B cells, DCs, and macrophages) and thymic epithelial cells. Induction of MHCII expression by IFNγ is also abolished. The loss of MHCII expression results in a severely compromised immune system.

The CD4$^+$ T cell population in *Mhc2ta* and *Rfx5* knockout mice is decreased at least tenfold (96–99). This strong reduction is a consequence of severely impaired positive selection, which results from the loss of MHCII expression on epithelial cells in the thymus. Surprisingly, the reduction in CD4$^+$ T cells is considerably less pronounced in the human disease; CD4$^+$ T cell counts are rarely reduced greater than two- to threefold in BLS patients (1, 3). The reason for this discrepancy between the human and mouse phenotypes is not clear. One plausible explanation is that positive selection in the human disease is compromised only partially because low levels of residual MHCII expression are retained in the thymus. Whether or not this explanation is valid remains to be determined because MHCII expression patterns in the thymus have been examined only in a few isolated cases (100, 101). A second possibility is that the CD4$^+$ T cells in BLS patients have escaped the normal thymic selection processes. They could for example have been selected on ligands other than MHCII molecules. In MHCII deficient mice, a large proportion of the residual CD4$^+$ T cells are CD1-restricted (102). Such alternative selection pathways could be more prominent in BLS patients. Interestingly, an analysis of the T cell repertoire in BLS patients has revealed minor alterations, suggesting that the CD4$^+$ T cells in these patients may indeed have been subjected to unusual selection mechanisms (103, 104).

The *Mhc2ta*−/− and *Rfx5*−/− mice exhibit residual MHCII expression in certain cell types (Table 3). This implies that there are alternative pathways for MHCII expression that bypass partially the strict requirement for RFX5 and/or CIITA

TABLE 3   Cell surface MHC expression in *Rfx5*−/− and *Mhc2ta*−/− mice

	MHCII expression	
Tissue/cell type	*Rfx5*−/−	*Mhc2ta*−/−
Thymic cortex	−	+ (Weak, patchy)
Thymic medulla	+ (Strong)	−
Naive B cells	−	−
IL4/LPS activated B cells	+ (Reduced 10 fold)	−
Germinal center B cells	Not determined	+ (Low level)
Macrophages − IFN-γ	−	−
Macrophages + IFN-γ	−	−
Splenic DCs	+ (15% of cells)	−
Bone marrow derived DCs	+ (5% of cells)	−
Lymph node DCs	Not determined	+ (Low level)
	MHCI expression	
T cells	Reduced 10 fold	Normal
B cells	Reduced 2−5 fold	Normal
IFNγ induced expression	Normal	Normal

(96, 97, 99). The precise pattern of residual MHCII expression differs between *Mhc2ta−/−* and *Rfx5−/−* mice (Table 3). Residual MHCII expression in the *Mhc2ta−/−* mice concerns mainly a subset of thymic epithelial cells, dendritic cells in the paracortex of lymph nodes, and B cells in the germinal centers of the spleen and lymph nodes. In contrast, *Rfx5−/−* mice retain strong MHCII expression on dendritic cells in the thymic medulla and significant, albeit weaker, expression on a fraction of splenic and bone marrow–derived dendritic cells. Low MHCII expression is also induced on *Rfx5−/−* B cells activated with LPS and/or IL-4. This difference in the residual expression pattern is surprising because the human disease is phenotypically homogeneous. Although low expression has been observed in cells from certain BLS patients, no distinctive residual expression pattern discriminating between patients lacking RFX5 and CIITA has been described (1–3). This discrepancy between the human disease and the mouse models could reflect species-specific differences in the function of the two MHCII regulatory genes. However, it is also possible that phenotypic differences in residual MHCII expression exist in the human disease as well but have escaped attention because not enough patients have been examined in detail.

PART 2: MOLECULAR BASIS FOR THE REGULATION OF MHCII EXPRESSION

The RFX DNA-Binding Complex

Elucidation of the molecular defects underlying BLS complementation groups B, C, and D demonstrated that RFX is a multimeric complex consisting of RFXANK, RFX5, and RFXAP, three unrelated subunits sharing no sequence homology (Figure 3) (31–34). The stoichiometry of the three subunits within the RFX complex remains to be determined. Co-immunoprecipitation experiments performed with nuclear extracts, as well as with recombinant proteins, have indicated that the RFX complex is preassembled in solution prior to binding to DNA (33, 105, 106). All three subunits are essential for assembly of RFX (33, 105, 106). A deficiency in any one of the three subunits results in the inability to assemble a functional complex, which explains the absence of RFX binding activity in cells from complementation groups B, C, and D. It is unlikely that RFX contains additional unidentified subunits because a complex indistinguishable from the native protein can be assembled in vitro from recombinant RFX5, RFXAP, and RFXANK (105, 106).

All three RFX subunits can be cross-linked to the DNA within the X box *cis*-acting sequence (107). It remains unknown how RFXAP and RFXANK contribute to binding of RFX. On the other hand, RFX5 contains a well-known DNA binding domain (DBD), called the RFX domain (32, 81, 82). The RFX domain has been identified in a variety of DNA-binding proteins having diverse regulatory functions in organisms ranging from yeast to human (81, 82, 108–110). The structure of the RFX domain of one member of the RFX family (RFX1) has recently been determined and shown to belong to the winged helix subfamily of the helix-turn-helix (HTH) proteins (111). Surprisingly, the RFX1 DBD binds DNA in a fashion radically different from that observed for all other known HTH proteins. Instead of relying on a recognition helix, the RFX1 DBD makes unprecedented use of a β-hairpin (called the wing) to recognize its binding site (111). The amino acids implicated in site-specific binding of the RFX1 DBD are strongly conserved in RFX5, implying that the latter interacts with its X box target site in a similar fashion (111).

Functionally essential domains within RFXANK, RFX5, and RFXAP have been defined (Figure 3) (105, 106, 112, 113) (W. Reith, unpublished data). The minimal essential region of RFXANK encompasses a C-terminal region containing a protein-protein interaction domain consisting of ankyrin repeats. This region is essential for assembly and binding of the RFX complex and for activation of MHCII promoters. All of the *RFXANK* mutations identified in BLS patients remove or affect the integrity of this minimal functional domain. The minimal region of RFX5 covers an internal segment containing the DBD and a proline rich region. This region is sufficient for assembly and binding of the RFX complex, cooperative binding with NF-Y (see below) and interaction with CIITA (see below). All of the *RFX5* mutations identified in BLS patients lead to deletion of the DBD and/or the proline rich region. In the case of RFXAP, the minimal region is restricted to a short C-terminal domain spanning a glutamine rich region. This region of RFXAP is sufficient for assembly and binding of the RFX complex and for activation of MHCII promoters. All of the mutations identified in BLS patients lead to the loss of this essential C-terminal region.

Several interesting features within the subunits of RFX appear to be dispensable for function (105, 106, 112, 113) (W Reith, unpublished data). RFXAP contains an N-terminal acidic region and a centrally placed basic region resembling a nuclear localization signal. Both of these regions can be removed without significantly affecting the function of RFXAP. The N-terminus of RFXANK contains an acidic region that has been suggested to be a PEST (proline/glutamic acid/serine/threonine) domain (34). PEST domains are frequently found in proteins that have short half-lives (114). Whether or not this region functions as a PEST domain remains to be determined. However, it is clearly not essential because it can be removed without eliminating the function of RFXANK.

RFX Promotes Assembly of an MHCII Enhanceosome Complex

One of the major roles of RFX is to promote stable binding of other transcription factors to MHCII promoters (Figure 5a). Strong evidence for this was first provided by DNAseI hypersensitivity studies and in vivo footprint experiments examining the occupation of MHCII promoter in B cells that express or lack RFX (64–66). All of the critical *cis*-acting sequences of MHCII promoters are occupied by their cognate DNA-binding proteins in RFX-positive B cells (wild-type cells and cells from BLS complementation group A) (Figure 4). In RFX-deficient B cells (BLS complementation groups B-D), on the other hand, MHCII promoters are bare (Figure 4) (64–66). This defect in occupation is not restricted to the X box target site of RFX. Instead, the X2 and Y boxes are also unoccupied, indicating that

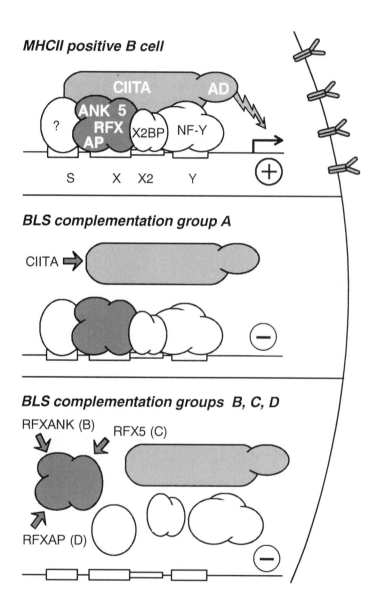

stable occupation of these sequences by their cognate DNA-binding factors is dependent on binding of RFX to the adjacent X box. Subsequent experiments explained this observation by demonstrating that RFX binds cooperatively (67–71, 115) with the Y box binding protein NF-Y (72) and the X2 box binding factor X2BP (67), which has recently been suggested to contain CREB (116) (Figure 5a). Cooperative binding interactions between these three proteins leads to the assembly of a remarkably stable higher order protein-DNA complex at MHCII promoters (67–71, 115).

In addition to enhancing stability, the cooperative interactions are also specific, thereby ensuring that the X, X2, and Y boxes are bound in vivo by RFX, X2BP (CREB), and NF-Y rather than by the multitude of other factors capable of binding to these sequences with comparatively low affinity in vitro. It is of particular relevance here that several other members of the X box binding family of proteins can bind to the X box in vitro, but fail to interact with X2BP or NFY, and thus fail to stabilize the multiprotein complex on MHCII promoters in vivo. These other X box binding proteins (RFX1 to RFX4) control other genes, by binding to X box sequences flanked by protein-binding motifs distinct from those found in MHCII promoters (81, 82, 108–110)

The higher order nucleoprotein complex that assembles at MHCII promoters has recently been coined the MHCII 'enhanceosome' (115). The requirement for the assembly of this enhanceosome explains the observation that the S, X, X2, and Y sequences function together as a single composite regulatory module in which correct spacing and stereospecific alignment is critical (71, 117, 118). Protein domains mediating cooperative binding interactions within the MHCII enhanceosome have begun to be defined. A region situated immediately downstream of the proline-rich segment of RFX5 mediates cooperative binding between RFX and

---

Figure 4 Molecular defects in the bare lymphocyte syndrome. A typical MHCII promoter containing the conserved S, X, X2, and Y sequences is depicted. The in vivo promoter occupancy and transcription status (+ or −) are shown for wild-type MHCII positive B cells and for B cells from BLS patients in complementation groups A, B, C, and D. Key transcription factors controlling promoter activity are indicated. RFX, X2BP, and NF-Y bind cooperatively to the X, X2, and Y sequences to form a highly stable nucleoprotein complex referred to as the MHCII enhanceosome. Proteins binding to the S box (?) remain poorly characterized. CIITA is a non-DNA-binding coactivator that is recruited to the promoter via protein-protein interactions with the DNA-binding components of enhanceosome. Proteins binding to the S (?), X (RFX), X2 (X2BP), and Y (NF-Y) boxes are all required for CIITA recruitment. CIITA activates transcription via N-terminal transcription activation domains (AD). The gene encoding CIITA is mutated in BLS patients in complementation group A. Mutations in CIITA do not affect assembly of the enhanceosome, and promoter occupation is consequently not modified. The genes that are defective in complementation groups B, C, and D, encode, respectively, the RFXANK, RFX5, and RFXAP subunits of RFX. In contrast to defects in CIITA, mutations in RFXANK, RFX5, or RFXAP disrupt assembly of the enhanceosome and thus lead to a bare promoter.

NF-Y (105). At the level of NF-Y, the minimal evolutionarily conserved regions comprising the DNA-binding domain are sufficient for cooperative binding with RFX (106). The regions within RFX and X2BP (CREB) that are implicated in their cooperative binding have not yet been mapped.

In addition to the crucial role of the MHCII enhanceosome in enhancing the stability and specificity of promoter occupation, it has very recently also been shown that this enhanceosome constitutes a platform onto which the transcriptional coactivator CIITA is recruited via protein-protein interactions (Figures 4 and 5, see above) (115). Association of CIITA with the MHCII enhanceosome

(a) cooperative binding with RFX

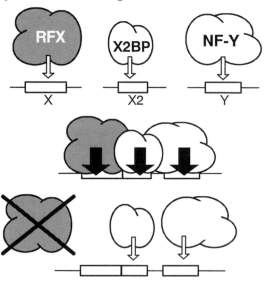

(b) protein-protein interactions with CIITA

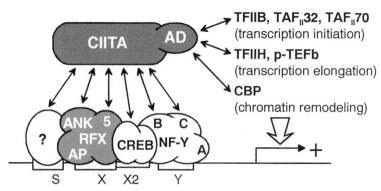

is mediated by synergistic contacts with multiple components of the enhanceosome, including factors binding to the S, X, X2, and Y sequences (see below) (112, 113, 115, 119).

The Non-DNA-Binding Coactivator CIITA

The gene encoding CIITA was isolated by virtue of its ability to correct the genetic defect in cell lines from BLS complementation group A (29). Although this genetic approach provided irrefutable evidence that CIITA is a crucial transactivator of MHCII genes, it provided frustratingly little information on how it achieves this. A considerable amount of effort has consequently been devoted to the elucidation of the mode of action of CIITA.

Several clues concerning the mode of action of CIITA are embedded in the primary sequence of the protein, which exhibits four major features of interest (Figure 2). First, the N terminus of the protein contains a region rich in acidic amino acids. Second, downstream of this acidic region lie three segments rich in proline, serine, and threonine (PST). Third, there is a centrally placed GTP binding domain that contains three characteristic sequences, a Walker A motif (also known as a P-loop) involved in nucleotide binding, a magnesium binding site, and a sequence that is believed to confer GTP binding specificity. Finally, there is a leucine rich repeat (LRR)–based protein-protein interaction motif near the C terminus of the protein. All four features are conserved between human and mouse CIITA and are necessary for the ability of the protein to activate MHCII promoters (120–125).

The acidic and PST regions found within the N-terminal portion of CIITA resemble the transcription activation domains typically found in mammalian transcription factors. Several observations support the notion that these regions of

←

Figure 5 Mode of action of RFX and CIITA. (*a*) RFX participates in cooperative binding interactions required for promoter occupation in vivo. (*Top*) When bound individually, RFX, X2BP, and NF-Y have only low affinity (thin open arrows) for their respective X, X2, and Y box target sites. (*Middle*) Their binding affinity is strongly enhanced (thick black arrows) when the three proteins bind cooperatively to the same MHCII promoter fragment. (*Bottom*) In RFX-deficient BLS cells, cooperative binding is lost, and the residual low binding affinity of X2BP and NF-Y are not sufficient for stable promoter occupation in vivo. (*b*) CIITA is a non-DNA-binding transcriptional coactivator that functions at MHCII promoters via protein-protein interactions. Tethering of CIITA to MHCII and related promoters requires protein-protein interactions (arrows) with an as yet poorly defined S box binding protein, the RFXANK and RFX5 subunits of RFX, an X2 box binding protein (CREB), and the B and C subunits of NF-Y. Once tethered to the promoter, CIITA is believed to activate transcription by recruiting (arrows) other factors via its N-terminal activation domains (AD). Candidate factors recruited by CIITA include TFIIB, $TAF_{II}32$, $TAF_{II}70$, TFIIH, p-TEFb, and CBP. The putative effects of these factors on transcription initiation, elongation, and chromatin remodeling are indicated.

CIITA actually serve as bona fide transcription activation domains (Figure 2). First, they are essential for the ability of CIITA to activate MHCII promoters, and their deletion generates dominant negative mutants of CIITA (120, 121, 123, 124, 126, 127). Second, the acidic region can function as an activation domain when it is grafted onto a heterologous DNA-binding protein such as GAL4 (124). Finally, the function of N-terminally deleted versions of CIITA can be partially rescued by fusing them to the activation domains of the transcription factors VP16 and TIF (124, 125).

At least three different mechanisms have been put forward to explain how the activation domains of CIITA stimulate transcription (Figure 5b). First, CIITA can interact with the general transcription factors TFIIB, hTAF$_{II}$32, and hTAF$_{II}$70, suggesting that it promotes transcription initiation by recruiting the general transcription machinery (128, 129). Second, CIITA has been proposed to enhance promoter clearance or transcription elongation by interacting with TFIIH or P-TEFb (129, 130). Third, CIITA may facilitate chromatin remodeling by recruiting the histone acetyltransferase CBP (131, 132). The latter mechanism could potentially explain why the accessibility of MHCII promoters to DNA-binding proteins is enhanced by CIITA in certain cell types (133, 134). These three mechanisms are not mutually exclusive, and CIITA could well function as a scaffold for the recruitment of several factors that activate transcription at different levels.

Very early on, it was recognized that CIITA does not activate transcription of MHCII genes by binding directly to the promoter DNA. This suggested that CIITA is a coactivator recruited to MHCII promoters by means of protein-protein interactions with one or more of the factors binding to the S, X, X2, and Y sequences (Figure 5b). Definitive evidence for this hypothesis has been provided only very recently (112, 113, 115, 119). Chromatin immunoprecipitation experiments have revealed that CIITA is indeed physically associated in vivo with MHCII promoters (115), both several different MHCII promoters (*HLA-DRA*, *HLA-DRB1*, and *HLA-DPB*) and the promoters of the *Ii* and *HLA-DM* genes (115). Furthermore, in vitro recruitment experiments have demonstrated that tethering of CIITA to MHCII promoters is mediated by multiple synergistic protein-protein interactions with components of the MHCII enhanceosome (Figure 5b). Factors bound to the S, X, X2, and Y boxes are all required for recruitment of CIITA (115). Yeast two-hybrid and coimmunoprecipitation experiments have shown that CIITA interacts directly with the RFXANK and RFX5 subunits of RFX, the B and C subunits of NF-Y, and CREB (Figure 5b) (112, 113, 119, 135).

Domains within CIITA that interact with the DNA bound factors have begun to be defined. It is clear that recruitment to the MHCII enhanceosome requires the C-terminal moiety of CIITA (Figure 2) (115). This is consistent with the earlier observation that the specificity of CIITA for MHCII promoters is conferred by its C-terminal portion (125). Moreover, domains mediating interactions with RFX5 and NF-YB have been mapped within this C-terminal region of CIITA (113).

The LRR region is also important because mutations disrupting this region in BLS patients reduce the CIITA-enhanceosome interaction (115). Results concerning the importance of the N-terminal portion of CIITA for recruitment are less coherent. A recent study has defined the N terminus of CIITA as being the region that mediates interactions with RFXANK and NF-YC (113). This is at odds with the observation that this region is actually dispensable for recruitment (115). In fact, dominant negative mutants of CIITA lacking the N-terminal activation domains actually bind better to the MHCII enhanceosome, suggesting that these dominant negative mutants are likely to function by blocking access of wild-type CIITA to the promoter (115). Further work will be required to reconcile these contradictory findings.

Three regions within CIITA have been implicated in nuclear localization (Figure 2). First, the C terminus of CIITA contains a 5-amino-acid motif resembling a nuclear localization signal (NLS) (136). This NLS motif is essential for nuclear localization of CIITA and can direct nuclear import in a manner that is independent of other CIITA sequences. A 24-amino-acid deletion removing this NLS in the BLS patient BLS-2 aborts nuclear import of CIITA (136). A second sequence implicated in nuclear import is the GTP-binding motif. Binding of GTP appears to be required for transport of CIITA into the nucleus (137). Finally, a detailed mutational analysis of the LRR region has shown that it is important for directing CIITA to the nucleus (119). It remains to be determined whether these three regions are redundant and function independently of each other, or if they act together in a concerted fashion. Whether the nuclear-cytoplasmic distribution of CIITA is regulated also remains an open question.

CIITA shares a similar architecture and a low level of sequence homology with a set of other proteins. All of these proteins contain a nucleotide-binding domain (NBD) coupled to a LRR domain situated near the C terminus (138, 139). These other proteins have functions very different from that of CIITA. They include the caspase recruitment protein Nod1 and certain plant disease resistance proteins (138, 139). Conservation of the NBD-LRR domain organization in proteins having very different functions is intriguing. It is tempting to speculate that the similar structure of these proteins reflects an as yet unknown analogy in their mode of action.

CIITA Is the Master Regulator of MHCII Expression

In contrast to the ubiquitous expression of the DNA-binding factors (including RFX) constituting the MHCII enhanceosome, expression of the *MHC2TA* gene is tightly regulated. In the majority of situations it is the expression of CIITA that dictates whether, and at what level, MHCII genes are expressed. The *MHC2TA* gene is therefore the master regulator of MHCII expression and hence has an essential immunomodulatory role. This conclusion has been firmly established by the following findings. First, the analysis of a large number of human and mouse cell lines and tissues has demonstrated that there is a strict correlation between MHCII and *MHC2TA* expression. Second, the majority of cell types do not express *MHC2TA* and are consequently MHCII-negative. Expression of the *MHC2TA* gene, and thus of MHCII, can be activated in such cells by stimulation with IFNγ (140, 141). This has been demonstrated in a variety of established cell lines, including fibroblasts, melanoma cells, and macrophages, and in several primary cell types such as mouse embryonic fibroblasts, peritoneal macrophages, microglia, and astrocytes (140–148). Transfection of MHCII-negative cells with CIITA expression vectors is generally sufficient to induce MHCII expression (140, 141, 149, 150). The latter point in particular emphasizes the fact that CIITA is both essential and sufficient, thereby justifying the notion that it represents the master regulator of MHCII expression. Third, experimental modulation of *MHC2TA* expression using a tetracycline inducible system has shown that the level of *MHC2TA* expression directly determines that of MHCII expression (151). Fourth, constitutive expression of MHCII in B cells and dendritic cells is sustained by constitutive expression of CIITA (29). Fifth, extinction of MHCII expression during the differentiation of B cells into mature plasma cells is caused by silencing of the *MHC2TA* gene (149, 152). Sixth, MHCII expression is induced upon activation of human T cells because the *MHC2TA* gene is switched on (A Muhlethaler-Mottet, B Mach, unpublished data). Activation of mouse T cells on the other hand does not turn on the *MHC2TA* gene, and hence MHCII expression is not induced (153). Seventh, repression of MHCII expression in trophoblast cells is caused by inhibition of *MHC2TA* expression (154, 155). Finally, an important emerging concept is that a variety of pathogens have developed the ability to inhibit CIITA expression—and thus MHCII expression—as a strategy to evade recognition by the immune system. Examples include cytomegalovirus (CMV) (156, 157), varicella-zoster virus (VZV) (158), *Mycobacterium bovis* (159) and chlamydia (160). This last point underlines the functional importance of CIITA as an essential immunomodulator.

Although the level of transcription of the *MHC2TA* gene is in the majority of situations the dominant factor dictating MHCII expression, other levels of regulation have also been reported. The modulatory effects of IFNβ and TNFα on IFNγ–induced MHCII expression act downstream of *MHC2TA* gene transcription (161–163). Moreover, weak or isotype specific MHCII expression has been observed in the absence of CIITA in certain mutant human cell lines (164) and in certain cell types in CIITA-deficient mice (Table 3) (96, 97). However, these examples of CIITA-independent MHCII expression remain exceptions, and the mechanisms involved are not yet understood.

Regulation of CIITA Expression

The fact that the expression pattern of MHCII genes is determined primarily by that of CIITA has motivated substantial interest in the mechanisms controlling transcription of the *MHC2TA* gene. A large (greater than 12 kb) and complex regulatory region containing several independent promoters controls transcription of *MHC2TA* (Figure 6a). Four promoters (pI, pII, pIII, and pIV) have been identified in the human gene, three of which (pI, pIII, and pIV) are also strongly conserved in the mouse gene (145). The usage of these promoters leads to the synthesis of distinct CIITA mRNAs (types I, III, and IV) containing alternative first exons spliced to a shared second exon (Figure 6a) (145). The study of the different *MHC2TA* promoters has demonstrated that it is their differential activity that ultimately determines the complex expression pattern of MHCII genes that is observed in vivo (145). This has been confirmed in several biological systems (144–147, 162, 165–167). Different cellular and functional specificities of MHCII expression have thus been allocated to distinct CIITA promoters, each one having a specific physiological relevance (Figure 6a).

In both humans and mice, pI is highly specific for DCs. Type I CIITA mRNA typically represents a preponderant fraction of the total CIITA mRNA found in various different DC preparations (145, 165). This is for instance the case for splenic and thymic DCs isolated ex vivo from the mouse, DCs derived from mouse bone marrow cultures and human monocyte–derived DCs (145, 165; W Reith, B Mach, unpublished data). However, pI is not the only promoter active in DCs; there is generally also a variable but significant fraction of type III CIITA mRNA (145; W Reith, unpublished data). Moreover, DC specificity of pI is not absolute; it is also used in mouse microglia and peritoneal macrophages following activation with IFNγ (165) (JM Waldburger, W Reith, manuscript in preparation). Type I transcripts contain an alternative first exon that contains a translation initiation codon and codes for a specific 94-amino-acid N-terminal extension of CIITA (Figure 6a) (145). CIITA protein isoforms containing this type I specific extension are detected in DCs (W Reith, B Mach, unpublished data).

PIII is used primarily in B cells (145, 147, 166, 167). Sequences important for B cell specificity of this promoter have been defined (166). It should however be mentioned that the B cell specificity of pIII is not absolute. It is for example also used in certain DC preparations (145; W Reith, unpublished data). An IFNγ–responsive enhancer has moreover been mapped upstream of pIII in the human gene (146). Type III CIITA mRNA contains an alternative first exon that contains a translation initiation codon and encodes a specific 17-amino-acid N-terminal extension (Figure 6a) (145). CIITA protein isoforms containing this type III specific extension are detected in B cells (W Reith, B Mach, unpublished data).

PIV is activated by IFNγ in a wide variety of established cell lines and primary cell types, including monocytes, macrophages, microglia, astrocytes, fibroblasts, and endothelial cells (143–147, 168). The function of pIV has been dissected in considerable detail, which has permitted the complete signal transduction pathway from the IFNγ receptor to MHCII expression to be elucidated (Figure 6b) (143–147, 168). IFNγ–induced activation of pIV relies on three *cis*-acting sequences (a GAS element, an IRF binding site, and an E box) that function together

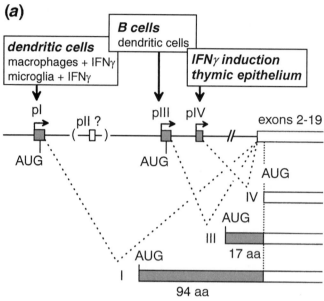

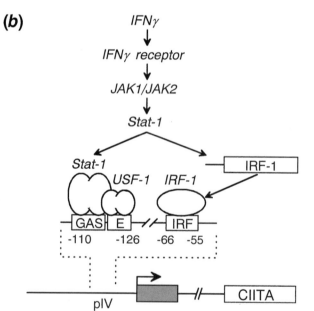

in synergy. The GAS and IRF sequences are bound, respectively, by STAT1 and IRF1 (144), two transcription factors that mediate IFNγ−induced gene expression in a variety of other systems (169–171). The relative contribution of STAT1 and IRF1 for pIV activation varies according to the cell type examined (146, 162). The E box is bound by USF1, a ubiquitously expressed transcription factor that binds cooperatively with STAT1 (144). Unlike the type I and III mRNAs, the type IV–specific exon does not contain a translation initiation codon and does therefore not encode an N-terminal extension (Figure 6a) (145). Translation of type IV CIITA mRNA is initiated at an initiation codon situated in the shared second exon (145).

To further refine the analysis of pIV usage we have excised it by gene targeting in mice (JM Waldburger, W Reith, manuscript in preparation). As expected, IFNγ−induced MHCII expression in pIV−/− mice is abolished in non–bone marrow–derived cells, including fibroblasts, astrocytes, hepatocytes, endothelial cells, and epithelial cells. Surprisingly, however, the excision of pIV does not eliminate MHCII expression in peritoneal macrophages and microglial cells following their activation with IFNγ. Thus, while pIV is essential for IFNγ−induced MHCII expression in non–bone marrow–derived cells, it is dispensable for MHCII expression in IFNγ−activated cells of the macrophage lineage. Enhanced MHCII expression in IFNγ−activated pIV−/− macrophages is due to the fact that pI is turned on in these cells. A second unexpected finding is that pIV−/− mice completely lack CIITA expression on epithelial cells of the thymic cortex. Since MHCII expression on these cells is essential for positive selection of CD4$^+$ thymocytes (7), pIV−/− mice have very low CD4$^+$ T cell counts.

Figure 6 Expression of the *MHC2TA* gene. (*a*) Several independent promoters drive transcription of the *MHC2TA* gene. Four promoters (pI, pII, pIII, pIV) have been identified in humans. Only three of these (pI, pIII, pIV) are conserved in the mouse. Usage of these promoters leads to the splicing (dashed lines) of alternative first exons to a shared second exon. Incorporation of exons I and III lead to the synthesis of type I and type III CIITA protein isoforms having specific N-terminal extensions of 94 and 17 amino acids, respectively. Translation of type IV CIITA is initiated at the AUG found in the shared second exon. The promoters exhibit different activities. pI is used primarily in human and mouse dendritic cells. It is also active in activated mouse macrophages and microglia. pIII is used mainly in B cells, but also to a variable extent in dendritic cells. pIV is essential for IFNγ−induced expression in non–bone marrow–derived cells, as well as for expression in thymic epithelial cells. (*b*) The entire signal transduction cascade mediating the induction of MHCII expression by IFNγ has been elucidated. Activation of Jak1 and Jak2 kinases by interaction of IFNγ with its receptor leads to the phosphorylation, dimerization, and nuclear import of STAT1. STAT1 binds cooperatively with USF-1 to a composite GAS/E box motif present in pIV of the *MHC2TA* gene. STAT1 also activates expression of IRF-1, which then binds to its cognate site in pIV. Activation of pIV by STAT1, USF-1, and IRF-1 leads to expression of CIITA, and thus to the induction of MHCII expression.

Induction of MHCII Expression: A Pathway Affected in Multiple Situations

pIV of the *MHC2TA* gene is turning out to be a privileged focal point for a growing number of influences that inhibit or abort MHCII expression, both under normal physiological situations and during the course of disease. First, a variety of cytokines known to inhibit IFNγ−induced MHCII expression, including TGFβ, L-4, IL-10, and IL-1β, have been shown to mediate their inhibitory effect by interfering with the induction of *MHC2TA* expression (142, 147, 168, 172, 173). Second, in trophoblast cells (154, 155) and in certain IFNγ unresponsive tumors (174, 175), the *MHC2TA* gene is refractory to induction by IFNγ. Third, the production of NO by activated macrophages inhibits IFNγ−induced activation of CIITA expression (176). Fourth, a number of pathogens, including cytomegalovirus (CMV) (156, 157), varicella-zoster virus (VZV) (158), *Mycobacterium bovis* (159) and Chlamydia (160) exhibit the ability to inhibit MHCII expression by interfering with the activation of CIITA expression. Finally, an emerging concept is that certain drugs can interfere with activation of MHCII expression. For instance, it has been shown very recently that the lipid lowering drugs statins inhibit IFNγ−induced CIITA expression (177). These various inhibitory effects likely converge on pIV of the *CIITA* gene, although evidence in support of this has been provided only for some of them (trophoblast cells, IL-1, TGFβ, CMV, Chlamydia, and statins) (142, 146, 147, 155–157, 160, 168, 172, 173).

So far, the molecular mechanisms underlying the inhibitory effect on activation of pIV by IFNγ have only been addressed in certain cases. In trophoblast cells, the lack of IFNγ inducibility of CIITA is due to methylation of pIV (155). The inhibition by CMV has been suggested to be due to enhanced proteasome-mediated degradation of Jak1, thereby limiting activation of Stat1 in response to IFNγ (156). Similarly, infection with VZV is associated with reduced levels of Stat1, Jak2, and IRF1, all of which would be expected to reduce induction of pIV (158). Finally, Chlamydia induces proteasome-mediated degradation of USF-1 (160), a ubiquitous transcription factor required for the activation of pIV (144). In addition to a reduction in the availability or activity of Stat1, USF1, or IRF1, other putative mechanisms could also be envisaged. A plausible target would, for example, be the cooperative binding interaction that takes place at pIV between Stat1 and IRF1 (144).

Specificity of RFX and CIITA

The clinical and immunological phenotypes of BLS patients in all four complementation groups can be explained by the absence of antigen presentation via MHCII molecules. This has been interpreted to indicate that RFX and CIITA are highly specific for the expression of the MHCII genes (4). The finding that RFX and CIITA are also required for expression of the genes encoding Ii, HLA-DM, and HLA-DO (14–19, 47) did not really challenge this specificity because these proteins are involved in the intercellular traffic and peptide loading of MHCII molecules. However, recent evidence has implicated RFX and CIITA in three other unrelated systems, demonstrating that their specificity for the MHCII system is not as tight as initially believed.

In addition to the profound deficiency in MHCII expression, a reduction in MHCI and $\beta 2$ microglobulin is observed on various cell types from many BLS patients (Table 1) (1). Moreover, a reduction in MHCI expression has also been observed in *Rfx5−/−* mice; cell surface levels of MHCI in *Rfx5−/−* mice are lowered tenfold in T cells and two- to fivefold in B cells (W Reith, unpublished data). Taken together, these observations suggest that RFX and CIITA contribute to the expression of MHCI genes. This has been confirmed directly by several studies (23, 25–27) (W Reith, unpublished data). First, it has been established that *MHCI* and *B2M* promoters contain a region showing homology to the MHCII regulatory module consisting of the S, X, X2, and Y sequences (23–27). Second, RFX and CIITA can transactivate *MHCI* and *B2M* promoters in transient transfection experiments (23, 25–27, 178, 179) (W Reith, unpublished data). Third, certain BLS cell lines show enhanced levels of MHCI expression once their genetic defect has been corrected (26). Finally, chromatin immunoprecipitation experiments have demonstrated that CIITA and RFX are physically associated with MHCI and *B2M* promoters in vivo (115).

The existence of an additional gene affected by CIITA has been revealed by the analysis of *Mhc2ta* knockout mice. Expression of IL-4 is the hallmark of Th2 cells, whereas this cytokine is normally not expressed by Th1 cells (180). Disruption of the *Mhc2ta* gene has been reported to lead to the aberrant activation of IL-4 expression in Th1 cells (181), suggesting that CIITA is required for repression of the *IL-4* gene in these cells. This is apparently not due to a direct effect of CIITA on the *IL-4* promoter. Instead, CIITA expressed in Th1 cells has been proposed to bind to and sequester the coactivator CBP, which is required for transcription of the *IL-4* gene (182).

An interesting role of CIITA in HIV infection has recently been documented (130, 183). Expression of CIITA in T cells enhances HIV-1 replication and transcriptional activity of the HIV-LTR (183). This finding is of particular interest because the primary cellular targets of HIV—activated human T cells and macrophages—express high levels of CIITA. The mechanism by which CIITA activates the HIV-LTR remains obscure.

The MHCII System as a Textbook Model for Regulation of Gene Expression

Thanks to elucidation of the BLS disease, the regulation of MHCII gene expression is one of the only mammalian transcriptional control systems that has been dissected genetically in detail (Figure 4). Moreover, several features make the regulation of MHCII genes a textbook model system for the regulation of gene expression. First, it represents an unprecedented paradigm for the role of gene-specific coactivators such as CIITA (Figure 5b). Second, it is among the few examples in which strong evidence for the involvement of a higher order enhanceosome complex has been provided (Figure 4 and 5A). Third, the MHCII system makes a very strong case for the key importance of combinatorial control mediated by cooperative protein-protein interactions. Such cooperative interactions are crucial at three levels in the MHCII system. At the MHCII promoter, the stability and specificity of enhanceosome assembly is strictly dependent on cooperative binding between at least three different DNA-binding factors, RFX, X2BP, and NF-Y (Figure 5a). The specificity of the coactivator CIITA for MHCII promoters is mediated by the combined effect of multiple weak protein-protein interactions with at least six different components of the DNA-bound enhanceosome complex (Figure 5b). Finally, the IFNγ–induced expression of CIITA is dependent on the cooperative binding of Stat1 and USF1 to a composite response element in pIV of the *MHC2TA* gene (Figure 6b). Taken together, these features make the MHCII system a valuable blueprint of widespread interest to the field of regulation of gene expression.

ACKNOWLEDGMENTS

We are indebted to all past and current members of the laboratory for their contributions to the work reviewed here. The work performed in the laboratory of the authors was supported by the Louis Jeantet Foundation, the Swiss National Science Foundation, the Gabriella Giorgi-Cavaglieri Foundation, the Ernst and Lucie Schmidheiny Foundation, the Roche Research Foundation and the Novartis Stiftung. The authors are particularly grateful to the Louis Jeantet Foundation (Geneva). B. M. was Louis Jeantet Professor of Molecular Genetics from 1991 to 1998, and throughout this period the Foundation provided generous support to his laboratory.

Visit the Annual Reviews home page at www.AnnualReviews.org

LITERATURE CITED

1. Klein C, Lisowska Grospierre B, LeDeist F, Fischer A, Griscelli C. 1993. Major histocompatibility complex class II deficiency: clinical manifestations, immunologic features, and outcome. *J. Pediatr.* 123:921–28

2. Reith W, Steimle V, Lisowska-Grospierre B, Fischer A, Mach B. 1999. Molecular basis of major histocompatibility class II deficiency, In *Primary Immunodeficiency Diseases, a Molecular and Genetic Approach*, ed. H Ochs, J Puck, E Smith, pp. 167–180. New York: Oxford Univ. Press

3. Griscelli C, Lisowska-Grospierre B, Mach B. 1993. Combined immunodeficiency with defective expression in MHC class II genes, In *Immunodeficiencies*, ed. FS Rosen, M Seligman, pp. 141–154. Chur, Switzerland: Harwood Academic

4. Mach B, Steimle V, Martinez-Soria E, Reith W. 1996. Regulation of MHC class II genes: lessons from a disease. *Annu. Rev. Immunol.* 14:301–31

5. Elhasid R, Etzioni A. 1996. Major histocompatibility complex class II deficiency: a clinical review. *Blood Rev.* 10:242–48

6. Trowsdale J. 1993. Genomic structure and function in the MHC. *Trends Genet.* 9:117–22

7. Viret C, Janeway CAJ. 1999. MHC and T cell development. *Rev. Immunogenet.* 1:91–104

8. Cresswell P. 1994. Assembly, transport, and function of MHC class II molecules. *Annu. Rev. Immunol.* 12:259–93

9. Guardiola J, Maffei A. 1993. Control of MHC class II gene expression in autoimmune, infectious, and neoplastic diseases. *Crit. Rev. Immunol.* 13:247–68

10. Benoist C, Mathis D. 1990. Regulation of major histocompatibility complex class II genes: X, Y and other letters of the alphabet. *Annu. Rev. Immunol.* 8:681–715

11. Glimcher LH, Kara CJ. 1992. Sequences and factors: a guide to MHC class-II transcription. *Annu. Rev. Immunol.* 10:13–49

12. Ting JP, Baldwin AS. 1993. Regulation of MHC gene expression. *Curr. Opin. Immunol.* 5:8–16

13. Boss JM. 1997. Regulation of transcription of MHC class II genes. *Curr. Opin. Immunol.* 9:107–13

14. Ting JP, Wright KL, Chin KC, Brickey WJ, Li G. 1997. The DMB promoter: delineation, in vivo footprint, trans-activation, and trans-dominant suppression. *J. Immunol.* 159:5457–62

15. Taxman DJ, Cressman DE, Ting JP. 2000. Identification of class II transcriptional activator-induced genes by representational difference analysis: discoordinate regulation of the DN alpha/DO beta heterodimer. *J. Immunol.* 165:1410–16

16. Westerheide SD, Louis-Plence P, Ping D, He XF, Boss JM. 1997. HLA-DMA and HLA-DMB gene expression functions through the conserved S-X-Y region. *J. Immunol.* 158:4812–21

17. Brown AM, Barr CL, Ting JP. 1991. Sequences homologous to class II MHC W, X, and Y elements mediate constitutive and IFN-gamma-induced expression of human

class II-associated invariant chain gene. *J. Immunol.* 146:3183–89

18. Brown AM, Wright KL, Ting JP. 1993. Human major histocompatibility complex class II-associated invariant chain gene promoter. Functional analysis and in vivo protein/DNA interactions of constitutive and IFN-gamma-induced expression. *J. Biol. Chem.* 268:26328–33

19. Tai AK, Zhou G, Chau K, Ono SJ. 1999. Cis-element dependence and occupancy of the human invariant chain promoter in CIITA-dependent and -independent transcription. *Mol. Immunol.* 36:447–60

20. Busch R, Mellins ED. 1996. Developing and shedding inhibitions: how MHC class II molecules reach maturity. *Curr. Opin. Immunol.* 8:51–58

21. Alfonso C, Karlsson L. 2000. Nonclassical MHC class II molecules. *Annu. Rev. Immunol.* 18:113–42

22. Cresswell P. 1996. Invariant chain structure and MHC class II function. *Cell* 84:505–7

23. Martin BK, Chin KC, Olsen JC, Skinner CA, Dey A, Ozato K, Ting JP. 1997. Induction of MHC class I expression by the MHC class II transactivator CIITA. *Immunity* 6:591–600

24. Riegert P, Andersen R, Bumstead N, Dohring C, Dominguez-Steglich M, Engberg J, Salomonsen J, Schmid M, Schwager J, Skjodt K, Kaufman J. 1996. The chicken beta 2-microglobulin gene is located on a non-major histocompatibility complex microchromosome: a small, G+C-rich gene with X and Y boxes in the promoter. *Proc. Natl. Acad. Sci. USA* 93:1243–48

25. Gobin SJ, Peijnenburg A, Keijsers V, van den Elsen PJ. 1997. Site alpha is crucial for two routes of IFN gamma-induced MHC class I transactivation: the ISRE-mediated route and a novel pathway involving CIITA. *Immunity* 6:601–11

26. Gobin SJ, Peijnenburg A, Van Eggermond M, van Zutphen M, van den Berg R, van den Elsen PJ. 1998. The RFX complex

is crucial for the constitutive and CIITA-mediated transactivation of MHC class I and beta2-microglobulin genes. *Immunity* 9:531–41

27. van den Elsen PJ, Peijnenburg A, van Eggermond MC, Gobin SJ. 1998. Shared regulatory elements in the promoters of MHC class I and class II genes. *Immunol. Today* 19:308–12

28. Steimle V, Mach B. 1995. Complementation cloning of mammalian transcriptional regulators: the example of MHC class II gene regulators. *Curr. Opin. Genet. Dev.* 5:646–51

29. Steimle V, Otten LA, Zufferey M, Mach B. 1993. Complementation cloning of an MHC class II transactivator mutated in hereditary MHC class II deficiency. *Cell* 75:135–46

30. Reith W, Satola S, Herrero Sanchez C, Amaldi I, Lisowska-Grospierre B, Griscelli C, Hadam MR, Mach B. 1988. Congenital immunodeficiency with a regulatory defect in MHC class II gene expression lacks a specific HLA-DR promoter binding protein, RF-X. *Cell* 53:897–906

31. Durand B, Sperisen P, Emery P, Barras E, Zufferey M, Mach B, Reith W. 1997. RFXAP, a novel subunit of the RFX DNA binding complex is mutated in MHC class II deficiency. *EMBO J.* 16:1045–55

32. Steimle V, Durand B, Barras E, Zufferey M, Hadam MR, Mach B, Reith W. 1995. A novel DNA binding regulatory factor is mutated in primary MHC class II deficiency (bare lymphocyte syndrome). *Genes Dev.* 9:1021–32

33. Masternak K, Barras E, Zufferey M, Conrad B, Corthals G, Aebersold R, Sanchez JC, Hochstrasser DF, Mach B, Reith W. 1998. A gene encoding a novel RFX-associated transactivator is mutated in the majority of MHC class II deficiency patients. *Nat. Genet.* 20:273–77

34. Nagarajan UM, Louis-Plence P, DeSandro A, Nilsen R, Bushey A, Boss JM. 1999. RFX-B is the gene responsible for

the most common cause of the bare lymphocyte syndrome, an MHC class II immunodeficiency. *Immunity* 10:153–62

35. Schuurmann RKB, Van Rood JJ, Vossen JM, Schellekens PTA, Feltkamp-Vroom TM, Doyer E, Gmelig-Meyling F, Visser HKA. 1979. Failure of lymphocyte-membrane HLA A and B expression in two siblings with combined immunodeficiency. *Clin. Immunol. Immunopathol.* 14:418–34

36. Griscelli C, Durandy A, Virelizier JL, Hors J, Lepage V, Colombani J. 1980. Impaired cell-to-cell interaction in partial combined immunodeficiency with variable expression of HLA antigens, In *Primary Immunodeficiencies*, ed. M Seligman, WH Hitzig, pp, 499–503. Amsterdam: Elsevier/North Holland

37. Kuis W, Roord J, Zegers BJM, Schuurmann RKB, Heijnen CJ, Baldwin WM, Goulmy E, Claas F, van de Griend RJ, Rijkers GT, Van Rood JJ, Vossen JM, Ballieux RE, Stoop RJ. 1981. Clinical and immunological studies in a patient with the "bare lymphocyte" syndrome, In *Bone Marrow Transplantation in Europe*, ed. JL Touraine, E Gluckman, C Griscelli, pp. 201–208. Amsterdam: Excerpta Medica

38. Hadam MR, Dopfer R, Dammer G, Peter HH, Schlesier M, Müller C, Niethammer D. 1984. Defective expression of HLA-D-region determinants in children with congenital agammaglobulinemia and malabsorption: a new syndrome, In *Histocompatibility Testing 1984*, ed. ED Albert, MP Baur, WR Mayr, pp. 645–650. Berlin Heidelberg: Springer-Verlag

39. Lisowska-Grospierre B, Durandy A, Virelizier JL, Fischer A, Griscelli C. 1983. Combined immunodeficiency with defective expression of HLA: modulation of an abnormal HLA synthesis and functional studies. *Birth Defects* 19:87–92

40. Touraine JL, Betuel H, Souillet G. 1978. Combined immunodeficiency disease associated with absence of cell surface HLA A and B antigen. *J. Pediatr.* 93:47–51

41. Touraine JL, Marseglia GL, Betuel H, Souillet G, Gebuhrer L. 1992. The bare lymphocyte syndrome. *Bone Marrow Transplant.* 9(Suppl 1):54–56

42. Rosen FS, Wedgwood RJ, Eibl M, et al. 1992. Primary immunodeficiency diseases: report of a WHO scientific group. *Immunodefic. Rev.* 3:195–236

43. Lisowska-Grospierre B, Fondaneche MC, Rols MP, Griscelli C, Fischer A. 1994. Two complementation groups account for most cases of inherited MHC class II deficiency. *Hum. Mol. Genet.* 3:953–58

44. Lisowska-Grospierre B, Charron DJ, de Preval C, Durandy A, Griscelli C, Mach B. 1985. A defect in the regulation of major histocompatibility complex class II gene expression in human HLA-DR negative lymphocytes from patients with combined immunodeficiency syndrome. *J. Clin. Invest.* 76:381–85

45. de Préval C, Lisowska-Grospierre B, Loche M, Griscelli C, Mach B. 1985. A trans-acting class II regulatory gene unlinked to the MHC controls expression of HLA class II genes. *Nature* 318:291–93

46. de Préval C, Hadam MR, Mach B. 1988. Regulation of genes for HLA class II antigens in cell lines from patients with severe combined immunodeficiency. *N. Engl. J. Med.* 318:1295–1300

47. Kern I, Steimle V, Siegrist C-A, Mach B. 1995. The two novel MHC class II transactivators RFX5 and CIITA both control expression of HLA-DM genes. *Int. Immunol.* 7:1295–99

48. Nocera A, Barocci S, Depalma R, Gorski J. 1993. Analysis of transcripts of genes located within the HLA-D region in B-cells from an HLA-severe combined immunodeficiency individual. *Hum. Immunol.* 38:231–34

49. Hume CR, Lee JS. 1989. Congenital immunodeficiencies associated with absence of HLA class II antigens on lymphocytes result from distinct mutations in trans-acting factors. *Hum. Immunol.* 26:288–309

50. Benichou B, Strominger JL. 1991. Class II-antigen-negative patient and mutant B-cell lines represent at least three, and probably four, distinct genetic defects defined by complementation analysis. *Proc. Natl. Acad. Sci. USA* 88:4285–88

51. Seidl C, Saraiya C, Osterweil Z, Fu YP, Lee JS. 1992. Genetic complexity of regulatory mutants defective for HLA class- II gene-expression. *J. Immunol.* 148:1576–84

52. Hasegawa SL, Riley JL, Sloan JH III, Boss JM. 1993. Protease treatment of nuclear extracts distinguishes between class II MHC X1 box DNA-binding proteins in wild-type and class II-deficient B cells. *J. Immunol.* 150:1781–93

53. Riley JL, Boss JM. 1993. Class II MHC transcriptional mutants are defective in higher order complex formation. *J. Immunol.* 151:6942–53

54. Durand B, Kobr M, Reith W, Mach B. 1994. Functional complementation of MHC class II regulatory mutants by the purified X box binding protein RFX. *Mol. Cell Biol.* 14:6839–47

55. Villard J, Lisowska-Grospierre B, Van den Elsen P, Fischer A, Reith W, Mach B. 1997. Mutation of RFXAP, a regulator of MHC class II genes, in primary MHC class II deficiency. *N. Engl. J. Med.* 337:748–53

56. Masternak K, Muhlethaler-Mottet A, Villard J, Peretti M, Reith W. 2000. Molecular genetics of the bare lymphocyte syndrome. *Rev. Immunogenet.* 2:In press

57. Accolla RS. 1983. Human B cell variants immunoselected against a single Ia antigen subset have lost expression in several Ia antigen subsets. *J. Exp. Med.* 157:1053–58

58. Gladstone P, Pious D. 1978. Stable variants affecting B cell alloantigens in human lymphoid cells. *Nature* 271:459–61

59. Brickey WJ, Wright KL, Zhu XS, Ting JP. 1999. Analysis of the defect in IFN-gamma induction of MHC class II genes in G1B cells: identification of a novel and functionally critical leucine- rich motif

(62-LYLYLQL-68) in the regulatory factor X 5 transcription factor. *J. Immunol.* 163:6622–30

60. Hauber I, Gulle H, Wolf HM, Maris M, Eggenbauer H, Eibl MM. 1995. Molecular characterization of major histocompatibility complex class II gene expression and demonstration of antigen-specific T cell response indicate a new phenotype in class II-deficient patients. *J. Exp. Med.* 181: 1411–23

61. Wolf HM, Hauber I, Gulle H, Thon V, Eggenbauer H, Fischer MB, Fiala S, Eibl MM. 1995. Twin boys with major histocompatibility complex class II deficiency but inducible immune responses. *N. Engl. J. Med.* 332:86–90

62. Douhan J III, Hauber I, Eibl MM, Glimcher LH. 1996. Genetic evidence for a new type of major histocompatibility complex class II combined immunodeficiency characterized by a dyscoordinate regulation of HLA-D alpha and beta chains. *J. Exp. Med.* 183:1063–69

63. Herrero Sanchez C, Reith W, Silacci P, Mach B. 1992. The DNA-binding defect observed in major histocompatibility complex class II regulatory mutants concerns only one member of a family of complexes binding to the X boxes of class II promoters. *Mol. Cell Biol.* 12:4076–83

64. Gönczy P, Reith W, Barras E, Lisowska-Grospierre B, Griscelli C, Hadam MR, Mach B. 1989. Inherited immunodeficiency with a defect in a major histocompatibility complex class II promoter-binding protein differs in the chromatin structure of the HLA-DRA gene. *Mol. Cell. Biol.* 9:296–302

65. Kara CJ, Glimcher LH. 1991. In vivo footprinting of MHC class II genes: bare promoters in the bare lymphocyte syndrome. *Science* 252:709–12

66. Kara CJ, Glimcher LH. 1993. Three in vivo promoter phenotypes in MHC class II deficient combined immunodeficiency. *Immunogenetics* 37:227–30

67. Moreno CS, Emery P, West JE, Durand B, Reith W, Mach B, Boss JM. 1995. Purified X2 binding protein (X2BP) cooperatively binds the class II MHC X box region in the presence of purified RFX, the X box factor deficient in the bare lymphocyte syndrome. *J. Immunol.* 155:4313–21

68. Reith W, Kobr M, Emery P, Durand B, Siegrist CA, Mach B. 1994. Cooperative binding between factors RFX and X2bp to the X and X2 boxes of MHC class II promoters. *J. Biol. Chem.* 269:20020–25

69. Louis-Plence P, Moreno CS, Boss JM. 1997. Formation of a regulatory factor X/X2 box-binding protein/nuclear factor-Y multiprotein complex on the conserved regulatory regions of HLA class II genes. *J. Immunol.* 159:3899–3909

70. Wright KL, Vilen BJ, Itoh Lindstrom Y, Moore TL, Li G, Criscitiello M, Cogswell P, Clarke JB, Ting JP. 1994. CCAAT box binding protein NF-Y facilitates in vivo recruitment of upstream DNA binding transcription factors. *EMBO J.* 13:4042–53

71. Reith W, Siegrist CA, Durand B, Barras E, Mach B. 1994. Function of major histocompatibility complex class II promoters requires cooperative binding between factors RFX and NF-Y. *Proc. Natl. Acad. Sci. USA* 91:554–58

72. Mantovani R. 1999. The molecular biology of the CCAAT-binding factor NF-Y. *Gene* 239:15–27

73. Accolla RS, Jotterand-Bellomo M, Scarpellino L, Maffei A, Carra G, Guardiola J. 1986. aIr-1, a newly found locus on mouse chromosome 16 encoding a transacting activator factor for MHC class II gene expression. *J. Exp. Med.* 164:369–74

74. Bono MR, Alcaide-Loridan C, Couillin P, Letouzé B, Grisard MC, Jouin H, Fellous M. 1991. Human chromosome 16 encodes a factor involved in induction of class II major histocompatibility antigens by interferon gamma. *Proc. Natl. Acad. Sci. USA* 88:6077–81

75. Chang CH, Flavell RA. 1995. Class II transactivator regulates the expression of multiple genes involved in antigen presentation. *J. Exp. Med.* 181:765–67

76. Bontron S, Steimle V, Ucla C, Mach B. 1997. Two novel mutations in the MHC class II transactivator CIITA in a second patient from MHC class II deficiency complementation group A. *Hum. Genet.* 99:541–46

77. Peijnenburg A, van den Berg R, Van Eggermond MJ, Sanal O, Vossen JM, Lennon AM, Alcaide-Loridan C, van den Elsen PJ. 2000. Defective MHC class II expression in an MHC class II deficiency patient is caused by a novel deletion of a splice donor site in the MHC class II transactivator gene. *Immunogenetics* 51:42–49

78. Quan V, Towey M, Sacks S, Kelly AP. 1999. Absence of MHC class II gene expression in a patient with a single amino acid substitution in the class II transactivator protein CIITA. *Immunogenetics* 49:957–63

79. Brown JA, He XF, Westerheide SD, Boss JM. 1995. Characterization of the expressed CIITA allele in the class II MHC transcriptional mutant RJ2.2.5. *Immunogenetics* 43:88–91

80. Moreno CS, Rogers EM, Brown JA, Boss JM. 1997. Regulatory factor X, a bare lymphocyte syndrome transcription factor, is a multimeric phosphoprotein complex. *J. Immunol.* 158:5841–48

81. Emery P, Durand B, Mach B, Reith W. 1996. RFX proteins, a novel family of DNA binding proteins conserved in the eukaryotic kingdom. *Nucleic Acids Res.* 24:803–7

82. Emery P, Strubin M, Hofmann K, Bucher P, Mach B, Reith W. 1996. A consensus motif in the RFX DNA binding domain and binding domain mutants with altered specificity. *Mol. Cell. Biol.* 16:4486–94

83. Villard J, Reith W, Barras E, Gos A, Morris MA, Antonarakis SE, van den Elsen PJ, Mach B. 1997. Analysis of mutations and chromosomal localisation of the gene encoding RFX5, a novel transcription factor affected in major histocompatibility complex class II deficiency. *Hum. Mutat.* 10:430–35

84. Peijnenburg A, van Eggermond MA, van den Berg R, Sanal Vossen JJ, van den Elsen PJ. 1999. Molecular analysis of an MHC class II deficiency patient reveals a novel mutation in the RFX5 gene. *Immunogenetics* 49:338–45

85. Peijnenburg A, Van Eggermond MJ, Gobin SJ, van den Berg R, Godthelp BC, Vossen JM, van den Elsen PJ. 1999. Discoordinate expression of invariant chain and MHC class II genes in class II transactivator-transfected fibroblasts defective for RFX5. *J. Immunol.* 163:794–801

86. Fondaneche MC, Villard J, Wiszniewski W, Jouanguy E, Etzioni A, Le Deist F, Peijnenburg A, Casanova JL, Reith W, Mach B, Fischer A, Lisowska-Grospierre B. 1998. Genetic and molecular definition of complementation group D in MHC class II deficiency. *Hum. Mol. Genet* 7:879–85

87. Wiszniewski W, Fondaneche MC, Lambert N, Masternak K, Picard C, Notarangelo L, Schwartz K, Bal J, Reith W, Alcaide C, de Saint B, Fischer A, Lisowska-Grospierre B. 2000. Founder effect for a 26-bp deletion in the RFXANK gene in North African major histocompatibility complex class II-deficient patients belonging to complementation group B. *Immunogenetics* 51:261–67

88. DeSandro A, Nagarajan UM, Boss JM. 1999. The bare lymphocyte syndrome: molecular clues to the transcriptional regulation of major histocompatibility complex class II genes. *Am. J. Hum. Genet.* 65:279–86

89. Klein C, Cavazzana-Calvo M, Le Deist F, Jabado N, Benkerrou M, Blanche S, Lisowska-Grospierre B, Griscelli C. 1995. Bone marrow transplantation in major histocompatibility complex class II deficiency: a single-center study of 19 patients. *Blood* 85:580–87

90. Canioni D, Patey N, Cuenod B, Benkerrou M, Brousse N. 1997. Major histocompatibility complex class II deficiency needs an early diagnosis: report of a case. *Pediatr. Pathol. Lab. Med.* 17:645–51

91. Ostrand-Rosenberg S, Thakur A, Clements V. 1990. Rejection of mouse sarcoma cells after transfection of MHC class II genes. *J. Immunol.* 144:4068–71

92. Ostrand-Rosenberg S, Clements VK, Thakur A, Cole GA. 1989. Transfection of major histocompatibility complex class I and class II genes causes tumour rejection. *J. Immunogenet.* 16:343–49

93. Panelli MC, Wang E, Shen S, Schluter SF, Bernstein RM, Hersh EM, Stopeck A, Gangavalli R, Barber J, Jolly D, Akporiaye ET. 1996. Interferon gamma (IFNgamma) gene transfer of an EMT6 tumor that is poorly responsive to IFNgamma stimulation: increase in tumor immunogenicity is accompanied by induction of a mouse class II transactivator and class II MHC. *Cancer Immunol. Immunother.* 42:99–107

94. Baskar S, Clements VK, Glimcher LH, Nabavi N, Ostrand-Rosenberg S. 1996. Rejection of MHC class II-transfected tumor cells requires induction of tumor-encoded B7-1 and/or B7-2 costimulatory molecules. *J. Immunol.* 156:3821–27

95. Martin BK, Frelinger JG, Ting JP. 1999. Combination gene therapy with CD86 and the MHC class II transactivator in the control of lung tumor growth. *J. Immunol.* 162:6663–70

96. Chang CH, Guerder S, Hong SC, van Ewijk W, Flavell RA. 1996. Mice lacking the MHC class II transactivator (CIITA) show tissue-specific impairment of MHC class II expression. *Immunity* 4:167–78

97. Williams GS, Malin M, Vremec D, Chang CH, Boyd R, Benoist C, Mathis D. 1998. Mice lacking the transcription factor CIITA–a second look. *Int. Immunol.* 10:1957–67

98. Itoh-Lindstrom Y, Piskurich JF, Felix NJ, Wang Y, Brickey WJ, Platt JL, Koller BH, Ting JP. 1999. Reduced IL-4-, lipopolysaccharide-, and IFN-gamma-induced MHC class II expression in mice lacking class II transactivator due to targeted deletion of the GTP-binding domain. *J. Immunol.* 163:2425–31

99. Clausen BE, Waldburger JM, Schwenk F, Barras E, Mach B, Rajewsky K, Forster I, Reith W. 1998. Residual MHC class II expression on mature dendritic cells and activated B cells in RFX5-deficient mice. *Immunity* 8:143–55

100. Schuurman HJ, van de Wijngaert FP, Huber J, Schuurman RK, Zegers BJ, Roord JJ, Kater L. 1985. The thymus in "bare lymphocyte" syndrome: significance of expression of major histocompatibility complex antigens on thymic epithelial cells in intrathymic T-cell maturation. *Hum. Immunol.* 13:69–82

101. Schuurman HJ, van de Wijngaert FP, Huber J, Zegers BJ, Schuurman RKB, Roord JJ, Kater L. 1985. The thymus in "bare lymphocyte" syndrome. *Adv. Exp. Med. Biol.* 186:921–28

102. Cardell S, Tangri S, Chan S, Kronenberg M, Benoist C, Mathis D. 1995. CD1-restricted CD4+ T cells in major histocompatibility complex class II-deficient mice. *J. Exp. Med.* 182:993–1004

103. van Eggermond MC, Rijkers GT, Kuis W, Zegers BJ, van den Elsen PJ. 1993. T cell development in a major histocompatibility complex class II-deficient patient. *Eur. J. Immunol.* 23:2585–91

104. Henwood J, van Eggermond MCJA, van Boxel-Dezaire AHH, Schipper R, den Hoedt M, Peijnenburg A, Sanal Ö, Ersoy F, Rijkers GT, Zegers BJM, Vossen JM, van Tol MJD, van den Elsen PJ. 1996. Human T cell repertoire generation in the absence of MHC class II expression results in a circulating CD4+CD8– population with altered physicochemical properties of complementarity-determining region 3. *J. Immunol.* 156:895–906

105. Villard J, Peretti M, Masternak K, Barras

E, Caretti G, Mantovani R, Reith W. 2000. A functionally essential domain of RFX5 mediates activation of MHC class II promoters by promoting cooperative binding between RFX and NF-Y. *Mol. Cell. Biol.* 20:3364–76

106. Caretti G, Cocchiarella F, Sidoli C, Villard J, Peretti M, Reith W, Mantovani R. 2000. Dissection of functional NF-Y-RFX cooperative interactions on the MHC class II Eα promoter. *J. Mol. Biol.* 302:539–52

107. Westerheide SD, Boss JM. 1999. Orientation and positional mapping of the subunits of the multicomponent transcription factors RFX and X2BP to the major histocompatibility complex class II transcriptional enhancer. *Nucleic Acids Res.* 27:1635–41

108. Huang M, Zhou Z, Elledge SJ. 1998. The DNA replication and damage checkpoint pathways induce transcription by inhibition of the Crt1 repressor. *Cell* 94:595–605

109. Katan-Khaykovich Y, Spiegel I, Shaul Y. 1999. The dimerization/repression domain of RFX1 is related to a conserved region of its yeast homologues Crt1 and Sak1: a new function for an ancient motif. *J. Mol. Biol.* 294:121–37

110. Schmitt EK, Kuck U. 2000. The fungal CPCR1 protein, which binds specifically to beta-lactam biosynthesis genes, is related to human regulatory factor X transcription factors. *J. Biol. Chem.* 275:9348–57

111. Gajiwala KS, Chen H, Cornille F, Roques BP, Reith W, Mach B, Burley SK. 2000. Structure of the winged-helix protein hRFX1 reveals a new mode of DNA binding. *Nature* 403:916–21

112. DeSandro AM, Nagarajan UM, Boss JM. 2000. Associations and interactions between bare lymphocyte syndrome factors. *Mol. Cell. Biol.* 20:6587–99

113. Zhu XS, Linhoff MW, Li G, Chin KC, Maity SN, Ting JP. 2000. Transcriptional scaffold: CIITA interacts with NF-Y, RFX, and CREB to cause stereospecific regulation of the class II major histocompatibility complex promoter. *Mol. Cell. Biol.* 20:6051–61

114. Rogers S, Wells R, Rechsteiner M. 1986. Amino acid sequences common to rapidly degraded proteins: the PEST hypothesis. *Science* 234:364–68

115. Masternak K, Muhlethaler-Mottet A, Villard J, Zufferey M, Steimle V, Reith W. 2000. CIITA is a transcriptional coactivator that is recruited to MHC class II promoters by multiple synergistic interactions with an enhanceosome complex. *Genes Dev.* 14:1156–66

116. Moreno CS, Beresford GW, Louis-Plence P, Morris AC, Boss JM. 1999. CREB regulates MHC class II expression in a CIITA-dependent manner. *Immunity* 10:143–51

117. Vilen BJ, Cogswell JP, Ting JP. 1991. Stereospecific alignment of the X and Y elements is required for major histocompatibility complex class II DRA promoter function. *Mol. Cell. Biol.* 11:2406–15

118. Vilen BJ, Penta JF, Ting JP-Y. 1992. Structural constraints within a trimeric transcriptional regulatory region: constitutive and interferon-g inducible expression of the HLA-DRA gene. *J. Biol. Chem.* 267:23728–34

119. Hake S, Masternak K, Kammerbauer C, Reith W, Steimle V. 2000. CIITA leucine-rich repeats control nuclear localization in vivo recruitment to the major histocompatibility complex (MHC) class II enhanceosome and MHC class II gene transactivation. *Mol. Cell. Biol.* 20:7716–25

120. Bontron S, Ucla C, Mach B, Steimle V. 1997. Efficient repression of endogenous major histocompatibility complex class II expression through dominant negative CIITA mutants isolated by a functional selection strategy. *Mol. Cell. Biol.* 17:4249–58

121. Brown JA, Rogers EM, Boss JM. 1998. The MHC class II transactivator (CIITA) requires conserved leucine charged domains for interactions with the conserved W box promoter element. *Nucleic Acids Res.* 26:4128–36

122. Chin KC, Li G, Ting JP. 1997. Activation and transdominant suppression of MHC class II and HLA-DMB promoters by a series of C-terminal class II transactivator deletion mutants. *J. Immunol.* 159:2789–94

123. Chin KC, Li GG, Ting JP. 1997. Importance of acidic, proline/serine/threonine-rich, and GTP-binding regions in the major histocompatibility complex class II transactivator: generation of transdominant-negative mutants. *Proc. Natl. Acad. Sci. USA* 94:2501–6

124. Riley JL, Westerheide SD, Price JA, Brown JA, Boss JM. 1995. Activation of class II MHC genes requires both the X box and the class II transactivator (CIITA). *Immunity* 2:533–43

125. Zhou H, Glimcher LH. 1995. Human MHC class II gene transcription directed by the carboxyl terminus of CIITA, one of the defective genes in type II MHC combined immune deficiency. *Immunity* 2:545–53

126. Yun S, Gustafsson K, Fabre JW. 1998. Suppression of human anti-porcine T-cell immune responses by major histocompatibility complex class II transactivator constructs lacking the amino terminal domain. *Transplantation* 66: 103–11

127. Zhou H, Su HS, Zhang X, Douhan J3, Glimcher LH. 1997. CIITA-dependent and -independent class II MHC expression revealed by a dominant negative mutant. *J. Immunol.* 158:4741–49

128. Fontes JD, Jiang B, Peterlin BM. 1997. The class II trans-activator CIITA interacts with the TBP-associated factor TAF II 32. *Nucleic Acids Res.* 25:2522–28

129. Mahanta SK, Scholl T, Yang FC, Strominger JL. 1997. Transactivation by CIITA, the type II bare lymphocyte syndrome-associated factor, requires participation of multiple regions of the TATA box binding protein. *Proc. Natl. Acad. Sci. USA* 94:6324–29

130. Kanazawa S, Okamoto T, Peterlin BM. 2000. Tat competes with CIITA for the binding to P-TEFb and blocks the expression of MHC class II genes in HIV infection. *Immunity* 12:61–70

131. Kretsovali A, Agalioti T, Spilianakis C, Tzortzakaki E, Merika M, Papamatheakis J. 1998. Involvement of CREB binding protein in expression of major histocompatibility complex class II genes via interaction with the class II transactivator. *Mol. Cell Biol.* 18:6777–83

132. Fontes JD, Kanazawa S, Jean D, Peterlin BM. 1999. Interactions between the class II transactivator and CREB binding protein increase transcription of major histocompatibility complex class II genes. *Mol. Cell. Biol.* 19:941–47

133. Wright KL, Chin KC, Linhoff M, Skinner C, Brown JA, Boss JM, Stark GR, Ting JP. 1998. CIITA stimulation of transcription factor binding to major histocompatibility complex class II and associated promoters in vivo. *Proc. Natl. Acad. Sci. USA* 95:6267–72

134. Villard J, Muhlethaler-Mottet A, Bontron S, Mach B, Reith W. 1999. CIITA-induced occupation of MHC class II promoters is independent of the cooperative stabilization of the promoter-bound multi-protein complexes. *Int. Immunol.* 11:461–69

135. Scholl T, Mahanta SK, Strominger JL. 1997. Specific complex formation between the type II bare lymphocyte syndrome-associated transactivators CIITA and RFX5. *Proc. Natl. Acad. Sci. USA* 94:6330–34

136. Cressman DE, Chin KC, Taxman DJ, Ting JP. 1999. A defect in the nuclear translocation of CIITA causes a form of type II bare

lymphocyte syndrome. *Immunity* 10:163–71

137. Harton JA, Cressman DE, Chin KC, Der CJ, Ting JP. 1999. GTP binding by class II transactivator: role in nuclear import. *Science* 285:1402–5

138. Erickson FL, Dinesh-Kumar SP, Holzberg S, Ustach CV, Dutton M, Handley V, Corr C, Baker BJ. 1999. Interactions between tobacco mosaic virus and the tobacco N gene. *Philos. Trans. R. Soc. Lond. B. Biol. Sci.* 354:653–58

139. Inohara N, Koseki T, del Peso L, Hu Y, Yee C, Chen S, Carrio R, Merino J, Liu D, Ni J, Nunez G. 1999. Nod1, an Apaf-1-like activator of caspase-9 and nuclear factor-kappaB. *J. Biol. Chem.* 274:14560–67

140. Steimle V, Siegrist C-A, Mottet A, Lisowska-Grospierre B, Mach B. 1994. Regulation of MHC class II expression by interferon-gamma mediated by the transactivator gene CIITA. *Science* 265:106–9

141. Chang CH, Fontes JD, Peterlin M, Flavell RA. 1994. Class II transactivator (CIITA) is sufficient for the inducible expression of major histocompatibility complex class II genes. *J. Exp. Med.* 180:1367–74

142. O'Keefe GM, Nguyen VT, Benveniste EN. 1999. Class II transactivator and class II MHC gene expression in microglia: modulation by the cytokines TGF-beta, IL-4, IL-13 and IL-10. *Eur. J. Immunol.* 29:1275–85

143. Dong Y, Rohn WM, Benveniste EN. 1999. IFN-gamma regulation of the type IV class II transactivator promoter in astrocytes. *J. Immunol.* 162:4731–39

144. Muhlethaler-Mottet A, Di Berardino W, Otten LA, Mach B. 1998. Activation of the MHC class II transactivator CIITA by interferon-γ requires cooperative interaction between Stat1 and USF-1. *Immunity* 8:157–66

145. Muhlethaler-Mottet A, Otten LA, Steimle V, Mach B. 1997. Expression of MHC class II molecules in different cellular and functional compartments is controlled by differential usage of multiple promoters of the transactivator CIITA. *EMBO J.* 16:2851–60

146. Piskurich JF, Linhoff MW, Wang Y, Ting JP. 1999. Two distinct gamma interferon-inducible promoters of the major histocompatibility complex class II transactivator gene are differentially regulated by STAT1, interferon regulatory factor 1, and transforming growth factor beta. *Mol. Cell Biol.* 19:431–40

147. Piskurich JF, Wang Y, Linhoff MW, White LC, Ting JP. 1998. Identification of distinct regions of 5' flanking DNA that mediate constitutive, IFN-gamma, STAT1, and TGF-beta-regulated expression of the class II transactivator gene. *J. Immunol.* 160:233–40

148. Lee YJ, Benveniste EN. 1996. Stat1 alpha expression is involved in IFN-gamma induction of the class II transactivator and class II MHC genes. *J. Immunol.* 157:1559–68

149. Silacci P, Mottet A, Steimle V, Reith W, Mach B. 1994. Developmental extinction of major histocompatibility complex class II gene expression in plasmocytes is mediated by silencing of the transactivator gene CIITA. *J. Exp. Med.* 180:1329–36

150. Sartoris S, Valle MT, Barbaro AL, Tosi G, Cestari T, D'Agostino A, Megiovanni AM, Manca F, Accolla RS. 1998. HLA class II expression in uninducible hepatocarcinoma cells after transfection of AIR-1 gene product CIITA: acquisition of antigen processing and presentation capacity. *J. Immunol.* 161:814–20

151. Otten LA, Steimle V, Bontron S, Mach B. 1998. Quantitative control of MHC class II expression by the transactivator CIITA. *Eur. J. Immunol.* 28:473–78

152. Sartoris S, Tosi G, De Lerma B, Cestari T, Accolla RS. 1996. Active suppression of the class II transactivator-encoding AIR-1 locus is responsible for the lack of major histocompatibility complex class II gene

expression observed during differentiation from B cells to plasma cells. *Eur. J. Immunol.* 26:2456–60

153. Chang CH, Hong SC, Hughes CC, Janeway CAJ, Flavell RA. 1995. CIITA activates the expression of MHC class II genes in mouse T cells. *Int. Immunol.* 7:1515–18

154. Morris AC, Riley JL, Fleming WH, Boss JM. 1998. MHC class II gene silencing in trophoblast cells is caused by inhibition of CIITA expression. *Am. J. Reprod. Immunol.* 40:385–94

155. Morris AC, Spangler WE, Boss JM. 2000. Methylation of class II trans-activator promoter IV: a novel mechanism of MHC class II gene control. *J. Immunol.* 164:4143–49

156. Miller DM, Rahill BM, Boss JM, Lairmore MD, Durbin JE, Waldman JW, Sedmak DD. 1998. Human cytomegalovirus inhibits major histocompatibility complex class II expression by disruption of the Jak/Stat pathway. *J. Exp. Med.* 187:675–83

157. Le Roy E, Muhlethaler-Mottet A, Davrinche C, Mach B, Davignon JL. 1999. Escape of human cytomegalovirus from HLA-DR-restricted CD4(+) T-cell response is mediated by repression of gamma interferon-induced class II transactivator expression. *J. Virol.* 73:6582–89

158. Abendroth A, Slobedman B, Lee E, Mellins E, Wallace M, Arvin AM. 2000. Modulation of major histocompatibility class II protein expression by varicella-zoster virus. *J. Virol.* 74:1900–7

159. Wojciechowski W, DeSanctis J, Skamene E, Radzioch D. 1999. Attenuation of MHC class II expression in macrophages infected with Mycobacterium bovis bacillus Calmette-Guerin involves class II transactivator and depends on the Nramp1 gene. *J. Immunol.* 163:2688–96

160. Zhong G, Fan T, Liu L. 1999. Chlamydia inhibits interferon gamma-inducible major histocompatibility complex class II expression by degradation of upstream stimulatory factor 1. *J. Exp. Med.* 189:1931–38

161. Lu HT, Riley JL, Babcock GT, Huston M, Stark GR, Boss JM, Ransohoff RM. 1995. Interferon (IFN) beta acts downstream of IFN-gamma-induced class II transactivator messenger RNA accumulation to block major histocompatibility complex class II gene expression and requires the 48-kD DNA-binding protein, ISGF3-gamma. *J. Exp. Med.* 182:1517–25

162. Nikcevich KM, Piskurich JF, Hellendall RP, Wang Y, Ting JP. 1999. Differential selectivity of CIITA promoter activation by IFN-gamma and IRF-1 in astrocytes and macrophages: CIITA promoter activation is not affected by TNF-alpha. *J. Neuroimmunol.* 99:195–204

163. Han Y, Zhou ZH, Ransohoff RM. 1999. TNF-alpha suppresses IFN-gamma-induced MHC class II expression in HT1080 cells by destabilizing class II trans-activator mRNA. *J. Immunol.* 163:1435–40

164. Douhan J, Lieberson R, Knoll JHM, Zhou H, Glimcher LH. 1997. An isotype-specific activator of major histocompatibility complex (MHC) class II genes that is independent of class II transactivator. *J. Exp. Med.* 185:1885–95

165. Suter T, Malipiero U, Otten L, Ludewig B, Muhlethaler-Mottet A, Mach B, Reith W, Fontana A. 2000. Dendritic cells and differential usage of the MHC class II transactivator promoters in the central nervous system in experimental autoimmune encephalitis. *Eur. J. Immunol.* 30:794–802

166. Ghosh N, Piskurich JF, Wright G, Hassani K, Ting JP, Wright KL. 1999. A novel element and a TEF-2-like element activate the major histocompatibility complex class II transactivator in B-lymphocytes. *J. Biol. Chem.* 274:32342–50

167. Lennon AM, Ottone C, Rigaud G, Deaven LL, Longmire J, Fellous M, Bono R, Alcaide-Loridan C. 1997. Isolation of a B-cell-specific promoter for the human class II transactivator. *Immunogenetics* 45:266–73

168. Rohn W, Tang LP, Dong Y, Benveniste EN. 1999. IL-1 beta inhibits IFN-gamma-induced class II MHC expression by suppressing transcription of the class II transactivator gene. *J. Immunol.* 162:886–96

169. Imada K, Leonard WJ. 2000. The jak-STAT pathway. *Mol. Immunol.* 37:1–11

170. Leonard WJ, O'Shea JJ. 1998. Jaks and STATs: biological implications. *Annu. Rev. Immunol.* 16:293–322

171. Harada H, Taniguchi T, Tanaka N. 1998. The role of interferon regulatory factors in the interferon system and cell growth control. *Biochimie* 80:641–50

172. Nandan D, Reiner NE. 1997. TGF-beta attenuates the class II transactivator and reveals an accessory pathway of IFN-gamma action. *J. Immunol.* 158:1095–1101

173. Lee YJ, Han Y, Lu HT, Nguyen V, Qin H, Howe PH, Hocevar BA, Boss JM, Ransohoff RM, Benveniste EN. 1997. TGF-beta suppresses IFN-gamma induction of class II MHC gene expression by inhibiting class II transactivator messenger RNA expression. *J. Immunol.* 158:2065–75

174. Blanck G. 1999. HLA class II expression in human tumor lines. *Microbes Infect.* 1:913–18

175. Kadota Y, Okumura M, Miyoshi S, Kitagawa-Sakakida S, Inoue M, Shiono H, Maeda Y, Kinoshita T, Shirakura R, Matsuda H. 2000. Altered T cell development in human thymoma is related to impairment of MHC class II transactivator expression induced by

176. Kielar ML, Sicher SC, Penfield JG, Jeyarajah DR, Lu CY. 2000. Nitric oxide inhibits INFgamma-induced increases in CIITA mRNA abundance and activation of CIITA dependent genes–class II MHC, Ii and H-2M. class II transactivator. *Inflammation* 24:431–45

177. Kwak B, Mulhaupt F, Myit S and Mach F. 2000. Statins as a newly recognized type of immunomodulator. *Nat. Med.* December 1, 2000.

178. Lefebvre S, Moreau P, Dausset J, Carosella ED, Paul P. 1999. Downregulation of HLA class I gene transcription in choriocarcinoma cells is controlled by the proximal promoter element and can be reversed by CIITA. *Placenta* 20:293–301

179. Girdlestone J. 2000. Synergistic induction of HLA class I expression by RelA and CIITA. *Blood* 95:3804–8

180. Murphy KM, Ouyang W, Farrar JD, Yang J, Ranganath S, Asnagli H, Afkarian M, Murphy TL. 2000. Signaling and transcription in T helper development. *Annu. Rev. Immunol.* 18:451–94:451–94

181. Gourley T, Roys S, Lukacs NW, Kunkel SL, Flavell RA, Chang CH. 1999. A novel role for the major histocompatibility complex class II transactivator CIITA in the repression of IL-4 production. *Immunity* 10:377–86

182. Sisk TJ, Gourley T, Roys S, Chang CH. 2000. MHC class II transactivator inhibits IL-4 gene transcription by competing with NF-AT to bind the coactivator CREB binding protein (CBP)/p300. *J. Immunol.* 165:2511–17

183. Saifuddin M, Roebuck KA, Chang C, Ting JP, Spear GT. 2000. Cutting edge: activation of HIV-1 transcription by the MHC class II transactivator. *J. Immunol.* 164:3941–45

Annu. Rev. Immunol. 2001. 19:375–96

THE IMMUNOLOGICAL SYNAPSE

Shannon K. Bromley[†], W. Richard Burack[†], Kenneth G. Johnson[†&], Kristina Somersalo[†], Tasha N. Sims[†], Cenk Sumen[#&], Mark M. Davis[#&], Andrey S. Shaw[†], Paul M. Allen[†], and Michael L. Dustin[†*]

[†]Department of Pathology and Immunology and [&]The Howard Hughes Medical Institute, Washington University School of Medicine, 660 S. Euclid Ave, St. Louis, Missouri 63110; e-mail: dustin@pathbox.wustl.edu
[#]Department of Immunology and Microbiology and [&]The Howard Hughes Medical Institute, Stanford University, Palo Alto, Callifornia 94305

Key Words   immunological synapse formation, membrane structure, T cell polarity, signaling pathways, cell adhesion

■ **Abstract**   The adaptive immune response is initiated by the interaction of T cell antigen receptors with major histocompatibility complex molecule-peptide complexes in the nanometer scale gap between a T cell and an antigen-presenting cell, referred to as an immunological synapse. In this review we focus on the concept of immunological synapse formation as it relates to membrane structure, T cell polarity, signaling pathways, and the antigen-presenting cell. Membrane domains provide an organizational principle for compartmentalization within the immunological synapse. T cell polarization by chemokines increases T cell sensitivity to antigen. The current model is that signaling and formation of the immunological synapse are tightly interwoven in mature T cells. We also extend this model to natural killer cell activation, where the inhibitory NK synapse provides a striking example in which inhibition of signaling leaves the synapse in its nascent, inverted state. The APC may also play an active role in immunological synapse formation, particularly for activation of naïve T cells.

INTRODUCTION

T cell activation requires sustained T cell receptor (TCR) interaction with MHC-peptide complexes in the immunological synapse (IS) between the T cell and antigen-presenting cell (APC) (1, 2). The required duration of signaling is on the order of hours, while the activating and inhibitory molecular interactions in the IS have half-lives on the order of seconds (3, 4). Imaging studies of the IS have revealed a remarkable organization that may help account for the longevity and specificity of signaling. The mature IS has been defined by the bull's eye arrangement of supramolecular activation clusters (SMACs) that form within a few minutes of T cell–APC contact (5–7). SMACs are detected by fluorescence microscopy and appear as increased densities of specific molecules (Figure 1; see color insert). The center of the bull's eye or cSMAC is enriched for TCR and MHC-peptide complexes. The ring of the bull's eye or pSMAC contains the integrin LFA-1 and its major counterreceptor ICAM-1. The cSMAC also includes the signaling molecules on the T cell cytoplasmic side of the IS, including protein kinase C θ (PKC θ) and the src family kinase lck. The T cell side of the pSMAC contains the integrin-associated cytoskeletal proteins including talin. The formation of the IS requires an intact T cell cytoskeleton and actually begins as an inverted structure with a central adhesion cluster surrounded by a ring of engaged TCR (5). The APC can be replaced by an artificial phospholipid bilayer. Therefore, activity of the APC is not absolutely required but may regulate IS formation. The final stage of IS formation is the stabilization of the central cluster of MHC-peptide complexes, which correlates with sustained parallel engagement of TCR by at least 60 MHC-peptide complexes. Maintenance of the stabilized IS for greater than 1 hr is well correlated with full T cell activation.

Physiological T cell activation can be divided into a series of temporal stages: T cell polarization, initial adhesion, IS formation (initial signaling), and IS maturation (sustained signaling) (5). The IS embodies a concept for understanding the high-order temporal and spatial cooperation of multiple biochemical and genetic elements known to be required for T cell activation. We discuss membrane organization at the outset due to the fundamental nature of this information and the need to incorporate recent advances in this area into an overview of how signaling complexes form in the IS. We then outline the temporal stages in formation of the IS and their relationship to signaling. The natural killer cell IS is presented as a showcase for the integration of positive and negative signals. Finally, evidence for an active role for the APC in IS formation is considered.

MEMBRANE RAFTS

Intrinsic Organization of the Plasma Membrane

Since our goal is to describe the highly organized structure that forms at the contact between T cell and APC, it is appropriate to first review concepts about preexisting structures within the plasma membrane. Cell biologists have long acknowledged that the plasma membrane is not homogenous (8, 9). This concept is currently associated with the word and concept of a raft. This topic has been extensively reviewed (10, 11). A particularly useful, broader, and more succinct overview of the subject is available (12). We focus on aspects that are most relevant to IS function.

The physical basis of rafts has been extensively discussed over many years as "membrane domains," and the process that produces them has been termed "lateral phase separation" (8, 9). Model membranes of pure phospholipids display a characteristic melting temperature with acyl chains ordered below and disordered above this temperature. In a membrane composed of several different types of phospholipids, the various lipids may not mix, and laterally segregated domains may form with relatively stable ordered and disordered regions. While the effect of cholesterol on membrane structure is variable depending on the specific lipid and its phase, it is generally true that cholesterol induces the formation of liquid-ordered structures, which segregate from disordered structures. These cholesterol induced liquid-ordered regions are enriched in cholesterol itself and appear to also include gangliosides like GM1 and the glycosylphosphatidylinositol (GPI) moieties of glycolipid anchored proteins that are incorporated into the liquid-ordered structures. Interestingly, the liquid-ordered structures are relatively insoluble in Triton X-100 detergent at low temperature, a property shared with biological rafts, which are also referred to as detergent-insoluble, glycolipid-enriched domains (DIGs) or glycosphingolipid enriched membranes (GEMs) (12). Hence, detergent insolubility of proteins is used as a biochemical marker for inclusion in rafts. The presence of many intrinsic membrane proteins in biological membranes may perturb or reinforce lipid packing and have a profound influence on the size and stability of lipid-based structures. The idea that proteins selectively associate with different lipid structures or may themselves organize lipid structures is central to the proposed roles of rafts in signaling and the IS.

EARLY EVIDENCE FOR RAFTS

T cell activation by cross-linking of rafts was described nearly a quarter century ago. These experiments were based on cholera toxin, a pentavalent molecule that binds with high affinity to GM1 and that upon further cross-linking induces capping of this lipid (13). Up to that point, capping had been a phenomenon performed using antibodies and related reagents to aggregate proteins (14). Capping of gangliosides suggested a "possible direct or indirect association between surface gangliosides and submembraneous cytoskeletal assemblies that control modulation of these surface components and may transmit stimuli to the interior of the cell" (15). Within the following decade, Spiegel and coworkers showed that cross-linking of gangliosides in thymocyte membranes resulted in their patching and induced DNA replication. The authors suggested "that gangliosides may self-associate in the plasma membrane, which may explain the basis for ganglioside redistribution and capping" (16).

A decade ago, two works appeared that seem to have set the stage for the current interest in rafts among cell biologists and immunologists. Brown & Rose indicated a role of lateral phase separation of glycosphingolipids and cholesterol in apical targeting of GPI-anchored proteins in polarized epithelial cells (17). Stefanova and coworkers demonstrated that lck could be co-immunoprecipitated with GPI-anchored proteins providing evidence for lipid-based structures spanning the plasma membrane (18). The wider impact of these ideas on several cell biological problems has been summarized (19).

Controversy over the Physical Nature of Rafts

The putative rafts are too small for visualization by light microscopy. The distribution of raft markers is homogenous in resting cells. For example, prior to exposing a mast cell line to its antigen, the Fc-receptor and GM1 are homogeneously distributed (20, 21). The same applies to the TCR and GM1 in studies of T cells (22). In general, cross-linking has been required to produce large enough aggregates to be visualized using epifluorescence microscopy.

A number of groups have attempted imaging methods that extend the resolution of fluorescence microscopy. Fluorescence resonance energy transfer (FRET) is sensitive to distances on the order of a few nanometers. Because FRET between GPI-anchored transferrin receptors interacted with natural ligands, Varma & Mayor concluded that rafts exist, but they are *smaller* than 70 nm in diameter (23). Using a similar approach and observing four distinct constructs interrogated with larger probes, Edidin and colleagues found no evidence of microdomains enriched in either GPI-anchored proteins or GM1 (24). These disparate results could be reconciled if the unperturbed rafts were indeed at a nanometer scale.

Baird and coworkers propose that prior to cross-linking, the rafts are sufficiently small that each contains a single molecule of the tyrosine kinase lyn or FcRε (20). Cross-linking the FcR creates a larger aggregate that can then recruit the small monomeric rafts, each containing a single molecule of lyn. This coalescence of rafts allows lyn to phosphorylate a large number of FcRs, thus allowing phosphorylation and signaling. The model reflects a much older concept of annular lipid, where rafts would represent the ability of specific proteins and lipoproteins to recruit a surround of liquid-ordered lipids that would then be predisposed to coalesce following either cross-linking or changes in conformation. Therefore, the initial size of rafts may be quite small, but the regulation of raft aggregation by cross-linking or lateral protein interactions in membranes is likely central in signaling and IS formation.

IMMUNOLOGICAL SYNAPSE FORMATION

T Cell Polarization and Initial Adhesion

Circulating T cells are rounded and nonpolarized, with a uniform radial distribution of membrane domains, receptors, and microvilli on the cell surface (25). These cells are relatively nonmotile and integrin adhesion molecules are maintained in a low-activity state (26). Thus, initial adhesion between the naive T cell and APC might require an innate signal that sets the stage for IS formation, for example, exposure to chemokines. T cells encounter chemokine gradients as they extravasate into lymph nodes and inflamed tissues. Therefore, T cells will be exposed to chemokines before they encounter APC.

Chemokine receptor signaling results in the rapid polarization of T lymphocytes. Exposure to a chemokine gradient induces the formation of a front end, or lamellapodium, and a back end, or uropod (25). Chemokine receptors are members of the serpentine family that link to heterotrimeric G proteins. Interestingly, chemokine receptor and TCR signaling share a number of components but differ greatly with respect to time. Effective chemokine signals are transient and determine the differential of signal strength as a function of time or distance. In contrast, TCR signals are maintained for hours and appear to integrate MHC-peptide and adhesion molecule signals to determine if they reach or exceed thresholds set during T cell differentiation.

Interaction with chemokines induces conformational changes in chemokine receptors that lead to the dissociation of the heterotrimeric G protein into active α (GTP bound) and $\beta\gamma$ subunits. While the role of rafts in G-protein signaling is not clear, it is interesting that $\beta\gamma$ subunits are prenylated, which favors exclusion from raft lipids, while the α subunit is acylated, which favors association with raft lipids (27). The time taken by the α subunit to hydrolyze GTP defines the time window of $\beta\gamma$ subunit activity. This time period is influenced by a regulator of G-protein signaling (RGS) proteins that act as GTPase activating proteins (GAPs) for the α subunits (28). In addition to this intrinsic timing mechanism, chemokine receptors are desensitized by G-protein receptor kinase/arrestin mechanisms acting on the receptor itself (29). The active $\beta\gamma$ subunits interact with phospholipase C (PLC) and phosphatidylinositol-3-kinase (PI-3K). PLCγ and PI-3K in turn activate protein kinase C (PKC) and generate ligands for pleckstrin homology (PH) domains, respectively. The Vav protooncogene and WASP, the protein deficient in the X-linked immunodeficiency Wiskott-Aldrich syndrome, have functionally relevant PH domains. Vav is a rho family guanine nucleotide exchange factor (GEF) that activates CDC42 and rac (30). WASP is activated by phosphatidylinositol (PtdIns)-4,5-bisphosphate and CDC42, and in turn WASP recruits and activates the ARP2/3 complex (31). The activated ARP2/3 complex nucleates new actin polymerization, a fundamental process for cell locomotion.

The response to chemokines is itself a polarized process. In granulocytes responding to a gradient of the chemoattractant fMLP, the PH domain of the Akt kinase, which interacts with phosphatidylinositol-3,4,5-trisphosphate, is transiently accumulated in the leading lamellipodium (32). Finally, neutrophils permeabilized after exposure to chemokine gradients demonstrated that new actin filaments were selectively generated at the edge of the cell near the chemoattractant source (33). These studies suggest that the leading edge of the migrating leukocyte is itself a specialized supramolecular compartment even before IS formation is initiated.

These changes at the leading edge of polarized lymphocytes lead to increased sensitivity to antigen. This has been directly demonstrated by studies in which polarized lymphocytes were contacted with APC on the leading membrane projections or on their uropods, where the leading edge was found to be greater than tenfold more sensitive than the uropod to antigen (34). The same signals that enhance actin polymerization at the leading edge are also implicated in integrin activation, possibly because integrin regulation requires coordinated actin polymerization. Enhanced integrin engagement at the leading edge may trigger actin-based protrusions tipped by TCR-enriched membranes that could form the basis of sensory contacts involved in MHC-peptide sampling and the initial stage of IS formation (35). An actin-based program for developing adhesion molecule–tipped protrusion has been vividly described for epithelial cell contacts (36). Conversely, the uropod is important as a site at which adhesive interactions are broken and as a depot for molecules that might inhibit interactions. For example, the mucin CD43 is sequestered in the uropod of polarized T cells, which may reduce the antiadhesive effects of this protein at the leading edge (25). Thus, polarization sets the stage for effective adhesion, TCR engagement, and IS formation.

ADHESION

Integrating signals delivered through multiple receptor systems is likely to be a key feature of the immunological synapse. Molecular segregation in the IS is a fundamental process in accomplishing integration. Topological models of T cell signaling predict that those molecules with large extracellular domains would be excluded from sites of TCR/peptide-MHC interactions due to the small distances between apposing membranes (~15 nm) (37). These close contact areas are established by adhesion molecules, which play an essential role in T cell activation. Close contacts may be achieved indirectly through cytoskeletal protrusions anchored to larger adhesion mechanisms like LFA-1 and ICAM-1 (5) or more directly by smaller adhesion receptor pairs like CD2 and CD58 that would work immediately beside the TCR. In agreement with this idea, increasing the size of the CD48 ligand for CD2 by adding additional Ig-like domains inhibits TCR engagement of MHC-peptide (38). Interestingly, both CD2 and its ligand CD48 are associated with rafts, as is the TCR (39). Depending upon the size of these structures, an initial close association of CD2 and TCR in rafts may explain the dominant negative effect of long forms of CD48, which may themselves be proximal to MHC molecules in rafts on the APC (40). The topological model is also consistent with observations that large mucin-like molecules including CD43 and CD45 are excluded from T cell/APC conjugates (41–43).

T CELL RECEPTOR SIGNALING

The mechanism of selective TCR triggering is a hotly debated area with three major models based on kinetic/oligomerization (44), conformational change (45), and kinetic/segregation (37). Current molecular data on IS formation cannot distinguish between these models, but it is certain that kinetic parameters are important. In particular, the off rate of the monomeric TCR-MHC/peptide interaction (46, 47) plays a decisive role in determining the final MHC density accumulated into the mature IS, and hence the extent of T cell activation (5). Likewise, the inhibitory effects of altered peptide ligands can manifest in a decreased MHC density in the cSMAC, consistent with a spoiler role where unproductive engagement of TCRs by antagonist peptide/MHC with fast off rates could dull the ability of the T cell to cluster MHC (48). Allosteric interactions may nevertheless have an impact on the stability of the central MHC cluster (49). Thermodynamic analysis of TCR/MHC-peptide binding has revealed a case for induced fit, which may explain the ability of excess TCR to scan through MHC complexes collected in the IS to differentiate signal from noise (50).

IS formation is a clear example where kinetics of interaction is linked to molecular segregation in formation of the SMACs; however, the very earliest signals leading to formation of these micron scale domains are not readily observed by conventional fluorescence microscopy. An added complication is that much of our knowledge of TCR signaling mechanisms is based on antibody cross-linking in T cell lines and hybridomas as the triggering event in the absence of any adhesion or contact organization. Thus, the following discussion combines information from multiple types of experiments with a goal of generating a coherent and testable model for how IS formation integrates the TCR signal with multiple additional signals to set a robust threshold for full T cell activation.

The first biochemical event that can be detected upon TCR/CD3-ligation is the lck-mediated phosphorylation of tyrosine residues within the immunoreceptor tyrosine-based activation motifs (ITAMs) of the invariant CD3 and ζ-chains, and the recruitment and activation of ZAP-70 (51). Activated ZAP-70 then phosphorylates a series of adapter proteins that lead to recruitment of PLC-γ, PI-3K, Itk, and Ras to the activated TCR complex. Tyrosine phosphorylation, calcium flux, and the generation of inositol phospholipids are proximal intracellular events following MHC-peptide recognition by the TCR, maximally occurring within 30 sec to 5 min following activation. This is the time frame in which the IS forms (5) and in which the T cell undergoes internal cytoskeletal rearrangements that align the secretory apparatus to the IS (1). The maturation of the IS into a stable structure continues well beyond this time frame into a range of sustained signaling important in T cell activation. TCR may be desensitized by a process of downregulation leading to a serial engagement of multiple TCR, followed by internalization and degradation (52). However, the IS may initiate a process of parallel engagement of multiple TCR in the cSMAC that may forestall internalization and promote a nucleus of sustained signaling (35). How is the IS formed, what are the intracellular signals that regulate cell polarization and de novo gene transcription, and how are these functions coordinated and/or interdependent? Recent progress in the dissection of T cell signaling mechanisms has greatly increased our understanding of how the T cell orchestrates signaling networks to regulate these processes.

Signaling, Rafts, and Segregation

The regulation of lck may be particularly responsive to membrane structure. Lck is an acylated protein that accumulates in DIGs and is visualized in aggregated rafts. In fact, membrane-bound lck that is excluded from DIGs is incapable of mediating full T cell activation (53). Lck is negatively regulated through the carboxyl-terminal tyrosine phosphorylation site (Y505), which mediates intramolecular binding to the SH2 domain that places the kinase in a closed conformation of decreased activity (54, 55). Conversely, a second site of tyrosine phosphorylation (Y394) found in the activation loop of the kinase domain is autophosphorylated to activate the kinase for substrate phosphorylation. Phosphorylation of inhibitory Y505 in lck is controlled by the opposing actions of the tyrosine kinase csk and by the tyrosine phosphatase CD45. Interestingly, Y394 of lck is also dephosphorylated by CD45, as well as by PEP (56, 57). CD45 is excluded from DIGs and from aggregated rafts (22, 58), whereas the CSK docking protein Cbp/PAG is an acylated transmembrane protein that is concentrated in DIGs (59). Cbp/PAG is dephosphorylated by an unknown phosphatase upon TCR engagement and releases CSK from the rafts. Thus, raft dynamics during activation may profoundly influence net activity of src family kinases and the initiation and maintenance of TCR signals.

Several groups have demonstrated that CD45 is excluded from the developing IS, and this is consistent with proposed models of signaling initiation whereby the exclusion of tyrosine phosphatases from membrane compartments is required for triggering the kinase cascade (37, 42, 43). The large ectodomain of CD45 may be responsible for this initial exclusion. Thus, in addition to its exclusion from low-density rafts, the location of CD45 may also be regulated by the size of its ectodomain through alternative splicing in a cell-specific manner (60). This model would permit a greater accessibility to the IS by the smaller rather than the larger isoforms. Accordingly, CD45 isoforms have differences in their effects on T cell activation (61). Imaging of CD45 with antibodies interacting with all isoforms demonstrates decreased CD45 in areas of ICAM-1/LFA-1 accumulation, possibly contributing to LFA-1 activation (62). However, a discreet pool of CD45 moves back into the central region of the mature IS, adjacent to the area of TCR/MHC engagement (43). In fact, the CD45 in this location appears to be in a previously undescribed cytoplasmic compartment near the cSMAC. The positive or negative roles of this CD45 movement are unknown, but it may provide a mechanism to sustain lck activity near engaged TCR.

The TCR is only weakly associated with DIGs both in nonstimulated Jurkat T cells and in thymocytes (63–65). Following TCR activation the association of TCR complexes with the DIG fraction increases. Particularly, the hyperphosphorylated P-p23 form of the ITAM rich ζ-chain is preferentially associated with DIGs as compared to the less phosphorylated P-p21 form. Conversely, little phosphorylated ζ-chain is found outside DIGs, consistent with the preferential phosphorylation of proteins within the rafts (63). Coreceptors CD4 and CD8 are strongly associated with DIGs and may play an important role in the initial alternations in the lipid and signaling environment of the TCR.

Once recruited to the ITAMs, ZAP-70 phosphorylates the Linker for activation of T cells (LAT), a 36/38 kDa transmembrane protein that is a critical docking molecule for a number of TCR effectors and is localized to DIGs (66, 67). Following phosphorylation by ZAP-70, LAT recruits directly and indirectly a number of signaling proteins to DIGs, including PLC-γ1, members of the Grb2/Gads/Grap adapter family, PI-3K, SLP-76, and Vav (66). The SH3 domains of the Grb2-adaptors are associated with the Ras GEF, Sos, and with SLP-76, and they serve to recruit these molecules to the cell membrane. Both LAT-deficient and Slp76-deficient Jurkat T cells are unable to initiate significant calcium signaling and

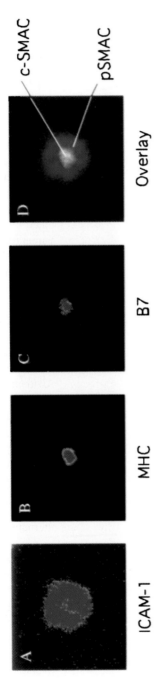

Figure 1 The mature immunological synapse. Patterns of LFA-1 (*A*), TCR (*B*), and CD28 (*C*) interaction in a functional synapse between a T cell and a supported planar bilayer containing Cy5-ICAM-1, Oregon Green- I-A^k,and Cy3-B7. All three markers are overlaid in panel D with the cSMAC and pSMAC labeled.

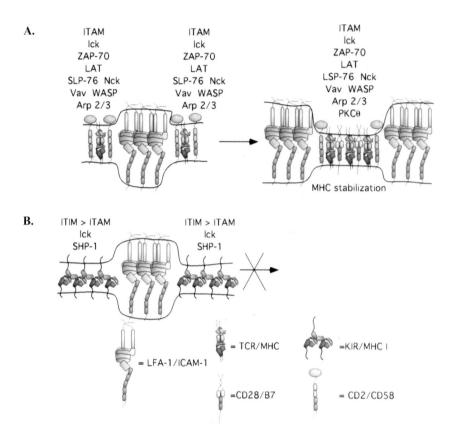

Figure 2 Model for signaling complex formation in the immunological synapse. (*A*) Formation of the T cell IS. Recruitment of PKC-θ is unique to the mature cSMAC. (*B*) Formation of the NK synapse arrested by inhibitory receptor signaling. The molecular pattern in an activating NK cell synapse is not known.

display poor NF-AT activation following TCR ligation, an effect that correlates with the abrogation of PLC-γ1 tyrosine phosphorylation (67).

Importantly, the activation and compartmentalization of a number of critical signaling molecules, including PLC-γ1, Itk, and Vav, are influenced by the interaction of their PH-domains with PtdIns lipids (68, 69). PtdIns-4,5-P_2 is highly enriched within low-density rafts of Jurkat T cells; hence the recruitment of PLC-γ1 to low-density rafts may juxtapose PLC-γ1 to its substrate (64). Similarly, the localization of PI-3K to the nucleated signaling complex catalyzes the conversion of PtdIns-4,5-P_2 to PtdIns-3,4,5-P_3, which is an essential regulator of Vav GEF activity and Itk kinase activity (68).

Following TCR ligation, tyrosine phosphorylated SLP-76 binds to the SH2 domain of Vav, and Vav itself becomes tyrosine phosphorylated, further increasing its GEF activity (70). Vav is important for the reorganization of the actin cytoskeleton. Antibody-mediated TCR capping is abrogated in T lymphocytes from Vav-deficient mice, although the tyrosine phosphorylation of proximal signaling components appears normal (71, 72). However, Vav-deficient T cells are unable to polymerize actin and fail to induce the association of ζ-chain to the cytoskeleton (72). The capping phenotype of Vav-deficient T cells correlates with the inhibition in T cell activation caused by the cytoskeletal inhibitor Cytochalasin D. Like Vav-deficient T cells, Cytochalasin D–treated T cells are unable to induce IL-2 gene transcription but are fully able to phosphorylate proximal signaling proteins following TCR ligation (71, 73). Consistent with this model, a recent study shows that vav-deficient T cells have defects in MHC clustering in T cell–APC contacts induced by superantigen (74). This demonstrates the important concept that the earliest TCR signaling events do not require cytoskeletal change, but instead lead to cytoskeletal rearrangements.

SLP-76, Vav, and Nck form a trimolecular complex, which itself binds to PAK and WASP, both mediators of cytoskeletal rearrangement. The colocalization of tyrosine phosphorylated Vav with Nck enables GTP-bound Rac and Cdc42 to bind and activate proteins implicated in cytoskeletal rearrangement, notably PAK and WASP (35, 75). In addition, SLP-76 provides a further link to the T cell cytoskeleton through the adaptor protein SLAP-130/Fyb (76). With SLP-76, SLAP-130/Fyb localizes to the interface between T cells and anti-CD3 coated beads and binds Evl, a member of the Ena/VASP family associated with actin-based projections and required for actin remodeling of the T cell cytoskeleton following T cell activation (77). These proteins collectively provide mechanisms for linking TCR signaling to actin cytoskeletal changes that are likely to be required for IS formation (35).

Sustaining the Signal: Quantitative or Qualitative?

The majority of T cell signaling mechanisms studied to date have been analyzed within the 15-min period concurrent with the formation of the IS, but little is known about the signals emanating from the mature IS at later times. Although by the time the IS is stabilized and the peak of phosphotyrosine signaling has subsided, detectable phosphorylation of tyrosine residues remains within the signaling cluster (42). The process of stabilization of the MHC-peptide cluster in the IS may signify the generation of signals both sustained and new.

Notably, PKCθ, but no other PKC isoform, translocates to the central region of the IS in the time frame of IS stabilization concordant with an increase in its catalytic activity (6, 78) (Figure 2, see color insert). Detectable recruitment of PKCθ to the cell membrane is observed only with T cell activation induced by agonist ligands; it does not occur with suboptimal partial or antagonist ligands (6). Recruitment of PKCθ may define the signaling threshold necessary to form a stable IS and fully activate the T cell. PKCθ is critically important for the regulation of IL-2 in T cells. The overexpression of PKCθ, but not PKCα, in T cell lines dramatically increases both AP-1 and NFκB activity following TCR ligation (79). The activation of Vav and signaling through JNK appear necessary for efficient PKCθ activation and translocation (80). The overexpression of Vav increases the amount of F-actin at the cell membrane and induces the specific recruitment of PKCθ to these patches, while dominant negative forms of Vav inhibit this translocation. Thus, the Vav/Rac pathway of T cell signaling appears to be critically required for the recruitment and activation of PKCθ, potentially forming a unique signal in the mature IS.

Costimulation

The two-signal model for T cell activation proposes that signal one is provided by the TCR/CD3 complex, while signal two is generated by engagement of T cell costimulatory receptors (81). The unification of the two signal model with the IS model is a current challenge in the field. Although numerous molecules have been implicated as costimulatory receptors, CD28 is the classical example.

It was proposed that CD28 activates the jun kinase, JNK, which is required for the induction of cytokine gene transcription (82). Experiments demonstrating trans-costimulation—in which the defective costimulatory activity of fixed APC could be restored by the addition of third party normal APC (83) or B7-transfected L cells (84)—bolsters this argument. However, coengagement of the TCR is still necessary. Furthermore, the ability to activate T cells from CD28-deficient mice demonstrates that CD28 is not absolutely required (85). In fact, double mutant mice lacking CD28 and CD2 are more impaired in T cell activation than are the corresponding single mutant mice (86). This suggests a degree of redundancy among adhesion/costimulation molecules. The only unique phenotypes associated with the CD28-deficient mice are the inability to respond to a wide range of peptide antigens, in contrast to lacking CD2 and LFA-1, which could only alter the quantitative aspects of the T cell response to a given MHC-peptide complex. These different attributes correlate with the location of these molecules in the immunological synapse; only CD28 is localized in the cSMAC, whereas CD2 and

LFA-1 are engaged in different subregions of the pSMAC (5) (Figure 1, see color insert). Therefore, CD28 is perfectly positioned to directly manipulate sustained TCR signals.

Coligation of TCR and CD28 or LFA-1 activates the actin-myosin-dependent transport (7) of receptors and lipid domains to IS. The coengagement of TCR and CD28 by antibodies on beads also triggers enhanced accumulation of GM1 at the interface, compared to engaging CD3 alone (87). This enhanced raft accumulation correlates with increased lck activation and degradation and increases in immediate and sustained tyrosine phosphorylation (87, 88). In comparison to TCR or CD28 engagement alone, coligation of TCR and CD28 results in the synergistic and sustained phosphorylation and membrane localization of Vav (88). CD28 may influence immediate and sustained TCR signaling by enhancing activation of PI-3K or lck or some combination of these effects (89). Thus, CD28 effects the earliest processes associated with TCR signaling and formation of the IS and is an ideal candidate for enhancing sustained engagement processes in the cSMAC.

Natural Killer Cell Synapse

Natural killer (NK) cells represent a newer frontier in the study of IS formation and extend the model beyond helper T cell interactions. Natural killer cells have large granular lymphocyte (LGL) morphology and play a role in the early protection against microbial infection and tumor cell invasion prior to development of adaptive immunity. They have the ability to lyse targets and also form part of both innate and adaptive immune responses (90). Most NK cells express the low-affinity (Fcγ) receptor type IIIA (CD16) that recognizes IgG-coated targets that can then be killed by antibody-dependent cell cytotoxicity (ADCC). In contrast, tumor- and virus-infected cells induce an innate immune response that integrates multiple signals from the target cells and utilizes invariant receptors. A central concept for NK cell killing is that they detect the absence of self-MHC molecules, the missing-self hypothesis (91). While this area is developing rapidly, the initial gestalt of the field provides a vivid example of how IS formation may play a central role in the integration of complex receptor information.

NK cells express two main types of innate recognition receptors (Table 1): activating receptors associate with ITAM-bearing polypeptide chains and inhibitory receptors with immunotyrosine base inhibitory motifs (ITIM). Activating NK receptors signal in much the same way as TCR, through a kinase cascade involving lck and Syk or Zap-70. These activating receptors are counteracted by the inhibitory receptors that recruit SHP-1 following phosphorylation of the ITIMs by src family kinases (92). The activation of the src family kinases is initiated by the activating receptors such that there is a sequential aspect to this process. SHP-1 extinguishes signaling through neighboring ITAMs. The key to this model is that the activating and inhibitory receptors are thoroughly intermixed in the IS.

TABLE 1 Human natural killer (NK) cell receptors involved in triggering or inhibition of cytotoxicity

	Ligand	Expression	Signaling	Components
Non-MHC specific activating receptors				
NCR				
NKp46	?	all	CD3ζ + FcR1γ	3 + 1 ITAM
NKp30	?	all	CD3ζ	3 ITAM
Nkp44	?	all IL2 act.	DAP12	
CD16	?/IgG Fc	all	CD3ζ FcR1γ	3 + 1 ITAM
NKRP-1 (= NK1.1)	?		FcR1γ	
Various adhesion receptors	variable	all	variable	
MHC specific activating receptors				
Immunoglobulins:				
KIR-S = NKR				
2DS1	HLA-Cw4	clonally	DAP12	1 ITAM
2DS2	HLA-Cw3	clonally	DAP12	1 ITAM
2DS3	HLA-Cw3 & Cw4	clonally	DAP12	1 ITAM
2DS4	?	clonally	DAP12	1 ITAM
2DS5	?	clonally	DAP12	1 ITAM
3DS1	HLA-Bw4	clonally	?	
ILT1 (= LIR7)		clonally	FcR1γ	1 ITAM
Lectin like receptors				
NKG2D	MICA	clonally	DAP10	PI3K docking site
NKG2C/CD94	HLA-E	clonally	DAP12	1 ITAM
MHC specific inhibitory receptors				
Immunoglobulins				
KIR-L				
2DL1 (= p58.1)	HLA-Cw4 group*	clonally	2 ITIM	
2DL2 (= p58.2)	HLA-Cw3 group*	clonally	2 ITIM	
2DL3	HLA-Cw3& Cw4	clonally	2 ITIM	
2DL4	HLA-G	all	1 ITIM	
3DL1 (= p70 & NKB1)	HLA-Bw4	clonally	2 ITIM	
3DL2 (= p140)	HLA-A3	clonally	4 ITIM	
ILT2 (= LIR-1& MIR-7 & CD85) (E, C) UL-18	HLA-A, -B, G	clonally	4 ITIM	
Lectin like				
NKG2A/CD94	HLA-E	clonally	1 ITIM	
Non-MHC specific inhibitory receptors				
LAIR-1 (= p40)	?		2 ITIM	
AIRM-1 (= p75)	Sialic acid		2 ITIM	
Irp60	?		2 ITIM	

*HLA-Cw3 group contains HLA-Cw1, -Cw3, -Cw7, Cw8 etc.
*HLA-Cw4 group contains HLA-Cw2, -Cw4, -Cw6, Cw15.

Non-MHC-Specific Receptors

Many adhesion and costimulatory molecules contribute to NK killing (e. g. LFA-1, CD2, 2B4) (Table 1). Antibodies to these molecules profoundly inhibit killing of target cells by NK cells (93). Some of these receptors would appear to be adhesion or costimulation structures; they may serve these roles in NK cells or alternatively may directly trigger killing. The ability of adhesion molecules to trigger killing may depend on the distribution of ligands. For example, ICAM-2, a ligand for LFA-1, appears to trigger NK cells when it is clustered on the uropod of target cells (94).

Natural cytotoxicity receptors (NCR) are recently described non-MHC-specific triggering receptors and include NKp46, NKp30, and NKp44. All resting human NK cells express NKp46 and NKp30; IL-2-activated cells also express NKp44 (95). The ligands for these molecules have not been identified.

MHC-Specific Receptors

There are two groups of activating receptors that bind specifically to HLA class I. Triggering killer inhibitory receptor-short (KIR-S) receptors are type I glycoproteins with Ig-like domains. Different NK-cell clones express various KIR-S receptors. One clone may express one to five KIR-S (96). The ligands of four KIR-S are known (97) (Table 1).

Another group of specific activating receptors are dimeric type II membrane proteins with C-type lectin domains. NKG2 is a receptor for stress-inducible MHC I–like molecule MICA (98). CD95/NKG2C is a receptor for HLA-E (99). In rodents, there are no KIRs. Instead, a family of C-type lectins of the Ly49 family fill this role (100).

Most HLA-specific activating receptors have inhibitory counterparts with the same specificity. Inhibitory receptors form three groups: six Ig-family KIR-L receptors with different specificities, one Ig family member ILT2, and the lectin-like NKG2A/CD95 (90). These molecules have cytoplasmic ITIMs (101). The crystal structure of KIR/MHC I complex shows that KIR and TCR footprints are different and recognition by KIR is also less allele-specific and less dependent on peptide than TCR/MHC class I recognition (102). The distance spanned by KIR/MHC class I is similar to that of the TCR/MHC interactions (<15 nm). Therefore, the topology of NK inhibitory interactions is consistent with interactions like that in the cSMAC of the helper T cell IS.

Interactions Between Receptors and Ligands

The affinity of the HLA-specific receptors is dependent on a peptide bound in the HLA groove. The Kd values of inhibitory KIR-Ls and inhibitory NKG2A/CD94 are approximately 10 μM with fast on and off rates, whereas the Kd for activating NKG2C/CD94 to the HLA-E ligand is more than 74 μM (103). The kinetics of the interactions of KIR and ligand are fast, faster than activating TCR/MHC interactions. From the crystal structure of KIR2DL2 in a complex with HLA-C3w, it can be concluded that there may be another binding site that can be connected to ligand-induced receptor aggregation (102).

Recently Davis et al described an inhibitory IS between an NK-cell line expressing KIR2D and a class I–transfected B cell line (104). In the NK cell IS, a ring of KIR/MHC interactions formed around the central LFA-1/ICAM-1 cluster, the opposite of the mature T cell IS (Figure 2, see color insert). Zn^{2+} modulates the negative signal of KIR2D when it binds to HLA-Cw4 or -Cw8. It was also demonstrated that MHC I clustering by KIR2DL may require Zn^{2+}, possibly to stabilize the clusters. It is not known what form the NK synapse takes when the activating signals outweigh the inhibitory signals. However, it is likely that the KIR/MHC ring of the inhibitory NK IS also contains engaged activating KIR, each surrounded by inhibitory receptors that recruit SHP-1 on demand.

ANTIGEN-PRESENTING CELLS: The Other Half of the Synapse

The IS is formed only in the context of MHC-peptide complexes on the APC. The APC plays a crucial and active role in the generation of the MHC-peptide complexes, but it is not as clear that the APC plays an active role once the MHC-peptide complexes are on the surface. The B cell cytoskeleton is apparently dispensable for IS formation by primed T cells (7). Nevertheless, different types of APC are functionally distinct, and their unique characteristics may include active contributions to IS formation. For example, dendritic cells (DC) activate naïve T cells most efficiently among APC, whereas a wider variety of APC can activate effector or memory T cells. Variations in molecule expression, membrane organization, antigen processing, and active responses of the APC to IS formation may define unique properties of each APC.

The general topic of antigen processing and determinant selection has been reviewed in detail (105, 106). Generally, antigen is separated in two pools to be presented by MHC molecules; class I presents antigens of intracellular origin to CD8 T cells, and class II presents antigens of extracellular origin to CD4 T cells. These pools are loaded with peptide in the endoplasmic reticulum and MIIC compartments, respectively, but appear to move to the surface in a common transport vesicle, the CIIV.

Dendritic Cells

DC encounter antigen in the periphery and then migrate to lymphoid organs where they present antigen in class I and II in the T cell area of the lymph node (107). Immature DC retain pools of MHC molecules intracellularly but express few MHC molecules on the surface until they are exposed to maturation signals. DC internalize antigen by macropincytosis and by using their C-type lectin and Fc receptors.

Upon maturation (in response to endotoxin, TNFα, or IL-1) (108) and entry into the lymph node T cell area, antigen is processed and mature MHC molecules are transported to the surface via CIIV compartments (109). The CIIV are in some manner associated with the actin cytoskeleton since latrunculin A blocks transport to the surface (110). With maturation, DC rearrange their cytoskeleton and increase their motility (111). The signals for CIIV fusion with the plasma membrane are not known, but it is interesting to consider that T cell contact may influence this process.

MHC at the Cell Surface

Interaction of MHC molecules with the cytoskeleton might control the mobility of MHC molecules and regulate IS formation. Class II diffusion rates are dependent on the cytoskeleton in some cell lines and on the cytoplasmic domain in I-A^k in fibroblast L cells, with cytoplasmic-tail deleted class II moving faster than wild type (112).

Superstructures of stimulatory molecules may efficiently present antigen to T cells. Fixed T and B lymphoma cells display coclustered class I and II on the cell surface (113) and could facilitate interactions between cells and influence signal transduction within a cell. The presence of the costimulatory molecules and the tetraspanin family members in the cluster also indicates a potential for a preformed complex of importance for T cell interactions (110, 114). These protein oligomers may be formed in the CIIV where class I, class II, and CD86 (B7-2) colocalize before class II appears at the DC surface (110). A role for cholesterol in formation of these clusters and the presence of GPI anchored proteins implicates a relationship of these structures to rafts in the APC membranes (110, 115). The grouping of MHC molecules has implications for signaling in the APC and for the nature of the ligand for the TCR. MHC class II preclustering in rafts enhances T cell activation (40). These MHC clusters may also transduce signals to the APC cytoskeleton upon receptor engagement. Induced association of the engaged MHC-ligands with the cytoskeleton could alter the dynamics of IS formation and may enhance signaling by promoting stabilization of the central cluster of engaged MHC molecules in the IS. The APC may also then display a degree of polarization of CIIV fusion with the plasma membrane, possibly delivering new complexes to existing IS to maintain these structures.

CONCLUSIONS

The IS is a dynamic structure that builds on pre-existing membrane organization in the form of small dynamic rafts in the context of a polarized lymphocyte to create a machinery for sustained T cell signaling. The stabilization of the central cluster of engaged MHC-peptide complexes is correlated with full T cell activation. The recruitment of PKCθ appears to be a marker for attainment of the stable IS. Natural killer cells appear to use a similar principle to measure the relative levels of positive and negative signals to identify infected or abnormal cells using a complex array of invariant receptors. Since APC differ in their ability to activate T cells at different stages of differentiation, it also is likely that at least some APC will engage in active processes to manipulate IS formation and stabilization. The potential for a role for rafts and cytoskeleton of the APC in the process of IS stabilization is particularly exciting. Future studies in this rich new area of research are likely to yield further insights as the high order organization of the IS is appreciated in greater detail.

ACKNOWLEDGMENTS

We thank Jerri Smith for assistance with the manuscript. We apologize to colleagues whose work could not be directly cited due to length limits.

Visit the Annual Reviews home page at www.AnnualReviews.org

LITERATURE CITED

1. Paul WE, Seder RA. 1994. Lymphocyte responses and cytokines. *Cell* 76:241–251
2. Norcross MA. 1984. A synaptic basis for T-lymphocyte activation. *Ann. Immunol. (Paris).* 135D:113–34
3. Matsui K, Boniface JJ, Steffner P, Reay PA, Davis MM. 1994. Kinetics of T-cell receptor binding to peptide/I-Ek complexes: correlation of the dissociation rate with T cell responsiveness. *Proc. Natl. Acad. Sci. USA* 91:12862–66
4. Iezzi G, Karjalainen K, Lanzavecchia A. 1998. The duration of antigenic stimulation determines the fate of naive and effector T cells. *Immunity* 8:89–95
5. Grakoui A, Bromley SK, Sumen C, Davis MM, Shaw AS, Allen PM, Dustin ML. 1999. The immunological synapse: A molecular machine controlling T cell activation. *Science* 285:221–27
6. Monks CR, Freiberg BA, Kupfer H, Sciaky N, Kupfer A. 1998. Three-dimensional segregation of supramolecular activation clusters in T cells. *Nature* 395:82–86
7. Wülfing C, Davis MM. 1998. A receptor/cytoskeletal movement triggered by costimulation during T cell activation. *Science* 282:2266–69

8. Klausner RD, Kleinfeld AM, Hoover RL, Karnovsky MJ. 1980. Lipid domains in membranes. Evidence derived from structural perturbations induced by free fatty acids and lifetime heterogeneity analysis. *J. Biol. Chem.* 255:1286–95
9. Karnovsky MJ, Kleinfeld AM, Hoover RL, Klausner RD. 1982. The concept of lipid domains in membranes. *J. Cell Biol.* 94:1–6
10. Langlet C, Bernard AM, Drevot P, He HT. 2000. Membrane rafts and signaling by the multichain immune recognition receptors. *Curr. Opin. Immunol.* 12:250–55
11. Janes PW, Ley SC, Magee AI, Kabouridis PS. 2000. The role of lipid rafts in T cell antigen receptor (TCR) signalling. *Semin. Immunol.* 12:23–34
12. Brown DA, London E. 2000. Structure and function of sphingolipid- and cholesterol-rich membrane rafts. *J. Biol. Chem.* 275:17221–24
13. Revesz T, Greaves M. 1975. Ligand-induced redistribution of lymphocyte membrane ganglioside GM1. *Nature* 257:103–6
14. Unanue ER, Perkins WD, Karnovsky MJ. 1972. Ligand-induced movement of

lymphocyte membrane macromolecules. I. Analysis by immunofluorescence and ultrastructural radioautography. *J. Exp. Med.* 136:885–906

15. Sela BA, Raz A, Geiger B. 1978. Antibodies to ganglioside GM1 induce mitogenic stimulation and cap formation in rat thymocytes. *Eur. J. Immunol.* 8:268–74

16. Spiegel S, Kassis S, Wilchek M, Fishman PH. 1984. Direct visualization of redistribution and capping of fluorescent gangliosides on lymphocytes. *J. Cell Biol.* 99:1575–81

17. Brown DA, Rose JK. 1992. Sorting of GPI-anchored proteins to glycolipid-enriched membrane subdomains during transport to the apical cell surface. *Cell* 68:533–44

18. Stefanova I, Horejsi V, Ansotegui IJ, Knapp W, Stockinger H. 1991. GPI-anchored cell-surface molecules complexed to protein tyrosine kinases. *Science* 254:1016–19

19. Simons K, Ikonen E. 1997. Functional rafts in cell membranes. *Nature* 387:569–72

20. Sheets ED, Holowka D, Baird B. 1999. Critical role for cholesterol in Lyn-mediated tyrosine phosphorylation of FcepsilonRI and their association with detergent-resistant membranes. *J. Cell Biol.* 145:877–87

21. Stauffer TP, Meyer T. 1997. Compartmentalized IgE receptor-mediated signal transduction in living cells. *J. Cell Biol.* 139:1447–54

22. Janes PW, Ley SC, Magee AI. 1999. Aggregation of lipid rafts accompanies signaling via the T cell antigen receptor. *J. Cell Biol.* 147:447–61

23. Varma R, Mayor S. 1998. GPI-anchored proteins are organized in submicron domains at the cell surface. *Nature* 394:798–801

24. Kenworthy AK, Petranova N, Edidin M. 2000. High-resolution FRET microscopy of cholera toxin B-subunit and GPI-anchored proteins in cell plasma membranes. *Mol. Biol. Cell.* 11:1645–55

25. Sanchez-Madrid F, del Pozo MA. 1999. Leukocyte polarization in cell migration and immune interactions. *Embo J.* 18:501–11

26. Kucik DF, Dustin ML, Miller JM, Brown EJ. 1996. Adhesion activating phorbol ester increases the mobility of leukocyte integrin LFA-1 in cultured lymphocytes. *J. Clin. Invest.* 97:2139–44

27. Moffett S, Brown DA, Linder ME. 2000. Lipid-dependent targeting of G proteins into rafts. *J. Biol. Chem.* 275:2191–98

28. Watson N, Linder ME, Druey KM, Kehrl JH, Blumer KJ. 1996. RGS family members: GTPase-activating proteins for heterotrimeric G-protein alpha-subunits. *Nature* 383:172–75

29. Orsini MJ, Parent JL, Mundell SJ, Benovic JL. 1999. Trafficking of the HIV coreceptor CXCR4. Role of arrestins and identification of residues in the c-terminal tail that mediate receptor internalization. *J. Biol. Chem.* 274:31076–86

30. Turner M, Mee PJ, Walters AE, Quinn ME, Mellor AL, Zamoyska R, Tybulewicz VL. 1997. A requirement for the Rho-family GTP exchange factor Vav in positive and negative selection of thymocytes. *Immunity* 7:451–60

31. Blanchoin L, Amann KJ, Higgs HN, Marchand JB, Kaiser DA, Pollard TD. 2000. Direct observation of dendritic actin filament networks nucleated by Arp2/3 complex and WASP/Scar proteins. *Nature* 404:1007–11

32. Servant G, Weiner OD, Herzmark P, Balla T, Sedat JW, Bourne HR. 2000. Polarization of chemoattractant receptor signaling during neutrophil chemotaxis. *Science* 287:1037–40

33. Weiner OD, Servant G, Welch MD, Mitchison TJ, Sedat JW, Bourne HR. 1999. Spatial control of actin polymerization during neutrophil chemotaxis. *Nat. Cell. Biol.* 1:75–81

34. Negulescu PA, Kraieva T, Khan A, Kerschbaum HH, Cahalan MD. 1996. Polarity

of T cell shape, motility, and sensitivity to antigen. *Immunity* 4:421–30

35. Dustin ML, Cooper JA. 2000. The actin cytoskeleton and the immunological synapse: molecular hardware for T cell signaling. *Nat. Immunol.* 1:23–29

36. Vasioukhin V, Bauer C, Yin M, Fuchs E. 2000. Directed actin polymerization is the driving force for epithelial cell-cell adhesion. *Cell* 100:209–19

37. van der Merwe PA, Davis SJ, Shaw AS, Dustin ML. 2000. Cytoskeletal polarization and redistribution of cell-surface molecules during T cell antigen recognition. *Semin. Immunol.* 12:5–21

38. Wild MK, Cambiaggi A, Brown MH, Davies EA, Ohno H, Saito T, van der Merwe PA. 1999. Dependence of T cell antigen recognition on the dimensions of an accessory receptor-ligand complex. *J. Exp. Med.* 190:31–41

39. Yashiro-Ohtani Y, Zhou XY, Toyo-Oka K, Tai XG, Park CS, Hamaoka T, Abe R, Miyake K, Fujiwara H. 2000. Non-CD28 costimulatory molecules present in T cell rafts induce T cell costimulation by enhancing the association of TCR with rafts. *J. Immunol.* 164:1251–59

40. Anderson HA, Hiltbold EM, Roche PA. 2000. Concentration of MHC class II molecules in lipid rafts facilitates antigen presentation. *Nat. Immunol.* 2:156–62

41. Sperling AI, Sedy JR, Manjunath N, Kupfer A, Ardman B, Burkhardt JK. 1998. TCR signaling induces selective exclusion of CD43 from the T cell-antigen-presenting cell contact site. *J. Immunol.* 161:6459–62

42. Leupin O, Zaru R, Laroche T, Muller S, Valitutti S. 2000. Exclusion of CD45 from the T-cell receptor signaling area in antigen-stimulated T lymphocytes. *Curr. Biol.* 10:277–80

43. Johnson KG, Bromley SK, Dustin ML, Thomas ML. 2000. A supramolecular basis for CD45 regulation during T cell activation. *Proc. Natl. Acad. Sci. USA* 97:10138–43

44. Reich Z, Boniface JJ, Lyons DS, Borochov N, Wachtel EJ, Davis MM. 1997. Ligand-specific oligomerization of T cell-receptor molecules. *Nature* 387:617–20

45. Janeway CA. 1995. Ligands for the T-cell receptor: hard times for avidity models. *Immunol. Today.* 16:209–55

46. Lyons DS, Lieberman SA, Hampl J, Boniface JJ, Chien Y, Berg LJ, Davis MM. 1996. A TCR binds to antagonist ligands with lower affinities and faster dissociation rates than to agonists. *Immunity* 5:53–61

47. Kersh EN, Shaw AS, Allen PM. 1998. Fidelity of T cell activation through multistep T cell receptor zeta phosphorylation. *Science* 281:572–75

48. Davis MM, Wulfing CW, Krummel MF, Savage PA, Xu J, Sumen C, Dustin ML, Chien YH. 2000. Visualizing T-cell recognition. *Cold Spring Harbor Symp. Quant. Biol.* 64:243–51

49. Alam SM, Davies GM, Lin CM, Zal T, Nasholds W, Jameson SC, Hogquist KA, Gascoigne NR, Travers PJ. 1999. Qualitative and quantitative differences in T cell receptor binding of agonist and antagonist ligands. *Immunity* 10:227–37

50. Boniface JJ, Reich Z, Lyons DS, Davis MM. 1999. Thermodynamics of T cell receptor binding to peptide-MHC: evidence for a general mechanism of molecular scanning. *Proc. Natl. Acad. Sci. USA* 96:11446–51

51. Kane LP, Lin J, Weiss A. 2000. Signal transduction by the TCR for antigen. *Curr. Opin. Immunol.* 12:242–49

52. Valitutti S, Müller S, Cella M, Padovan E, Lanzavecchia A. 1995. Serial triggering of many T-cell receptors by a few peptide-MHC complexes. *Nature* 375:148–51

53. Kabouridis PS, Magee AI, Ley SC. 1997. S-acylation of LCK protein tyrosine kinase is essential for its signalling function in T lymphocytes. *Embo J.* 16:4983–98

54. Sicheri F, Moarefi I, Kuriyan J. 1997. Crystal structure of the Src family kinase Hck. *Nature* 385:602–9

55. Ostergaard HL, Shackelford DA, Hurley TR, Johnson P, Hyman R, Sefton BM, Trowbridge IS. 1989. Expression of CD45 alters phosphorylation of the lck-encoded tyrosine protein kinase in murine lymphoma T-cell lines. *Proc. Natl. Acad. Sci. USA* 86:8959–63

56. D'Oro U, Ashwell JD. 1999. Cutting edge: the CD45 tyrosine phosphatase is an inhibitor of Lck activity in thymocytes. *J. Immunol.* 162:1879–83

57. Seavitt JR, White LS, Murphy KM, Loh DY, Perlmutter RM, Thomas ML. 1999. Expression of the p56(Lck) Y505F mutation in CD45-deficient mice rescues thymocyte development. *Mol. Cell. Biol.* 19:4200–8

58. Rodgers W, Rose JK. 1996. Exclusion of CD45 inhibits activity of p56lck associated with glycolipid-enriched membrane domains. *J. Cell Biol.* 135:1515–23

59. Kawabuchi M, Satomi Y, Takao T, Shimonishi Y, Nada S, Nagai K, Tarakhovsky A, Okada M. 2000. Transmembrane phosphoprotein Cbp regulates the activities of Src-family tyrosine kinases. *Nature* 404:999–1003

60. Thomas ML, Lefrancois L. 1988. Differential expression of the leucocyte-common antigen family. *Immunol. Today* 9:320–26

61. Novak TJ, Farber D, Leitenberg D, Hong SC, Johnson P, Bottomly K. 1994. Isoforms of the transmembrane tyrosine phosphatase CD45 differentially affect T cell recognition. *Immunity* 1:109–19

62. Thomas ML, Brown EJ. 1999. Positive and negative regulation of Src-family membrane kinases by CD45. *Immunol. Today* 20:406–11

63. Montixi C, Langlet C, Bernard AM, Thimonier J, Dubois C, Wurbel MA, Chauvin JP, Pierres M, He HT. 1998. Engagement of T cell receptor triggers its recruitment to low-density detergent-insoluble membrane domains. *Embo J.* 17:5334–48

64. Xavier R, Brennan T, Li Q, McCormack C, Seed B. 1998. Membrane compartmentation is required for efficient T cell activation. *Immunity* 8:723–32

65. Zhang W, Trible RP, Samelson LE. 1998. LAT palmitoylation: its essential role in membrane microdomain targeting and tyrosine phosphorylation during T cell activation. *Immunity* 9:239–46

66. Zhang W, Sloan-Lancaster J, Kitchen J, Trible RP, Samelson LE. 1998. LAT: the ZAP-70 tyrosine kinase substrate that links T cell receptor to cellular activation. *Cell* 92:83–92

67. Zhang W, Irvin BJ, Trible RP, Abraham RT, Samelson LE. 1999. Functional analysis of LAT in TCR-mediated signaling pathways using a LAT-deficient Jurkat cell line. *Int. Immunol.* 11:943–50

68. August A, Sadra A, Dupont B, Hanafusa H. 1997. Src-induced activation of inducible T cell kinase (ITK) requires phosphatidylinositol 3-kinase activity and the Pleckstrin homology domain of inducible T cell kinase. *Proc. Natl. Acad. Sci. USA* 94:11227–32

69. Han J, Luby-Phelps K, Das B, Shu X, Xia Y, Mosteller RD, Krishna UM, Falck JR, White MA, Broek D. 1998. Role of substrates and products of PI 3-kinase in regulating activation of Rac-related guanosine triphosphatases by Vav. *Science* 279:558–60

70. Tuosto L, Michel F, Acuto O. 1996. p95vav associates with tyrosine-phosphorylated SLP-76 in antigen-stimulated T cells. *J. Exp. Med.* 184:1161–66

71. Holsinger LJ, Graef IA, Swat W, Chi T, Bautista DM, Davidson L, Lewis RS, Alt FW, Crabtree GR. 1998. Defects in actin-cap formation in Vav-deficient mice implicate an actin requirement for lymphocyte signal transduction. *Curr. Biol.* 8:563–72

72. Fischer KD, Kong YY, Nishina H, Tedford

K, Marengere LE, Kozieradzki I, Sasaki T, Starr M, Chan G, Gardener S, Nghiem MP, Bouchard D, Barbacid M, Bernstein A, Penninger JM. 1998. Vav is a regulator of cytoskeletal reorganization mediated by the T-cell receptor. *Curr. Biol.* 8:554–62

73. Valitutti S, Dessing M, Aktories K, Gallati H, Lanzavecchia A. 1995. Sustained signalling leading to T cell activation results from prolonged T cell receptor occupancy. Role of T cell actin cytoskeleton. *J. Exp. Med.* 181:577–84

74. Wülfing C, Bauch A, Crabtree GR, Davis MM. 2000. The Vav exchange factor is an essential regulator in the actin-dependent receptor translocation to the lymphocyte-antigen presenting cell interface. *Proc. Natl. Acad. Sci. USA* 97:10150–55

75. Bubeck Wardenburg J, Pappu R, Bu JY, Mayer B, Chernoff J, Straus D, Chan AC. 1998. Regulation of PAK activation and the T cell cytoskeleton by the linker protein SLP-76. *Immunity* 9:607–16

76. Musci MA, Hendricks-Taylor LR, Motto DG, Paskind M, Kamens J, Turck CW, Koretzky GA. 1997. Molecular cloning of SLAP-130, an SLP-76-associated substrate of the T cell antigen receptor-stimulated protein tyrosine kinases. *J. Biol. Chem.* 272:11674–77

77. Krause M, Sechi AS, Konradt M, Monner D, Gertler FB, Wehland J. 2000. Fyn-binding protein (Fyb)/SLP-76-associated protein (SLAP), Ena/Vasodilator-stimulated prosphoprotein (VASP) proteins and the Arp2/3 complex link T cell receptor (TCR) signaling to the actin cytoskeleton. *J. Cell Biol.* 149:181–94

78. Baier G, Baier-Bitterlich G, Meller N, Coggeshall KM, Giampa L, Telford D, Isakov N, Altman A. 1994. Expression and biochemical characterization of human protein kinase C-theta. *Eur. J. Biochem.* 225:195–203

79. Sun Z, Arendt CW, Ellmeier W, Schaeffer EM, Sunshine MJ, Gandhi L, Annes J, Petrzilka D, Kupfer A, Schwartzberg PL, Littman DR. 2000. PKC-θ is required for TCR-induced NK-κB activation in mature but not immature T lymphocytes. *Nature* 404:402–7

80. Villalba M, Coudronniere N, Deckert M, Teixeiro E, Mas P, Altman A. 2000. A novel functional interaction between Vav and PKCtheta is required for TCR-induced T cell activation. *Immunity* 12:151–60

81. Schwartz RH. 1990. A cell culture model for T lymphocyte clonal anergy. *Science* 248:1349–56

82. Su B, Jacinto E, Hibi M, Kallunki T, Karin M, Ben-Neriah Y. 1994. JNK is involved in signal integration during costimulation of T lymphocytes. *Cell* 77:727–36

83. Jenkins MK, Ashwell JD, Schwartz RH. 1988. Allogeneic non-T spleen cells restore the responsiveness of normal T cell clones stimulated with antigen and chemically modified antigen-presenting cells. *J. Immunol.* 140:3324–30

84. Ding L, Shevach EM. 1994. Activation of CD4+ T cells by delivery of the B7 costimulatory signal on bystander antigen-presenting cells (trans-costimulation). *Eur. J. Immunol.* 24:859–66

85. Shahinian A, Pfeffer K, Lee KP, Kundig TM, Kishihara K, Wakeham A, Kawai K, Ohashi PS, Thompson CB, Mak TW. 1993. Differential T cell costimulatory requirements in CD28-deficient mice. *Science* 261:609–12

86. Green JM, Karpitskiy V, Kimzey SL, Shaw AS. 2000. Coordinate regulation of T cell activation by CD2 and CD28. *J. Immunol.* 164:3591–95

87. Viola A, Schroeder S, Sakakibara Y, Lanzavecchia A. 1999. T lymphocyte costimulation mediated by reorganization of membrane microdomains. *Science* 283:680–82

88. Tuosto L, Acuto O. 1998. CD28 affects the earliest signaling events generated by TCR engagement. *Eur. J. Immunol.* 28:2131–42

89. Holdorf AD, Green JM, Levin SD, Denny MF, Straus DB, Link V, Changelian

PS, Allen PM, Shaw AS. 1999. Proline residues in CD28 and the Src homology (SH)3 domain of Lck are required for T cell costimulation. *J. Exp. Med.* 190:375–84

90. Long EO, Rajagopalan S. 2000. HLA class I recognition by killer cell Ig-like receptors. *Semin. Immunol.* 12:101–8

91. Ljunggren HG, Karre K. 1990. In search of the 'missing self': MHC molecules and NK cell recognition. *Immunol. Today* 11:237–44

92. Binstadt BA, Brumbaugh KM, Dick CJ, Scharenberg AM, Williams BL, Colonna M, Lanier LL, Kinet JP, Abraham RT, Leibson PJ. 1996. Sequential involvement of Lck and SHP-1 with MHC-recognizing receptors on NK cells inhibits FcR-initiated tyrosine kinase activation. *Immunity* 5:629–38

93. Lanier LL. 1998. Follow the leader: NK cell receptors for classical and nonclassical MHC class I. *Cell* 92:705–7

94. Helander TS, Carpen O, Turunen O, Kovanen PE, Vaheri A, Timonen T. 1996. ICAM-2 redistributed by ezrin as a target for killer cells. *Nature* 382:265–68

95. Bottino C, Biassoni R, Millo R, Moretta L, Moretta A. 2000. The human natural cytotoxicity receptors (NCR) that induce HLA class I-independent NK cell triggering. *Hum. Immunol.* 61:1–6

96. Valiante NM, Uhrberg M, Shilling HG, Lienert-Weidenbach K, Arnett KL, D'Andrea D, Phillips JH, Lanier LL, Parham P. 1997. Functionally and structurally distinct NK cell receptor repertoires in the peripheral blood of two human donors. *Immunity* 7:739–51

97. Vales-Gomez M, Reyburn H, Strominger J. 2000. Molecular analyses of the interactions between human NK receptors and their HLA ligands. *Hum. Immunol.* 61:28–38

98. Bauer S, Groh V, Wu J, Steinle A, Phillips JH, Lanier LL, Spies T. 1999. Activation of NK cells and T cells by NKG2D, a receptor for stress-inducible MICA. *Science* 285:727–29

99. Lopez-Botet M, Carretero M, Bellon T, Perez-Villar JJ, Llano M, Navarro F. 1998. The CD94/NKG2 C-type lectin receptor complex. *Curr. Topics Microbiol. Immunol.* 230:41–52

100. Yokoyama WM, Daniels BF, Seaman WE, Hunziker R, Margulies DH, Smith HR. 1995. A family of murine NK cell receptors specific for target cell MHC class I molecules. *Semin. Immunol.* 7:89–101

101. Tomasello E, Blery M, Vely E, Vivier E. 2000. Signaling pathways engaged by NK cell receptors: double concerto for activating receptors, inhibitory receptors and NK cells. *Semin. Immunol.* 12:139–47

102. Boyington JC, Motyka AS, Schuck P, Brooks AG, Sun PD. 2000. Crystal structure of an NK cell immunoglobulin-like receptor in complex with its class I MHC ligand. *Nature* 405:537–43

103. Vales-Gomez M, Reyburn HT, Erskine RA, Lopez-Botet M, Strominger JL. 1999. Kinetics and peptide dependency of the binding of the inhibitory NK receptor CD94/NKG2-A and the activating receptor CD94/NKG2-C to HLA-E. *EMBO J.* 18:4250–60

104. Davis DM, Chiu I, Fassett M, Cohen GB, Mandelboim O, Strominger JL. 1999. The human natural killer cell immune synapse. *Proc. Natl. Acad. Sci. USA* 96:15062–67

105. Wubbolts R, Neefjes J. 1999. Intracellular transport and peptide loading of MHC class II molecules: regulation by chaperones and motors. *Immunol. Rev.* 172:189–208

106. York IA, Goldberg AL, Mo XY, Rock RL. 1999. Proteolysis and class I major histocompatibility complex antigen presentation. *Immunol. Rev.* 172:49–66

107. Bancereau J, Steinman RM. 1998. Dendritic cells and the control of immunity. *Nature* 392:245–52

108. Roake JA. 1995. Pathways of dendritic

cell differentiation and development. *Eye* 9:161–66

109. Inaba K, Turley S, Iyoda T, Yamaide F, Shimoyama S, Reis e Sousa C, Germain RN, Mellman I, Steinman RM. 2000. The formation of immunogenic major histocompatibility complex class II-peptide ligands in lysosomal compartments of dendritic cells is regulated by inflammatory stimuli. *J. Exp. Med.* 191:927–36

110. Turley SJ, Inaba K, Garrett WS, Ebersold M, Unternaehrer J, Steinman RM, Mellman I. 2000. Transport of peptide-MHC class II complexes in developing dendritic cells. *Science* 288:522–27

111. Winzler C, Rovere P, Rescigno M, Granucci F, Penna G, Adorini L, Zimmermann VS, Davoust J, Ricciardi-Castagnoli P. 1997. Maturation stages of mouse dendritic cells in growth factor-dependent long-term cultures. *J. Exp. Med.* 185:317–28

112. Wade WF, Freed JH, Edidin M. 1989. Translational diffusion of class II major histocompatibility complex molecules is constrained by their cytoplasmic domains. *J. Cell. Biol.* 109:3325–3331

113. Jenei A, Varga S, Bene L, Matyus L, Bodnar A, Bacso Z, Pieri C, Gaspar R Jr, Farkas T, Damjanovich S. 1997. HLA class I and II antigens are partially co-clustered in the plasma membrane of human lymphoblastoid cells. *Proc. Natl. Acad. Sci. USA* 94:7269–74

114. Szollosi J, Horejsi V, Bene L, Angelisova P, Damjanovich S. 1996. Supramolecular complexes of MHC class I, MHC class II, CD20, and tetraspan molecules (CD53, CD81, and CD82) at the surface of a B cell line JY. *J. Immunol.* 157:2939–46

115. Vereb G, Matko J, Vamosi G, Ibrahim SM, Magyar E, Varga S, Jenei A, Gaspar R Jr, Waldmann TA, Damjanovich S. 2000. Cholesterol-dependent clustering of IL-2R alpha and its colocalization with HLA and CD48 on T lymphoma cells suggest their functional association with lipid rafts. *Proc. Natl. Acad. Sci. USA* 97:6013–18

Annu. Rev. Immunol. 2001. 19:397–421

CHEMOKINE SIGNALING AND FUNCTIONAL RESPONSES: The Role of Receptor Dimerization and TK Pathway Activation

Mario Mellado, José Miguel Rodríguez-Frade, Santos Mañes and Carlos Martínez-A.

Department of Immunology and Oncology, Centro Nacional de Biotecnología/CSIC, UAM Campus de Cantoblanco, E-28049 Madrid, Spain; e-mail: cmartineza@cnb.uam.es

Key Words JAK/STAT pathway, cell mobility, HIV-1 coreceptors

■ **Abstract**   A broad array of biological responses, including cell polarization, movement, immune and inflammatory responses, and prevention of HIV-1 infection, are triggered by the chemokines, a family of structurally related chemoattractant proteins that bind to specific seven-transmembrane receptors linked to G proteins. Here we discuss one of the early signaling pathways activated by chemokines, the JAK/STAT pathway. Through this pathway, and possibly in conjunction with other signaling pathways, the chemokines promote changes in cellular morphology, collectively known as polarization, required for chemotactic responses. The polarized cell expresses the chemokine receptors at the leading cell edge, to which they are conveyed by rafts, a cholesterol-enriched membrane fraction fundamental to the lateral organization of the plasma membrane. Finally, the mechanisms through which the chemokines promote their effect are discussed in the context of the prevention of HIV-1 infection.

CHEMOKINES

The chemokines are a family of low-molecular-weight proteins involved in leukocyte activation and migration. The two main groups, the CXC or α chemokines and the CC or β chemokines, differ in their structural properties and in their chromosomal location. Most chemokines exhibit four conserved cysteines in specific positions. The CXC family is characterized by an amino acid positioned between the first and second cysteines, whereas in the CC family these two cysteines are located side by side. Two minor families have been described; one has lost the first and third cysteines, is represented by lymphotactin, and is known as C or γ chemokines. The other, the CX3C or δ family, exhibits three amino acids between the first two cysteines and is represented by fractalkine or neurotactin (1–3).

Since the description of the first chemokine (PF4) in 1961, many different chemoattractant cytokines have been characterized. Their role in migration and their specificity for various leukocyte subsets have been characterized in detail. Significant advances have been made in recent years in understanding the role of chemokines (4) in inflammatory diseases (5), hematopoiesis, angiogenesis, metastasis, tumor rejection (6), Th1/Th2 responses (7, 8), and HIV-1 infection. This last case, that is, the neutralizing effect of chemokines on HIV-1 infection and the characterization of chemokine receptors as HIV-1 coreceptors, has triggered new studies of chemokines and their mechanism of action (9–11). Future directions in chemokine research include the characterization of chemokine antagonists, which will open up therapeutic opportunities for autoimmune diseases, transplantation, and immune deficiencies (12).

CHEMOKINE RECEPTORS

Chemokines exert their effects by interaction with seven-transmembrane, G protein–coupled receptors (GPCR) present in the membrane of the target cell. All of these receptors are comprised of approximately 350 amino acids and a molecular weight around 40 kDa. The extracellular domain consists of the N-terminus and three extracellular loops that act in concert to bind the chemokine ligand. The intracellular region is composed of three loops and the C-terminus, which also collaborate to transduce the chemokine signal. Based on their amino acid sequences, chemokine receptors belong to the class A rhodopsin-like family. Although similar to other seven-transmembrane receptors, the chemokine receptors share certain structural features, such as the highly conserved DRYLAIV amino acid sequence in the second intracellular loop (13).

As is the case for the chemokines, the receptors can also be grouped into four major families, CR, CCR, CXCR, and CX3CR, which interact with the C, CC, CXC, and CX3C chemokines, respectively. Their structural similarity has aided in the identification of new chemokine receptors, in many cases even before the ligand is described. The HIV-1 coreceptor CXCR4 was cloned several years ago, for example, and designated LESTR at the time; it was classified as a putative chemokine receptor based on its similarity to IL-8 receptors and to CCR1 and CCR2 (14).

Several caveats must be considered when chemokine signaling is being evaluated. First of all, chemokine receptor expression on the cell surface is highly variable; that is, although mRNA may be found in a cell, it does not always correspond to functional receptor expression but corresponds rather to an internal pool in many cases. Second, the use of GFP fusion proteins and tagged receptors, which substitute for the lack of appropriate receptors, have limited the study of chemokine signaling to transfected cells; their use may also alter both expression and signaling in these modified receptors. The lack of reliable chemokine-specific reagents has impeded characterization of the biochemical pathways associated with chemokine responses, although a number of recently produced chemokine receptor–specific monoclonal antibodies are now helping to elucidate some of the chemokine-triggered intracellular signals. Much of the information we have today about chemokine signaling has been deduced mainly from available information on GPCR signaling. Known pathways for other GPCR that have been studied include G protein coupling, JAK/STAT, as well as both tyrosine and Ser/Thr kinases (15–17).

SIGNALING THROUGH CHEMOKINE RECEPTORS

Chemokine Receptor Dimerization and Activation of the Tyrosine Kinase Pathway

Despite substantial recent advances in our understanding of chemotaxis, the precise mechanism through which cells respond to a chemotactic gradient remains unclear. Leukocyte motion involves several phenomena, including changes in cell shape, changes in integrin affinity, and integrin recycling at the cell's leading edge (18). These events appear to be mediated by phosphorylation signals triggered through chemokine receptors, although the signal transduction machinery implicated has only begun to be elucidated (15). Figure 1 (see color insert) shows a scheme illustrating the main signaling pathways described to date; these pathways are activated following ligand binding to chemokine receptors and lead to a number of important cellular consequences including gene expression, cell polarization, and chemotaxis. All GPCR share a core domain consisting of the seven transmembrane helices; conformational changes in this domain are believed to be responsible for receptor activation. Similar conformational changes can be elicited by a wide variety of ligands including light, Ca^{2+}, pheromones, and small molecules (amino acids, amines, nucleotides, prostaglandins, peptides) or proteins (glycoproteins, interleukins, chemokines), suggesting the existence of a large variety of molecular mechanisms that induce such activation (19). GPCR may exist in equilibrium between two conformational states, active and inactive; the presence of an agonist would drive this balance toward the active state, whereas an antagonist would favor the inactive form. Like other GPCR, some if not all chemokine receptors initiate their ligand-induced signaling cascades by receptor dimerization (20–22).

Our laboratory has concentrated its efforts on understanding the mechanisms behind the activation of the tyrosine kinase pathway by chemokines, as well as its biological significance. We thus focus here on the study of ligand-mediated chemokine receptor dimerization, a phenomenon that has been observed in many receptor families, including the seven-transmembrane GPCR.

Chemokine receptor dimerization was first demonstrated for CCR2, the MCP-1 receptor. The similarity among chemokine receptors, including conservation of the DRY motif, nonetheless suggests that dimerization and JAK/STAT pathway activation are not exclusive to CCR2 but are found for other chemokine receptors, including members of the CCR and CXCR families. This is the case for CCR5 and

CXCR4, both of which induce activation of different JAK/STAT family members. In the CCR5-transfected HEK-293 cell response to RANTES, CCR5 is rapidly tyrosine phosphorylated, and JAK1, but not JAK2 or JAK3, associates with the receptor (21). JAK1 association in response to RANTES promotes STAT5b transcriptional factor association to the receptor, as well as its activation. Activation of STAT transcriptional factors was also seen in T cells after RANTES and MIP-1α stimulation (23); in this case, STAT1 and STAT3 are implicated, both of which induce expression of the STAT-inducible proto-oncogene c-fos. In addition, SDF-1α promotes rapid activation and association of JAK1 and JAK2 to the CXCR4. This activation promotes STAT1, 2, 3, and 5b association to the CXCR4, followed by its activation (22).

In the CCR2, tyrosine Y139 in the DRY motif has been identified as the primary target for JAK2-mediated CCR2b receptor phosphorylation (16). A CCR2b mutant receptor in which this residue has been replaced by phenylalanine (CCR2bY139F) retains its capacity to form homodimers in response to MCP-1 stimulation, but it shows impairment of Gα_i association to CCR2b and thus of G$_i$-mediated effects such as calcium mobilization and chemotaxis. This is a direct consequence of the lack of CCR2b phosphorylation and JAK2 activation. When CCR2bY139F is coexpressed with wild-type CCR2b in HEK-293 cells, these cells are unable to signal in response to MCP-1. This is because of the inability of the CCR2bY139F mutant to be phosphorylated on Tyr, rendering it unable to recruit and trigger JAK2 phosphorylation and association to the receptor, impeding G$_i$ activation. This shows that CCR2bY139F acts as a CCR2b dominant negative mutant, blocking chemokine responses by its ability to form nonproductive complexes with partners containing the functional domain, demonstrating the significance of dimerization in chemokine responses. These data also show that, in the absence of JAK activation, chemokine signaling through chemokine receptors does not occur, as confirmed by the observation that G protein–mediated signaling events are blocked by JAK kinase inhibitors (16).

Although reports of chemokine receptor dimerization and chemokine-mediated JAK/STAT activation are relatively recent, several lines of evidence suggest that GPCR dimers may have an important role in signaling (24). Examples include the chimeric α2-adrenergic-m3-muscarinic receptors (25), as well as the angiotensin (AT1) (26), V2-vasopressin (27), β2-adrenergic (28), δ-opioid (29), mGluR5 (30), and calcium-sensing receptors (31). It is interesting to note that, as for the chemokine receptors, this activation is apparently independent of G protein–related events (32).

In another member of the seven-transmembrane receptor family, the response to GABA requires heterodimerization of the GBR1 and GBR2 receptors (33–35). Physical interaction between GBR1 and GRB2 appears to be essential for the activation of potassium channels. More recently, another group of GPCR, the opioid receptors, were shown to undergo heterodimerization (36). In this case, there is clear biochemical and pharmacological evidence for the heterodimerization of two functional opioid receptors, κ and δ. Heterodimerization of these two receptors causes synergistic agonist binding and potentiates the biological signal, although there are no biochemical data to explain this heterodimer-triggered synergistic response. A similar observation has been recently made for the dopamine and the somatostatin receptors (37).

Both the dimerization of chemokine receptors and the extensive sequence identity among some of them strongly suggest that chemokine receptors may heterodimerize. In fact, chemokine receptor heterodimerization could be the mechanism by which individuals with the CCR2V64I allele show delayed AIDS progression (11). As for other GPCR, chemokine receptor heterodimerization would have important functional consequences, including increases in the sensitivity of some responses (37) or initiation of signaling events not triggered by individual chemokines, such as specific recruitment of non-G_i proteins (38).

Activation of Chemokine Receptor-Associated G Proteins

The classical view of chemoattractant receptor signaling requires activation of the G protein pathway after chemokine binding. The majority of these responses are inhibited by PTX treatment, indicating that members of the G_i protein family are the primary transduction partners associated with the receptors (13, 39) (Figure 1, see color insert). Physical association of $G\alpha_i$ to several chemokine receptors has been described; these include CXCR1 (40), CCR2 (16), CCR5 (21), and CXCR4 (22), following activation by IL-8, MCP-1, RANTES, and SDF-1α, respectively. Signaling studies of the CC chemokine receptors in transfected HEK-293 cells revealed potent, agonist-dependent inhibition of adenylyl cyclase and mobilization of intracellular calcium, consistent with receptor coupling to $G\alpha_i$ (41). In some studies, PTX did not completely block the calcium response, suggesting that chemokine receptors may couple to G proteins other than G_i, such as G_q or G_{16}, depending on the chemokine receptor studied; this indicates that receptor/G protein pairings may be cell type–specific (42, 43). Although chemokine responses in many leukocytes require G_i activation, leukocytes express G_i-coupled receptors that are not known to induce chemotaxis (44). It thus appears that G_i activation, although necessary, is not sufficient for chemotaxis. The role of G_i may thus be due to the indirect effect of $G\alpha_i$ sequestration of $G\beta\gamma$ subunits, which has been described to prevent the chemotactic response (45–47). A direct effect of $G\alpha_i$ on some other signaling pathway cannot be ruled out.

Following activation by the chemokine-triggered receptor, the heterotrimeric $G\alpha\beta\gamma$ protein dissociates into the $G\beta\gamma$ subunit complex and the GTP-bound $G\alpha_i$ subunit. $G\alpha_i$ binds the receptor, probably by interaction with one or more intracellular loop regions (42); this is a consequence of conformational changes promoted in the chemokine receptor by ligand binding, Janus kinase association, and tyrosine phosphorylation of the receptor. Both events, receptor association and subunit dissociation, initiate independent intracellular signaling responses by acting on distinct effector molecules.

The $G\beta\gamma$ subunits trigger PLC activation (48) leading to formation of inositol triphosphate [$Ins(1,4,5)P_3$] and diacylglycerol (DAG). Through binding to its specific receptor in the endoplasmic reticulum, $Ins(1,4,5)P_3$ mobilizes Ca^{2+} from intracellular stores. Acting in conjunction with Ca^{2+}, DAG activates various protein kinase C (PKC) isoforms; PKC then activates a cascade of signal transduction events both intracytoplasmically and within the nucleus. $G\beta\gamma$ also acts as a docking protein, providing an interface for the GPCR, which would facilitate GPCR interaction in diverse signaling pathways. This is the case for the coupling of the G protein–coupled receptor kinases (GRK) (49), which are involved in chemokine receptor desensitization (see below).

CC chemokines also activate phospholipase A_2 (PLA_2) and the release of arachidonic acid in human monocytes (50, 51). Arachidonic acid seems to be involved in or at least closely associated with the chemotactic response; in fact, PLA_2 inhibitors decrease chemokine-induced monocyte migration in a concentration-dependent manner (52). Phospholipase D (PLD) activation by chemokines has been reported (53), although its significance is speculative and details of its regulation in leukocytes remain to be elucidated.

Shutdown of G protein–activated signals is dependent on $G\alpha$ subunit GTPase activity. The slow hydrolysis of GTP to guanosine diphosphate (GDP), which remains protein-bound, promotes dissociation of the $G\alpha$ subunit from effectors and reassociation with the $G\beta\gamma$ subunit. The slow intrinsic rate of GTP hydrolysis by $G\alpha$ proteins is regulated by interactions with GTPase-activating proteins (GAP). There is a large, newly discovered family of GAP for $G\alpha$ proteins, known as regulators of G protein signaling, or RGS proteins, which act as negative regulators of G protein signaling (54, 55) by interacting directly with $G\alpha$ so that it cannot interact with effectors or with $G\beta\gamma$ (56). It is not yet known how RGS are regulated in vivo, nor has their role in chemokine signaling been demonstrated, although it has been shown that the CXCR2 receptor can specifically interact with the PDZ domain of RGS12 (55) and that RGS1 desensitizes a variety of chemotactic receptors, such as those of N-fMLP and leukotrienes B4 and C5 (57).

The classical view of chemokine signaling involving G proteins is more complex than expected. Although some chemokine-mediated responses are clearly linked to $G\alpha_i$ proteins, other effects appear to be mediated by other G proteins or by $G\beta\gamma$ subunit release. Further studies may elucidate the role of the distinct G proteins in chemokine signaling and the functional consequences.

Chemokines Trigger Phosphatidylinositol 3-Kinase (PI3K) Activation

PI3K activity is rapidly stimulated by chemoattractants (58, 59) (see also Figure 1, color insert) SDF-1α activates PI3K and induces p85 association to CXCR4 (60). This results in the generation of 3-phosphorylated lipids that act as second messengers for downstream effectors such as PKC, AKT, and Ras pathways (61). This activation has been implicated in integrin adhesiveness, cell migration, and polarization (62). In PI3Kγ KO mice, it has recently been shown that migration in response to chemoattractants is impaired but not eliminated, suggesting that this specific G protein–activated PI3K subtype is important in, but not essential to, chemotaxis (63). In fact, the major effect of PI3K inhibition in neutrophils appears to be blockade of NADPH oxidase activity (63–65), although it is also involved in cytoskeletal change phenomena necessary for polarization (58, 60). Some studies suggest that the p85 subunit SH2 domain may be required for its association with the tyrosine-phosphorylated p125[FAK] (66). Furthermore, the association between p125[FAK] and the activated CCR5 receptor has been shown using CCR5-transfected cells (21). Signaling through the CCR5 receptor leads to phosphorylation and activation of a recently discovered FAK family protein kinase, Pyk2 (also known as RAFTK or CAK-β) (67, 68). This activation results in downstream modulation of the JNK/SAPK kinase system. Activation of the FAK kinases by chemokines acting through CCR5 results in phosphorylation of the cytoskeletal protein paxillin and its association to this receptor.

Recent studies in whole human PBL reveal that inhibition of PI3K activity by chemical compounds or by overexpression of its dominant negative form prevent the polarization of adhesion molecules and of several cytoskeletal elements such as the protein moesin of the ezrin/radexin/moesin (ERM) complex. These data indicate that PI3K activation induces polarization of adhesion molecules (60). Other PI3K effectors include the low-molecular-weight GTPases, such as Rho, Rac, and Cdc42, which participate in regulation of the actin cytoskeleton and cell adhesion through specific targets (69, 70).

In conclusion, PI3K activity is an important mediator of chemotactic responses. Although all PI3K isoforms generate intracellular messengers such as PIP3, a general signal for migration responses, further studies are required to obtain a more complete view of their individual contributions in the variety of events that lead to cell migration.

Ser/Thr Phosphorylation of Chemokine Receptors

Lymphocyte trafficking is a complex process controlled by a vast array of molecules. These cells must be able to detect minimal changes in chemoattractant gradients; for this, cells probably employ an on-off mechanism in which chemokine receptor desensitization may be an important step. Little is known of the regulatory mechanisms in the cellular response to chemokines, or of the role of desensitization in lymphocyte migration. For a large number of related GPCR, rapid desensitization appears to involve agonist-promoted receptor phosphorylation by members of the GRK family (71). GRK-mediated phosphorylation of Ser/Thr residues in the carboxyl tail and/or intracellular loops of GPCR increases affinity for arrestin-type proteins, the binding of which prevents any further coupling between the receptor and G proteins (72). Following chemokine stimulation, receptors of both CXC and CC chemokine families are phosphorylated at multiple serine residues in the C-terminal domain by GRK enzymes (73–78). This phosphorylation is similar to that observed for several other GPCR and is critical in receptor function, as it mediates receptor desensitization and internalization into vesicular compartments. This phosphorylation was first described for CCR2 (73, 78) and later extended to other chemokine receptors (79–81) that, following ligand-induced activation, form a macromolecular complex with GRK and the regulatory protein β-arrestin. Variations in GRK family member use by receptors appear to reflect GRK availability in the cells employed rather than a specific GRK–chemokine receptor relationship.

During the GRK2-mediated desensitization process, both GRK2 catalytic activity and the CCR2b C-terminal domain Ser/Thr residues are critical. Coexpression of GRK2 and CCR2 blocks MCP-1-induced responses. When a CCR2 receptor mutant lacking Ser/Thr residues in the carboxyl tail was expressed, the MCP-1-induced signal was not inhibited by GRK2 coexpression (78). This critical role for GRK kinase in CCR2 deactivation was also shown when the CCR2 receptor was coexpressed with a dominant-negative mutant of GRK2 (82); the cellular response to a second MCP-1 challenge was equivalent to the original response (73). A similar response to ligand challenge was observed by expressing a truncated C-terminal form of the CXCR2 receptor or a receptor mutated in Ser and Thr residues (80, 81). The active role of β-arrestin in receptor internalization is indicated by the fact that dominant negative mutants of this protein block CXCR1 internalization (83).

Synaptic vesicle recycling and endocytosis of many receptors, including GPCR, require the GTPase activity of dynamin (84). Coexpression of CXCR2 or CXCR1 with a dominant negative dynamin mutant inhibits receptor internalization (83, 85), and RANTES promotes a transient association between dynamin and CCR5 in the clathrin vesicles that mediate internalization (79). Figure 2 (see color insert) shows the sequence of chemokine signaling events that leads to receptor internalization.

As for other GPCR, the turning off of chemokine receptors thus requires the participation of different molecules, including GRK, arrestin, clathrin, and dynamin; this leads to receptor internalization to the endosome, where the receptor will be dephosphorylated and either recycled to the cell surface or degraded. This process may have a more direct role, as it has been suggested for other GPCR that internalization is needed to activate specific signaling cascades (86, 87).

Activation of the MAP Kinase Cascade

MAP kinases (MAPK), also known as extracellular signal-regulated kinases (ERK), are activated by phosphorylation of Tyr/Thr residues (88, 89) and regulate several different proteins, including oncogenic transcription factors and protein kinases. MAPK activation of PLA2 (90) and cytoskeletal elements (91) suggests a specific role for this signaling cascade in chemokine-induced cellular responses. Stimulation of human neutrophils with f-MLP activates Ras (92), which initiates the MAPK cascade by binding to the Ser/Thr kinase Raf. Ras translocates Raf from the cytoplasm to the plasma membrane (93), where it is activated through interactions with members of the 14-3-3 protein family (94, 95). Both Raf and MEKK, another MAP kinase, phosphorylate and activate MAPK (59, 96).

PTX treatment blocks chemokine activation of the MAPK cascade in neutrophils, indicating that the activation of this kinase is a process mediated via G_i. With COS-7-transfected cells and transient MAPK coexpression with GPCR, activated $G\alpha_i$ subunits failed to mimic receptor stimulation of MAPK activity, evidence of the active role of $G\beta\gamma$ dimers in this signaling pathway. Under different experimental conditions, MAPK activation by $G\beta\gamma$ subunits required neither PLC-β nor PKC activation but was blocked by dominant interfering mutants of Ras (97, 98); $G\beta\gamma$ subunits induced accumulation of the GTP-bound, active form of Ras.

Chemokine activation of MAPK has a number of functional consequences. As MAPK can phosphorylate and activate transcription factors (99), chemokines may be involved in regulation of gene expression through this pathway (Figure 1, see color insert). Furthermore, MAPK phosphorylates and activates cytoplasmic PLA2, leading to release of arachidonic acid and phospholipid (100). Arachidonic acid–induced leukotriene production is essential for actin polymerization (101). These data also indicate a chemokine-induced pathway involving MAPK and cPLA2 that may regulate cytoskeletal changes necessary for cell migration. In any case, this function may not be critical, as the p38-MAPK inhibitor SK&F 86002 has no significant effect on chemokine-mediated chemotaxis or chemokinesis (102).

CHEMOKINE-TRIGGERED BIOLOGICAL RESPONSES

Cell Polarization: Chemokine Receptor Expression at the Leading Cell Edge

Cell migration has a crucial role in a wide variety of biological phenomena. It is of particular importance for leukocyte function and in the inflammatory response. For a cell to begin to migrate, the acquisition of a polarized morphology that allows cell locomotion appears to be required. This morphology is also involved in a number of other processes, such as cell differentiation, vectorial transport of molecules across cell layers, induction of the immune response, and recognition and binding of APC by T cells. Cytolytic T lymphocytes and natural killer (NK) cells maintain a polarized phenotype when bound to their targets, and they initiate the polarized secretion of cytolytic granules, which are required for proper cell-killing function (103, 104).

Chemokines and other chemotactic cytokines induce T, B, and NK cell as well as phagocyte polarization (103–106). One of the earliest events in chemoattractant-induced leukocyte polarization is a change in cell distribution of filamentous F-actin, from a radial symmetrical pattern to concentration in specific cell regions. As a consequence, two differentiated areas are established in the cell, the leading edge and the uropod. The uropod, which is not observed in other migrating eukaryotic cells, is a pseudopod-like projection that represents a specialized structure with important motility and adhesion functions. The leading cell edge concentrates several receptors, including the $\alpha v\beta 3$ integrin, receptors for classic chemoattractants such as the fMLP receptor, and chemokine receptors such as CCR2, CCR5, and CXCR4 in lymphocytes. The redistribution of chemokine receptors to the leading edge is triggered by several chemotactic factors and by cytokines such as IL-2 and IL-15. In migrating cells, a number of adhesion molecules are concentrated in the uropod, among them ICAM, L-selectin, PSGL-1, Mac-1, and CD43. The presence of these molecules in the uropod promotes the binding of other cells, enhancing leukocyte recruitment and transendothelial migration (18).

The presence of chemokine receptors at the leading cell edge implies the establishment of endogenous polarity but also the specialization of this cell domain to detect the chemoattractant gradient. Cell polarization thus correlates with orientation toward the chemoattractant source. The signal transduction molecules coupled to the activated chemokine receptors also localize at the advancing front of the cell. Chemokine activation of G_i protein signaling events at the stimulated edge of chemotactic cells has also been described in other models (107); this led to the proposal of a model in which receptor activation at the stimulated cell edge recruits molecules that signal the cytoskeleton directly. Some evidence indicates recruitment of the pleckstrin homology domain of the AKT protein kinase to the leading edge of neutrophils activated by chemoattractant molecules, in a process requiring one or more Rho guanosine triphosphatases (108). The Rho family of GTPases has a major role in regulating the actin cytoskeleton, which organizes membrane protrusion and focal adhesion, and in regulating cell polarity during leukocyte migration. The mechanisms through which Rho GTPases exert their effects have not been completely elucidated, although some actin-binding proteins may be the effectors (109, 110).

Chemokines also induce NK cell polarization and redistribution both of adhesion molecules to the uropod and of chemokine receptors to the leading cell edge. This observation assigns chemokines an important role in the NK cell cytotoxic response (104, 111). The leading edge is involved in target cell adhesion, in granule release during cytotoxic phenomena, and in directing cell migration, whereas the uropod has functions related to leukocyte recruitment. The formation of NK-target cell conjugates induces the release of chemokines responsible for NK cell migration, an effect that is mimicked by in vitro activation of NK cells.

The morphological asymmetry characteristic of polarized lymphocytes reflects the spatial rearrangement of several molecules, including cytoskeletal proteins, membrane receptors, and signaling molecules. Lymphocyte polarization is essential not only for cell migration, but also in leukocyte effector functions such as T helper cell interactions with antigen-presenting cells, as well as during target cell recognition and killing by NK and cytotoxic T cells.

Chemokine Receptors Are Transported to the Leading Cell Edge in Rafts

The redistribution of chemokine receptors and the associated trimeric G proteins at the leading edge of the moving cell correlates with the acquisition of a migrating phenotype. The mechanisms involved in chemokine receptor transport to the

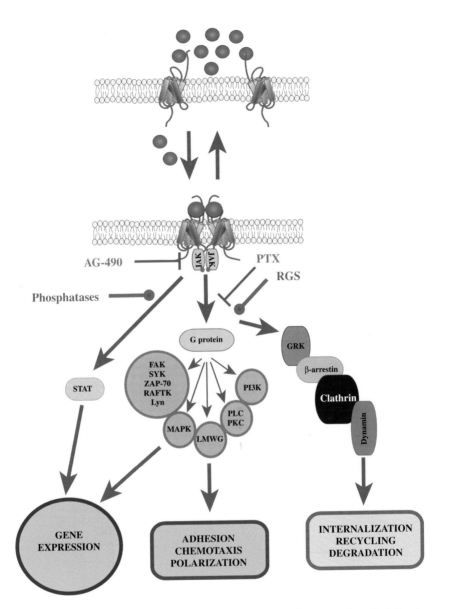

Figure 1 Schematic model showing the signaling pathways activated following chemokine binding to receptors. The figure shows some of the molecules involved in these pathways and the effects they promote. Selected regulatory molecules and the steps they affect are depicted.

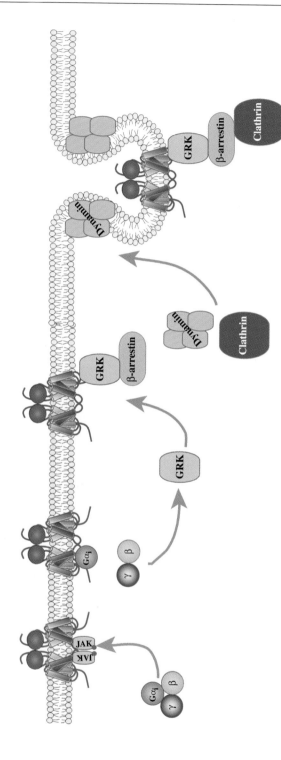

Figure 2 Chemokines induce receptor desensitization and internalization. Chemokine receptor desensitization is initiated by ligand binding and includes association of GRK molecules, receptor phosphorylation and association of β-arrestin. Internalization of chemokine receptors occurs in clathrin vesicles, which require the GTPase activity of dynamin.

Infection

Blocking infection

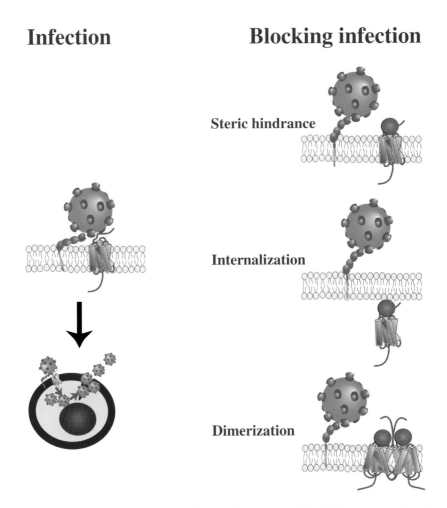

Figure 3 Postulated models by which chemokines may inhibit HIV-1 infection. The figure shows a schematic representation of the current models that explain inhibition of HIV-1 infection by chemokines, steric hindrance, receptor internalization and receptor dimerization.

leading edge has only recently come to be understood. Cell polarization may be considered the final result of complex mechanisms that establish and maintain functionally specialized domains in the plasma membrane during cell migration. Favoring this view, the signals that trigger and maintain asymmetric chemokine receptor redistribution in leukocytes appear to be independent of the polarization-inducing agent used (103, 112). This suggests that cell asymmetry is not the consequence of chemoattractant receptor distribution but that protein redistribution is the final result of the polarization process.

Migrating cells are not the only cells that segregate proteins into specific plasma membrane regions. In polarized cell types such as neurons or epithelial cells, distinct plasma membrane domains (apical and basolateral compartments for epithelia, and axon and dendrites for neurons) differ strongly in lipid and protein composition (113, 114). It is proposed that the asymmetric distribution of membrane proteins among apical and basolateral membranes (for epithelia) or axon and dendrites (for neurons) is achieved by specific co-sorting with glycosphingolipids in vesicular carriers (114–116). According to this model, specific membrane proteins clustered with glycosphingolipids and cholesterol-enriched membrane rafts in the trans-Golgi network (TGN) would be delivered preferentially to the apical membrane or to the axon (117). In nonpolarized cells such as BHK, CHO, or 3T3 fibroblasts, several membrane proteins are also delivered with glycosphingolipids in vesicular carriers from the TGN to the cell surface (118–120). These protein-lipid complexes are conserved on the surface of living cells (121, 122), where they are viewed as moving platforms of highly ordered membrane that transport specific proteins. Because of their lateral and rotational mobility, lipid rafts are fundamental in the lateral organization of the proteins anchored to the plasma membrane (123).

Several lines of recent evidence suggest that segregation between raft and non-raft proteins in unstimulated cells is crucial in distributing specialized molecules to specific locations during cell polarization (124). First, chemokine receptors associate with membrane raft microdomains, and receptor asymmetry parallels the preferential leading edge redistribution of other raft-linked molecules, including GM1, glycosylphosphatidyl inositol-anchored green fluorescent protein (GFP-GPI), and ephrinB1; conversely, proteins not located in rafts are distributed homogeneously over the cell surface. Second, modification of proteins such that they do not associate with rafts inhibits their asymmetric redistribution in polarized cells. Indeed, the non–raft-associated mutant ephrinB1ΔC (125) is distributed homogeneously in the plasma membrane of migrating cells, whereas raft-associated ephrinB1wt redistributes to the leading edge of polarized cells. Third, the protein redistribution is not restricted to molecules with functional significance, as redistribution of GFP-GPI and chemokine receptors to the leading edge occurs simultaneously. This result highlights that raft association is the pivotal determinant for the redistribution of proteins to the leading edge of polarized cells, and so the result supports the observation that asymmetric chemokine receptor distribution to the leading cell edge is a phenomenon that reflects the cell polarization process.

Cell asymmetry thus appears to be dependent on protein association with rafts; disruption of raft structure, and hence function, would render cells unable to achieve a polarized phenotype. Raft function can be abrogated by chemical sequestration of cholesterol from the membrane (120). Cholesterol depletion impedes chemokine-induced cell polarization and inhibits cell chemotaxis, which can be restored by replenishing the plasma membrane with cholesterol (124). Cholesterol depletion does not, however, inhibit chemoattractant-mediated early signaling or recruitment of the signaling-associated receptor complex. Collectively, these results indicate that raft integrity is required for the acquisition of front-rear polarity and, consequently, for cell motility. Since cholesterol depletion treatment abolishes the association of chemokine receptors with raft membrane microdomains (124), these findings suggest that chemoattractants engage all the signaling machinery necessary to induce cell polarization, using the lipid rafts as platforms.

Chemokines Prevent HIV-1 Infection

In the mid-1990s, the protective role of chemokines in HIV-1 infection was described (126), as was the fact that chemokine receptors, in conjunction with CD4, could act as HIV-1 coreceptors (127). Today we know that T-tropic HIV-1 strains use CXCR4 as a coreceptor, whereas CCR5 is the entry cofactor for M-tropic isolates (128). An important advance in understanding the role of chemokine receptors as HIV-1 receptors was the identification of a CCR5 polymorphism that renders homozygous individuals highly resistant to viral infection (129, 130). This polymorphism is a 32-base-pair deletion (ccr5-Δ32) that results in the production of a truncated receptor molecule not expressed on the cell surface; ccr5-Δ32 homozygous individuals are thus resistant to infection by M-tropic HIV-1 viral strains (129). In addition to CXCR4 and CCR5, other receptors show limited coreceptor activity, as is the case of CCR2, CCR3, CCR8, CCR9, CXCR3, or the orphans Bonzo and BOB (10, 131). This discovery provided new perspectives on fundamental aspects of HIV-1 transmission and pathogenesis, and it suggests fresh approaches for the development of anti-AIDS therapies. Nonetheless, current understanding of the events triggered by chemokine or virus interaction with chemokine receptors is based on observations made using different, not always comparable methods. This, and the variable expression of chemokine receptors depending on cell line, donor, and activation method employed, renders both chemokine signaling and its implications in HIV-1 infection a complex although promising field.

HIV-1 entry into a cell is a multistep process that involves high-affinity interaction with CD4, which is thought to trigger the conformational changes (132) needed for subsequent interaction with chemokine receptors (133). The coreceptors represent new players in the fusion process, leading to more complex models involving multiple protein-protein interactions and conformational changes. Several chemokine receptor regions have been implicated in this interaction, based on receptor chimeras, point mutation studies, comparison of chemokine receptor homologues from different species, and analysis of the blocking activity of chemokine analogues and anti-chemokine receptor antibodies. Although the results are extremely complex and sometimes contradictory, certain conclusions can be drawn. In the CCR5, there is a clear role for the N-terminal region and one of the extracellular loops in the maintenance of viral infection (134, 135). For CXCR4, the N-terminal region does not have such a critical part in viral interaction; the extracellular loops account for most of the residues involved in binding with the viral *env* proteins. The transmembrane regions also influences activity, however, probably affecting the display of the extracellular regions.

Several mechanisms have been postulated by which chemokines inhibit HIV-1 infection (136–139), as illustrated in Figure 3 (see color insert). One, the so-called steric hindrance model, holds that chemokine binding to its receptor blocks interaction of the HIV-1-env/CD4 complex with the receptor. Results of experiments using modified chemokines that are antagonists in functional assays such as chemotaxis indicate that this may be a mode of blockage (138, 139). Nonetheless, earlier studies indicate that the CCR5 domains involved in chemokine ligand specificity and in coreceptor usage for various HIV-1 strains are not identical (140). Whereas N-terminal-specific mAb block gp120-CCR5 binding very efficiently, antibodies specific for the second extracellular loop are more potent in preventing viral infection.

Another model suggests that chemokines induce chemokine receptor desensitization and internalization, preventing viral interaction with and infection of the target cell; evidence for this mode of action has also been reported (137). This model allowed generation of potent chemokine agonists that induce receptor internalization, preventing HIV-1 infection. This is the case of an N-terminally modified RANTES protein, aminooxypentane-RANTES (AOP-RANTES), a potent inhibitor of infection by M-tropic HIV-1 strains in monocytes and lymphocytes (139). AOP-RANTES treatment results in a rapid decrease in surface CCR5 expression in these cells (79, 139).

The third possibility is that the receptor undergoes a conformational change after chemokine binding, giving rise to a structure no longer recognized by the virus. A conformational change, dimerization, indeed follows chemokine or antibody binding; this may in turn impede the interaction between HIV-1 gp120 and the chemokine receptor (141). Indeed, monoclonal antibodies have been described that block HIV-1 infection with no detectable CCR5 activation and that trigger receptor dimerization (141).

Receptor dimerization has also been used to explain certain cases of resistance to HIV-1 infection. Thus, several studies describe CCR2V64I, a CCR2-related polymorphism (142) characterized by a conservative valine-to-isoleucine change at position 64 in the first CCR2 transmembrane domain, a region with complete amino acid sequence identity to CCR5. The allele is found in all ethnic groups tested with frequencies ranging from 10%–25% (143). Although CCR2V64I has no effect on initial HIV transmission, studies show that seroconvertors bearing the CCR2V64I allele progress to AIDS significantly more slowly (2–4 years) than do CCR2 wild-type HIV-1 seroconvertors (142). There is nonetheless substantial doubt that the CCR2V64I mechanism of action involves CCR2 directly, as this coreceptor is used by relatively few HIV-1 isolates in vitro and has not been consistently demonstrated to mediate HIV-1 infection in primary cells (144). Although it is suggested that CCR2V64I is linked to another polymorphism that affects CCR5 expression or function, there is thus far no evidence to support this hypothesis. An association has been found between the CCR2V64I genotype and reduced CXCR4 levels on healthy donor PBMC (145). A means by which this mutation prevents disease progression has recently been proposed, as the ability of CCR2V64I to form heterodimers with CCR5 and CXCR4, impairs the ability of both R5 and X4 HIV-1 strains to infect target cells (11).

Raft Integrity Is Required for HIV-1 Infection

HIV-1 infection depends on multiple intermolecular interactions at the cell surface that occur sequentially. Accumulated evidence indicates that membrane rafts are fundamental in the lateral organization of the plasma membrane (123). This organization is achieved because laterally diffusing lipid rafts can eventually coalesce with other rafts at the cell surface but not with other lipids encompassing a different membrane conformation. Certain membrane proteins are specifically raft-associated, whereas others are selectively excluded from these microdomains. This bulk separation of membrane-associated proteins between raft and non-raft membrane phases determines that only proteins sharing a preference for the same lipid environment will copatch into tightly associated domains, following stimulation that induces aggregation of membrane markers. This is of the utmost relevance, since HIV-1 infection activates lateral cell surface associations whose mechanisms nonetheless remain elusive. Interestingly, both HIV-1 receptors, that is, CD4 and the chemokine receptors, partition preferentially in membrane rafts (124, 146). Moreover, permissive molecules that favor HIV-1 infection, such as CD44 and CD28, are found in and mediate reorganization of lipid rafts in living cells (147). Physicochemical studies of gp120 interaction with defined glycosphingolipids (GSL) (148, 149) and inhibition of HIV-1 in vitro infection after treatment of cells with anti-GSL antibodies (149) suggest that raft components may also be important in HIV-1 infection.

Evidence suggests that raft preference by both chemokine receptors and CD4 is essential for fusion of the HIV-1 envelope and the cell membrane, probably by enabling gp120-induced lateral association of CD4 and CXCR4 (150). Functional raft disruption caused by the decrease in cellular GSL or cholesterol levels abolishes HIV-1 infection. Since GSL and cholesterol are both basic components of lipid rafts, the inhibitory effect of these lipids may be mediated by impeding lateral diffusion of the HIV-1 co-receptors CD4 and CXCR4 or CCR5, a multimolecular organization critical for viral entry. This suggests that cell envelope fusion requires integrity of rafts bearing CD4 and CXCR4 or CCR5 receptors to enable viral infection in the target cell.

This and the recently described budding of HIV-1 in rafts (151) point to chemokine receptors in membrane rafts as a possible target for new strategies to prevent and/or block HIV-1 infection. Such a therapeutic approach would be suitable for both X4 and R5 viral strains, and it would obviate the problem of resistance mutants generated using current treatments. The observation that chemokines trigger higher molecular organization of chemokine receptors, affecting their presence in rafts, may be an important step in this direction.

CONCLUDING REMARKS

Chemokines are the principal chemotactic factors implicated in the regulation of leukocyte traffic as well as in establishing lymphoid organ architecture. They regulate lymphocyte precursor entry into primary lymphoid organs as well as mature lymphocyte migration to secondary lymphoid organs, where following activation, they are responsible for triggering functional immune responses. The chemokines implicated in these activities constitute the homeostatic chemokines. Another large subset of chemokines appears to provoke inflammatory cell migration into tissues: the so-called inflammatory chemokines. Both chemokine subsets mediate their function by interacting with specific receptors belonging to the family of seven-transmembrane, G protein–coupled receptors, expressed on the leukocyte surface.

Much information is available on the biochemical pathways activated by this large receptor family, but recent studies of signaling by chemokine and other ligands show that they also activate a tyrosine kinase pathway that shares many components with the biochemical pathway activated by the cytokine receptors: recruitment of the JAK and STAT transcriptional factors that trigger gene expression following nuclear translocation. As in the cytokine responses, activation of this pathway appears to depend on ligand-mediated receptor homodimerization. These findings open up a new pathway not only for intervention in chemokine responses, especially in those cases aimed at preventing tissue infiltration, but also for exploring the now obvious connection between chemokine and cytokine responses.

One of the most prominent biological functions of chemokines is to trigger chemotaxis. Chemokines elicit a chemotactic response through the activation of trimeric G_i proteins and the subsequent $G\beta\gamma$ dimer release from the trimeric $G\alpha_i\beta\gamma$ complex. It is suggested that $G\beta\gamma$ dimers may function as a cell guidance system in eukaryotic cells. A cell moving along a chemotactic gradient acquires and maintains spatial as well as functional asymmetry between two opposite sides of the cell, the front and the rear. Chemokines may control the acquisition of front-rear polarity by triggering molecular rearrangements that lead to cellular asymmetry, such as relocalization of chemoattractant receptors to the leading cell edge and redistribution of adhesion receptors. The asymmetric distribution of chemokine receptors may thus be pivotal to the specific localization of the $G\beta\gamma$ guidance system at the cell leading edge.

An intriguing question is how cells engage these chemotactic signals at the cell front. It has been proposed that membrane proteins are selectively delivered to specialized cell surfaces in polarized neurons and epithelial cells by the clustering of specific proteins with glycosphingolipid and cholesterol-enriched membrane platforms, the raft microdomains. In nonpolarized cells, these rafts are homogeneously distributed over the cell surface; following chemoattractant stimulation, the membrane rafts and the specific membrane proteins associated to them redistribute preferentially to the leading edge. Membrane proteins excluded from rafts remain homogeneously distributed. Raft association appears to be a general requirement for G protein–coupled chemoattractant receptor migration to the leading edge; indeed, both heterotrimeric G proteins and chemokine receptors associate with membrane raft microdomains. Chemokine receptor polarization parallels the preferential redistribution to the leading edge of other raft-linked molecules, including those with no functional relevance in the polarization process. Disruption of chemokine receptor association with lipid rafts impedes cell polarization and inhibits chemotaxis. The lateral organization imposed by membrane raft microdomains is therefore fundamental to the engagement of all chemotactic signals at the proper cell location.

Finally, the identification of chemokine receptors as the HIV-1 receptors has opened up new horizons for understanding HIV-1 infection and for the development of rational approaches to its prevention. Chemokines block infection through a mechanism apparently independent of chemokine receptor signaling and downregulation, in which receptor di/oligomerization appears to cause the detachment of CD4. This process may be mediated by differential co-receptor expression on rafts, since raft disorganization also prevents HIV-1 infection. This mechanism of chemokine signaling via receptor di/oligomerization is implicated at the initial stages of many critical physiological and pathological processes. This perspective of chemokine immunobiology will provide a clearer comprehension of these conditions, possibly leading to new orientations toward the treatment of many inflammatory and infectious diseases.

ACKNOWLEDGMENTS

We would like to thank Dr. Jens Stein for critical reading of the manuscript and Catherine Mark for editorial assistance. We also thank Drs. Antonio J. Vila-Coro, Emilia Mira, and Rosa Ana Lacalle, as well as Silvia Fernández, Ana M. Martín de Ana, and Concepción Gómez-Moutón for much of the work that contributed to this review. This work was partially supported by grants from the CICyT, European Union/FEDER, and the Comunidad Autónoma de Madrid. The Department of Immunology and Oncology was founded and is supported by the Spanish Research Council (CSIC) and by the Pharmacia Corporation.

Visit the Annual Reviews home page at www.AnnualReviews.org

LITERATURE CITED

1. Baggiolini M. 1998. Chemokines and leukocyte traffic. *Nature* 392:565–68
2. Rollins BJ. 1997. Chemokines. *Blood* 90: 909–28
3. Schall TJ, Bacon KB. 1994. Chemokines, leukocyte trafficking and inflammation. *Curr. Opin. Immunol.* 6:865–73
4. Rossi D, Zlotnik A. 2000. The biology of

chemokines and their receptors. *Annu. Rev. Immunol.* 18:217–42

5. Murdoch C, Finn A. 2000. Chemokine receptors and their role in inflammation and infectious diseases. *Blood* 95:3032–43

6. Wang JM, Deng X, Gong W, Su S. 1998. Chemokines and their role in tumor growth and metastasis. *J. Immunol. Methods* 220:1–17

7. Bonecchi R, Bianchi G, Panina-Bordignon P, D'Ambrosio D, Lang R, Borsatti A, Sozzani S, Allavena P, Gray PA, Mantovani A, Sinigaglia F. 1998. Differential expression of the chemokine receptors and chemotactic responsiveness of type 1 T helper clones (Th1s) and Th2s. *J. Exp. Med.* 187:129–34

8. Sallusto F, Mackay CR, Lanzavecchia A. 2000. The role of chemokine receptors in primary, effector, and memory immune responses. *Annu. Rev. Immunol.* 18:593–620

9. Cairns JS, D'Souza MP. 1998. Chemokines and HIV-1 second receptors: the therapeutic connection. *Nat. Med.* 4:563–68

10. Berger EA, Murphy PM, Farber JM. 1999. Chemokine receptors as HIV-1 coreceptors: roles in viral entry, tropism, and disease. *Annu. Rev. Immunol.* 17:657–700

11. Mellado M, Rodríguez-Frade JM, Vila-Coro AJ, Martín de Ana A, Martínez-A C. 1999. Chemokine control of HIV-1 infection. *Nature* 400:723–24

12. Baggiolini M, Moser B. 1997. Blocking chemokine receptors. *J. Exp. Med.* 186:1189–91

13. Murphy PM. 1994. The molecular biology of leukocyte chemoattractant receptors. *Annu. Rev. Immunol.* 12:593–633

14. Loetscher M, Geiser T, O'Reilly T, Zwahlen R, Baggiolini M, Moser B. 1994. Cloning of a human seven-transmembrane domain receptor, LESTR, that is highly expressed in leukocytes. *J. Biol. Chem.* 269:232–37

15. Bokoch GM. 1995. Chemoattractant signaling and leukocyte activation. *Blood* 86:1649–60

16. Mellado M, Rodríguez-Frade JM, Aragay A, del Real G, Martín AM, Vila-Coro AJ, Serrano A, Mayor Jr F, Martínez-A C. 1998. The chemokine MCP-1 triggers JAK2 kinase activation and tyrosine phosphorylation of the CCR2b receptor. *J. Immunol.* 161:805–13

17. Pelchen-Matthews A, Signoret N, Klasse PJ, Fraile-Ramos A, Marsh M. 1999. Chemokine receptor trafficking and viral replication. *Immunol. Rev.* 168:33–49

18. Sánchez-Madrid F, del Pozo MA. 1999. Leukocyte polarization in cell migration and immune interactions. *EMBO J.* 18:501–11

19. Bockaert J, Pin JP. 1999. Molecular tinkering of G protein-coupled receptors: an evolutionary success. *EMBO J.* 18:1723–29

20. Rodríguez-Frade JM, Vila-Coro AJ, Martín de Ana A, Albar JP, Martínez-A C, Mellado M. 1999. The chemokine monocyte chemoattractant protein-1 induces functional responses through dimerization of its receptor CCR2. *Proc. Natl. Acad. Sci. USA* 96:3628–33

21. Rodríguez-Frade JM, Vila-Coro A, Martin de Ana A, Nieto M, Sánchez-Madrid F, Proudfoot AEI, Wells TNC, Martínez-A C, Mellado M. 1999. Similarities and differences in RANTES- and (AOP)-RANTES-triggered signals: implications for chemotaxis. *J. Cell. Biol.* 144:755–65

22. Vila-Coro AJ, Rodríguez-Frade JM, Martín de Ana A, Moreno-Ortíz MC, Martínez-A C, Mellado M. 1999. The chemokine SDF-1α triggers CXCR4 receptor dimerization and activates the JAK/STAT pathway. *FASEB J.* 13:1699–1710

23. Wong M, Fish EN. 1998. RANTES and MIP-1α activate STATs in T cells. *J. Biol. Chem.* 273:309–14

24. Salahpour A, Angers S, Bouvier M. 2000. Functional significance of oligomerization of G-protein-coupled receptors. *Trends Endocrin. Metab.* 11:163–68

25. Maggio R, Vogel Z, Wess J. 1993.

Coexpression studies with mutant muscarinic/adrenergic receptors provide evidence for intermolecular "cross-talk" between G protein-linked receptors. *Proc. Natl. Acad. Sci. USA* 90:3103–7

26. Monnot C, Bihoreau C, Conchon S, Curnow KM, Corvol P, Clauser E. 1996. Polar residues in the transmembrane domain of the type 1 angiotensin II receptor are required for binding and coupling. Reconstitution of the binding site by coexpression of two deficient mutants. *J. Biol. Chem.* 271:1507–13

27. Zhu X, Wess J. 1998. Truncated V2 vasopressin receptors as negative regulators of wild-type V2 receptor function. *Biochemistry* 37:15773–84

28. Hebert TE, Loisel TP, Adam L, Ethier N, Onge SS, Bouvier M. 1998. Functional rescue of a constitutively desensitized beta2AR through receptor dimerization. *Biochem. J.* 330:287–93

29. Cvejic S, Devi LA. 1997. Dimerization of the delta opioid receptor: implication for a role in receptor internalization. *J. Biol. Chem.* 272:26959–64

30. Romano C, Yang WL, O'Malley KL. 1996. Metabotropic glutamate receptor 5 is a disulfide-linked dimer. *J. Biol. Chem.* 271:28611–16

31. Bai M, Trivedi S, Brown EM. 1998. Dimerization of the extracellular calcium-sensing receptor (CaR) on the cell surface of CaR-transfected HEK293 cells. *J. Biol. Chem.* 273:23605–10

32. Williams JG. 1999. Serpentine receptors and STAT activation: more than one way to twin a STAT. *Trends Biochem. Sci.* 24:333–34

33. White JH, Wise A, Main MJ, Green A, Fraser NJ, Disney GH, Barnes AA, Emson P, Foord SM, Marshall FH. 1998. Heterodimerization is required for the formation of a functional GABA(B) receptor. *Nature* 396:679–82

34. Kaupmann K, Malitschek B, Schuler V, Heid J, Froestl W, Beck P, Mosbacher J,

Bischoff S, Kulik A, Shigemoto R, Karschin A, Bettler B. 1998. GABA(B)-receptor subtypes assemble into functional heteromeric complexes. *Nature* 396:683–87

35. Kuner R, Kohr G, Grunewald S, Eisenhardt G, Bach A, Kornau HC. 1999. Role of heteromer formation in GABAB receptor function. *Science* 283:74–77

36. Jordan BA, Devi LA. 1999. G-protein-coupled receptor heterodimerization modulates receptor function. *Nature* 399:697–700

37. Rocheville M, Lange DC, Kumar U, Patel SC, Patel RC, Patel YC. 2000. Receptors for dopamine and somatostatin: formation of hetero-oligomers with enhanced functional activity. *Science* 288:154–57

38. George SR, Fan T, Xie Z, Tse R, Tam V, Varghese G, O'Dowd BF. 2000. Oligomerization of the μ and δ-opioid receptors. Generation of novel functional properties. *J. Biol. Chem.* 275:26128–35

39. Frade JM, Mellado M, Lind P, Gutierrez-Ramos JC, Martínez-A C. 1997. Characterization of the CCR2 chemokine receptor. Functional CCR2 receptor expression on B cells. *J. Immunol.* 159:5576–84

40. Damaj BB, McColl SR, Neote K, Songquing N, Ogborn KT, Hebert CA, Naccache PH. 1996. Identification of G protein binding sites of the human interleukin-8 receptors by functional mapping of the intracellular loops. *FASEB J.* 12:1426–34

41. Myers SJ, Wong LM, Charo IF. 1995. Signal transduction and ligand specificity of the human monocyte chemoattractant protein-1 receptor in transfected embryonic kidney cells. *J. Biol. Chem.* 270:5786–92

42. Arai H, Charo IF. 1996. Differential regulation of G-protein-mediated signaling by chemokine receptors. *J. Biol. Chem.* 271:21814–19

43. Al-Aoukaty A, Schall TJ, Maghazachi AA. 1996. Differential coupling of CC

chemokine receptors to multiple heterotrimeric G proteins in human interleukin-2-activated natural killer cells. *Blood* 87:4255–60

44. Carolan EJ, Casale TB. 1993. Effects of neuropeptides on neutrophil migration through noncellular and endothelial barriers. *J. Allergy Clin. Immunol.* 92:589–98

45. Arai H, Tsou CL, Charo IF. 1997. Chemotaxis in a lymphocyte cell line transfected with C-C chemokine receptor 2B: evidence that directed migration is mediated by $\beta\gamma$ dimers released by activation of $G\alpha_i$-coupled receptors. *Proc. Natl. Acad. Sci. USA* 94:14495–94

46. Neptune ER, Bourne HR. 1997. Receptors induce chemotaxis by releasing the $\beta\gamma$ subunit of G_i, not by activating G_q or G_s. *Proc. Natl. Acad. Sci. USA* 94:14489–94

47. Lin CH, Duncan JA, Kozasa T, Gilman AG. 1998. Sequestration of G protein $\beta\gamma$ subunit complex inhibits receptor-mediated endocytosis. *Proc. Natl. Acad. Sci. USA* 95:5057–60

48. Jiang H, Kuang Y, Wu Y, Surcka A, Simon MI, Wu D. 1996. Pertussis toxin-sensitive activation of phospholipase C by the C5a and fMet-Leu-Phe receptors. *J. Biol. Chem.* 27:13430–34

49. Wu G, Benovic JL, Hildebrandt JD, Lanier SM. 1998. Receptor docking sites for G-protein $\beta\gamma$ subunits. Implications for signal regulation. *J. Biol. Chem.* 273:7197–7200

50. Locati M, Zhou D, Luini W, Evangelista V, Mantovani A, Sozzani S. 1994. Rapid induction of arachidonic acid release by monocyte chemotactic protein-1 and related chemokines. Role of calcium influx, synergism with platelet-activating factor and significance for chemotaxis. *J. Biol. Chem.* 269:4746–53

51. Dennis EA. 1994. Diversity of group types, regulation, and function of phospholipase A2. *J. Biol. Chem* 269:13057–60

52. Locati M, Lamorte G, Luini W, Introna M, Bernasconi S, Mantovani A, Sozzani S.

1996. Inhibition of monocyte chemotaxis to C-C chemokines by antisense oligonucleotide for cytosolic phospholipase A2. *J. Biol. Chem.* 271:6010–16

53. Bacon KB, Schall TJ, Dairaghi DJ. 1998. RANTES activation of phospholipase D in Jurkat T cells: requirement of GTP-binding proteins ARF and RhoA. *J. Immunol.* 160:1894–1900

54. Berman DM, Gilman AG. 1998. Mammalian RGS proteins: barbarians at the gate. *J. Biol. Chem.* 273:1269–72

55. de Vries L, Farquhar MG. 1999. RGS proteins: more than just GAPs for heterotrimeric G proteins. *Trends Cell Biol.* 9:138–44

56. Sowa ME, He W, Wensel TG, Lichtarde O. 2000. A regulator of G protein signaling interaction surface linked to effector specificity. *Proc. Natl. Acad. Sci. USA* 97:1483–88

57. Denecke B, Meyerdierks A, Bottger EC. 1999. RGS1 is expressed in monocytes and acts as a GTPase-activating protein for G-protein-coupled chemoattractant receptors. *J. Biol. Chem.* 274:26860–68

58. Turner L, Ward SG, Westwick J. 1995. RANTES-activated human T lymphocytes. A role for phosphoinositide 3-kinase. *J. Immunol.* 155:2437–44

59. Ganju RK, Brubaker SA, Meyer J, Dutt P, Yang Y, Qin S, Newman W, Groopman JE. 1998. The α-chemokine, stromal cell-derived factor-1α, binds to the transmembrane G-protein-coupled CXCR-4 receptor and activates multiple signal transduction pathways. *J. Biol. Chem.* 273:23169–75

60. Vicente-Manzanares M, Rey M, Jones DR, Sancho D, Mellado M, Rodríguez-Frade JM, del Pozo MA, Yañez-Mo M, Martín de Ana AM, Martínez-A C, Mérida I, Sánchez-Madrid F. 1999. Involvement of phosphatidylinositol 3-kinase in stromal cell-derived factor-1 alpha-induced lymphocyte polarization and chemotaxis. *J. Immunol.* 163:4001–12

61. Shimizu Y, Hunt III SW. 1996. Regulating

integrin-mediated adhesion: one more function for PI3-kinase? *Immunol. Today* 17:565–73

62. Dekker LV, Segal AW. 2000. Signals to move cells. *Science* 287:982–85

63. Li Z, Jiang H, Xie W, Zhang Z, Smrcka AV, Wu D. 2000. Roles of PLC-β2 and -β3 and PI3Kγ in chemoattractant-mediated signal transduction. *Science* 287:1046–49

64. Sasaki T, Irie-Sasaki J, Jones R, Oliveira-dos Santos A, Standford W, Bolon B, Wakeman A, Itie A, Bouchard D, Kozier-adki I, Joza N, Mak T, Osashi P, Suzuki A, Penninger J. 2000. Function of PI3Kγ in thymocyte development, T cell activation, and neutrophil migration. *Science* 287:1040–46

65. Hirsch E, Katanaev V, Garlanda C, Azzolino O, Pirola L, Silengo C, Sozzani S, Mantovani A, Altruda F, Wymann M. 2000. Central role for G protein-coupled phosphoinositide 3-kinase γ in inflammation. *Science* 287:1049–53

66. Chen HC, Guan JL. 1994. Association of focal adhesion kinase with its potential substrate phosphatidylinositol 3-kinase. *Proc. Natl. Acad. Sci. USA* 91:10148–52

67. Ganju RK, Dutt P, Wu L, Newman W, Avraham H, Avraham S, Groopman J. 1998. β-chemokine receptor CCR5 signals via the novel tyrosine kinase RAFTK. *Blood* 91:791–97

68. Dikic I, Dikic I, Schlessinger J. 1998. Identification of a new Pyk2 isoform implicated in chemokine and antigen receptor signaling *J. Biol. Chem.* 273:14301–8

69. Serrados JM, Nieto M, Sánchez-Madrid F. 1999. Cytoskeletal rearrangement during migration and activation of T lymphocytes. *Trends Cell Biol.* 9:228–32

70. Kaibuchi K, Kuroda S, Amano M. 1999. Regulation of the cytoskeleton and cell adhesion by the Rho family of GTPases in mammalian cells. *Annu. Rev. Biochem.* 68:459–80

71. Lefkowitz RJ. 1993. G protein-coupled receptor kinases. *Cell* 74:409–12

72. Bohm SK, Grady EF, Bunnett NW. 1997. Regulatory mechanisms that modulate signalling by G protein-coupled receptors. *Biochem. J.* 322:1–18

73. Aragay A, Frade JMR, Mellado M, Serrano A, Martínez-A C, Mayor Jr F. 1998. MCP-1-induced CCR2b receptor desensitization by the G protein-coupled receptor kinase-2. *Proc. Natl. Acad. Sci. USA* 95:2985–90

74. Yang W, Wang D, Richmond A. 1999. Role of clathrin-mediated endocytosis in CXCR2 sequestration, resensitization, and signal transduction. *J. Biol. Chem.* 274:11328–33

75. Tardif M, Mery L, Brouchon L, Boulay F. 1993. Agonist-dependent phosphorylation of N-formylpeptide and activation peptide from the fifth component of C (C5a) chemoattractant receptors in differentiated HL60 cells. *J. Immunol.* 150:3534–45

76. Ali H, Richardson RM, Tomhave ED, Didsbury JR, Snyderman R. 1993. Differences in phosphorylation of formylpeptide and C5a chemoattractant receptors correlate with differences in desensitization. *J. Biol. Chem.* 268:24247–54

77. Prossnitz ER, Kim CM, Benovic JL, Ye RD. 1995. Phosphorylation of the N-formylpeptide receptor carboxyl terminus by the G protein-coupled kinase GRK2. *J. Biol. Chem.* 270:1130–37

78. Franci C, Gosling J, Tsou CL, Coughlin SR, Charo IF. 1996. Phosphorylation by a G protein-coupled kinase inhibits signaling and promotes internalization of the monocyte chemoattractant protein-1 receptor. Critical role of carboxyl-tail serines/threonines in receptor function. *J. Immunol.* 157:5606–12

79. Vila-Coro AJ, Mellado M, Martín de Ana A, Martínez-A C, Rodríguez-Frade JM. 1999. Characterization of RANTES- and aminooxypentane-RANTES-triggered desensitization signals reveals differences in

recruitment of the G protein-coupled receptor complex. *J. Immunol.* 163:3037–44

80. Oppermann M, Mack M, Proudfoot AEI, Olbrich H. 1999. Differential effects of CC chemokines on CC chemokine receptor 5 (CCR5) phosphorylation and identification of phosphorylation sites on the CCR5 carboxyl terminus. *J. Biol. Chem.* 274:8875–85

81. Mueller SG, White JR, Schraw WP, Lam V, Richmond A. 1997. Ligand-induced desensitization of the human CXC chemokine receptor-2 is modulated by multiple serine residues in the carboxyl-terminal domain of the receptor. *J. Biol. Chem.* 272:8207–14

82. Kong G, Penn R, Benovic JL. 1994. A β-adrenergic receptor kinase dominant negative mutant attenuates desensitization of the β2-adrenergic receptor. *J. Biol. Chem.* 269:13084–87

83. Barlic J, Khandaker MH, Mahon E, Andrews J, De Vries ME, Mitchell GB, Rahimpour R, Tan CM, Ferguson SSG, Kelvin DJ. 1999. β-arrestins regulate interleukin-8-induced CXCR1 internalization. *J. Biol. Chem.* 274:16287–94

84. Schmid S, McNiven M, De Camilli P. 1998. Dynamin and its partners: progress report. *Curr. Opin. Cell Biol.* 10:504–2

85. Yang W, Wang D, Richmond A. 1999. Role of clathrin-mediated endocytosis in CXCR2 sequestration, resensitization, and signal transduction. *J. Biol. Chem.* 274:11328–3

86. Pierce KL, Maudsley S, Daaka Y, Luttrell LM, Lefkowitz RJ. 2000. Role of endocytosis in the activation of the extracellular signal-regulated kinase cascade by sequestering and nonsequestering G protein-coupled receptors. *Proc. Natl. Acad. Sci. USA* 97:1489–90

87. Maudsley S, Pierce KL, Zamah AM, Miller WE, Ahn S, Daaka Y, Lefkowitz RJ, Luttrell LM. 2000. The beta(2)-adrenergic receptor mediates extracellular signal-regulated kinase activation via assembly of a multi-receptor complex with the epidermal growth factor receptor. *J. Biol. Chem.* 275:9572

88. Rossomando AJ, Sanghera JS, Marsden LA, Weber MJ, Pelech SL, Sturgill TW. 1991. Biochemical characterization of a family of serine/threonine protein kinases regulated by tyrosine and serine/threonine phosphorylations. *J. Biol. Chem.* 266:20270–75

89. Nel AE, Pollack S, Landreth G, Ledbetter JA, Hultin L, Williams K, Katz R, Akerley B. 1990. CD-3-mediated activation of MAP-2 kinase can be modified by ligation of the CD4 receptor. Evidence for tyrosine phosphorylation during activation of this kinase. *J. Immunol.* 145:971–79

90. Nemenoff RA, Winitz S, Qian NX, Van Putten V, Johnson GL, Heasley LE. 1993. Phosphorylation and activation of a high molecular weight form of phospholipase A2 by p42 microtubule-associated protein 2 kinase and protein kinase C. *J. Biol. Chem.* 268:1960–64

91. Gotoh Y, Nishida E, Matsuda S, Shiina N, Kosako H, Shiokawa K, Akiyama T, Ohta K, Sakai H. 1991. *In vitro* effects on microtubule dynamics of purified *Xenopus* M phase-activated MAP kinase. *Nature* 349:251–54

92. Coffer PJ, Geijsen N, M'rabet L, Schweizer RC, Maikoe T, Raaijmakers JA, Lammers JW, Koenderman L. 1998. Comparison of the roles of mitogen-activated protein kinase kinase and phosphaditidylinositol 3-kinase signal transduction in neutrophil effector function. *Biochem. J.* 329:121–30

93. Leevers SJ, Paterson HF, Marshall CJ. 1994. Requirement for Ras in Raf activation is overcome by targeting Raf to the plasma membrane. *Nature* 369:411–14

94. Freed E, Symons M, Macdonald SG, McCormick F, Ruggieri R. 1994. Binding of 14-3-3 proteins to the protein kinase Raf and effects on its activation. *Science* 265:1713–16

95. Irie K, Gotoh Y, Yashar BM, Errede B,

Nishida E, Matsumoto K. 1994. Stimulatory effects of yeast and mammalian 14-3-3 proteins on the Raf protein kinase. *Science* 265:1716–19

96. Venkatakrishnan G, Salgia R, Groopman JE. 2000. Chemokine receptors CXCR-1/2 activate mitogen-activated protein kinase via the epidermal growth factor receptor in ovarian cancer cells. *J. Biol. Chem.* 275:6868–75

97. Koch WJ, Hawes BE, Allen LF, Lefkowitz RJ. 1994. Direct evidence that G_i-coupled receptor stimulation of mitogen-activated protein kinase is mediated by $G\beta\gamma$ activation of p21ras. *Proc. Natl. Acad. Sci. USA* 91:12706–10

98. Crespo P, Xu N, Simonds WF, Gutkind JS. 1994. Ras-dependent activation of MAP kinase pathway mediated by G-protein $\beta\gamma$ subunits. *Nature* 369:418–20

99. Hill CS, Treisman R. 1995. Transcriptional regulation by extracellular signals: mechanisms and specificity. *Cell* 80:199–211

100. Durstin M, Durstin S, Molski TFP, Becker EL, Sha'afi RI. 1994. Cytoplasmic phospholipase A2 translocates to membrane fraction in human neutrophils activated by stimuli that phosphorylate mitogen-activated protein kinase. *Proc. Natl. Acad. Sci. USA* 91:3142–46

101. Peppelenbosch MP, Tertoolen LG, Hage WJ, De Laat SW. 1993. Epidermal growth factor-induced actin remodeling is regulated by 5-lipoxygenase and cyclooxygenase products. *Cell* 74:565–75

102. Knall C, Worthen GS, Johnson GL. 1997. Interleukin 8-stimulated phosphatidylinositol-3-kinase activity regulates the migration of human neutrophils independent of extracellular signal-regulated kinase and p38 mitogen-activated protein kinases. *Proc. Natl. Acad. Sci. USA* 94:3052–57

103. Nieto M, Frade JMR, Sancho D, Mellado M, Martínez-A C, Sánchez-Madrid F. 1997. Polarization of the chemokine receptors to the leading edge during lymphocyte migration. *J. Exp. Med.* 186:153–58

104. Nieto M, Navarro F, Pérez-Villar JJ, del Pozo MA, González-Amaro R, Mellado M, R-Frade JM, Martínez-A C, López-Botet M, Sánchez-Madrid F. 1998. Roles of chemokines and receptor polarization in NK-target cell interactions. *J. Immunol.* 161:3330–39

105. Vicente-Manzanares M, Montoya MC, Mellado M, Frade JMR, del Pozo MA, Nieto M, Ortíz de Landázuri M, Martínez-A C, Sánchez-Madrid F. 1998. The chemokine SDF-1α triggers chemotactic responses and induces cell polarization in human B lymphocytes. *Eur. J. Immunol.* 28:2197–2207

106. Alonso-Lebrero JL, Serrador JM, Domínguez-Jiménez C, Barreiro O, Luque A, del Pozo MA, Snapp K, Kansas G, Schwartz-Albiez R, Furthmayr H, Lozano F, Sánchez-Madrid F. 2000. Polarization and interaction of adhesion molecules P-selectin glycoprotein ligand I and intercellular adhesion molecule 3 with moesin and ezrin in myeloid cells. *Blood* 95:2413–19

107. Parent CA, Blacklocks BJ, Froehlich WM, Murphy DB, Devreotes PN. 1998. G protein sigaling events are activated at the leading edge of chemotactic cells. *Cell* 95:81–91

108. Servant G, Weiner OD, Herzmark P, Balla T, Sedat JW, Bourne HR. 2000. Polarization of chemoattractant receptor signaling during neutrophil chemotaxis. *Science* 287:1037–40

109. Hall A. 1998. Rho GTPases and the actin cytoskeleton. *Science* 279:509–14

110. Reif K, Cantrell DA. 1998. Networking Rho family GTPases in lymphocytes. *Immunity* 8:395–401

111. Loetscher P, Seitz M, Clark-Lewis I, Baggliolini M, Moser B. 1996. Activation of NK cells by CC chemokines, chemotaxis,

Ca2+ mobilization, and enzyme release. *J. Immunol.* 156:322–27

112. McKay D, Kusel J, Wilkinson P. 1991. Studies of chemotactic factor-induced polarity in human neutrophils. Lipid mobility, receptor redistribution and the time-sequence of polarization. *J. Cell Sci.* 100: 473–79

113. Rodríguez-Boulan E, Nelson WJ. 1989. Morphogenesis of the polarized epithelial phenotype. *Science* 245:718–25

114. Dotti C, Simons K. 1990. Polarized sorting of viral glycoproteins to the axon and dendrites of hippocampal neurons in culture. *Cell* 62:63–72

115. Simons K, Wandinger-Ness A. 1990. Polarized sorting in epithelia. *Cell* 62:207–10

116. Ledesma M, Brügger B, Bünning C, Wieland F, Dotti C. 1999. Maturation of the axonal plasma membrane requires upregulation of sphingomyelin synthesis and formation of protein-lipid complexes. *EMBO J.* 18:1761–71

117. Brown D, Rose J. 1992. Sorting of GPI-anchored proteins to glycolipid-enriched membrane subdomains during transport to the apical cell surface. *Cell* 68:533–44

118. Müsch A, Xu H, Shields D, Rodríguez-Boulan E. 1996. Transport of vesicular stomatitis virus to the cell surface is signal mediated in polarized and nonpolarized cells. *J. Cell Biol.* 133:543–58

119. Yoshimori T, Keller P, Roth M, Simons K. 1996. Different biosynthetic transport routes to the plasma membrane in BHK and CHO cells. *J. Cell Biol.* 133:247–56

120. Keller P, Simons K. 1998. Cholesterol is required for surface transport of influenza virus hemagglutinin. *J. Cell Biol.* 140:1357–67

121. Friedrichson T, Kurzchalia T. 1998. Microdomains of GPI-anchored proteins in living cells revealed by crosslinking. *Nature* 394:802–5

122. Varma R, Mayor S. 1998. GPI-anchored proteins are organized in submicron domains at the cell surface. *Nature* 394:798–801

123. Harder T, Scheiffele P, Verkade P, Simons K. 1998. Lipid domain structure of the plasma membrane revealed by patching of membrane components. *J. Cell Biol.* 141:929–42

124. Mañes S, Mira E, Gómez-Moutón C, Lacalle RA, Keller P, Labrador JP, Martínez-A C. 1999. Membrane raft microdomains mediate front-rear polarity in migrating cells. *EMBO J.* 18:6211–20

125. Brückner K, Labrador J, Scheiffele P, Herb A, Seeburg P, Klein R. 1999. EphrinB ligands recruit GRIP family PDZ adaptor proteins into raft membrane microdomains. *Neuron* 22:511–24

126. Cocchi F, DeVico AL, Garzino-Demo A, Arya SK, Gallo RC, Lusso P. 1995. Identification of RANTES, MIP-1α, and MIP-1β as the major HIV-suppressive factors produced by CD8+ T cells. *Science* 270:1811–15

127. Feng Y, Broder CC, Kennedy PE, Berger EA. 1996. HIV-1 entry cofactor: functional cDNA cloning of a seven-transmembrane G protein-coupled receptor. *Science* 272:872–77

128. Littman DR. 1998. Chemokine receptors: keys to AIDS pathogenesis. *Cell* 93:677–80

129. Liu R, Paxton WA, Choe S, Ceradini D, Martin SR, Horuk R, MacDonald ME, Stuhlmann H, Koup RA, Landau NR. 1996. Homozygous defect in HIV-1 coreceptor accounts for resistance of some multiply-exposed individuals to HIV-1 infection. *Cell* 86:367–77

130. Samson M, Libert F, Doranz BJ, Rucker J, Liesnard C, Farber C-M, Saragosti S, Lapouméroulie C, Cognaux J, Forceille C, Muyldermans G, Verhofstede C, Burtonboy G, Georges M, Imai T, Rana S, Yi Y, Smyth RJ, Collman RG, Doms RW, Vassart G, Parmentier M. 1996. Resistance to HIV-1 infection in Caucasian individuals bearing mutant alleles of the

CCR-5 chemokine receptor gene. *Nature* 382:722–25

131. Zhang L, Huang Y, Chen Z, Guo Y, Wu S, Kunstman KJ, Brown RC, Phair JP, Neumann AU, Ho DD, Wolinsky SM. 1998. Chemokine coreceptor usage by diverse primary isolates of human immunodeficiency virus type 1. *J. Virol.* 72:9307–12

132. Wyatt R, Sodroski J. 1998. The HIV-1 envelope glycoproteins: fusogens, antigens, and immunogens. *Science* 280:1884–88

133. Horuk R. 1999. Chemokine receptors and HIV-1: the fusion of two major research fields. *Immunol. Today* 20:89–94

134. Horuk R. 1994. Molecular properties of the chemokine receptor family. *TIPs* 15:159–65

135. Doms RW, Peiper SC. 1997. Unwelcomed guests with master keys: how HIV uses chemokine receptors for cellular entry. *Virology* 235:179–90

136. Amara A, Le Gall S, Schwartz O, Salamero J, Montes M, Loetscher P, Baggiolini M, Virelizier J-L, Arenzana-Seisdedos F. 1997. HIV coreceptor downregulation as antiviral principle: SDF-1α-dependent internalization of the chemokine receptor CXCR4 contributes to inhibition of HIV replication *J. Exp. Med.* 186:139–46

137. Mack M, Luckow B, Nelson PJ, Cihak J, Simmons G, Clapham PR, Signoret N, Marsh M, Stangassinger M, Borlat F, Wells TNC, Schlöndorff D, Proudfoot AEI. 1998. Aminooxypentane-RANTES induces CCR5 internalization but inhibits recycling: a novel inhibitory mechanism of HIV infectivity. *J. Exp. Med.* 187:1215–24

138. Arenzana-Seisdedos F, Virelizier J-L, Rousset D, Clark-Lewis I, Loetscher P, Moser B, Baggiolini M. 1996. HIV blocked by chemokine antagonist. *Nature* 383:400

139. Simmons G, Clapham PR, Picard L, Offord RE, Rosenkilde MM, Schwartz TW, Busser R, Wells TNC, Proudfoot AEI. 1997. Potent inhibition of HIV-1 infectivity in macrophages and lymphocytes by a novel CCR5 antagonist. *Science* 276:276–79

140. Rucker J, Samson M, Doranz BJ, Libert F, Berson JF, Yi Y, Smyth RJ, Collman RG, Broder CC, Vassart G, Doms RW, Parmentier M. 1996. Regions of the β-chemokine receptors CCR5 and CCR2b that determine HIV-1 cofactor specificity. *Cell* 87:437–46

141. Vila-Coro AJ, Mellado M, Martín de Ana A, Lucas P, del Real G, Martínez-A C, Rodríguez-Frade JM. 2000. HIV-1 infection through the CCR5 receptor is blocked by receptor dimerization. *Proc. Natl. Acad. Sci. USA* 97:3388–93

142. Smith MW, Dean M, Carrington M, Winkler C, Huttley GA, Lomb DA, Goedert JJ, O'Brien TR, Jacobson LP, Kaslow R, Buchbinder S, Vittinghoff E, Vlahov D, Hoots K, Hilgartner MW, O'Brien SJ. 1997. Contrasting genetic influence of CCR2 and CCR5 variants on HIV-1 infection and disease progression. Hemophilia Growth and Development Study (HGDS), Multicenter AIDS Cohort Study (MACS), Multicenter Hemophilia Cohort Study (MHCS), San Francisco City Cohort (SFCC), ALIVE Study. *Science* 277:959–65

143. Smith MW, Dean M, Carrington M, Winkler C, Huttley GA, Lomb DA, Goedert JJ, O'Brien TR, Jacobson LP, Kaslow R, Buchbinder S, Vittinghoff E, Vlahov D, Hoots K, Hilgartner MW, O'Brien SJ. 1997. Contrasting genetic influence of CCR2 and CCR5 variants on HIV-1 infection and disease progression. *Nat. Med.* 277:959–66

144. Frade JM, Llorente M, Mellado M, Alcamí J, Gutierrez-Ramos JC, Zaballos A, del Real G, Martínez-A C. 1997. The amino-terminal domain of the CCR2 chemokine receptor acts as coreceptor for HIV-1 infection. *J. Clin. Invest.* 100:1–6

145. Lee B, Doranz BJ, Rana S, Yi Y, Mellado M, Frade JMR, Martínez-A C, O'Brien SJ, Dean M, Coleman RG, Doms R. 1998. Influence of the CCR2-V64I polymorphism on HIV-1 coreceptor activity and chemokine receptor function of CCR2b, CCR3, CCR5 and CXCR4. *J. Virology* 72:7450–58

146. Xavier R, Brennan T, Li Q, McCormack C, Seed B. 1998. Membrane compartmentalization is required for efficient T cell activation. *Immunity* 8:723–32

147. Viola A, Schroeder S, Sakakibara Y, Lanzavecchia A. 1999. T lymphocyte costimulation mediated by reorganization of membrane microdomains. *Science* 283:680–82

148. Hammache D, Yahi N, Maresca M, Pieroni G, Fantini J. 1999. Human erythrocyte glycosphingolipids as alternative cofactors for human immunodeficiency virus type 1 (HIV-1) entry: evidence for CD4-induced interactions between HIV-1 gp120 and reconstituted membrane microdomains of glycosphingolipids (Gb3 and GM3). *J. Virol.* 73:5244–48

149. Harouse J, Bhat S, Spitalnik S, Laughlin M, Stefano K, Silberberg D, González-Scarano F. 1991. Inhibition of entry of HIV-1 in neural cell lines by antibodies against galactosyl ceramide. *Science* 253:320–23

150. Mañes S, del Real G, Lacalle RA, Lucas P, Gómez-Moutón C, Sánchez-Palomino S, Delgado R, Alcamí J, Mira E, Martínez-A C. 2000. Membrane raft microdomains mediate lateral assemblies required for HIV-1 infection. *EMBO Rep.* 1:190–96

151. Nguyen D, Hildreth J. 2000. Evidence for budding of human immunodeficiency virus type 1 selectively from glycolipid-enriched membrane lipid rafts. *J. Virol.* 74:3264–72

Annu. Rev. Immunol. 2001. 19:423–74

INTERLEUKIN-18 REGULATES BOTH TH1 AND TH2 RESPONSES

Kenji Nakanishi,[1, 2, 3, 4] Tomohiro Yoshimoto,[1, 2, 3] Hiroko Tsutsui,[1] and Haruki Okamura[1, 2, 3]

[1]Department of Immunology and Medical Zoology, [2]Laboratory of Host Defenses, Institute for Advanced Medical Sciences, Hyogo College of Medicine, Nishinomiya, Hyogo 663-8501, Japan; e-mail: nakaken@hyo-med.ac.jp
[3]Core Research for Evolutional Science and Technology of Japan Science and Technology Corporation, Tokyo, 101-0062, Japan

Key Words Th1-mediated immune responses, Th2-mediated immune responses, host defense, pathogenesis

■ **Abstract** Although interleukin-18 is structurally homologous to IL-1 and its receptor belongs to the IL-1R/Toll-like receptor (TLR) superfamily, its function is quite different from that of IL-1. IL-18 is produced not only by types of immune cells but also by non-immune cells. In collaboration with IL-12, IL-18 stimulates Th1-mediated immune responses, which play a critical role in the host defense against infection with intracellular microbes through the induction of IFN-γ. However, the overproduction of IL-12 and IL-18 induces severe inflammatory disorders, suggesting that IL-18 is a potent proinflammatory cytokine that has pathophysiological roles in several inflammatory conditions. IL-18 mRNA is expressed in a wide range of cells including Kupffer cells, macrophages, T cells, B cells, dendritic cells, osteoblasts, keratinocytes, astrocytes, and microglias. Thus, the pathophysiological role of IL-18 has been extensively tested in the organs that contain these cells. Somewhat surprisingly, IL-18 alone can stimulate Th2 cytokine production as well as allergic inflammation. Therefore, the functions of IL-18 in vivo are very heterogeneous and complicated. In principle, IL-18 enhances the IL-12-driven Th1 immune responses, but it can also stimulate Th2 immune responses in the absence of IL-12.

INTRODUCTION

IL-18 is a new member of the IL-1 family (1–13). IL-18 is produced as a biologically inactive precursor, and active IL-18 is secreted after cleavage with caspase-1 or with other caspases (6, 14–16). IL-1β is processed by the same pathways (6, 15, 17, 18). The IL-18 receptor (R) system and its signal transduction pathway are analogous to those of the IL-1R (19–23). Recently, Toll-like receptors (TLRs) have been identified that utilize a signaling pathway shared with IL-1R/IL-18R (24–32). Thus, the IL-18/IL-18R system may be regarded as a very primitive immune system capable of stimulating innate immunity. However, originally discovered as a factor that induces IFN-γ production from Th1 cells in the presence of IL-12, IL-18 can act on Th1 cells, nonpolarized T cells, NK cells, B cells, and dendritic cells to produce IFN-γ in the presence of IL-12 (1–4, 10, 13, 33–36). Moreover, to our surprise, IL-18 without help from IL-12 has the potential to induce IL-4 and IL-13 production in T cells, NK cells, mast cells, and basophils (37–39). Therefore, IL-18 has the capacity to stimulate innate immunity and both Th1- and Th2-mediated responses. Representative examples that manifest important physiological roles of IL-18 are observed in host defense (12). The source of IL-18 has been initially demonstrated to be LPS-activated and *Propionibacterium acnes* (*P. acnes*)-elicited Kupffer cells. But we know now that IL-18 mRNA is expressed in a wide range of cells, including Kupffer cells, macrophages, T cells, B cells, dendritic cells, osteoblasts, keratinocytes, astrocytes, and microglias. Thus, IL-18, in addition to being an important regulator of both innate and acquired immune response, may play an important role in the non-immune system. Here we review the recent advances in the study of the pathophysiological roles of IL-18.

MOLECULAR STRUCTURE OF IL-18

Discovery of IL-18

In vitro secretion of IFN-γ from Th1 cells is induced by stimulation with Ag or immobilized anti-CD3 (40). Moreover, injection of Ag, anti-CD3, PPD, or staphylococcal enterotoxin A (SEA) into *P. acnes*-primed mice induced high levels of IFN-γ production by stimulation of T cells (41), suggesting that *P. acnes* treatment induced Th1 cells in vivo. Surprisingly, injection of lipopolysaccharide (LPS) could induce comparable levels of IFN-γ in these *P. acnes*-treated mice or Bacillus Calmette-Guerin (BCG)-infected mice. The rodent is generally resistant to bacterial endotoxin LPS. Heat-killed *P. acnes* or live BCG are substances that sensitize cells to LPS. Therefore, *P. acnes*-pretreated mice were highly susceptible to LPS, and most of them died of lethal shock or, if surviving, later suffered from acute liver injury (42, 43). Since IL-12 is produced by macrophages in response to LPS (44), we first assumed that LPS-stimulated macrophages produce IL-12 that stimulates naive T cells to develop into Th1 cells and activates NK cells to produce IFN-γ in vivo. Indeed, the sera from *P. acnes*-primed and LPS-challenged mice contained high levels of IL-12. However, addition of the sera could induce IFN-γ production from anti-CD3-stimulated T cells more strikingly than did addition of excess IL-12, suggesting the presence of another IFN-γ-inducing factor(s) in the sera (2).

Molecular Structure of IL-18

IL-18 was purified from the sera or the extracts of liver tissues of mice that had been sequentially treated with *P. acnes* and LPS (2). The resultant material is a single peptide chain with a molecular weight of 18,000 and a pI of 4.8 (1). Isolated murine and human IL-18 cDNAs encode novel proteins consisting of 192 and 193 amino acids, respectively. Human IL-18 cDNA showed 65% homology with that of murine IL-18 (45). Both mouse and human IL-18 lack the usual leader sequence necessary for the secretion of IL-18 from the cell membrane but instead contain an unusual leader sequence including 35 amino acids at its N-terminus.

Like IL-1β, IL-18 is synthesized as a 24-kDa precursor protein, which is then enzymatically cleaved to an 18 kDa mature IL-18 protein (1, 6, 14–16). The murine IL-18 peptide has a 12% homology to murine IL-1α and 19% to murine IL-1β when analyzed by the fold recognition method (46). Homologies between the amino acid sequences for human IL-18 and human IL-1α, and those for human IL-18 and human IL-1β, are only 15% and 18%, respectively. Nevertheless, IL-18 shows similarity to IL-1β in its three-dimensional structure of β-pleated sheets forming a barrel configuration, indicating that the conserved protein structure among these cytokines, evidenced by the positions of the β-pleated sheets, is important for receptor binding to their receptor. The function of murine IL-18 is different from that of murine IL-1β. Several studies revealed that IL-18 shares biological properties with IL-12, such as induction of IFN-γ production and stimulation of NK cell activity. Despite their functional similarity, IL-18 is structurally unrelated to IL-12.

GENE AND ITS REGULATION

Macrophages including Kupffer cells were first shown to express high levels of IL-18 mRNA (1, 47, 48). Succeeding studies revealed that IL-18 mRNA is also constitutively expressed in many cell types, in sharp contrast to the requirement for appropriate stimulation for induction of mRNA for other cytokines (e.g., IL-12 p40, IL-1β). The murine IL-18 gene is composed of 7 exons, and exons 1 and 2 are noncoding (49). There are at least two distinct promoters (49). The promoter activity upstream of exon 2 is constitutively high, whereas that upstream of exon 1 is upregulatable by activation with LPS, presumably resulting in constitutive expression of mRNA for IL-18. Both promoters are TATA-less and G+C poor type, both characteristically observed in a wide spectrum of cell types. In contrast, most other cytokines have promoters that contain TATA boxes. This may explain why IL-18 is expressed in various cell types including not only macrophages but also non-immune cells. As an NF-κB recognition sequence is located in the promoter region of the IL-18 gene, NF-κB was suggested to be involved in upregulation of IL-18 gene expression.

Recently, the regulatory elements of both IL-18 promoters have been investigated by 5'-serial deletions and site-directed mutation (50). These studies revealed that an IFN consensus sequence binding protein (ICSBP) binding site is critical for the activity of the promoter upstream of exon 1 and that a PU.1 binding site is essential for the promoter upstream of exon 2. ICSBP, a member of the interferon regulatory factor (IRF) family, is constitutively expressed in the nuclei of immune competent cells including macrophages (51) and is upregulated by IFN-γ or IFN-α/β (52). Since ICSBP-deficient mice show impaired Th1 cell responses due to defective IL-12 production, ICSBP is an essential transcription factor for IL-12, particularly IL-12 p40 production (53, 54). PU.1, one of the transcription factors participating in myelopoiesis, is expressed exclusively in myeloid cells and B cells and is upregulated by IFN-γ or LPS (55–57). Therefore, IL-18 gene expression may be upregulated by direct stimulation with microbe products such as LPS, or by cytokines such as IFN-α/β and IFN-γ (49, 57). Most cytokine genes contain many copies of an RNA-destabilizing element that shortens the half-life of the cytokine mRNA (58). In contrast, the IL-18 gene has none or only one RNA-destabilizing element, resulting in an unusually stable expression of IL-18. This may explain why IL-18 is constitutively and intracellularly stored, but as the biologically inactive precursor (1, 14), in various cell types including not only macrophages but also non-immune cells. Biologically active, mature IL-18 secretion is regulated by intracellular processing machinery.

The human IL-18 gene is located on chromosome 11q22.2–22.3, closely linked to the DRD2 (dopamine receptor D2) locus (59). The relative gene order is ATM–IL-18–DRD2–THY1, which is the same as that of murine IL-18 (60). Preliminary experiments on nonobese diabetic (NOD) mice, a mouse model for spontaneous insulin-dependent diabetes mellitus, revealed that the murine IL-18 gene localizes on chromosome 9 within the *Idd2* interval, which implicates IL-18 as a NOD susceptibility gene (60).

PRODUCTION AND PROCESSING OF IL-18

IL-18 is produced not only by cells in the immune system but also by non-immune cells. IL-18 is synthesized as a precursor protein (proIL-18) and is processed by intracellular cysteine protease, caspase-1. However, recent studies revealed the presence of other processing mechanisms for proIL-18, as described below.

Producing Cells

Murine macrophages, such as Kupffer cells, splenic macrophages, alveolar macrophages, peritoneal exudate cells, and microglia, secrete functional IL-18 only after activation with appropriate stimuli (1, 48, 61–66). In contrast, human peripheral blood mononuclear cells (PBMCs) can secrete proIL-18 under normal conditions (67), suggesting that human proIL-18 from PBMCs may be cleaved into mature IL-18 extracellularly (6). Murine and human dendritic cells constitutively express IL-18 mRNA and produce mature IL-18 (68). Epidermal cells, particularly keratinocytes, can secrete IL-18, along with IL-12, in response to stimulation with contact allergens (69). However, keratinocytes do not have caspase-1 under normal conditions (70), suggesting that IL-18 secretion by keratinocytes might be induced in a caspase-1-independent manner, presumably extracellularly by proteinase-3.

Intestinal epithelial cells express IL-18 (71). Airway epithelia also express IL-18 (72). Osteoblastic stromal cells produce IL-18, which acts on T cells to promote the release of GM-CSF and IFN-γ. This GM-CSF acts independently of IFN-γ on osteoclast precursors to inhibit the generation of osteoclast-like multinucleated cells (73). Expression of IL-18 mRNA is also induced in the glucocorticoid (GC)-producing cells of the adrenal cortex by acute cold stress possibly via ACTH and independently of GC (74, 75). Therefore, in contrast to the anti-inflammatory action of GCs, IL-18 may have an immunostimulatory role during acute stress. IL-18 secretion is also detected in the central nervous system (65, 66) and endocrine system (74, 75). Moreover, IL-18 and IL-18R can be detected in the brain of normal adult rats (76). These reports allow us to hypothesize that IL-18, like IL-1β, may play an important role in connecting the immune system to the endocrine and nervous systems.

Intrinsic IL-18 Processing

IL-18 has structural homology to IL-1. Caspase-1 is a member of the caspase family and cleaves both proIL-1β and proIL-18 after an aspartic acid (14, 15, 61). Serum levels of IL-18, IL-1β, and IFN-γ were markedly increased in LPS-challenged *P. acnes*-primed wild-type mice. In contrast, these increases were abrogated in *P. acnes*-primed caspase-1-deficient mice after LPS challenge, suggesting that caspase-1 plays a critical role in induction of IL-18-dependent IFN-γ production both in vitro and in vivo (14). Moreover, we have found that transgenic mice overexpressing human caspase-1 in their keratinocytes, that constitutively express proIL-18 and proIL-1β, contained relatively high serum levels of mature IL-18 and very low serum levels of mature IL-1β (77).

Caspase-1 is detectable in many cell types including T cells, neutrophils, and macrophages (78, 79). Like other caspases, caspase-1 is also produced as a biologically inactive form. Precursor caspase-1 is a protein of 45 kDa and becomes the mature form consisting of p10 and p20 subunits after cleavage with caspase-11 (80) or autoproteolytically (81). LPS reportedly has the capacity to induce the activation of caspase-1 in mouse and human macrophage cell lines (14, 82) (Figure 1).

The mechanism underlying LPS-stimulated caspase-1 activation has not been fully characterized. Recently, some members of the Toll-like receptor (TLR) family were discovered to be signaling receptors for LPS (83). The signaling pathway stemming from TLRs is shared with that of the IL-1R and IL-18R (25, 24), although no adaptor molecule that physically links TLRs to caspase-1 has yet been identified. Recently, MyD88 was identified as an adaptor molecule required for LPS signaling through TLR (11, 25–29). We have found that Kupffer cells from TLR4-deficient mice do not secrete IL-18, but those from MyD88-deficient mice can secrete biologically active IL-18, indicating that LPS-induced caspase-1-dependent IL-18 secretion does require TLR4 but not MyD88 (83a) (Figure 1).

Caspase-1-dependent IL-18 processing can also be demonstrated by using virus-infected human macrophages (84). GM-CSF-treated macrophages secrete mature

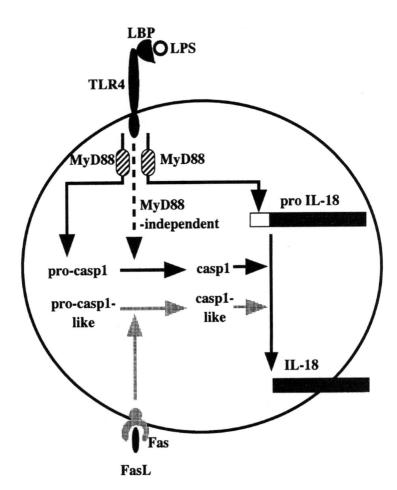

Figure 1 IL-18 secretion from macrophages. IL-18 is synthesized as a 24-kDa precursor (proIL-18), which is cleaved into 18-kDa mature IL-18 by active form caspase-1 (casp1) or casp1-like enzymes induced by stimulation with LPS or FasL, respectively. After TLR4 is activated by LPS via LPS-binding protein (LBP), casp1 is activated independently of MyD88, whereas LPS-induced accumulation of pro-caspase-1 and proIL-18 requires MyD-88-dependent signaling (83). LPS-induced activation of casp1 leads to secretion of biologically active IL-18 (14, 15). Upon stimulation with FasL, caspase other than caspase-1, termed casp1-like, might be activated to cleave proIL-18 into active IL-18, resulting in IL-18 secretion (16).

IL-18 and IL-1β when infected in vitro with Sendai virus or influenza A (84). This is completely inhibited by caspase-1 inhibitors. Thus, some viral infection causes IL-18 secretion from macrophages in a caspase-1-dependent manner. However, caspase-1-independent secretion of IL-1β has also been recently demonstrated (18). Thioglicolate-induced murine peritoneal exudate neutrophils secrete IL-1β after stimulation with Fas ligand (FasL). This was observed in the absence of caspase-1. We also observed that both Kupffer cells and splenic macrophages from *P. acnes*-primed caspase-1-deficient mice secreted active IL-18 after stimulation with membrane-associated FasL or soluble FasL (16) (Figure 1). This was suppressed by caspase inhibitors, indicating that IL-18 is secreted by FasL-stimulated macrophages in caspase other than caspase-1-dependent fashion. Caspase-4 has the capacity to cleave proIL-18 after the Asp^{35} residue, the same site used by caspase-1. However, the efficiency of IL-18 processing by caspase-4 is one hundredth or thousandth that of caspase-1 (14). Caspase-3 can also cleave IL-18, either proIL-18 or mature IL-18, but at another site, between Asp^{69} and Ile^{70}, resulting in the accumulation of biologically inactive products (14, 85). Thus, caspase-3 may act as a functional scavenger for mature IL-18 (85).

Since overproduction of IL-18 and/or IL-1β is responsible for tissue injury, the prolonged production of this cytokine may be harmful. Nitric oxide (NO) can directly suppress the action of caspase-1, thereby preventing IL-1β and IL-18 secretion (86). This downregulation of caspase-1 by NO may be important for the protection of tissues from inflammatory damage induced by IL-18 or IL-1β. Regulation of caspase-1 activity via an endogenous inhibitor has also been studied. Serine protease inhibitor (serpin) PI-9 accounts for this activity. As this molecule was demonstrated in human vascular smooth muscle cells and its activity inversely correlates with the level of production of IL-1β and IL-18, PI-9 may be involved in vascular atherogenesis (87).

Exogenous Pathway of IL-18 Processing

Recently, proteinase-3 was shown to cleave proIL-18, but presumably at a different cutting site(s) from that of caspase-1 (6). Supernatants of proIL-18 incubated with recombinant proteinase-3 have IFN-γ-inducing activity. Proteinase-3 is a serine protease of 29 kDa localized in the azulophil granules of neutrophils and monocytes and in the cytoplasm of endothelial cells (88–91). After being appropriately activated, for example by phagocytosis or stimulation with TNF-α, proteinase-3 is secreted following their degranulation and translocates onto the cell surface to exert its enzymatic action (89).

IL-18 RECEPTOR

IL-1R/TLR Superfamily

The IL-18R system is very similar to the IL-1R system. Two different receptors for IL-1 have been identified, and all components of both receptors are members of the Ig superfamily. The type I IL-1R (IL-1R1) is expressed on almost all cell types and is associated with the IL-1R accessory protein (IL-1RAcP), which is homologous to IL-1R1 (17). As IL-1RAcP does not bind IL-1 directly, the expression of IL-1R1 mainly determines the IL-1 responsiveness of a given cell. The type II IL-1R (IL-1R2) is expressed mainly on B cells, and its major function is to act as a decoy receptor. The cytoplasmic portion of IL-1R1 is homologous to that of a *Drosophila* cell surface Toll protein (92). In *Drosophila*, Toll plays a role in development, and several Toll-like receptors are essential for its antifungal response (93). Toll is a transmembrane receptor containing the extracellular domain with leucine rich repeats and a cytoplasmic domain highly homologous to those of the IL-1R family members (24). Engagement of Toll activates the transcription factor Dorsal, a homologue of NF-κB. Recently, mammalian homologs of Toll have been identified and designated as Toll-like receptors (TLRs). The signaling pathway of the TLR family activates NF-κB via MyD88 and IRAK, molecules shared with the IL-1R/IL-18R signaling pathway (29–32,94,95). The mammalian TLR family is believed to participate in innate immunity as a pattern recognition receptor, which recognizes pathogen-associated molecular patterns (PAMPs) (95). LPS, a major component of the Gram-negative bacterial cell wall, is one of the PAMPs. LPS is recognized by TLR-4 in the mouse (26, 28, 96). TLR-2 is involved in the activation by lipoproteins, peptidoglycan, and lipoteichoic acid, but not by LPS (28). We do not know whether IL-1, IL-18, and PAMPs take advantage of the common signaling pathway shared by IL-1R, IL-18R, and TLRs.

Structure of IL-18R

The IL-18 binding receptor was purified from a Hodgkin's disease cell line (L428 cells) using a monoclonal antibody that inhibits IL-18 binding to L428. Its N-terminal and internal amino acid sequences all matched those of human IL-1Rrp, which had been published as an orphan receptor belonging to the IL-1R family (19, 97). COS-1 cells transfected with hIL-1Rrp cDNA showed low-affinity IL-18 binding capacity (Kd 46 nM) (19). A novel member of the IL-1R family, with the highly conserved IL-1R hallmark domains, was also cloned (23). Based on its homology to IL-1R AcP, it is termed an IL-1R-AcP–like protein (AcPL). AcPL itself does not directly bind IL-18, but its coexpression is essential for activation of NF-κB and c-Jun N-terminal kinase (JNK) in response to IL-18 (23). Furthermore, a dominant-negative form of AcPL specifically inhibited IL-18 signaling. Thus, IL-18R consists of a ligand-binding subunit, IL-1Rrp, and a signal-transducing subunit, AcPL. As the ligand-binding and signaling components of complex forms of receptors are often termed α chain and β chain, respectively, we termed IL-1Rrp and AcPL as IL-18Rα and IL-18Rβ, respectively (Figure 2).

Murine IL-18Rα is 65% homologous to human IL-18Rα in overall amino acid sequence. It is related to murine IL-1R AcP (31% homology); to murine T1/ST2 (30% homology), an orphan receptor of the IL-1R family specifically expressed on Th2 cells and to murine IL-1R1 (27% homology) (97, 98–98b). The cytoplasmic domains exhibit slightly greater sequence homology (36%–44%) than the

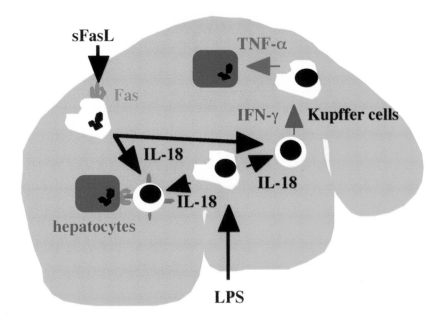

Figure 5 Acute hepatitis induced by LPS or soluble FasL.
When LPS is administered into *P. acnes*-primed mice, LPS-activated Kupffer cells secrete IL-18 that induces both FasL expression and IFN-γ production in hepatic lymphocytes. Subsequently, hepatocytes are killed by FasL-expressed lymphocytes and TNF-α produced by Kupffer cells upon stimulation with IFN-γ (48). Administration of soluble FasL induces IL-18 secretion by Fas-expressing *P. acnes*-elicited Kupffer cells, which evokes chain reactions shown in the case of LPS-induced hepatitis (16).

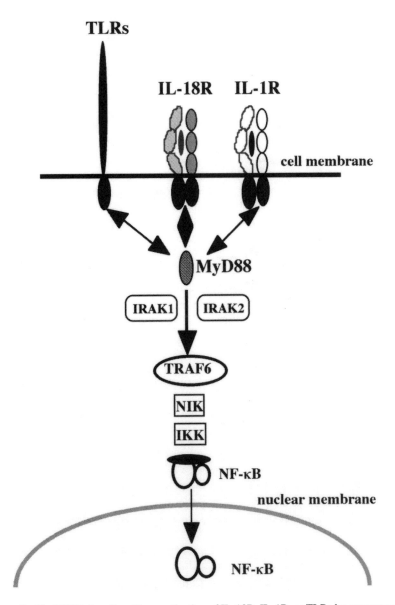

Figure 2   IL-1/TLR signaling. Upon activation of IL-18R, IL-1R, or TLRs by corresponding ligands, MyD88 is recruited by each cytoplasmic domain. MyD88 relays a signal from
phosphorylation of IRAK or IRAK2 to intranuclear translocation of NF-κB (24, 32).

extracellular portions (20%–27%) (97). Murine IL-18Rβ shows homology of 25% to IL-1R1, 27% to IL-1 AcP, and 26% to IL-18Rα, respectively (23). Human IL-18Rα maps to chromosome 2q13–21, where genes encoding IL-1α, IL-1β, IL-1R antagonist (IL-1RA), IL-1R1, and IL-1R2 are located (59, 97). On the other hand, human IL-18 maps to chromosome 11q22, closely linked to DRD2. Therefore, genes for IL-18 ligand and IL-18R map to different chromosomes.

Regulation of IL-18R Expression

IL-18 and IL-12 synergistically exert their IFN-γ-inducing activities in T cells and NK cells, whereas each cytokine alone is much less active. This synergism is mediated by the induction of IL-18Rα on naive T cells by IL-12 and by subsequent reciprocal upregulation of IL-12Rβ2 by IL-18 (34, 98c). The role of IL-18Rα was determined by generation of IL-18Rα-deficient mice (20). Naive T cells, when stimulated with Ag and IL-12, develop into Th1 cells, which express both high- and low-affinity IL-18R and produce IFN-γ in response to IL-18 (20, 34). In contrast, Th1 cells from IL-18Rα-deficient mice do not bind IL-18 or activate NF-κB or JNK upon stimulation with IL-18. These results revealed IL-18Rα as an IL-18 binding component on Th1 cells (20). Consequently, a high level of IL-18R is selectively expressed on Th1 cells but not on Th2 cells, which instead express T1/ST2 (98–98b). Therefore, IL-18R or T1/ST2 expression can be a useful surface marker for Th1 cells and Th2 cells, respectively. NK cells freshly isolated from spleen or liver constitutively express IL-18R, as well as IL-12Rβ2, and both IL-18 and IL-12 augment NK activity independently of each other (99).

IL-18Rα mRNA is detectable in various organs of mice including thymus, spleen, liver, lung, intestine, colon, placenta, prostate, and heart. However, it is not detectable in brain, kidney, skeletal muscle, and pancreas (97). In addition to the above organs, weak expression of IL-18Rα mRNA is observed in the testis and ovary. IL-18Rα is also detected in myeloid, monocytoid, erythroid, and megakaryocytic cell lines (100). Thus, IL-18Rα mRNA is widely, but not universally, distributed, although it is still unknown which cell types express IL-18R and how IL-18R expression is regulated in these IL-18Rα mRNA-expressing tissues.

IL-18 Binding Protein

Recently, IL-18 binding protein (BP) was demonstrated in the urine of healthy individuals (101, 102) and was purified by using IL-18-coupled beads. It is secreted in soluble form because IL-18 BP lacks a transmembrane domain. Human IL-18 BP can bind to murine IL-18, suggesting no species specificity. IL-18 BP can block binding of mature IL-18 to its authentic receptor, IL-18R, resulting in the inhibition of IL-18-induced IFN-γ production (101, 103). Therefore, IL-18BP may be a soluble decoy receptor, functionally similar to the membrane-associated IL-1R2. Recently, it has been reported that IL-18 BP consists of 6 isoforms, resulting from mRNA splicing. Some of them have biological activity but the others lack it (104). IL-18 BP is highly homologous to the proteins encoded by several poxviruses but not to IL-1 or IL-1R (101). Indeed, it has been reported that molluscum contagiosum virus, a common human poxvirus, encodes a family of IL-18 BP homologous proteins, and that the proteins can inhibit IL-18-induced IFN-γ production and NK cell or CTL activity in a dose-dependent manner (105–107). Thus, some poxviruses suppress the action and secretion of host-derived mature IL-18 and IL-1β by production of IL-18 BP homologues as well as Crm A, a potent inhibitor of caspase-1 (105–108).

Murine IL-18 BP is 65.7% identical at the amino acid level to human IL-18 BP. There is no apparent homology of IL-18 BP with any other cytokine or cytokine receptor (23). The gene for IL-18 BP is localized on chromosome 11q13 (101).

IL-18R-Mediated Signaling Pathway

IL-18R shares a signal transducing pathway with IL-1R (21, 109, 110) (Figure 2), because the cytoplasmic regions of the receptors for IL-1 and IL-18 are homologous to each other and to members of the Toll family (17, 32). IL-18R does not activate the JAK/STAT signaling pathway in Th1 cells (109). IL-1-induced signal transduction is initiated by ligand-mediated association of IL-1R1 and AcP through their extracellular domains. A complex of IL-1R1 and AcP recruits MyD88, which provides a platform for IRAK. The requirement of each molecule for IL-1 and IL-18 signal transduction has been demonstrated by the analysis of mice deficient in individual molecules (20, 25, 30, 111). Spleen cells from IL-18Rα-deficient mice, MyD88-deficient mice, or IRAK-deficient mice do not respond to stimulation with IL-18 or with IL-1. MyD88 has an amino acid sequence highly homologous to the Toll/IL-1R (TIR) domain, a cytoplasmic portion highly conserved in the IL-1R/TLR superfamily (24). MyD88 does not contain the transmembrane portion but possesses the death domain at its amino terminus. The targeted disruption of the MyD88 gene results in the abolition of signaling by both IL-1 and IL-18 (25). T cell proliferation and induction of acute phase proteins from the liver in response to IL-1 were abrogated. Furthermore, IL-18-induced increases in the production of IFN-γ and NK cell activity were also impaired. IRAK autophosphorylates and dissociates from the receptor complex and subsequently interacts with TNFR-associated factor-6 (TRAF6), which then relays the signal via NF-κB-induced kinase (NIK) to two IκB kinases (IKK-1 and IKK-2), leading to the formation of activated NF-κB (p65 homodimer or p65/p50 heterodimer). Recently, IRAK-deficient mice have been shown to have a defective response to stimulation with IL-1 and IL-18 similar to that in MyD88-deficient mice (25, 30, 111). Significant defects in JNK induction and partial impairment in NF-κB activation were found in IRAK-deficient Th1 cells and NK cells (30, 111).

Thus, the IRAK/TRAF6 signaling pathway is apparently a major one. However, there is another distinct signaling pathway for IL-18. IL-18 signaling is suggested to be mediated by mitogen-activated protein kinase (MAPK). Protein tyrosine kinase, as well as src kinase LCK, is activated in Th1 cells stimulated with IL-18 (112). A recent study demonstrated the importance of the MAPK pathway in

IL-18-mediated activation of NK cells (113). Cells of the human NK cell line NK92 express IL-18Rα/β and IL-18 BP. IL-18 activates STAT3 but not STAT5 in them. IL-18 also activates MAPK p44^{erk-1} and p42^{erk-21}. As IL-18-augmented cytolytic activity was suppressed by specific inhibitors of MAPK pathways, this pathway is essential for IL-18-induced cytolysis augmentation in NK92 cells. IL-18 can induce IFN-γ mRNA, but secretion of its protein product requires costimulation with IL-2. The MAPK pathway is also involved in induction of IFN-γ.

BIOLOGICAL FUNCTIONS

IL-18 was originally discovered as a factor that induces IFN-γ production from Th1 and NK cells, particularly in the presence of IL-12 (1–4). But recent studies by ourselves and others clearly revealed that IL-18, without help from IL-12, induces the production of Th2 cytokines from T cells, NK cells, and basophils/mast cells (13, 37–39, 114). We summarize the wide spectrum of actions of IL-18 on lymphoid cells in vitro and in vivo (Figure 3).

Induction of IFN-γ Production by IL-12 and IL-18

In general, IFN-γ production by T cells depends on TCR-mediated T cell activation. However, a combination of IL-12 and IL-18 synergistically induces IFN-γ production by T cells without TCR engagement (33, 34, 115–117). This ability is neither enhanced by additional stimulation with immobilized anti-CD3 nor inhibited by cyclosporin A, a potent inhibitor for activation by signaling through TCR (34, 117). Thus, TCR-mediated T cell activation is not essential for synergistic induction of IFN-γ production by IL-12 and IL-18. However, TCR engagement is essential for induction of Th1 cells, because when T cells were stimulated with IL-12 and IL-18 in the presence or absence of anti-CD3, only T cells stimulated with anti-CD3 developed into Th1 cells (34, 109). IL-18 also acts on CD8^{+} T cells and, in combination with IL-12, synergistically induces IFN-γ production in CD8^{+} T cells. Moreover, similar to their synergistic action on T cells, IL-12

Figure 3 Pleiotropic action of IL-18. IL-18 is a peculiar cytokine that regulates both innate immunity and acquired immunity. Both IL-12 and IL-18 are produced by macrophages and synergize for IFN-γ product from NK cells, T cells, and B cells. IL-18 acts on Th1 cells to produce IFN-γ, IL-2, and GM-CSF. IFN-γ from Th1 cells, NK cells, and B cells stimulates macrophages to produce TNF-α, nitric oxide (NO), and reactive oxygen intermediates (ROI), leading to eradication of intracellular microbes (181–183). However, their excess production often induces severe tissue injury. Furthermore, IL-18 stimulates NK cells and CD8^{+} T cells to show cytotoxic activity, leading to killing virus-infected cells or tumor cells. Importantly, IFN-γ from IL-12 and IL-18 stimulated B cells inhibits IgE production but increases IgG production, suggesting the potentiality of therapeutic usage of IL-12 and IL-18 for the treatment of allergic disorders (33, 39, 271).

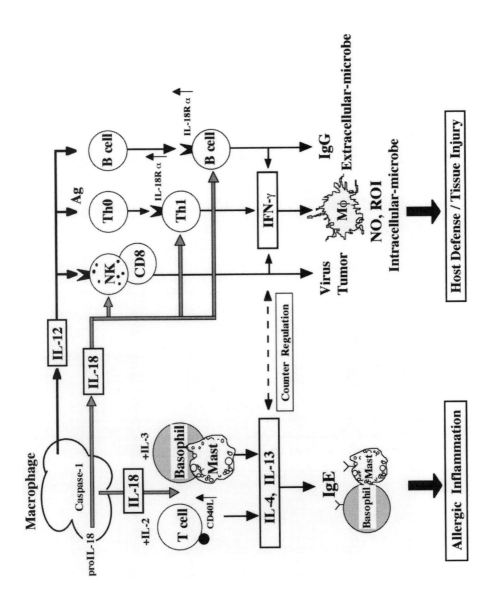

and IL-18 synergistically induce IFN-γ in NK cells (118–120). Interestingly, IL-12 alone can also induce IFN-γ in murine splenocytes, whereas a specific inhibitor of caspase-1 or anti-IL-18 Ab strongly reduces their IFN-γ production, suggesting that IL-12-induced IFN-γ production may be principally dependent on processing of proIL-18 by activated caspase-1 (121).

Human T cells also require both IL-12 and IL-18 for maximal production of IFN-γ (45, 116, 122, 123). Human CD4$^+$ T cells (CD4$^+$CD45RA$^+$ T cells) increase IL-18Rα expression after being stimulated with IL-12 and show dose-dependent production of IFN-γ and proliferation in response to IL-18α (116, 124). Thus, IL-18Rα can be a useful differentiation marker for human Th1 cells. Interestingly, simultaneous or sequential stimulation of human T cells with IL-12 and IL-1 also induces IFN-γ production by T cells, suggesting the possibility that IL-1 is also an IFN-γ-inducing factor in humans (116).

Synergistic Induction of IFN-γ at the Transcriptional Level

The IFN-γ promoter has consensus sequences for NF-κB and AP-1, as well as a cyclosporin A–sensitive NFAT binding site, an intronic enhancer region (C3), and a STAT-4 binding site (122, 125–127). IL-18 activates the IRAK-TRAF6 pathway, resulting in both the activation, AP-1 via JNK and translocation of NF-κB (21, 25, 30, 109–111, 122, 128) into the nucleus, where they bind to specific regulatory DNA sequences in the promoter of the IFN-γ gene (129). IL-12 activates STAT4, a member of the STAT family, and AP-1; these in combination activate the IFN-γ promoter (126). NF-κB recognition sequence is located at -786 to -776 of the IFN-γ gene regulatory region (designated as KBB site) (130). Mutation or deletion of the AP-1- and STAT4-binding sites renders human CD4$^+$ T cells unable to transactivate the IFN-γ gene upon combined stimulation with IL-12 and IL-18 (122). Moreover, the simultaneous activation of NF-κB and STAT4 is also involved in synergistic IFN-γ production from the human myelomonocytic cell line by IL-12 and IL-18 (130). Therefore, the synergistic action of IL-12 and IL-18 results from the orchestrated action of these transcription factors (4, 34, 109, 117, 122).

Effect of IL-18 on Th1 Cells

IL-18 by itself induces only a small amount of IFN-γ in anti-CD3-stimulated Th1 cells. This is also the case for IL-12. But combined stimulation with IL-12 and IL-18 synergistically induces IFN-γ in anti-CD3-stimulated Th1 cells (1, 33, 34, 109, 115, 131–133). Therefore, IL-18 is critically involved in IFN-γ production in Th1 cells in collaboration with IL-12. Besides this induction of IFN-γ production from Th1 cells, IL-18 selectively enhances FasL-mediated cytotoxicity of cloned murine Th1 cells. Furthermore, IL-18 acts as a costimulant for Th1 cells to augment IL-2, GM-CSF, and IL-2Rα production, and it induces cell proliferation, whereas IL-18 has no effect on Th2 clones (20, 34, 109, 133). IL-18Rα is selectively expressed on the surface of Th1 cells but not of Th2 cells

(34, 109, 131), suggesting that the difference in IL-18 responsiveness between Th1 and Th2 cells might result from their differential expression of IL-18Rα (20, 34, 109). Furthermore, IL-18Rα expression can be considered as a cell surface marker distinguishing Th1 cells from Th2 cells (Figure 3).

IL-12 is a major determinant of development of naive T cells into IL-18Rα-expressing Th1 cells in vitro (34, 98b). The essential role of IL-12 in Th1 cell development in vivo has been well established using IL-12-deficient or STAT4-deficient mice (134, 135). Although IL-18 is a potent IFN-γ-inducing factor, IL-18 by itself, unlike IL-12, cannot induce Th1 cell differentiation but rather accelerates it in vitro (8, 34, 109, 136). This action of IL-18 is also proved in vivo by the comparison of Th1 cell differentiation abilities among IL-18-deficient, IL-12-deficient, and double knockout mice upon in vivo treatment with *P. acnes*, a potent in vivo inducer of Th1 cell responses (137). *P. acnes*-primed T cells from IL-18-deficient mice show lesser defects in a shift to Th1 cell than do those from IL-12-deficient mice. Nevertheless, Th1 cell-amplifying activity of IL-18 may contribute to some microbial clearances, in which Th1 cell response is essential (12).

Upregulatory Effect of IL-18 on Cytotoxic Activities

IL-18 directly upregulates cytotoxic activities of NK cells and cytotoxic T cells (1, 45, 99, 120, 138–143). NK cells as well as CD8$^+$ T cells exert their cytocidal action by utilizing perforin, FasL, and TNF-related apoptosis-inducing ligand (TRAIL) (120, 144, 145). IL-18 upregulates perforin-dependent cytotoxic activity and FasL expression but does not enhance TRAIL expression (120, 139, 141). Perforin is a potent pore-forming molecule against target cell membrane (146). FasL induces apoptosis in Fas-expressing target cells (53, 120, 147, 148). TRAIL was recently identified as a third cytotoxic machine responsible for the apoptotic death of a wide variety of tumor cell lines expressing TRAIL receptors (144, 145). Although IL-18 and IL-12 synergistically induce IFN-γ production, they do not synergize for their upregulation of cytotoxic activities of effector cells. This may indicate that the activation of a signal-transducing system for IFN-γ production is not the same as that for perforin and granzyme-mediated cytotoxicity.

Like IL-12 (134), IL-18 is important for the functional development of NK cells (137). As compared with wild-type mice, IL-18-deficient or IL-18Rα-deficient mice have almost the same number of NK cells but show reduced cytolytic activity against NK cell targets (20, 137). Their NK activity, however, is enhanced by exogenous IL-12, IL-18, and IL-2 to the same level as that of wild-type NK cells. This was also the case for IL-12-deficient NK cells (134, 137). Therefore, IL-12 and IL-18 exert these actions on NK cells independent of each other.

Effect of IL-18 on B Cells and Macrophages

B cells produce IgG1 and IgE when stimulated with anti-CD40 and IL-4. We showed that a combination of IL-12 and IL-18 induces anti-CD40-activated highly purified murine B cells to produce IFN-γ, which inhibits IL-4-dependent IgE and IgG1 production and enhances IgG2a production (33). We also showed that B cells obtained from normal mice could develop into IFN-γ-producing cells in IFN-γ-deficient host mice in response to in vivo treatment with IL-12 and IL-18, indicating that B cells act as regulatory cells in the immune response. An intrinsic role of IL-12 and IL-18 in IgE responses was reported using the SJL mouse, which manifests poor IgE production upon helminth infection (149). B cells obtained only by depletion of T cells from SJL spleen cells failed to proliferate and to produce IgE and IgG1 in response to LPS plus IL-4. This diminished IgE production in vitro was restored by anti-IL-12, which was enhanced by additional treatment with anti-IL-18 antibody, suggesting that SJL macrophages contaminated in the B cell preparation might produce IL-12 and IL-18 in response to LPS (149).

Interestingly, macrophages derived from murine bone marrow can also produce a large amount of IFN-γ when stimulated with IL-12 and IL-18 (150). Moreover, murine microglia cells not only produce but also respond to IL-18 (66). Dendritic cells produce IFN-γ when stimulated with IL-12 and IL-18 (36). Thus, the macrophage is a potent inducer of IFN-γ production from T cells, NK cells, and B cells by production of IL-12 and IL-18, but it also produces IFN-γ in response to these cytokines, suggesting a unique pathway of autocrine macrophage activation (150).

Induction of IL-4 and IL-13 Production by IL-18

As the biological action of IL-18 was investigated in the presence of IL-12, IL-18 was originally regarded as a factor that induced IFN-γ. However, recent studies have revealed that naive T cells express a low level of IL-18Rα and produce IL-13 and GM-CSF in response to IL-18, particularly in collaboration with IL-2 (37). More recently, we have discovered that naive CD4$^+$ T cells cultured with IL-2 and IL-18 without TCR engagement for 4 days expressed CD40L and produced a large amount of IL-13 and a small amount of IL-4 (38). Additional stimulation with anti-CD3 augmented their capacity to produce these Th2 cytokines. Furthermore, these activated T cells developed into Th2 cells. However, naive CD4$^+$ T cells stimulated with the same protocol but in addition with anti-IL-4 for 4 days developed into Th1 but not into Th2 cells, suggesting that IL-18 has the potential to induce Th2 cells in an IL-4-dependent manner (Figure 4). Moreover, we have recently demonstrated that basophils and mast cells derived from bone marrow cells incubated with IL-3 for 10 days expressed IL-18Rα and produced large amounts of IL-4 and IL-13 in response to stimulation with IL-3 and IL-18 (39). As mast cells and basophils are major inducers and effectors of allergic inflammation, IL-18 might be critically involved in the induction of allergic inflammation. Histamine, a chemical mediator produced by mast cells and basophils, stimulates the production of IL-18 in PBMCs (151). As IL-18 in combination with IL-3 stimulates basophils and mast cells to produce histamine (39), there may be a positive feedback regulation between histamine and

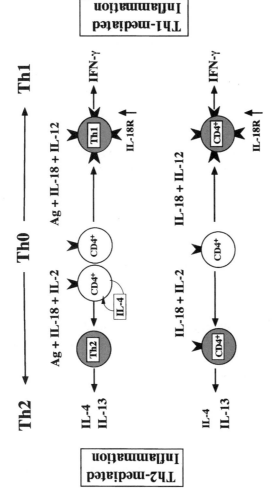

Figure 4 IL-18 stimulates Th1 or Th2 response depending on its cytokine milieu. Although naive CD4$^+$ T cells weakly express IL-18R, they cannot produce IFN-γ when stimulated with Ag and/or IL-18. However, they produce a large amount of IFN-γ in response to IL-12 and IL-18. Additional Ag stimulation has no effect on this response, suggesting that TCR engagement is not essential for induction of IFN-γ. But TCR engagement is a prerequisite condition for induction of Th1 cells. Neither IL-2 nor IL-18 induces a significant amount of IL-4 and IL-13 in naive T cells, while the combination induces naive T cells to produce IL-4 and IL-13. Additional stimulation with Ag not only increases their IL-4 production but also causes them to develop into Th2 cells (38).

IL-18 (151). Interestingly, histamine also stimulates the production of IL-18 and IFN-γ from PBMCs without induction of IL-12 (151). Therefore, histamine is unique in triggering an IL-18-initiated cytokine cascade without inducing IL-12 production.

Dual Regulatory Roles of IL-18 in IgE Production

As described above, in combination with IL-12, IL-18 is a potent inducer of IFN-γ production and can augment Th1 responses both in vitro and in vivo. Indeed, administration of a mixture of IL-12 and IL-18 completely inhibited IgE production induced by infection with a helminth, a prototype pathogen for in vivo Th2 responses (33). Furthermore, this treatment abolishes the capacity of basophils to produce IL-4 and IL-13 in response to stimulation either with IL-3 and IL-18 or with FcεR cross-linkage (39). This inhibitory effect of IL-18 on helminth-induced accumulation of IgE is completely dependent on IFN-γ, because the administration of IL-12 and IL-18 did not produce these effects in helminth-infected IFN-γ-deficient mice (33). Interestingly, injection of a mixture of IL-12 and IL-18 rather increased serum IgE levels in helminth-infected or anti-IgD-injected IFN-γ-deficient mice (33, 39). However, administration of IL-18 alone enhanced Th2 cytokine production, eosinophilia, and the IgE response in helminth-infected or anti-IgD-injected mice or a ragweed allergy mouse model (39, 152). More surprisingly, IL-18 alone has the capacity to induce IgE accumulation in vivo. Daily administration of IL-18 caused a striking, dose-dependent increase in serum IgE levels in vivo (38, 114, 152). This IL-18-induced IgE accumulation in vivo is completely dependent on the IL-4/IL-4R system but not on IL-13 (38, 114). Furthermore, transgenic mice overexpressing human caspase-1 in keratinocytes, which have high serum levels of mature IL-18, spontaneously develop chronic dermatitis with high serum levels of IgE and IgG1. Disruption of IL-18 or STAT6, an essential element for signal transduction by IL-4, resulted in decreased serum IgE and IgG1 in caspase-1 transgenic mice, indicating that IL-18- and IL-4-mediated signaling are involved in their spontaneous elevation of IgE and IgG1 (38). These results indicate that IL-18 has the potential to initiate Th2 cell development.

IL-18 may also play an important role in the effector limb of allergic responses. Both airway epithelial cells (72) and keratinocytes (69, 153), important targets in asthma and atopic dermatitis, respectively, constitutively express IL-18. Stimulation of IL-18-processing enzymes such as caspase-1 would cause the release of IL-18, which in turn might result in induction of IL-4/IL-13 in the airway and the skin in an IgE-independent manner, where they may directly induce allergic inflammatory responses. These findings suggest that caspase-1/IL-18 is a potential target in the effort to develop agents that regulate allergic inflammatory responses and provide new insight into potential mechanisms through which Th2 responses may become dominant in an individual.

Intermezzo: A Story Behind Our Keystone Finding That IL-18 Has the Capacity to Differentiate Naive CD4$^+$ T Cells Into Th2 Cells

In this short section, we would like to disclose the inside story about how we came upon the idea that IL-18 may play a role as a Th2-developing factor. IL-18 was discovered as a potent IFN-γ-inducing factor in 1995. The initial reports primarily had characterized IL-18 as a factor involved in inflammatory immune responses. A couple of years after the discovery of IL-18, when we and others had intensively studied the biological functions of IL-18 as a Th1-related cytokine and proinflammatory cytokine, we chanced to see that caspase-1 transgenic mice with severe chronic dermatitis scratched out even their ulcerative skin lesions (77). This strongly impressed upon us that mature IL-18 might be involved in atopic immune responses. Indeed, studies revealed that the transgenic mice contained high serum levels of IgE as well as biologically active IL-18 (77). To confirm the involvement of IL-18 in the elevation of serum IgE, we crossed the transgenic mice with IL-18-deficient or STAT6-deficient mice. IL-18-deficient or STAT6-deficient caspase-1 transgenic mice decreased their serum IgE partly and completely, respectively. These results encouraged us to examine whether IL-18 had the capacity to differentiate naive CD4$^+$ T cells into Th2 cells, maturing into the study recently reported (38).

PROTECTIVE ROLE OF IL-18 IN HOST DEFENSE

Microbes can be classified into intracellular and extracellular types. In general, intracellular microbes are expelled by cell-mediated immunity, whereas extracellular microbes evoke humoral immunity. Since IFN-γ stimulates macrophages and B cells to produce oxygen radicals and Ig, respectively (Figure 3), IL-18 is expected to play an important role in host defenses against various infectious microbes. Th1 cells are generally associated with resistance to infection with intracellular microbes by production of IFN-γ, whereas Th2 cells are associated with progressive infection. Protection against intracellular microbes is critically dependent on the function of NK cells at an early stage and on Th1 cell development in later stages. Because activation of these cells is induced by the action of IL-12 and IL-18, we assumed that IL-18 along with IL-12 participates in microbe clearance. Furthermore, IL-18 directly activates CD8$^+$ T cells (138, 143), which play a central role in viral clearance. We briefly summarize the protective role of IL-18 in host defense, including surveillance against tumor generation.

Bacterial Infection

Mycobacterium avium (*M. avium*) is an intracellular microorganism that infects and multiplies within macrophages. In a mouse model of infection, genetically susceptible BALB/c mice show decreased expression of IL-12 and IL-18 associated with a diminished IFN-γ/Th1 response. In contrast, resistant DBA/2 mice exhibited increased expression of IL-12, IL-18, and IFN-γ (154), indicating a good correlation between clearance of *M. avium* and levels of IL-12, IL-18, and IFN-γ. Indeed, IL-18-deficient C57BL/6 mice manifested more severe infection, and the pathological changes were significantly suppressed by treatment with exogenous IL-18 (155). PBMCs from patients infected with *M. tuberculosis* showed a decreased capacity to produce IL-12, IL-18, and IFN-γ in response to mycobacterial antigen compared with PBMCs from PPD-reactive healthy individuals, suggesting a contribution of IL-18 to a protective Th1 cytokine response (156). Furthermore, injection of DNA encoding IL-18 into the skin enhances both humoral and T cell-mediated responses upon mycobacterial infection (156a). However, a recent study also indicated that PBMCs from patients with active tuberculosis showed significantly enhanced production of IL-18 and IL-10 after 96 h of stimulation with mycobacterial antigen (157). Indeed, significantly increased serum levels of IL-18 and IFN-γ were found in patients with pulmonary tuberculosis as compared with those in healthy controls (158). Therefore, IL-18 appears to be important for protective immunity to *M. tuberculosis* infection. However, its exact protective role is still uncertain.

Leprosy is an infectious disease in which the balance between Th1 and Th2 cells plays a critical role in determination of disease progression and clinical outcome (159). At one extreme, tuberculoid leprosy (TL) patients are resistant to infection by local production of IFN-γ. In contrast, lepromatous leprosy (LL) patients have high specific titers but weak cell-mediated immune response because their lesions produce IL-4. Thus, Th1- or Th2-deviated immune responses to intracellular microbes are believed to play a critical role in the character of the lesions. In animal models, IL-12 administration resulted in a significant reduction of bacterial counts in mice infected with *M. leprae*. Furthermore, the combination of IL-18 and IL-12 afforded stronger protection in these models (160). These results suggested that a combined effect of IL-12 and IL-18 in promoting *M. leprae*-specific Th1 responses is an essential effector mechanism for *M. leprae* clearance in the host.

However, a study using patients infected with *M. leprae* disclosed a complicated role of IL-18 in mediating pathological changes. IL-18 mRNA expression was higher in lesions from TL patients as compared with LL patients, and monocytes from the TL patients showed increased expression of IL-18 mRNA in response to *M. leprae* in vitro (161). Exogenous IL-18 augmented *M. leprae*-induced IFN-γ in NK cells and T cells from TL patients but not from LL patients in vitro, while IL-4 production was not elevated. Moreover, anti-IL-12 Ab partially inhibited *M. leprae*-induced release of IFN-γ in the presence of IL-18, suggesting a combined effect of IL-12 and IL-18 in promoting *M. leprae*-specific Th1 responses.

Unexpectedly, the serum level of IL-18 in patients with LL is much higher than that in patients with TL (38), although serum levels of IL-12 are within normal levels in both types of patients. Thus, IL-18 may be an important determinant of the development of Th2 cells, which are characteristic of LL, and of the lesions and clinical course of *M. leprae* infections. At least, serum IL-18 levels correlate well with the activity of leprosy. However, as noted above, the level of IL-18 mRNA in leprosy lesions of patients with LL is lower than that of patients with TL. At present we do not know how to reconcile the discrepant results of these two studies. Although it is well documented that infection with intracellular microbes often induces simultaneous production of IL-12 and IL-18 by macrophages, this observation may suggest that there are some circumstances in which IL-18 is made without IL-12 and that IL-18 is involved in polarization of naive T cells into Th2 cells.

In a model of *Salmonella typhimurium* infection, the protective role of IL-18 is also demonstrated by treatment of mice with anti-IL-18 Ab or administration of IL-18 into infected mice (162). Endogenous IL-18 is also involved in the defense against infection with *Yersinia enterocolitica* (62). In these models, IL-18 protected them from lethality in an IFN-γ-dependent manner. The importance of caspase-1-dependent processing of IL-1β and IL-18 for host defense against *Shigella flexneri* (*S. flexneri*), the etiological agent of bacillary dysentery, is also revealed by infection of caspase-1-deficient mice with *S. flexneri* (163). *S. flexneri* induces apoptosis in macrophages, which requires and activates caspase-1, resulting in the release of bioactive IL-1β and IL-18 (163). Caspase-1-deficient mice infected with *S. flexneri* do not develop the acute inflammation characteristic of shigellosis and are unable to resolve the bacterial infection. Furthermore, supplementation with IL-1β and/or IL-18 established that IL-1β and IL-18 are both required to mediate inflammation in *S. flexneri* infections (163).

Th1 cells are also important in protective immunity against chlamydiae, intracellular bacteria. Because epithelial cells constitutively express IL-18 mRNA and pro-IL-18, the effects of *Chlamydia trachomatis* (*C. trachomatis*) infection of human epithelial cell lines on IL-18 secretion were investigated (164). *C. trachomatis* infection causes cells to secrete mature IL-18. In contrast to epithelial cell lines, fibroblast cell lines constitutively expressed much lower levels of pro-IL-18 and did not secrete mature IL-18 after chlamydial infection even though caspase-1 was activated. Taken together, the results suggest that a chlamydia infection induces mature IL-18 secretion through caspase-1 activation in infected epithelial cells.

Fungal Infection

IL-18 also exerts antifungal activity against *Cryptococcus neoformans* (*C. neoformans*), an intracellularly parasitized fungus. Peritoneal exudate cells incubated with IL-18, together with IL-12, suppress the growth of *C. neoformans* (165, 166). The effect is dependent on both IFN-γ production by NK cells and NO production by macrophages, suggesting that IL-18 plays an important role in innate immunity against *C. neoformans* in collaboration with IL-12. Furthermore, administration of IL-18 or a combination of subtherapeutic doses of IL-12 and IL-18 showed a significant protective effect by upregulation of IFN-γ production but downregulation of IL-4 production. The protective effect of these cytokines was mediated by IL-18-induced IFN-γ production from NK cells and T cells, but not from CD4$^+$ T cells, in the lung during the early period of the infection (166–168). In particular, IL-18 contributes well to host resistance to *C. neoformans* infection by induction of IFN-γ production from NK cells, but not through Th1 cell differentiation, when IL-12 synthesis is deficient (169).

Viral Infection

In addition to its potent induction of IFN-γ, IL-18 alone activates CD8$^+$ T cells, which play a central role in viral clearance, suggesting a role of IL-18 in viral infection. A protective effect of IL-18 against infection with herpes simplex virus (HSV) was shown in a mouse model (170). Administration of IL-18 to mice before the infection remarkably improved their survival rates through upregulated IFN-γ-induced NO induction in a T cell- and B cell-independent manner. The effect was also exerted in athymic nude mice and SCID mice, suggesting that IL-18 augments innate immunity. Infection with influenza A virus resulted in accumulation of IFN-α/β, TNF-α, IL-1β, and IL-18, whereas the production of IL-12 was not detected (171). Virus-infected macrophage-derived IL-18 synergized with IFN-α/β produced by the same cells to induce a rapid IFN-γ production by T cells, consequently leading to a possible induction of Th1 immune responses. The in vivo antiviral effect of IL-18 was also investigated in a mouse model of vaccinia virus infection (172). Intraperitoneal injection of IL-18 significantly suppressed pock formation on the tails of BALB/c mice inoculated with vaccinia virus. Interestingly, several viruses including poxviruses have been reported to encode putative proteins highly homologous to IL-18 BP, which binds IL-18 and blocks its biological activity (101, 103, 104). A remarkable feature of poxvirus infection in humans is multiple small skin lesions, which contain a large number of virus particles but lack inflammatory cell infiltrates, suggesting inhibition of IL-18 by poxvirus-encoded proteins may attenuate the inflammatory antiviral response partly owing to the blockade of IL-18-induced accumulation of a chemokine, IL-8 (173, 174).

IL-18 induces HIV replication. In vitro experiments using the monocytic cell line U1 containing HIV-1 copies have demonstrated increased HIV-1 production after stimulation with proinflammatory cytokines, such as IL-1 and TNF-α, or after exposure to IL-6 (175). IL-18 also increases HIV-1 production by U1 cells (176). In addition, treatment with TNF-binding protein or a neutralizing anti-IL-6 mAb reduced IL-18-stimulated HIV-1 production, suggesting a role for IL-18 in HIV-1 pathogenesis. It has been reported that as compared with PBMCs from uninfected control donors, PBMCs from HIV-1-infected individuals produced very similar levels of TNF-α and IL-1β, more IL-4, and less IL-12 p70 when challenged with *Staphylococcus aureus* in vitro (177). However, at this moment, the production of IL-18 by HIV-infected patients remains unclear.

Protozoan Infection

Leishmania major (*L. major*) is an example of intracellular protozoa. Cutaneous inoculation of *L. major* induces in most inbred mouse strains a localized lesion that heals spontaneously, resulting in acquisition of resistance to reinfection. However, some strains are susceptible to this infection as manifested by a fatal visceral illness. CD4$^+$ T cells from an infected resistant strain contain high levels of IFN-γ but little IL-4, whereas those from an infected susceptible strain contain inverse levels of each cytokine (178, 179). Healing of lesions caused by *L. major* infection requires the induction and expansion of Th1 cells, leading to IFN-γ-induced iNOS-mediated NO production, a critical effector molecule involved in clearance of *L. major* (180). Since IL-12 and IL-18 synergize for IFN-γ production, we and others investigated the importance of IL-18 in *L. major* clearance (181–183). Neither IL-12 nor IL-18 alone induced wound healing, whereas the combination completely protected from *L. major*-infection-induced footpad swelling in an NO-dependent manner. Furthermore, these recovered mice acquired protective immunity against *L. major* reinfection (182). Treatment with neutralizing anti-IL-18 antibody markedly reduced their resistance to *L. major* infection by downregulation of IFN-γ production, leading to diminished NO production upon *L. major* infection. Moreover, compared with their wild-type littermates, IL-18-deficient mice on the resistant background clearly developed larger lesions during the early phase of infection but eventually resolved (182, 183). Thus, IL-18 may play an important role in early control of *L. major* infection but is not critically involved in host immunity, because IL-18-deficient mice eventually recovered from the infection by the development of Th1 cells (182, 183).

Recently, a recombinant leishmania protein, LeIF, was shown to stimulate Th1 responses and protect BALB/c mice from *L. major* in an IL-12- and IL-18-dependent manner (184). Since the production of IFN-γ by LeIF-stimulated SCID splenocytes is suppressed by addition of neutralizing antibody to IL-12 or IL-18 in a dose-dependent manner, vaccination with LeIF stimulates macrophages to produce IL-12 and IL-18 for protection.

IFN-γ, produced after infection with *Trypanosoma cruzi* (*T. cruzi*), has been shown to be crucial in the determination of resistance or susceptibility. Using the in situ hybridization technique, it has been shown that the mRNAs for IL-12 p40 and IL-18 were induced in the spleen by a parasitic infection and were at a high level during infection with *T. cruzi* (185). The transcript for IL-18 was produced earlier during infection and declined until day 38, when IFN-γ and IL-12 p40 transcripts were optimally expressed. Therefore, *T. cruzi* induces strong IL-12 and IL-18 gene expression in vivo, correlating with IFN-γ production.

Tumor Regression

Recently, tumor-associated macrophages have been highlighted because of their potent ability to release antitumor cytokines, such as IL-12, TNF-α, and IL-18 (186). Similar to IL-12, IL-18 stimulates cytotoxic activity of NK cells and CD8$^+$

T cells. Therefore, IL-18 as well as IL-12 has been expected to be a target for tumor immunotherapy. In fact, many investigators have reported antitumor action of IL-18 against various types of tumor cell lines in vivo. Intraperitoneal administration of IL-18 inhibits growth of Meth A sarcoma inoculated into syngeneic mice by activation of NK cells, although IL-18 by itself has no inhibitory action against tumor cell growth in vitro (187, 188). Furthermore, surviving mice became resistant to rechallenge with Meth A sarcoma by the generation of tumor-specific cytotoxic CD4$^+$ T cells. The antitumor effect of IL-18 is also revealed by gene transfer experiments (189, 190). A mouse neuroblastoma cell line transfected with retroviral constructs designed to express mature IL-18 is rejected when inoculated into syngeneic mice, whereas parental tumor cells lacking IL-18 are highly tumorigenic. Furthermore, IL-18 and B7.1 (CD80) transfected tumor cells have synergistic antitumor effects against B16 murine melanoma (191). In addition, the same IL-18-expressing tumor cells are tumorigenic when inoculated into CD4$^+$ and/or CD8$^+$ T cell-depleted mice, indicating that the antitumor action of IL-18 is T cell-dependent (190). The antitumor effect of IL-18 has also been shown against mouse glioma cells, an effect that is reduced after depletion of NK cells (192). Transfection of retroviral or adenoviral vectors encoding mature IL-18 into a fibrosarcoma cell line results in loss of tumorigenicity. This effect is enhanced by simultaneous transfection with an IL-12-expressing vector (189). However, the antitumor effect of exogenous IL-18 on a melanoma cell line and a sarcoma cell line is independent of endogenous IL-12 or IFN-γ (193). Interestingly, the antitumor effect of IL-18 is distinct from that of IL-12 (194). Administration of IL-18 and IL-12 equally inhibits growth of CL8-1, a murine melanoma cell line, in mice. However, exogenous IL-18 did not prove antitumorigenic on CL8-1-bearing *gld/gld* mice lacking functional FasL, whereas IL-12 showed an equal antitumor effect on them compared with wild-type mice. In contrast, hepatic lymphocytes from IL-12-treated perforin-deficient mice do not show augmented cytolytic activity, whereas those from IL-18-treated perforin-deficient mice display enhanced killing action as compared with those from IL-12-treated wild-type mice, suggesting that IL-18 exerts its antitumor action through upregulation of FasL-mediated tumoricidal activity but that the IL-12 antitumor effect is completely dependent on perforin-mediated killing. Since IL-18 is constitutively expressed in intestinal epithelial cells (71), carcinoma of epithelial cell origin seems to be relatively benign for the host. However, IL-18 positive colon cancer cell lines do not contain its processing enzyme caspase-1, resulting in their acquisition of malignancy (195).

There is one report that soluble products from B16 melanoma cells stimulate hepatic sinusoidal endothelial cells (HSE) to release TNF-α, IL-1β, and IL-18, which upregulates the expression of vascular cell adhesion molecules on HSE, promoting cancer cell adhesion on HSE and metastasis to the liver (196). Furthermore, B16B10 melanoma cells, which express both IL-18 and IL-18R, increase FasL expression and intracellular reactive oxygen intermediate (ROI) levels in an autocrine manner. Thus, endogenous IL-18 in melanoma cells may help them to evade the host immune system by regulating the expression of FasL as well as ROI (197). Thus, a careful manipulation of IL-18 may be required for practical immunotherapy (196).

Antitumor action of IL-18 is demonstrated also to be due to its inhibitory effect on angiogenesis (198, 199). In vitro, IL-18 inhibits fibroblast growth-factor-induced proliferation of capillary endothelial cells. Exogenous IL-18 also suppresses fibroblast growth-factor-induced corneal neovascularization. Administration of IL-18 leads to inhibition of fibrosarcoma growth accompanied by hypovascularization. Combination therapy using IL-12- and IL-18-expressing tumor cells shows more efficacy in tumor regression. Therefore, IL-18, particularly in combination with IL-12, may become a potent antitumor agent.

Recently, synergistic antitumor effects of IL-12 and IL-18 have been reported by many investigators (200–205). Murine bladder cancer cell line MBT2 is introduced by the IL-12 gene, resulting in lack of tumorigenesis. Systemic administration of IL-18 does not inhibit growth of inoculated parental tumor cells. However, coinoculation of parental MBT2 cells with IL-12-expressing MBT2 cells suppresses parental tumor cell growth. Furthermore, exogenous administration of IL-18 synergistically inhibits parental tumor cell growth in an IFN-γ-dependent manner when inoculated with IL-12-expressing MBT2 cells (200). Synergistic inhibition of tumor growth is observed by combinational gene therapy using IL-12, proIL-18 and its cleaving enzyme, caspase-1 (201). This effect is mediated by the activation of CD8$^+$ T cells and accumulated IFN-γ.

PATHOLOGICAL ROLES OF IL-18

As described above, IL-18 contributes well to the host defenses. However, overproduction of IL-18, especially in association with IL-12, is harmful because IL-18 is a powerful proinflammatory cytokine with a wide-spectrum potentiality covering not only the immune system but also the non-immune system (73, 74, 206–209). In this section, we describe multiple pathological roles of IL-18, particularly focusing on its roles in immune disturbances such as autoimmune diseases and inflammatory disorders.

Autoimmune Diseases

Insulin-Dependent Diabetes Mellitus (IDDM)   IDDM is accepted to occur under autoimmune T cell-mediated circumstances. The NOD mouse is a good model for human IDDM. NOD mice spontaneously manifest progressive insulitis characterized by destruction of islet β cells, insulin-producing cells, resulting in diabetes with further growth. Genetic comparison between NOD and diabetes-resistant mice reveals several NOD-specific polymorphisms in MHC genes. This is also the case for patients with IDDM (210–213). Recently, it has been shown that transgenic mice bearing human diabetogenic MHC class II and lacking endogenous mouse MHC class II spontaneously develop diabetes (214, 215). Furthermore, T cells from the transgenic mouse could respond to insulin and glutamic acid decarboxylase (GAD), putative islet autoantigens, and diabetes was shown to be transferable to nondiabetic mice by adoptive transfer of the T cells (215). These islet autoantigens were recognized and targeted by diabetogenic CD8$^+$ T cells from young NOD mice that have not yet developed diabetes (216), suggesting that both insulin and GAD may be autoantigens responsible for human IDDM. Endogenously accumulated cytokines have been reported to affect disease activity (217). TNF-α/TNF-αR and IFN-γ/IFN-γR are profoundly involved in the development of diabetes (218, 219). By contrast, Th2-related cytokines IL-10 and IL-4 protect against development of diabetes (220, 221).

IL-18 has been reported to be associated with the development of diabetes in NOD mice. The gene encoding IL-18 maps to the *idd2* susceptibility locus, which is one of the genes involved in the development of diabetes in NOD, suggesting a possible contribution of IL-18 in Th1-mediated autoimmunity (60). Indeed, mRNA for IL-18 increased in pancreata of even pre-onset NOD mice after administration of the diabetes-inducing agent cyclophosphamide, suggesting IL-18 as a diabetes-relating molecule in mice. The levels of IL-18 as well as of IL-12 and TNF-α in pancreatic islets were elevated after induction of diabetes in the transgenic mice that express the TCR from a diabetogenic CD4$^+$ T cell clone derived from NOD mice (222). Unexpectedly, however, IL-18 supplements rather delayed diabetes development in NOD mice (223). NOD mice increased IL-4 mRNA in their pancreata after IL-18 treatment, suggesting exogenous IL-18 may skew the process of islet infiltrating T cells into IL-4-producing cells. These apparently conflicting results may give us a clue about involvement of IL-18 in Th2 responses (37, 38). More recently, IL-13, a downstream cytokine of IL-18, was reported capable of preventing IDDM in NOD (224). Establishment of IL-18-deficient NOD mice will clarify the role of endogenous IL-18 in the development of IDDM.

Multiple Sclerosis (MS)   Multiple sclerosis is a human autoimmune disease of the central nervous system (CNS). Inflammatory changes extending to the myelin sheath cause demyelination, resulting in the blockade of nerve conduction. Disease symptoms of MS vary corresponding to the site of demyelination and may produce visual, motor, and sensory disturbances (225). Patients with MS exhibit T cells specific for CNS-derived autoantigens, myelin sheath components that include myelin basic protein (MBP) (226). Experimental autoimmune encephalomyelitis (EAE) is an animal model of MS. EAE mice do not spontaneously develop limb paralysis, but this is induced by administration with the myelin sheath components. EAE is caused by MBP-specific CD4$^+$ T cells secreting Th1 cytokines, particularly IFN-γ and TNF-α. Transgenic mice that express the TCR gene of the encephalitogenic CD4$^+$ T cell clone derived from EAE mice spontaneously manifest signs of nervous disturbances (227). As in the case of IDDM, susceptible MHC class II genes associated with MS have been clarified. This is also the case for EAE models. In fact, susceptibility to EAE differs widely among mice with various MHC backgrounds (210, 213).

IL-18 is involved in EAE development. The brain cells of EAE-induced rats express high levels of IL-18 mRNA levels at the onset and during the course of EAE (228). The administration of neutralizing anti-IL-18 partially protects rats from EAE and is accompanied by the downregulated Th1 response of autoantigen-specific T cells. Although IL-18 alone cannot produce Th1 cells (109), endogenously accumulated IL-18 in the EAE course may contribute to the acquisition of responsiveness to IL-12, a pivotal cytokine responsible for development of EAE, by upregulation of expression of IL-12Rβ2, an inducible subunit of the receptor for IL-12 (212, 229, 230). Demyelinating brain lesions from patients with MS also express IL-18 mRNA as well as IFN-γ mRNA, accompanied by the preferential distribution of Th1 cells determined by expressing Th1-deviated chemokine receptors, such as CCR5 and CXCR3 (231). Furthermore, caspase-1 mRNA levels in PBMCs from the patients with MS were reported to be elevated compared with those from healthy volunteers (232). The importance of caspase-1 in EAE development is also demonstrated by using caspase-1-deficient mice and treatment with caspase-1 inhibitors (233). Therefore, caspase-1 and its product, mature IL-18, are profoundly involved in EAE and MS, possibly providing a new therapeutic strategy for the disease.

Rheumatoid Arthritis (RA)   Rheumatoid arthritis is a common autoimmune disease in joints. RA is thought to be a Th1-associated disease. However, we do not know how the Th1 deviation is induced in RA, although in vitro study suggests an important role for IL-12-producing macrophages in the synovium (234, 235). It has recently been reported that a high level of IL-18 was observed in the synovial fluid from patients with RA (236). DBA/1 mice injected with type II collagen (CII) in complete Freund's adjuvant (FA) develop arthritis (CIA) with many similarities to human RA, providing an experimental animal model of RA. As with the other autoimmune diseases described above, the susceptibility to the disease is associated with particular MHC genes (213). Transgenic mice bearing human arthritogenic MHC class II are highly susceptible to CIA. In contrast, transgenic mice expressing the nonarthritogenic haplotype show a much lower incidence of CIA. In this animal model, IL-18 was shown to be produced by macrophages but not by T cells in the synovium, whereas IL-18R is expressed on both synovial macrophages and T cells, suggesting a possible involvement of IL-18 in CIA. Recently, IL-18 was reported to enhance CIA in DBA/1 mice injected with CII in incomplete FA (237). Coadministration of IL-18 changed this low-grade arthritis seen in DBA/1 mice treated with CII in incomplete FA to arthritis indistinguishable from that in mice treated with CII in complete FA. Treatment with IL-12 or IL-18 alone promotes CIA, which is enhanced further by treatment with combined IL-12 and IL-18. IL-18-treated mice produce more TNF-α and IL-6 through direct effects of IL-18 on macrophages, but less IFN-γ, compared to mice treated with IL-12. Furthermore, mice treated with IL-18 or IL-18 plus IL-12 produce markedly more IgG1 and

IgG2a anti-collagen Ab compared with controls, whereas IL-12 treatment only leads to an enhanced IgG2a response. The possible role of IL-18 with IL-12 in the synovium of RA may be as a potent inducer of TNF-α, IL-6, and IFN-γ by locally accumulated T cells that sustain the inflammatory response in the joints.

Inflammatory Tissue Damage

Liver Diseases We recently reviewed the roles of IL-18 in liver injury (10). Thus, we briefly summarize them here. IL-18 was initially described as a molecule responsible for liver injury in the mice sequentially treated with *P. acnes* and LPS (1). IL-18 induces acute liver injury in mice by induction of hepatotoxic factors such as TNF-α and FasL (48) (Figure 5, see color insert). Indeed, administration of neutralizing anti-IL-18 completely protects mice from this endotoxin-induced liver injury, and IL-18-deficient mice are resistant to this liver injury (1, 48, 238).

IL-18 is also a pivotal factor in inducing soluble FasL-induced acute liver injury. Liver parenchymal cells have been reported to express Fas under normal conditions (147, 148). When agonistic anti-Fas mAb was administered into normal mice, all the mice promptly died of fulminant hepatitis (239). The mechanism underlying this anti-Fas-induced lethal liver injury is demonstrated to be caused by a direct action of anti-Fas inducing apoptosis in Fas-expressing liver parenchymal cells. In contrast, soluble FasL, which is shed from FasL-expressing lymphocytes (240), does not cause any liver damage in normal mice, whereas *P. acnes*-primed mice die from massive liver injury following administration of soluble FasL (241). As recently shown, Kupffer cells do not express Fas under normal conditions, whereas *P. acnes*-elicited Kupffer cells express Fas, the activation of which by membrane-anchored or soluble FasL leads to secretion of biologically active IL-18 in a caspase other than caspase-1-dependent manner. IL-18 secreted from FasL-activated *P. acnes*-elicited Kupffer cells raises chain reactions of hepatic proinflammatory cytokines started by IFN-γ, and it also augments endogenous FasL expression on hepatic immune competent cells. This positive loop between IL-18 secretion and the activation of FasL seems to lead to acute liver injury (16) (Figure 5). ConA hepatitis is modeled in a T cell-dependent liver injury mouse, where it is mediated by multiple factors including the activation of Fas/FasL system, accumulation of hepatocidal cytokines such as IFN-γ and TNF-α, and the induction of IL-4. Recently, IL-18 has been shown to play a role in ConA hepatitis (242, 243). NO-aspirin derivatives in a dose-dependent fashion protected against liver damage induced by ConA by inhibiting caspases involved in the processing and maturation of IL-1β and IL-18 (242).

IL-18 has been reported to accumulate in hepatic lesions of actual human liver diseases. The patients with chronic hepatitis caused by infection with hepatitis C virus (HCV), which by itself is not cytopathic for liver parenchymal cells (unlike hepatocytopathic hepatitis A virus), have increased numbers of activated Kupffer cells and elevated IL-18 and IFN-γ levels in their liver (244). Although the role of accumulated IL-18 in the liver of patients with chronic HCV hepatitis is unclear, the levels of IFN-γ in their liver specimen are well correlated with those of IL-18, suggesting a role of IL-18 in upregulating Th1-mediated intrahepatic immune response in chronic HCV hepatitis (244). IL-18 also plays a role in progressive inflammation in bilialy atresia (245). The liver specimens from the patients with bilialy atresia contain increased numbers of activated Kupffer cells. In addition, their serum IL-18 levels are elevated. Interestingly, after liver transplantation, serum levels of IL-18 are downregulated. Thus, as expected from early studies, IL-18 appears to play a role in human liver injury.

Graft-Versus-Host Disease (GVHD)   Although bone marrow transplantation is a potent therapeutic for malignant hematological disorder, incidentally occurring acute GVHD (aGVHD) still represents a major side effect that causes fatal tissue damage to the gastrointestinal tract, liver, and skin (246). aGVHD is mediated by grafted T cells after their development into Th1 cells and alloreactive CTLs, presumably initiated by endogenous IL-12 and TNF-α, respectively (247, 248). Indeed, both CD4$^+$ and CD8$^+$ T cells from aGVHD mice produce potent cytocidal molecules, IFN-γ and FasL, leading to severe tissue injury. IL-18, an upstream cytokine for both IFN-γ and FasL, is upregulated in patients with aGVHD (249–251). Serum IL-18 levels parallel the disease activity, providing us with IL-18 as a good diagnostic indicator for aGVHD (249). Further study is needed to conclude that IL-18, like IL-12 (246), also participates in the initiation of the disease.

By contrast, chronic GVHD (cGVHD) is a systemic autoimmune disease. cGVHD is characterized by the accumulation of autoantibodies and upregulated serum levels of IgG1 and IgE in association with Th2 polarization of alloreactive T cells (252). IL-12 has the potential to convert cGVHD into aGVHD (253). Like IL-12, exogenous IL-18 also inhibits cGVHD by induction of IFN-γ and, with IL-12, synergistically inhibits in vitro IgG1 production by causing both T cells and B cells to produce IFN-γ (254). It is important that exogenous IL-18 inhibits cGVHD-induced upregulation of IgE and IgG1 levels as well as elevation of serum IgG antinuclear Abs, possibly by induction of donor-derived anti-host CTLs and IFN-γ production, without causing a GVHD-like syndrome reported for IL-12 treatment (253, 255). We need further study to know how endogenous IL-18 is involved in the initiation and development of aGVHD and how exogenous IL-18 determines the development of alloreactive Th1 cells in cGVHD.

Crohn's Disease   Crohn's disease is a chronic inflammatory disorder characterized by granulomatous inflammation in the gastrointestinal tract. The lesions of Crohn's disease are characterized by Th1-deviated T cells and accumulation of IL-12 (256–258). A recent short-term study of chimeric monoclonal Ab against TNF-α disclosed a significant efficacy of this Ab for induction of remission from the active stage in patients, suggesting an important role of TNF-α in development of this disease (259). Recently, IL-18 expression has been reported in association with active caspase-1 in lesions of patients with Crohn's disease, by studies with RT-PCR, immunochemistry, Western blotting, and functional assay (260, 261).

Lamina propria mononuclear cells freshly isolated from the lesions of Crohn's disease patients expressed a high amount of IL-18 mRNA.

Immunohistochemically, IL-18 is expressed in scattered inflammatory cells, including macrophages (histiocytes) and mononuclear cells, in the lamina propria. Immunoblotting assay reveals an active form of IL-18 in the lesions. In addition to upregulation of active IL-18, an active form of caspase-1 was observed in lesions of Crohn's disease, suggesting possible accumulation of active IL-18 through processing by active caspase-1. Mucosal macrophages from the lesions have capacity to release several kinds of cytokines, including IL-12, IL-18, IL-1, and TNF-α (262). IL-18 as well as IL-12 was also located in lesions of a mouse colitis model, in HLA-B27/β2 microglobulin transgenic mice (263). More recently, direct evidence has demonstrated involvement of IL-18 in colitis (264, 265). Daily treatment with IL-18 and IL-12 induces severe body weight loss accompanied by diarrhea, hemorrhagic colitis, and mortality in mice. Besides these adverse effects, these mice also manifested splenomegaly, fatty liver, and thymic atrophy (265). Although most of these symptoms are similar to those in LPS-induced lethal mice, IL-18/IL-12-treated mice did not show increased serum levels of TNF-α, a molecule causing lethality in LPS-treated mice (265). Induction of fatty liver was abrogated in IFN-γ-deficient mice, the majority of which showed mortality and severe pulmonary edema (265). The depletion of T cells and NK cells does not prevent IL-18/IL-12-induced weight loss, indicating that the effect of these cytokines does not require either T cells or NK cells (264). Recently, IFN-γ was shown to be only partly involved in colitis induced by hapten (266). Both wild-type mice and IFN-γ R1-deficient mice lose equivalent amounts of body weight after induction of hapten colitis. Histological features of hapten-induced colitis in IFN-γ R1-deficient mice are comparable to those in wild-type mice. Therefore, IL-18 appears to play a role in the development of inflammatory bowel diseases.

Systemic Inflammatory Disease   Sepsis is still a fatal disease occasionally following severe illness, such as malignant tumor, open thoracic surgery, and trauma. LPS produced by all Gram-negative bacteria activates macrophages to release cytokines that are potentially lethal. Recently, IL-18 was demonstrated to be involved in the determination of lethality in systemic endotoxemia (267). When wild-type mice were given a high dose of LPS from *Escherichia coli* (*E. coli*) or *Salmonella typhimurium* (*S. typhimurium*), all the mice died within 5 days after challenge. However, pretreatment with neutralizing anti-IL-18 completely protected mice from the mortality caused by the administration of LPS from *E. coli* and partly from mortality from *S. typhimurium*. Anti-IL-18 treatment reduced neutrophil accumulation in liver or lung in both cases. Interestingly, the mechanism underlying protection by anti-IL-18 was distinct in part. Anti-IL-18 suppressed the serum increase of IFN-γ but not TNF-α, levels by *E. coli* LPS challenge, whereas the inverse effect was observed in the case of challenge by *S. typhimurium* LPS. IL-18-deficient mice showed reduced response to LPS-induced lethality (268). In LPS-injected IL-18-deficient mice, IFN-γ production was abrogated, whereas induction of TNF-α, and IL-12 was not affected, suggesting the importance of IL-18 in LPS-induced IFN-γ production and lethality. This study's results appeared to conflict with the experimental results shown by Sakao et al (238). They reported that IL-18-deficient mice were highly susceptible to lethality induced by sequential administration of heat-killed *P. acnes* and *E. coli* LPS. Although the outcome after LPS administration is quite different between these two models, the role of IL-18 after LPS challenge is equivalent in both models. IL-18 has two different aspects in *P. acnes*/LPS-induced lethal shock. IL-18 in the priming phase induced by *P. acnes* treatment downregulates the sensitivity of *P. acnes*-primed mice to LPS, although the mechanism is unknown. In contrast, IL-18 in LPS phase upregulates host inflammatory response to LPS (238). Therefore, IL-18 may act in two distinct roles, as angel or devil, in the *P. acnes* priming phase and the LPS challenge phase, respectively.

CNS regulates systemic inflammatory responses to LPS through humoral mechanisms. A recent study indicates that acetylcholine, the principal vagal neurotransmitter, significantly attenuates the release of TNF, IL-1β, IL-6, and IL-18, but not the anti-inflammatory cytokine IL-10, in LPS-stimulated human macrophage cultures. Furthermore, direct electrical stimulation of the peripheral vagus nerve in vivo during lethal endotoxemia in rats inhibited TNF synthesis in liver, attenuated peak serum TNF amounts, and prevented the development of shock, indicating the presence of a parasympathetic anti-inflammatory pathway by which CNS modulates systemic inflammatory responses to LPS (269).

Allergic Disorders   Asthma is a chronic inflammatory airway disease characterized by local infiltration with allergen-specific Th2 cells. CD4$^+$ T cells accumulated in the inflammatory lesion play a role in promoting the disease by production of Th2 cytokines (270). Atopic asthma is induced in Ag-sensitized mice by nasal challenge with the same Ag. Hofstra et al have shown that IL-12/IL-18 treatment can inhibit the development of Th2 cells, which is associated with decreased IgE levels, inhibition of airway hyperresponsiveness, and eosinophilic infiltration in a mouse model of allergic asthma (271). Recently, new therapeutic approaches have been introduced, such as oligodeoxynucleotides containing CpG motifs, chitin particles composed by N-acetyl-D-glucosamine polymer, and heat-killed *Listeria monocytogenes*, a Gram-positive intracellular bacterium (272–274). These substances exert their actions by means of endogenous upregulation of IL-12 and IL-18, as we have suggested (33). Taken together, IL-12 plus IL-18 is a powerful combination in treatment to prevent IgE production in vivo.

However, very recently, IL-18 has been demonstrated to play complicated roles in this murine asthma model. Deletion of IL-18 by continuous administration of neutralizing anti-IL-18 before sensitization with Ag or by genetically homologous recombination results in elevated levels of pulmonary-infiltrated eosinophils, an important indicator of disease activity (275, 276). Furthermore, administration of IL-18 at times of nasal challenges into IL-18-deficient mice reduced the number of eosinophils in the lung (275). However, intratracheal administration of IL-18 at nasal challenge enhanced eosinophil infiltration in the pulmonary lesion through induction of eotaxin, a potent chemotactic factor for eosinophils, accompanied by the elevation of Th2 cytokine expression in the lung (152, 276, 277). Moreover, administration of IL-18 during sensitization with Ag induced increases in serum levels of Ag-specific IgE and in Th2 cytokine production by Ag-specific splenocytes, as compared to mice not treated with IL-18 (152). Although IL-18 administered intraperitoneally at challenge reduces eosinophils (276), IL-18 administered intratracheally increases eosinophils (152). Furthermore, our recent study indicates that atopic patients have high levels of IL-18 in their sera (T Tanaka et al, unpublished observation). Thus, IL-18 plays an important role in induction of allergic disorders, although it may play distinct roles depending on its immunological environment and the route of administration in atopic asthma.

Others   IL-18 has been shown to be involved in skin diseases. Keratinocytes express IL-18 as well as IL-1β but lack caspase-1 under normal conditions (69, 70). They secrete biologically active IL-18 when stimulated by the contact sensitizer, dinitrochlorobenzene, in association with the activation of caspase-1 (153). IL-18 locally secreted may induce IFN-γ production from the dendritic epidermal T cells (278), particularly in collaboration with IL-12 produced by Langerhans cells (279), presumably leading to inflammatory skin reaction (278). Recently, IL-18 was also shown to be involved in cutaneous wound repair (280).

IL-18 levels are upregulated in the lesions of osteoarthritis. Osteoarthritis is an inflammatory disease in the joint, in which IL-1β is demonstrated to be a major catabolic cytokine responsible for articular destruction (281). Recently, IL-18 was demonstrated to be also involved in the pathogenesis of this disease (282). Articular chondrocytes isolated from healthy organ donors can secrete biologically active IL-18 in response to IL-1β that induces activation of caspase-1 (283). IL-18 inhibits TGF-β-induced proliferation of chondrocytes and upregulates expression of effector molecules such as NO, cyclooxygenase, IL-6, and stromelysin, and it increases glycosaminoglycans release in vitro (283). The joint lesion of osteoarthritis reveals colocalization of active caspase-1 and IL-18 as well as IL-1β, suggesting a possible role of IL-18 in the development of osteoarthritis (282). Although IL-18 acts as a proinflammatory cytokine, it also plays somewhat complicated roles; IL-18 directly suppressed angiogenesis (199) and inhibited osteoclast formation through GM-CSF production (73). Thus, IL-18 is deeply involved in bone metabolism.

IL-12 upregulates the production of vascular permeability factor (VPF), a candidate causing minimal-change nephrotic syndrome (284). Recently, IL-18 was reported to selectively increase the production of VPF from T cells synergistically with IL-12. T cells from symptomatic patients with minimal-change nephrotic syndrome produced much more VPF than those from healthy individuals and from asymptomatic patients, suggesting a possible involvement of overproduction of VPF, induced by IL-12 and IL-18, in this nephrotic syndrome (284, 285).

Hemorrhage and endotoxemia are important risk factors for the development of acute lung injury. IL-18 was recently shown to be involved in acute lung injury (286). IL-18 mRNA is increased in the lung after hemorrhage or endotoxemia. However, IL-18 protein, IL-12 mRNA, and caspase-1 expression are detectable only in the case of endotoxemia but not of hemorrhage, although both treatments induce IFN-γ expression in the liver, suggesting that IL-18 might play a role in modulating the development of acute lung injury after endotoxemia but not after hemorrhage (286).

PERSPECTIVES

IL-18 was discovered as a factor that induces IFN-γ production from Th1 cells. But IL-18, without help from IL-12, induces Th2 cells by induction of IL-4 production from naive T cells. Thus, IL-18 has the potential to stimulate both Th1 and Th2 responses. IL-18 is unique because it produces completely opposite effects depending on the presence or absence of IL-12. The molecular mechanism of the synergistic induction of IFN-γ by IL-12 and IL-18 as well as IL-18-mediated IL-4 production needs to be elucidated. Such elucidation will provide us a novel and powerful tool to control the Th1/Th2 balance at the transcriptional level. Because IL-18 is synthesized as a precursor molecule that becomes active after cleavage with caspase-1 or caspase-1-like enzymes, these converting enzymes might be useful therapeutic targets. The exponential increase in the number of publications concerning IL-18 since its discovery five years ago suggests the importance of IL-18 not only in the immune system but also in other systems such as the endocrine, nervous, and vascular systems.

ACKNOWLEDGMENTS

These studies are supported by a Hitech Research Center grant and by grants including those for scientific research on priority areas (367, 386) from the Ministry of Education, Science and Culture of Japan. The authors express our sincere thanks to Drs. Shizuo Akira, Hitoshi Mizutani, and William E. Paul for their great help in all stages of the work and to Hayashibara Biochemical Laboratories for providing us with reagents.

Visit the Annual Reviews home page at www.AnnualReviews.org

LITERATURE CITED

1. Okamura H, Tsutsui H, Komatsu T, Yutsudo M, Hakura A, Tanimoto T, Torigoe K, Okura T, Nukada Y, Hattori K, et al. 1995. Cloning of a new cytokine that induces IFN-γ production by T cells. *Nature* 378:88–91

2. Okamura H, Nagata K, Komatsu T, Tanimoto T, Nukata Y, Tanabe F, Akita K, Torigoe K, Okura T, Fukuda S. 1995. A novel costimulatory factor for gamma interferon induction found in the liver of mice causes

endotoxic shock. *Infect. Immun.* 63:3966–72

3. Okamura H, Tsutsui H, Kashiwamura S, Yoshimoto T, Nakanishi K. 1998. Interleukin-18: a novel cytokine that augments both innate and acquired immunity. *Adv. Immunol.* 70:281–312

4. Okamura H, Kashiwamura S, Tsutsui H, Yoshimoto T, Nakanishi K. 1998. Regulation of interferon-γ production by IL-12 and IL-18. *Curr. Opin. Immunol.* 10:259–64

5. Dinarello CA, Novick D, Puren AJ, Fantuzzi G, Shapiro L, Muhl H, Yoon DY, Reznikov LL, Kim SH, Rubinstein M. 1998. Overview of interleukin-18: more than an interferon-gamma inducing factor. *J. Leukoc. Biol.* 63:658–64

6. Fantuzzi G, Dinarello CA. 1999. Interleukin-18 and interleukin-1β: two cytokine substrates for ICE (caspase-1). *J. Clin. Immunol.* 19:1–11

7. Dinarello CA. 1998. Interleukin-1, interleukin-1 receptors and interleukin-1 receptor antagonist. *Int. Rev. Immunol.* 16:457–99

8. Dinarello CA. 1999. IL-18: a Th1-inducing, proinflammatory cytokine and new member of the IL-1 family. *J. Allergy Clin. Immunol.* 103:11–24

9. Dinarello CA. 1999. Interleukin-18. *Methods* 19:123–32

10. Tsutsui H, Matsui K, Okamura H, Nakanishi K. 2000. Pathophysiological roles of interleukin-18 for inflammatory liver diseases. *Immunol. Rev.* 174:192–209

11. Akira S. 2000. The role of IL-18 in innate immunity. *Curr. Opin. Immunol.* 12:59–63

12. Nakanishi K, Yoshimoto T, Kashiwamura S-I, Tsutsui H, Okamura H. 2000. Potentiality of interleukin-18 as a useful reagent for the treatment of infectious diseases. In *Cytokine Therapeutics in Infectious Diseases*, ed. SM Holland. Philadelphia: Lippincott Williams & Wilkins. In press

13. Nakanishi K, Yoshimoto T, Tsutsui H, Okamura H. 2000. Interleukin-18 is a unique cytokine that stimulates both Th1 and Th2 responses depending on its cytokine milieu. *Cytokine Growth Factor Rev.* In press

14. Gu Y, Kuida K, Tsutsui H, Ku G, Hsiao K, Fleming MA, Hayashi N, Higashino K, Okamura H, Nakanishi K, Kurimoto M, Tanimoto T, Flavell RA, Sato V, Harding MW, Livingston DJ, Su MS. 1997. Activation of interferon-γ inducing factor mediated by interleukin-1β converting enzyme. *Science* 275:206–9

15. Ghayur T, Banerjee S, Hugunin M, Butler D, Herzog L, Carter A, Quintal L, Sekut L, Talanian R, Paskind M, Wong W, Kamen R, Tracey D, Allen H. 1997. Caspase-1 processes IFN-γ-inducing factor and regulates LPS-induced IFN-γ production. *Nature* 386:619–23

16. Tsutsui H, Kayagaki N, Kuida K, Nakano H, Hayashi N, Takeda K, Matsui K, Kashiwamura S-I, Hada T, Akira S, Yagita H, Okamura H, Nakanishi K. 1999. Caspase-1-independent, Fas/Fas ligand-mediated IL-18 secretion from macrophages causes acute liver injury in mice. *Immunity* 11:359–67

17. Dinarello CA. 1996. Biologic basis for interleukin-1 in disease. *Blood* 87:2095–2147

18. Miwa K, Asano M, Horai R, Iwakura Y, Nagata S, Suda T. 1998. Caspase-1-independent IL-1β release and inflammation induced by the apoptosis inducer Fas ligand. *Nat. Med.* 4:1287–92

19. Torigoe K, Ushio S, Okura T, Kobayashi S, Taniai M, Kunikata T, Murakami T, Sanou O, Kojima H, Fujii M, Ohta T, Ikeda M, Ikegami H, Kurimoto M. 1997. Purification and characterization of the human interleukin-18 receptor. *J. Biol. Chem.* 272:25737–42

20. Hoshino K, Tsutsui H, Kawai T, Takeda K, Nakanishi K, Takeda Y, Akira S. 1999. Generation of IL-18 receptor-deficient mice: evidence for IL-1 receptor-related

protein as an essential IL-18 binding receptor. *J. Immunol.* 162:5041–44

21. Kojima H, Takeuchi M, Ohta T, Nishida Y, Arai N, Ikeda M, Ikegami H, Kurimoto M. 1998. Interleukin-18 activates the IRAK-TRAF6 pathway in mouse EL-4 cells. *Biochem. Biophys. Res. Commun.* 244:183–86

22. Okamura H, Tsutsui H, Kashiwamura S-I, Yoshimoto T, Nakanishi K. 2000. IL-18 receptor. In *The Cytokine Reference*, ed. JJ Oppenheim, M Feldmann, SK Duram, T Hirano, J Vilcek, NA Nicola, pp. 1065–9 London: Academic. In press

23. Born TL, Thomassen E, Bird TA, Sims JE. 1998. Cloning of a novel receptor subunit, AcPL, required for interleukin-18 signaling. *J. Biol. Chem.* 273:29445–50

24. O'Neill LA, Greene C. 1998. Signal transduction pathways activated by the IL-1 receptor family: ancient signaling machinery in mammals, insects, and plants. *J. Leukoc. Biol.* 63:650–57

25. Adachi O, Kawai T, Takeda K, Matsumoto M, Tsutsui H, Sakagami M, Nakanishi K, Akira S. 1998. Targeted disruption of the MyD88 gene results in loss of IL-1- and IL-18-mediated function. *Immunity* 9:143–50

26. Hoshino K, Takeuchi O, Kawai T, Sanjo H, Ogawa T, Takeda Y, Takeda K, Akira S. 1999. Toll-like receptor 4 (TLR4)-deficient mice are hyporesponsive to lipopolysaccharide: evidence for TLR4 as the *Lps* gene product. *J. Immunol.* 162:3749–52

27. Kawai T, Adachi O, Ogawa T, Takeda K, Akira S. 1999. Unresponsiveness of MyD88-deficient mice to endotoxin. *Immunity* 11:115–22

28. Takeuchi O, Hoshino K, Kawai T, Sanjo H, Takada H, Ogawa T, Takeda K, Akira S. 1999. Differential roles of TLR2 and TLR4 in recognition of Gram-negative and Gram-positive bacterial cell wall components. *Immunity* 11:443–51

29. Takeuchi O, Takeda K, Hoshino K, Adachi O, Ogawa T, Akira S. 2000. Cellular responses to bacterial cell wall components are mediated through MyD88-dependent signaling cascades. *Int. Immunol.* 12:113–17

30. Kanakaraj P, Ngo K, Wu Y, Angulo A, Ghazal P, Harris CA, Siekierka JJ, Peterson PA, Fung LW. 1999. Defective interleukin (IL)-18-mediated natural killer and T helper cell type 1 responses in IL-1 receptor-associated kinase (IRAK)-deficient mice. *J. Exp. Med.* 189:1129–38

31. Swantek JL, Tsen MF, Cobb MH, Thomas JA. 2000. IL-1 Receptor-associated kinase modulates host responsiveness to endotoxin. *J. Immunol.* 164:4301–6

32. O'Neill LA, Dinarello CA. 2000. The IL-1 receptor/toll-like receptor superfamily: crucial receptors for inflammation and host defense. *Immunol. Today* 21:206–9

33. Yoshimoto T, Okamura H, Tagawa YI, Iwakura Y, Nakanishi K. 1997. Interleukin 18 together with interleukin 12 inhibits IgE production by induction of interferon-γ production from activated B cells. *Proc. Natl. Acad. Sci. USA* 94:3948–53

34. Yoshimoto T, Takeda K, Tanaka T, Ohkusu K, Kashiwamura S, Okamura H, Akira S, Nakanishi K. 1998. IL-12 up-regulates IL-18 receptor expression on T cells, Th1 cells, and B cells: synergism with IL-18 for IFN-γ production. *J. Immunol.* 161:3400–7

35. Okamura H, Tsutsui H, Kashiwamura S-I, Yoshimoto T, Nakanishi K. 2000. Interleukin 18. In *The Cytokine Reference*, ed. JJ Oppenheim, M Feldmann, SK Duram, T Hirano, J Vilcek, NA Nicola, pp. 337–50. London: Academic. In press

36. Fukao T, Matsuda S, Koyasu S. 2000. Synergistic effects of IL-4 and IL-18 on IL-12-dependent IFN-γ production by dendritic cells. *J. Immunol.* 164:64–71

37. Hoshino T, Wiltrout RH, Young HA. 1999. IL-18 is a potent coinducer of IL-13 in NK and T cells: a new potential role for IL-18 in modulating the immune response. *J. Immunol.* 162:5070–77

38. Yoshimoto T, Mizutani H, Tsutsui H, Noben-Trauth N, Yamanaka K, Tanaka M, Izumi S, Okamura H, Paul WE, Nakanishi K. 2000. IL-18 induction of IgE: dependence on CD4$^+$ T cells, IL-4 and STAT6. *Nat. Immunol.* 1:132–37

39. Yoshimoto T, Tsutsui H, Tominaga K, Hoshino K, Okamura H, Akira S, Paul WE, Nakanishi K. 1999. IL-18, although antiallergic when administered with IL-12, stimulates IL-4 and histamine release by basophils. *Proc. Natl. Acad. Sci. USA.* 96:13962–66

40. Farrar M, Schreiber R. 1993. The molecular cell biology of interferon-γ and its receptor. *Annu. Rev. Immunol.* 11:571–93

41. Wada M, Okamura H, Nagata K, Shimoyama T, Kawada Y. 1985. Cellular mechanisms *in vivo* production of gamma interferon induced by lipopolysaccharide in mice infected with *Mycobacterium bovis* BCG. *J. Interferon Res.* 5:431–43

42. Yoshimoto T, Nakanishi K, Hirose K, Hiroishi K, Okamura H, Takemoto Y, Kanamaru A, Hada T, Tamura T, Kakishita E, Higashino K. 1992. High serum IL-6 level reflects susceptible status of the host to endotoxin and IL-1/tumor necrosis factor. *J. Immunol.* 148:3596–3603

43. Tsutsui H, Mizoguchi Y, Morisawa S. 1992. Importance of direct hepatocytolysis by liver macrophages in experimental fulminant hepatitis. *Hepato-Gastroenterology* 39:553–59

44. Trinchieri G. 1995. Interleukin-12: a proinflammatory cytokine with immunoregulatory functions that bridge innate resistance and antigen-specific and adaptive immunity. *Annu. Rev. Immunol.* 13:251–76

45. Ushio S, Namba M, Okura T, Hattori K, Nukada Y, Akita K, Tanabe F, Konishi K, Micallef M, Fujii M, Torigoe K, Tanimoto T, Fukuda S, Ikeda M, Okamura H, Kurimoto M. 1996. Cloning of the cDNA for human IFN-γ-inducing factor, expression in *Escherichia coli*, and studies on the biologic activities of the protein. *J. Immunol.* 156:4274–79

46. Bazan JF, Timans JC, Kastelein RA. 1996. A newly defined interleukin-1? *Nature* 379:591

47. Matsui K, Yoshimoto T, Tsutsui H, Hyodo Y, Hayashi N, Hiroishi K, Kawada N, Okamura H, Nakanishi K, Higashino K. 1997. *Propionibacterium acnes* treatment diminishes CD4$^+$ NK1.1$^+$ T cells but induces type I T cells in the liver by induction of IL-12 and IL-18 production from Kupffer cells. *J. Immunol.* 159:97–106

48. Tsutsui H, Matsui K, Kawada N, Hyodo Y, Hayashi N, Okamura H, Higashino K, Nakanishi K. 1997. IL-18 accounts for both TNF-α- and Fas ligand-mediated hepatotoxic pathways in endotoxin-induced liver injury in mice. *J. Immunol.* 159:3961–67

49. Tone M, Thompson SA, Tone Y, Fairchild PJ, Waldmann H. 1997. Regulation of IL-18 (IFN-γ-inducing factor) gene expression. *J. Immunol.* 159:6156–63

50. Kim Y-M, Kang H-S, Paik S-G, Pyun K-H, Anderson KL, Torbett BE, Choi I. 1999. Roles of IFN consensus sequence binding protein and PU.1 in regulating IL-18 gene expression. *J. Immunol.* 163:2000–7

51. Nelson Y, Kannno Y, Hong C, Contursi C, Fujita T, Fowlkes BJ, O'Connell E, Hu-Li J, Paul WE, Jankovic D. 1996. Expression of IFN regulatory factor family proteins in lymphocytes. Induction of Stat-1 and IFN consensus sequence binding protein expression by T cell activation. *J. Immunol.* 156:3711–20

52. Sharf R, Meraro D, Azriel A, Thornton AM, Ozato K, Petricoin EF, Larner AC, Schaper F, Hauser H, B-ZL 1997. Phosphorylation events modulate the ability of interferon consensus sequence binding protein to interact with interferon regulatory factors and to bind DNA. *J. Biol. Chem.* 272:9785–92

53. Trinchieri G. 1998. Interleukin-12; a cytokine at the interface of inflammation and immunity. *Adv. Immunol.* 70:83–243
54. Wu C-Y, Maeda H, Contursi C, Ozato K, Seder RA. 1999. Differential requirement of IFN consensus sequence binding protein for the production of IL-12 and induction of Th1-type cells in response to IFN-γ. *J. Immunol.* 162:807–12
55. Moulton KS, Semple K, Wu H, Glass CK. 1994. Cell-specific expression of the macrophage scavenger receptor gene is dependent on PU.1 and a composite AP-1/ets motif. *Mol. Cell. Biol.* 14:4408–18
56. Borras FE, Loberas J, Maki RA, Celada A. 1995. Repression of I-Aβ gene expression by the transcription factor PU.1. *J. Biol. Chem.* 270:24385–91
57. Shackelford R, Adams DO, Johnson SP. 1995. IFN-γ and lipopolysaccharide induce DNA binding of transcription factor PU.1 in murine tissue macrophages. *J. Immunol.* 154:1374–82
58. Cosman D. 1987. Control of messenger RNA stability. *Immunol. Today* 8:16–18
59. Nolan K, Greaves D, Waldmann H. 1998. The human interleukin 18 gene IL-18 maps to 11q22.2-q22.3, closely linked to the DRD2 gene locus and distinct from mapped IDDM loci. *Genomics* 51:161–63
60. Rothe H, Jenkins NA, Copeland NG, Kolb H. 1997. Active stage of autoimmune diabetes is associated with the expression of a novel cytokine, IGIF, which is located near *Idd2*. *J. Clin. Invest.* 99:469–74
61. Fantuzzi G, Puren AJ, Harding MW, Livingston DJ, Dinarello CA. 1998. Interleukin-18 regulation of interferon-γ production and cell proliferation as shown in interleukin-1β-converting enzyme (caspase-1)-deficient mice. *Blood* 91:2118–25
62. Bohn E, Sing A, Zumbihl R, Bielfeldt C, Okamura H, Kurimoto M, Heesemann J, Autenrieth IB. 1998. IL-18 (IFN-γ-inducing factor) regulates early cytokine production in, and promotes resolution of, bacterial infection in mice. *J. Immunol.* 160:299–307
63. Shibata Y, Foster LA, Kurimoto M, Okamura H, Nakamura RM, Kawajiri K, Justice JP, Van SM, Myrvik QN, Metzger WJ. 1998. Immunoregulatory roles of IL-10 in innate immunity: IL-10 inhibits macrophage production of IFNγ -inducing factors but enhances NK cell production of IFN-γ. *J. Immunol.* 161:4283–88
64. Sanchez-Bueno A, Verkhusha V, Tanaka Y, Takikawa O, Yoshida R. 1996. Interferon-γ-dependent expression of inducible nitric oxide synthase, interleukin-12, and interferon-γ-inducing factor in macrophages elicited by allografted tumor cells. *Biochem. Biophys. Res. Commun.* 224:555–63
65. Conti B, Park LC, Calingasan NY, Kim Y, Kim H, Bae Y, Gilson G, Joh TH. 1999. Cultures of astrocytes and microglia express interleukin 18. *Brain Res. Mol. Brain. Res.* 67:46–52
66. Prinz M, Hanisch UK. 1999. Murine microglial cells produce and respond to interleukin-18. *J. Neurochem.* 72:2215–18
67. Puren AJ, Fantuzzi G, Dinarello CA. 1999. Gene expression, synthesis, and secretion of interleukin 18 and interleukin 1β are differentially regulated in human blood mononuclear cells and mouse spleen cells. *Proc. Natl. Acad. Sci. USA* 96:2256–61
68. Stoll S, Jonuleit H, Schmitt E, Muller G, Yamauchi H, Kurimoto M, Knop J, Enk AH. 1998. Production of functional IL-18 by different subtypes of murine and human dendritic cells (DC): DC-derived IL-18 enhances IL-12-dependent Th1 development. *Eur. J. Immunol.* 28:3231–39
69. Stoll S, Muller G, Kurimoto M, Saloga J, Tanimoto T, Yamauchi H, Okamura H, Knop J, Enk AH. 1997. Production of IL-18 (IFN-γ-inducing factor) messenger RNA and functional protein by murine keratinocytes. *J. Immunol.* 159:298–302
70. Mizutani H, Black R, Kupper TS. 1991. Human keratinocytes produce but do not

process pro-interleukin-1 (IL-1) β. *J. Clin. Invest.* 87:1066–71

71. Takeuchi M, Nishizaki Y, Sano O, Ohta T, Ikeda M, Kurimoto M. 1997. Immunohistochemical and immuno-electron-microscopic detection of interferon-γ-inducing factor (interleukin-18) in mouse intestinal epithelial cells. *Cell Tissue Res.* 289:499–507

72. Cameron LA, Taha RA, Tsicopoulos A, Kurimoto M, Olivenstein R, Wllaert B, Minshall EM, Hamid QA. 1999. Airway epithelium expresses interleukin-18. *Eur. Respir. J.* 14:553–59

73. Udagawa N, Horwood NJ, Elliott J, Mackay A, Owens J, Okamura H, Kurimoto M, Chambers TJ, Martin TJ, Gillespie MT. 1997. Interleukin-18 (interferon-γ-inducing factor) is produced by osteoblasts and acts *via* granulo-cyte/macrophage colony-stimulating factor and not *via* interferon-γ to inhibit osteoclast formation. *J. Exp. Med.* 185:1005–12

74. Conti B, Jahng JW, Tinti C, Son JH, Joh TH. 1997. Induction of interferon-γ inducing factor in the adrenal cortex. *J. Biol. Chem.* 272:2035–37

75. Conti B, Sugama S, Kim Y, Tinti C, Kim H, Baker H, Volpe B, Attardi B, Joh T. 2000. Modulation of IL-18 production in the adrenal cortex following acute ACTH or chronic corticosterone treatment. *Neuroimmunomodulation* 8:1–7

76. Wheeler RD, Culhane AC, Hall MD, Pickering-Brown S, Rothwell NJ, Luheshi GN. 2000. Detection of the interleukin 18 family in rat brain by RT-PCR. *Brain Res. Mol. Brain Res.* 77:290–93

77. Yamanaka K, Tanaka M, Tsutsui H, Kupper TS, Asahi K, Okamura H, Nakanishi K, Sazuki M, Kayagaki N, Black RA, Miller DK, Nakashima K, Shimizu M, Mizutani H. 2000. Skin-specific caspase-1 transgenic mice show cutaneous apoptosis and pre-endotoxin shock condition with a high serum level of IL-18. *J. Immunol.* 165:997–1003

78. Cerretti DP, Kozlosky CJ, Mosley B, Nelson N, Vaan Ness K, Greenstreet TA, March CJ, Kronheim SR, Druck T, Cannizzaro LA, Huebner K, Black RA. 1992. Molecular cloning of the interleukin-1β converting enzyme. *Science* 256:97–100

79. Singer II, Scott S, Chin J, Bayne EK, Limjuco G, Weidner J, Miller DK, Chapman K, Kostura MJ. 1995. The interleukin-1β-converting enzyme (ICE) is localized on the eternal cell surface membranes and in the cytoplasmic ground substance of human monocytes by immuno-electron microscopy. *J. Exp. Med.* 182:1447–59

80. Wang S, Miura M, Jung Y-K, Zhu H, Li E, Yuan J. 1998. Murine caspase-11, an ICE-interacting protease, is essential for the activation of ICE. *Cell* 92:501–9

81. Ramage P, Cheneval D, Chvei M, Graff P, Hemmig R, Heng R, Kocher HP, Mackenzie A, Memmert K, Revesz L, Wishart W. 1995. Expression, refolding, and autocatalytic proteolytic processing of the interleukin-1β-converting enzyme precursor. *J. Biol. Chem.* 270:9378–83

82. Schumann RR, Belka C, Reuter D, Lamping N, Kirschning CJ, Wever JR, Pfeil D. 1998. Lipopolysaccharide activates caspase-1 (interleukin-1-converting enzyme) in cultured monocytic and endothelial cells. *Blood* 91:577–84

83. Ulevitch RJ. 1999. Endotoxin opens the *Toll* gates to innate immunity. *Nat. Med.* 5:144–45

83a. Seki E, Tsutsui H, Nakano H, Tsuji NM, Hoshino K, Adachi O, Adachi K, Futatsugi S, Kuida K, Takeuchi O, Okamura H, Fujimoto J, Akira S, Nakanishi K. 2001. LPS induced IL-18 secretion from murine Kupffer cells independently of MyD88 that is critically involved in induction of production of IL-12 and IL-1β. *J. Immunol.* In press

84. Pirhonen J, Sareneve T, Kurimoto M, Julkunen I, Matikainen S. 1999. Virus

infection activates IL-1β and IL-18 production in human macrophages by a caspase-1-dependent pathway. *J. Immunol.* 162:7322–29

85. Akita K, Ohtsuki T, Nakada Y, Tanimoto T, Namba M, Okura T, Takakura-Yamamoto R, Torigoe K, Gu Y, -S. SMS, Jujii M, Satoh-Itoh M, Yamamoto K, Kohno K, Ikeda M, Kurimoto M. 1997. Involvement of caspase-1 and caspase-3 in the production and processing of mature human interleukin 18 in monocytic THP.1 cells. *J. Biol. Chem.* 272:26595–603

86. Kim YM, Talanian RV, Li J, Billiar TR. 1998. Nitric oxide prevents IL-1β and IFN-γ-inducing factor (IL-18) release from macrophages by inhibiting caspase-1 (IL-1β-converting enzyme). *J. Immunol.* 161:4122–28

87. Young JL, Sukhova GK, Foster D, Kisiel W, Libby P, Schonbeck U. 2000. The serpin proteinase inhibitor 9 is an endogenous inhibitor of interleukin-1β-converting enzyme (caspase-1) activity in human vascular smooth muscle cells. *J. Exp. Med.* 191:1535–44

88. Mayet W-J, Csernok E, Szymkowiak C, Gross WL, Myer zum Büschenfelde HK. 1993. Human endothelial cells express proteinase 3, the target antigen of anticytoplasmic antibodies in Wegener's granulomatosis. *Blood* 82:1221–29

89. Ernst CM, Schmitt W, Bainton DF, Gross WL. 1994. Activated neutrophils express proteinase 3 on their plasma membrane *in vitro* and *in vivo*. *Clin. Exp. Immunol.* 95:244–50

90. Bergenfeldt M, Axelsson L, Ohlsson K. 1992. Release of neutrophil proteinase 4 (3) and leukocyte elastase during phagocytosis and their interaction with proteinase inhibitors. *Scand. J. Clin. Lab. Invest.* 52:823–29

91. Henshaw TJ, Malone CC, Gabay JE, Williams JRC. 1994. Elevations of neutrophil proteinase 3 in serum of patients with Wegener's granulomatosis and polyarteritis nodosa. *Arthritis Rheum.* 37:104–12

92. Hashimoto C, Hudson KL, Anderson KV. 1988. The Toll gene of *Drosophila*, required for dorsal-ventral embryonic polarity, appears to encode a trans membrane protein. *Cell* 52:269–79

93. Lemaitre B, Reichhart JM, Hoffmann JA. 1997. *Drosophila* host defense: differential induction of antimicrobial peptide genes after infection by various classes of microorganisms. *Proc. Natl. Acad. Sci. USA* 94:14614–19

94. Muzio M, Natoli G, Saccani S, Levrero M, Mantovani A. 1998. The human toll signaling pathway: divergence of NF-κB and JNK/SAPK activation upstream of tumor necrosis factor-associated factor 6 (TRAF6). *J. Exp. Med.* 187:2097–2101

95. Medzhitov R, Preston-Hurburt P, Janeway CA Jr. 1998. Innate immunity: the virtues of a nonclonal system of recognition. *Cell* 91:295–98

96. Wong PMC, Kang A, Chen H, Yuan Q, Fan P, Sultzer BM, Kan YW, Chung S-C. 1999. Lps^d/Ran of endotoxin-resistant C3H/HeJ. mice is defective in mediating lipopolysaccharide endotoxin responses. *Proc. Natl. Acad. Sci. USA* 96:11543–48

97. Parnet P, Garka KE, Bonnet TP, Dower SK, Sim JE. 1996. IL-1RrP is a novel receptor-like molecule similar to the type I interleukin-1 receptor and its homologues T1/ST2 and IL-1R AcP. *J. Biol. Chem.* 271:3967–70

98. Hoshino K, Kashiwamura S, Kuribayashi K, Kodama T, Tsujimura T, Nakanishi K, Matsuyama T, Takeda K, Akira S. 1999. The absence of interleukin 1 receptor-related T1/ST2 does not affect T helper cell type 2 development and its effector function. *J. Exp. Med.* 190:1541–47

98a. Löhning M, Stroehmann A, Coyle AJ, Grogan JL, Lin S, Gutierrez-Ramos J-C, Levinson D, Radbruch A, Kamradt T. 1998. T1/ST2 is preferentially expressed on murine Th2 cells, independent of interleukin 4, interleukin 5, and interleukin 10, and important for Th2 effector function. *Proc. Natl. Acad. Sci. USA* 95:6930–35

98b. Xu D, Chan WL, Leung BP, Huang F-p, Wheeler R, Piedrafita D, Robinson JH, Liew FY. 1998. Selective expression of a stable cell surface molecule on type 2 but not type 1 helper T cells. *J. Exp. Med.* 187:787–94

98c. Chang JT, Segal BM, Nakanishi K, Okamura H, Shevach EM. 2000. The costimulatory effect of IL-18 on the induction of antigen-specific IFN-γ production by resting T cells is IL-12 dependent and is mediated by up-regulation of the IL-12 receptor β2 subunit. *Eur. J. Immunol.* 30:1113–19

99. Hyodo Y, Matsui K, Hayashi N, Tsutsui H, Kashiwamura S, Yamauchi H, Hiroishi K, Takeda K, Tagawa Y, Iwakura Y, Kayagaki N, Kurimoto M, Okamura H, Hada T, Yagita H, Akira S, Nakanishi K, Higashino K. 1999. IL-18 upregulates perforin-mediated NK activity without increasing perforin messenger RNA expression by binding to constitutively expressed IL-18 receptor. *J. Immunol.* 162:1662–68

100. Nakamura S, Otani T, Okura R, Ijiri Y, Motoda R, Kurimoto M, Orita K. 2000. Expression and responsiveness of human interleukin-18 receptor (IL-18R) on hematopoietic cell lines. *Leukemia* 14:1052–59

101. Novick D, Kim SH, Fantuzzi G, Reznikov LL, Dinarello CA, Rubinstein M. 1999. Interleukin-18 binding protein: a novel modulator of the Th1 cytokine response. *Immunity* 10:127–36

102. Aizawa Y, Akita K, Taniai M, Torigoe K, Mori T, Nishida Y, Ushio S, Nukada Y, Tanimoto T, Ikegami H, Ikeda M, Kurimoto M. 1999. Cloning and expression of interleukin-18 binding protein. *FEBS Lett.* 445:338–42

103. Reznikov LL, Kim S-H, Westcott JY, Frishman J, Fantuzzi G, Novick D, Rubinstein M, Dinarello CA. 2000. IL-18 binding protein increases spontaneous and IL-1-induced prostaglandin production *via* inhibition of IFN-γ. *Proc. Natl. Acad. Sci. USA* 97:2174–79

104. Kim S-H, Eisenstein M, Reznikov L, Fantuzzi G, Novick D, Rubinstein M, Dinarello CA. 2000. Structural requirements of six naturally occurring isoforms of the IL-18 binding protein to inhibit IL-18. *Proc. Natl. Acad. Sci. USA* 97:1190–95

105. Xiang Y, Moss B. 1999. IL-18 binding and inhibition of interferon γ induction by human poxvirus-encoded proteins. *Proc. Natl. Acad. Sci. USA* 96:11537–42

106. Born TL, Morrison LA, Esteban DJ, VandenBos T, Thebeau LG, Chen N, Spriggs MK, Sims JE, Buller RM. 2000. A poxvirus protein that binds to and inactivates IL-18, and inhibits NK cell response. *J. Immunol.* 164:3246–54

107. Smith VP, Bryant NA, Alcami A. 2000. Ectromelia, vaccinia and cowpox viruses encode secreted interleukin-18-binding proteins. *J. Gen. Virol.* 5:1223–30

108. Ray CA, Black RA, Kronheim SR, Greenstreet TA, Sleath PR, Salvesen GS, Pciup DJ. 1992. Viral inhibition of inflammation: cowpox virus encodes an inhibitor of the interleukin-1β converting enzyme. *Cell* 69:597–604

109. Robinson D, Shibuya K, Mui A, Zonin F, Murphy E, Sana T, Hartley SB, Menon S, Kastelein R, Bazan F, O'Garra A. 1997. IGIF does not drive Th1 development but synergizes with IL-12 for interferon-gamma production and activates IRAK and NF-κB. *Immunity* 7:571–81

110. Matsumoto S, Tsuji TK, Aizawa Y, Koide K, Takeuchi M, Ohta T, Kurimoto M. 1997. Interleukin-18 activates NF-κB in murine T helper type 1 cells. *Biochem. Biophys. Res. Commun.* 234:454–57

111. Thomas JA, Allen JL, Tsen M, Dubnicoff

T, Danao J, Liao XC, Cao Z, Wasserman SA. 1999. Impaired cytokine signaling in mice lacking the IL-1 receptor-associated kinase. *J. Immunol.* 163:978–84

112. Tsuji TK, Matsumoto S, Koide K, Takeuchi M, Ikeda M, Ohta T, Kurimoto M. 1997. Interleukin-18 induces activation and association of p56 (*lck*) and MAPK in a murine TH1 clone. *Biochem. Biophys. Res. Commun.* 237:126–30

113. Kalina U, Kauschat D, Koyama N, Nuernberger H, Ballas K, Koschmieder S, Bug G, Hofman W-K, Hoelzer D, Ottmann OG. 2000. IL-18 activates STAT3 in the natural killer cell line 92, augments cytotoxic activity, and mediates IFN-γ production by the stress kinase p38 and by the extracellular regulated kinases p44^{erk-1} and p42^{erk-21}. *J. Immunol.* 165:1307–13

114. Hoshino T, Yagita H, Ortldo RH, Young HA. 2000. *In vivo* administration of IL-18 can induce IgE production through Th2 cytokine induction and up-regulation of CD40 ligand (CD154) expression on CD4$^+$ T cells. *Eur. J. Immunol.* 30:1998–2006

115. Ahn HJ, Maruo S, Tomura M, Mu J, Hamaoka T, Nakanishi K, Clark S, Kurimoto M, Okamura H, Fujiwara H. 1997. A mechanism underlying synergy between IL-12 and IFN-γ-inducing factor in enhanced production of IFN-γ. *J. Immunol.* 159:2125–31

116. Tominaga K, Yoshimoto T, Torigoe K, Kurimoto M, Matsui K, Hada T, Okamura H, Nakanishi K. 2000. IL-12 synergizes with IL-18 or IL-1β for IFN-γ production from human T cells. *Int. Immunol.* 12:151–60

117. Yang J, Murphy TL, Ouyang W, Murphy KM. 1999. Induction of interferon-γ production in Th1 CD4$^+$ T cells: evidence for two distinct pathways for promoter activation. *Eur. J. Immunol.* 29:548–55

118. Tomura M, Zhou XY, Maruo S, Ahn HJ, Hamaoka T, Okamura H, Nakanishi K, Tanimoto T, Kurimoto M, Fujiwara H.

1998. A critical role for IL-18 in the proliferation and activation of NK1.1$^+$ CD3$^-$ cells. *J. Immunol.* 160:4738–46

119. Hunter CA, Timans J, Pisacane P, Menon S, Cai G, Walker W, Aste AM, Chizzonite R, Bazan JF, Kastelein RA. 1997. Comparison of the effects of interleukin-1α, interleukin-1β and interferon-γ-inducing factor on the production of interferon-γ by natural killer. *Eur. J. Immunol.* 27:2787–92

120. Tsutsui H, Nakanishi K, Matsui K, Higashino H, Okamura Y, Miyazawa Kaneda K. 1996. Interferon-γ-inducing factor up-regulates Fas ligand-mediated cytotoxic activity of murine natural killer cell clones. *J. Immunol.* 157:3967–73

121. Fantuzzi G, Reed DA, Dinarello CA. 1999. IL-12-induced IFN-γ is dependent on caspase-1 processing of the IL-18 precursor. *J. Clin. Invest.* 104:761–67

122. Barbulescu K, Becker C, Schlaak JF, Schmitt E, Meyer zum Büschenfelde K, Neurath MF. 1998. IL-12 and IL-18 differentially regulate the transcriptional activity of the human IFN-γ promoter in primary CD4$^+$ T lymphocytes. *J. Immunol.* 160:3642–47

123. Leite-de-Moraes MC, Hameg A, Arnould A, Machavoine F, Koezuka Y, Schneider E, Herbelin A, Dy M. 1999. A distinct IL-18-induced pathway to fully activate NK T lymphocytes independently from TCR engagement. *J. Immunol.* 163:5871–76

124. Kunikata T, Torigoe K, Ushio S, Okura T, Ushio C, Yamauchi H, Ikeda M, Ikegami H, Kurimoto M. 1998. Constitutive and induced IL-18 receptor expression by various peripheral blood cell subsets as determined by anti-hIL-18R monoclonal antibody. *Cell Immunol.* 189:135–43

125. Sica A, Dorman L, Viggiano V, Cippitelli M, Ghosh P, Rice N, Young HA. 1997. Interaction of NF-κB and NFAT with the interferon-γ promoter. *J. Biol. Chem.* 272:30412–20

126. Xu X, Sun Y-L, Hoey T. 1996. Co-operative DNA binding and sequence-selective recognition conferred by the STAT amino-terminal domain. *Science* 273:794–97

127. Szabo SJ, Jacobson NG, Dighe AS, Gubler U, Murphy KM. 1995. Developmental commitment to the Th2 lineage by extinction of IL-12 signaling. *Immunity* 2:665–75

128. Thomassen E, Bird TA, Renshaw BR, Kennedy MK, Sims JE. 1998. Binding of interleukin-18 to the interleukin-1 receptor homologous receptor IL-1RrP1 leads to activation of signaling pathways similar to those used by interleukin-1. *J. Interferon Cytokine Res.* 18:1077–88

129. Baeuerle PA, Henkel T. 1994. Function and activation of NF–κB in the immune system. *Annu. Rev. Immunol.* 12:141–79

130. Kojima H, Aizawa Y, Yanai Y, Nagaoka K, Takeuchi M, Ohta T, Ikegami H, Ikeda M, Kurimoto M. 1999. An essential role for NF-κB in IL-18-induced IFN-γ expression in KG-1 cells. *J. Immunol.* 162:5063–69

131. Xu D, Chan WL, Leung BP, Hunter D, Schulz K, Carter RW, McInnes IB, Robinson JH, Liew FY. 1998. Selective expression and functions of interleukin 18 receptor on T helper (Th) type 1 but not Th2 cells. *J. Exp. Med.* 188:1485–92

132. Micallef MJ, Ohtsuki T, Kohno K, Tanabe F, Ushio S, Namba M, Tanimoto T, Torigoe K, Fujii M, Ikeda M, Fukuda S, Kurimoto M. 1996. Interferon-γ-inducing factor enhances T helper 1 cytokine production by stimulated human T cells: synergism with interleukin-12 for interferon-gamma production. *Eur. J. Immunol.* 26:1647–51

133. Kohno K, Kataoka J, Ohtsuki T, Suemoto Y, Okamoto I, Usui M, Ikeda M, Kurimoto M. 1997. IFN-γ-inducing factor (IGIF) is a costimulatory factor on the activation of Th1 but not Th2 cells and exerts its ef-

fect independently of IL-12. *J. Immunol.* 158:1541–50

134. Magram J, Connaughton SE, Warrier RR, Carvajal DM, Wu C-Y, Ferrante J, Stewart C, Sarmiento U, Faherty DA, Gately MK. 1996. IL-12-deficient mice are defective in IFN-γ production and type 1 cytokine responses. *Immunity* 4:471–81

135. Kaplan MH, Sun YL, Hoey T, Grusby MJ. 1996. Impaired IL-12 responses and enhanced development of Th2 cells in Stat4-deficient mice. *Nature* 382:174–77

136. Murphy KM. 1998. T lymphocyte differentiation in the periphery. *Curr. Opin. Immunol.* 10:226–32

137. Takeda K, Tsutsui H, Yoshimoto T, Adachi O, Yoshida N, Kishimoto T, Okamura H, Nakanishi K, Akira S. 1998. Defective NK cell activity and Th1 response in IL-18-deficient mice. *Immunity* 8:383–90

138. Okamoto I, Kohno K, Tanimoto T, Ikegami H, Kurimoto M. 1999. Development of CD8+ effector T cells is differentially regulated by IL-18 and IL-12. *J. Immunol.* 162:3202–11

139. Dao T, Ohashi K, Kayano T, Kurimoto M, Okamura H. 1996. Interferon-γ-inducing factor, a novel cytokine, enhances Fas ligand-mediated cytotoxicity of murine T helper 1 cells. *Cell. Immunol.* 173:230–35

140. Dao T, Mehal WZ, Crispe IN. 1998. IL-18 augments perforin-dependent cytotoxicity of liver NK-T cells. *J. Immunol.* 161:2217–22

141. Kayagaki N, Yamaguchi N, Nakayama M, Takeda K, Akiba H, Tsutsui T, Okamura H, Nakanishi K, Okumura K, Yagita H. 1999. Expression and function of TNF-related apoptosis-inducing ligand (TRAIL) on murine activated NK cells. *J. Immunol.* 163:1906–13

142. Kayagaki N, Yamaguchi N, Nakayama M, Kawasaki A, Akiba H, Okumura K, Yagita H. 1999. Involvement of TNF-related apoptosis-inducing ligand in

human CD4$^+$ T cell-mediated cytotoxicity. *J. Immunol.* 162:2639–47

143. Kohyama M, Saijyo K, Hayasida M, Yasugi T, Kurimoto M, Ohno T. 1998. Direct activation of human CD8$^+$ cytotoxic T lymphocytes by interleukin-18. *Jpn. J. Cancer Res.* 89:1014–16

144. Wiley SR, Schooley K, Smolak PJ, Din WS, Huang C-P, Nicholl JK, Sutherland GR, Smith TD, Rauch C, Smith CA, Goodwin RG. 1995. Identification and characterization of a new member of the TNF family that induces apoptosis. *Immunity* 3:673–82

145. Griffith TS, Lynch DH. 1998. TRAIL: a molecule with multiple receptors and control mechanisms. *Curr. Opin. Immunol.* 10:559–63

146. Kägi D, Ledermann B, Bürki K, Zinkernagel RM, Hengartner H. 1996. Molecular mechanisms of lymphocyte-mediated cytotoxicity and their role in immunological protection and pathogenesis *in vivo*. *Annu. Rev. Immunol.* 14:207–32

147. Nagata S, Golstein P. 1995. The Fas death factor. *Science* 267:1449–56

148. Nagata S. 1997. Apoptosis by death factor. *Cell* 88:355–65

149. Yoshimoto T, Nagai N, Ohkusu K, Ueda H, Okamura H, Nakanishi K. 1998. LPS-stimulated SJL macrophages produce IL-12 and IL-18 that inhibit IgE production *in vitro* by induction of IFN-γ production from CD3^{int}IL-2Rβ^+ T cells. *J. Immunol.* 161:1483–92

150. Munder M, Mallo M, Eichmann K, Modolell M. 1998. Murine macrophages secrete interferon γ upon combined stimulation with interleukin (IL)-12 and IL-18: a novel pathway of autocrine macrophage activation. *J. Exp. Med.* 187:2103–8

151. Kohka H, Nishibori M, Iwagaki H, Nakaya H, Yoshino T, Kobashi K, Saaeki K, Tanaka N, Akagi T. 2000. Histamine is a potent inducer of IL-18 and IFN-γ

in human peripheral blood mononuclear cells. *J. Immunol.* 164:6640–46

152. Wild JS, Sigounas A, Sur N, Siddiqui MS, Alam R, Kurimoto M, Sur S. 2000. IFN-γ-inducing factor (IL-18) increases allergic sensitization, serum IgE, Th2 cytokines, and airway eosinophilia in a mouse model of allergic asthma. *J. Immunol.* 164:2701–10

153. Naik SM, Cannon G, Burbach GJ, Singh SR, Swerlick RA, Wilcox JN, Ansel JC, Caughman SW. 1999. Human keratinocytes constitutively express interleukin-18 and secrete biologically active interleukin-18 after treatment with pro-inflammatory mediators and dinitrochlorobenzene. *J. Invest. Dermatol.* 113:766–72

154. Kobayashi K, Nakata N, Kai M, Kasama T, Hanyuda Y, Hatano Y. 1997. Decreased expression of cytokines that induce type 1 helper T cell/interferon-γ responses in genetically susceptible mice infected with *Mycobacterium avium*. *Clin. Immunol. Immunopathol.* 85:112–16

155. Sugawara I, Yamada H, Kaneko H, Mizuno S, Takeda K, Akira S. 1999. Role of interleukin-18 (IL-18) in mycobacterial infection in IL-18-gene-disrupted mice. *Infect. Immun.* 67:2585–89

156. Yankayalapati R, Wizel B, Weis SE, Samten B, Girard WM, Barnes PF. 2000. Production of interleukin-18 in human tuberculosis. *J. Infect. Dis.* 182:234–39

156a. Kremer L, Dupré L, Wolowczuk I, Locht C. 1999. In vivo immunomodulation following intradermal injection with DNA encoding IL-18. *Am. Assoc. Immunol.*

157. Song CH, Kim HJ, Park JK, Lim JH, Kim UO, Kim JS, Paik TH, Kim KJ, Suhr JW, Jo EK. 2000. Depressed interleukin-12 (IL-12), but not IL-18, production in response to a 30- or 32-kilodalton mycobacterial antigen in patients with active pulmonary tuberculosis. *Infect. Immun.* 68:4477–84

158. Yamada G, Shijubo N, Shigehara K, Okamura K, Kurimoto M, Abe S. 2000. Increased levels of circulating interleukin-18 in patients with advanced tuberculosis. *Am. J. Respir. Crit. Care Med.* 161:1786–89

159. Salgame P, Abrams JS, Clayberger C, Goldstein H, Convit J, Modlin RL, Bloom BR. 1991. Differing lymphokine profiles of functional subsets of human CD4 and CD8 T cell clones. *Science* 254:279–82

160. Kobayashi K, Kai M, Gidoh M, Nakata N, Endoh M, Singh RP, Kasama T, Saito H. 1998. The possible role of interleukin (IL)-12 and interferon-gamma-inducing factor/IL-18 in protection against experimental *Mycobacterium leprae* infection in mice. *Clin. Immunol. Immunopathol.* 88:226–31

161. Garcia VE, Uyemura K, Sieling PA, Ochoa MT, Morita CT, Okamura H, Kurimoto M, Rea TH, Modlin RL. 1999. IL-18 promotes type 1 cytokine production from NK cells and T cells in human intracellular infection. *J. Immunol.* 162:6114–21

162. Mastroeni P, Clare S, Khan S, Harrison JA, Hormaeche CE, Okamura H, Kurimoto M, Dougan G. 1999. Interleukin 18 contributes to host resistance and gamma interferon production in mice infected with virulent *Salmonella typhimurium*. *Infect. Immun.* 67:478–83

163. Sansonetti PJ, Phalipon A, Arondel J, Thirumalai K, Banerjee S, Akira S, Takeda K, Zychlisky A. 2000. Caspase-1 activation of IL-1β and IL-18 are essential for *Shigella flexneri*-induced inflammation. *Immunity* 12:581–90

164. Lu H, Shen C, Brunham RC. 2000. *Chlamydia trachomatis* infection of epithelial cells induces the activation of caspase-1 and release of mature IL-18. *J. Immunol.* 165:1463–69

165. Zhang T, Kawakami K, Qureshi MH, Okamura H, Kurimoto M, Saito A. 1997. Interleukin-12 (IL-12) and IL-18 syner-gistically induce the fungicidal activity of murine peritoneal exudate cells against *Cryptococcus neoformans* through production of gamma interferon by natural killer cells. *Infect. Immun.* 65:3594–99

166. Qureshi MH, Zhang T, Koguchi Y, Nakashima K, Okamura H, Kurimoto M, Kawakami K. 1999. Combined effects of IL-12 and IL-18 on the clinical course and local cytokine production in murine pulmonary infection with *Cryptococcus neoformans*. *Eur. J. Immunol.* 29:643–49

167. Kawakami K, Qureshi MH, Koguchi Y, Zhang T, Okamura H, Kurimoto M, Saito A. 1999. Role of TNF-α in the induction of fungicidal activity of mouse peritoneal exudate cells against *Cryptococcus neoformans* by IL-12 and IL-18. *Cell Immunol.* 193:9–16

168. Brummer E. 1999. Human defenses against *Cryptococcus neoformans*: an update. *Mycopathologia* 143:121–25

169. Kawakami K, Koguchi Y, Qureshi MH, Miyazato A, Yara S, Kinjo Y, Iwakura Y, Takeda K, Akira S, Kurimoto M, Saito A. 2000. IL-18 contributes to host resistance against infection with *Cryptococcus neoformans* in mice with defective IL-12 synthesis through induction of IFN-γ production by NK cells. *J. Immunol.* 165:941–47

170. Fujioka N, Akazawa R, Ohashi K, Fujii M, Ikeda M, Kurimoto M. 1999. Interleukin-18 protects mice against acute herpes simplex virus type 1 infection. *J. Virol.* 73:2401–9

171. Sareneva T, Matikainen S, Kurimoto M, Julkunen I. 1998. Influenza A virus-induced IFN-α/β and IL-18 synergistically enhance IFN-γ gene expression in human T cells. *J. Immunol.* 160:6032–38

172. Tanaka-Kataoka M, Kunikata T, Takayama S, Iwaki K, Ohashi K, Ikeda M, Kurimoto M. 1999. *In vivo* antiviral effect of interleukin 18 in a

mouse model of vaccinia virus infection. *Cytokine* 11:593–99

173. Puren AJ, Razeghi P, Fantuzzi G, Dinarello CA. 1998. Interleukin-18 enhances lipopolysaccharide-induced interferon*γ* production in human whole blood cultures. *J. Infect. Dis.* 178:1830–34

174. Puren AJ, Fantuzzi G, Gu Y, Su MS, Dinarello CA. 1998. Interleukin-18 (IFN gamma-inducing factor) induces IL-8 and IL-1 *β* via TNF *α* production from non-CD14$^+$ human blood mononuclear cells. *J. Clin Invest.* 101:711–21

175. Poli G, Kinter AL, Justement JS, Bressler P, Kehrl JH, Fauci AS. 1992. Retinoic acid mimics transforming growth factor *β* in the regulation of human immunodeficiency virus expression in monocytic cells. *Proc. Natl. Acad. Sci. USA* 89:2689–93

176. Shapiro L, Puren AJ, Barton HA, Novick D, Peskind RL, Shenkar R, Gu Y, Su MS, Dinarello CA. 1998. Interleukin 18 stimulates HIV type 1 in monocytic cells. *Proc. Natl. Acad. Sci. USA* 95:12550–55

177. Chehimi J, Starr SE, Frank I, D'Andrea A, Ma X, MacGregor RR, Sennelier J, Trinchieri G. 1994. Impaired interleukin 12 production in human immunodeficiency virus-infected patients. *J. Exp. Med.* 179:1361–66

178. Sher A, Coffman R. 1992. Regulation of immunity to parasites by T cells and T cell-derived cytokines. *Annu. Rev. Immunol.* 10:385–409

179. Heinzel FP, Sadick MD, Mutha S, Locksley RM. 1991. Production of interferon-*γ*, IL-2, IL-4, and IL-10 by CD4$^+$ lymphocytes *in vivo* during healing and progression of murine leishmaniasis. *Proc. Natl. Acad. Sci. USA* 88:7011–15

180. Diefenbach A, Schindler H, Donhause N, Lorenz E, Laskay T, MacMicking J, Röllinghoff M, Gresser I, Bogdan C. 1998. Type 1 interferon (IFN*α*/*β*) and type 2 nitric oxide synthase regulate the innate immune response to a protozoan parasite. *Immunity* 8:77–87

181. Wei XQ, Leung BP, Niedbala W, Piedrafita D, Feng GJ, Sweet M, Dobbie L, Smith AJ, Liew FY. 1999. Altered immune responses and susceptibility to *Leishmania major* and *Staphylococcus aureus* infection in IL-18-deficient mice. *J. Immunol.* 163:2821–28

182. Ohkusu K, Yoshimoto T, Takeda K, Ogura T, Kashiwamura S-I, Iwakura Y, Akira S, Okamura H, Nakanishi K. 2000. Potentiality of interleukin-18 as a useful reagent for treatment and prevention of *Leishmania major* infection. *Infect. Immun.* 68:2449–56

183. Monteforte GM, Takeda K, Rodriguez-Sosa M, Akira S, David JR, Satoskar AR. 2000. Genetically resistant mice lacking IL-18 gene develop Th1 response and control cutaneous *Leishmania major* infection. *J. Immunol.* 164:5890–93

184. Skeiky YA, Kennedy M, Kaufman D, Borges MM, Guderian JA, Scholler JK, Ovendale PJ, Picha KS, Morrissey PJ, Grabstein KH, Campos NA, Reed SG. 1998. LeIF: a recombinant Leishmania protein that induces an IL-12-mediated Th1 cytokine profile. *J. Immunol.* 161:6171–79

185. Meyer zum Büschenfelde KH, Cramer S, Trumpfheller C, Fleischer B, Frosch S. 1997. *Trypanosoma cruzi* induces strong IL-12 and IL-18 gene expression *in vivo*: correlation with interferon-gamma (IFN-*γ*) production. *Clin. Exp. Immunol.* 110:378–85

186. Wahl LM, Kleinman HK. 1998. Tumor-associated macrophages as targets for cancer therapy. *J. Natl. Cancer Inst.* 90:1583–84

187. Micallef MJ, Yoshida K, Kawai S, Hanaya T, Kohno K, Arai S, Tanimoto T, Torigoe K, Fujii M, Ikeda M, Kurimoto M. 1997. *In vivo* anti-tumor effects of murine interferon-*γ*-inducing factor/interleukin-18 in mice

bearing syngeneic Meth A sarcoma malignant ascites. *Cancer Immunol. Immunother.* 43:361–67

188. Micallef MJ, Tanimoto T, Kohno K, Ikeda M, Kurimoto M. 1997. Interleukin 18 induces the sequential activation of natural killer cells and cytotoxic T lymphocytes to protect syngeneic mice from transplantation with Meth A sarcoma. *Cancer Res.* 57:4557–63

189. Osaki T, Hashimoto W, Gambotto A, Okamura H, Robbins PD, Kurimoto M, Lotze MT, Tahara H. 1999. Potent antitumor effects mediated by local expression of the mature form of the interferon-γ inducing factor, interleukin-18 (IL-18). *Gene Ther.* 6:808–15

190. Heuer JG, Tucker-McClung C, Hock RA. 1999. Neuroblastoma cells expressing mature IL-18, but not proIL-18, induce a strong and immediate antitumor immune response. *J. Immunother.* 22:324–35

191. Cho D, Kim TG, Lee W, Hwang YI, Cho HI, Han H, Kwon O, Kim D, Park H, Houh D. 2000. Interleukin-18 and the costimulatory molecule B7-1 have a synergistic anti-tumor effect on murine melanoma; implication of combined immunotherapy for poorly immunogenic malignancy. *J. Invest. Dermatol.* 114:928–34

192. Kikuchi T, Akasaki Y, Joki T, Abe T, Kurimoto M, Ohno T. 2000. Antitumor activity of interleukin-18 on mouse glioma cells. *J. Immunother.* 23:184–89

193. Osaki T, Peron JM, Cai Q, Okamura H, Robbins PD, Kurimoto M, Lotze MT, Tahara H. 1998. IFN-γ-inducing factor/IL-18 administration mediates IFN-γ- and IL-12-independent antitumor effects. *J. Immunol.* 160:1742–49

194. Hashimoto W, Osaki T, Okamura H, Robbins PD, Kurimoto M, Nagata S, Lotze MT, Tahara H. 1999. Differential antitumor effects of administration of recombinant IL-18 or recombinant IL-12 are mediated primarily by Fas-Fas ligand-

and perforin-induced tumor apoptosis, respectively. *J. Immunol.* 163:583–89

195. Pagés F, Berger A, Henglein B, Piqueras B, Danel C, Zinzindohoue F, Thiounn N, Cugnenc PH, Fridman WH. 1999. Modulation of interleukin-18 expression in human colon carcinoma: consequences for tumor immune surveillance. *Int. J. Cancer* 84:326–30

196. Vidal-Vanaclocha F, Fantuzzi G, Mendozaa L, Fuentes AM, Agasagasti MJ, Martin J, Caarraascal T, Walsh P, Reznikov LL, Kim SH, Novick D, Rubinstein M, Dinarello CA. 2000. IL-18 regulates IL-1β-dependent hepatic melanoma metastasis *via* vascular cell adhesion molecule-1. *Proc. Natl. Acad. Sci. USA* 97:734–39

197. Cho D, Song H, Kim YM, Houh D, Hur DY, Park H, Yoon D, Pvun KH, Lee WJ, Kurimoto M, Kim YB, Kim YS, Choi I. 2000. Endogenous interleukin-18 modulates immune escape of murine melanoma cells by regulating the expression of Fas ligand and reactive oxygen intermediates. *Cancer Res.* 60:2703–9

198. Coughlin CM, Salhany KE, Wysocka M, Aruga E, Kurzawa H, Chang AE, Hunter CA, Fox JC, Trinchieri G, Lee W. 1998. Interleukin-12 and interleukin-18 synergistically induce murine tumor regression which involves inhibition of angiogenesis. *J. Clin. Invest.* 101:1441–52

199. Cao R, Famebo J, Kurimoto M, Cao Y. 2000. Interleukin-18 acts as an angiogenesis and tumor suppresser. *FASEB J.* 13:2195–2202

200. Yamanaka K, Hara I, Nagai H, Miyake Gohji K, Micallef MJ, Kurimoto M, Arakawa S, Kamidono S. 1999. Synergistic antitumor effects of interleukin-12 gene transfer and systemic administration of interleukin-18 in a mouse bladder cancer model. *Cancer Immunol. Immunother.* 48:297–302

201. Oshikawa K, Shi F, Rakhmilevich AL, Sondel PM, Mahvi DM, Yang NS. 1999.

Synergistic inhibition of tumor growth in a murine mammary adenocarcinoma model by combinational gene therapy using IL-12, pro-IL-18, and IL-1β converting enzyme cDNA. *Proc. Natl. Acad. Sci. USA* 96:13351–56

202. O'Donnell MA, Luo Y, Chen X, Szilvasi A, Hunter SE, Clinton SK. 1999. Role of IL-12 in the induction and potentiation of IFN-γ in response to Bacillus Calmette-Guerin. *J. Immunol.* 163:4246–52

203. Nagai H, Hara I, Horikawa T, Fujii M, Kurimoto M, Kamidono S, Ichihashi M. 2000. Antitumor effects on mouse melanoma elicited by local secretion of interleukin-12 and their enhancement by testament with interleukin-18. *Cancer Invest.* 18:206–13

204. Hara I, Nagai H, Miyake H, Yamanaka K, Hara S, Micallef MJ, Kurimoto M, Gohji K, Arakawa S, Ichihashi M, Kamidono S. 2000. Effectiveness of cancer vaccine therapy using cells transduced with the interleukin-12 gene combined with systemic interleukin-18 administration. *Cancer Gene Ther.* 7:83–90

205. Tasaki K, Yoshida Y, Maeda T, Miyauchi M, Kawamura K, Takenaga K, Yamamoto H, Kouzu T, Asano T, Ochiai T, Sakiyama S, Tagawa M. 2000. Protective immunity is induced in murine colon carcinoma cells by the expression of interleukin-12 or interleukin-18, which activate type 1 helper T cells. *Cancer Gene Ther.* 7:247–54

206. Gillespie MT, Horwood NJ. 1998. Interleukin-18: perspectives on the newest interleukin. *Cytokine Growth Factor Rev.* 9:109–16

207. Horwood NJ, Udagawa N, Elliott J, Grail D, Okamura H, Kurimoto M, Dunn AR, Martin T, Gillespie MT. 1998. Interleukin 18 inhibits osteoclast formation *via* T cell production of granulocyte macrophage colony-stimulating factor. *J. Clin. Invest.* 101:595–603

208. Martin TJ, Romas E, Gillespie MT. 1998. Interleukins in the control of osteoclast differentiation. *Crit. Rev. Eukaryot. Gene Express.* 8:107–23

209. Culhane AC, Hall MD, Rothwell NJ, Luheshi GN. 1998. Cloning of rat brain interleukin-18 cDNA. *Mol. Psychiatry* 3:362–66

210. Taneja V, David CS. 1999. HLA class II transgenic mice as models of human diseases. *Immunol. Rev.* 169:67–79

211. McDevitt HO. 1998. The role of MHC class II molecules in susceptibility and resistance to autoimmunity. *Curr. Opin. Immunol.* 10:677–81

212. McDuffie M. 1998. Genetics of autoimmune diabetes in animal models. *Curr. Opin. Immunol.* 10:704–9

213. Abraham RS, David CS. 2000. Identification of HLA-class-II-restricted epitopes of autoantigens in transgenic mice. *Curr. Opin. Immunol.* 12:122–29

214. Mora C, Wong FS, Chang C-H, Flavell RA. 1999. Pancreatic infiltration but not diabetes occurs in the relative absence of MHC class II-restricted CD4 T cells: studies using NOD/CIITA-deficient mice. *J. Immunol.* 162:4576–88

215. Wen L, Wong FS, Tang J, Chen N-Y, Altieri M, David C, Flavell R, Sherwin R. 2000. *In vivo* evidence for the contribution of human histocompatibility leukocyte antigen (HLA)-DQ molecules to the development of diabetes. *J. Exp. Med.* 191:97–104

216. Wong FS, Janeway CA Jr. 1999. Insulin-dependent diabetes mellitus and its animal models. *Curr. Opin. Immunol.* 11:643–47

217. Wong FS, Dittel BN, Janeway CA Jr. 1999. Transgenes and knockout mutations in animal models of type 1 diabetes and multiple sclerosis. *Immunol. Rev.* 169:93–106

218. Wang B, André I, Gonzaalez A, Katz JD, Aguet M, Benoist C, Matis D. 1997. Interferon-γ impacts at multiple points during the progression of autoimmune

diabetes. *Proc. Natl. Acad. Sci. USA* 94:13844–49

219. Pakala SV, Chivetta M, Kelly CB, Katz JD. 1999. In autoimmune diabetes transition from benign to pernicious insulitis requires an islet cell response to tumor necrosis factor α. *J. Exp. Med.* 189:1053–62

220. Hammond KJL, Poulton LD, Palmisano LJ, Silveira PA, Godfrey DI, Baxer A. 1998. α/β-T cell receptor (TCR)⁺ CD4⁻CD8⁻ (NKT) thymocytes prevent insulin-dependent diabetes mellitus in nonobese diabetic (NOD)/Li mice by the influence of interleukin (IL)-4 and/or IL-10. *J. Exp. Med.* 187:1047–56

221. Suri A, Katz JD. 1999. Dissecting role of CD4⁺T cells in autoimmune diabetes through the use of TCR transgenic mice. *Immunol. Rev.* 169:55–56

222. André-Schmutz I, Hindelang C, Benoist C, Mathis D. 1999. Cellular and molecular changes accompanying the progression from insulitis to diabetes. *Eur. J. Immunol.* 29:245–45

223. Rothe H, Hausmann A, Casteels K, Okamura H, Kurimoto M, Burkart V, Mathieu C, Kolb H. 1999. IL-18 inhibits diabetes development in nonobese diabetic mice by counterregulation of Th1-dependent destructive insulitis. *J. Immunol.* 163:1230–36

224. Zaccone P, Phillips J, Conget I, Gomis R, Haskins K, Minty A, Bendtzen K, Cooke A, Nicoletti F. 1999. Interleukin-13 prevents autoimmune diabetes in NOD mice. *Diabetes* 48:1522–28

225. Steinman L. 1996. Multiple sclerosis: a coordinated immunological attack against myelin in the central nervous system. *Cell* 85:299–302

226. Olsson T, Zhi WW, Hojeberg B, Kostulas V, Jiang YP, Anderson G, Ekre HP, Link H. 1990. Autoreactive T lymphocytes in multiple sclerosis determined by antigen-induced secretion of interferon-γ. *J. Clin. Invest.* 86:981–85

227. Lafaille JJ, Nagashima K, Katsuki M, Tonegawa S. 1994. High incidence of spontaneous autoimmune encephalomyelitis in immunodeficient and anti-myelin basic protein T cell receptor transgenic mice. *Cell* 78:399–408

228. Wildbaum G, Youssef S, Grabie N, Karin N. 1998. Neutralizing antibodies to IFN-γ-inducing factor prevent experimental autoimmune encephalomyelitis. *J. Immunol.* 161:6368–74

229. Shevach EM, Chang JT, Segal BM. 1999. The critical role of IL-12 and the IL-12Rβ2 subunit in the generation of pathogenic autoreactive Th1 cells. *Springer Semin. Immunopathol.* 21:249–62

230. Leonard JP, Waldburger KE, Goldman SJ. 1995. Prevention of experimental autoimmune encephalomyelitis by antibodies against interleukin 12. *J. Exp. Med.* 181:381–86

231. Balashov KE, Rottman JB, Weiner HL, Hancock WW. 1999. CCR5⁺ and CXCR3⁺ T cells are increased in multiple sclerosis and their ligands MIP-1alpha and IP-10 are expressed in demyelinating brain lesions. *Proc. Natl. Acad. Sci. USA* 96:6873–78

232. Furlan R, Filippi M, Bergami A, Rocca MA, Martinelli V, Poliani PL, Grimaldi LM, Desina G, Comi G, Matino G. 1999. Peripheral levels of caspase-1 mRNA correlate with disease activity in patients with multiple sclerosis; a preliminary study. *J. Neurol. Neurosurg. Psychiatry* 67:785–88

233. Furlan R, Martino G, Galbiati F, Poliani PL, Smiroldo S, Bergami A, Desinaa G, Comi G, Flavell R, Su M, Adorini L. 1999. Caspase-1 regulates the inflammatory process leading to autoimmune demyelination. *J. Immunol.* 163:2403–9

234. Feldmann F, Brennan FM, Mini RN. 1996. Role of cytokines in rheumatoid arthritis. *Annu. Rev. Immunol.* 14:397–440

235. Dayer JM. 1999. Interleukin-18, rheumatoid arthritis, and tissue destruction. *J. Clin. Invest.* 104:1337–39

236. Gracie JA, Forsey RJ, Chan WL, Gilmour A, Leung BP, Greer MR, Kennedy K, Carter R, Wei XQ, Field M, Foulis A, Liew FY, McInnes IB. 1999. A proinflammatory role for IL-18 in rheumatoid arthritis. *J. Clin. Invest.* 104:1393–401

237. Leung BP, McInnes IB, Esfandiari E, Wei X-q, Liew FY. 2000. Combined effects of IL-12 and IL-18 on the induction of collagen-induced arthritis. *J. Immunol.* 164:6495–502

238. Sakao Y, Takeda K, Tsutsui H, Kaisho T, Nomura F, Okamura H, Nakanishi K, Akira S. 1999. IL-18-deficient mice are resistant to endotoxin-induced liver injury but highly susceptible to endotoxin shock. *Int. Immunol.* 11:471–80

239. Ogasawara J, Watanabe-Fukunaga R, Adachi M, Matsuzawa A, Kasuga T, Kitamura Y, Nagata S. 1993. Lethal effect of the anti-Fas antibody in mice. *Nature* 364:806–9

240. Tanaka M, Suda T, Haze K, Nakamura N, Sato K, Kimura F, Motoyoshi K, Mizuki M, Tagawa S, Ohga S, Hatake K, Drummond AH, Nagata S. 1996. Fas ligand in human serum. *Nat. Med.* 2:317–22

241. Tanaka M, Suda T, Yatomi T, Nakamura N, Nagata S. 1997. Lethal effect of recombinant human Fas ligand in mice pretreated with *Propionibacterium acnes*. *J. Immunol.* 158:2303–9

242. Fiorucci S, Santucci L, Antonelli E, Distrutti E, Del Sero G, Morelli O, Romani L, Federici B, Del Soldato P, Morelli A. 2000. NO-aspirin protects from T cell-mediated liver injury by inhibiting caspase-dependent processing of Th1-like cytokines. *Gastroenterology* 118:404–12

243. Faggioni R, Jones-Carson J, Reed DA, Dinarello CA, Feingold KR, Grunfeld C, Fantuzzi G. 2000. Leptin-deficient (*ob/ob*) mice are protected from T cell-mediated hepatotoxicity: role of tumor necrosis factor α and IL-18. *Proc. Natl. Acad. Sci. USA* 97:2367–72

244. McGuinness PH, Painter D, Davies S, McCaughan GW. 2000. Increases in intrahepatic CD68 positive cells, MAC387 positive cells, and proinflammatory cytokines (particularly interleukin 18) in chronic hepatitis C infection. *Gut* 46:260–69

245. Urushihara N, Iwagaki H, Yagi T, Kohka H, Kobashi K, Morimoto Y, Yoshino T, Tanimoto T, Kurimoto M, Tanaka N. 2000. Elevation of serum interleukin-18 levels and activation of Kupffer cells in biliary atresia. *J. Pediatr. Surg.* 35:446–49

246. Krenger W, Ferrara JLM. 1996. Graft-versus-host disease and the Th1/Th2 paradigm. *Immunol. Res.* 15:50–73

247. Williamson E, Garside P, Andrew Bradley I, More IAR, Mowat A. 1997. Neutralizing IL-12 during induction of murine acute graft-versus-host disease polarizes the cytokine profile toward a Th2-type alloimmune response and confers long term protection from disease. *J. Immunol.* 159:1208–15

248. Hill GR, Tshima T, Rebel VI, Krijanovski OI, Cooke KR, Brinson YS, Ferrara JLM. 2000. The p55 IFN-α receptor plays a critical role in T cell alloreactivity. *J. Immunol.* 164:656–63

249. Fujimori Y, Takatsuka H, Takemoto Y, Hara H, Okamura H, Nakanishi K, Kakishita E. 2000. Elevated interleukin (IL)-18 levels during acute graft-versus-host disease after allogeneic bone marrow transplantation. *Br. J. Haematol.* 109:652–57

250. Hu HZ, Li GL, Lim YK, Chan SH, Yap EH. 1999. Kinetics of interferon-gamma secretion and its regulatory factors in the early phase of acute graft-versus-host disease. *Immunology* 98:379–85

251. Nakamura H, Komatsu K, Ayaki M, Kawamoto S, Murakami M, Uoshima N,

Yagi T, Hasegawa T, Yasumi M, Karasuno T, Teshima H, Hiraoka A, Masaoka T. 2000. Serum levels of soluble IL-2 receptor, IL-12, IL-18, and IFN-γ in patients with acute graft-versus-host disease after allogeneic bone marrow transplantation. *J. Allergy Clin. Immunol.* 106:45–50

252. Via CS, Shearer GM. 1988. T-cell interactions in autoimmunity: insights from a murine model of graft-versus-host disease. *Immunol. Today* 9:207–13

253. Via CS, Rus V, Gately MK, Finkelman FD. 1994. IL-12 stimulates the development of acute graft-versus-host disease in mice that normally would develop chronic, autoimmune graft-versus-host disease. *J. Immunol.* 153:4040–47

254. Lauwerys BR, Renauld JC, Houssiau FA. 1999. Inhibition of *in vitro* immunoglobulin production by IL-12 in murine chronic graft-vs-host disease: synergism with IL-18. *Eur. J. Immunol.* 28:2017–24

255. Okamoto I, Kohno K, Tanimoto T, Iwaki K, Ishihara T, Akamatsu S, Ikegami H, Kurimoto M. 2000. IL-18 prevents the development of chronic graft-versus-host disease in mice. *J. Immunol.* 164:6067–74

256. Davidson NJ, Leach MW, Fort MM, Thompson-Snipes L, Kühn R, Müller W, Berg DJ, Rennick DM. 1996. T helper cell 1-type CD4$^+$ T cells, but not B cells, mediate colitis in interleukin 10-deficient mice. *J. Exp. Med.* 184:241–51

257. Monteleone G, Biancone L, Marasco R, Morrone G, Marasco O, Luzza F, Pallone F. 1997. Interleukin 12 is expressed and actively released by Crohn's disease intestinal lamina propria mononuclear cells. *Gastroenterol.* 112:1169–78

258. Parronchi P, Romagnani P, Annunziato F, Sampognaro F, Becchio A, Giannarini L, Maggi E, Pupilli C, Tonelli F, Romagnani S. 1997. Type 1 T-helper cell predominance and interleukin-12 expression in the gut of patients with Crohn's disease. *Am. J. Pathol.* 150:823–32

259. Targan SR, Hanauer SB, Deventer SJH,

Mayer L, Present DH, Baraakman T, DeWoody KL, Schaible TF, Rutgeerts PJ. 1997. A short-term study of chimeric monoclonal antibody cA2 to tumor necrosis factor α for Crohn's disease. *N. Engl. J. Med.* 337:1029–35

260. Pizarro TT, Michie MH, Bents M, Woraratanadharm J, Smith MF Jr, Foley E, Moskaluk CA, Bickston SJ, Cominelli F. 1999. IL-18, a novel immunoregulatory cytokine, is up-regulated in Crohn's disease: expression and localization in intestinal mucosal cells. *J. Immunol.* 162:6829–35

261. Monteleone G, Trapasso F, Parrello T, Biancone L, Stella A, Iuliano R, Luzza F, Fusco A, Pallone F. 1999. Bioactive IL-18 expression is up-regulated in Crohn's disease. *J. Immunol.* 163:143–47

262. Mahida YR. 2000. The key role of macrophages in the immunopathogenesis of inflammatory bowel disease. *Inflamm. Bowel Dis.* 6:21–33

263. Sartor RB. 2000. Colitis in HLA-B27/β2 microglobulin transgenic rats. *Int. Rev. Immunol.* 19:39–50

264. Nakamura S, Otani T, Ijiri Y, Motoda R, Kurimoto M, Orita K. 2000. IFN-γ-dependent and -independent mechanisms in adverse effects caused by concomitant administration of IL-18 and IL-12. *J. Immunol.* 164:3330–36

265. Chikano S, Sawada K, Shimoyama T, Kashiwamura S-I, Sugihara A, Sekikawa K, Terada N, Nakanishi K, Okamura H. 2000. IL-18 and IL-12 induce intestinal inflammation and fatty liver in mice in an IFN-γ-dependent manner. *Gut* 779–86

266. Camoglio L, te Velde AA, de Boer A, ten Kate FJ, Kopf M, van Deventer SJ. 2000. Hapten-induced colitis associated with maintained Th1 and inflammatory responses in IFN-γ receptor-deficient mice. *Eur. J. Immunol.* 30:1486–95

267. Netea MG, Fantuzzi G, Kullberg BJ, Stuyt RJL, Pulido EJ, McIntyre RCJ, Joosten LAB, Van der Meer JWM, Dinarello CA.

2000. Neutralization of IL-18 reduces neutrophil tissue accumulation and protects mice against *Escherichia coli* and *Salmonella typhimurium* endotoxemia. *J. Immunol.* 164:2644–49

268. Hockholzer P, Lipford GB, Wagner H, Pfeffer K, Heeg K. 2000. Role of interleukin-18 (IL-18) during lethal shock: decreased lipopolysaccharide sensitivity but normal superantigen reaction in IL-18-deficient mice. *Infect. Immun.* 68:3502–8

269. Borovikova LV, Ivanova S, Zhang M, Yang H, Botchkina GH, Vatkins LR, Wang H, Abumrad N, Eaton JW, Tracey KJ. 2000. Vagus nerve stimulation attenuates the systemic inflammatory response to endotoxin. *Nature* 405:458–62

270. Robinson DS, Hamid Q, Ying A, Tsicopoulus A, Barkans J, Bentley AM, Corrigan C, Durham SR, Kay AB. 1992. Th2-like bronchoalveolar T-lymphocyte population in atopic asthma. *N. Engl. J. Med.* 326:298–304

271. Hofstra CL, Van AI, Hofman G, Kool M, Nijkamp FP, Van Oosterhout A. 1998. Prevention of Th2-like cell responses by coadministration of IL-12 and IL-18 is associated with inhibition of antigen-induced airway hyperresponsiveness, eosinophilia, and serum IgE levels. *J. Immunol.* 161:5054–60

272. Bohle B, Jahn-Schmid B, Maurer D, Kraft D, Ebner C. 1999. Oligodeoxynucleotides containing CpG motifs induce IL-12, IL-18 and IFN-γ production in cells from allergic individuals and inhibit IgE synthesis *in vitro*. *Eur. J. Immunol.* 29:2344–53

273. Hansen G, Yeung VP, Berry G, Umetsu DT, DeKruyff RH. 2000. Vaccination with heat-killed Listeria as adjuvant reverses established allergen-induced airway hyperreactivity and inflammation: role of CD8$^+$ T cells and IL-18. *J. Immunol.* 164:223–30

274. Shibata Y, Foster LA, Bradfield JF,

Myrvik QN. 2000. Oral administration of chitin down-regulates serum IgE levels and lung eosinophilia in the allergic mouse. *J. Immunol.* 164:1314–21

275. Kodama T, Matsuyama T, Kuribayashi K, Nishioka Y, Sugita M, Akira S, Nakanishi K, Okamura H. 2000. IL-18 deficiency selectively enhances allergen-induced eosinophilia in mice. *J. Allergy Clin. Immunol.* 105:45–53

276. Campbell E, Kunkel SL, Strieter RM, Lukacs NW. 2000. Differential roles of IL-18 in allergic airway disease: induction of eotaxin by resident cell populations exacerbates eosinophils accumulation. *J. Immunol.* 164:1096–102

277. Kumano K, Nakao A, Nakajima H, Hayashi F, Kurimoto M, Okamura H, Saito Y, Iwamoto I. 1999. Interleukin-18 enhances antigen-induced eosinophil recruitment into the mouse airways. *Am. J. Respir. Crit. Care Med.* 160:873–78

278. Sugaya M, Nakamura K, Tamaki K. 1999. Interleukin 18 and 12 synergistically upregulate interferon-γ production by murine dendritic epidermal T cells. *J. Invest. Dermatol.* 113:350–54

279. Lamont AG, Adorini L. 1996. IL-12: a key cytokine in immune regulation. *Immunol. Today* 17:214–17

280. Kämpfer H, Kalina U, Muhl H, Pfeilschifter J, Frank S. 1999. Counterregulation of interleukin-18 mRNA and protein expression during cutaneous wound repair in mice. *J. Invest. Dermatol.* 113:369–74

281. Pelletier JP. 1999. The influence of tissue cross-talking on OA progression: role of nonsteroidal antiinflammatory drugs. *Osteoarthritis Cartilage* 7:374–76

282. Saha N, Moldovan F, Tardif G, Pelletier JP, Cloutier JM, Martel-Pelletier J. 1999. Interleukin-1β-converting enzyme/caspase-1 in human osteoarthritic tissues: localization and role in the maturation of interleukin-1β and interleukin-18. *Arthritis Rheum.* 42:1577–87

283. Olee T, Hashimoto S, Quach J, Lotz M. 1999. IL-18 is produced by articular chondrocytes and induces proinflammatory and catabolic responses. *J. Immunol.* 162:1096–100

284. Matsumoto K, Kanmatsuse K. 2000. Interleukin-18 and interleukin-12 synergize to stimulate the production of vascular permeability factor by T lymphocytes in normal subjects and in patients with minimal-change nephrotic syndrome. *Nephron* 85:127–33

285. Heslan J-M, Branellec AI, Pilatte Y, Lang P, Lagrue G. 1991. Differentiation between vascular permeability factor and IL-2 in lymphocyte supernatants from patients with minimal-change nephrotic syndrome. *Clin. Exp. Immunol.* 86:157–62

286. Arndt PG, Fantuzzi G, Abraham E. 2000. Expression of interleukin-18 in the lung after endotoxemia or hemorrhage-induced acute lung injury. *Am. J. Respir. Cell Mol. Biol.* 22:708–13

Annu. Rev. Immunol. 2001. 19:475–96

MULTIPLE VIRAL STRATEGIES OF HTLV-1 FOR DYSREGULATION OF CELL GROWTH CONTROL

Mitsuaki Yoshida

Banyu Tsukuba Research Institute, Tsukuba, Ibaraki 300-2611, Japan;
e-mail: yoshimx@banyu.co.jp

Key Words adult T cell leukemia, p16INK4, cell cycle activation, Rb pathway, transcriptional coactivators

■ **Abstract** The human T cell leukemia virus-1 (HTLV-1) is a retrovirus that causes adult T cell leukemia (ATL) and neurological disorder, the tropical spastic paraparesis (HAM/TSP). The pathogenesis apparently results from the pleiotropic function of Tax protein, which is a key regulator of viral replication. Tax exerts (*a*) trans-activation and -repression of transcription of different sets of cellular genes through binding to groups of transcription factors and coactivators, (*b*) dysregulation of cell cycle through binding to inhibitors of CDK4/6, and (*c*) inhibition of some tumor suppressor proteins. These effects on a wide variety of cellular targets seem to cooperate in promoting cell proliferation. This is an effective viral strategy to amplify its proviral genome through replication of infected cells; ultimately it results in cell transformation and leukemogenesis.

INTRODUCTION

Proliferation and differentiation of eukaryotic cells are triggered by extracellular signals and are regulated downstream of signal transduction. Accumulation of genetic alterations controlling these regulatory systems is thought to be the origin of cancers. Infection with tumor virus is equivalent to the genetic alteration integrating the viral genome into the host cell DNA.

Human tumor viruses including human T cell leukemia viruses, Epstein-Barr virus, human papillomavirus, and human hepatitis B and C viruses provide unique systems to study the mechanisms of human cancers. They also provide useful strategies for diagnosis, treatment, and prevention of the specific cancers. Among these, human T cell leukemia virus type 1 (HTLV-1) is unique both because it is a retrovirus (1, 2) and also because it acts in the etiology of leukemogenesis (3, 4) and a myelopathy, HAM/TSP (5, 6). HTLV-1 causes adult T cell leukemia (ATL), which is a malignancy of CD4-positive T cells; it frequently has an abnormal nucleus and high level of expression of interleukin 2 receptor α subunit. HTLV-1 does not efficiently replicate in vivo and is transmitted through infected T cells in breast milk (from mother to child), in semen (from male to female), and in blood (transfusion).

0732-0582/01/0407-0475$14.00

As the result of its natural infection pattern, HTLV-1 and the associated diseases appear in familial and local aggregation and are clustered in Southern Japan, South America, Central Africa, and South-East Asia. The lifelong risk for ATL among an infected population is 3%–5%, but no effective therapy is yet available.

Unlike acute leukemia viruses of animal origin, HTLV-1 has no typical oncogene derived from the cellular genome, but rather it has an extra sequence of 1.6 kb (called pX region) in the 3′ terminal region of its genome (7). The pX region codes for several proteins including Tax (8, 9), Rex (10, 11), p21X-III (10), p12 (12), and others (13) by combination of the reading frames and alternative splicing (14, 15). Expression of retroviral genomes is generally regulated by *cis*-acting elements in the long terminal repeat (LTR). The *cis*-acting elements of HTLV-1 are uniquely regulated by a *trans*-acting factor, Tax, encoded by the pX region (16–18). Thus, Tax is essential for the effective replication of HTLV-1. Tax is also believed to contribute to its pathogenesis through its capacity to immortalize primary T cells (19), to transform rodent fibroblasts (20, 21), and to induce tumors in transgenic mice expressing Tax (22, 23). This proposal is consistent with its pleiotropic, biochemical, and cellular functions.

In this review, the molecular biology of Tax is summarized, focusing on the possible mechanisms of host-cell regulation. The effects of Tax cover transcriptional activation of a specific set of cellular genes, *trans*-repression of another set of genes, and cell cycle promotion through inactivation of different types of tumor suppressor proteins. The target molecules are CREB, CREM, NF-κB, IκB, SRF, and CBP/p300 for activation, E47, p53, and CBP/p300 for repression, and p16INK4a, p15INK4b, p18INK4c, and hDlg for cell cycle promotion. Such pleiotropic effects of Tax protein seem to be the viral strategy to induce effective proliferation of infected cells to amplify its proviruses, which in turn immortalize and transform the infected cells. In addition to Tax, HTLV-1 expresses other minor proteins such as p12 (12, 14) and p35 (13) as a result of alternative splicing of the same region of the viral genome. These minor proteins are not covered in this review, although some of these related proteins also have the capacity to modulate cellular function and are required for in vivo replication (24).

ONCOGENIC ROLE OF TAX PROTEIN

The original prediction for viral involvement in leukemogenesis was made based on the finding of provirus integration in leukemic cells of ATL patients: Every ATL cell contained the proviral genome integrated in its chromosomal DNA, and the integration sites were clonal within individuals, indicating that leukemic cells originated from a single infected T cell (25). However, the sites were not common among patients (26). Therefore, the *cis*-acting effect of the LTR (long terminal repeat) of integrated proviruses seems unlikely to be the mechanism for ATL. Consequently, a *trans*-acting viral factor, Tax, has been proposed to be pivotal in the viral pathogenicity.

Independent from these in vivo studies, cell biology research demonstrated the oncogenic capacity of Tax: introduction of expression vector of Tax immortalized primary CD4-positive T cells (27); transfection of a Tax-expressing vector transformed Rat-1 and NIH3T3 to proliferate in suspension in soft agar (20); and furthermore, the vector transformed even primary rat fibroblasts in cooperation with ras oncogene (21). Transgenic mice carrying the tax gene under the control of the LTR developed tumors, although they were of mesenchymal origin (22). Mice with tax gene under the T cell–specific promoter developed leukemia/lymphoma (23), although it was not similar to ATL. All these in vitro findings clearly indicate the oncogenic capacity of Tax in vivo.

PLEIOTROPIC FUNCTION OF TAX

Tax is a 40-kDa protein mainly localized in the nucleus and originally identified as a *trans*-activator of viral gene expression responding to the 21-bp enhancer in the LTR (17, 16). Transcriptional regulation is the most critical step in retroviral replication; thus, studies initially focused on this function. Then this function of Tax was found to enhance expression of cellular oncogenes, growth factors, and some of their receptors, and more attention was directed to understanding the mechanism of cellular gene activation. Meanwhile, some other genes were found to be repressed by Tax, including tumor suppressor genes; therefore, research became more focused on *trans*-repression than *trans*-activation with respect to the leukemogenesis. This direction was further accelerated by the finding that Tax binds directly to and inhibits some tumor suppressor proteins. These functions of Tax not only induce abnormal cell proliferation, which may lead to malignant transformation, but they also increase the mutation rate or apoptotic resistance, although these mechanisms are not well understood.

Transcriptional Activation

Transcriptional activation is basically achieved by two independent mechanisms: The first is the binding of Tax to enhancer-binding proteins on the DNA such as CREB, NF-κB, and SRF, and the second is the inhibition or destabilization of inhibitors of transcription factors such as IκB (28). The first is a general mechanism for three different enhancers and explains well how Tax is able to respond to structurally unrelated enhancers. The second is specific to activation of NF-κB in the cytoplasm (Figure 1). These mechanisms are briefly reviewed in the following section, then their pathological significance is discussed.

CREB and CREM   To activate the viral LTR, Tax requires at least two copies of the 21-bp enhancer containing an imperfect CRE (cAMP-responsive element), to which binds cyclic AMP response element binding protein (CREB) (29, 30), cyclic AMP response element modulator (CREM) (29), activating transcription factors (ATFs) (31), Tax-responsive element binding proteins (TREB), and 21-bp

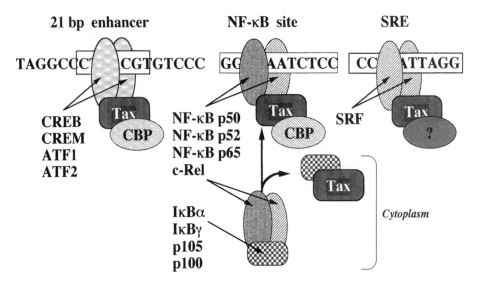

Figure 1   Activation of transcription. Tax binds to transcription factors such as CREB, NF-κB, and SRF and activates them or binds to IκBα and induces its instability.

binding proteins (HEBs; 32). The CREB and CREM proteins bind to Tax protein on the 21-bp enhancer without specific phosphorylation.

In normally regulated cells, CREB is phosphorylated by protein kinase A upon stimulation of the cell (33), and the phosphorylation of CREB allows its binding to a transcriptional activator, CBP (34, 35). The CBP thus associated with DNA would acetylate histone through its histone-acetylating activity (36–38), resulting in opening the nucleosome structure around the transcriptional site (39), thus leading to activation of transcription. Thus, CRE-dependent transcription becomes signal dependent. On the other hand, Tax was found to bind to CBP (40); therefore, Tax would be able to bridge between CREB and CBP without specific phosphorylation of CREB. This abnormal interaction of CREB-Tax-CBP would be able to explain the constitutive activation of the 21-bp enhancer in HTLV-1-infected cells (41, 42).

However, we have previously reported that the consensus sequence of the CRE is not *trans*-activated by Tax, and a unique but small flanking sequence upstream of the CRE is required (43); therefore, it is postulated that some other mechanism or factor is involved. This puzzle is still not well solved, but thus far different observations have been reported. Adya et al (44) reported that CREB protein, bound to the viral 21-bp enhancer but not to the consensus CRE, is able to undergo conformational change in the presence of Tax; thus, the complex on the DNA element is stabilized. On the other hand, Nyborg et al (45) claimed that Tax has to interact with 21-bp enhancer DNA directly for *trans*-activation. Recently, PCAF (p300/CBP-associated factor), a transcriptional coactivator (46), was reported to interact with Tax and *trans*-activate transcription in a histone-acetyltransferase-independent manner (47, 48). It is not clear whether PCAF is involved in the 21-bp-specific *trans*-activation; however, further studies on Tax-induced *trans*-activation would elucidate more complete features of CREB-mediated transcription.

hGli2   At least two copies of the viral 21-bp enhancer are required for efficient activation by Tax in reconstituted promoter systems. Despite this principle, a series of deletion mutagenesis of the LTR indicated that an LTR fragment containing a single copy of the third 21-bp is highly activated by Tax (49, 50). Analyzing this phenomenon, we identified another sequence termed TRE-2 (Tax-responsive element-2) adjacent to the third copy of the 21-bp as an additional element responsible for the activation. A newly identified protein, hGli2, binds to TRE-2 (51), and the binding of hGli2 to TRE-2 is essential for Tax-mediated *trans*-activation of one copy of the 21-bp enhancer. It has been revealed that hGli2 binding to TRE-2 enhanced the recruitment of CREB onto the adjacent element 21-bp (52). The recruited CREB would now be able to bind to Tax to activate transcription similarly to the *trans*-activation through two copies of the 21-bp enhancer.

NF-κB Activation of NF-κB   HTLV-1-infected T cell lines frequently produce various lymphokines such as interleukin-6 (IL-6), granulocyte macrophage colony stimulating factor (GM-CSF), tumor necrosis factor β (TNFβ), and others (53). One of the characteristics of ATL cells is overexpression of the alpha subunit of the IL-2 receptor (IL-2Rα) (54). This overexpression or overproduction is mediated by activation of a transcription factor family NF-κB. The interaction of NF-κB with Tax was originally identified by immunoprecipitation of an NF-κB precursor, p105, with anti-Tax antibodies from HTLV-1-infected cell extracts (55). It is now well established that Tax binds to NF-κB family proteins including NF-κB p50, p65, c-Rel (56, 57), and NF-κB-2 (lyt10; 58) and activates the NF-κB-dependent transcription.

The NF-κB proteins bind to p300 (59, 60, 61), similarly to the interaction of CREB and CBP (discussed above). Therefore, a mechanism similar to activation of CRE-dependent transcription through Tax-CREB interaction has been predicted for the activation of NF-κB-dependent transcription by Tax (41). Abnormally high expression of IL-2Rα on ATL cells might also be explained by this mechanism (62).

Inactivation of IκB   In unstimulated cells, NF-κB proteins are held up in the cytoplasm as an inactive complex with IκB (63). Stimulatory signals phosphorylate IκB and destabilize it, resulting in release from the inactive complex and nuclear translocation of the active form of NFκB, thus enhancing NF-κB-dependent transcription. Therefore, HTLV-1-infected cells require an additional mechanism for NF-κB activation by Tax in the nucleus. This mechanism is the binding of Tax to IκBα, which results in destabilization of IκBα and nuclear transloca-tion of NFκB (64, 65). In addition to the simple binding of Tax to IκB, activation of cytokine-inducible kinases, IKKα and IKKβ, was reported to result in con-stitutive phosphorylation and degradation followed by nuclear translocation of NF-κB (66). Therefore, two independent processes appear to be involved in acti-vation of NFκB. This is evidence that Tax also functions in the cytoplasm.

SRF (Serum Response Factor)   For the *trans*-activation of the immediate early nuclear oncogenes, c-fos and c-egr, Tax binds to a serum responsive factor (p67^{SRF}) (67, 56) on SRE. Biologically inactive mutants of Tax did not bind to p67^{SRF}, indi-cating that the complex formation is important for *trans*-activation. It is uncertain which transcriptional coactivator is involved in this activation.

Transcriptional Repression

When the Tax-mediated *trans*-activation was actively investigated, an opposite function, *trans*-repression, was described in the expression of DNA polymerase β (68). The mechanism of the *trans*-repression, however, has not been well charac-terized until recently. The finding regarding *trans*-repression of Tax on p18INK4c gene, a family member of the inhibitors of cycline-dependent kinase, and the effect on p53 revealed the linkage between *trans*-repression and leukemogenesis.

P18INK4c is an inhibitor of CDK4, a member of tumor suppressor gene p16INK4a, and is thus able to arrest the cell at G1 phase of the cell cycle. We found downregulation of the promoter activity of p18INK4 by Tax expression (69, 70); the so-called E-Box element in the p18INK4 gene is responsible for the *trans*-repression. An E-Box-binding protein, E47, showed no interaction with Tax (42). This finding suggested a mechanistic correlation between *trans*-activation and *trans*-repression through interaction of Tax with CBP/p300 (40), which is able to interact with CREB and also with E47 (see Figure 2).

Transcriptional Coactivators, CBP/p300   A reporter plasmid carrying the E-Box sequence was activated by cotransfection of E-47 and p300, and the enhanced expression was efficiently *trans*-repressed by Tax (42). E47 is an E-Box binding protein, and p300 is a member of the transcriptional co-activator family, CBP/p300 (71, 72). The binding of E47 to the E-Box DNA was not affected by Tax, but asso-ciation of p300 with the E47-DNA complex was decreased by Tax. The decrease of p300 association was correlated with *trans*-repression and also correlated with the formation of Tax-p300 complex (42), clearly indicating that Tax binds to p300 and interferes with the integration of p300 into the E47-E-Box complex, thus re-sulting in downregulation of transcription. This conclusion implies that Tax and transcription factors compete with coactivators CBP/p300, and their expression levels and affinity to CBP/p300 affect the efficiency of transcription; that is, the cascade of Tax in transcriptional repression is unexpectedly wide in its targets and highly variable in its effectiveness.

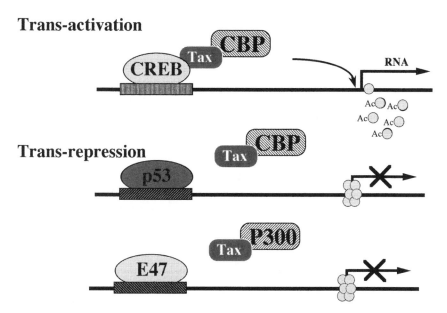

Figure 2 Proposed mechanisms for *trans*-activation and *trans*-repression by HTLV-1 Tax. Tax binds to CBP/p300 and either accelerates interaction with CREB or interferes with interaction with p53 or E47.

Transcription Factor p53 Recently, it has been reported that p53-dependent transcription is repressed by Tax protein (73, 74). The p53-dependent transcription requires binding of the p53-CBP complex to the p53-binding site of the reporter (75). Similarly to the case of p18INK4c promoter, CBP binding to p53 on the p53-binding site was effectively inhibited by Tax binding to CBP (42). Therefore, the same mechanism as that for E-Box-mediated *trans*-repression has been proposed, namely, Tax binding to CBP interferes with the interaction of CBP with p53 on the DNA (76, 77).

Other mechanisms have also been reported for the repression of p53-mediated transcription. In HTLV-1-infected cells, Ser-15 of p53 is hyperphosphorylated and p53 is inactive in interaction with transcription factor TFIID, although it is active in sequence-specific DNA binding (78). Although the mechanism for hyperphosphorylation is not elucidated, apparently the mechanism for the inactivation of p53 is categorically different from the events on specific DNA element. Another finding is NF-κB-dependent inactivation of p53 (79). According to this report, Tax inactivation of p53 correlates with NF-κB activation but not with CBP/p300 squelching. Interestingly, Tax failed to inactivate p53 in NF-κB p65 knockout mouse embryo fibroblasts (79). Redundancy and cross-talk of regulatory pathways are operating, and the viral infection seems able to modify these pathways through a single protein, Tax.

Unified Principle for Trans-Activation and Trans-Repression

To molecular biologists, it is an interesting question how a single protein is able to activate one set of gene expression and to repress another set. After finding transcriptional coactivators, CBP/p300, as the common factors between the opposite responses to Tax function, we proposed a unified principle for the *trans*-activation and -repression: "Tax binds to CBP/p300, and when Tax in the Tax-CBP/p300 has high affinity to transcription factors, the interaction would result in *trans*-activation, but when Tax in the protein complex has no affinity to transcription factors, the interaction would result in *trans*-repression" (42; see Figure 2). In fact, Tax was confirmed to recruit CBP/p300 efficiently into enhancer-transcription factor complex when Tax has affinity to the transcription factor (42). The effects of Tax in this unified principle would depend on the affinity of Tax to CBP/p300 in transactivation and also on the competing ability of transcription factors with Tax to CBP/p300 in *trans*-repression. Particularly in *trans*-repression, the competing capacity would be greatly affected by the affinity of transcription factors to CBP/p300 (72) and by the expression levels of the transcription factors; it would thus be highly variable. Competition with low levels of CBP/p300 (80) would take place not only with Tax but also among transcription factors. However, the full situation seems to be more complex, since histone acetyltransferase-independent *trans*-activation has been described even in the CBP/p300-dependent transcription system (47).

Inhibition of Tumor Suppressor Proteins

Independently from transcriptional regulation, Tax was found to interact with negative regulators of cycline-dependent kinases, inhibitors of CDK4 (INK4) (19, 81). A typical member of the INK4 family is $p16^{INK4a}$, which is also known to be a tumor suppressor gene in many types of human tumors (82). When the negative function of $p16^{INK4a}$ is impaired, CDK4/6 is activated and phosphorylates Rb, a tumor-suppressor protein. Hyperphosphorylated Rb then releases E2F as an active form, a family of transcription factors, and then activates expression of various genes required for progression of cells from G1 to S phase (83, 84). The clue for $p16^{INK4a}$ as a Tax target came from the binding domain of IκB for Tax, the ankyrin motif, which is also contained in the INK4 family proteins (85). $P16^{INK4a}$ is an effective target of Tax protein.

p16INK4a and p15INK4b, Cell Cycle Regulators   The binding of Tax to p16-INK4a was demonstrated in vitro using GST-p16INK4a and also in vivo using cotransfection followed by immunoprecipitation (81). The binding of Tax to p16INK4a inhibited its negative function on CDK4/6 and thus rescued the kinase activity from the inhibition by p16INK4a (81; see Figure 3). A mutant of Tax, D320, which binds to Tax, also restored the kinase activity, but another mutant that does not bind to Tax was unable to do so. The effect of Tax binding to p16INK4a on cell proliferation was examined using a cell line U2OS that lacks the

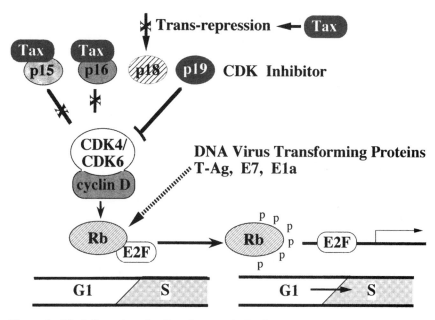

Figure 3 Viral disruption of cell cycle control. Tax binds to p16INK4a and p15INK4b and inactivates their function; on the other hand, Tax *trans*-represses p18INK4c expression. The signaling pathway includes Rb, which is targeted by DNA tumor viruses.

p16^{INK4a} gene but retains the wild-type Rb. The results indicated that the binding of Tax to p16INK4a was able to activate CDK4/6 and phosphorylated Rb and then to induce G1/S phase transition of the target cells (81).

Exactly the same results were obtained with p15INK4b, another member of the INK4 family; therefore, both p16INK4a and p15INK4b are functionally knocked out by Tax protein (70). These two genes are recognized as tumor suppressor genes, MTS-1 and -2, and are frequently deleted in human cancer cells (82). Therefore, the Tax-induced functional inactivation of these two INK4 family proteins might mimic the effect of deletion of these genes in cancer cells, strongly suggesting involvement of this mechanism in ATL development.

hDlg Which Associates with APC A yeast two hybrid system using Tax as a bait was used to isolate a human counterpart of Dlg, a drosophila tumor suppressor gene (86). hDlg is a signaling molecule downstream of the Wnt/Frizzle pathway (87) and interacts with the C-terminus of a tumor suppressor protein, APC (88). Tax was found to bind to the same domain, PDZ domain, of hDlg in vitro and also in vivo (89, 90); therefore, the C-terminus of Tax and APC compete with the same site of the hDlg molecule (86). Furthermore, Tax-expression induced hyperphosphorylation of hDlg, as demonstrated by slower migration in gel electrophoresis (86). The Tax mutant at the C-terminus, which cannot bind to hDlg, did not induce slower migration of the band; thus, Tax binding to hDlg is responsible for the induction of hyperphosphorylation. Through these two effects of Tax, binding competition with APC and hyperphosphorylation of hDlg, Tax is able to induce cell growth. BrUdR incorporation assay into newly synthesized DNA demonstrated that binding of Tax to hDlg is able to perturb the cytostatic effect of hDlg and to promote abnormal proliferation of cells. However, here, one may argue that APC is a tumor suppressor gene of the colon, but not of lymphocytes. In such discussion, it is noteworthy that APC and hDlg are significantly expressed in normal T cells (T Suzuki, M Yoshida, unpublished observation); thus, these interactions might have some roles in T cells, although they are not well understood.

Functional Similarities of Tax and Transforming Proteins of DNA Tumor Viruses

Viral oncogenes are not required for retroviral replication; however, Tax is essential for gene expression and replication of HTLV-1. The physiological significance of Tax is thus in contrast to the retroviral oncogenes, but rather similar to the transforming proteins of DNA tumor viruses (84). T antigens of SV40 and poliomavirus, E1A of adenoviruses, and E6/7 of papillomaviruses are all required for viral replication and also modify cellular regulation through multiple mechanisms.

Similarities are also pointed out in the cellular targets and/or targeted signaling pathway. Tax inactivates p16INK4a and p15INK4b, inhibitors of CDK4/6, which are upstream of Rb targeted by the transforming proteins of DNA tumor viruses, T-Ag, E1A, and E7 (see Figure 3). That is, retrovirus HTLV-1 and DNA tumor viruses knock out the same signaling pathway although targeting different components (84). The targeting hDlg is also shared among Tax 86, E6 of high-risk HPV (89, 91), and E4 9ORF1 protein of adenoviruses (89). CBP/p300 also interacts with T-Ag and E1A (92–94).

It is surprising to recognize that developmentally unrelated viruses target such similar molecules and signaling pathways among the many regulatory mechanisms. A possible explanation may reside in the key function of the targets; that is, they are critical for normal regulation of cell proliferation; therefore, modulation of these pathways is the most effective strategy to induce unregulatable cell growth. Irrespective of viral evolution, tumor viruses that acquired the most effective strategy for their replication could have survived until today. If this hypothesis is accepted, then it can be further deduced that these signaling molecules play key roles in fibroblastic and lymphoid tissues.

Another surprising aspect is the reason retrovirus and DNA virus should share the targets for their replication. In general, retroviruses require transcription, and DNA viruses require DNA replication as a critical replicative process. The reason why HTLV-1 adopted the strategy to enhance proliferation of infected cells might be as follows: HTLV-1 adopted the strategy to repress its own replication to survive under strong pressure of immunosurveillance in humans. To achieve this, HTLV-1 would have acquired a negative regulator, Rex, downregulating viral gene expression (not discussed sufficiently in this review; see Ref. 95) and HTLV-1 replication become transient, maintained at low levels and mostly latent in vivo (96). Therefore, replication of the host cells into which its genome was integrated would be required to amplify the viral genome, similar to DNA tumor viruses enhancing cellular DNA replication.

Domains for Tax Interaction

Tax now appears to interact with many proteins, and certainly, more will be found. However, the interacting domains of Tax protein are not well defined thus far. Only some mutants were informative. For example, d3 (55) and M22 (97) mutating at the N-terminal region do not bind to CREB, but do bind to NF-κB; and mutant M47 97 substituting at the C-terminal region binds to CREB, but not to NF-κB. These mutants clearly indicate that the domains for these interactions are not identical, but data are not adequate to define the whole feature of the domains. For binding to CBP/p300, a region around amino acid residues 82 to 89 was proposed to be important (98).

On the other hand, the interacting domains of the target proteins have been defined in some cases: a basic region adjacent to the leucine zipper structure of CREB (99), Rel-homology domain of NF-κB (57), ankyrin motifs of IκB (85), KIX domain of CBP (100), PDZ domain of hDlg (89, 86), and others. No significant homology has been identified among the primary amino acid sequences of these domains, apparently suggesting that the binding domains for Tax might be arranged by protein folding, but nothing certain is known in this respect.

COOPERATION AND CROSS-TALK OF PLEIOTROPIC FUNCTIONS OF TAX

Tax protein functions at different levels, activating and repressing transcription, and inhibiting cell cycle regulators and tumor suppressor proteins. Why is Tax so pleiotropic? Are only some of these effects associated with malignant transformation? There is no definite answer to these question today, but interesting and suggestive discussion is possible.

Cell Proliferation

Tax targets for *trans*-activation are lymphokines such as IL-6 (101), GM-CSF (102), and TGFβ (103), lymphokine receptors such as IL-2 receptor α (62), and nuclear oncogenes such as c-*fos* (104), c-*egr*, and c-*jun* (105). These genes are *trans*-activated independently through NF-κB and SRF but are mostly growth-promoting genes; thus, this *trans*-activation would be cooperative for efficient proliferation of infected cells. Furthermore, the genes *trans*-repressed by Tax include p18INK4c (70), Lck (106), a tyrosine kinase that downregulates T cell stimulation, and NF-1 (107), a tumor suppressor protein of neurofibroblastoma.

Interestingly, these are mostly growth-retarding genes; thus, these *trans*-repression mechanisms would again cooperate with each other and also with *trans*-activation of other sets of genes for efficient proliferation of infected cells (Figure 4).

Furthermore, other effects of Tax on tumor suppressor proteins such as p16-INK4a, p15 (81, 108), cyclin D3 (19), and hDlg (89, 86) result in abnormal promotion of the cell cycle, which frequently links to malignant transformation. After all, most of the genes targeted by Tax through categorically different mechanisms seem to cooperate to promote cell proliferation. A surprising aspect is that a single protein, Tax, is able to affect so many targets, mostly directed to cell proliferation. Such a situation is unlikely to be a coincidental selection of targets by Tax; this therefore suggests a few possible molecules that coordinate divergent and redundant regulatory machinery for cell proliferation and differentiation. Tax may mimic these putative molecules.

Cell Cycle Check Point, Mutation, and Apoptosis

Tax affects genes the functions of which are not directly linked to cell proliferation. One is *trans*-repression of DNA polymerase β (68), a key enzyme for DNA repair. DNA polymerase β is involved in repair of damaged DNA; therefore, *trans*-repression of this gene might result in higher frequency of mutation in host cells.

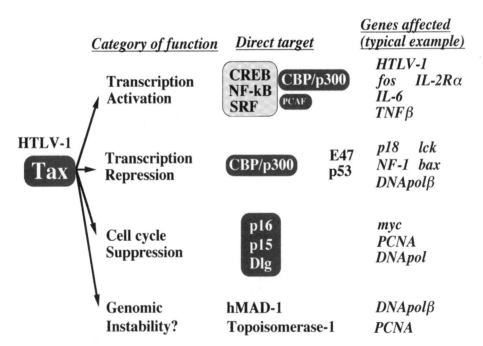

Figure 4   Pleiotropic function of Tax. Four different categories of Tax function and their direct targets and final target genes are summarized.

Other possible mechanisms for higher mutation rate have also been proposed: direct inhibition of topoisomerase I by Tax (109) and *trans*-activation by Tax of PCNA gene (cellular proliferating cell nuclear antigen (110). As expected from these molecular analyses, a mutagenic effect of Tax on host cell chromosomes was directly demonstrated (111, 112). Thus, Tax expression and modulation of DNA polymerase β, topoisomerase I, and/or PCNA predispose cells to accumulation of DNA damage and contribute to malignant conversion of infected cells.

In relation to DNA damage and its repair, attention should be focused on the Tax effects on p53. *Trans*-repression of p53-dependent transcription is particularly notable (73, 74, 42). In addition to this *trans*-repression, inactivation of p53 through phosphorylation of Ser-15 (78) and NF-κB-dependent inactivation of p53 (79) have been described. The details are not known yet, but it is apparent that activation of kinase, activation of NF-κB, and *trans*-repression of p53-dependent transcription all cooperate to abolish the cell cycle check point function of p53, thus leading cells to accumulation of DNA mutations in cells. Continuous disposition of infected cells to such a situation would accelerate malignant transformation and thus progression to ATL.

Cell cycle processes are inspected at checkpoints and allowed to progress only when the scheduled processes are verified. Thus, once the checkpoint system faces any problem, undesired cells can go through their cell cycle and proliferate, fixing the abnormality. Tax of HTLV-1 was described to bind to the human homolog (HsMAD1) of yeast mitotic checkpoint protein MAD1 (113). HsMAD1 is a component of the mitotic checkpoint system that prevents anaphase and commitment to cellular division until chromosomal alignment is properly completed. Therefore, abrogation of the mitotic checkpoint function of HsMAD1 may be linked to abnormal cell division and accumulation of chromosomal abnormalities. These cells are triggered to undergo apoptosis. Tax protein, however, is able to prevent apoptosis that arises from suppression of p53 function through activation of NF-κB and *trans*-activation of Bcl-X (114) or expression of XIAP (X-chromosome-linked inhibitor of apoptosis) protein (115). Other possible mechanisms include repression of bax gene expression (116).

In summary, most of the pleiotropic functions of Tax protein cooperate in promoting cell proliferation, accumulation of DNA damage, and avoiding apoptosis of abnormal cells infected with HTLV-1.

TRANSIENT OR RARE EXPRESSION OF TAX IN VIVO AND ATL DEVELOPMENT

As discussed in the previous sections, the pleiotropic function of Tax cooperates to promote proliferation of HTLV-1-infected cells; therefore, these would be the early mechanism of ATL development in vivo. Consistent with the prediction, infected cells in vivo are random in their clonality. However, leukemic cells are always monoclonal at their proviral integration site within an individual patient.

Apparently, Tax alone is not sufficient for the clonal expansion of infected cells, but nothing is known about such genetic event(s). Even for the early mechanism, the expression level of Tax has been thought to be too low; that is, the expression can be detected only by PCR and is absolutely negative in over 95% of infected cells. Such low expression is observed in both leukemic and nonleukemic cells. However, once cells are taken out and put into culture, these cells initiate viral gene expression as rapidly as a few hours after cultivation. Such extremely low expression of Tax is always a target of discussion in the application of in vitro observations to ATL development.

Continuous expression of the viral antigens would not be possible since such cells would be rejected by the host immune response; therefore, expression has to be transient, otherwise infected cells would not be able to survive in vivo. Therefore, it is reasonable to predict that a certain level of Tax is transiently expressed in a limited population of infected cells at one time and in another cell population at another time. For example, a small number of infected cells could be stimulated to express Tax, and its expression would be diminished soon by feedback regulation by Rex and then become latent for a while. Different specificity of stimulation would induce Tax expression in a different population of T cells. During transient expression of Tax, a cell proliferation would be efficiently enhanced in a given population through multiple mechanisms. Such a situation would take place in carriers repeatedly for a long period, even after clonal expansion of infected cells (Figure 5). During the early stage, cell growth–promoting effects would be significant in increasing the cell population for malignant transformation, but in the later

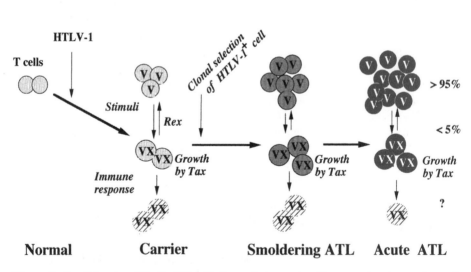

Figure 5 Possible roles of Tax in ATL initiation and progression. Tax promotes abnormal growth of a small population of infected cells where it is expressed, increases the cell population for transformation, and also promotes cell growth even after progression of infected cells toward more malignancy. V: HTLV-infected cell; VX: HTLV-expressing cell.

stages, functions related to accumulation of mutations and prevention of apoptosis may have more significance. In this respect, Tax is able to function as a tumor initiator as well as a tumor promoter.

For example, Tax inhibits tumor suppressor protein p16INK4a during its transient expression; thus, cells can undergo abnormal growth with the wild-type expression of p16INK4a. In fact, HTLV-1-infected T cell lines mostly maintain p16INK4a genes, although all uninfected T cell lines do not. Even though this is true in infected cells, deletion of p16INK4a in infected cells would allow more efficient proliferation than that by Tax-induced functional inhibition; therefore, once p16INK4a deletion is taking place in infected cells, the cells would progress more easily to ATL cells. Therefore, the finding that some ATL patients have deletion of p16INK4a gene 117 can be explained without any difficulty.

Finally, it should be emphasized that Tax alone is apparently not sufficient to explain the final leukemia. It is still necessary to identify second, third, or even further molecular events during the progression of ATL for the full understanding of ATL.

Visit the Annual Reviews home page at www.AnnualReviews.org

LITERATURE CITED

1. Seiki M, Hattori S, Yoshida M. 1982. Human adult T-cell leukemia virus: molecular cloning of the provirus DNA and the unique terminal structure. *Proc. Natl. Acad. Sci. USA* 79:6899–902

2. Poeisz BJ, Ruscetti RW, Gazdar AF, Bunn PA, Minna JD, Gallo RC. 1980. Detection and isolation of the C retrovirus from fresh and cultured lymphocytes of a patient with T cell lymphoma. *Proc. Natl. Acad. Sci. USA* 77:7415–19

3. Yoshida M, Miyoshi I, Hinuma Y. 1982. Isolation and characterization of retrovirus from cell lines of human adult T-cell leukemia and its implication in the disease. *Proc. Natl. Acad. Sci. USA* 79:2031–35

4. Hinuma Y, Nagata K, Hanaoka M, Nakai M, Matsumoto T, Kinoshita KI, Shirakawa S, Miyoshi I. 1981. Adult T-cell leukemia: antigen in an ATL cell line and detection of antibodies to the antigen in human sera. *Proc. Natl. Acad. Sci. USA* 78:6476–80

5. Osame M, Usuku K, Izumo S, Ijichi N, Amitani H, Igata A, Matsumoto M, Tara M. 1986. HTLV-I associated myelopathy, a new clinical entity [letter]. *Lancet* 1:1031–32

6. Gessain A, Barin F, Vernant JC, Gout O, Maurs L, Calender A, de The G. 1985. Antibodies to human T-lymphotropic virus type-I in patients with tropical spastic paraparesis. *Lancet* 2:407–10

7. Seiki M, Hattori S, Hirayama Y, Yoshida M. 1983. Human adult T-cell leukemia virus: complete nucleotide sequence of the provirus genome integrated in leukemia cell DNA. *Proc. Natl. Acad. Sci. USA* 80:3618–22

8. Kiyokawa T, Seiki M, Imagawa K, Shimizu F, Yoshida M. 1984. Identification of a protein (p40x) encoded by a unique sequence pX of human T-cell leukemia virus type I. *Gann* 75:747–51

9. Lee TH, Coligan JE, Sodroski JG, Haseltine WA, Salahuddin SZ, Wong-Staal F, Gallo RC, Essex M. 1984. Antigens encoded by the 3′-terminal region of human T-cell leukemia virus: evidence for a functional gene. *Science* 226:57–61

10. Kiyokawa T, Seiki M, Iwashita S, Imagawa K, Shimizu F, Yoshida M. 1985. p27x-III and p21x-III, proteins encoded by the pX sequence of human T-cell leukemia virus type I. *Proc. Natl. Acad. Sci. USA* 82:8359–63

11. Dokhelar MC, Pickford H, Sodroski J, Haseltine WA. 1989. HTLV-I p27rex regulates gag and env protein expression. *J. Acquir. Immune Defic. Syndr.* 2:431–40

12. Franchini G, Mulloy JC, Koralnik IJ, Lo Monico A, Sparkowski JJ, Andresson T, Goldstein DJ, Schlegel R. 1993. The human T-cell leukemia/lymphotropic virus type I p12I protein cooperates with the E5 oncoprotein of bovine papillomavirus in cell transformation and binds the 16-kilodalton subunit of the vacuolar H+ ATPase. *J. Virol.* 67:7701–4

13. Koralnik IJ, Gessain A, Klotman ME, Lo Monico A, Berneman ZN, Franchini G. 1992. Protein isoforms encoded by the pX region of human T-cell leukemia/lymphotropic virus type I. *Proc. Natl. Acad. Sci. USA* 89:8813–17

14. Ciminale V, Pavlakis GN, Derse D, Cunningham CP, Felber BK. 1992. Complex splicing in the human T-cell leukemia virus (HTLV) family of retroviruses: novel mRNAs and proteins produced by HTLV type I. *J. Virol.* 66:1737–45

15. Seiki M, Hikikoshi A, Taniguchi T, Yoshida M. 1985. Expression of the pX gene of HTLV-I: general splicing mechanism in the HTLV family. *Science* 228:1532–34

16. Fujisawa J, Seiki M, Kiyokawa T, Yoshida M. 1985. Functional activation of the long terminal repeat of human T-cell leukemia virus type I by a trans-acting factor. *Proc. Natl. Acad. Sci. USA* 82:2277–81

17. Sodroski JG, Rosen CA, Haseltine WA. 1984. Trans-acting transcriptional activation of the long terminal repeat of human T lymphotropic viruses in infected cells. *Science* 225:381–85

18. Seiki M, Inoue J, Takeda T, Hikikoshi A, Sato M, Yoshida M. 1985. The p40x of human T-cell leukemia virus type I is a transacting activator of viral gene transcription. *Jpn. J. Cancer Res.* 76:1127–31

19. Neuveut C, Low KG, Maldarelli F, Schmitt I, Majone F, Grassmann R, Jeang KT. 1998. Human T-cell leukemia virus type 1 Tax and cell cycle progression: role of cyclin D-cdk and p110Rb. *Mol. Cell. Biol.* 18:3620–32

20. Tanaka A, Takahashi C, Yamaoka S, Nosaka T, Maki M, Hatanaka M. 1990. Oncogenic transformation by the tax gene of human T-cell leukemia virus type I in vitro. *Proc. Natl. Acad. Sci. USA* 87:1071–75

21. Pozzatti R, Vogel J, Jay G. 1990. The human T-lymphotropic virus type I tax gene can cooperate with the ras oncogene to induce neoplastic transformation of cells. *Mol. Cell. Biol.* 10:413–17

22. Nerenberg M, Hinrichs SH, Reynolds RK, Khoury G, Jay G. 1987. The tat gene of human T lymphotropic virus type I induces mesenchymal tumors in transgenic mice. *Science* 237:1324–29

23. Grossman WJ, Kimata JT, Wong FH, Zutter M, Ley TJ, Ratner L. 1995. Development of leukemia in mice transgenic for the tax gene of human T-cell leukemia virus type I. *Proc. Natl. Acad. Sci. USA* 92:1057–61

24. Kerkhofs P, Heremans H, Burny A, Kettmann R, Willems L. 1998. In vitro and in vivo oncogenic potential of bovine leukemia virus G4 protein. *J. Virol.* 72:2554–59

25. Yoshida M, Seiki M, Yamaguchi K, Takatsuki K. 1984. Monoclonal integration of human T-cell leukemia provirus in all primary tumors of adult T-cell leukemia suggests causative role of human T-cell leukemia virus in the disease. *Proc. Natl. Acad. Sci. USA* 81:2534–37

26. Seiki M, Eddy R, Shows TB, Yoshida M. 1984. Nonspecific integration of the

HTLV provirus genome into adult T-cell leukaemia cells. *Nature* 309:640–42

27. Grassmann R, Berchtold S, Radant I, Alt M, Fleckenstein B, Sodroski JG, Haseltine WA, Ramstedt U. 1992. Role of human T-cell leukemia virus type 1 X region proteins in immortalization of primary human lymphocytes in culture. *J. Virol.* 66:4570–75

28. Yoshida M. 1993. HTLV-1 Tax: regulation of gene expression and disease. *Trends Microbiol.* 1:131–35

29. Suzuki T, Fujisawa JI, Toita M, Yoshida M. 1993. The trans-activator tax of human T-cell leukemia virus type 1 (HTLV-1) interacts with cAMP-responsive element (CRE) binding and CRE modulator proteins that bind to the 21-base-pair enhancer of HTLV-1. *Proc. Natl. Acad. Sci. USA* 90:610–14

30. Zhao LJ, Giam CZ. 1992. Human T-cell lymphotropic virus type I (HTLV-I) transcriptional activator, Tax, enhances CREB binding to HTLV-I 21-base-pair repeats by protein-protein interaction. *Proc. Natl. Acad. Sci. USA* 89:7070–74

31. Hai TW, Liu F, Coukos WJ, Green MR. 1989. Transcription factor ATF cDNA clones: an extensive family of leucine zipper proteins able to selectively form DNA-binding heterodimers [published erratum appears in *Genes Dev.* 1990 Apr; 4(4):682]. *Genes Dev.* 3:2083–90

32. Beraud C, Lombard-Platet G, Michal Y, Jalinot P. 1991. Binding of the HTLV-I Tax1 transactivator to the inducible 21 bp enhancer is mediated by the cellular factor HEB1. *EMBO J.* 10:3795–3803

33. Gonzalez GA, Yamamoto KK, Fischer WH, Karr D, Menzel P, Biggs Wd, Vale WW, Montminy MR. 1989. A cluster of phosphorylation sites on the cyclic AMP-regulated nuclear factor CREB predicted by its sequence. *Nature* 337:749–52

34. Chrivia JC, Kwok RP, Lamb N, Hagiwara M, Montminy MR, Goodman RH. 1993. Phosphorylated CREB binds specifically to the nuclear protein CBP. *Nature* 365:855–59

35. Kwok RP, Lundblad JR, Chrivia JC, Richards JP, Bachinger HP, Brennan RG, Roberts SG, Green MR, Goodman RH. 1994. Nuclear protein CBP is a coactivator for the transcription factor CREB. *Nature* 370:223–26

36. Bannister AJ, Kouzarides T. 1996. The CBP co-activator is a histone acetyltransferase. *Nature* 384:641–43

37. Ogryzko VV, Schiltz RL, Russanova V, Howard BH, Nakatani Y. 1996. The transcriptional coactivators p300 and CBP are histone acetyltransferases. *Cell* 87:953–59

38. Yang XJ, Ogryzko VV, Nishikawa J, Howard BH, Nakatani Y. 1996. A p300/CBP-associated factor that competes with the adenoviral oncoprotein E1A. *Nature* 382:319–24

39. Munshi N, Merika M, Yie J, Senger K, Chen G, Thanos D. 1998. Acetylation of HMG I(Y) by CBP turns off IFN beta expression by disrupting the enhanceosome. *Mol. Cell.* 2:457–67

40. Kwok RP, Laurance ME, Lundblad JR, Goldman PS, Shih H, Connor LM, Marriott SJ, Goodman RH. 1996. Control of cAMP-regulated enhancers by the viral transactivator Tax through CREB and the coactivator CBP. *Nature* 380:642–46

41. Bex F, Yin MJ, Burny A, Gaynor RB. 1998. Differential transcriptional activation by human T-cell leukemia virus type 1 Tax mutants is mediated by distinct interactions with CREB binding protein and p300. *Mol. Cell. Biol.* 18:2392–405

42. Suzuki T, Uchida-Toita M, Yoshida M. 1999. Tax protein of HTLV-1 inhibits CBP/p300-mediated transcription by interfering with recruitment of CBP/p300 onto DNA element of E-box or p53 binding site. *Oncogene* 18:4137–43

43. Fujisawa J, Toita M, Yoshida M. 1989. A unique enhancer element for the trans activator (p40tax) of human T-cell leukemia virus type I that is distinct from cyclic

AMP- and 12-O-tetradecanoylphorbol-13-acetate-responsive elements. *J. Virol.* 63: 3234–39

44. Adya N, Zhao LJ, Huang W, Boros I, Giam CZ. 1994. Expansion of CREB's DNA recognition specificity by Tax results from interaction with Ala-Ala-Arg at positions 282-284 near the conserved DNA-binding domain of CREB. *Proc. Natl. Acad. Sci. USA* 91:5642–46

45. Lenzmeier BA, Giebler HA, Nyborg JK. 1998. Human T-cell leukemia virus type 1 Tax requires direct access to DNA for recruitment of CREB binding protein to the viral promoter. *Mol. Cell. Biol.* 18:721–31

46. Puri P, Sartorelli V, Yang X, Hamamori Y, Ogryzko V, Howard B, Kedes L, Wang J, Grassmann A, Nakatani Y. 1997. Differential roles of p300 and PCAF acetyltransferases in muscle differentiation. *Mol. Cell.* 1:35–45

47. Jiang H, Lu H, Schitz R, Pise-Masison C, Ogryzko V, Nakatani Y, Brady J. 1999. PCAF interacts with tax and stimulates tax transactivation in a histone acetyltransferase-independent manner. *Mol. Cell. Biol.* 19:8136–45

48. Harrod R, Kuo Y, Tang Y, Yao Y, Vassilev A, Nakatani Y, Giam C. 2000. p300 and p300/cAMP-responsive element-binding protein associated factor interact with human T-cell lymphotropic virus type-1 Tax in a multi-histone acetyltransferase/activator-enhacer complex. *J. Biol. Chem.* 275:11852–57

49. Brady J, Jeang KT, Duvall J, Khoury G. 1987. Identification of p40x-responsive regulatory sequences within the human T-cell leukemia virus type I long terminal repeat. *J. Virol.* 61:2175–81

50. Tanimura A, Teshima H, Fujisawa J, Yoshida M. 1993. A new regulatory element that augments the Tax-dependent enhancer of human T-cell leukemia virus type 1 and cloning of cDNAs encoding its binding proteins. *J. Virol.* 67:5375–82

51. Tanimura A, Dan S, Yoshida M. 1998.

Cloning of novel isoforms of the human Gli2 oncogene and their activities to enhance tax-dependent transcription of the human T-cell leukemia virus type 1 genome. *J. Virol.* 72:3958–64

52. Dan S, Tanimura A, Yoshida M. 1999. Interaction of Gli2 with CREB protein on DNA elements in the long terminal repeat of human T-cell leukemia virus type 1 is responsible for transcriptional activation by tax protein. *J. Virol.* 73:3258–63

53. Yoshida M. 1995. HTLV-1 oncoprotein Tax deregulates transcription of cellular genes through multiple mechanisms. *J. Cancer Res. Clin. Oncol.* 121:521–28

54. Teshigawara K, Maeda M, Nishino K, Nikaido T, Uchiyama T, Tsudo M, Wano Y, Yodoi J. 1985. Adult T leukemia cells produce a lymphokine that augments interleukin 2 receptor expression. *J. Mol. Cell. Immunol.* 2:17–26

55. Hirai H, Fujisawa J, Suzuki T, Ueda K, Muramatsu M, Tsuboi A, Arai N, Yoshida M. 1992. Transcriptional activator Tax of HTLV-1 binds to the NF-kappa B precursor p105. *Oncogene* 7:1737–42

56. Suzuki T, Hirai H, Fujisawa J, Fujita T, Yoshida M. 1993. A trans-activator Tax of human T-cell leukemia virus type 1 binds to NF-kappa B p50 and serum response factor (SRF) and associates with enhancer DNAs of the NF-kappa B site and CArG box. *Oncogene* 8:2391–97

57. Suzuki T, Hirai H, Yoshida M. 1994. Tax protein of HTLV-1 interacts with the Rel homology domain of NF-kappa B p65 and c-Rel proteins bound to the NF-kappa B binding site and activates transcription. *Oncogene* 9:3099–3105

58. Murakami T, Hirai H, Suzuki T, Fujisawa J, Yoshida M. 1995. HTLV-1 Tax enhances NF-kappa B2 expression and binds to the products p52 and p100, but does not suppress the inhibitory function of p100. *Virology* 206:1066–74

59. Gerritsen ME, Williams AJ, Neish AS,

Moore S, Shi Y, Collins T. 1997. CREB-binding protein/p300 are transcriptional coactivators of p65. *Proc. Natl. Acad. Sci. USA* 94:2927–32

60. Perkins ND, Felzien LK, Betts JC, Leung K, Beach DH, Nabel GJ. 1997. Regulation of NF-kappaB by cyclin-dependent kinases associated with the p300 coactivator. *Science* 275:523–27

61. Zhong H, Voll RE, Ghosh S. 1998. Phosphorylation of NF-kappa B p65 by PKA stimulates transcriptional activity by promoting a novel bivalent interaction with the coactivator CBP/p300. *Mol. Cell.* 1:661–71

62. Inoue J, Seiki M, Taniguchi T, Tsuru S, Yoshida M. 1986. Induction of interleukin 2 receptor gene expression by p40x encoded by human T-cell leukemia virus type 1. *EMBO J.* 5:2883–88

63. Baeuerle PA. 1991. The inducible transcription activator NF-kappa B: regulation by distinct protein subunits. *Biochim. Biophys. Acta* 1072:63–80

64. Suzuki T, Hirai H, Murakami T, Yoshida M. 1995. Tax protein of HTLV-1 destabilizes the complexes of NF-kappa B and I kappa B-alpha and induces nuclear translocation of NF-kappa B for transcriptional activation. *Oncogene* 10:1199–1207

65. Maggirwar SB, HarhaJ E, Sun SC. 1995. Activation of NF-kappa B/Rel by Tax involves degradation of I kappa B alpha and is blocked by a proteasome inhibitor. *Oncogene* 11:993–98

66. Li X, Murphy K, Palka K, Surabhi R, Gaynor R. 1999. The human T-cell leukemia virus type-1 Tax protein regulates the activity of the IkappaB kinase complex. *J. Biol. Chem.* 274:34417–24

67. Fujii M, Tsuchiya H, Chuhjo T, Akizawa T, Seiki M. 1992. Interaction of HTLV-1 Tax1 with p67SRF causes the aberrant induction of cellular immediate early genes through CArG boxes. *Genes Dev.* 6:2066–76

68. Jeang KT, Widen SG, Semmes OJt, Wilson S. H. 1990. HTLV-I trans-activator protein,

tax, is a trans-repressor of the human beta-polymerase gene. *Science* 247:1082–84

69. Hirai H, Roussel MF, Kato JY, Ashmun RA, Sherr CJ. 1995. Novel INK4 proteins, p19 and p18, are specific inhibitors of the cyclin D-dependent kinases CDK4 and CDK6. *Mol. Cell. Biol.* 15:2672–81

70. Suzuki T, Narita T, Uchida-Toita M, Yoshida M. 1999. Down-regulation of the INK4 family of cyclin-dependent kinase inhibitors by tax protein of HTLV-1 through two distinct mechanisms. *Virology* 259:384–91

71. Eckner R, Yao TP, Oldread E, Livingston DM. 1996. Interaction and functional collaboration of p300/CBP and bHLH proteins in muscle and B-cell differentiation. *Genes Dev.* 10:2478–90

72. Lundblad JR, Kwok RP, Laurance ME, Harter ML, Goodman RH. 1995. Adenoviral E1A-associated protein p300 as a functional homologue of the transcriptional coactivator CBP. *Nature* 374:85–88

73. Mulloy JC, Kislyakova T, Cereseto A, Casareto L, LoMonico A, Fullen J, Lorenzi MV, Cara A, Nicot C, Giam C. 1998. Human T-cell lymphotropic/leukemia virus type 1 tax abrogates p53- induced cell cycle arrest and apoptosis through its CREB/ATF functional domain. *J. Virol.* 72:8852–60

74. Pise-Masison CA, Choi KS, Radonovich M, Dittmer J, Kim SJ, Brady JN. 1998. Inhibition of p53 transactivation function by the human T-cell lymphotropic virus type 1 Tax protein. *J. Virol.* 72:1165–70

75. Lill NL, Grossman SR, Ginsberg D, DeCaprio J, Livingston DM. 1997. Binding and modulation of p53 by p300/CBP coactivators. *Nature* 387:823–27

76. Van Orden K, Giebler H, Lemasson I, Gonzales M, Nyborg J. 1999. Binding of p53 to the KIX domain of CREB binding protein. A potential link to human T-cell leukemia virus type 1-associated leukemogenesis. *J. Biol. Chem.* 274:26321–28

77. Ariumi Y, Kaida A, Lin J, Hirota M,

Masui O, Yamaoka S, Taya Y, Shimo-tohno K. 2000. HTLV-1 tax oncoprotein represses the p53-mediated trans-activation function through coactivator CBP sequestration. *Oncogene* 19:1491–99

78. Pise-Masison C, Radonovich M, Sakaguchi K, Appella E, Brady J. 1998. Phosphorylation of p53: a novel pathway for p53 inactivation in human T-cell lymphotropic virus type 1-transformed cells. *J. Virol.* 72:6348–55

79. Pise-Masison C, Mahieux R, Jiang H, Ashcroft M, Radonovich M, Duvall J, Guillerm C, Brady J. 2000. Inactivation of p53 by human T-cell lymphotropic virus type 1 Tax requires activation of the NF-kappaB pathway and is dependent on p53 phosphorylation. *Mol. Cell. Biol.* 20:3377–86

80. Parry GC, Mackman N. 1997. Role of cyclic AMP response element-binding protein in cyclic AMP inhibition of NF-kappaB-mediated transcription. *J. Immunol.* 159:5450–56

81. Suzuki T, Kitao S, Matsushime H, Yoshida M. 1996. HTLV-1 Tax protein interacts with cyclin-dependent kinase inhibitor p16INK4A and counteracts its inhibitory activity towards CDK4. *EMBO J.* 15:1607–14

82. Kamb A, Gruis NA, Weaver-Feldhaus J, Liu Q, Harshman K, Tavtigian SV, Stockert E, Day R Sr, Johnson BE, Skolnick MH. 1994. A cell cycle regulator potentially involved in genesis of many tumor types. *Science* 264:436–40

83. Hinds PW, Weinberg RA. 1994. Tumor suppressor genes. *Curr. Opin. Genet. Dev.* 4:135–41

84. Nevins JR. 1992. E2F: a link between the Rb tumor suppressor protein and viraloncoproteins. *Science* 258:424–29

85. Hirai H, Suzuki T, Fujisawa J, Inoue J, Yoshida M. 1994. Tax protein of human T-cell leukemia virus type I binds to the ankyrin motifs of inhibitory factor kappa B and induces nuclear translocation of transcription factor NF-kappa B proteins for transcriptional activation. *Proc. Natl. Acad. Sci. USA* 91:3584–88

86. Suzuki T, Ohsugi Y, Uchida-Toita M, Akiyama M, Yoshida M. 1999. Tax oncoprotein of HTLV-1 binds to the human homologue of Drosophila discs large tumor suppressor protein, hDLG, and perturbs its function in cell growth control. *Oncogene* 18:5967–72

87. Woods DF, Bryant PJ. 1991. The discs-large tumor suppressor gene of Drosophila encodes a guanylate kinase homolog localized at septate junctions. *Cell* 66:451–64

88. Matsumine A, Ogai A, Senda T, Okumura N, Satoh K, Baeg GH, Kawahara T, Kobayashi S, Okada M, Toyoshima K. 1996. Binding of APC to the human homolog of the Drosophila discs large tumor suppressor protein. *Science* 272:1020–23

89. Lee SS, Weiss RS, Javier RT. 1997. Binding of human virus oncoproteins to hDlg/SAP97, a mammalian homolog of the Drosophila discs large tumor suppressor protein. *Proc. Natl. Acad. Sci. USA* 94:6670–75

90. Rousset R, Fabre S, Desbois C, Bantignies F, Jalinot P. 1998. The C-terminus of the HTLV-1 Tax oncoprotein mediates interaction with the PDZ domain of cellular proteins. *Oncogene* 16:643–54

91. Kiyono T, Hiraiwa A, Fujita M, Hayashi Y, Akiyama T, Ishibashi M. 1997. Binding of high-risk human papillomavirus E6 oncoproteins to the human homologue of the Drosophila discs large tumor suppressor protein. *Proc. Natl. Acad. Sci. USA* 94:11612–16

92. Arany Z, Newsome D, Oldread E, Livingston DM, Eckner R. 1995. A family of transcriptional adaptor proteins targeted by the E1A oncoprotein. *Nature* 374:81–84

93. Eckner R, Ludlow JW, Lill NL, Oldread E, Arany Z, Modjtahedi N, DeCaprio JA, Livingston DM, Morgan JA. 1996. Association of p300 and CBP with simian virus 40

large T antigen. *Mol. Cell. Biol.* 16:3454–64

94. Lundblad JR, Kwok RP, Laurance ME, Harter ML, Goodman RH. 1995. Adenoviral E1A-associated protein p300 as a functional homologue of the transcriptional co-activator CBP. *Nature* 374:85–88

95. Hidaka M, Inoue J, Yoshida M, Seiki M. 1988. Post-transcriptional regulator (rex) of HTLV-1 initiates expression of viral structural proteins but suppresses expression of regulatory proteins. *EMBO J.* 7:519–23

96. Kinoshita T, Shimoyama M, Tobinai K, Ito M, Ito S, Ikeda S, Tajima K, Shimotohno K, Sugimura T. 1989. Detection of mRNA for the tax1/rex1 gene of human T-cell leukemia virus type I in fresh peripheral blood mononuclear cells of adult T-cell leukemia patients and viral carriers by using the polymerase chain reaction. *Proc. Natl. Acad. Sci. USA* 86:5620–24

97. Smith MR, Greene WC. 1990. Identification of HTLV-I tax trans-activator mutants exhibiting novel transcriptional phenotypes [published errata appear in *Genes Dev.* 1991 Jan; 5(1):150 and 1995 Sep 15;9(18):2324]. *Genes Dev.* 4:1875–85

98. Harrod R, Tang Y, Nicot C, Lu HS, Vassilev A, Nakatani Y, Giam CZ. 1998. An exposed KID-like domain in human T-cell lymphotropic virus type 1 Tax is responsible for the recruitment of coactivators CBP/p300. *Mol. Cell. Biol.* 18:5052–61

99. Yin MJ, Paulssen E, Seeler J, Gaynor RB. 1995. Chimeric proteins composed of Jun and CREB define domains required for interaction with the human T-cell leukemia virus type 1 Tax protein. *J. Virol.* 69:6209–18

100. Giebler HA, Loring JE, van Orden K, Colgin MA, Garrus JE, Escudero KW, Brauweiler A, Nyborg JK. 1997. Anchoring of CREB binding protein to the human T-cell leukemia virus type 1 promoter: a molecular mechanism of Tax transactivation. *Mol. Cell. Biol.* 17:5156–64

101. Muraoka O, Kaisho T, Tanabe M, Hirano T. 1993. Transcriptional activation of the interleukin-6 gene by HTLV-1 p40tax through an NF-kappa B-like binding site. *Immunol. Lett.* 37:159–65

102. Miyatake S, Seiki M, Yoshida M, Arai K. 1988. T-cell activation signals and human T-cell leukemia virus type I-encoded p40x protein activate the mouse granulocyte-macrophage colony-stimulating factor gene through a common DNA element. *Mol. Cell. Biol.* 8:5581–87

103. Kim SJ, Kehrl JH, Burton J, Tendler CL, Jeang KT, Danielpour D, Thevenin C, Kim KY, Sporn MB, Roberts AB. 1990. Transactivation of the transforming growth factor beta 1 (TGF-beta 1) gene by human T lymphotropic virus type 1 tax: a potential mechanism for the increased production of TGF-beta 1 in adult T cell leukemia. *J. Exp. Med.* 172:121–29

104. Fujii M, Sassone-Corsi P, Verma IM. 1988. c-fos promoter trans-activation by the tax1 protein of human T-cell leukemia virus type I. *Proc. Natl. Acad. Sci. USA* 85:8526–30

105. Fujii M, Tsuchiya H, Chuhjo T, Minamino T, Miyamoto K, Seiki M. 1994. Serum response factor has functional roles both in indirect binding to the CArG box and in the transcriptional activation function of human T-cell leukemia virus type I Tax. *J. Virol.* 68:7275–83

106. Lemasson I, Robert-Hebmann V, Hamaia S, Duc Dodon M, Gazzolo L, Devaux C. 1997. Transrepression of lck gene expression by human T-cell leukemia virus type 1-encoded p40tax. *J. Virol.* 71:1975–83

107. Feigenbaum L, Fujita K, Collins FS, Jay G. 1996. Repression of the NF1 gene by Tax may explain the development of neurofibromas in human T-lymphotropic virus type 1 transgenic mice. *J. Virol.* 70:3280–85

108. Low KG, Dorner LF, Fernando DB, Grossman J, Jeang KT, Comb MJ. 1997. Human T-cell leukemia virus type 1 Tax releases cell cycle arrest induced by p16INK4a. *J. Virol.* 71:1956–62

109. Suzuki T, Uchida-Toita M, Andoh T, Yoshida M. 2000. HTLV-1 tax oncoprotein binds to DNA topoisomerase I and inhibits its catalytic activity. *Virology* 270:291–98

110. Kao S, Marriott S. 1999. Disruption of nucleotide excision repair by the human T-cell leukemia virus type 1 Tax protein. *J. Virol.* 73:4299–304

111. Miyake H, Suzuki T, Hirai H, Yoshida M. 1999. Trans-activator Tax of human T-cell leukemia virus type 1 enhances mutation frequency of the cellular genome. *Virology* 253:155–61

112. Philpott S, Buehring G. 1999. Defective DNA repair in cell with human T-cell leukemia/bovine leukemia viruses: role of tax gene. *J. Natl. Cancer Inst.* 91:933–42

113. Jin DY, Spencer F, Jeang KT. 1998. Human T cell leukemia virus type 1 oncoprotein Tax targets the human mitotic checkpoint protein MAD1. *Cell* 93:81–91

114. Tsukahara T, Kannagi M, Ohashi T, Kato H, Arai M, Nunez G, Iwanaga Y, Yamamoto N, Ohtani K, Fujii M. 1999. Induction of Bcl-x(L) expression by human T-cell leukemia virus type 1 Tax through NF-kappaB in apoptosis-resistant T-cell transfectants with Tax. *J. Virol.* 73:7981–87

115. Kawakami A, Nakashima T, Sakai H, Urayama S, Yamasaki S, Hida A, Tsuboi M, Nakamura H, Ida H, Migita K. 1999. Inhibition of caspase cascade by HTLV-1 tax through induction of NF-kappaB nuclear translocation. *Blood* 94:3847–54

116. Brauweiler A, Garrus JE, Reed JC, Nyborg JK. 1997. Repression of bax gene expression by the HTLV-1 Tax protein: implications for suppression of apoptosis in virally infected cells. *Virology* 231:135–40

117. Hangaishi A, Ogawa S, Imamura N, Miyawaki S, Miura Y, Uike N, Shimazaki C, Emi N, Takeyama K, Hirosawa S. 1996. Inactivation of multiple tumor-suppressor genes involved in negative regulation of the cell cycle, MTS1/p16INK4A/CDKN2, MTS2/p15INK4B, p53, and Rb genes in primary lymphoid malignancies. *Blood* 87:4949–58

Annu. Rev. Immunol. 2001. 19:497–521

Calcium Signaling Mechanisms in T Lymphocytes

Richard S Lewis

*Department of Molecular and Cellular Physiology and Program in Immunology,
Stanford University School of Medicine, Stanford, California 94305;
e-mail: rslewis@stanford.edu*

Key Words   T cell activation, store-operated calcium channel, IP_3 receptor, calcium ATPase, mitochondria, calcium oscillations

■ **Abstract**   Elevation of intracellular free Ca^{2+} is one of the key triggering signals for T-cell activation by antigen. A remarkable variety of Ca^{2+} signals in T cells, ranging from infrequent spikes to sustained oscillations and plateaus, derives from the interactions of multiple Ca^{2+} sources and sinks in the cell. Following engagement of the T cell receptor, intracellular channels (IP_3 and ryanodine receptors) release Ca^{2+} from intracellular stores, and by depleting the stores trigger prolonged Ca^{2+} influx through store-operated Ca^{2+} (CRAC) channels in the plasma membrane. The amplitude and dynamics of the Ca^{2+} signal are shaped by several mechanisms, including K^+ channels and membrane potential, slow modulation of the plasma membrane Ca^{2+}-ATPase, and mitochondria that buffer Ca^{2+} and prevent the inactivation of CRAC channels. Ca^{2+} signals have a number of downstream targets occurring on multiple time scales. At short times, Ca^{2+} signals help to stabilize contacts between T cells and antigen-presenting cells through changes in motility and cytoskeletal reorganization. Over periods of minutes to hours, the amplitude, duration, and kinetic signature of Ca^{2+} signals increase the efficiency and specificity of gene activation events. The complexity of Ca^{2+} signals contains a wealth of information that may help to instruct lymphocytes to choose between alternate fates in response to antigenic stimulation.

INTRODUCTION

The elevation of intracellular free Ca^{2+} ($[Ca^{2+}]_i$) is an essential triggering signal for T cell activation by antigen and other stimuli that cross-link the T cell antigen receptor (TCR) (1–3). Over the past decade significant progress has been made in identifying and characterizing the biochemical and cellular mechanisms that generate these signals (Figure 1; see color insert). The binding of antigen/MHC complexes to the TCR triggers the recruitment of a series of tyrosine kinases and substrates to the TCR/CD3 complex, ultimately resulting in the phosphorylation and activation of phospholipase C-γ (PLCγ) (4, 5). PLCγ cleaves PIP$_2$ in the plasma membrane to generate diacylglycerol, which activates protein kinase C (PKC) and ras-dependent pathways, and 1,4,5-inositol trisphosphate (IP$_3$), which causes entry of Ca^{2+} to cytosol from two sources: the endoplasmic reticulum (ER) and the extracellular space. In most cases, Ca^{2+} influx must be maintained for 1–2 h to efficiently drive cell activation events that lead to interleukin-2 (IL-2) expression (6, 7), a commitment point beyond which further T cell activation becomes antigen independent (8). This requirement for sustained signaling arises largely from the need to keep Nuclear Factor of Activated T cells (NFAT), a key transcriptional regulator of the IL-2 gene and other cytokine genes, in the nucleus (9) and to keep NFAT in a transcriptionally active state (10).

We owe much of our current understanding of the nature of Ca^{2+} signals in T cells to the development of Ca^{2+}-dependent dyes and microscopic imaging techniques that enable the time course of [Ca^{2+}]$_i$ to be measured in single T cells. Imaging studies have revealed a remarkable variety of T cell responses to TCR engagement, ranging from [Ca^{2+}]$_i$ transients to repetitive oscillations to sustained elevations spanning a concentration range of $\sim$200 nM to >1 μM (7, 11–17). This complexity serves to illustrate graphically that the Ca^{2+} signal is not a binary switch, but that it contains in principle a wealth of information. Studies of a variety of naïve T cells, cloned T cells, T cell hybridomas, and transformed T cell lines suggest that the character of Ca^{2+} response is strongly influenced by, among other things, the type of T cell and its state of maturation as well as the APC and the characteristics of the antigen. Some of these same factors are known to influence the outcome of TCR occupancy and guide cells towards activation, anergy, or death. Thus, the character of the Ca^{2+} signal may well contribute to the type of instructions that are transmitted through the TCR in a particular immunological context (18).

This review is presented in two parts. The first section focuses on the molecular and cellular mechanisms that generate Ca^{2+} signals in T cells and ways in which they may interact to generate complexity. The second section considers the downstream consequences of Ca^{2+} signaling, in particular the influence of signal complexity on gene expression. The emphasis is on T cells, although selected examples from B cells and other nonlymphoid cells are also discussed where appropriate.

MOLECULAR MECHANISMS
OF CALCIUM SIGNAL GENERATION

Cellular calcium signals result from the interaction of multiple Ca^{2+} sources and sinks. The large number of participants in Ca^{2+} signal generation contributes complexity, reliability, and abundant opportunities for signal modulation through other pathways. This section summarizes our current understanding of the major transport mechanisms that regulate $[Ca^{2+}]_i$ in T cells, drawing from recent studies of T cells and other non-excitable cells.

Initiating the Response: Ca^{2+} Release From Intracellular Stores

IP_3 generated subsequent to TCR stimulation binds to receptors in the endoplasmic reticulum (ER) membrane, opening Ca^{2+} channels that release Ca^{2+} to the cytosol (19, 20). Release is a highly cooperative process, owing to both the binding of multiple IP_3 molecules to the tetrameric receptor and to positive feedback by Ca^{2+} released from the ER (21, 22). The end result is that release generates a rapid transient that reaches a peak concentration of $\sim$500 nM but returns to the baseline of $\sim$100 nM within $\sim$100 sec. Lymphocytes express multiple isoforms of the IP_3 receptor (IP3R); Jurkat T cells and DT40 B cells express IP3R-1, -2, and -3, while thymocytes and splenocytes express only IP3R-2 and -3 (23, 24). The three receptor isoforms differ in their regulation by Ca^{2+} and their sensitivity to IP_3, which may have important implications for function in vivo. In the presence of IP_3, IP3R-1 is rapidly activated and slowly inactivated by Ca^{2+} (25, 26). In contrast, IP3R-2 is more effectively activated by IP_3 and Ca^{2+} (27, 28), and neither IP3R-2 nor -3 are inactivated by Ca^{2+} (27, 29). The different Ca^{2+} signaling patterns supported by each type of receptor have been elegantly demonstrated in a series of DT40 double-knockout cell lines (28). In cells stimulated through the B cell receptor, IP3R-2 and, to a lesser extent, IP3R-1 support $[Ca^{2+}]_i$ oscillations. However, IP3R-3-expressing cells exhibit only a single Ca^{2+} spike, similar to other cells in which this isoform is dominant (29). Thus, the specific combination of expressed IP3R isoforms may bias the cell toward particular patterns of Ca^{2+} signaling.

The role of the IP3R in Ca^{2+} release during T cell activation was tested by suppressing it in Jurkat cells through stable expression of antisense IP3R-1 cDNA (30). In these cells, anti-CD3-evoked Ca^{2+} release was suppressed in parallel with IP3R-1 immunoreactivity, indicating that release requires functional IP3R. However, the specific role of the IP3R-1 isoform was difficult to determine, because a later study showed the antisense cDNA also partially suppressed IP3R-2 and -3 (31). Functional redundancy has been clearly demonstrated in DT40 IP3R-knockout cells, where deletion of any IP3R alone has no detectable effect on BCR-stimulated release, and deletion of all three isoforms is required to prevent Ca^{2+} release (32).

The activity of the IP3R may be increased during the early phase of T cell activation by fyn (24, 33). The IP3R is phosphorylated on tyr tyrosine within several minutes after stimulation with anti-CD3, and phosphorylation by fyn in vitro enhances IP3R opening in response to IP_3 in bilayer experiments. Consistent with these results T cells from $fyn^{-/-}$ mice show reduced Ca^{2+} release (34) and a two thirds reduction in IP3R phosphorylation in response to anti-CD3 (33). However, at this point how much of the Ca^{2+} signaling defect is also due to a decrease in IP_3 or the activity of other kinases downstream of fyn is not clear.

Although the experiments discussed above indicate that IP_3 receptors are necessary for antigen-triggered Ca^{2+} release, they do not prove sufficiency. One unexplained puzzle is that Ca^{2+} signaling by Ca^{2+} release-activated Ca^{2+} (CRAC) channels is prolonged for >1 hr following TCR engagement (35), even though average IP_3 levels return to near basal levels within 10 min (20, 36). This discrepancy might be explained if local IP_3 production remains sufficiently high to keep Ca^{2+} stores near the plasma membrane depleted and thereby sustains CRAC channel activity; such an idea is plausible given that membrane-proximal stores are thought to be preferentially involved in activating Ca^{2+} entry through CRAC channels (discussed below). An alternative possibility introduced by Guse and colleagues is that the ryanodine receptor (RyR), another ER Ca^{2+} release channel, also contributes to Ca^{2+} release in T cells through the action of the second messenger cyclic ADP-ribose (cADPR) (37–39). Several types of evidence support this notion. Jurkat cells express the type 3 RyR (39), and cADPR releases Ca^{2+} from stores of permeabilized or microinjected Jurkat cells (37, 38). Treatment of Jurkat cells with anti-CD3 elicits a threefold increase in cytosolic cADPR, which lasts for >60 min and is associated with increased activity of a soluble ADP-ribosyl cyclase (39). Increasing doses of a membrane permeant inhibitor of cADPR, 7-deaza-8-Br-cADPR, progressively increase the latency of the $[Ca^{2+}]_i$ rise and shorten its duration. A pharmacological inhibitor of IP3R completely blocks the Ca^{2+} response when applied before stimulation but not when applied several minutes later. Together these results support the idea that cADPR acts together with IP_3 to initiate the response but acts alone at later times to sustain it (39). Does a cADPR also function in normal T cells? Although a cADPR inhibitor suppresses activation of human peripheral T cells in vitro at levels that affect Ca^{2+} signaling in Jurkat (39), T cell proliferation appears normal in $RyR3^{-/-}$ mice (40). Further work will be needed to resolve these discrepancies and to describe the molecular pathway connecting the TCR to activation of ADP-ribosyl cyclase.

In contrast to many other types of nonexcitable cells, Ca^{2+} release in T cells makes a relatively small contribution to the total Ca^{2+} signal compared to that of Ca^{2+} influx (11, 12, 41). Thus, a major function of Ca^{2+} release in T cells is to serve as a sensitive trigger for controlling a much larger flux of Ca^{2+} across the plasma membrane. A more prominent role for Ca^{2+} release is certainly possible, particularly at low levels of TCR occupancy. However, the contribution of stores to the Ca^{2+} signal is often hard to determine, as blocking influx to isolate the release component also prevents refilling of stores, leading rapidly to their exhaustion. Additional roles have been implicated for IP3R-1 and IP3R-3 in controlling susceptibility to dexamethasone-induced apoptosis, based on the protective effects of suppressing either receptor with antisense cDNA (31, 42, 43). The basis for these effects is not known.

Sustaining the Response: Ca^{2+} Entry Through Store-Operated Ca^{2+} Channels

In many cells including lymphocytes, IP_3 evokes a biphasic elevation of $[Ca^{2+}]_i$ due to Ca^{2+} release from stores followed by influx across the plasma membrane (44). Putney was the first to show in exocrine cells that influx is triggered by the depletion of stores rather than by IP_3 directly, as it can occur long after IP_3 levels have returned to basal values, provided that stores are kept in a depleted state. This and other results gave rise to the capacitative Ca^{2+} entry hypothesis, whereby store depletion causes store-operated Ca^{2+} channels in the plasma membrane to open, facilitating store refilling (45). A hallmark of store-operated channels is activation by receptor-independent stimuli that empty the ER Ca^{2+} store. Effective stimuli include thapsigargin (TG), a selective inhibitor of SERCA Ca^{2+} pumps in the ER (46); ionomycin, a lipophilic ionophore that transports Ca^{2+} out of the ER; and intracellular Ca^{2+} chelators, which interfere with Ca^{2+} reuptake by the stores (47, 48). Patch-clamp studies in many cell types have distinguished different classes of store-operated channels (SOCs) (47, 48). The class found in T cells is the Ca^{2+} release-activated Ca^{2+} (CRAC) channel, named for a similar channel originally found in mast cells (49). It is distinguished from other SOCs primarily by its extremely high Ca^{2+} selectivity, but it also exhibits a number of other features described below that comprise a characteristic "fingerprint" for its identification.

Several lines of evidence strongly support the idea that CRAC channels are solely responsible for Ca^{2+} influx during T cell activation. First, the Ca^{2+} currents induced by TCR cross-linking and by passive store depletion (using TG or intracellular EGTA or BAPTA) are identical in terms of ion selectivity, conductance, Ca^{2+}-dependent inactivation, and block by heavy metals (50, 51). Second, stimulation of the TCR with lectins or antibodies does not further increase Ca^{2+} influx or Ca^{2+} current in T cells whose stores are already depleted with TG (51–53). Third, SKF 96365 or nanomolar amounts of La^{3+} block I_{CRAC} in parallel with the $[Ca^{2+}]_i$ rise and induction of T cell activation markers (54, 55). Finally, in patients with a severe immunodeficiency, nonresponsive T cells displayed a specific defect in Ca^{2+} influx associated with the absence of I_{CRAC} (56). Likewise, in Jurkat mutants selected specifically for the absence of store-operated Ca^{2+} entry, TCR stimulation with anti-CD3 evokes Ca^{2+} release but not influx (57). A recent imaging study has shown that I_{CRAC} channels are also likely to be the sole Ca^{2+} influx pathway operating during delivery of the lethal hit by cytotoxic T cells (58).

Additional Ca^{2+} influx pathways can be activated independently of the TCR in T cells. For example, integrins activate influx in Jurkat cells (59), and hypoosmotic cell swelling and ATP acting upon purinergic receptors trigger two different modes of Ca^{2+} influx in murine thymocytes (60, 61). These pathways appear to be distinct from CRAC channels, but their roles in T cell physiology are not yet well understood. In additional to other specific functions, they may affect thresholds for signaling through the TCR by contributing to the overall rise in $[Ca^{2+}]_i$.

The Mechanism of CRAC Channel Selectivity   Practically all the current flowing through CRAC channels is carried by Ca^{2+}, even though Na^+ is normally present at $\sim$75-fold excess in the extracellular medium. Hoth and Penner showed that CRAC channels select for Ca^{2+} over monovalent cations by a ratio of $>1000:1$, an exquisite degree of selectivity matched only by that of L-type voltage-gated Ca^{2+} (Ca_V) channels (62, 63). Recent studies show several other similarities in permeation properties. Like Ca_V channels CRAC channels require extracellular Ca^{2+} to attain their selectivity for Ca^{2+}; when extracellular divalent cations (Ca^{2+}, Mg^{2+}) are lowered to micromolar levels, CRAC channels conduct monovalent ions efficiently (62, 64, 65). Under these conditions, CRAC channels conduct organic cations up to a diameter of $\sim$0.55 nm, implying a pore size similar to that of Ca_V channels (65). Finally, both channels have similar sensitivities to block by internal and external H^+. These results indicate that the pore region of the CRAC channel may be similar to that of cloned Ca_V channels, a characteristic that may be useful in identifying candidates for the CRAC channel gene(s) through sequence database analysis. The high Ca^{2+} selectivity of CRAC channels ensures that they conduct Ca^{2+} into the cell with maximum efficiency, avoiding excessive membrane depolarization that could undermine the driving force for Ca^{2+} entry.

Single CRAC Channels: New Insights into Activation   During whole-cell recording from Jurkat cells with a low-Ca^{2+} intracellular solution to deplete stores and a divalent free extracellular solution to allow Na^+ to permeate CRAC channels, Kerschbaum & Cahalan observed single CRAC channel openings with a conductance of 36–40 pS (66). Surprisingly, the gradual induction of the whole-cell current occurred as a series of small current steps corresponding to single CRAC channels, each with an open probability close to 1. Thus, it appears that the gradual emptying of the stores triggers the all-or-none activation of an increasing number of channels. This unusual characteristic may provide clues to the activation mechanism (see below). Although the single-channel CRAC conductance has not been measured in the presence of Ca^{2+}, an estimate of 1–2 pS in 20 mM Ca^{2+} has been made by scaling the Na^+-channel conductance by the ratio of the whole-cell Na^+ and Ca^{2+} current amplitudes ($\sim$25). The ratio of whole-cell and single-channel Na^+ currents provides an estimate of only 100–400 for the number of CRAC channels per Jurkat T cell, implying that the channel is a relatively rare protein. Single-channel recording of CRAC currents in excised patches is likely to be a powerful approach to studies of regulatory mechanisms.

Indirect Regulation of CRAC Channels by IP_3   The effects of IP_3 on I_{CRAC} activity in intact cells is critical for understanding Ca^{2+} signaling through PLC-coupled pathways such as the TCR. In whole-cell recordings from RBL cells, Parekh et al reported that activation of I_{CRAC} by IP_3 in the recording pipette was highly nonlinear, exhibiting "all-or-none" behavior at a threshold concentration of IP_3 (67). Such a threshold effect may be explained by the explosive nature of Ca^{2+}

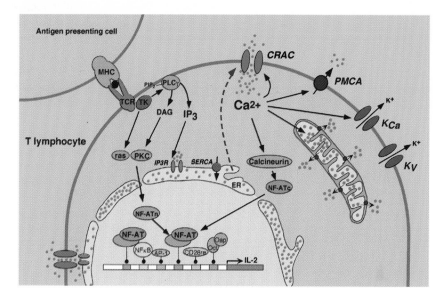

Figure 1 Overview of Ca^{2+} signaling pathways in T cells. IP$_3$ releases Ca^{2+} from the ER, and the resultant depletion of Ca^{2+} stores activates CRAC channels through an unknown mechanism indicated by the dashed line. Ca^{2+} entering the cell inhibits CRAC channels, activates K$_{Ca}$ channels, upregulates PMCA activity, and activates calcineurin, which dephosphorylates NFAT to allow its translocation to the nucleus. Mitochondria take up Ca^{2+} near CRAC channels to prevent their inactivation, and redistribute it to other sites in the cell.

release by IP_3 (see above). In addition, higher concentrations of IP_3 were needed to activate I_{CRAC} than to trigger Ca^{2+} release, suggesting that CRAC channels are controlled by a subset of stores with low apparent IP_3 sensitivity. This hypothesis has been invoked to explain how store release becomes uncoupled from Ca^{2+} influx in Itk- or Btk-deficient lymphocytes, in which $PLC\gamma$ activity is partially suppressed (see below). The idea that a specialized subset of stores residing close to the plasma membrane controls CRAC channel activity has important implications for the behavior of these channels during T cell activation. However, it is important to note that the high intracellular EGTA used in most whole-cell studies may affect CRAC channel behavior. Subsequent work has shown high intracellular EGTA may interfere with store refilling, tending to make the I_{CRAC} response less graded with $[IP_3]$ (68). In fact, in experiments with minimal buffering, μM levels of IP_3 do not detectably activate I_{CRAC} at all, possibly because of efficient refilling of stores near the plasma membrane (68, 69). These experiments underscore the complexity of interactions between Ca^{2+} release, Ca^{2+} influx, and Ca^{2+} reuptake, and they suggest the need for conducting electrophysiological studies under more physiological conditions.

Regulation of CRAC Channel Activity by Calcium   Several modes of Ca^{2+}-dependent regulation of I_{CRAC} are known (for reviews, see 47, 70). As expected for any store-operated channel, CRAC channels deactivate in response to store refilling, a process that occurs over tens of seconds (71, 72). CRAC channels also exhibit two types of store-independent inactivation. Rapid inactivation over a time scale of tens of milliseconds results from local accumulation of intracellular Ca^{2+} (49, 73, 74). By comparing the abilities of "fast" (BAPTA) and "slow" (EGTA) cytosolic Ca^{2+} buffers to block inactivation, Zweifach and Lewis estimated that the location of the fast inactivation site is ~ 3 nm from the pore, suggesting a site on the CRAC channel itself or an associated protein (73). A second type of Ca^{2+}-dependent inactivation occurs over tens of seconds. In whole-cell recordings from Jurkat cells treated with TG to permanently empty the stores, I_{CRAC} slowly inactivates by about 50% as $[Ca^{2+}]_i$ rises above ~ 200 nM to micromolar levels (71). The inactivation is Ca^{2+}-dependent, as it is largely blocked by loading the cell with 12 mM EGTA to prevent the rise in $[Ca^{2+}]_i$, but the underlying mechanism is unknown.

Slow store-independent inactivation of I_{CRAC} is seemingly at odds with the ability of the T cells to maintain high plateaus of $[Ca^{2+}]_i$ for periods of tens of minutes following stimulation through the TCR or by TG. This paradox may be resolved by the recent finding that mitochondria can prevent I_{CRAC} inactivation (75). Addition of mitochondrial substrates and ATP to the intracellular whole-cell recording solution ("energized" whole-cell conditions) blocks slow inactivation of I_{CRAC}. Inactivation is also absent in perforated-patch recording, a relatively noninvasive recording method that, unlike whole-cell recording, does not deplete the cell of metabolic substrates. Addition of mitochondrial inhibitors (CCCP, antimycin A1, and oligomycin) unmasks Ca^{2+}-dependent inactivation of I_{CRAC} in both perforated-patch and "energized" whole-cell recording modes. Thus, functional mitochondria prevent slow inactivation from occuring in intact Jurkat cells, enabling the cells to maintain a high rate of Ca^{2+} entry over long periods (discussed below).

Toward a Molecular Description of Store-Operated Calcium Entry

Considerable effort has been focused on elucidating the molecular mechanism of store-operated Ca^{2+} entry. These efforts have concentrated on two main areas: identifying the genes that encode SOCs and understanding how store depletion leads to channel activation. Identifying SOC genes through heterologous expression has been especially challenging because all of the commonly used expression systems express an endogenous SOC, and biochemical approaches have been hindered by a lack of high-affinity ligands or blockers. [For additional background on the search for SOC genes and activation mechanisms, see the previous reviews (47, 48, 76, 77).] Here I focus on recent results most directly relevant to the CRAC channel.

TRP Homologs as Candidate CRAC Genes   The best current candidates for SOC genes are mammalian homologs of the *Drosophila trp* gene. TRP is found in *Drosophila* photoreceptors, where it was originally thought to function as a store-operated channel, but many subsequent studies have challenged that hypothesis (for review, see 77a). Seven mammalian members of this gene family have been cloned and overexpressed heterologously in a variety of nonlymphoid mammalian cell lines. Most of the cDNAs (e.g. TRP1, TRP3, and TRP6) are associated with relatively nonselective currents, and some are not gated by store depletion but rather by Ca^{2+}, G proteins, or diacylgycerol (TRP3, TRP6). Hence, these TRPs are believed to be unlikely to encode the CRAC channel. However, many cells express multiple endogenous TRPs, and the product of an exogenous cDNA may recombine with variable stoichiometry with endogenous subunits or form nonphysiological homomultimers, thereby creating channels with variable and/or abnormal properties. Thus, when tested by overexpression experiments, the lack of Ca^{2+} selectivity or insensitivity to store depletion does not necessarily rule out a role for any particular TRP in helping to make an endogenous CRAC channel. One way to avoid this problem is to change the expression level of an endogenous TRP and measure the resulting change in I_{CRAC}. Taking this approach, Philipp et al (78) found that bovine adrenal cortical (SBAC) cells abundantly express TRP4 protein (and to a much lesser extent TRP1) and display a highly selective CRAC-like Ca^{2+} current. After transfection with TRP4 antisense cDNA, TRP4 protein and I_{CRAC} are downregulated in parallel. These studies provide the best current evidence for a TRP encoding part of a CRAC channel; however, the authors note that TRP4 is expressed at a lower level in Jurkat and not detectably in RBL cells, both of which have a much larger CRAC conductance than SBAC cells. Moreover, another study found that TRP4 expressed heterologously in HEK cells was neither store-operated nor Ca^{2+}-selective (78a). These discrepancies will have to be explained before any particular TRP can be assigned to the CRAC channel in T cells.

The Elusive Activation Mechanism of CRAC Channels   There is general agreement that IP_3 opens CRAC channels by depleting stores rather than directly affecting the channel. For example, I_{CRAC} is activated by TG and by intracellular Ca^{2+} buffers (neither of which induces a rise in IP_3) (49–51), even in the presence of high concentrations of heparin that would be expected to block binding of background levels of IP_3 to its receptor (49, 79). I_{CRAC} is also activated by TPEN, a membrane permeant Ca^{2+} chelator that reduces ER $[Ca^{2+}]$ directly (72, 91). It is generally agreed that the activation signal is a local one, as Ca^{2+} influx is spatially restricted close to the location of depleted stores in *Xenopus* oocytes (80, 81). Indirect evidence also suggests that stores near the plasma membrane are preferentially involved in CRAC channel activation, in part based on the ability of cortical actin polymerization to reversibly inhibit the activation of SOCs in smooth muscle and HEK293 cells (82, 83; but see also 84).

What is the message that links store depletion to channel activation? Three general models have been most widely studied. In the diffusible messenger model, store depletion releases a molecule that diffuses to the plasma membrane to activate I_{CRAC}. A critical test of such a messenger is to show that it can activate I_{CRAC} even when the stores remain full. The original calcium influx factor (CIF) isolated from the cytosol of activated Jurkat cells (85) lacked this property (86). Subsequent work identified an extract of TG-treated Jurkat cells that activated Ca^{2+} influx when injected into oocytes, although the interpretation was complicated by the fact that the influx differed from oocyte I_{CRAC} in its sensitivity to block by La^{3+} (87). A similar activity was obtained from the cytosol of *pmr1* mutant yeast that lack the PMR1 Ca^{2+}-ATPase and have an elevated uptake of Ca^{2+}. When applied to Jurkat cells through the recording pipette, CIF accelerated I_{CRAC} activation relative to activation by EGTA alone. However, the Ca^{2+} content of the stores was not assessed. Recently, CIF was shown to rapidly activate a 3-pS store-operated channel in excised membrane patches from vascular smooth muscle (88). Although it is too early to say whether CIF directly activates CRAC channels, the ability to detect single CRAC channels in the absence of extracellular divalent ions (66) may enable tests of this idea using patches from T cells.

A second proposal involves depletion-activated insertion of the CRAC channel or its activator into the plasma membrane. This type of mechanism was proposed originally on the basis of inhibition of I_{CRAC} activation by primaquine (89) and $GTP\gamma S$ (90), both of which are known to nonspecifically inhibit secretion. More recent support comes from experiments of Yao et al (91) in which activation of I_{CRAC} in *Xenopus* oocytes was inhibited by botulinum toxin A and by dominant-negative truncated SNAP-25 peptides, both of which are well known to inhibit the function of SNAP-25 in membrane fusion. This is an attractive hypothesis, as insertion of new channels might explain the stepwise nature of I_{CRAC} activation seen in the single-channel experiments of Kerschbaum and Cahalan (see above). However, inhibitory effects on I_{CRAC} required hours of preincubation, and several other clostridial neurotoxins that inhibit secretion by cleaving SNAREs had no effect. These issues may be resolved by applying a larger number of SNARE-specific inhibitors and by defining the sites at which they act in the assembly and/or the function of the Ca^{2+} entry pathway.

A third possible mechanism for SOC activation is a "conformational coupling" model in which depletion-induced changes in IP3R conformation elicit the opening of SOCs through a direct physical coupling between the two channels (92). This model is supported by the ability of IP_3 receptors in microsomes as well as cytosolic IP3R fragments to activate TRP3 channels in patches from TRP3-transfected HEK293 cells (93, 94). Sites of association between TRP3 and IP3R have been identified through coimmunoprecipitation studies, and overexpression of IP3R peptides containing these regions can partially enhance or suppress endogenous store-operated Ca^{2+} entry in HEK cells (95). Together, these studies support the idea that TRP3 is gated through an interaction with IP_3 receptors. However, extrapolating these results to CRAC channels is tenuous because TRP3 does not behave like a true store-operated channel (83), and unlike the CRAC channel, it directly requires IP_3 for activity (93, 94). The ability of 2-APB, a noncompetitive inhibitor of IP_3 receptor function, to inhibit native store-operated Ca^{2+} entry in HEK cells has been cited as support for the conformational coupling model (83). However, more recent results suggest that 2-APB inhibits CRAC channels directly (95a). The major argument against conformational coupling comes from experiments on DT40 cells in which all three IP3R isoforms have been knocked out by homologous recombination. In these cells, TG continued to activate a normal level of Ca^{2+} influx (32). As DT40 cells display I_{CRAC} (D Bautista & R Lewis, unpublished data), it seems likely that IP_3 receptors are not needed for CRAC-channel gating.

Modulation of Ca^{2+} Entry Through CRAC Channels

Membrane potential as well as endogenous inhibitors of CRAC channels can have potent effects on Ca^{2+} influx in T cells, with potentially important consequences for T cell responsiveness. This section focuses on recent studies of the modulatory roles of K^+ channels and sphingolipids.

Several types of K^+ channels have the ability to modulate the rate of Ca^{2+} entry through CRAC channels by hyperpolarizing the membrane, which increases the total driving force for Ca^{2+} entry (for review, see 3, 96). K^+ channels in human T cells include the voltage-gated channel Kv1.3, a charybdotoxin-insensitive Kv channel, and the Ca^{2+}-activated K^+ channel, IKCa1.

Scorpion venom–derived toxins have provided powerful tools for dissecting the roles of K^+ channels in Ca^{2+} signaling and T cell activation. Toxins that specifically block Kv1.3 with nanomolar affinity, such as margatoxin and noxiustoxin, cause depolarization, reduce the $[Ca^{2+}]_i$ rise, and inhibit activation in vitro (97, 98; for review, see 3). In vivo administration of margatoxin inhibits delayed type hypersensitivity and the response to an allogeneic challenge in miniswine (99), supporting the idea that K^+-channel blockers may offer significant therapeutic value as immuno-suppressants (96). Similar effects may be expected from endogenous K^+-channel blockers; in fact, normal suppression of the maternal immune response against the fetus has been ascribed to inhibition of K^+ channels by placental progesterone (99a).

In contrast, the lack of a specific, high-affinity blocker of K_{Ca} channels has until recently precluded analogous tests of the role of K_{Ca} channels. Wulff et al (100) have recently synthesized a derivative of clotrimazole, TRAM-34, that selectively blocks IKCa1 with a K_d of 20–25 nM without inhibiting cytochrome P450 enzymes (a side effect of the parent compound). TRAM-34 inhibits ^3H-thy incorporation in human T cells stimulated through the TCR. It is interesting that the sensitivity to the drug depends on the history of the cell; EC_{50} was ~10 μM for naïve cells, which express few K_{Ca} channels (reflecting a nonspecific effect) but only 100 nM–1 μM for cells that had been previously activated and allowed to become quiescent. Such preactivation evokes a 25-fold upregulation of IKCa1 in human T cells (101); thus, the results suggest that K_{Ca} channels may play a role primarily in the reactivation of memory cells rather than in the initial activation of naïve cells.

These results are generally consistent with the idea that K^+ channels affect activation through effects on $[Ca^{2+}]_i$. It is reasonable to assume that K^+ channel blockers inhibit activation through depolarization and its effect on Ca^{2+} influx, but the sufficiency of the observed changes in potential to account for the changes in $[Ca^{2+}]_i$, and for the changes in $[Ca^{2+}]_i$ to explain the inhibition of cell activation, needs to be tested.

Blockade of CRAC channels by sphingolipids may also inhibit T cell activation, and this may play a role in the immune escape of tumor cells expressing high levels of CD95L (Fas ligand) in vivo. Engagement or cross-linking of FAS95 in lymphocytes potently inhibits I_{CRAC} and TG- or TCR-triggered Ca^{2+} entry (101a). The effect requires the expression of acidic sphingomyelinase (ASM), which is activated by CD95 stimulation to produce ceramide and its metabolite, sphingosine. These lipid messengers are known to block I_{CRAC} in RBL cells and T cells (101a,b). Anti-CD95 inhibits IL-2 synthesis in apoptosis-resistant Jurkat cells stimulated through the TCR, but the inhibition can be overcome with Ca^{2+} ionophore. Thus, these results suggest that the blockade of I_{CRAC} is responsible for the anergic response in vitro and raise the intriguing possibility that sphingolipids could act as potent immunosuppressants in vivo through their effects on CRAC channels.

Mechanisms for Calcium Clearance in T Cells

Despite the greater attention given to Ca^{2+} sources in T cell signaling, mechanisms that remove Ca^{2+} from the cytosol also exert a powerful influence over the amplitude, duration, and dynamics of the net Ca^{2+} signal. Sarco-endoplasmic reticulum Ca^{2+}-ATPases (SERCA) pump Ca^{2+} from the cytosol into the ER. Their contribution in human T cells to the rate of clearance of cytosolic Ca^{2+} following a rise is minimal (41); however, SERCA form a significant part of the Ca^{2+} signaling network in T cells by accumulating Ca^{2+} in the ER, thereby enabling

Ca^{2+} transients via IP_3-induced release and controlling store-operated Ca^{2+} entry. Human T cells and T cell lines express primarily two isoforms, SERCA 2b and SERCA 3 (102, 103), whose expression changes with activation. Treatment with ionomycin and phorbol ester causes SERCA 2b to increase twofold, while SERCA 3 decreases by $\sim$90% over a period of 1–3 days (102). The functional consequences of these changes are not known, but they are likely to depend on the subcellular localization of the different SERCA isoforms and their relation to stores involved in gating CRAC channels.

Calcium Pumps in the Plasma Membrane   Plasma membrane Ca^{2+}-ATPases (PMCA) provide the dominant mechanism for Ca^{2+} clearance in human T cells and Jurkat, although Na^+/Ca^{2+} exchange also contributes in human T cells (12, 104, 105). Following a rise in $[Ca^{2+}]_i$ PMCA activity increases with a biphasic time course. A rapid increase is simply explained by increased binding of Ca^{2+} to the pump's transport site. However, a several-fold further increase occurs over tens of seconds when $[Ca^{2+}]_i$ rises above several hundred nanomolar (106) (D Bautista, M Hoth, & R Lewis, unpublished results). This modulation reverses slowly with a time constant of 400 sec after $[Ca^{2+}]_i$ returns to baseline, giving the pumps a "memory" of the $[Ca^{2+}]_i$ rise. The predominant isoform expressed in Jurkat cells, PMCA 4b, contains an autoinhibitory C-terminal cytoplasmic domain with modified IQ motifs; binding of Ca^{2+}-calmodulin slowly relieves the inhibition in vitro, suggesting a molecular mechanism for modulation (107, 108). Phosphorylation of the C-terminal domain by PKC also relieves inhibition, which may explain the enhancement of Ca^{2+} clearance in Jurkat cells by phorbol esters (109). These studies suggest that modulation of PMCA by multiple pathways can contribute to Ca^{2+} signal processing in T cells. Modulation by Ca^{2+} enables the pumps to act as a high-pass filter, minimally attenuating brief Ca^{2+} transients but reducing the size of prolonged $[Ca^{2+}]_i$ rises. In this way, PMCA modulation contributes to the overshoot of $[Ca^{2+}]_i$ during the typical biphasic Ca^{2+} response, as shown in erythrocytes (110) and endothelial cells (111, 111b). Modulation also increases the dynamic range of sustained Ca^{2+} signaling in T cells; by slowly upregulating activity, the pump can adjust its activity to match the Ca^{2+} influx rate and achieve a steady $[Ca^{2+}]_i$ plateau even at micromolar levels of $[Ca^{2+}]_i$, which are far above the K_M for the pump ($\sim$200 nM). In this way, PMCA modulation contributes to both the dynamics and the stability of Ca^{2+} signaling in T cells.

Mitochondria: New Members of the Ca^{2+} Signaling Network in T Cells

In addition to their roles in ATP synthesis and apoptosis, mitochondria have become widely recognized over the past decade as important regulators of Ca^{2+} signaling in a wide variety of cells (112, 113). Mitochondrial uptake of Ca^{2+} through a uniporter in the inner membrane is driven by the large negative mitochondrial membrane potential, and the accumulated Ca^{2+} is released slowly through Na^+-dependent and -independent exchangers (114). Recent studies show that mitochondria have several important actions that are relevant to T cell activation and function. They act as Ca^{2+} buffers, taking up Ca^{2+} during periods of activity and slowly releasing it later (115). Thus, they reduce the size of Ca^{2+} peaks, but they prolong the return of $[Ca^{2+}]_i$ to baseline. The effects of this buffering action on downstream targets in T cells have not been explored. However, delaying the return of $[Ca^{2+}]_i$ to baseline could act to potentiate Ca^{2+}-dependent responses to a subsequent $[Ca^{2+}]_i$ rise, as occurs during post-tetanic potentiation of synaptic transmission in neurons (116). An additional consequence of Ca^{2+} uptake by mitochondria is to couple production of ATP to metabolic need. Ca^{2+} uptake by mitochondria under physiological conditions activates mitochondrial dehydrogenases, boosting production of NADH and ATP (117, 118). This effect may be an important part of readying the T cell for the increased metabolic demands of RNA and protein synthesis that accompany cell cycle entry and other activation events (119).

An unexpected new role for mitochondria has recently emerged in T cells, where they act to maintain high sustained rates of Ca^{2+} influx through CRAC channels (115, 119b). In T cells stimulated with TG or anti-CD3, agents that depolarize mitochondria (CCCP or antimycin A1 + oligomycin) and thereby prevent them from taking up Ca^{2+} cause $[Ca^{2+}]_i$ to fall within minutes from a high plateau of $\sim1\ \mu M$ to a low one of 300–400 nM (115). Similar effects are produced by Na^+ depletion, a maneuver that inhibits Ca^{2+} release from mitochondria by inhibiting Na^+/Ca^{2+} exchange. These changes in $[Ca^{2+}]_i$ are associated with a 50% decrease in accumulation of NFAT in the nucleus, indicating that the ability of mitochondria to sustain a high rate of $[Ca^{2+}]_i$ entry is significant for T cell activation (75). The effects may be explained by observations that mitochondria localized close to CRAC channels take up Ca^{2+} (115), which prevents its accumulation at sites that cause CRAC channel inactivation (see above; also see 75). The inhibitory effect of Na^+ depletion suggests that Ca^{2+} release is also necessary for maintaining a high rate of entry, possibly through activation of K_{Ca} channels and membrane hyperpolarization. This is a testable hypothesis according to which mitochondria act as a local sink, taking up Ca^{2+} near CRAC channels and redistributing it more diffusely to other sites in the cell.

Complex Behaviors Arise from Interacting Parts of the Ca^{2+} Signaling Machine

The large number of Ca^{2+} sources and sinks described above interact in lymphocytes to produce a variety of Ca^{2+} responses, ranging from isolated transients to sustained oscillations and elevated plateaus. An understanding of how these various patterns are produced will require more detailed information not only on the basic properties of the underlying components but also on their spatial distributions within the cell.

One example involves $[Ca^{2+}]_i$ oscillations in T cells, which result from a variety of "physiologic" stimuli (e.g. antigen presentation, TCR cross-linking with mAbs or lectins), and "nonphysiologic" stimuli (e.g. low doses of TG or ionomycin) and are mostly driven by fluctuations in Ca^{2+} influx through CRAC channels (11, 12, 41). The common feature of these stimuli is that they all partially activate CRAC channels through partial depletion of intracellular stores. Under these conditions, delays between store emptying and I_{CRAC} activation as well as store refilling and I_{CRAC} deactivation will tend to make I_{CRAC} oscillate. Additional factors such as periodic changes in membrane potential induced by K^+ channels (120) and modulation of PMCA activity (106) are also expected to contribute to the time course of Ca^{2+} fluxes. Once these basic processes become more fully characterized, it should be possible to apply a well-constrained quantitative model to understand the contributions of each to the generation of oscillations and other complex signaling patterns.

Another example of complex interactions among Ca^{2+} signaling elements involves the action of Tec-family tyrosine kinases. Knockout of Itk in T cells reduces Ca^{2+} influx but not Ca^{2+} release triggered through antigen receptors (121). An even more dramatic uncoupling of release from influx is seen in B cells following $Fc\gamma RII$ receptor stimulation (122), which inhibits recruitment of Btk to the plasma membrane (123). In both cases $PLC\gamma$ is less efficiently stimulated and IP_3 levels are reduced, consistent with a role for Tec-family kinases in $PLC\gamma$ activation. The selective inhibition of Ca^{2+} influx does not appear to involve inhibition of the store-operated Ca^{2+} entry per se, as the response to TG is normal (121). Instead, a possible explanation is that if CRAC activation stores comprise a small subset of total Ca^{2+} stores and have a higher IP_3 threshold for release then a partial decline in IP_3 may preferentially inhibit influx (121, 123). Further tests of this hypothesis will require a greater understanding of the Ca^{2+} signaling microenvironment that includes $PLC\gamma$, CRAC channels, stores, IP_3 receptors, and pumps.

DECODING THE CALCIUM SIGNAL: Making the Most of a Multifunctional Messenger

Given the diverse Ca^{2+} signals that are observed in T cells, it is natural to ask how they are related to subsequent events in the cell's response. Among the many effects of Ca^{2+}, I focus here on downstream events occurring on two overlapping time scales: relatively rapid changes in motility and cytoskeletal structure occurring over seconds to minutes, and more protracted programs of gene expression occurring over minutes to hours. Recent work suggests that the complexity of Ca^{2+} signals in lymphocytes may contribute to both the efficiency and the selectivity of T cell responses.

Calcium Signals Optimize T Cell Contact With the Antigen-Presenting Cell

In order to generate efficiently the sustained signals necessary for cell activation, T cells must change from an actively motile state to an immobile one after they have encountered a cell presenting the correct antigen. When cloned T cells or hybridoma T cells interact with APCs in vitro, $[Ca^{2+}]_i$ rises within ~30 sec, and shortly after this they round up and stop crawling (13, 124). Ca^{2+} appears to be sufficient to induce this behavior, as ionomycin and TG effect similar changes independently of the TCR (13, 124). The $[Ca^{2+}]_i$ rise also seems to be necessary insofar as high K^+ and BAPTA/AM loading prevent the $[Ca^{2+}]_i$ rise and reversibly block the stopping reaction in T hybridoma cells (124). Ca^{2+} appears to be less effective at stopping naïve T cells in contact with APCs, which continue to extend and retract lamellapodia after the $[Ca^{2+}]_i$ rise (125). Accordingly, a Ca^{2+}-independent stop signal has been implicated in the interaction of naïve transgenic mouse T cells with Ag/MHC (126), suggesting that multiple signals may cooperatively affect shape and motility in naïve cells. Ca^{2+} appears to stabilize the contact zone between naïve T cells and APCs, but it is not required for cytoskeletal changes involved in the initial formation of a productive contact (125). Consistent with these data, Wülfing and Davis have shown by blocking the $[Ca^{2+}]_i$ rise pharmacologically that it is needed for reorientation of the cortical actin cytoskeleton to the contact zone, an event that may be involved in stabilization by bringing additional coreceptors to the zone (127). An interesting question is to what extent local rather than global changes in $[Ca^{2+}]_i$ serve to facilitate these changes in cell polarity. Studies of the localization of Ca^{2+} channels and pumps during formation of T cell-APC contacts may shed light on this issue.

Complex Ca^{2+} Signals Increase the Efficiency and Specificity of Transcription in B and T Cells

A major unresolved question in cell signaling is how a messenger like Ca^{2+} with its large number of downstream targets (2) can be used in cells to elicit selective responses. Studies of murine B cells show that the amplitude and duration of Ca^{2+} signals controls specific subsets of Ca^{2+}-sensitive transcription factors and that this may be involved in maintaining tolerance to self antigen. In naïve HEL-specific transgenic B cells, exposure to HEL evokes a biphasic $[Ca^{2+}]_i$ rise, consisting of a large transient followed by a smaller, persistent plateau. This response is accompanied by rapid activation of transcriptional regulators NFAT, NFκB, and c-Jun N-terminal kinase (JNK) (128). Using ionomycin to simulate the spike and plateau phases of the Ca^{2+} response separately in the presence of phorbol ester, Dolmetsch et al showed that the spike activates NFκB and JNK selectively, whereas the low plateau activates only NFAT (128). This selectivity arises because NFκB and JNK have a relatively low Ca^{2+} sensitivity but long persistence of activity after Ca^{2+} removal, whereas NFAT has higher Ca^{2+} sensitivity but is rapidly reversible. These different Ca^{2+} requirements may help explain the pattern of transcription factor activation in tolerant B cells. In B cells from animals expressing HEL as a self-antigen, the presence of low tolerizing levels of HEL elicits low-amplitude $[Ca^{2+}]_i$ oscillations that are sufficient to activate nuclear translocation of NFAT, but acute exposure to higher levels of HEL fails to elicit the large Ca^{2+} spike and correspondingly fails to activate NFκB or JNK (129). One implication of these studies is that the pattern of gene expression characteristic of the tolerant state may be controlled through the amplitude and duration of the Ca^{2+} signal.

Given the widespread occurrence of $[Ca^{2+}]_i$ oscillations in T cells and many other cells, an essential question is whether oscillations confer any advantage in terms of signaling or whether they are simply the inevitable consequence of multiple feedback pathways involved in $[Ca^{2+}]_i$ regulation. In a first attempt to address this question, Negulescu et al (7) stimulated T hybridoma cells with anti-CD3 and compared NFAT-dependent *lacZ* expression in oscillating and nonoscillating cells. Though there was a tendency for cells with larger and more frequent spikes to be lacZ$^+$, the cell-to-cell variability was large, and it was difficult to rule out effects due to parallel signaling pathways initiated through the TCR. Two later studies adopted more reductionist approaches to focus specifically on the role of Ca^{2+}. Li et al (130) photoreleased a constant total amount of IP$_3$ in RBL cells using different temporal patterns, and they found that pulses of IP$_3$ with a period of $\sim$60 sec, close to the natural period of $[Ca^{2+}]_i$ oscillations in T cells, was most efficient in stimulating NFAT. Dolmetsch et al (131) applied TG to tonically activate CRAC channels in Jurkat cells, followed by extracellular Ca^{2+} pulses to create controlled $[Ca^{2+}]_i$ oscillations of various sizes. At low average $[Ca^{2+}]_i$ (below $\sim$200 nM), oscillations appear to be more effective than a steady $[Ca^{2+}]_i$ rise of the same average value at activating NFAT-dependent transcription. Oscillations lose their advantage at higher levels of stimulation. Both of these studies imply that $[Ca^{2+}]_i$ oscillations increase the efficiency of detecting weak stimuli and hence may help to maximize the sensitivity of T cells to low doses of antigen.

Oscillations also help to encode the specificity of Ca^{2+}-dependent gene expression. In experiments on Jurkat cells stimulated with controlled $[Ca^{2+}]_i$ oscillations and phorbol ester, transcription factors that regulate IL-2 expression differed in their dependence on oscillation frequency; NFAT and Oct-1/Oap required rapid oscillations ($>$1 per 400 sec), whereas NFκB could be activated significantly even by spikes as infrequent as one every 30 min (131). These differences may reflect the specific deactivation kinetics for each factor, as noted above. Importantly, intact promoters for the IL-2 gene (with NFAT, Oct/Oap, and NFκB sites) and the IL-8 gene (with an NFκB site but no NFAT or Oct/Oap) show a similar divergence in frequency sensitivity. These results suggest that specific combinations of transcription factors may enable $[Ca^{2+}]_i$ oscillations to activate particular subsets of Ca^{2+}-dependent genes in a frequency-encoded manner.

These studies constitute an essential first step in demonstrating that lymphocyte Ca^{2+} signals are much more than a binary switch and that they can transmit specific information embedded in their duration, amplitude, and kinetics. Important challenges for the future include identifying the full complement of genes that respond to specific patterns of Ca^{2+} signaling and relating this information back to the Ca^{2+} signals and patterns of gene expression that occur as lymphocytes respond to stimuli in vivo. In addition, it will be important to know not only how the signals are specified but also what biochemical effectors and networks act to decode them.

FUTURE PERSPECTIVES

A rather large number of pathways are now known to participate in the generation of Ca^{2+} signals in T cells following contact with antigen. Interactions among these help to generate a diversity of complex Ca^{2+} signaling patterns, which may transmit specific types of information to the cell. Though substantial progress has been made in cloning some of the molecules involved in Ca^{2+} signaling, identifying the molecular basis of the CRAC channel and its mechanism of regulation by store content remains a central but elusive goal. The spatial distributions of Ca^{2+} sources and sinks in T cells are also largely unknown, but they may be critical in establishing specific interactions that control patterns of Ca^{2+} signaling. The fine structure of Ca^{2+} signals appears to change as T cells mature and as mature cells undergo further differentiation to become Th1, Th2, or memory cells (14, 17, 132, 133). Thus, an important long-range goal will be to bring Ca^{2+} signaling studies to the in vivo level to ask what types of signals accompany differentiation and functional responses in the lymphocyte's native environment and to what extent these signals serve an instructive or a permissive role.

ACKNOWLEDGMENT

I would like to thank Dr. Markus Hoth for contributing the diagram depicted in Figure 1.

Visit the Annual Reviews home page at www.AnnualReviews.org

LITERATURE CITED

1. Weiss A, Imboden JB. 1987. Cell surface molecules and early events involved in human T lymphocyte activation. *Adv. Immunol.* 41:1–38

2. Premack BA, Gardner P. 1992. Signal transduction by T-cell receptors: mobilization of Ca and regulation of Ca-dependent effector molecules. *Am. J. Physiol.* 263:C1119–40

3. Lewis RS, Cahalan MD. 1995. Potassium and calcium channels in lymphocytes. *Annu. Rev. Immunol.* 13:623–53

4. Qian D, Weiss A. 1997. T cell antigen receptor signal transduction. *Curr. Opin. Cell Biol.* 9:205–12

5. van Leeuwen JE, Samelson LE. 1999. T cell antigen-receptor signal transduction. *Curr. Opin. Immunol.* 11:242–48

6. Karttunen J, Shastri N. 1991. Measurement of ligand-induced activation in single viable T cells using the *lacZ* reporter gene. *Proc. Natl. Acad. Sci. USA* 88:3972–76

7. Negulescu PA, Shastri N, Cahalan MD. 1994. Intracellular calcium dependence of gene expression in single T lymphocytes. *Proc. Natl. Acad. Sci. USA* 91:2873–77

8. Crabtree GR. 1989. Contingent genetic regulatory events in T lymphocyte activation. *Science* 243:355–61

9. Timmerman LA, Clipstone NA, Ho SN, Northrop JP, Crabtree GR. 1996. Rapid shuttling of NF-AT in discrimination of Ca^{2+} signals and immunosuppression. *Nature* 383:837–40

10. Rao A, Luo C, Hogan PG. 1997. Transcription factors of the NFAT family: regulation and function. *Annu. Rev. Immunol.* 15:707–47

11. Lewis RS, Cahalan MD. 1989. Mitogen-induced oscillations of cytosolic Ca^{2+} and transmembrane Ca^{2+} current in human leukemic T cells. *Cell Regul.* 1:99–112

12. Donnadieu E, Bismuth G, Trautmann A. 1992. Calcium fluxes in T lymphocytes. *J. Biol. Chem.* 267:25864–72

13. Donnadieu E, Bismuth G, Trautmann A. 1994. Antigen recognition by helper T cells elicits a sequence of distinct changes of their shape and intracellular calcium. *Curr. Biol.* 4:584–95

14. Verheugen JA, Le Deist F, Devignot V, Korn H. 1997. Enhancement of calcium signaling and proliferation responses in activated human T lymphocytes. Inhibitory effects of K^+ channel block by charybdotoxin depend on the T cell activation state. *Cell Calcium* 21:1–17

15. Wülfing C, Rabinowitz JD, Beeson C, Sjaastad MD, McConnell HM, Davis MM. 1997. Kinetics and extent of T cell activation as measured with the calcium signal. *J. Exp. Med.* 185:1815–25

16. Delon J, Bercovici N, Raposo G, Liblau R, Trautmann A. 1998. Antigen-dependent and -independent Ca^{2+} responses triggered in T cells by dendritic cells compared with B cells. *J. Exp. Med.* 188:1473–84

17. Freedman BD, Liu QH, Somersan S, Kotlikoff MI, Punt JA. 1999. Receptor avidity and costimulation specify the intracellular Ca^{2+} signaling pattern in CD4$^+$ CD8$^+$ thymocytes. *J. Exp. Med.* 190:943–52

18. Berridge MJ, Bootman MD, Lipp P. 1998. Calcium—a life and death signal. *Nature* 395:645–48

19. Imboden JB, Stobo JD. 1985. Transmembrane signalling by the T cell antigen receptor. Perturbation of the T3-antigen receptor complex generates inositol phosphates and releases calcium ions from intracellular stores. *J. Exp. Med.* 161:446–56

20. Guse AH, Roth E, Emmrich F. 1993. Intracellular Ca^{2+} pools in Jurkat T-lymphocytes. *Biochem. J.* 291:447–51

21. Iino M, Endo M. 1992. Calcium-dependent immediate feedback control of inositol 1,4,5-trisphosphate-induced Ca^{2+} release. *Nature* 360:76–78

22. Bezprozvanny I, Ehrlich BE. 1995. The inositol 1,4,5-trisphosphate (InsP$_3$) receptor. *J. Membr. Biol.* 145:205–16

23. Sugiyama T, Furuya A, Monkawa T, Yamamoto-Hino M, Satoh S, Ohmori K, Miyawaki A, Hanai N, Mikoshiba K, Hasegawa M. 1994. Monoclonal antibodies distinctively recognizing the subtypes of inositol 1,4,5-trisphosphate receptor: application to the studies on inflammatory cells. *FEBS Lett.* 354:149–54

24. Harnick DJ, Jayaraman T, Ma Y, Mulieri P, Go LO, Marks AR. 1995. The human type 1 inositol 1,4,5-trisphosphate receptor from T lymphocytes. Structure, localization, and tyrosine phosphorylation. *J. Biol. Chem.* 270:2833–40

25. Bezprozvanny I, Watras J, Ehrlich BE. 1991. Bell-shaped calcium-response curves of Ins(1,4,5)P$_3$- and calcium-gated channels from endoplasmic reticulum of cerebellum. *Nature* 351:751–54

26. Finch EA, Turner TJ, Goldin SM. 1991. Calcium as a coagonist of inositol 1,4,5-trisphosphate-induced calcium release. *Science* 252:443–46

27. Ramos-Franco J, Fill M, Mignery GA. 1998. Isoform-specific function of single inositol 1,4,5-trisphosphate receptor channels. *Biophys. J.* 75:834–39

28. Miyakawa T, Maeda A, Yamazawa T,

Hirose K, Kurosaki T, Iino M. 1999. Encoding of Ca^{2+} signals by differential expression of IP_3 receptor subtypes. *EMBO J.* 18:1303–8

29. Hagar RE, Burgstahler AD, Nathanson MH, Ehrlich BE. 1998. Type III $InsP_3$ receptor channel stays open in the presence of increased calcium. *Nature* 396:81–84

30. Jayaraman T, Ondriasova E, Ondrias K, Harnick DJ, Marks AR. 1995. The inositol 1,4,5-trisphosphate receptor is essential for T-cell receptor signaling. *Proc. Natl. Acad. Sci. USA* 92:6007–11

31. Jayaraman T, Marks AR. 1997. T cells deficient in inositol 1,4,5-trisphosphate receptor are resistant to apoptosis. *Mol. Cell. Biol.* 17:3005–12

32. Sugawara H, Kurosaki M, Takata M, Kurosaki T. 1997. Genetic evidence for involvement of type 1, type 2 and type 3 inositol 1,4,5-trisphosphate receptors in signal transduction through the B-cell antigen receptor. *EMBO J.* 16:3078–88

33. Jayaraman T, Ondrias K, Ondriasova E, Marks AR. 1996. Regulation of the inositol 1,4,5-trisphosphate receptor by tyrosine phosphorylation. *Science* 272:1492–94

34. Appleby MW, Gross JA, Cooke MP, Levin SD, Qian X, Perlmutter RM. 1992. Defective T cell receptor signaling in mice lacking the thymic isoform of p59*fyn*. *Cell* 70:751–63

35. Donnadieu E, Cefai D, Tan YP, Paresys G, Bismuth G, Trautmann A. 1992. Imaging early steps of human T cell activation by antigen-presenting cells. *J. Immunol.* 148:2643–53

36. Guse AH. 1998. Ca^{2+} signaling in T-lymphocytes. *Crit. Rev. Immunol.* 18:419–48

37. Guse AH, da Silva CP, Emmrich F, Ashamu GA, Potter BV, Mayr GW. 1995. Characterization of cyclic adenosine diphosphate-ribose-induced Ca^{2+} release in T lymphocyte cell lines. *J. Immunol.* 155:3353–59

38. Guse AH, Berg I, da Silva CP, Potter BV, Mayr GW. 1997. Ca^{2+} entry induced by cyclic ADP-ribose in intact T-lymphocytes. *J. Biol. Chem.* 272:8546–50

39. Guse AH, da Silva CP, Berg I, Skapenko AL, Weber K, Heyer P, Hohenegger M, Ashamu GA, Schulze-Koops H, Potter BV, Mayr GW. 1999. Regulation of calcium signalling in T lymphocytes by the second messenger cyclic ADP-ribose. *Nature* 398:70–73

40. Takeshima H, Ikemoto T, Nishi M, Nishiyama N, Shimuta M, Sugitani Y, Kuno J, Saito I, Saito H, Endo M, Iino M, Noda T. 1996. Generation and characterization of mutant mice lacking ryanodine receptor type 3. *J. Biol. Chem.* 271:19649–52

41. Dolmetsch RE, Lewis RS. 1994. Signaling between intracellular Ca^{2+} stores and depletion-activated Ca^{2+} channels generates $[Ca^{2+}]_i$ oscillations in T lymphocytes. *J. Gen. Physiol.* 103:365–88

42. Khan AA, Soloski MJ, Sharp AH, Schilling G, Sabatini DM, Li SH, Ross CA, Snyder SH. 1996. Lymphocyte apoptosis: mediation by increased type 3 inositol 1,4,5-trisphosphate receptor. *Science* 273:503–7

43. Marks AR. 1997. Intracellular calcium-release channels: regulators of cell life and death. *Am. J. Physiol.* 272:H597–605

44. Berridge MJ. 1993. Inositol trisphosphate and calcium signalling. *Nature* 361:315–25

45. Putney JW Jr. 1990. Capacitative calcium entry revisited. *Cell Calcium* 11:611–24

46. Thastrup O, Dawson AP, Scharff O, Foder B, Cullen PJ, Drobak BK, Bjerrum PJ, Christensen SB, Hanley MR. 1989. Thapsigargin, a novel molecular probe for studying intracellular calcium release and storage. *Agents Actions* 27:17–23

47. Parekh AB, Penner R. 1997. Store depletion and calcium influx. *Physiol. Rev.* 77:901–30

48. Lewis RS. 1999. Store-operated calcium channels. *Adv. Second Messenger Phosphoprotein Res.* 33:279–307

49. Hoth M, Penner R. 1992. Depletion of

intracellular calcium stores activates a calcium current in mast cells. *Nature* 355:353–56

50. Zweifach A, Lewis RS. 1993. Mitogen-regulated Ca^{2+} current of T lymphocytes is activated by depletion of intracellular Ca^{2+} stores. *Proc. Natl. Acad. Sci. USA* 90:6295–99

51. Premack BA, McDonald TV, Gardner P. 1994. Activation of Ca^{2+} current in Jurkat T cells following the depletion of Ca^{2+} stores by microsomal Ca^{2+}-ATPase inhibitors. *J. Immunol.* 152:5226–40

52. Mason MJ, Garcia-Rodriguez C, Grinstein S. 1991. Coupling between intracellular Ca^{2+} stores and the Ca^{2+} permeability of the plasma membrane. Comparison of the effects of thapsigargin, 2,5-di-(tert-butyl)-1,4-hydroquinone, and cyclopiazonic acid in rat thymic lymphocytes. *J. Biol. Chem.* 266:20856–62

53. Sarkadi B, Tordai A, Homolya L, Scharff O, Gárdos G. 1991. Calcium influx and intracellular calcium release in anti-CD3 antibody-stimulated and thapsigargin-treated human T lymphoblasts. *J. Membr. Biol.* 123:9–21

54. Chung SC, McDonald TV, Gardner P. 1994. Inhibition by SK&F 96365 of Ca^{2+} current, IL-2 production and activation in T lymphocytes. *Br. J. Pharmacol.* 113:861–68

55. Aussel C, Marhaba R, Pelassy C, Breittmayer JP. 1996. Submicromolar La^{3+} concentrations block the calcium release-activated channel, and impair CD69 and CD25 expression in CD3- or thapsigargin-activated Jurkat cells. *Biochem. J.* 313:909–13

56. Partiseti M, Le Deist F, Hivroz C, Fischer A, Korn H, Choquet D. 1994. The calcium current activated by T cell receptor and store depletion in human lymphocytes is absent in a primary immunodeficiency. *J. Biol. Chem.* 269:32327–35

57. Fanger CM, Hoth M, Crabtree GR, Lewis RS. 1995. Characterization of T cell

mutants with defects in capacitative calcium entry: genetic evidence for the physiological roles of CRAC channels. *J. Cell Biol.* 131:655–67

58. Zweifach A. 2000. Target-cell contact activates a highly selective capacitative calcium entry pathway in cytotoxic T lymphocytes. *J. Cell Biol.* 148:603–14

59. Weismann M, Guse AH, Sorokin L, Broker B, Frieser M, Hallmann R, Mayr GW. 1997. Integrin-mediated intracellular Ca^{2+} signaling in Jurkat T lymphocytes. *J. Immunol.* 158:1618–27

60. Ross PE, Cahalan MD. 1995. Ca^{2+} influx pathways mediated by swelling or stores depletion in mouse thymocytes. *J. Gen. Physiol.* 106:415–44

61. Ross PE, Ehring GR, Cahalan MD. 1997. Dynamics of ATP-induced calcium signaling in single mouse thymocytes. *J. Cell Biol.* 138:987–98

62. Hoth M, Penner R. 1993. Calcium release-activated calcium current in rat mast cells. *J. Physiol.* 465:359–86

63. Hoth M. 1995. Calcium and barium permeation through calcium release-activated calcium (CRAC) channels. *Pflügers Arch.* 430:315–22

64. Lepple-Wienhues A, Cahalan MD. 1996. Conductance and permeation of monovalent cations through depletion-activated Ca^{2+} channels (I_{CRAC}) in Jurkat T cells. *Biophys. J.* 71:787–94

65. Kerschbaum HH, Cahalan MD. 1998. Monovalent permeability, rectification, and ionic block of store-operated calcium channels in Jurkat T lymphocytes. *J. Gen. Physiol.* 111:521–37

66. Kerschbaum HH, Cahalan MD. 1999. Single-channel recording of a store-operated Ca^{2+} channel in Jurkat T lymphocytes. *Science* 283:836–39

67. Parekh AB, Fleig A, Penner R. 1997. The store-operated calcium current I_{CRAC}: nonlinear activation by $InsP_3$ and dissociation from calcium release. *Cell* 89:973–80

68. Glitsch MD, Parekh AB. 2000. Ca^{2+} store dynamics determines the pattern of activation of the store-operated Ca^{2+} current I_{CRAC} in response to $InsP_3$ in rat basophilic leukaemia cells. *J. Physiol.* 523:283–90

69. Huang Y, Takahashi M, Tanzawa K, Putney JW Jr. 1998. Effect of adenophostin A on Ca^{2+} entry and calcium release-activated calcium current (I_{crac}) in rat basophilic leukemia cells. *J. Biol. Chem.* 273:31815–21

70. Lewis RS, Dolmetsch RE, Zweifach A. 1996. Positive and negative regulation of depletion-activated calcium channels by calcium. *Soc. Gen. Physiol. Ser.* 51:241–54

71. Zweifach A, Lewis RS. 1995. Slow calcium-dependent inactivation of depletion-activated calcium current. Store-dependent and -independent mechanisms. *J. Biol. Chem.* 270:14445–51

72. Hofer AM, Fasolato C, Pozzan T. 1998. Capacitative Ca^{2+} entry is closely linked to the filling state of internal Ca^{2+} stores: a study using simultaneous measurements of I_{CRAC} and intraluminal $[Ca^{2+}]$. *J. Cell Biol.* 140:325–34

73. Zweifach A, Lewis RS. 1995. Rapid inactivation of depletion-activated calcium current (I_{CRAC}) due to local calcium feedback. *J. Gen. Physiol.* 105:209–26

74. Fierro L, Parekh AB. 1999. Fast calcium-dependent inactivation of calcium release-activated calcium current (CRAC) in RBL-1 cells. *J. Membr. Biol.* 168:9–17

75. Hoth M, Button DC, Lewis RS. 2000. Mitochondrial control of calcium-channel gating: a mechanism for sustained signaling and transcriptional activation in T lymphocytes. *Proc. Natl. Acad. Sci. USA* 97:10607–12

76. Putney JW Jr., Bird GS. 1993. The inositol phosphate-calcium signaling system in nonexcitable cells. *Endocr. Rev.* 14:610–31

77. Putney JW Jr., McKay RR. 1999. Capacitative calcium entry channels. *Bioessays* 21:38–46

77a. Montell C. 1998. TRP trapped in fly signaling web. *Curr. Opin. Neurobiol.* 8:389–97

78. Philipp S, Trost C, Warnat J, Rautmann J, Himmerkus N, Schroth G, Kretz O, Nastainczyk W, Cavalie A, Hoth M, Flockerzi V. 2000. TRP4 (CCE1) is part of native calcium release activated Ca^{2+} -like channels in adrenal cells. *J. Biol. Chem.* 275:23965–72

78a. Schaefer M, Plant TD, Obukhov AG, Hofmann T, Gudermann T, Schultz G. 2000. Receptor-mediated regulation of the nonselective cation channels TRPC4 and TRPC5. *J. Biol. Chem.* 275:17517–26

79. Fierro L, Parekh AB. 1999. On the characterisation of the mechanism underlying passive activation of the Ca^{2+} release-activated Ca^{2+} current I_{CRAC} in rat basophilic leukaemia cells. *J. Physiol.* 520:407–16

80. Petersen CC, Berridge MJ. 1996. Capacitative calcium entry is colocalised with calcium release in Xenopus oocytes: evidence against a highly diffusible calcium influx factor. *Pflügers Arch.* 432:286–92

81. Jaconi M, Pyle J, Bortolon R, Ou J, Clapham D. 1997. Calcium release and influx colocalize to the endoplasmic reticulum. *Curr. Biol.* 7:599–602

82. Patterson RL, van Rossum DB, Gill DL. 1999. Store-operated Ca^{2+} entry: evidence for a secretion-like coupling model. *Cell* 98:487–99

83. Ma HT, Patterson RL, van Rossum DB, Birnbaumer L, Mikoshiba K, Gill DL. 2000. Requirement of the inositol trisphosphate receptor for activation of store-operated Ca^{2+} channels. *Science* 287:1647–51

84. Ribeiro CM, Reece J, Putney JW Jr. 1997. Role of the cytoskeleton in calcium signaling in NIH 3T3 cells. An intact cytoskeleton is required for agonist-induced $[Ca^{2+}]_i$ signaling, but not for capacitative calcium entry. *J. Biol. Chem.* 272:26555–61

85. Randriamampita C, Tsien RY. 1993.

Emptying of intracellular Ca^{2+} stores releases a novel small messenger that stimulates Ca^{2+} influx. *Nature* 364:809–14

86. Gilon P, Bird GJ, Bian X, Yakel JL, Putney JW Jr. 1995. The Ca^{2+}-mobilizing actions of a Jurkat cell extract on mammalian cells and *Xenopus laevis* oocytes. *J. Biol. Chem.* 270:8050–55

87. Csutora P, Su Z, Kim HY, Bugrim A, Cunningham KW, Nuccitelli R, Keizer JE, Hanley MR, Blalock JE, Marchase RB. 1999. Calcium influx factor is synthesized by yeast and mammalian cells depleted of organellar calcium stores. *Proc. Natl. Acad. Sci. USA* 96:121–26

88. Trepakova ES, Csutora P, Hunton DL, Marchase RB, Cohen RA, Bolotina VM. 2000. Calcium influx factor directly activates store-operated cation channels in vascular smooth muscle cells. *J. Biol. Chem.* 275:26158–63

89. Somasundaram B, Norman JC, Mahaut-Smith MP. 1995. Primaquine, an inhibitor of vesicular transport, blocks the calcium-release-activated current in rat megakaryocytes. *Biochem. J.* 309:725–29

90. Fasolato C, Hoth M, Penner R. 1993. A GTP-dependent step in the activation mechanism of capacitative calcium influx. *J. Biol. Chem.* 268:20737–40

91. Yao Y, Ferrer-Montiel AV, Montal M, Tsien RY. 1999. Activation of store-operated Ca^{2+} current in Xenopus oocytes requires SNAP-25 but not a diffusible messenger. *Cell* 98:475–85

92. Berridge MJ. 1995. Capacitative calcium entry. *Biochem. J.* 312:1–11

93. Kiselyov K, Xu X, Mozhayeva G, Kuo T, Pessah I, Mignery G, Zhu X, Birnbaumer L, Muallem S. 1998. Functional interaction between InsP3 receptors and store-operated Htrp3 channels. *Nature* 396:478–82

94. Kiselyov K, Mignery GA, Zhu MX, Muallem S. 1999. The N-terminal domain of the IP3 receptor gates store-operated hTrp3 channels. *Mol. Cell* 4:423–29

95. Boulay G, Brown DM, Qin N, Jiang M, Dietrich A, Zhu MX, Chen Z, Birnbaumer M, Mikoshiba K, Birnbaumer L. 1999. Modulation of Ca^{2+} entry by polypeptides of the inositol 1,4, 5- trisphosphate receptor (IP3R) that bind transient receptor potential (TRP): evidence for roles of TRP and IP3R in store depletion-activated Ca^{2+} entry. *Proc. Natl. Acad. Sci. USA* 96:14955–60

95a. Braun F-J, Broad LM, Armstrong DL, Putney JW Jr. 2000. Stable activation of single CRAC-channels in divalent cation-free solutions. *J. Biol. Chem.* In press

96. Cahalan MD, Chandy KG. 1997. Ion channels in the immune system as targets for immunosuppression. *Curr. Opin. Biotech.* 8:749–56

97. Leonard RJ, Garcia ML, Slaughter RS, Reuben JP. 1992. Selective blockers of voltage-gated K^+ channels depolarize human T lymphocytes: mechanism of the antiproliferative effect of charybdotoxin. *Proc. Natl. Acad. Sci. USA* 89:10094–98

98. Lin CS, Boltz RC, Blake JT, Nguyen M, Talento A, Fischer PA, Springer MS, Sigal NH, Slaughter RS, Garcia ML, Kaczorowski GJ, Koo GC. 1993. Voltage-gated potassium channels regulate calcium-dependent pathways involved in human T lymphocyte activation. *J. Exp. Med.* 177:637–45

99. Koo GC, Blake JT, Talento A, Nguyen M, Lin S, Sirotina A, Shah K, Mulvany K, Hora D Jr., Cunningham P, Wunderler DL, McManus OB, Slaughter R, Bugianesi R, Felix J, Garcia M, Williamson J, Kaczorowski G, Sigal NH, Springer MS, Feeney W. 1997. Blockade of the voltage-gated potassium channel Kv1.3 inhibits immune responses in vivo. *J. Immunol.* 158:5120–28

99a. Ehring GR, Kerschbaum HH, Eder C, Neben AL, Fanger CM, Khoury RM, Negulescu PA, Cahalan MD. 1998. A nongenomic mechanism for progesterone mediated immunosuppression:

Inhibition of K^+ channels, Ca^{2+} signaling, and gene expression in T lymphocytes. *J. Exp. Med.* 188:1593–612

100. Wulff H, Miller MJ, Hänsel W, Grissmer S, Cahalan MD, Chandy KG. 2000. Design of a potent and selective inhibitor of the intermediate-conductance Ca^{2+}-activated K^+ channel, IKCa1: a potential immunosuppressant. *Proc. Natl. Acad. Sci. USA* 97:8151–56

101. Grissmer S, Nguyen AN, Cahalan MD. 1993. Calcium-activated potassium channels in resting and activated human T lymphocytes. Expression levels, calcium dependence, ion selectivity, and pharmacology. *J. Gen. Physiol.* 102:601–30

101a. Lepple-Wienhues A, Belka C, Laun T, Jekle A, Walter B, Wieland U, Welz M, Heil L, Kun J, Busch G, Weller M, Bamberg M, Gulbins E, Lang F. 1999. Stimulation of CD95 (Fas) blocks T lymphocyte calcium channels through sphingomyelinase and sphingolipids. *Proc. Natl. Acad. Sci. USA* 96:13795–13800

101b. Mathes C, Fleig A, Penner R. 1998. Calcium release-activated calcium current (I_{CRAC}) is a direct target for sphingosine. *J. Biol. Chem.* 273:25020–30

102. Launay S, Bobe R, Lacabaratz-Porret C, Bredoux R, Kovacs T, Enouf J, Papp B. 1997. Modulation of endoplasmic reticulum calcium pump expression during T lymphocyte activation. *J. Biol. Chem.* 272:10746–50

103. Poch E, Leach S, Snape S, Cacic T, MacLennan DH, Lytton J. 1998. Functional characterization of alternatively spliced human SERCA3 transcripts. *Am. J. Physiol.* 275:C1449–58

104. Balasubramanyam M, Kimura M, Aviv A, Gardner JP. 1993. Kinetics of calcium transport across the lymphocyte plasma membrane. *Am. J. Physiol.* 265:C321–27

105. Donnadieu E, Trautmann A. 1993. Is

there a Na^+/Ca^{2+} exchanger in macrophages and in lymphocytes? *Pflügers Arch.* 424:448–55

106. Bautista DM, Lewis RS. 1999. Modulation of plasma membrane calcium-ATPase studied with a calcium-clamp technique. *Biophys. J.* 76:A379

107. Penniston JT, Enyedi A. 1998. Modulation of the plasma membrane Ca^{2+} pump. *J. Membr. Biol.* 165:101–9

108. Caride AJ, Elwess NL, Verma AK, Filoteo AG, Enyedi A, Bajzer Z, Penniston JT. 1999. The rate of activation by calmodulin of isoform 4 of the plasma membrane Ca^{2+} pump is slow and is changed by alternative splicing. *J. Biol. Chem.* 274:35227–32

109. Balasubramanyam M, Gardner JP. 1995. Protein kinase C modulates cytosolic free calcium by stimulating calcium pump activity in Jurkat T cells. *Cell Calcium* 18:526–41

110. Scharff O, Foder B, Skibsted U. 1983. Hysteretic activation of the Ca^{2+} pump revealed by calcium transients in human red cells. *Biochim. Biophys. Acta* 730:295–305

111. Sedova M, Blatter LA. 1999. Dynamic regulation of $[Ca^{2+}]_i$ by plasma membrane Ca^{2+}-ATPase and Na^+/Ca^{2+} exchange during capacitative Ca^{2+} entry in bovine vascular endothelial cells. *Cell Calcium* 25:333–43

111b. Snitsarev VA, Taylor CW. 1999. Overshooting cytosolic Ca^{2+} signals evoked by capacitative Ca^{2+} entry result from delayed stimulation of a plasma membrane Ca^{2+} pump. *Cell Calcium* 25:409–17

112. Babcock DF, Hille B. 1998. Mitochondrial oversight of cellular Ca^{2+} signaling. *Curr. Opin. Neurobiol.* 8:398–404

113. Duchen MR. 1999. Contributions of mitochondria to animal physiology: from homeostatic sensor to calcium signalling and cell death. *J. Physiol.* 516:1–17

114. Gunter TE, Pfeiffer DR. 1990. Mechanisms by which mitochondria transport calcium. *Am. J. Physiol.* 258:C755–86

115. Hoth M, Fanger CM, Lewis RS. 1997. Mitochondrial regulation of store-operated calcium signaling in T lymphocytes. *J. Cell Biol.* 137:633–48

116. Tang Y, Zucker RS. 1997. Mitochondrial involvement in post-tetanic potentiation of synaptic transmission. *Neuron* 18:483–91

117. Hajnóczky G, Robb-Gaspers LD, Seitz MB, Thomas AP. 1995. Decoding of cytosolic calcium oscillations in the mitochondria. *Cell* 82:415–24

118. Jouaville LS, Pinton P, Bastianutto C, Rutter GA, Rizzuto R. 1999. Regulation of mitochondrial ATP synthesis by calcium: evidence for a long-term metabolic priming. *Proc. Natl. Acad. Sci. USA* 96:13807–12

119. Buttgereit F, Burmester GR, Brand MD. 2000. Bioenergetics of immune functions: fundamental and therapeutic aspects. *Immunol. Today* 21:192–99

119b. Makowska A, Zablocki K, Duszynski J. 2000. The role of mitochondria in the regulation of calcium influx into Jurkat cells. *Eur. J. Biochem.* 267:877–84

120. Verheugen JA, Vijverberg HP. 1995. Intracellular Ca^{2+} oscillations and membrane potential fluctuations in intact human T lymphocytes: role of K^+ channels in Ca^{2+} signaling. *Cell Calcium* 17:287–300

121. Liu KQ, Bunnell SC, Gurniak CB, Berg LJ. 1998. T cell receptor-initiated calcium release is uncoupled from capacitative calcium entry in Itk-deficient T cells. *J. Exp. Med.* 187:1721–27

122. Choquet D, Partiseti M, Amigorena S, Bonnerot C, Fridman WH, Korn H. 1993. Cross-linking of IgG receptors inhibits membrane immunoglobulin-stimulated calcium influx in B lymphocytes. *J. Cell Biol.* 121:355–63

123. Scharenberg AM, Kinet JP. 1998. PtdIns-3,4,5-P3: a regulatory nexus between tyrosine kinases and sustained calcium signals. *Cell* 94:5–8

124. Negulescu PA, Krasieva TB, Khan A, Kerschbaum HH, Cahalan MD. 1996. Polarity of T cell shape, motility, and sensitivity to antigen. *Immunity* 4:421–30

125. Delon J, Bercovici N, Liblau R, Trautmann A. 1998. Imaging antigen recognition by naive $CD4^+$ T cells: compulsory cytoskeletal alterations for the triggering of an intracellular calcium response. *Eur. J. Immunol.* 28:716–29

126. Dustin ML, Bromley SK, Kan Z, Peterson DA, Unanue ER. 1997. Antigen receptor engagement delivers a stop signal to migrating T lymphocytes. *Proc. Natl. Acad. Sci. USA* 94:3909–13

127. Wülfing C, Davis MM. 1998. A receptor/cytoskeletal movement triggered by costimulation during T cell activation. *Science* 282:2266–69

128. Dolmetsch RE, Lewis RS, Goodnow CC, Healy JI. 1997. Differential activation of transcription factors induced by Ca^{2+} response amplitude and duration. *Nature* 386:855–58

129. Healy JI, Dolmetsch RE, Timmerman LA, Cyster JG, Thomas ML, Crabtree GR, Lewis RS, Goodnow CC. 1997. Different nuclear signals are activated by the B cell receptor during positive versus negative signaling. *Immunity* 6:419–28

130. Li W, Llopis J, Whitney M, Zlokarnik G, Tsien RY. 1998. Cell-permeant caged InsP$_3$ ester shows that Ca^{2+} spike frequency can optimize gene expression. *Nature* 392:936–41

131. Dolmetsch RE, Xu K, Lewis RS. 1998. Calcium oscillations increase the efficiency and specificity of gene expression. *Nature* 392:933–36

132. Tanchot C, Guillaume S, Delon J,

Bourgeois C, Franzke A, Sarukhan A, Trautmann A, Rocha B. 1998. Modifications of CD8$^+$ T cell function during in vivo memory or tolerance induction. *Immunity* 8:581–90

133. Fanger CM, Neben AL, Cahalan MD. 2000. Differential Ca^{2+} influx, K$_{Ca}$ channel activity, and Ca^{2+} clearance distinguish Th1 and Th2 lymphocytes. *J. Immunol.* 164:1153–60

Annu. Rev. Immunol. 2001. 19:523–63

THE DESIGN OF VACCINES AGAINST *HELICOBACTER PYLORI* AND THEIR DEVELOPMENT

Giuseppe Del Giudice[1], Antonello Covacci[1], John L. Telford[1], Cesare Montecucco[2], and Rino Rappuoli[1]

*IRIS Research Center, Chiron SpA, Via Fiorentina 1, 53100 Siena, Italy[1];
e-mail: giuseppe_del_giudice@chiron.it; and Department of Biomedical Sciences,
University of Padova, 35121, Padova, Italy[2]*

Key Words *Helicobacter pylori*, vaccines, mucosal immunity, adjuvants, animal models

■ **Abstract** *Helicobacter pylori* is a gram negative, spiral, microaerophylic bacterium that infects the stomach of more than 50% of the human population worldwide. It is mostly acquired during childhood and, if not treated, persists chronically, causing chronic gastritis, peptic ulcer disease, and in some individuals, gastric adenocarcinoma and gastric B cell lymphoma. The current therapy, based on the use of a proton-pump inhibitor and antibiotics, is efficacious but faces problems such as patient compliance, antibiotic resistance, and possible recurrence of infection. The development of an efficacious vaccine against *H. pylori* would thus offer several advantages. Various approaches have been followed in the development of vaccines against *H. pylori*, most of which have been based on the use of selected antigens known to be involved in the pathogenesis of the infection, such as urease, the vacuolating cytotoxin (VacA), the cytotoxin-associated antigen (CagA), the neutrophil-activating protein (NAP), and others, and intended to confer protection prophylactically and/or therapeutically in animal models of infection. However, very little is known of the natural history of *H. pylori* infection and of the kinetics of the induced immune responses. Several lines of evidence suggest that *H. pylori* infection is accompanied by a pronounced Th1-type CD4+ T cell response. It appears, however, that after immunization, the antigen-specific response is predominantly polarized toward a Th2-type response, with production of cytokines that can inhibit the activation of Th1 cells and of macrophages, and the production of proinflammatory cytokines. The exact effector mechanisms of protection induced after immunization are still poorly understood. The next couple of years will be crucial for the development of vaccines against *H. pylori*. Several trials are foreseen in humans, and expectations are that most of the questions being asked now on the host-microbe interactions will be answered.

0732-0582/01/0407-0523$14.00

INTRODUCTION

From Serendipity to Commonplace

Helicobacter pylori belongs to the long list of emerging microorganisms that have popped out of the Pandora's box in the past thirty years. *H. pylori* exists alongside other bacteria (e.g. *Legionella pneumophila*) and viruses (e.g. HIV, HCV, rotaviruses) that cause a huge burden of mortality and morbidity and that had not been recognized until recently. The discovery by Bizzozero at the end of 1800 of spiral bacteria in the stomach of dogs went unnoticed (1). We had to wait almost a century before spiral, gram-negative, flagellated, microaerophilic bacteria were identified in the stomach of humans (2, 3) and finally recognized as the cause of peptic ulcer and gastric cancer.

The serendipidous discovery of *H. pylori* was followed by the observation that colonization of gastric mucosa (and/or of other organs such as intestine and liver) with *Helicobacter* species is a very common event in several animal species (4), with *H. pylori* specialized in infecting humans and some nonhuman primates (5). The commonness of the gastric colonization with urease-producing gram-negative spiral bacteria is underlined by the fact that more than 50% of the human population worldwide is infected with *H. pylori* (6). This prevalence is much higher in developing countries, where 90% or more of the population usually acquires the infection early in life (7). The prevalence of *H. pylori* infection increases with age, which is attributed to a birth cohort effect (8), though constant acquisition over time during adulthood has also been hypothesized (9). The vast majority of infections are acquired in childhood, in both developing and developed countries (10, 11, 12), most probably transmitted by the mother to the child (13). Most infections persist for life (supported by the same colonizing strain) (14), unless eradication is achieved.

Still open is the question of transmission of *H. pylori*. The involvement of pets in transmission is extremely unlikely (15). The finding of contaminated water supplies (16) and sheep milk (17) may represent a consequence of bacterial shedding from infected people, rather than an actual source of infection. The fecal-oral route has been invoked; however, it is not clear yet whether *H. pylori* would actually be able to survive the normal transit through the intestine. Oral-oral transmission has also been proposed (6). Recent data from *H. pylori*–infected adults, however, have shown that *H. pylori* is cultivable from pharmacologically induced vomiting and/or diarrhea (18). Similar results have been obtained in children with spontaneous vomitus (19). Vomiting and diarrhea may thus represent the vehicles for transmission of *H. pylori*, especially in environments with low socioeconomic conditions and/or at pediatric ages when these events are very common.

15%–20% of infected individuals will eventually develop severe gastroduodenal diseases. Given the wide distribution of this infection, it is estimated that each year at least 7 million cases of *H. pylori*–induced diseases occur worldwide (20). These diseases, which in most instances develop several years after colonization, range from peptic ulcer disease to adenocarcinoma of the distal stomach (antral region), and gastric mucosa-associated lymphoid tissue (MALT) lymphoma.

Rationale for Vaccine Development

The current treatment of *H. pylori*–symptomatic patients consists of the daily administration of a proton pump inhibitor and two antibiotics for one to two weeks. This treatment leads to eradication of the infection in 80%–90% of cases (21). Notwithstanding its validity, the antibiotic treatment poses several difficulties. First, the high number of tablets to be taken every day may reduce the compliance of the patients. Second, the kind and the amounts of antibiotics used can lead to side effects, such as abdominal pain, nausea, diarrhea, etc (22), which may limit the usefulness of the treatment. Third, *H. pylori* strains resistant to the most commonly used antibiotics (e.g. clarythromycin, metronidazole, ampicillin) are increasingly being reported (23). Active research is currently devoted to the discovery of new antibiotics and new therapeutic agents with the ultimate goal of avoiding the development of drug resistance. In addition, several studies in developed countries have shown that reinfection rates are low (~1%) in adults and children successfully treated with the antibiotics (24, 25). However, rates of reinfection are much higher in areas where *H. pylori* is endemic (26). Finally, a treatment is given only to patients with gastrointestinal symptoms. Clearly, asymptomatic *H. pylori* patients remain at risk of developing chronic gastritis and eventually gastric cancer.

Most of the drawbacks of the pharmacological treatment could be overcome by the availability of efficacious vaccines and even more of vaccines able to work both prophylactically and therapeutically. An anti-*H. pylori* vaccine would be especially useful in less developed countries, where *H. pylori* infection is much more prevalent and can negatively influence the growth of very young children (27), and where the high cost of the pharmacological treatments can be afforded by only a few.

Currently, various academic groups and private companies are pursuing the objective of developing vaccines against *H. pylori*, following different approaches. Some are based on traditional procedures that were followed for other vaccines: An oral inactivated whole-cell vaccine preparation has been tested in a phase I trial in human volunteers (see below); outer membrane vesicles are also being proposed as potential vaccines. More efforts, however, are being devoted to the development of vaccines based on defined *H. pylori* antigens. Some of these antigens are being identified by bioinformatics analysis of the sequences of the genomes of two strains of *H. pylori* (28, 29, 30). However, most of the antigens under consideration as potential vaccines were identified in the pregenomic era (4, 31), based on their abundance and/or on their involvement in pathogenesis.

In this review, we discuss those molecules that allow the bacterium to establish a dialogue with its host and that are considered as promising antigens for vaccine development. The experimental models of *H. pylori* infection in which most of these antigens are tested prophylactically and/or therapeutically are briefly outlined. We analyze the aspects of the immune response(s) induced by the natural infection that may be the basis of the gastric pathology or of the protective immunity induced by vaccination. We conclude with current information available on the testing of some of these constructs in humans.

VIRULENCE FACTORS THAT MAKE THE DIALOGUE POSSIBLE

Urease

To reach its unique ecological niche, *H. pylori* must survive passage through the low pH stomach lumen and enter the mucus layer covering the epithelial cells, where the pH is closer to neutrality owing to the unique permeability properties of the mucus to protons and bicarbonate anions. *H. pylori* is itself very sensitive to low pH (32) but resistant to acidic conditions in the presence of urea. This resistance results from its high amounts of urease (5%–10% of the total protein content), which converts gastric urea into ammonia and CO_2, thus effectively buffering its surface. Urease is a nickel-containing hetero-oligomeric enzyme consisting of six 27-kDa UreA subunits and six 62-kDa UreB subunits (33). Urease may play additional roles in the pathogenesis of *H. pylori* infection, including adhesion and stimulation of inflammatory cells.

Urease-negative *H. pylori* strains are unable to colonize the stomach of gnotobiotic piglets (34, 35), demonstrating the role of this enzyme in the colonization. Urease may favor the survival of *H. pylori* also by providing ammonia as a source of nitrogen for the production of glutamine from glutamate (36), though the relative importance of ammonia as a nutrient for amino acid synthesis in the general metabolism of *H. pylori* is not clear. Urease may intervene directly and/or indirectly in the induction of tissue damage in the stomach (37). *H. pylori* releases urease via autolysis; the protein may then attach to the bacterial surface (38) or diffuse in the surrounding gastric tissues (39). It is not clear, however, whether this protein represents a major target of local immune responses. Despite its abundance, antibody response to urease in chronically infected individuals living in areas of high transmission is not frequent (40). Furthermore, urease-specific $CD4^+$ T cell clones are found at very low frequency in gastric lymphocytes isolated from *H. pylori*–infected individuals, even from those with the most severe gastric pathologies (41, 42). Nonetheless, urease is widely investigated as a potential antigen for the development of prophylactic and therapeutic vaccines against *H. pylori* infection.

Vacuolating Cytotoxin (VacA)

The existence of a toxin in *H. pylori* was defined several years ago following the observation that bacterial culture supernatants induced cytoplasmic vacuoles in eukaryotic cells (43). The protein was therefore called vacuolating cytotoxin

(VacA). It was purified and then its sequence was determined (44, 45). It is produced as a cytosolic precursor of 140 kDa consisting of four domains. The N-terminal, 33 residues-long signal sequence drives the transport of the toxin to the periplasm. The second domain, of 37 kDa, is essential for the toxic activity of VacA; the deletion of a few residues from the N-terminus inactivates the toxin (46, 47). The third domain, of 58 kDa, is responsible for the binding of the toxin to the target cells (48). The C-terminal region mediates the translocation of the toxin from the periplasm to the bacterial surface, where it is released in the medium as a 95-Da protein. VacA readily associates into flower-shaped oligomers made of 6 or 7 subunits (49, 50). Oligomeric VacA is poorly active and, at least in vitro, requires exposure to acidic or alkaline media to dissociate into highly toxic monomers (51, 52). VacA also induces superficial erosions of gastric epithelial cells when administered orally to mice (45). To exert its toxic activity, VacA binds to target cells through its p58 moiety (53) to RPTP-β recently identified as its cellular receptor (54). After insertion into the membane, VacA forms transmembrane anion-selective channels that are believed to support an osmotically driven swelling and fusion of late endosomal compartments and lysosomes (52). Indeed, vacuole formation is strictly dependent on an active rab7 (55), a member of the family of small GTP-binding proteins believed to control vesicle trafficking inside the cell.

Vacuolization causes alteration in cell trafficking and endosomal protein degradation that may be very relevant to pathogenesis as well as to survival of the bacterium itself. Indeed, VacA-induced vacuoles do not retain the activities of late endosomes. For example, VacA profoundly affects the processing of antigens in antigen-presenting cells, resulting in a reduced generation of peptides able to bind to MHC class II antigens and to stimulate antigen-specific CD4$^+$ T cell clones (56). It is not clear which outcome in T cell stimulation in vivo this effect may have. Studies at T cell clonal level in *H. pylori*–infected subjects have shown that VacA-specific CD4$^+$ T cells at gastric level are found at a low frequency (41). Moreover, immunosuppressive events on induction of virus-specific CD8$^+$ T cells have been observed in mice experimentally infected with *H. pylori*, which became unable to control a challenge with recombinant vaccinia virus (57). It remains unclear, however, whether these in vivo phenomena can be ascribed to VacA. In addition, in vacuolated cells, precursors of acid hydrolases are impaired in their journey from the trans-Golgi compartment to lysosomes, and therefore substantial amounts are released in the medium (58). Should the same happen in vivo, these hydrolase precursors would be released and activated in the apical acidic compartment with ensuing degradation of the protecting mucus film. This would reduce the life span of epithelial cells exposed to a harsher environment and would favor bacterial growth by increasing the uptake of nutrients.

Afflux of ions and nutrients to *H. pylori* is also favored by VacA, either soluble (59) or bound to the bacteria (60), by increasing the permeability of polarized epithelial cell monolayers. An increased apical secretion of anions and the observed increase of short circuit current (61) taking place in the duodenum and intestine may contribute to the diarrhea observed in some children with acute infection with *H. pylori* (62, 63).

The amino acid sequence of VacA is well conserved. However, two regions exhibit some variability. The first is the "s" (signal) region, for which four alleles have been identified (s1a, s1b, s1c, and s2). The other is the "m" (mid) region within the p58 moiety of the toxin, for which two alleles (m1 and m2) have been identified (64, 65). Until recently it was believed that VacA with the m2 phenotype was nontoxic, because it did not induce vacuolization of HeLa cells (44, 66). This observation did not fit with the clinical observation that both m1 and m2 *H. pylori* strains were equally associated with severe forms of gastric pathology (67). We have shown that m2 VacA induces vacuoles in other cell lines in vitro (RK-13) and in primary human gastric epithelial cells (68). This finding implies that the "m" region is involved in the interaction with the VacA receptor and that the two alleles have evolved to adapt to polymorphic receptors. Antibodies raised against one allele after experimental immunization of animals or natural infection of humans recognize the other allele although at a lower extent (68, 69). It is not known, however, whether this limited recognition may affect the induction of immunity against both allelic forms of VacA after immunization. One may expect that the immune response to the conserved region containing the functional domain of VacA results in an efficient immunity against the bacterium.

CagA and cag Pathogenicity Island (PAI)

Initial studies on different isolates of *H. pylori* showed that strains from individuals with most severe gastric pathologies (i.e. peptic ulcer, gastric cancer) produced VacA and an antigen encoded by a gene called cytotoxin-associated gene (*cagA*). Strains from individuals with less severe gastric pathologies (i.e. chronic gastritis) were more frequently devoid of VacA activity and did not express CagA (70, 71, 72). The most virulent strains were referred to as type I strains, whereas the less virulent strains were referred to as type II strains (72). It is now known that both type I and type II strains express the *vacA* gene and that the vast majority of them produce an active cytotoxin, though in variable amounts. The major difference between the two types of strains resides in their ability to express (type I) or not to express (type II) CagA. Interest in this protein was generated by the observation that the antibody response to CagA appeared to correlate with the severity of the *H. pylori*–induced gastric pathology (73, 74). This observation was later extended, and CagA is now considered an immunodominant antigen and a marker of disease (75, 76).

The genetic difference between type I and type II strains is more complex than expected. By comparing several type I versus II *H. pylori* strains, we discovered that the *cagA* gene resides in a 40 kb fragment of DNA present in type I, but not in type II strains (77). This region, called *cag*, represents a pathogenicity island (PAI) with genetic and structural characteristics similar to the PAIs of other pathogens, such as enteropathogenic *E. coli*, *Agrobacterium tumefaciens*, *Bordetella pertussis*, etc (31). The *H. pylori* PAI includes 31 genes and may contain an insertion sequence (IS605) encoding two transposases that can disrupt in different manners the integrity of the PAI, leading to a heterogeneous mutilation of the PAI (77). The majority (70%–80%) of the clinical isolates of *H. pylori* from individuals living in developed countries express CagA. In some countries like Japan or Korea, the frequency of CagA positive strains can even reach 100% (78, 79, 80, 81).

By analogy with other bacteria, at least part of the genes in the *H. pylori* PAI encode a type IV secretion machinery specialized in the active transfer of molecules into the eukaryotic cells (31). The fact that the *H. pylori* PAI is operative was suggested by the observation that *cag* PAI positive (type I) strains, but not isogenic mutants deprived of it, were able to induce the production of IL-8 by epithelial cells (77, 82), activation of NF-κB complexes, remodeling of cytoskeleton with formation of pedestals (82), activation of the transcription factor AP-1, expression of proto-oncogenes *c-jun* and *c-fos* (83), etc. It was originally observed that *cag* PAI induced the tyrosine-phosphorylation of a protein of 140 kDa (82, 84). The 140-kDa protein originally thought to be of host origin is instead CagA that, following tyrosine phosphorylation, triggers the *cag* PAI-mediated phenomena mentioned above (85, 86, 87, 88, 89).

Taken together, these observations suggest that, after translocation into the host cell cytosol and phosphorylation, CagA induces a number of morphological and functional cell changes (90). The inoculation of CagA into epithelial cells may account for the high immunogenicity of this protein during infection with *H. pylori* (73, 74, 91), at both the humoral and cellular level. CD4$^+$ T cell clones isolated from gastric biopsies from individuals chronically infected with *H. pylori* are very frequently specific for CagA, whereas urease-specific or VacA-specific T cell clones are rarely isolated (41, 42). Finally, it would be interesting to determine whether CagA or other *cag* PAI injected material could be responsible for the polarization of the immune response toward a Th1 type functional phenotype frequently observed both in *H. pylori*–infected individuals (41, 42, 92, 93, 94, 95) and in experimentally infected animals (96, 97, 98).

Neutrophil Activating Protein (NAP)

One almost invariable pathological finding in biopsies from *H. pylori*–infected stomachs is the infiltration by neutrophils and mononuclear cells (99). Although the kinetics of this infiltration has not been clarified yet, and possibly different waves of infiltration of inflammatory cells take place during the chronic development of the infection, neutrophil infiltration is very likely to contribute substantially to the epithelial damage during the different stages of *H. pylori* infection (100, 101). Different factors can contribute to the recruitment of neutrophils (and mononuclear cells) to the site of *H. pylori* infection. The *H. pylori*–induced release of IL-8 promotes the recruitment of neutrophils and other inflammatory cells at the level of gastric lesions. Successful eradication of *H. pylori* infection in humans is accompanied by the disappearance of the neutrophil infiltrate and, at the same time, of detectable levels of IL-8, but not of other cytokines such as IL-6 (102).

Other specific and nonspecific factors can contribute to the migration of phagocytes in the stomach and to their activation during *H. pylori* infection. Proteins
present in soluble extracts of *H. pylori* were known to induce migration and activation of neutrophils and other inflammatory cells (103, 104, 105, 106, 107). A
protein capable of inducing neutrophil adhesion to endothelial cells was identified (108), and later purified and sequenced (109, 110). It is a 15-kDa protein
with a strong tendency to oligomerize (109). This protein was termed neutrophil-
activating protein (NAP) because of its ability to induce the production of reactive
oxygen intermediates (ROI) by neutrophils (109). More recently, using a recombinant protein expressed in *Bacillus subtilis*, we showed that NAP is a four-helix
bundle protein that forms regular dodecamers with a central hole (110a) and that is
structurally but not functionally similar to the DNA binding protein Dps of *E. coli*
(111). The dodecamer binds iron and is very resistant to thermal and chemical
treatments (110a). NAP is chemotactic for neutrophils and monocytes and is a
strong inducer for the production of ROI, an activity potentiated by IFN-γ and by
TNF-α (112).

NAP is highly conserved among *H. pylori* strains (113), though its level of
expression varies, and NAP is not regulated by heavy metals, including iron, or by
stress (109; Dundon et al, in preparation). Available data suggest that NAP is an
important target antigen for the immune response during infection with *H. pylori*,
and that infected subjects mount an antibody response to it at a given moment after
infection with *H. pylori* (112, 114). It will be important to understand the potential
role of the immune response to this protein in the host-microbe relationship.

Other Antigens

Space limitations do not allow us to discuss in detail all other antigens that have
been involved in the pathogenesis of the *H. pylori* infection and of the *H. pylori*-
induced diseases. Among these, however, are flagellins, adhesins, heat shock proteins, LPS, various enzymes, etc (reviewed in 4, 31, 37). The involvement of these
antigens has been inferred in most instances with isogenic knockout mutants and
determination of their inability to adhere to eukaryotic cells in vitro or to colonize
the gastric mucosa in some animal models. In a few cases, their importance has
been implied following successful experiments of protection in animals, mainly
mice. In most cases, however, detailed biochemical and physiological investigations are still missing. These would provide a precise understanding of the pathogenetic events triggered by these antigens in the induction of *H. pylori*–associated
diseases.

ANIMAL MODELS OF *H. PYLORI* INFECTION

The need for animal models of infection was clear immediately after *H. pylori*
was found to be associated with severe gastric diseases. Most of our knowledge
of the infection derives from studies in subjects with chronic infection, in other

terms, years or even decades after the first colonization with the bacterium, leaving the early stages of infection still poorly understood. These early stages are known through the two cases of self-infection carried out during the 1980s (115, 116), a few cases of accidental infections occurring for professional reasons (117), a limited number of acute infections during the pediatric age (118), and more recently some volunteers experimentally infected with a CagA-negative *H. pylori* strain (119). Animal models reproducing the different aspects of the pathology and the immune response induced by *H. pylori* would be extremely helpful in understanding the kinetics of the interactions between the bacterium and the host. Animal models are also very useful in the search for antimicrobial therapies, in the analysis in vivo of potential virulence factors, in the dissection of the immune responses during infection or after immunization, and in providing baseline information for the development of vaccines against *H. pylori*.

Up to now, there is no ideal animal model, reproducing all the different aspects of infection and disease as they are seen in humans, also because we do not know all the aspects of the infection as they kinetically appear in humans. However, animal models represent a necessary tool to select potential vaccine candidates. In the following section, we very briefly summarize the characteristics of the more common animal models, commenting on their relevance to the research on vaccine development.

Mice and Other Rodents

The first successful colonization of the stomach of mice with *Helicobacter* species was reported in 1990 by A. Lee using germ-free mice and *H. felis* (120), a bacterium that spontaneously infects cats. The use of this model became very popular, and several studies of immunization were carried out in mice then challenged with *H. felis*. This was made possible by the fact that the antigens tested as potential vaccine candidates at that time [i.e. urease (121) and heat shock proteins (122, 123)] are conserved in the two species. However, *H. felis* has a biology quite different from that of *H. pylori*, and data on infection with this species may not be relevant to pathogenesis of *H. pylori* infection. For example, *H. felis* does not attach to gastric epithelial cells and does not contain any toxin equivalent to VacA nor genes equivalent to CagA or PAI (72).

The first reproducible model of infection of immunocompetent mice (the outbred CD1 strain) with *H. pylori* was developed in our laboratories (124). To adapt *H. pylori* strains to the mouse stomach, very fresh clinical isolates were used with several in vivo passages in the mouse, after isolation and reinoculation. This model reproduces several aspects of the human infection. For example, type I (*cag+*) strains induce more severe lesions (e.g. superficial erosions, cell infiltration in the lamina propria) than type II (*cag−*) strains (124). This model has been used to investigate the role of some virulence factors, such as VacA, CagA, and urease in gastric colonization and inflammation (125). In addition, the gastric pathology in this model is much more severe in C57BL/6 than in BALB/c mice (4), suggesting a role of the host immune response in the outcome of the local gastric lesions. This infection extends chronically for at least one year with the appearance in the gastric mucosa of several lymphocytic infiltrates that organize in very well-structured lymphoid follicles (126).

Other laboratories have now adapted other strains of *H. pylori* to infect mice, both positive and negative for the *cag* PAI (127, 128). These models have been used to investigate several aspects of the *H. pylori*-host interactions and the possibility of selecting potential vaccine candidates for further development.

Successful colonization with *H. pylori* has been reported in rats (129), guinea pigs (130), and Mongolian gerbils (131, 132, 133). However, these models have not been exploited in the research for *H. pylori* vaccines, probably because they are less convenient than the mouse model, and also because of the limitation of specific reagents as in the case of gerbils. The Mongolian gerbils have received much attention after they were shown to develop gastric atrophy and intestinal metaplasia, following infection with *H. pylori*, with eventual development of gastric adenocarcinoma in one third of the infected animals (134). Mongolian gerbils may become a precious tool to investigate the bacterial and host factors intervening in the *H. pylori*-induced gastric cancer.

Gnotobiotic Pigs

The first in vivo demonstration of urease as a virulence factor derived from the infection studies carried out in gnotobiotic piglets (34, 35). This model has been also used to show the possibility of mixed infections with type I and type II *H. pylori* strains (135) and the role of flagellins in the colonization (136). This model faces, however, limitations both at the pathological level since histological lesions differ from those observed in humans, and for the complex logistics required to house and follow any gnotobiotic animals.

Monkeys

Besides humans, *H. pylori* can spontaneously infect some nonhuman primates. In some colonies 60% of rhesus monkeys have been infected at the age of 2 years, and 90% at the age of 11 years or more (137), with pathological changes very similar to those observed in humans (5). However, the cost of the animals and the high rates of spontaneous infection seriously limit the use of this model at large scale. Therapeutic vaccination protocols have been carried out with varying success in this model.

H. mustelae in Ferrets

Ferrets are naturally infected with *H. mustelae* and develop chronic lymphocytic gastritis and ulcers (138). Such a virulence may be mediated by a CagA-like element (139). The infection is susceptible to antibiotic treatment and induces specific immune responses. Although unpractical, interesting results related to vaccine development and to the immunity following infection have been obtained in this model and are mentioned later.

Cats and Dogs

Natural infection of cats with *H. pylori* has been reported in one colony (140, 141). They develop a lymphocytic antral gastritis, but with few neutrophils infiltrating the antral mucosa. The infection with a *cag-vac+ H. pylori* strain becomes chronic after three years of follow up (142). Natural infection of dogs with *H. pylori* has not been reported. Although suggested that pets may represent a source of infection and that *H. pylori* infection in some epidemiological settings may be a zoonosis, available data are against this possibility (15) and rather support anthroponosis for *H. pylori* infection in pets (143).

Experimental infection of gnotobiotic Beagle dogs was demonstrated in 1990 (144). Recently, we have shown that experimental infection with *H. pylori* can be established in conventional Beagle dogs (145), using a mouse-adapted strain of *H. pylori*. This model allows one to follow up the animals without the need of necropsy, as in the case of smaller animals. We could show very early infiltration of the gastric mucosa with neutrophils (accompanied by increased expression of IL-8), which are then replaced by mononuclear cells. One month after infection, lymphoid cells infiltrating the mucosa organize to form macroscopically evident follicular structures, mainly at the antral level, with peripheral CD4$^+$ cells surrounding a germinal center–like structure rich in CD21$^+$ (B) cells (146). Interestingly, acutely infected dogs showed clinical symptoms, such as vomiting and diarrhea (145), which very closely resemble those observed in the few cases of acute infections reported in humans (115, 116, 119). Potential vaccine formulations are now being tested in this model for both prophylactic and therapeutic vaccinations.

FEASIBILITY OF THE VACCINE APPROACH TO PREVENT AND CURE CHRONIC INFECTION

Tables 1 and 2 summarize most of the studies carried out in animals (mostly in mice) showing the feasibility of both prophylactic and therapeutic vaccinations against *H. pylori*. Considering the strictly extracellular localization of *H. pylori* at the gastric mucosal level, particular emphasis has been given to oral immunization. More recently, other mucosal routes of immunization as well as the parenteral routes were considered. In the studies pursuing the oral route of vaccination in the mouse, antigens are given together with a suitable mucosal adjuvant [such as cholera toxin (CT), *E. coli* heat-labile enterotoxin (LT) or their nontoxic mutants] three or more times at different time intervals. Mice are then challenged with an *H. pylori* strain adapted to the mouse. The efficacy of vaccination is evaluated microbiologically, by counting the number of cultures from each stomach, and/or

TABLE 1 Prophylactic vaccination against *H. pylori* in different animal models

Animal models	H. pylori antigen(s)	Adjuvant/Vector	Route(*)	Challenge with	Reference
Mice	Whole-cell preparations	CT	os	*H. felis*	148, 149, 150, 151, 186, 190
		LT	os	*H. pylori*	4, 124, 147
		LTK63	os	*H. pylori*	147
		CTB	os	*H. felis*	190
	Urease or subunits	CT	os	*H. felis*	151, 164, 186
		LT	os	*H. felis*	165, 168
		LT	os	*H. pylori*	124, 166, 167
		LTK63	os	*H. pylori*	147
		LT, CT	i.n.	*H. felis*	173
		LT	rectal	*H. pylori*	166
		LT, LTB	s.c.	*H. pylori*	176
		QS21, Bay	s.c.	*H. pylori*	167, 175
		alum	s.c.	*H. pylori*	167
		CT	i.n.	*H. heilmannii*	174
		S. typhimurium	i.n.	*H. pylori*	170
		S. typhimurium	os	*H. pylori*	169
	GroEL	CT	os	*H. felis*	185
	GroES	CT	os	*H. felis*	185, 186
	GroEL	LTK63	os	*H. pylori*	unpublished
	GroES + UreB	CT	os	*H. felis*	185
	GroEL peptide	Freund's	i.p.	*H. pylori*	187

	Antigen	Adjuvant	Route	Challenge	References
	VacA (native)	LT, LTK63	os	*H. pylori*	4, 124, 147
	VacA (native + formaldehyde)	LTK63	os	*H. pylori*	184
	VacA (p95)	LT, LTK63	os	*H. pylori*	147
	VacA (p58 or p37)	LTK63	os	*H. pylori*	147
	VacA + Urease	LT, LTK63	os	*H. pylori*	147
	CagA	LT, LTK63	os	*H. pylori*	147
	CagA	LTK63	i.n.	*H. pylori*	unpublished
	CagA fragment A17/12	LT, LTK63	os	*H. pylori*	147
	NAP	LTK63	os	*H. pylori*	112
	Catalase	CT	os	*H. pylori*	188
	Outer Membrane Vesicles	CT	os	*H. pylori*	157, 159, 160
	Lpp20	CT	os	*H. pylori*	159, 161
	L7/L12 ribosomal protein	CT	os	*H. pylori*	161
	Unidentified proteins	CT	os	*H. pylori*	161
	50/52 kDa antigen	Freund's	IPP	*H. pylori*	189
Gnotobiotic piglets	Whole-cell preparations	none	os, i.p.	*H. pylori*	34
		LT	os	*H. pylori*	192
		Freund's	s.c., i.p.	*H. pylori*	192
Monkeys	Urease	LT + Bay or alum	os + i.m.	*H. pylori*	179
		LT or Bay	os or i.m.	*H. pylori*	182

(*) Os: oral (mostly intragastric); i.n.: intranasal; s.c.: subcutaneous; i.p.: intraperitoneal; i.m.: intramuscular; IPP: intra-Payer's patches

TABLE 2   Therapeutic vaccination against *H. pylori* in different animal models

Animal models	H. pylori antigen(s)	Adjuvant	Route(*)	Infection with	References
Mice	Whole-cell preparations	CT	os	*H. felis*	152, 153
		LTK63	os	*H. pylori*	126
	UreB	CT	os	*H. felis*	97, 171
		CT	i.n.	*H. heilmannii*	174
	Urease	LT	os	*H. pylori*	172
		QS21; Bay	s.c.	*H. pylori*	172
		CT	i.n.	*H. heilmannii*	174
	VacA (native)	LTK63	os	*H. pylori*	126
	VacA (p95)	LTK63	os	*H. pylori*	126
	CagA	LTK63	os	*H. pylori*	126
Ferrets	Whole-cell preparations	MDP	os	*H. mustelae*	195
	Urease	CT	os	*H. mustelae*	177
Monkeys	Whole-cell preparations	DC Chol	i.m.	*H. heilmannii*	181
	Urease	LT	os	*H. pylori*	178, 180

(*) Os: oral (mostly intragastric); i.n.: intranasal; s.c.: subcutaneous; i.m.: intramuscular

by rapid urease test. Depending on the strain employed, protection has been considered as a statistically significant reduction (one or more orders of magnitudes) in the number of countable colonies or, with our mouse model using the SPM326 strain for challenge, as complete absence of detectable colonies (124, 147). The read out for efficacy remains the same in the therapeutic mode of vaccination (126).

Whole-Cell Vaccines

The first approach of vaccination proved efficacious prophylactically (Table 1) and therapeutically (Table 2) against *H. pylori* (or *H. felis*) employed lysates of bacteria or chemically inactivated whole-cell bacteria given orally together with CT or LT as mucosal adjuvants (4, 124, 126, 147–153). Protection using crude antigen preparations of *H. pylori* is very efficient, often reaching 100%. However, such an approach faces serious limitations. Crude whole-cell vaccines would encounter quality control and regulatory problems related to the quality and the reproducibility of lot preparations. More importantly, whole-cell preparations would include the entire antigenic repertoire of the bacteria, including the LPS, which contain epitopes such as those of the Lewis blood group shared with the self and expressed at the surface of the majority of human cells, including gastric epithelial cells. Sera from chronically infected individuals (154, 155) and experimentally infected animals (155) can contain antibodies cross-reacting with Lewis epitopes and with gastric epithelial and parietal cells. At least part of the gastric pathology observed during chronic infection with this bacterium may result from molecular mimicry with different antigens expressed by gastric cells, such as Lewis antigens, H+/K+ ATP pump, etc (156). Although this possibility has not been formally proven in humans, it would be difficult for a vaccine based on whole-cell bacteria to pass the ethical considerations concerning proof of their safety. Nevertheless, a phase I trial has been carried out in volunteers using whole-cell *H. pylori* preparations given orally along with a still-toxic mutant of LT (see below).

Outer Membrane Vesicles (OMV)

As other gram-negative bacteria, by blebbing of the outer membrane *H. pylori* releases OMV, which contain LPS, porins (157), and other antigens, including the vacuolating toxin VacA (157, 158) and the Lpp20 lipoprotein (159), an 18–20 kDa conserved antigen. Purified OMV protect mice against a challenge with *H. pylori* (160). Protection may be mediated by the Lpp20 because antibody response to this antigen was consistently present in protected mice (159) and because immunization of mice with purified native or recombinant Lpp20 antigen conferred protection against *H. pylori* challenge (159, 161). However, other antigens, such as VacA (124, 147), may contribute to the protection provided by OMV. Finally, if OMV from *H. pylori* behave in vivo as in the case of OMV from other gram negative bacteria, such as *Neisseria meningitidis* group B, one can reasonably expect that most of the immune response induced following immunization would be driven by porins, that, as in the case of group B meningococci, are highly variable and induce an exquisite strain-specific immunity (162).

Antigen-Based Vaccines

The most promising approaches for the development of vaccines against *H. pylori* infection and diseases are based on the use of defined antigens. These approaches are discussed below.

Urease   This antigen has drawn the attention of most researchers (see Tables 1 and 2 and related references), a vast program of vaccine development based on urease is currently in progress, and some trials have been already carried out in humans. The fact that urease is by far the most abundant protein of *H. pylori* (5% to 10% of the protein content), its role in colonization and its potential involvement in some of the pathogenetic events leading to colonization and infection (37), provided the rationale of using this antigen as a vaccine candidate. In addition, the conservation of urease among the different species of the *Helicobacter* genus (121) has also allowed the use of this protein in animal models employing *Helicobacter* species different from *H. pylori*.

Oral immunization with urease (as a ureB subunit or as holoenzyme) associated together with mucosal adjuvants such as CT or LT, or with nontoxic mutants of LT developed in our laboratories (163), has been extensively shown to be protective against infection with *H. felis* (151, 164, 165) and with *H. pylori* (124, 147, 166–168). Protection was also shown after oral (169) or intranasal immunization (170) with attenuated strains of *Salmonella typhimurium* expressing urease. Oral therapeutic vaccination of mice with urease also strongly reduces or fully suppresses the colonization of the gastric mucosa with *H. felis* (97, 171) or with *H. pylori* (172). In addition, successful protection against *Helicobacter* spp. has been shown in mice after intranasal and rectal immunization (166, 173, 174). A significant reduction in the number of *H. pylori* colonizing the stomach was also observed in mice immunized systemically with urease and defined adjuvants suitable for parenteral immunization (167, 175). Along this line, significant protection was also obtained when urease adjuvanted with wild-type LT was given systemically (176).

The feasibility of the therapeutic approach of vaccination using urease was also shown in ferrets, which are naturally infected with *H. mustelae*. Infected animals immunized orally with purified *H. pylori* urease plus CT as adjuvant exhibited a reduced gastritis as compared to controls; in addition, in 30% of immunized animals the *H. mustelae* infection was eradicated (177).

These very promising results with urease in mice and in ferrets have been only partially reproduced in monkeys. A significant reduction in the number of bacteria colonizing the stomach was reported in the rhesus monkeys therapeutically immunized orally with urease (at doses as high as 40 milligrams) with 25 μg of LT as the adjuvant (178). The best results were obtained in rhesus monkeys primed by oral immunization and then boosted by intramuscular immunization (179). In another therapeutic vaccination experiment, oral immunization with urease did not affect the bacterial load at the gastric level; however, some immunized monkeys exhibited some reduction in the level of gastritis (180). As in the mice, also in monkeys systemic immunization with urease and appropriate adjuvants decreased the number of *H. heilmannii* colonizing the stomach in two thirds of the cynomolgus monkeys (181). The prophylactic vaccination studies, however, were carried out in monkeys not immunologically naive, since they were previously spontaneously infected with *H. pylori* and then cured with antibiotics (178, 179). When similar experiments were repeated (4 mg of urease plus 100 μg of wild-type LT) in rhesus monkeys that had never been infected with *H. pylori* before, no effect at all was observed on gastric bacterial colonization nor on gastric pathological changes (182).

VacA, CagA, and NAP   Immunity induced against bacterial virulence factors is known to protect humans against relevant infections; some of these proteins are now part of new vaccines. The best example is provided by the new acellular pertussis vaccines that contain chemically or genetically detoxified pertussis toxin (PT), responsible for most of the toxic effects observed during pertussis, by filamentous hemagglutinin (FHA) that mediates adhesion to epithelial cells, and by pertactin, a 69-kDa protein with adhesion properties (183). Following this line of reasoning, we envisaged the possibility of achieving protection in our mouse model (124) using *H. pylori* antigens strongly involved in the pathogenesis of *H. pylori* infection such as VacA, CagA, or NAP. Recombinant VacA, native VacA, and formaldehyde-inactivated native VacA given orally with either wild-type LT or with the fully nontoxic mutant LTK63 (124, 147, 184) completely prevented gastric colonization with the VacA+/CagA+ *H. pylori* strain SPM362. Protection was antigen specific because immunization with VacA did not prevent gastric colonization with a VacA-negative strain (147). Similar regimens of immunization with VacA fully eradicated an already established infection with *H. pylori* (126). In the same set of experiments, therapeutic immunization with recombinant VacA successfully protected mice against a rechallenge with *H. pylori* (126), showing that antigen-specific immunological memory was induced by oral vaccination.

Prophylactic and therapeutic protection can also been achieved with CagA following oral (126, 147) or intranasal (unpublished) immunization with the LTK63 nontoxic LT mutant as an adjuvant. Interestingly, in the experiments of intranasal immunization, increasing the dose of CagA increased the levels of specific serum antibodies but did not improve the level of protection, suggesting that no correlation between protection and antigen-specific antibody titers, in agreement with results obtained in other *H. pylori* models (see below).

More recently we also showed that a recombinant form of the *H. pylori* NAP prevented colonization of the stomach after challenge with *H. pylori* (112). These results suggest that neutralization of the chemotactic effect of this protein and of the neutrophil/monocyte activating properties can prevent colonization and/or survival of *H. pylori* in the gastric environment.

Other Antigens   Other *H. pylori* antigens have been reported that, following mucosal immunization of mice, can confer protection against infection with *H. pylori*. Among these, a few years ago particular attention was focused on heat shock proteins (185, 186). More recently a conserved epitope of the hsp60 was shown to protect mice against *H. pylori* following intraperitoneal immunization with a peptide reproducing this epitope that was given with Freund's adjuvants (187). It remains difficult to consider as feasible immunizations with proteins that are highly conserved phylogenetically and have the intrinsic risk of inducing immune responses cross-reacting with their human homologues.

Also antigens such as catalase (188), Lpp20 (159, 161), 50/59 kDa (189), and others not yet well characterized (161) confer prophylactic protection to mice against *H. pylori*, though in most cases available data are still limited. One can reasonably expect that in the near future work based on the information derived from the *H. pylori* genome will deliver other antigens as potential vaccine candidates.

Antigen- and Adjuvant-Related Requirements for Protection

From the results summarized above, some conclusions can been drawn on the general requirements that antigens, adjuvants, and formulations should (or should not) have to protect animals against *H. pylori*.

Native Structure/Conformation of the Antigen   Work carried out with urease and with VacA and NAP (see Tables 1 and 2 for specific references) show that protection in mice is achieved with recombinant urease devoid of enzymatic activity, recombinant VacA without vacuolating activity, or recombinant NAP expressed as a fusion protein with GST and not assembled as a dodecamer. These data strongly suggest that the effector mechanism(s) induced following immunization with these molecules do not rely on their native structure. Such a hypothesis is in agreement with the results showing that antibodies (at least those directed against conformational epitopes and functional enzymatic sites) do not appear to play a major role in the effector arm of the immune response against *H. pylori* induced by oral immunization with whole-cell bacterial extracts or with urease (see below).

Length of the Antigen   Both VacA and CagA confer protection against *H. pylori*. However, protection is not achieved when mice are immunized with fragments of these molecules. Immunization with recombinant proteins reproducing the two moieties of VacA (p37 and p58), or with a recombinant fragment of CagA (A17/12) that is the major target of antibody response in animals and humans (74), do not protect against *H. pylori* (147, Table 1). This suggests that structures encompassing the different moieties of VacA and CagA are essential in inducing protection against the infection. One can also hypothesize that full-length proteins would contain the entire set of B and T cell epitopes able to induce protective immune responses. The situation is different for urease and hsp60. In fact, immunization with the recombinant B subunit alone is still able to protect mice both prophylactically and therapeutically (Tables 1 and 2). Moreover, a short peptide from the hsp60 was shown to be protective in mice (187). In the absence of knowledge of the mechanisms underlying protection against *H. pylori*, it is not possible to determine why the whole-length structure is needed for some antigens, but not for others.

Holotoxin Structure of the Mucosal Adjuvant   To achieve significant levels of protection in animal models, strong mucosal adjuvants are required, such as CT, LT, or the fully nontoxic LT mutant LTK63 (124, 147, Table 1). Oral immunization with urease did not confer protection to mice against *H. felis* when the antigen was given together with the B subunit of LT (190). Although conflicting data have been obtained following parenteral immunization with urease and LTB subunit (176), these data suggest that strong mucosal adjuvants are required for protection, either by quantitatively increasing the antigen-specific immune response or by qualitatively favoring polarization toward protective immune response (see below). The poor protective effects of LTB-adjuvanted urease mucosal vaccines are in agreement with the poor adjuvanticity of LTB as compared to holotoxins both in their wild-type form or as nontoxic mutants (163, 191). The major limitation of these data resides in the fact that in most instances these mucosal adjuvants are not directly compared in the same sets of experiments.

Route of Immunization   In the early work to prove the feasibility of vaccination against *H. pylori*, immunization via the oral route was considered essential; thus, most of the work has utilized this route of immunization. It is clear now that significant levels of protection (mainly intended as significant reduction in the bacterial load at the gastric level) is achieved using other mucosal routes (such as nasal and rectal) (166) or the parenteral route. The latter has been proven efficacious both in mice (167, 175, 176) and monkeys (179, 181), using whole-cell extracts or urease with different adjuvant preparations. This mode of immunization has not been equally successful in other models such as in gnotobiotic pigs (192) and in monkeys (182). The parenteral immunization would offer practical advantages of vaccine formulation over the mucosal routes, with the need of lower amounts of antigens. On the other hand, it is unlikely that the parenteral route would offer the advantage offered by the mucosal immunization in inducing immune responses at the site of infection. It remains to be determined whether the parenteral route of immunization would also be able to protect humans against *H. pylori*.

Gastric Pathology   Some reports have shown that following prophylactic or therapeutic immunizations of animals with whole-cell extracts or with urease, animals can develop a gastritis due to the immunization (151, 164, 174, 193). The exact mechanisms underlying the development of this gastritis are not known. Post-immunization gastritis may be immune-mediated and could represent an antigen-specific Th1 type response, such as a DTH, taking place of the gastric level (96). Indeed, some of these pathological events in the gastric mucosa can be reproduced by passive transfer of spleen T lymphocytes into *H. pylori*–infected SCID mice (194). It is not clear whether these phenomena represent transient expression of inflammatory events leading to tissue repair following infection and cure. Conversely, in some experiments the pathological gastric changes may have been caused by inappropriate immunization regimens. This was shown in ferrets immunized with antigen together with an inappropriate mucosal adjuvant, such as MDP, that worsened the gastric disease in infant ferrets (195). In experiments of therapeutic immunization carried out in our laboratories using CagA or VacA, we never observed any post-immunization gastritis; instead, immunization clearly favored the disappearance of those gastric pathological changes that became chronic in unimmunized, control mice (126).

Association of Antigens   Studies of immunization with a mixture of antigens are limited. In the mouse model of infection, oral immunization of hsp plus urease B subunit (185) or VacA plus urease (147) appears to improve the level of protection as compared to that with mice immunized with single antigens. The statistical power of this improvement is however not clear because good levels of protection are also achieved with one antigen alone. The failure of protection reported in humans with urease alone (see below) and the observation in other models, such as pertussis, that increased protection is achieved by using three antigens together, strongly suggest that the association of two or more antigens will be required for final formulation of a *H. pylori* vaccine. The use of more than one antigen in the vaccine would increase the chances of protecting against a number of strains higher than that covered by a single antigen.

DOES *H. PYLORI* INFECTION EVOKE PROTECTIVE IMMUNITY?

Natural infection with *H. pylori* induces vigorous antibody and cellular immune responses at both systemic and mucosal levels. The vast majority of infected individuals have detectable levels of antibodies in the serum, and these have been exploited for the development of noninvasive tools for diagnosis of *H. pylori* infection (196). In addition, *H. pylori*–infected individuals, both asymptomatic and with peptic ulcer, exhibit a high frequency of antibody secreting cells (ASC) producing antigen-specific IgA or IgM antibodies in biopsies taken from antrum and corpus (197). However, *H. pylori* causes an infection of the stomach that, if not treated, persists chronically, eventually leading to serious complications like peptic ulcers and gastric cancer. It is then logical to conclude that natural infection with *H. pylori* does not induce protective immunity. Indeed, two studies in ferrets naturally or experimentally infected with *H. mustelae* showed that animals successfully cured with antibiotic treatment were still fully susceptible to reinfection with *H. mustelae* and that this infection remained chronic (198, 199). In developed countries, a limited though sizeable (∼1%) number of individuals treated for *H. pylori* infection are reinfected every year (24, 25). In less developed countries, such as Peru, however, 40 out of 55 treated individuals became reinfected by 8 months after full drug treatment (26). This epidemiological observation could imply that natural immunity may be strain-specific, thus not preventing colonization with other strains. Conversely, one cannot rule out that in some instances these "reinfections" were instead recrudescence of a partially eradicated infection.

A small number of children and adults infected with *H. pylori* spontaneously revert to a negative serology, which may suggest a spontaneous eradication of the infection (200), mediated at least partly by specific immune mechanisms. It is possible, however, that the current widespread nonspecific use of antibiotics may affect the potential contribution of naturally acquired immunity in this phenomenon of spontaneous *H. pylori* clearance (201). In the absence of a precise knowledge of the natural history of the *H. pylori* infection and of the immune responses it induces at the difference stages of its progression, one cannot exclude the possibility that naturally induced immune responses may influence at least partly the progression and/or the clinical outcomes of the infection, depending also upon the genetic characteristics of the hosts. For the time being, we can conclude that immune responses to *H. pylori* represent more a flag of current or previous infection or, in the best case, more a marker of disease (as for anti-CagA antibody response) than a marker of immune protection. This suggests that *H. pylori* infection resembles other chronic bacterial and viral diseases, such as tuberculosis, HIV infection, HCV infection, etc.

IS THE GASTRIC PATHOLOGY INDUCED BY *H. PYLORI* MEDIATED BY THE SPECIFIC IMMUNE RESPONSE?

Most of our present knowledge of *H. pylori* infection comes from studies carried out in adults chronically infected for decades. If several bacterium-related factors (e.g. *cag* PAI) have been identified as crucial virulence factors, it is not clear which host-related (immune) factors are required for successful colonization and development of gastric pathology. The first unanswered question is where the priming of the immune response takes place after infection with *H. pylori*. The absence of lymphoid structures comparable to the intestinal Peyer's patches and of professional cells able to take up antigens and microorganisms, such as M cells, indicate that the stomach mucosa may not be the priming site (202). Furthermore, under normal conditions, the gastric mucosa does not contain antigen-presenting cells nor lymphoid cells; in addition, gastric epithelial cells do not express MHC class II molecules (203). However, gastric epithelial cell lines and freshly isolated epithelial cells constitutively express B7-1 and B7-2 costimulatory molecules (204). Upregulation of MHC class II and of B7-2 molecules by gastric epithelial cells has been reported in *H. pylori*–infected patients with chronic gastritis (204), as well as an increase of monocytes and of activated (HLA-DR-positive) macrophages in the lamina propria (101, 205). These observations suggest that, during chronic infection with *H. pylori*, gastric epithelial cells may function as antigen-presenting cells for CD4[+] cells, thus favoring, together with locally produced pro-inflammatory cytokines, local pathological changes.

Biopsies from patients chronically infected with *H. pylori* consistently show an important infiltration in the lamina propria and in the epithelium of lymphocytes with the CD3[+] CD4[+] phenotype (95). These lymphocytes are mostly TCR $\alpha\beta+$ (206); they exhibit an activated/memory phenotype (CD45RO+, IL-2R+) (95) and organize to form lymphoid follicles consisting of B lymphocytes surrounded by mostly CD4[+] cells (207). These lymphoid structures can become macroscopically evident, are considered pathognomonic of *H. pylori* infection, and have been hypothesized to represent the sites wherefrom MALT lymphoma originate (208, 209). CD8[+] lymphocytes represent a minority of the lymphoid cells infiltrating the gastric mucosa of *H. pylori* chronically infected patients (95). In animal models, lymphoid cell infiltration of the gastric mucosa represents a relatively early event. In the Beagle dog model of infection, well-structured gastric lymphoid follicles appear already 4 weeks after infection, with CD4+ cells surrounding clusters of B (CD21+) lymphocytes (146). These follicles become then macroscopically visible, giving a nodular aspect to the gastric surface at endoscopy, and they persist chronically (145, 146).

CD4+ lymphocytes from peripheral blood and from gastric epithelium and lamina propria of *H. pylori*-infected individuals proliferate in an antigen-specific fashion, in the presence of crude extracts of *H. pylori* or in the presence of specific antigens, such as urease, hsp60, CagA, VacA (41, 42, 92, 210, 211), etc. The higher cloning efficiency of CD4+ lymphocytes from the gastric mucosa, as compared with that of cells from peripheral blood (41), strongly suggests that antigen-specific CD4+ cells tend to accumulate at the site of gastric colonization by both active recruitment and locally induced proliferation.

Several lines of evidence obtained from naturally infected individuals and from experimentally infected animals have shown that CD4+ lymphocytes infiltrating the gastric mucosa exhibit a very pronounced pro-inflammatory (Th1-type) phenotype. The number of IFN-γ producing T cells at the gastric level is significantly increased in *H. pylori*–infected subjects (or animals) as compared to uninfected controls (93–95, 97, 98, 212–214). Similar results have been obtained with TGF-β (94). On the contrary, it has always been very difficult to detect IL-4–producing cells and IL-4–specific mRNA in biopsies from *H. pylori*–infected individuals (41, 93, 95). The preferential activation of Th1-type CD4+ T cells by *H. pylori* was also shown at the clonal level (41, 42, 92). IFN-γ producing T cell clones were more frequently originated than Th0 clones from biopsies of *H. pylori*–infected individuals. In addition, the frequency of Th1-type T cell clones was significantly higher in individuals with peptic ulcer as compared to individuals without peptic ulcer. It is noteworthy that most of these Th1 clones of gastric origin were specific for CagA, and that a very limited number of clones were specific for other *H. pylori* antigens, such as urease or VacA (42). It is not clear yet why a very abundant antigen, such as urease, is so poorly immunogenic at T cell level, as compared to CagA, which is comparatively less expressed by replicating bacteria. In any case, these data are in agreement with those at antibody level showing that anti-urease antibodies are inconsistently found in naturally infected individuals (40). In addition, anti-CagA antibodies are very frequently detected in subjects infected with CagA+ *H. pylori* strains, and these antibodies increase with the severity of *H. pylori*–mediated diseases, representing thus a potential marker for disease (74, 75, 76, 91). The recent finding that CagA is injected into the epithelial cells by the molecular syringe encoded by the genes of the *cag* PAI (85–89) offers a fascinating working hypothesis not only to explain the toxic effects of CagA in the eukaryotic cells but also to explain the high immunogenicity of this protein. Conversely, the presence of CagA in the cytoplasmic compartment may favor the induction of antigen-specific MHC class I–restricted CD8+ T cells that may contribute to the inflammatory process triggered by the infection through the production of IFN-γ and/or other pro-inflammatory cytokines.

The preferential activation of Th1-type CD4$^+$ cells has also been confirmed in mice experimentally infected with *H. pylori* or with *H. felis* (96, 97). Passive transfer of spleen cells from *H. felis*–infected mice into naive mice induced a severe gastric pathology once the recipients were challenged with the bacterium (96). In addition, Th-regulated IgG isotypes are more abundantly produced during *H. pylori* infection both in mice (126) and in Beagle dogs (145). Similarly, a preferential Th1-type cell activation has also been described in rhesus monkeys infected with *H. pylori* (98). In the *H. felis* murine model of infection, the gastric pathology is significantly more severe in IL-10 knockout animals, as compared to their wild-type littermates (215). These data strongly suggest that, in the Helicobacter infection, IL-10 intervenes by inhibiting the synthesis of pro-inflammatory cytokines by Th1 cells and by activated macrophages, as shown in vitro. Similarly, a more severe gastric inflammation was observed in IL-4 gene–decifient mice infected with *H. pylori*, as compared to the infection observed in mice lacking the IFN-γ gene (216).

From these data it can be concluded that the *H. pylori*–induced disease in experimental animals and possibly in chronically infected individuals is associated with a Th1-type cell response. This would cause an increased production of IL-12 (214), IFN-γ, and other pro-inflammatory cytokines and chemokines (217), with an enhanced activation of macrophages and polymorphonuclear cells that would lead to tissue lesions through the production of reactive oxygen radicals and nitric oxide (103–107). Some *H. pylori* antigens, such as NAP, induce chemotaxis and activation of monocytes and neutrophils, with a synergistic effect of IFN-γ and TNF-α (109, 112). In addition, local gastric lesions could also be induced by the induction of apoptosis of epithelial cells, which could be mediated by the increased expression of Fas/Fas ligand induced by TNF-α or other cytokines (218, 219, 220). On the contrary, Th2 type responses (e.g. through IL-10) could participate in limiting the pathological consequences of this infection, either directly or indirectly by deactivating IL-12 and/or IFN-γ triggered inflammatory phenomena.

WHAT DOES THEN A PROTECTIVE IMMUNE RESPONSE LOOK LIKE?

Based on the above discussion, *H. pylori* causes a chronic infection and never induces protective immunity; in addition, *H. pylori*-induced gastric disease is mediated by pro-inflammatory immune responses. It remains to understand how mucosal or systemic immunization can induce protection against *H. pylori*, prophylactically and therapeutically.

A first hypothesis was that locally produced antibodies, either IgA (165) or IgG (186), mediated protection by favoring killing by neutrophils or monocytes through bacterial opsonization (221) or by neutralizing the bacterial toxic activity of VacA (222). This was supported by two observations: Preincubation of *H. felis* with IgG or IgA monoclonal antibodies against urease suppressed the ability of the bacteria to infect mice (223), and passively transferred IgA monoclonal antibody conferred protection against a challenge with *H. felis* (149).

However, experiments carried out later showed that protection against *Helicobacter* infection could also be achieved by oral immunization in IgA-deficient mice (224). These data are in agreement with those showing that protection against influenza virus can also be achieved in IgA-deficient mice (225), and with those showing that humans with primary IgA antibody deficiency do not suffer from a more severe *H. pylori*–mediated gastric pathology as compared to fully immunocompetent individuals (226). All these data strongly speak against a major role of IgA in the protective immune response against *H. pylori*. The role of antibodies in the effector mechanisms induced by oral or systemic vaccination against *H. pylori* was even more seriously questioned when several groups demonstrated (153, 167, 227) that prophylactic or therapeutic protection against *H. pylori* or *H. felis* could be achieved by immunization with whole-cell preparations or purified antigens of μ-MT mice (228), which are totally unable to produce any antibody. These same studies and others have also shown that protection in mice requires, instead of antibodies, the presence of an intact MHC class II-restricted CD^+ T cell compartment (167, 229). It remains to decipher the fine mechanisms through which *H. pylori*–specific $CD4^+$ lymphocytes mediate protection.

A logical hypothesis (although perhaps simplistic) is that after immunization the antigen-specific response is predominantly polarized toward a Th2-type response, with production of cytokines (such as IL-10) with the ability to inhibit the activation of Th1 cells and of macrophages with the production of pro-inflammatory cytokines. This possibility is supported by the finding that immunization fails to confer protection to IL-4 knockout mice (230). In addition, Saldinger et al. (97) showed that, following infection with *H. felis*, high levels of IFN-γ are produced by antigen-specific spleen $CD4^+$ T lymphocytes. After therapeutic immunization with urease B subunit plus CT as adjuvant, the levels of IL-4 constantly increased after each immunization, while those of IFN-γ decreased. Concomitantly, mice mounted an urease B-specific IgG response with a predominant Th1-regulated IgG1 isotype. These data show that immunization can drive the immune response toward a polarized Th2-type functional phenotype. This polarization could well be mediated by adjuvants. Indeed, CT has the ability to activate IL-5 producing $CD4^+$ T lymphocytes (231). This polarization could also be favored by other mucosal adjuvants, such as LT and nontoxic LT mutants (191), already shown to behave as strong adjuvants for *H. pylori* antigens in mice (124, 126, 147, 176). In addition, systemic adjuvants such as aluminium salts are very well known to preferentially induce Th2-type immune responses (232).

Though the polarization of the immune response toward a Th2 type is the key element required to achieve protection against *H. pylori*, it still remains to be formally proven whether it is induced by the adjuvants employed or by other factors. It is clear that the mechanism(s) of development of the immune-mediated protection against *H. pylori* is far from being understood. This opens the way to a fascinating area of research. The knowledge of the immunological parameters that correlate with protection is of paramount importance for the clinical trials that are planned in the next few years. This knowledge would probably have helped in better designing the few trials of *H. pylori* vaccination that have been carried out so far in volunteers.

STUDIES CARRIED OUT IN HUMANS

Very few trials in humans have been carried out so far with anti-*H. pylori* vaccine candidates. We can infer that these trials have not been particularly successful, showing that a significant amount of work still remains to be performed to optimize vaccine formulation and delivery of these vaccines.

Therapeutic Vaccination with Urease and LT

The most detailed study in humans was conducted in *H. pylori*–infected volunteers (233). The subjects were immunized with urease, given orally at very high doses (20, 60, or 180 mg four times weekly) together with the *E. coli* LT wild type (5 μg). If the antigen was well tolerated, as previously shown in a safety trial in the absence of any adjuvants (234), the LT was not. In fact, diarrhea was induced by the wild-type LT adjuvant in 16 out of 24 volunteers (66%), with numbers of episodes not influenced by the dose of urease. Volunteers receiving the highest doses of urease (60 or 180 mg) had a significant increase of the anti-urease serum IgA titers and of the circulating IgA antibody secreting cells versus the controls. The anti-urease antibody titers did not correlate with the reduction in the gastric bacterial load. Eradication was never observed, and paradoxically, reduction in the number of colonies was more evident in the group of volunteers receiving the lowest dose of urease (20 mg). Finally, immunization with urease did not contribute to the amelioration of the gastritis score evaluated after antibiotic treatment of the volunteers (233).

Several factors may have determined the failure of this therapeutic trial. First, it could be that higher doses of mucosal adjuvants are required to enhance the immunogenicity of the vaccine. This would never be achieved with the fully toxic LT, which was already diarrheogenic at doses as low as 5 μg. One may speculate that nontoxic LT mutants (163) would be better suited for mucosal delivery of these vaccines. Very little is known about the precise requirements for antigen-specific priming at the mucosal level in general, and at the gastrointestinal level in particular. It is then possible that the formulation of antigen plus adjuvant could enormously influence the outcome of the response, both quantitatively and qualitatively. Second, it could also be that, despite the positive results in the animals, urease is not a protective immunogenic vaccine component in humans. Third, it may well be that a single antigen is not enough to protect against *H. pylori*. Although there is evidence with *Borrelia burgdorferi* that one single recombinant antigen (OspA) is efficacious in protecting against Lyme disease (235, 236), experience with acellular vaccines against pertussis suggests that a better efficacy is obtained when more than one antigen is used in the vaccine (183). Finally, one could speculate that the effector mechanisms to be induced for an efficacious therapeutic vaccination are different from those required for prophylaxis. Despite major efforts in the past decades, no therapeutic vaccines are available so far, although great hopes currently exist for therapeutic HBV vaccine, herpes vaccines, and cancer vaccines. Thus, at the present time one cannot rule out that an orally delivered urease-based vaccine may show some efficacy in a prophylactic mode of vaccination, although this remains to be proven.

Phase I Trial with Attenuated *Salmonella typhi*–Expressing Urease

In a phase I trial carried out to evaluate the immunogenicity of urease expressed by a *Salmonella typhi* strain attenuated by deletion of the *phoP/phoQ* genes (237), anti-*Salmonella* LPS antibodies were detected. However, none of the volunteers developed any detectable antibody response (either systemic nor mucosal) against urease, not even the three volunteers who received one oral boosting dose of 60 mg of recombinant urease together with 2.5 μg of wild-type *E. coli* LT as a mucosal adjuvant (two of these three volunteers had diarrhea).

Phase I Trial with Whole-Cell Vaccine

A phase I trial with oral whole-cell *H. pylori* vaccine has also been conducted recently (238). The whole-cell preparation was given three times to *H. pylori*-negative and to *H. pylori*-positive volunteers together with the LTR192G, an LT mutant that had been shown to retain most of the intrinsic toxicity of the wild-type LT (reviewed in 191). Doses as high as 10^{10} bacteria induced detectable levels of *H. pylori*–specific systemic and mucosal (salivary and fecal) antibody titers and antibody-secreting cells in circulating blood and gastric biopsies, which were more pronounced in *H. pylori*–positive subjects. Interestingly, 25 μg of the LTG192R caused diarrhea in six volunteers. This study did not report whether immunization with the whole-cell vaccine induced antibodies cross-reacting with epitopes also expressed by human cells. In addition, the effect of oral vaccination of *H. pylori*–positive subjects on gastric colonization with *H. pylori* was not reported.

Challenge Trials

Therapeutic trials of vaccination could turn out to be particularly difficult due to problems intrinsic to this approach. Prophylactic vaccination faces problems related to the low incidence of *H. pylori* infection in developed countries. Trials require large numbers of subjects and a long follow up to determine efficacy of a vaccine. As a consequence, it is likely that future prophylactic *H. pylori* vaccines will be tested in areas with high transmission rates, as in less developed countries, in order to obtain information on efficacy in a reasonable period of time. An alternative approach has recently been undertaken by developing models of experimental infection with *H. pylori* in volunteers. This approach offers two undeniable advantages. First, in this model one could investigate the early stages of infection, which, in the vast majority of cases of *H. pylori* infection, are undiagnosed; thus it would offer the possibility to better understand the pathogenesis of the infection. Second, it would represent a unique tool to test the prophylactic efficacy of vaccine constructs within a short time frame, as already done with other bacterial vaccines, such as those against *S. typhi, Shigella* spp, *Vibrio cholerae*, ETEC, etc (239). A first experimental infection of volunteers has been carried out with a *cag*-negative *H. pylori* strain (119). Most of the infected volunteers experienced clear clinical symptoms, such as vomiting, diarrhea, abdominal cramps, etc, confirming the results of the two experiments of self-infection carried out earlier (115, 116). These symptoms appeared 3–6 days after challenge and resolved within two weeks. An early infiltration of the gastric mucosa with neutrophils was evident despite the fact that this strain was lacking *cag*, suggesting that factors other than the *cag*-mediated induction of IL-8 can mediate early recruitment and activation of neutrophils in the sites of *H. pylori* colonization. One of these factors could well be NAP, as we have recently shown (112), an antigen that is well conserved in all the strains of *H. pylori* (113). It will be interesting to see in the very near future whether the vaccine candidates under development will be able to confer protection in this experimental model of human infection with *H. pylori*.

CONCLUSIONS

The last decade has seen impressive progress toward understanding of the genetics of *H. pylori* and deciphering some of the virulence factors involved in the pathogenetic events at the basis of *H. pylori* colonization and *H. pylori*–mediated pathology. The complete sequences of the genomes of two *H. pylori* strains offer a unique tool to identify genes important in the host-microbe interaction. However, relatively little is still known of the natural history of the infection and of the immune responses evoked by *H. pylori* infection. Current knowledge comes from studies of adults chronically infected for several years. It is hoped that in the near future more studies will focus on children and on the early events of this infection. This would offer a big opportunity to investigate the different aspects of the immune response that up to now have remained quite sketchy. In the absence of knowledge of the aspects of the immune responses induced by natural infection, it is hard to define which of these aspects may correlate with protection. We are now facing a situation in which we have antigens and formulations that confer (partial or complete) protection in animal models, without knowing through which immune mechanisms this protection is achieved. The next couple of years will be crucial for the development of vaccines against *H. pylori*: Several trials are foreseen in humans, and a big hope remains that most of the questions we are asking now on the host-microbe interactions will be answered. This would allow the preparation of vaccines against *H. pylori* infection and against its most dangerous complications, such as the development of gastric cancer.

ACKNOWLEDGMENT

The authors are grateful to C Mallia for manuscript editing.

Visit the Annual Reviews home page at www.AnnualReviews.org

LITERATURE CITED

1. Bizzozero G. 1893. Über die schlauch-förmingen Drüsen des Magendarmkanals und die Beziehungen ihres Epithels zu dem Oberflächenepithel der Schleimhaut. *Arch. Mikrosk. Anat.* 42:82
2. Marshall BJ. 1983. Unidentified curved bacilli on gastric epithelium in active chronic gastritis. *Lancet* i:1273–275
3. Warren JR. 1983. Unidentified curved bacilli on gastric epithelium in active chronic gastritis. *Lancet* i:1273
4. Ghiara P, Covacci A, Telford JL, Rappuoli R. 1996. *Helicobacter pylori*: pathogenic determinants and strategies for vaccine design. In *Concepts in Vaccine Development*, ed. SHE Kaufmann, pp. 459–496. Berlin/New York: Walter de Gruyter
5. Dubois A, Fiala N, Heman-Ackah LM, Drazek ES, Tarnawski A. 1994. Natural gastric infection with *Helicobacter pylori* in monkeys. *Gastroenterology* 106:1405–17
6. Mitchell HM. 1999. The epidemiology of *Helicobacter pylori*. *Curr. Top. Microbiol. Immunol.* 241:11–30
7. Thomas JE, Dale A, Harding M, Coward WA, Cole TJ, Weaver LT. 1999. *Helicobacter pylori* colonization in early life. *Pediatr. Res.* 45:218–23
8. Cullen DJE, Collins BJ, Christiansen KJ, Epis J, Warren JR. 1993. When is *Helicobacter pylori* infection acquired? *Gut* 34:1681–82
9. Veldhuyze van Zanten SJO, Pollak PT, Best

LM, Bezanson GS, Marrier T. 1994. Increasing prevalence of *Helicobacter pylori* infection with age—continuous risk of infection in adults rather than cohort effect. *J. Infect. Dis.* 169:434–37
10. Neale KR, Logan RP. 1995. The epidemiology and transmission of *Helicobacter pylori* in children. *Aliment. Pharmacol. Ther.* 9(Suppl. 2):77–84
11. Rothenbacher D, Bode G, Berg G, Knwyer U, Gonser T. 1999. *Helicobacter pylori* among preschool children and their parents: evidence of parent-child transmission *J. Infect. Dis.* 179:398–402
12. Rotenbacher D, Inceoglu J, Bode G, Brenner H. 2000. Acquisition of *Helicobacter pylori* infection in a high-risk population occurs within the first 2 years of life. *J. Pediatr.* 136:744–48
13. Malaty HM, Kumagai T, Tanaka E, Ota H, Kiyosawa K. 2000. Evidence from a nine-year birth cohort study in Japan of transmission pathways of *Helicobacter pylori* infection. *J. Clin. Microbiol.* 38:1971–73
14. Miehlke S, Thomas R, Gutierrez O, Graham DY, Go MF. 1999. DNA fingerprinting of single colonies of *Helicobacter pylori* from gastric cancer patients suggests infection with a single predominant strain. *J. Clin. Microbiol.* 37:245–47
15. Bode G, Rothenbacher D, Brenner H, Adler G. 1998. Pets are not a risk factor

for *Helicobacter pylori* infection in young children: results of a population-based study in Southern Germany. *Pediatr. Infect. Dis. J.* 17:909–12

16. Hulten K, Han SW, Enroth H, Klein PD, Opekun AR. 1996. *Helicobacter pylori* in the drinking water in Peru. *Gastroenterology* 110:1031–35

17. Dore MP, Sepulveda AR, Osato MS, Realdi G, Graham DY. 1999. *Helicobacter pylori* in sheep milk. *Lancet* 354:132

18. Parsonnet J, Shmuely H, Haggerty T. 1999. Fecal and oral shedding of *Helicobacter pylori* from healthy infected adults. *JAMA* 282:2240–45

19. Leung WK, Siu KLK, Kwok CKL, Chan SY, Sung R, Sung JJY. 1999. Isolation of *Helicobacter pylori* from vomitus in children and its implication in gastro-oral transmission. *Am. J. Gastroenterol.* 94:2881–84

20. Parsonnet J. 1998. *Helicobacter pylori*: the size of the problem. *Gut* 43(Suppl. 1):S6–S9

21. Unge P. 1999. Antibiotic treatment of *Helicobacter pylori* infection. *Curr. Top. Microbiol. Immunol.* 241:261–300

22. Bell GD, Powell K, Burridge SM, Pallecaros A, Jones PH. 1992. Experience with "triple" anti-*Helicobacter* eradication therapy: side effects and the importance of testing the pre-treatment bacterial isolate for metronidazole resistance. *Aliment. Pharmacol. Ther.* 6:427–35

23. Graham DY. 1998. Antibiotic resistance in *Helicobacter pylori*: implications for therapy. *Gastroenterology* 115:1272–77

24. Forbes GM, Glaser ME, Cullen DJ, Warren JR, Christiansen KJ. 1994. Duodenal ulcer treatment with *Helicobacter pylori* eradication: seven year follow-up. *Lancet* 343:258–60

25. Rowland M, Kumar D, Daly L, O'Connor P, Vaughan D, Drumm B. 1999. Low rates of *Helicobacter pylori* reinfection in children. *Gastroenterology* 117:336–41

26. Ramirez-Ramos A, Gilman RH, Leon-Barua R, Recavarren-Arce S, Watanabe J. 1997. Rapid recurrence of *Helicobacter pylori* infection in Peruvian patients after successful eradication. Gastrointestinal Physiology Working Group of the Universidad Peruana Cayetano Heredia and the Johns Hopkins University. *Clin. Infect. Dis.* 25:1027–31

27. Dale A, Thomas JE, Darboe MK, Coward WA, Harding M, Weaver LT. 1998. *Helicobacter pylori* infection, gastric acid secretion, and infant growth. *J. Pediatr. Gastroenterol. Nutr.* 26:393–97

28. Tomb JF, White O, Kerlavage AR, Clayton RA, Sutton GG. 1997. The complete genome sequence of the gastric pathogen *Helicobacter pylori*. *Nature* 388:539–47

29. Alm RA, Ling LSL, Moir DT, King BL, Brown ED. 1999. Genomic sequence comparison of two unrelated isolates of the human gastric pathogen *Helicobacter pylori*. *Nature* 397:176–180

30. Alm RA, Bina J, Andrews BM, Doig P, Hancock REW, Trust TJ. 2000. Comparative genomics of *Helicobacter pylori*: analysis of the outer membrane protein families. *Infect. Immun.* 68:4155–68

31. Covacci A, Telford JL, Del Giudice G, Parsonnet J, Rappuoli R. 1999. *Helicobacter pylori*, virulence and genetic geography. *Science* 284:1328–33

32. Bauerfeind P, Garner R, Dunn BE, Mobley HLT. 1997. Synthesis and activity of *Helicobacter pylori* urease and catalase at low pH. *Gut* 40:25–30

33. Mobley HLT, Island MD, Hausinger RP. 1995. Molecular biology of ureases. *Microbiol. Rev.* 59:451–80

34. Eaton KA, Brooks CL, Morgan DR, Krakowka S. 1991. Essential role of urease in pathogenesis of gastritis induced by *Helicobacter pylori* in gnotobiotic pigs. *Infect. Immun.* 59:2470–75

35. Eaton KA, Krakowka S. 1994. Effect of gastric pH on urease-dependent colonization of gnotobiotic piglets by *Helicobacter pylori*. *Infect. Immun.* 62:3604–7

36. Hazell SL, Mendz GL. 1993. The metabolism and enzymes of *Helicobacter pylori*: function and potential virulence effects. In *Helicobacter pylori: Biology and Clinical Practice*, ed. CS Goodwin, BW Worsley, pp. 115–142. London: CRC Press

37. McGee DJ, Mobley HLT. 1999. Mechanisms of *Helicobacter pylori* infection: bacterial factors. *Curr. Top. Microbiol. Immunol.* 241:155–80

38. Phadnis SH, Parlow MH, Levy M, Ilver D, Caulkins CM. 1996. Surface localization of *Helicobacter pylori* urease and heat shock protein homolog requires bacterial autolysis. *Infect. Immun.* 64:905–12

39. Dunn BE, Vakil NB, Schneider BG, Miller MM, Zitzer JB. 1997. Localization of *Helicobacter pylori* urease and heat shock protein in human gastric biopsies. *Infect. Immun.* 65:1181–88

40. Leal-Herrera Y, Torres J, Perez-Perez G, Gomez A, Monath T. 1999. Serologic IgG response to urease in *Helicobacter pylori*-infected persons from Mexico. *Am. J. Trop. Med. Hyg.* 60:587–92

41. D'Elios MM, Manghetti M, De Carli M, Costa F, Baldari CT. 1997. T helper 1 effector cells specific for *Helicobacter pylori* in the gastric antrum of patients with peptic ulcer disease. *J. Immunol.* 158:962–67

42. D'Elios MM, Manghetti M, Almerigogna F, Amedei A, Costa F. 1997. Different cytokine profile and antigen-specificity repertoire in *Helicobacter pylori*-specific T cell clones from the antrum of chronic gastritis patients with or without peptic ulcer. *Eur. J. Immunol.* 27:1751–55

43. Leunk RD, Johnson PT, David BC, Kraft WG, Morgan DR. 1988. Cytotoxin activity in broth-culture filtrates of *Campylobacter pylori*. *J. Med. Microbiol.* 26:93–99

44. Cover TL, Tummuru MKR, Cao P, Thompson SA, Blaser MJ. 1994. Divergence of genetic sequences for the vacuolating cytotoxin among *Helicobacter pylori* strains. *J. Biol. Chem.* 269:10566–73

45. Telford JL, Ghiara P, Dell'Orco M, Comanducci M, Burroni D. 1994. Purification and characterization of the vacuolating toxin from *Helicobacter pylori*. *J. Exp. Med.* 179:1653–58

46. de Bernard M, Burroni D, Papini E, Rappuoli R, Telford J, Montecucco C. 1998. Identification of the *Helicobacter pylori* VacA toxin domain in the cell cytosol. *Infect. Immun.* 66:6014–16

47. Ye D, Willhite DC, Blanke SR. 1999. Identification of the minimal intracellular domain of the *Helicobacter pylori* vacuolating toxin. *J. Biol. Chem.* 274:9277–82

48. Reyrat JM, Lanzavecchia S, Lupetti S, de Barbard M, Pagliaccia C. 1999. 3D structure and location in the holotoxin holigomer of the 58 kDa cell binding subunit of the *Helicobacter pylori* cytotoxin. *J. Biol. Mol.* 290:459–70

49. Lupetti P, Heuser JE, Manetti R, Massari P, Lanzavecchia S. 1996. Oligomeric and subunit structure of the *Helicobacter pylori* vacuolating cytotoxin. *J. Cell Biol.* 133:801–7

50. Cover TL, Hanson PI, Heuser JE. 1997. Acid-induced dissociation of VacA, the *Helicobacter pylori* vacuolating cytotoxin, reveals its pattern of assembly. *J. Cell Biol.* 138:759–69

51. de Bernard M, Papini E, de Filippis V, Gottardi E, Telford J. 1995. Low pH activates the vacuolating toxin of *Helicobacter pylori*, which becomes acid and pepsin resistant. *J. Biol. Chem.* 270:23937–40

52. Molinari M, Galli C, Norais N, Telford JL, Rappuoli R. 1997. Vacuoles induced by *Helicobacter pylori* toxin contain both late endosomal and lysosomal markers. *J. Biol. Chem.* 272:25339–44

53. Massari P, Manetti R, Burroni D, Nuti S, Norais N. 1998. Binding of *Helicobacter pylori* cytotoxin to target cells. *Infect. Immun.* 66:3981–84

54. Padilla PI, Wada A, Yahiro K, Kimura M, Niidome T. 2000. Morphologic differentiation of HL-60 cells is associated

with appearance of RPTPβ and induction of *Helicobacter pylori* VacA sensitivity. *J. Biol. Chem.* 275:15200–6

55. Papini E, Satin B, Bucci C, de Bernard M, Telford JL. 1997. The small GTP binding protein rab7 is essential for cellular vacuolation induced by *Helicobacter pylori* cytotoxin. *EMBO J.* 16:15–24

56. Molinari M, Salio M, Galli C, Norais N, Rappuoli R. 1998. Selective inhibition of Ii-dependent antigen presentation by *Helicobacter pylori* toxin VacA. *J. Exp. Med.* 187:135–40

57. Shirai M, Arichi T, Nakazawa T, Berzofsky JA. 1998. Persistent infection by *Helicobacter pylori* down-modulates virus-specific CD8+ cytotoxic T cell response and prolongs viral infection. *J. Infect. Dis.* 177:72–80

58. Satin B, Norais N, Telford J, Rappuoli R, Murgia M. 1997. Effect of *Helicobacter pylori* vacuolating toxin on maturation and extracellular release of procathepsin D and on epidermal growth factor degradation. *J. Biol. Chem.* 272:25022–28

59. Papini E, Satin B, Norais N, de Barbard M, Telford JL. 1998. *Helicobacter pylori* vacuolating toxin increases the permeability of polarized epithelial cells monolayers. *J. Clin. Invest.* 102:813–20

60. Pelicic V, Reyrat JM, Sartori L, Pagliaccia C, Rappuoli R. 1999. *Helicobacter pylori* VacA cytotoxin associated to bacteria increases epithelial permeability independently of its vacuolating activity. *Microbiology* 145:2043–50

61. Guarino A, Bisceglia M, Canani RB, Boccia MC, Malardo G. 1998. Enterotoxic effect of the vacuolating toxin produced by *Helicobacter pylori* in Caco-2 cells. *J. Infect. Dis.* 178:1373–78

62. Sullivan PB, Thomas JE, Wight DG, Neale G, Estham EJ. 1990. *Helicobacter pylori* in Gambian children with chronic diarrhoea and malnutrition. *Arch. Dis. Child.* 65:189–91

63. Luzzi I, Covacci A, Censini S, Pezzella C,

Crotti D. 1996. Detection of a vacuolating cytotoxin in stools from children with diarrhea. *Clin. Infect. Dis.* 23:101–6

64. Reyrat JM, Pelicic V, Papini E, Montecucco C, Rappuoli R, Telford JL. 1999. Towards deciphering the *Helicobacter pylori* cytotoxin. *Mol. Microbiol.* 34:197–204

65. Ji X, Fernandez T, Burroni D, Pagliaccia C, Atherton JC. 2000. Cell specificity of *Helicobacter pylori* cytotoxin is determined by a short region in the polymorphic midregion. *Infect. Immun.* 68:3754–57

66. Wang HJ, Kuo CH, Yeh AA, Chang PC, Wang WC. 1998. Vacuolating toxin production in clinical isolates of *Helicobacter pylori* with different *vacA* genotypes. *J. Infect. Dis.* 178:207–12

67. Go MF, Cissell L, Graham DY. 1998. Failure to confirm association of *vacA* gene mosiacism with duodenal ulcer disease. *Scand. J. Gastroenterol.* 33:132–36

68. Pagliaccia C, de Bernard M, Lupetti P, Ji X, Burroni D. 1998. The m2 form of *Helicobacter pylori* cytotoxin has cell type-specific vacuolating activity. *Proc. Natl. Acad. Sci. USA* 95:10212–17

69. Perez-Perez GI, Peek RM Jr, Atherton JC, Blaser MJ, Cover TL. 1999. Detection of anti-VacA antibody responses in serum and gastric juice samples using type s1/m1 and s2/m2 *Helicobacter pylori* VacA antigens. *Clin. Diagn. Lab. Immunol.* 6:489–93

70. Covacci A, Censini S, Bugnoli M, Petracca R, Burroni D. 1993. Molecular characterization of the 128-kDa immunodominant antigen of *Helicobacter pylori* associated with cytotoxicity and duodenal ulcer. *Proc. Natl. Acad. Sci. USA* 90:5791–95

71. Tummuru MK, Cover TL, Blaser MJ. 1993. Cloning and expession of a high-molecular-mass major antigen of *Helicobacter pylori*: evidence of linkage to cytotoxin production. *Infect. Immun.* 61:1799–1809

72. Xiang ZY, Censini S, Bayeli PF, Telford JL, Figura N. 1995. Analysis and expression of VacA and CagA virulence factors

in 43 strains of *Helicobacter pylori* reveals that clinical isolates can be divided into two major types and that CagA is not necessary for expression of the vacuolating cytotoxin. *Infect. Immun.* 63:94–98

73. Cover TL, Dooley CP, Blaser MJ. 1990. Characterization of and human serologic response to proteins in *Helicobacter pylori* broth culture supernatants with vacuolizing cytotoxin activity. *Infect. Immun.* 58:603–10

74. Xiang ZY, Bugnoli M, Ponzetto A, Morgando A, Figura N. 1993. Detection in an enzyme immunoassay of an immune response to a recombinant fragment of the 128 kilodalton protein (CagA) of *Helicobacter pylori. Eur. J. Clin. Microbiol. Infect. Dis.* 12:739–45

75. Parsonnet J, Friedman GD, Orentreich N, Vogelman H. 1997. Risk for gastric cancer in people with CagA positive or CagA negative *Helicobacter pylori* strains. *Gut* 40:297–301

76. Webb PM, Crabtree JE, Forman D. 1999. Gastric cancer, cytotoxin-associated gene A-positive *Helicobacter pylori* and serum pepsinogens: an international study, the Eurogast Study Group. *Gastroenterology* 116:269–76

77. Censini S, Lange C, Xiang Z, Crabtree JE, Ghiara P. 1996. *cag*, a pathogenicity island of *Helicobacter pylori*, encodes type I-specific and disease-associated virulence factors. *Proc. Natl. Acad. Sci. USA* 93:14648–53

78. Weel JF, van der Hulst RW, Gerrits Y, Roorda P, Feller M. 1996. The interrelationship between cytotoxin-associated gene A, vacuolating cytotoxin, and *Helicobacter pylori*-related diseases. *J. Infect. Dis.* 173:1771–75

79. Atherton JC, Tham KT, Peek RM Jr, Cover TL, Blaser MJ. 1996. Density of *Helicobacter pylori* infection in vivo as assessed by quantitative culture and histology. *J. Infect. Dis.* 174:552–56

80. Maeda S, Ogura K, Yoshida H, Kanai F,

Ikenoue T. 1998. Major virulence factors, VacA and CagA, are commonly positive in *Helicobacter pylori* isolates in Japan. *Gut* 42:338–43

81. Park SM, Park J, Kim JG, Cho HD, Cho JH. 1998. Infection with *Helicobacter pylori* expressing the *cagA* gene is not associated with an increased risk of developing peptic ulcer diseases in Korean patients. *Scand. J. Gastroenterol.* 33:923–27

82. Segal ED, Lange C, Covacci A, Tompkins LS, Falkow S. 1997. Induction of host signal transduction pathways by *Helicobacter pylori. Proc. Natl. Acad. Sci. USA* 94:7595–99

83. Meyer-ter-Vehn T, Covacci A, Kist M, Pahl HL. 2000. *Helicobacter pylori* activates mitogen-activated protein kinase cascades and induces expression of the proto-oncogenes c-fos and c-jun. *J. Biol. Chem.* 275:16064–72

84. Glocker E. Lange C, Covacci A, Bereswill S, Kist M, Pahl HL. 1998. Proteins encoded by the *cag* pathogenicity island of *Helicobacter pylori* are required for NF-•B activation. *Infect. Immun.* 66:2346–48

85. Segal ED, Cha J, Lo J, Falkow S, Tompkins LS. 1999. Altered states: involvement of phosphorylated CagA in the induction of host cellular growth changes by *Helicobacter pylori. Proc. Natl. Acad. Sci. USA* 96:14559–64

86. Asahi M, Azuma T, Ito S, Ito Y, Suto H. 2000. *Helicobacter pylori* CagA protein can be tyrosine phosphorylated in gastric epithelial cells. *J. Exp. Med.* 191:593–602

87. Stein M, Rappuoli R, Covacci A. 2000. Tyrosine phosphorylation of *Helicobacter pylori* CagA antigen after *cag*-driven host cell translocation. *Proc. Natl. Acad. Sci. USA* 97:1263–68

88. Odenbreit S, Puls J, Sedlmaier B, Gerland E, Fischer W, Haas R. 2000. Translocation of *Helicobacter pylori* CagA into gastric epithelial cells by type IV secretion. *Science* 287:1497–1500

89. Backert S, Ziska E, Brinkmann V, Zimny-Arndt U, Fauconnier A. 2000. Translocation of the *Helicobacter* CagA protein in gastric epithelial cells by a type IV secretion apparatus. *Cell. Microbiol.* 2:155–64

90. Covacci A, Rappuoli R. 2000. Tyrosine-phosphorylated bacterial proteins: Trojan horses for the host cell. *J. Exp. Med.* 191:587–92

91. Cover TL, Glupczynski Y, Lage AP, Burette A, Tummuru MKR. 1995. Serology detection of infection with cagA+ *Helicobacter pylori* strains. *J. Clin. Microbiol.* 33:1496–1500

92. Di Tommaso A, Xiang ZY, Bugnoli M, Pileri P, Figura N. 1996. *Helicobacter pylori*-specific CD4+ T-cell clones from peripheral blood and gastric biopsies. *Infect. Immun.* 63:1102–6

93. Sommer F, Faller G, Konturek P, Kirchner T, Hahn EG. 1998. Antrum and corpus mucosa-infiltrating CD4+ lymphocytes in *Helicobacter pylori* gastritis display a Th1 phenotype. *Infect. Immun.* 66:5543–46

94. Lindholm C, Quiding-Jarbrink M, Lonroth H, Hamlet A, Svennerholm AM. 1998. Local cytokine response in *Helicobacter pylori* infected subjects. *Infect. Immun.* 66:5964–71

95. Bamford KB, Fan X, Crowe SE, Leary JF, Gourley WK. 1998. Lymphocytes in the human gastric mucosa during *Helicobacter pylori* infection have a T helper cell 1 phenotype. *Gastroenterology* 114:482–92

96. Mohammadi M, Czinn S, Redline R, Nedrud J. 1996. *Helicobacter*-specific cell-mediated immune responses display a predominant Th1 phenotype and promote a delayed-type hypersensitivity response in the stomachs of mice. *J. Immunol.* 156:4729–38

97. Saldinger PF, Porta N, Launois P, Louis JA, Wanders GA. 1998. Immunization of BALB/c mice with *Helicobacter* urease B induces a T helper 2 response absent in *Helicobacter* infection. *Gastroenterology* 115:891–97

98. Mattapallil JJ, Dandekar S, Canfield DR, Solnick JV. 2000. A predominant Th1 type of immune response is induced early during acute *Helicobacter pylori* infection in rhesus macaques. *Gastroenterology* 118:307–15

99. Suzuki M, Mori M, Miyayama A, Iwai N, Tsunematsu N. 1997. Enhancement of neutrophil infiltration in the corpus after failure of *Helicobacter pylori* eradication. *J. Clin. Gastroenterol.* 25:S222–S228

100. Davies GR, Banatvala N, Collins CE, Sheaff MT, Abdi Y. 1994. Relationship between infective load of *Helicobacter pylori* and reactive oxygen metabolite production in antral mucosa. *Scand. J. Gastroenterol.* 29:419–24

101. Fiocca R, Luinetti O, Villani L, Chiaravalli AM, Capella C, Solcia E. 1994. Epithelial cytotoxicity, immune responses, and inflammatory components of *Helicobacter pylori* gastritis. *Scand. J. Gastroenterol.* 205 (Suppl.):11–21

102. Ando T, Kusugami K, Ohsuga M, Ina K, Shinoda M. 1998. Differential normalization of mucosal interleukin-8 and interleukin-6 activity after *Helicobacter pylori* eradication. *Infect. Immun.* 66:4742–47

103. Mai UE, Perez-Perez GI, Wahl LM, Wahl SM, Blaser MJ, Smith PD. 1991. Soluble surface proteins from *Helicobacter pylori* activate monocytes/macrophages by lipopolysaccharide-independent mechanism. *J. Clin. Invest.* 87:894–900

104. Mai UE, Perez-Perez GI, Allen JB, Wahl SM, Blaser MJ, Smith PD. 1992. Surface proteins from *Helicobacter pylori* exhibit chemotactic activity for human leukocytes and are present in gastric mucosa. *J. Exp. Med.* 175:517–25

105. Craig PM, Territo MC, Karnes WE, Walsh JH. 1992. *Helicobacter pylori* secretes

a chemotactic factor for monocytes and neutrophils. *Gut* 33:1020–23

106. Nielsen H, Andersen LP. 1992. Chemotactic activity of *Helicobacter pylori* sonicate for human polymorphonuclear leukocytes and monocytes. *Gut* 33:738–42

107. Nielsen H, Andersen LP. 1992. Activation of human phagocyte oxidative metabolism by *Helicobacter pylori*. *Gastroenterology* 103:1747–53

108. Yoshida N, Granger DN, Evans DJ Jr, Evans DG, Graham DY. 1993. Mechanisms involved in *Helicobacter pylori*-induced inflammation. *Gastroenterology* 105:1431–40

109. Evans DJ Jr, Evans DG, Takemura T, Nakano H, Lampert HC. 1995. Characterization of a *Helicobacter pylori* neutrophil-activating protein. *Infect. Immun.* 63:2213–20

110. Evans DJ Jr, Evans DG, Lampert HC, Nakano H. 1995. Identification of four new prokaryotic bacterioferritins, from *Helicobacter pylori, Anabaena variabilis, Bacillus subtilis and Treponema pallidum*, by analysis of gene sequences. *Gene* 153:123–27

110a. Tonello F, Dundon WG, Satin B, Molinari M, Tognon G. 1999. The *Helicobacter pylori* neutrophil-activating protein is an iron-binding protein with dodecameric structure. *Mol. Microbiol.* 34:238–46

111. Grant RA, Filman DJ, Finkel SE, Kolter R, Hogle JM. 1998. The crystal structure of Dps, a ferritin homolog that binds and protects DNA. *Nature Struct. Biol.* 5:294–303

112. Satin B, Del Giudice G, Della Bianca V, Dusi S, Laudanna C. 2000. The neutrophil-activating protein (HP-NAP) of *Helicobacter pylori* is a protective antigen and a major virulence factor. *J. Exp. Med.* 191:1567–76

113. Dundon WG, Guidotti S, Covacci A, Rappuoli R, Montecucco C. 2000. Suit-

ability of the neutrophil activating protein (HP-NAP) as a vaccine candidate. *FEMS Microbiol. Immunol. Lett.* In press

114. Kimmel B, Bosserhoff A, Frank R, Gross R, Goebel W, Beier D. 2000. Identification of immunodominant antigens from *Helicobacter pylori* and evaluation of their reactivities with sera from patients with different gastroduodenal pathologies. *Infect. Immun.* 68:915–20

115. Marshall BJ, Armstrong JA, McGechie DB, Glancy RJ. 1985. Attempt to fulfil Koch's postulates for pyloric Campylobacter. *Med. J. Aust.* 142:436–39

116. Morris A, Nicholson G. 1987. Ingestion of *Campylobacter pyloridis* causes gastritis and raised resting gastric pH. *Am. J. Gastroenterol.* 82:192–99

117. Sobala GM, Crabtree JE, Dixon MF, Schorah CJ, Taylor JD. 1991. Acute *Helicobacter pylori* infection: clinical features, local and systemic immune response, gastric mucosal histology, and gastric juice ascorbic acid concentrations. *Gut* 32:1415–18

118. Mitchell JD, Mitchell HM, Tobias V. 1992. Acute *Helicobacter pylori* infection in an infant, associated with gastric ulceration and serological evidence of intrafamilial transmission. *Am. J. Gastroenterol.* 87:382–86

119. Graham DY, Opekun AR, Osato MS, El Zimaity HMT, Cadoz M. 1999. *H. pylori* vaccine development in humans: challenge model. In *Third Annual Winter* H. Pylori *Workshop*, Orlando, FL, February 26–27, 1999, Poster no. 54

120. Lee A, Fox JG, Otto G, Murphy J. 1990. A small animal model of human *Helicobacter pylori* active chronic gastritis. *Gastroenterology* 99:1315–23

121. Ferrero RL, Labigne A. 1993. Cloning, expression, and sequencing of *Helicobacter felis* urease genes. *Mol. Microbiol.* 9:323–33

122. Macchia G, Massone A, Burroni D, Covacci A, Censini S, Rappuoli R. 1993.

The Hsp60 of *Helicobacter pylori*: structure and immune response in patients with gastroduodenal diseases. *Mol. Microbiol.* 9:645–52

123. Suerbaum S, Thiberge J, Kansau I, Ferrero RL, Labigne A. 1994. *Helicobacter pylori* hspA-hspB heat-shock gene cluster: nucleotide sequence, expression, putative function and immunogenicity. *Mol. Microbiol.* 14:959–74

124. Marchetti M, Aricò B, Burroni D, Figura N, Rappuoli R, Ghiara P. 1995. Development of a mouse model of *Helicobacter pylori* infection that mimics human disease. *Science* 267:1655–58

125. Ghiara P, Marchetti M, Blaser MJ, Tummuru MKR, Cover TL. 1995. Role of the *Helicobacter pylori* virulence factors vacuolating cytotoxin, CagA and urease in a mouse model of disease. *Infect. Immun.* 63:4154–60

126. Ghiara P, Rossi M, Marchetti M, Di Tommaso A, Vindigni C. 1997. Therapeutic intragastric vaccination against *Helicobacter pylori* in mice eradicates an otherwise chronic infection and confers protection against reinfection. *Infect. Immun.* 65:4996–5002

127. Kleanthous H, Tibbitts T, Bakios TJ, Georgokopoulos K, Myers G. 1995. In vivo selection of a highly adapted *H. pylori* isolate and the development of a *H. pylori* model for studying vaccine efficacy. *Gut* 37:A94

128. Lee A, O'Rourke J, De Ungria MC, Robertson B, Daskalopoulos G, Dixon MF. 1997. A standardized mouse model of *Helicobacter pylori* infection. *Gastroenterology* 112:1386–97

129. Li H, Kalies I, Mellgård, Helander HF. 1998. A rat model of chronic *Helicobacter pylori* infection. Studies of epithelial cell turnover and gastric ulcer healing. *Scand. J. Gastroenterol.* 33:370–78

130. Shomer NH, Dangler CA, Whary MT, Fox JG. 1998. Experimental *Helicobacter pylori* infection induces antral gastritis and gastric mucosa-associated lymphoid tissue in guinea pigs. *Infect. Immun.* 66:2614–18

131. Hirayama F, Takagi S, Kusuhara H, Iwao E, Yokoyama Y, Ikeda Y. 1996. Induction of gastric ulcer and intestinal metaplasia in Mongolian gerbils infected with *Helicobacter pylori*. *J. Gastroenterol.* 31:755–57

132. Honda S, Fujioka T, Tokieda M, Gotoh T, Nishizono A, Nasu M. 1998. Gastric ulcer, atrophic gastritis, and intestinal metaplasia caused by *Helicobacter* infection in Mongolian gerbils. *Scand. J. Gastroenterol.* 33:454–60

133. Wirth HP, Beins MH, Yang M, Tham KT, Blaser MJ. 1998. Experimental infection of Mongolian gerbils with wild-type and mutants *Helicobacter pylori* strains. *Infect. Immun.* 66:4856–66

134. Watanabe T, Tada M, Nagai H, Sasaki S, Nakao M. 1998. *Helicobacter pylori* induces gastric cancer in Mongolian gerbils. *Gastroenterology* 115:642–48

135. Akopyants NS, Eaton KA, Berg DE. 1995. Adaptive mutation and cocolonization during *Helicobacter pylori* infection of gnotobiotic piglets. *Infect. Immun.* 63:116–21

136. Eaton KA, Suerbaum S, Josenhans C, Krakowka S. 1996. Colonization of gnotobiotic piglets by *Helicobacter pylori* deficient in two flagellin genes. *Infect. Immun.* 64:2445–48

137. Dubois A, Berg DE. 1997. The nonhuman primate model for *H. pylori* infection. In *Methods in Molecular Medicine*. Helicobacter pylori *Protocols*, ed. CL Clayton, HTL Mobley, pp. 253–69. Totowa, NJ: Humana

138. Fox JG, Correa P, Taylor NS, Lee A, Otto G. 1990. *Helicobacter mustelae*-associated gastritis in ferrets. An animal model of *Helicobacter pylori* gastritis in humans. *Gastroenterology* 99:352–61

139. Andrutis KA, Fox JG, Schauer DB, Shames B, Yan L. 1995. Identification of a *cagA* gene in *Helicobacter mustelae* strains. *Gut* 37 (Suppl. 1):A30

140. Handt LK, Fox JG, Stalis IH, Rufo R, Lee G. 1995. Characterization of feline *Helicobacter pylori* strains and associated gastritis in a colony of domestic cats. *J. Clin. Microbiol.* 33:2280–89

141. Fox JG, Batchelder M, Marini R, Yan L, Handt L. 1995. *Helicobacter pylori*-induced gastritis in the domestic cat. *Infect. Immun.* 63:2674–81

142. Esteves MI, Schrenzel MD, Marini RP, Taylor NS, Xu S. 2000. *Helicobacter pylori* gastritis in cats with long-term natural infection as a model of human disease. *Am. J. Pathol.* 156:709–21

143. El-Zaatari FAK, Woo JS, Badr A, Osato MS, Serna H. 1997. Failure to isolate *Helicobacter pylori* from stray cats indicate that *H. pylori* in cats may be an anthroponosis — an animal infection with a human pathogen. *J. Med. Microbiol.* 46:372–76

144. Radin MJ, Eaton KA, Krakowka S, Morgan DR, Lee A. 1990. *Helicobacter pylori* gastric infection in gnotobiotic beagle dogs. *Infect. Immun.* 58:2606–12

145. Rossi G, Rossi M, Vitali CG, Fortuna D, Burroni D. 1999. A conventional beagle dog model for acute and chronic infection with *Helicobacter pylori*. *Infect. Immun.* 67:3112–20

146. Rossi G, Fortuna D, Pancotto L, Renzoni G, Taccini E. 2000. Immunohistochemical study of the lymphocyte populations infiltrating the gastric mucosa of beagle dogs experimentally infected with *Helicobacter pylori*. *Infect. Immun.* 68:4769–72

147. Marchetti M, Rossi M, Giannelli V, Giuliani MM, Pizza M. 1998. Protection against *Helicobacter pylori* infection in mice by intragastric vaccination with *H. pylori* antigens is achieved using a non-toxic mutant of *E. coli* heat-labile enterotoxin (LT) as adjuvant. 16:33–37

148. Czinn SJ, Nedrud JG. 1991. Oral immunization against *Helicobacter pylori*. *Infect. Immun.* 59:2359–63

149. Czinn SJ, Cai A, Nedrud JG. 1993. Protection of germ-free mice from infection by *Helicobacter felis* after active oral or passive IgA immunization. *Vaccine* 11:637–42

150. Chen M, Lee A, Hazell S. 1992. Immunisation against gastric Helicobacter infection in a mouse/*Helicobacter felis* model. *Lancet* 339:1120–21

151. Michetti P, Corthésy-Theulaz I, Davin C, Haas R, Vaney AC. 1994. Immunization of BALB/c mice against *Helicobacter felis* infection with *Helicobacter pylori* urease. *Gastroenterology* 107:1002–11

152. Doidge C, Gust I, Lee A, Buck F, Hazell S, Manne U. 1994. Therapeutic immunization against *Helicobacter* infection. *Lancet* 343:914–15

153. Sutton P, Wilson J, Kosaka T, Wolowczuk I, Lee A. 2000. Therapeutic immunization against *Helicobacter pylori* infection in the absence of antibodies. *Immunol. Cell. Biol.* 78:28–30

154. Negrini R, Lisato L, Zanella I, Cavazzini L, Gullini S. 1991. *Helicobacter pylori* infection induces antibodies cross-reacting with human gastric mucosa. *Gastroenterology* 101:437–45

155. Appelmelk BJ, Simoons-Smit I, Negrini R, Moran AP, Aspinall GO. 1996. Potential role of molecular mimicry between *Helicobacter pylori* lipopolysaccharide and host Lewis blood group antigens in autoimmunity. *Infect. Immun.* 64:2031–40

156. Appelmelk BJ, Negrini R, Moran AP, Kuipers EJ. 1997. Molecular mimicry between *Helicobacter pylori* and the host. *Trends Microbiol.* 5:70–73

157. Keenan J, Day T, Neal S, Cook B, Perez-Perez G. 2000. A role for the

bacterial outer membrane in the pathogenesis of *Helicobacter pylori* infection. *FEMS Microbiol. Lett.* 182:259–64

158. Sommi P, Ricci V, Fiocca R, Necchi V, Romano M. 1998. Persistence of *Helicobacter pylori* VacA toxin and vacuolating potential in cultured gastric epithelial cells. *Am. J. Physiol.* 38:G681–688

159. Keenan J, Oliaro J, Domigan N, Potter H, Aitken G. 2000b. Immune response to an 18-kilodalton outer membrane antigen lipoprotein 20 as a *Helicobacter pylori* vaccine candidate. *Infect. Immun.* 68:3337–43

160. Keenan J, Allardyce RA, Bangshaw PF. 1998. Lack of protection following immunization with *Helicobacter pylori* outer membrane vesicles highlights antigenic differences between *H. felis* and *H. pylori*. *FEMS Microbiol. Lett.* 161:21–27

161. Hocking D, Webb E, Radcliff F, Rothel L, Taylor S. 1999. Isolation of recombinant protective *Helicobacter pylori* antigens. *Infect. Immun.* 67:4713–19

162. Milagres LG, Gorla MCA, Sacchi CT, Rodrigues MM. 1998. Specificity of bactericidal antibody response to serogroup B meningococcal strains in Brazilian children after immunization with an outer membrane vaccine. *Infect. Immun.* 66:4755–61

163. Giuliani MM, Del Giudice G, Giannelli V, Dougan G, Douce G. 1998. Mucosal adjuvanticity and immunogenicity of LTR72, a novel mutant of *Escherichia coli* heat-labile enterotoxin with partial knockout of ADP-ribosyltransferase activity. *J. Exp. Med.* 187:1123–32

164. Ferrero RL, Thiberge JM, Huerre M, Labigne A. 1994. Recombinant antigens prepared from the urease subunits of *Helicobacter* spp: evidence of protection in a mouse model of gastric infection. *Infect. Immun.* 62:4981–89

165. Lee CK, Weltzin R, Thomas WD Jr, Kleanthous H, Ermak TH. 1995. Oral immunization with recombinant *Helicobacter pylori* urease induces secretory IgA antibodies and protects mice from challenge with *Helicobacter felis*. *J. Infect. Dis.* 172:161–72

166. Kleanthous H, Myers GA, Georgakopoulos KM, Tibbitts TJ, Ingrassia JW. 1998. Rectal and intranasal immunizations with recombinant urease induce distinct local and serum immune responses in mice and protect against *Helicobacter pylori* infection. *Infect. Immun.* 66:2879–86

167. Ermak TH, Giannasca PJ, Nichols R, Myers GA, Nedrud J. 1998. Immunization of mice with urease vaccine affords protection against *Helicobacter pylori* infection in the absence of antibodies and is mediated by MHC class II-restricted responses. *J. Exp. Med.* 188:2277–88

168. Myers GA, Ermak TH, Georgakopoulos K, Tibbitts T, Ingrassia J. 1999. Oral immunization with recombinant *Helicobacter pylori* urease confers long-lasting immunity against *Helicobacter felis* infection. *Vaccine* 17:1394–1403

169. Gomez-Duarte OG, Lucas B, Yan Z, Panthel K, Haas R, Meyer TF. 1998. Urease subunits A and B delivered by attenuated *Salmonella typhimurium* vaccine strain protects mice against gastric colonization by *Helicobacter pylori*. *Vaccine* 16:460–71

170. Corthésy-Theulaz IE, Hopkins S, Bachmann D, Saldinger PF, Porta N. 1998. Mice are protected from *Helicobacter pylori* infection by nasal immunization with attenuated *Salmonella typhimurium phoPc* expressing urease A and B subunits. *Infect. Immun.* 66:581–86

171. Corthésy-Theulaz I, Porta N, Glauser M, Saraga E, Vaney AC. 1995. Oral immunization with *Helicobacter pylori* urease B subunit as a treatment against *Helicobacter* infection in mice. *Gastroenterology* 109:115–21

172. Guy B, Hessler C, Fourage S, Robki B, Quentin Millet MJ. 1999. Comparison

between targeted and untargeted systemic immunizations with adjuvanted urease to cure *Helicobacter pylori* infection in mice. *Vaccine* 17:1130–35

173. Weltzin R, Kleanthous H, Guirakhoo F, Monath TP, Lee CK. 1997. Novel intranasal immunization techniques for antibody induction and protection of mice against gastric *Helicobacter felis* infection. *Vaccine* 15:370–76

174. Dieterich C, Bouzourène H, Blum AL, Corthésy-Theulaz IE. 1999. Urease-based mucosal immunization against *Helicobacter heilmannii* infection induces corpus atrophy in mice. *Infect. Immun.* 67:6206–9

175. Guy B, Hessler C, Fourage S, Haensler J, Vialon-Lafay E. 1998. Systemic immunization with urease protects mice against *Helicobacter pylori* infection. *Vaccine* 16:850–56

176. Weltzin R, Guy B, Thomas WD Jr, Giannasca PJ, Monath TP. 2000. Parenteral adjuvant activities of *Escherichia coli* heat-labile toxin and its B subunit for immunization of mice against gastric *Helicobacter pylori* infection. *Infect. Immun.* 68:2775–82

177. Cuenca R, Blanchard TG, Czinn SJ, Nedrud JG, Monath TP. 1996. Therapeutic immunization against *Helicobacter mustelae* in naturally infected ferrets. *Gastroenterology* 110:1770–75

178. Lee CK, Soike K, Hill J, Georgakopoulos K, Tibbitts T. 1999a. Immunization with recombinant *Helicobacter pylori* urease decreases colonization levels following experimental infection of rhesus monkeys. *Vaccine* 17:1493–1505

179. Lee CK, Soike K, Giannasca P, Hill J, Weltzin R. 1999b. Immunization of rhesus monkeys with a mucosal prime, parenteral boost strategy protects against infection with *Helicobacter pylori*. *Vaccine* 17:3072–82

180. Dubois A, Lee CK, Kleanthous H, Mehlman PT, Monath T. 1998. Immunization against natural *Helicobacter pylori* infection in nonhuman primates. *Infect. Immun.* 66:4340–46

181. Guy B, Hessler C, Fourage S, Lecoindre P, Chevalier M. 1997. Mucosal, systemic, or combined therapeutic immunization in cynomolgus monkeys naturally infected with *Gastrospirillum hominis*-like organisms. *Vaccine Res.* 6:141–50

182. Solnick JV, Canfield DR, Hansen LM, Torabian SZ. 2000. Immunization with recombinant *Helicobacter pylori* urease in specific-pathogen-free rhesus monkeys (*Macaca mulatta*). *Infect. Immun.* 68:2560–65

183. Rappuoli R. 1997. Rational design of vaccines. *Nature Med.* 3:374–76

184. Manetti R, Massari P, Marchetti M, Magagnoli C, Nuti S. 1997. Detoxification of *Helicobacter pylori* cytotoxin. *Infect. Immun.* 65:4615–19

185. Ferrero RL, Thiberge JM, Kansau I, Wuscher N, Huerre M, Labigne A. 1995. The GroES homolog of *Helicobacter pylori* confers protective immunity against mucosal infection in mice. *Proc. Natl. Acad. Sci. USA* 92:6499–6503

186. Ferrero RL, Thieberge JM, Labigne A. 1997. Local immunoglobulin G antibodies in the stomach may contribute to immunity against *Helicobacter* infection in mice. *Gastroenterology* 113:185–94

187. Yamaguchi H, Osaki T, Kai M, Taguchi H, Kamiya S. 2000. Immune response against a cross-reactive epitope on the heat shock protein 60 homologue of *Helicobacter pylori*. *Infect. Immun.* 68:3448–54

188. Radcliff FJ, Hazell SL, Kolesnikow T, Doidge C, Lee A. 1997. Catalase, a novel antigen for *Helicobacter pylori* vaccination. *Infect. Immun.* 65:4668–74

189. Dunkley ML, Harris SJ, McCoy RJ, Musicka MJ, Eyers FM. 1999. Protection against *Helicobacter pylori* infection by intestinal immunisation with a 50/52-kDa

subunit protein. *FEMS Immunol. Med. Microbiol.* 24:221–25

190. Blanchard TG, Lycke N, Czinn SJ, Nedrud JG. 1998. Recombinant cholera toxin B subunit is not an effective mucosal adjuvant for oral immunization of mice against *Helicobacter felis. Immunology* 93:22–27

191. Rappuoli R, Pizza M, Douce G, Dougan G. 1999. Structure and mucosal adjuvanticity of cholera and *Escherichia coli* heat-labile enterotoxins. *Immunol. Today* 20:493–500

192. Eaton KA, Ringler SS, Krakowka S. 1998. Vaccination of gnotobiotic piglets against *Helicobacter pylori. J. Infect. Dis.* 178:1399–1405

193. Pappo J, Thomas WD Jr, Kabok Z, Taylor NS, Murphy JC, Fox JG. 1995. Effect of oral immunization with recombinant urease on murine *Helicobacter felis* gastritis. *Infect. Immun.* 63:1246–52

194. Eaton KA, Ringler SS, Danon SJ. 1999. Murine splenocytes induce severe gastritis and delayed-type hypersensitivity and suppress bacterial colonization in *Helicobacter pylori*-infected SCID mice. *Infect. Immun.* 67:4594

195. Whary MT, Palley LS, Batchelder M, Murphy JC, Yan L. 1997. Promotion of ulcerative duodenatis in young ferrets by oral immunization with *Helicobacter mustelae* and muramyl dipeptide. *Helicobacter* 2:65–77

196. Herbrink P, van Doorn LJ. 2000. Serological methods for diagnosis of *Helicobacter pylori* infection and monitoring of eradication therapy. *Eur. J. Clin. Microbiol. Infect. Dis.* 19:164–73

197. Mattsson A, Quiding-Jarbrink M, Lonroth H, Hamlet A, Ahlstedt I, Svennerholm A. 1998. Antibody-secreting cells in the stomachs of symptomatic and asymptomatic *Helicobacter pylori* subjects. *Infect. Immun.* 66:2705–12

198. Czinn SJ, Bierman JC, Diters RW, Blanchard TJ, Leunk RD. 1996. Characteriza-

tion and therapy of experimental infection by *Helicobacter mustelae* in ferrets. *Helicobacter* 1:43–51

199. Batchelder M, Fox J, Hayward A, Yan L, Shames B. 1996. Natural and experimental *Helicobacter mustelae* reinfection following successful antimicrobial eradication in ferrets. *Helicobacter* 1:34–42

200. Kumagai T, Malaty HM, Graham DY, Hosogaya S, Misawa K. 1998. Acquisition versus loss of *Helicobacter pylori* infection in Japan: results from an 8-year birth cohort study. *J. Infect. Dis.* 178:717–21

201. Rothenbacher D, Bode G, Adler G, Brenner H. 1998. History of antibiotic treatment and prevalence of *H. pylori* infection among children: results of a population-based study. *J. Clin. Epidemiol.* 51:267–71

202. Neutra MR, Pringault E, Kraehenbuhl JP. 1996. Antigen sampling across epithelial barriers and induction of mucosal immune responses. *Annu. Rev. Immunol.* 14:275–300

203. Valnes K, Huitfeldt HS, Brandtzaeg P. 1990. Relation between T cell number and epithelial HLA class II expression quantified by image analysis in normal and inflamed gastric mucosa. *Gut* 31:647–52

204. Ye G, Barrera C, Fan X, Gourley WK, Crowe SE. 1997. Expression of B7-1 and B7-2 costimulatory molecules by human gastric epithelial cells. Potential role of CD4+ T cell activation during *Helicobacter pylori* infection. *J. Clin. Invest.* 99:1628–36

205. Archimandritis A, Sougioultzis S, Foukas PG, Tzivras M, Davaris P, Moutsopoulos HM. 2000. Expression of HLA-DR, costimulatory molecules B7-1, B7-2, intercellular adhesion molecule-1 (ICAM-1) and Fas ligand (FasL) on gastric epithelial cells in *Helicobacter pylori* gastritis. Influence of *H. pylori* eradication. *Clin. Exp. Immunol.* 119:464–71

206. Hatz RA, Meimarakis G, Bayerdorffer

E, Stolte M, Kirchner T, Enders G. 1996. Characterization of lymphocytic infiltrates in *Helicobacter pylori*-associated gastritis. *Scand. J. Gastroenterol.* 31:222–28

207. Terres AM, Pajares JM. 1998. An increased number of follicles containing activated CD69+ helper T cells and proliferating CD71+ B cells are found in *H. pylori*-infected gastric mucosa. *Am. J. Gastroenterol.* 93:579–83

208. Genta RM, Hamner HW, Graham DY. 1993. Gastric lymphoid follicles in *Helicobacter pylori* infection: frequency, distribution, and response to triple therapy. *Hum. Pathol.* 24:577–83

209. Mukhopadhyay P. 1999. Gastric cancer and lymphoma. *Curr. Top. Microbiol. Immunol.* 241:57–69

210. Sharma SA, Miller GG, Perez-Perez GI, Gupta RS, Blaser MJ. 1994. Humoral and cellular immune recognition of *Helicobacter pylori* proteins are not concordant. *Clin. Exp. Immunol.* 97:126–32

211. Sharma SA, Miller GG, Peek RA Jr, Perez-Perez G, Blaser MJ. 1997. T-cell, antibody, and cytokine responses to homologs of the 60-kilodalton heat shock protein in *Helicobacter pylori* infection. *Clin. Diagn. Lab. Immunol.* 4:440–46

212. Karttunen R, Karttunen T, Ekre HP, MacDonald TT. 1995. Interferon gamma and interleukin 4 secreting cells in the gastric antrum in *Helicobacter pylori* positive and negative gastritis. *Gut* 36:341–45

213. Karttunen RA, Karttunen TJ, Yosufi MM, el-Zimaity HM, Graham DY, el-Zaatari FA. 1997. Expression of mRNA for interferon-gamma, interleukin-10, and interleukin-12 (p40) in normal gastric mucosa and in mucosa infected with *Helicobacter pylori*. *Scand. J. Gastroenterol.* 32:22–27

214. Haeberle HA, Kubin M, Bamford KB, Garofalo R, Graham DY. 1997. Differential stimulation of interleukin-12 (IL-12) and IL-10 by live and killed *Heli-*

cobacter pylori in vitro and association of IL-12 production with gamma interferon-producing T cells in the human gastric mucosa. *Infect. Immun.* 65:4229–35

215. Berg DJ, Lynch NA, Lynch RG, Mauricella DM. 1998. Rapid development of severe hyperplastic gastritis with gastric epithelial dedifferentiation in *Helicobacter felis*-infected IL-10−/− mice. *Am. J. Pathol.* 152:1377–86

216. Smythies LE, Waites KB, Lindsey JR, Harris PR, Ghiara P, Smith PD. 2000. *Helicobacter pylori*-induced mucosal inflammation is Th1 mediated and exacerbated in IL-4, but not IFN-γ, gene-deficient mice. *J. Immunol.* 165:1022–29

217. Yamaoka Y, Kita M, Kodama T, Sawai N, Tanahashi T. 1998. Chemokines in the gastric mucosa in *Helicobacter pylori* infection. *Gut* 42:609–17

218. Jones NL, Day AS, Jennings HA, Sherman PM. 1999. *Helicobacter pylori* induces gastric epithelial cell apoptosis in association with increased Fas receptor expression. *Infect. Immun.* 67:4237–42

219. Houghton J, Macera-Bloch LS, Harrison L, Kim KH, Korah RM. 2000. Tumor necrosis factor alpha and interleukin 1β up-regulate gastric mucosal Fas antigen expression in *Helicobacter pylori* infection. *Infect. Immun.* 68:1189–95

220. Wang J, Fan X, Lindholm C, Bennett M, O'Connoll J. 2000. *Helicobacter pylori* modulates lymphoepithelial cell interactions leading to epithelial cell damage through Fas/Fas ligand interactions. *Infect. Immun.* 68:4303–11

221. Tosi MF, Czinn SJ. 1990. Opsonic activity of specific human IgG against *Helicobacter pylori*. *J. Infect. Dis.* 162:156–62

222. Cover TL, Cao P, Murphy UK, Sipple MS, Blaser MJ. 1992. Serum neutralizing antibody response to the vacuolating cytotoxin of *Helicobacter pylori*. *J. Clin. Invest.* 90:913–18

223. Blanchard TG, Czinn SJ, Maurer R, Thomas WD, Soman G, Nedrud JG.

1995. Urease-specific monoclonal antibodies prevent *Helicobacter felis* infection in mice. *Infect. Immun.* 63:1394–99

224. Nedrud J, Blanchard T, Czinn S, Harriman G. 1996. Orally-immunized IgA deficient mice are protected against *H. felis* infection. *Gut* 39 (Suppl. 2):A45

225. Mbawuike IN, Pacheco S, Acuna CL, Switzer KC, Zhang Y, Harriman GR. 1999. Mucosal immunity to influenza without IgA: an IgA knockout mouse model. *J. Immunol.* 162:2530–37

226. Bogstedt AK, Nava S, Wadstrom T, Hammarstrom L. 1996. *Helicobacter pylori* infection in IgA deficiency: lack of role for the secretory immune system. *Clin. Exp. Immunol.* 105:202–4

227. Blanchard TG, Czinn SJ, Redline RW, Sigmund N, Harriman G, Nedrud JG. 1999. Antibody-independent protective mucosal immunity to gastric Helicobacter infection in mice. *Cell. Immunol.* 191: 84

228. Kitamura D, Rose J, Kuehn R, Rajewski K. 1991. A B cell-deficient mouse by targeted disruption of the membrane exon of the immunoglobulin μ chain gene. *Nature* 350:423–26

229. Pappo J, Torrey D, Castriota L, Saviainen A, Kabok Z, Ibraghimov A. 1999. *Helicobacter pylori* infection in immunized mice lacking major histocompatibility complex class I and class II functions. *Infect. Immun.* 67:337–41

230. Radcliff FJ, Ramsay AJ, Lee A. 1996. Failure of immunization against *Helicobacter* infection in IL-4 deficient mice: evidence for a Th2 immune response as the bias for protective immunity. *Gastroenterology* 110:A997

231. Marinaro M, Staats HF, Hiroi T, Jackson RJ, Coste M. 1995. Mucosal adjuvant effect of cholera toxin in mice results from induction of T helper 2 (Th2) cells and IL-4. *J. Immunol.* 155:4621–29

232. Del Giudice G. 1992. New carriers and adjuvants in the development of vacciners. *Curr. Opin. Immunol.* 4:454–59

233. Michetti P, Kreiss C, Kotloff K, Porta N, Blanco JL. 1999. Oral immunization with urease and *Escherichia coli* heat-labile enterotoxin is safe and immunogenic in *Helicobacter pylori*-infected adults. *Gastroenterology* 116:804–12

234. Kreiss C, Buclin T, Cosma M, Corthésy-Theulaz I, Michetti P. 1996. Safety of oral immunization with recombinant urease in patients with *Helicobacter pylori* infection. *Lancet* 347:1630–31

235. Steere AC, Sikand VK, Meurice F, Parenti DL, Fikrig E. 1998. Vaccination against Lyme disease with recombinant *Borrelia burgdorferi* outer-surface lipoprotein A with adjuvant. Lyme disease vaccine study group. *N. Engl. J. Med.* 339:209–15

236. Sigal LH, Zahradnik JM, Lavin P, Patella SJ, Bryant G. 1998. A vaccine consisting of recombinant *Borrelia burgdorferi* outer-surface protein A to prevent Lyme disease. Recombinant outer-surface protein A Lyme disease vaccine study consortium. *N. Engl. J. Med.* 339:216–22

237. Di Petrillo MD, Tibbetts T, Kleanthous H, Killeen KP, Hohmann EL. 2000. Safety and immunogenicity of *phoP/phoQ*-deleted *Salmonella typhi* expressing *Helicobacter pylori* urease in adult volunteers. *Vaccine* 18:449–59

238. Kotloff K, Losonsky G, Wasserman S, Walker R. 1999. Safety and immunogenicity of a *Helicobacter pylori* vaccine in human volunteers. In Third Annual Winter *H. Pylori* Workshop, Orlando, FL, February 26–27, 1999, Poster no. 63

239. Levine MM. 1998. Experimental challenge studies in the development of vaccines for infectious diseases. *Dev. Biol. Stand.* 95:169–74

Annu. Rev. Immunol. 2001. 19:565–94

CTLA-4-MEDIATED INHIBITION IN REGULATION OF T CELL RESPONSES: Mechanisms and Manipulation in Tumor Immunotherapy

Cynthia A. Chambers,[1]* Michael S. Kuhns,[2]* Jackson G. Egen,*[2] and James P. Allison*[2]

[1]*University of Massachusetts Medical School, Worcester, Massachusetts 01655*

[2]*Howard Hughes Medical Institute, University of California, Berkeley Department of Molecular and Cell Biology, and the Cancer Research Laboratory, Berkeley, California 94720; e-mail: jallison@uclink4.berkeley.edu*

Key Words   cytotoxic T lymphocyte antigen-4 (CTLA-4), CD28, costimulation, T cell activation, T cell regulation

■ **Abstract**   The T cell compartment of adaptive immunity provides vertebrates with the potential to survey for and respond specifically to an incredible diversity of antigens. The T cell repertoire must be carefully regulated to prevent unwanted responses to self. In the periphery, one important level of regulation is the action of costimulatory signals in concert with T cell antigen-receptor (TCR) signals to promote full T cell activation. The past few years have revealed that costimulation is quite complex, involving an integration of activating signals and inhibitory signals from CD28 and CTLA-4 molecules, respectively, with TCR signals to determine the outcome of a T cell's encounter with antigen. Newly emerging data suggest that inhibitory signals mediated by CTLA-4 not only can determine whether T cells become activated, but also can play a role in regulating the clonal representation in a polyclonal response. This review primarily focuses on the cellular and molecular mechanisms of regulation by CTLA-4 and its manipulation as a strategy for tumor immunotherapy.

INTRODUCTION

The first definitive experimental demonstration that T cell antigen receptor (TCR) engagement was insufficient for T cell activation came from the work of Jenkins & Schwartz in the late 1980s (1). They clearly demonstrated that T cell clones that received only a TCR signal did not become activated but were induced into a state of antigen-specific unresponsiveness, or anergy. They showed that a second signal was required and that this costimulatory signal was provided

---

*These authors contributed equally and are listed in alphabetical order.

0732-0582/01/0407-0565$14.00   **565**

exclusively by a cell surface ligand restricted to cells which, for want of a better term, are called professional antigen-presenting cells (APC). Cells with potent costimulatory activity included dendritic cells, activated macrophages, and activated B cells. It was subsequently shown that naïve T cells had a similar requirement for these costimulatory signals in order to produce IL-2 and progress through the cell cycle. This requirement of T cells for costimulation, together with the sharp restriction of the costimulatory ligands to professional APC, was proposed to be a mechanism for maintenance of peripheral T cell tolerance. These observations and ideas naturally provoked considerable interest in the identity of the costimulatory molecules that could suffice, in addition to antigen receptor signals, to allow full activation of naïve T cells and prevent induction of anergy in T cell clones.

CD28 AND CTLA-4: Positive and Negative Costimulators

A considerable literature has developed demonstrating that interactions between the cell surface molecule CD28 and its counter receptor B7 on antigen presenting cells are the major, if not the only, source of costimulatory signals in the sense of the original definition (2). While the term costimulatory has in recent years come to be used as a general term to describe molecules whose engagement enhances T cell responses, it appears that many of these have their effect at later stages in the immune response by influencing cell survival, cytokine production, or other aspects important in elaboration, but not necessarily the initiation, of T cell responses. However, these do not fit the strict definition of signals that, in addition to TCR signals, influence IL-2 production and proliferation. This review focuses on the roles of the classical costimulatory molecules, one positive (CD28) and one inhibitory (CTLA-4; CD152), with a particular emphasis on the regulation of the early stages of the immune response by inhibitory costimulation. Further, it gives some examples of manipulation of these signals in the development of novel strategies for tumor immunotherapy.

The suggestion that CD28 may play an important role in costimulation came from in vitro experiments showing that its engagement could enhance IL-2 (3, 4). Subsequently it was shown that intact anti-CD28 antibodies could prevent the induction of anergy in T cell clones stimulated by chemically fixed APC, whereas Fab fragments of anti-CD28 resulted in induction of hyporesponsiveness in T cell clones stimulated by intact APC (5). In addition, anti-CD28 antibodies are sufficient to provide costimulation to naïve CD4$^+$ T cells stimulated by planar membranes containing purified MHC molecules (6). Engagement of the CD28 ligands B7-1 (CD80) and B7-2 (CD86) is critical for costimulation (7, 8). Antibodies to B7-1 or B7-2 diminished, and a combination of anti-B7-1 plus B7-2 or a CTLA-4-Ig fusion protein (see below) efficiently blocked T cell responses in a variety of in vitro and in vivo settings (9). Finally, evidence from knockout mice also demonstrated the importance of CD28/B7 interactions in T cell responses. While CD28$^{-/-}$ mice retained the ability to reject some viruses, most T cell responses were severely impaired (10). Subsequent work showed that the determining factor in responses that occur in the absence of CD28 may be the persistence of TCR signaling: repeated administration of antigenic peptides over a 48-h period supported responses in the absence of CD28, but in the absence of this sustained stimulation, T cells from CD28$^{-/-}$ mice failed to respond productively (11). The phenotype of B7-1/B7-2 double knockout mice was quite clear—T cell responses were essentially absent (12).

Very early in the story it became apparent that CD28 was not the only player. A homologue of CD28 named cytotoxic T lymphocyte antigen-4 (CTLA-4) had been previously identified in a subtractive approach directed toward identifying gene products important in the function of cytotoxic T lymphocytes (13). However, even after recognition of the important role of CD28 in costimulation, the role of CTLA-4 remained obscure. It was apparent that the molecules were not only homologous and genetically linked, but shared several intriguing properties, including genomic organization and the presence of a motif, MYPPY, that was implicated as important in ligand binding by CD28 (14). It was also shown that a soluble version of the CTLA-4 ectodomain fused to an immunoglobulin tail (CTLA-4-Ig), like CD28, bound to both B7-1 and B7-2 (15). In fact, binding of both B7-1 and B7-2 by CTLA-4 was of considerably higher affinity than that of CD28, by a factor of 50–2000-fold, depending on the method of analysis (14, 16). Unlike CD28, CTLA-4 mRNA was not readily detectable in naïve resting T cells but was induced by activation (13). Given that CD28 is constitutively expressed by all T cells and seemed to be sufficient and necessary for costimulation, an obvious and intriguing question was the biological role of a second receptor for B7 that was inducible and had an even higher affinity (17).

The role of CTLA-4 in the regulation of T cell responses began to become apparent with the generation of specific monoclonal antibodies. The early reports showed that CTLA-4 antibodies (providing cross-linking was not possible) did not costimulate T cells stimulated via the T cell receptor only, but could enhance proliferation and IL-2 production by cells stimulated by anti-CD3 along with anti-CD28 (18, 19). These findings, together with the observation that anti-B7 antibodies also had the effect of enhancing responses of T cells activated by anti-CD3 along with anti-CD28, suggested that the enhancement was a result of removal of inhibitory signals rather than provision of auxiliary costimulatory signals. This conclusion was also supported by the fact that co-cross-linking of CTLA-4 with CD28 and TCR antibodies resulted in an inhibition of T cell activation in vitro. Finally, the fact that anti-CD28 antibodies inhibited, whereas anti-CTLA-4 antibodies enhanced, T cell responses in vivo suggested that these reagents were blocking costimulatory and inhibitory signals, respectively (20, 21).

CTLA-4$^{-/-}$ Mice: The Importance of Brakes

The most dramatic evidence of the inhibitory function of CTLA-4 came from the knockout mice (22–24). CTLA-4-deficient mice develop a fatal lymphoproliferative disorder. T cell activation is detectable within 5–6 days after birth, and the mice die at 18–28 days of age due to lymphocytic infiltration into nonlymphoid tissues. This phenotype is one of the most aggressive lymphoproliferative disorders reported in gene-targeted mice. CTLA-4$^{-/-}$ mice die much earlier than those with defects in apoptotic pathways (*lpr* or *gld* mice) (25), cytokine signaling such as in mice with a T cell–specific defect in TGFβ signal transduction (26, 27), or targeted deletion of the inhibitory molecule PD-1 (28). The absence of CTLA-4 results in virtually all of the peripheral T cells displaying an activated phenotype (CD69$^+$, CD25$^+$, CD44^{hi}, CD45RB^{lo}, CD62L^{lo}) (22, 23) and an approximately fourfold increase in the proportion of T cells in cell cycle, as detected by BrdU incorporation, compared to age-matched littermate controls (29). T cells proliferate spontaneously for several days in vitro and secrete a variety of cytokines including IL-2, -4, -6, -3, and GM-CSF (22, 23). The absence of CTLA-4 appears to affect the CD4$^+$ and CD8$^+$ T cell subsets differentially, with CD4$^+$ T cells being preferentially activated at the onset of the lymphoproliferation (29). Although it has not been formally demonstrated, indirect evidence indicates that TCR/MHC engagement is necessary for the polyclonal T cell activation, including the down-regulation of the TCR expression levels on the T cells (22, 23), upregulation of CD69, and increased levels of phosphorylation of CD3ζ (30, 31). CD28/B7 interactions are also required for CTLA-4$^{-/-}$ T cell activation, since CTLA-4-Ig treatment from birth or the genetic absence of B7 ligands prevent T cell activation (29, 32–34). This is reversible, since cessation of CTLA-4Ig treatment results in the T cells rapidly becoming activated (32). The phenotype of the T cells and the failure to detect any defect in apoptosis suggest that there is continuous activation of the CTLA-4-deficient T cells in vivo.

One possible origin of the phenotype observed in the CTLA-4$^{-/-}$ mice is a defect in central tolerance (22, 23). Failure to negatively select thymocytes expressing TCRs with a high affinity for self-MHC and/or self-peptide would permit the emigration of highly autoreactive T cells to the periphery. However, thymocyte development appears normal in CTLA-4$^{-/-}$ mice expressing an unmanipulated repertoire (24), as well as in CTLA-4$^{-/-}$ mice bearing MHC class I- or class II-restricted transgenic TCRs (35–38). These results suggest that there is no defect in thymocyte development but rather that CTLA-4 is necessary for the regulation of peripheral T cell tolerance and homeostasis.

The lymphadenopathy that occurs in CTLA-4$^{-/-}$ mice appears to be initiated by CD4$^+$ T cells that are preferentially activated in young CTLA-4 $^{-/-}$ mice. Depletion of CD4$^+$ T cells from birth prevented the onset of lymphoproliferation (29). Restriction of the TCR repertoire by the introduction of MHC class II–restricted TCR transgenes delays, but does not prevent, the development of lymphoproliferative disease (37, 38). A predominant role for CD4$^+$ T cells in the lymphadenopathy was also supported by introduction of MHC class I–restricted TCR transgenes (35, 36). CTLA-4$^{-/-}$ mice bearing the HY, 2C, or an LCMV-specific TCR developed lymphoproliferative disorder that was a result of activation and expansion not of the predominant CD8$^+$ population, but rather of CD4$^+$ cells that presumably expressed endogenous TCR. Further restriction of the TCR repertoire in the CD4$^+$ T cells by introduction of the *rag-1* null mutation into the AND TCR Tg$^+$

CTLA-4$^{-/-}$ mice resulted in a considerable delay in the onset of, but did not prevent CD4$^+$ T cell activation (39).

TCR transgenic T cells from CTLA-4-deficient mice have been used to examine the role of CTLA-4 in the regulation of peptide-specific T cell responses. Naïve CD4$^+$ T cells from AND Tg$^+$Rag$^{-/-}$CTLA-4$^{-/-}$ mice had a moderately enhanced proliferative response upon primary stimulation as compared to comparable cells from wild-type mice (37). Upon restimulation of resting, previously activated T cells, however, there was a much more dramatic increase in the magnitude of the response of the CTLA-4-deficient T cells. This enhanced response was evident at the level of proliferation, bulk cytokine secretion, and frequency of cytokine secreting T cells (37). In both cases, the differences were more pronounced at the high end of the dose response. An increased secondary response in the absence of CTLA-4 was also observed in the proliferative and cytokine responses of 4-day blasts of CD4$^+$ T cells expressing the DO.11.10 TCR (38).

A role for CTLA-4 in regulation of CD8$^+$ T cell responses has been controversial. The observations that naïve CD8$^+$ T cells from CTLA-4$^{-/-}$ mice bearing a transgene specific for an MHC class I–restricted epitope of LCMV have no alterations in response to primary peptide stimulation in vitro or in the ability to resolve LCMV infection in vivo led to the proposal that CTLA-4 does not regulate CD8$^+$ T cell responses (40). However, the results in this system may not reflect all situations. For example, the response of wild-type and CTLA-4-deficient T cells bearing the 2C TCR are essentially identical upon primary stimulation in vitro. However, upon secondary stimulation the CTLA-4-deficient cells exhibit a marked increase in the magnitude of both the proliferative and cytokine responses, an effect that was most pronounced at the high end of the dose response curve (36). As is discussed below, experiments using CTLA-4 blockade in vivo also support a direct role in the regulation of CD8$^+$ T cell responses.

These results suggest two features of CTLA-4 regulation of T cell responses. First, consistent with the fact that it is expressed by both CD4$^+$ and CD8$^+$ T cells, CTLA-4 can play a role in attenuating the response of both. Second, the observation that the effects of the absence of CTLA-4 are most evident in secondary responses suggests that the activational history of the T cell will influence the role of CTLA-4. It is unclear if this simply occurs due to the fact that previously activated T cells express higher basal levels of CTLA-4 compared to naïve T cells (41, 42) and/or if previously activated T cells are more responsive to CTLA-4 signals. Differential sensitivity of T cells to CTLA-4-mediated costimulation would have obvious implications for the generation and maintenance of memory T cells, and the induction of memory responses.

CTLA-4 Regulates Cell Cycle Progression, Not Cell Death

Taken together, these data provide a strong case for CTLA-4 as a crucial negative regulator of T cell responses in the periphery. The process by which this regulation occurs is clearly distinct from activation-induced cell death. An early experiment cross-linking CTLA-4 on human T cell clones suggested that CTLA-4 inhibits

T cell responses by inducing apoptosis (43). Similarly, cross-linking CTLA-4 on mouse ConA T cell blasts was reported to induce apoptosis (44). Conversely, there is no evidence that CTLA-4 ligation in conjunction with TCR and CD28 cross-linking on resting murine T cells induces apoptosis (45–48). Further, CTLA-4 ligation does not alter the CD28-mediated upregulation of survival factor bcl-x (49), arguing against apoptosis induction being the major mechanism of CTLA-4 inhibition. In addition, no defect in Fas/FasL-mediated apoptosis has been observed in T cells deficient in CTLA-4 (22, 50). It seems likely that the induction of apoptosis in experiments utilizing human T cell blasts and clones may have been an indirect result of cytokine deprivation as a result of CTLA-4-mediated inhibition of IL-2 secretion, rather than direct induction of apoptosis.

The fact that CTLA-4 deficiency is lethal relatively early in life and that the Fas pathway is intact indicates that CTLA-4 can play a critical role in limiting T cell expansion. CTLA-4 has effects on at least two aspects of activation that have critical relevance to proliferation. The first is on IL-2 production. CD28 costimulation enhances IL-2 production both at the level of transcription and mRNA stabilization (51, 52). Extensive ligation of CTLA-4 under suboptimal conditions of stimulation by TCR plus CD28 can result in inhibition of IL-2 production, probably at the level of transcription (45, 46, 53). CTLA-4 ligation does not prevent IL-2 from causing degradation of the cell cycle inhibitor $p27^{kip}$, but does inhibit TCR-induced production of cdk4, cdk6, and cyclin D3, all of which are required for G0/G1 progression (53). Thus CTLA-4 can limit expansion not only by reducing production of an important growth factor, but also by inhibiting TCR-mediated induction and assembly of essential components of the cell cycle machinery.

THE CELL BIOLOGY OF COSTIMULATION

Protein trafficking and localization during the process of T cell activation is thought to play a major role in the ability of a protein to regulate the T cell response. The finding that CTLA-4 and CD28 deliver opposing signals to the T cell yet bind the same ligands on APCs suggests that a balance may exist between the signals generated by these two molecules. Shifting this balance in one direction or another could influence to what extent an individual T cell becomes activated. It is likely that one mechanism of controlling the function of CTLA-4 and CD28 involves their differential trafficking to the T cell–APC interface, where these molecules interact with their B7 ligands.

While CTLA-4 and CD28 are homologous molecules, they have very different lifestyles (for brief reviews, see 17). CD28 is constitutively expressed on the surface of T cells, with levels increasing slightly upon activation. CTLA-4 is not readily detectable in naïve T cells but is rapidly upregulated upon T cell activation. CTLA-4 mRNA can be readily detected within 1 h of TCR engagement and peaks at about 24–36 h (54). CTLA-4 is not readily detectable at the cell surface until 24–48 h after activation (18). However, an accurate assessment of the kinetics of CTLA-4 protein expression is complicated by the fact that it is not primarily expressed at the cell surface.

Surface expression of CTLA-4 is tightly regulated as a result of the presence of a tyrosine-based intracellular localization motif in its cytoplasmic tail (55). This motif results in both the rapid endocytosis of CTLA-4 from the cell surface to endosomal compartments, as well as the targeting of at least some CTLA-4 to the lysosomes for degradation (56, 57). It is unclear whether endocytosed CTLA-4 can recycle back to the surface or if this represents a terminal pathway for the protein. Through the use of a yeast-two-hybrid screen to search for proteins that bound to the unphosphorylated tail of CTLA-4, several groups demonstrated an association with the medium subunit of the clathrin-coated pit adaptor complex, AP2, thus providing a mechanism for CTLA-4 cellular localization (58–61). CTLA-4 expression on the T cell surface is stabilized and increased by tyrosine phosphorylation of the endocytosis motif, which inhibits AP2 association. It is noteworthy that the intracellular portion of CTLA-4 is 100% conserved among many different species of animals, suggesting that control of intracellular trafficking may be extremely important for its function. Indeed, a recent report proposed that the T cell lymphoproliferative disorder in the human disease Chediak-Higashi syndrome was a result of defective CTLA-4 trafficking and localization (62).

It has been reported that upon antibody cross-linking CD28 may also associate with PI3K and be shuttled into intracellular compartments to be degraded and/or recycled (63). However, since CD28 cell surface expression does not vary markedly following T cell activation, the functional importance of this internalization is unclear (42, 64).

Upon focal engagement of the TCR by antibody-coated beads, slides, or allogeneic cells, the bulk of intracellular CTLA-4 within an activated cell is reorganized toward sites facing TCR engagement (65). This finding is not unexpected given experiments showing reorganization of the microtubule organizing center, and all of its associated membrane structures, toward sites facing T cell interactions with APC (66). However, whether the localization of intracellular CTLA-4 beneath the T cell-APC contact site is accompanied by surface expression and phosphorylation-induced surface stabilization of CTLA-4 remains unclear. In addition, the source of CTLA-4 that localizes to the T cell–APC interface is unknown. Long-lasting intracellular stores of CTLA-4 may be rapidly mobilized to the T cell–APC interface upon antigen encounter, as well as newly translated CTLA-4 leaving the *trans*-Golgi Network.

MOLECULAR MECHANISMS OF COSTIMULATION

Despite considerable interest and effort, the mechanisms by which CD28 and CTLA-4 exert their effects remain poorly understood. Several models for CD28 signal transduction have been proposed. An extensive and detailed discussion of the literature is beyond the scope of this review, but the proposed pathways for CD28 costimulation can be grouped into three broad categories. Based on the identification of unique CD28-responsive elements in the IL-2 promoter, it has been proposed that CD28 utilizes a signaling pathway distinct from that of the TCR and induces a unique transcription factor (67). Alternatively, it has been proposed that CD28-mediated signals converge distally with the TCR signaling pathways, possibly at the level of JUN-kinase (68) and synergize in the induction of multiple transcription factors. Based on visualization of T cell activation by a number of laboratories (69–72), there is a new and growing appreciation for the physical changes that occur spatially during T cell activation. The plasma membrane reorganizes to form cholesterol-rich rafts of proteins involved in T cell signaling (73), and CD28 may play a critical role in recruitment of these rafts to the T cell/APC interface (72). Collectively these observations have led to a new model of T cell activation. In this model, the CD28 and TCR-mediated signals intersect proximally and act synergistically to enhance the TCR signaling pathway.

Examination of the consequences of CTLA-4-ligation in conjunction with TCR and CD28-mediated signals have provided data consistent with this model of the integration of TCR and costimulatory signals. A number of proteins known to play a role in various signaling pathways including TCR signals have been reported to bind to CD28 and CTLA-4 cytoplasmic tails (74). However, controversy over the proteins and the potential substrates involved in the biochemical signal transduction pathways for costimulatory molecules remains. The details of the mechanism or mechanisms by which CTLA-4 inhibition occurs are even more unclear. Several possibilities have been proposed including direct effects on phosphorylation levels and/or indirect effects due to competition with CD28 for ligand, sequestration of signaling molecules, or disruption of signaling complexes.

The observation that many proteins known to be involved in T cell signaling were hyperphosphorylated in CTLA-4$^{-/-}$ T cells led to the notion that CTLA-4 might decrease CD3/CD28-mediated phosphorylation by the recruitment of phosphatases (31). One candidate was the protein tyrosine phosphatase SHP-1, which is involved in transducing inhibitory signals initiated by NK receptors (75). SHP-1 binds to a phosphorylated polypeptide of the CTLA-4 cytoplasmic tail (61). However, normal levels of SHP-1 are not required for CTLA-4-mediated inhibition (76). Another protein tyrosine phosphatase, SHP-2, associates with the cytoplasmic tail of CTLA-4 and it has been proposed that catalytically active SHP-2 binds to the SH2-binding domain (YxxM motif) in the CTLA-4 cytoplasmic tail (30, 31) following phosphorylation of the motif by the src family kinase p56^{lck} (60, 77). However, there is conflicting data regarding whether SHP-2 binds directly to CTLA-4 (30, 78) and, if so, whether there is a requirement for phosphorylation of the YxxM tyrosine (30, 31, 61, 77, 78). Further, SHP-2 was reported to bind to phosphorylated peptides corresponding to the cytoplasmic tails of CD28 as well as CTLA-4 in pull-down assays (61). Thus, while the accumulated data suggests a role for SHP-2 in signaling, its role in CTLA-4-mediated inhibition remains to be definitively established.

Several other proteins have been reported to associate with CTLA-4. JAK2 associates with the proline-rich box1-like domain of the cytoplasmic tail of

CTLA-4, and this kinase may phosphorylate the tyrosine in the YxxM motif of the CTLA-4 tail (79). Most recently it has been reported that the serine/threonine phosphatases PP2A and PP6 bind to the phosphorylated YxxM motif of CTLA-4 and to the similar motif in the CD28 cytoplasmic tail (80). What proteins are required for CTLA-4 signal transduction remains unclear. Because the phosphorylation status of the tyrosine in the YxxM motif also regulates CTLA-4 intracellular localization, it has been difficult to separate the regulation of CTLA-4 intracellular trafficking versus signal transduction.

Despite the confusion concerning the specific role of the YxxM motif, and the identity and the role of proteins involved, some evidence implicating a role for tyrosine phosphatase activity has been reported. CTLA-4 cross-linking on recently activated T cell blasts resulted in a decrease in the level of tyrosine phosphorylation of proximal T cell signaling molecules such as CD3ζ (30). This offers a compelling scenario for CTLA-4 mediated inhibitionn of proximal steps in TCR signaling. CTLA-4 cross-linking was also found to inhibit downstream activation events including the phosphorylation of ERK and JUN-N-terminal kinase (30, 81). Identification of potential substrates for the tyrosine and serine/threonine phosphatases, and how these proteins function in the integration of CTLA-4, CD28, and TCR signal transduction, awaits further experiments but offers interesting possibilities.

Evidence that CTLA-4 might function at least in part by competing with CD28 for B7 ligands and thereby acting as an indirect attenuator of costimulatory signals comes from both in vitro and in vivo systems. Experiments utilizing T cell transfectants of CTLA-4 with mutations or truncations suggest that the CTLA-4 cytoplasmic tail is not always necessary for the inhibitory function of CTLA-4 (82–84). Competition may be most effective when B7 levels are low, but direct signaling through the tail seems to be necessary if B7 levels are high (83). Constitutive expression of high levels of a tailless CTLA-4 mutant on the cell surface delayed but did not prevent T cell activation and lymphoproliferation in CTLA-4$^{-/-}$ mice, indicating that competition for B7 ligands is not sufficient for normal CTLA-4 function (85).

CTLA-4 may also function by physically disturbing the assembly or organization of molecules in the synapse. This could occur by sequestration of proteins involved in signal transduction away from the immunological synapse, thereby reducing the resultant signaling. An alternative mechanism is suggested by the recently solved structures of B7-1 and CTLA-4 (86, 87). Both molecules are dimers, and the structures suggest that one CTLA-4 homodimer may bind two B7 molecules and form a very stable multimeric complex. This mode of binding, combined with the higher avidity of CTLA-4 than CD28 for B7 molecules, leads to the suggestion that the formation of stable CTLA-4/B7 lattices in the immunological synapse may disrupt the organized assembly of key components involved in the generation of TCR/CD28 signals (86, 87). The possibility of disruption of the synapse as a method of inhibition is especially intriguing, and could account for many of the functional observations.

A final possibility for an indirect mode of action of CTLA-4 is that CTLA-4 engagement costimulates the secretion of inhibitory cytokines, such as TGFβ (48). This more global and indirect effect is discussed below.

A schematic representation of trafficking and possible signal transduction mechanisms is shown in Figure 1 (see color insert).

DYNAMIC INTEGRATION OF TCR AND COSTIMULATORY SIGNALS

As previously discussed, CD28 is constitutively expressed on T cells, whereas CTLA-4 appears after activation. Because of this, and perhaps as a result of our innate appreciation for symmetry, the idea arose that CD28 engagement allowed initiation, while CTLA-4 provided for termination of immune responses (87g). Surprisingly, the majority of the in vitro data has demonstrated an inhibitory role for CTLA-4 in the early stages of T cell activation. A summary of the effects of CTLA-4 ligation on early events in T cell activation are summarized in Table 1. As can be seen, IL-2 production, expression of early markers such as CD69 and CD25, and a number of other aspects of activation are inhibited upon CTLA-4 cross-linking. These events take place within hours of T cell activation with anti-CD3 and CD28. In fact, the inhibition of the induction of IL-2 transcription was detected 4 h after stimulation (53). This suggests either that there is a physiologically relevant intracellular pool of CTLA-4 present in naïve T cells or that protein expression is induced rapidly upon activation.

Appreciation for the possibility that CTLA-4 can inhibit early stages of T cell activation has led to the development of models that stress that the dynamic interplay of costimulatory and TCR signals depends on the activation state of the T cell as well as the activation state of the antigen-presenting cell (88). Such a model is shown in Figure 2 (see color insert). As in the classical two-signal model, an encounter of a naïve T cell with a cell expressing appropriate MHC/antigen complex but lacking B7 does not result in activation of the T cell owing to lack of costimulation. The cells receiving a TCR signal in the absence of CD28-mediated costimulation may be rendered anergic. However, engagement of the TCR can lead to rapid induction and/or mobilization of small amounts of CTLA-4. Under conditions where there is an incompletely activated APC expressing only low amounts of B7, CTLA-4 could, by virtue of its higher affinity, outcompete CD28 for B7 and/or deliver inhibitory signals. This could effectively raise the threshold of CD28 and/or TCR signals needed for full activation. However, when a T cell encounters an antigen on a fully activated antigen-presenting cell expressing high amounts of B7, the scant amount of CTLA-4 induced after TCR engagement would become limiting. This would leave B7 available to engage CD28, allowing costimulation, IL-2 production, and proliferation of the T cells. One consequence of this activation would be further induction of CTLA-4, which could serve to terminate the response or attenuate it in more subtle ways, e.g. by limiting the burst size of the activated T cell.

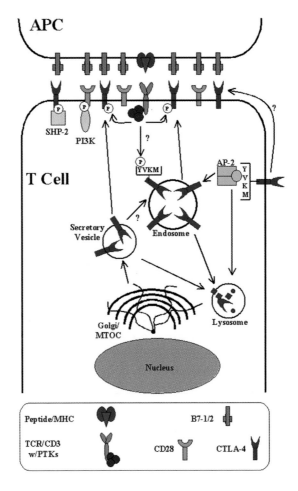

Figure 1 Protein trafficking of CTLA-4 in T cells. Newly translated CTLA-4 emerging from the Golgi apparatus in secretory vesicles may traffic to endosomal compartments or directly to the cell surface. Upon TCR stimulation, the Microtubule Organizing Center (MTOC) relocates to a site facing the APC, thereby polarizing associated compartments such as endosomes and the Golgi apparatus. This allows for directed secretion of CTLA-4 to the T cell-APC interface. Once at the interface the intracellular localization motif of CTLA-4 may be phosphorylated by protein tyrosine kinases (PTKs) associated with the TCR, resulting in surface-stabilization of CTLA-4 by inhibiting association with the clathrin-coated pit adaptor protein AP-2. This phosphorylated CTLA-4 may then interact with SH2 domain containing proteins such as the phosphatase SHP-2 and/or physically disrupt the assembly of molecules at the immunological synapse. Alternatively, unphosphorylated CTLA-4 will associate with AP-2 and enter the endosomal pathway where it may recycle back to the T cell surface or traffic to lysosomes for degradation. Further complexities of CTLA-4 trafficking are shown.

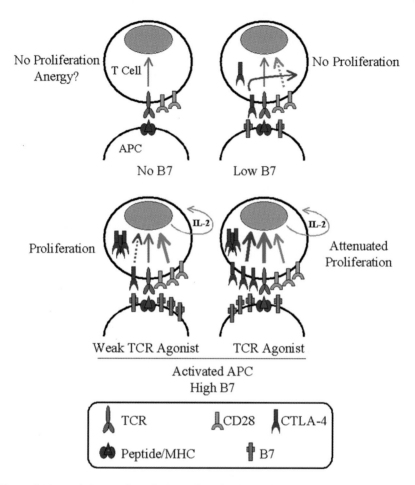

Figure 2 Dynamic integration of TCR and costimulatory signals. The contribution of signals generated by the T cell antigen receptor (TCR), CD28, and CTLA-4 depends on the activation state of the T cell as well as the nature and activation state of the antigen presenting cell (APC). TCR engagement in the absence of B7 expression by an APC, does not result in proliferation and may induce anergy. However, if the T cell encounters an APC expressing low levels of B7, rapidly induced CTLA-4 can compete with CD28 for B7 binding and/or deliver inhibitory signals which prevent T cell activation. Under conditions where the APC is activated and expressing high levels of B7, CD28 costimulation may dominate and activation proceeds. However, this results in induction and/or mobilization of CTLA-4 that may be proportional to the strength of the TCR signal, resulting in differential inhibition. Importantly, the proliferation of T cells receiving agonist signals may still be greater than cells receiving weak agonist signals due to differences in the ability of these ligands to induce T cell activation. Therefore, TCR signals may directly regulate the balance between activating and inhibitory costimulatory signals thereby determining the outcome of T cell interactions with APC.

For the purposes of a reductionist and admittedly oversimplified discussion, it is useful to consider the impact of CTLA-4 expression and function under two extreme situations: (*a*) Where B7 levels are low and TCR signals are weak, the amount of CTLA-4 induced is low but may be sufficient to minimize costimulation and prevent activation. Under these conditions CTLA-4 may set a threshold for activation. (*b*) Where B7 levels are high and TCR signals strong, the higher levels of CTLA-4 induced after activation may be able to attenuate the response of activated cells at relatively early stages of the response (Figure 2, see color insert).

Threshold Model

There are two scenarios in which CTLA-4 may play a role in establishing a threshold for CD28 and/or TCR signals needed for activation of naïve T cells. Both presume that low levels of CTLA-4 pre-exist or can be rapidly induced in naïve T cells upon engagement of the TCR and CD28. Due to the exponential expansion of T cells that follows activation, CTLA-4 need only have a very subtle effect on T cell activation threshold to have a large impact on the magnitude of the T cell response in vivo.

The first scenario suggests a role for CTLA-4 in maintaining peripheral tolerance of T cells with specificity for tissue-specific antigens that are not expressed in the thymus and have not been deleted as a consequence of negative selection. This is essentially the same context in which the two-signal model originally proposed that the absence of costimulatory ligands from all but very specialized APC would provide a fail-safe mechanism for self-tolerance (1). CTLA-4 may provide additional level of regulation to ensure peripheral tolerance by preventing activation when a T cell encounters a normal self-antigen in the context of low B7, as discussed above. This scenario may explain the observation that CTLA-4 blockade or deficiency accelerates the onset and severity of insulitis and diabetes in nonobese diabetic (NOD) mice expressing a transgenic $\alpha\beta$ TCR cloned from an islet-β-cell-specific CD4$^+$ T cell clone isolated from a NOD mouse (89, 90). T cells bearing this TCR are efficiently selected, rather than deleted in the thymus, demonstrating that central tolerance is not effective for T cells with this specificity. The observation that blockade or loss of CTLA-4 dramatically accelerates disease in this model system is a testament to the significance of CTLA-4 in limiting autoreactive T cells bearing TCRs specific to autoantigens. It is possible that CTLA-4 could also similarly regulate T cell activation in response to low levels of foreign antigens in the absence of inflammation-mediated upregulation of B7 on activated APC.

The second scenario deals with the regulation of the response of T cells to tonic signaling by self-peptide/MHC interactions. The idea that T cells are regularly stimulated by such signals was initially suggested by the observation that the TCRζ chain is partially phosphorylated in freshly isolated, unstimulated T cells (91). These continuous TCR interactions with self-peptide/MHC provide important signals to the T cells, although there is some controversy about whether these are necessary for T cell survival, homeostasis, or readiness for activation (92–94).

Some of these tonic interactions, under conditions of low levels of CD28/B7 interaction, might be sufficiently stimulatory to lead to the activation of CD4$^+$ T cells and the induction and/or mobilization of CTLA-4. Based on the analysis of the CTLA-4$^{-/-}$ mice and the kinetic properties of CTLA-4 and CD28 interactions with B7 molecules, we have speculated that CTLA-4 might prevent the signals generated by these interactions from leading to full activation of CD4$^+$ T cells but would enable the T cells to receive partial signals (29). Full T cell activation could be prevented by mechanisms described earlier. In this scenario, due to limiting B7 levels, competition for ligand may be the primary mechanism of action, and CTLA-4 will predominantly affect the CD28-mediated signals. Thus, we propose that CTLA-4 is involved in maintaining naïve CD4$^+$ T cells and previously activated T cells in a resting state.

This model is supported by several observations with the CTLA-4$^{-/-}$ mice. First, the expansion of T cells that occurs in these mice is polyclonal, as assessed by Vβ repertoire analysis and TCR α and β CDR3 spectratyping (22, 24, 95). This suggests that the expansion may not be a result of a failure to terminate responses to a few environmental pathogens. It is also consistent with the observation that the phenotype of the mice is independent of the peripheral peptide repertoire. For example, H-2M$\alpha^{-/-}$ mice display a very restricted peptide repertoire that seems to be entirely of self-origin (96, 97). Despite the restricted peptide repertoire, CD4$^+$CTLA-4$^{-/-}$ T cells become activated in H-2M$\alpha^{-/-}$ mice (CA Chambers, JP Allison, unpublished results). Results of experiments using transgenes to restrict the TCR repertoire are mixed. The results from mice expressing restricted TCR repertoires are consistent with there being an initial preferential activation of CD4$^+$ T cells in vivo (35–37). However, there is a lag in the development of the phenotype and expansion is primarily of CD4$^+$ MHC class II–restricted TCR Tg$^+$ and T cells expressing endogenous TCR chains (36, 38). In mice that also bear the *rag*-1$^{-/-}$ mutation, T cell activation is delayed longer, and there is no dramatic lymphoproliferation (39). This result is on first glance not consistent with the threshold scenario. However, it is unclear whether this effect is due to defects in the RAG-1$^{-/-}$ mice, such as alterations in the splenic and lymph node architecture. Finally, the threshold model would predict that an alternative source of a dominant inhibitory signal should rescue the phenotype. Consistent with this, Ly49A expression on CTLA-4$^{-/-}$ T cells delays and reduces lymphoproliferation and T cell activation in the presence of the appropriate MHC class I allele (98).

Attenuation Model

The scenarios presented above would occur primarily when T cells are weakly stimulated under conditions of limited B7. The dynamic integration model holds that when B7 levels are high, CD28-mediated costimulation overwhelms the inhibitory effects of low levels of CTLA-4, allowing T cell activation to proceed. However, CTLA-4 can have an effect on regulating early T cell responses primed by activated APCs when B7 levels are high.

Regulation of T cell responses primed under inflammatory conditions by CTLA-4 has been demonstrated in in vivo systems using anti-CTLA-4 antibodies or Fab fragments to disrupt CTLA-4/B7 interactions. The first report employed an adoptive transfer system to study a monoclonal $CD4^+$ T cell response primed with the agonist ligand in adjuvant (20). Blockade of CTLA-4 resulted in increased numbers of transferred cells at the peak of the response. The kinetics of expansion and contraction were similar between anti-CTLA-4 and control treated animals, suggesting that CTLA-4 may have affected the expansive phase but did not affect termination of the response. This study did not distinguish between effects on the proliferative capacity or the frequency of responders in the transferred pool, or both. Nevertheless, the data demonstrated a role for CTLA-4 in regulating the magnitude of a T cell response to a strong agonist signal under inflammatory conditions.

CTLA-4 also regulates antigen-specific polyclonal T cell responses. Experimental autoimmune encephalomyelitis (EAE), a murine model system of multiple sclerosis (MS), has been widely used for these studies. EAE is induced in susceptible strains by immunization of animals with myelin sheath-derived proteins or peptide antigens in adjuvant. This primes autoreactive $CD4^+$ T cells that differentiate to a Th1 phenotype and mediate demyelination. Blockade of CTLA-4 enhances disease (99–101) and is associated with an increased frequency of inflammatory lesions in the CNS (101), enhanced secretion of pro-inflammatory cytokines (99, 100), and increased proliferative responses to antigen stimulation in vitro (99). CTLA-4 also plays a critical role in regulating relapsing EAE mediated by T cell responses to myelin epitopes distinct from the disease-inducing epitope (99, 102). This process of relapse by epitope spreading was enhanced if CTLA-4 was blocked during the initial priming or the acute phase of disease. Enhanced relapse was also associated with increased in vitro proliferation to the relapse-associated antigens (102).

Blockade of CTLA-4 in tumor models has provided additional evidence for a role of CTLA-4 in attenuation of antigen-specific polyclonal T cell responses. As is discussed in more detail below, rejection of weakly immunogenic tumors can be accomplished by concomitant administration of anti-CTLA-4 along with tumor vaccines expressing GM-CSF, presumably by enhancing T cell cross-priming by activated host APC (103–105). Interestingly, anti-CTLA-4/tumor vaccine treatment resulted in tissue-specific autoimmunity in the melanoma and prostate systems (104, 105). CTLA-4 blockade also enhances $CD8^+$ T cell responses primed in vivo by GM-CSF activated peptide-pulsed dendritic cells, even in the absence of helper T cells (106).

The mechanisms by which CTLA-4 regulates polyclonal T cell responses in the systems discussed above are likely to be complex. In the context of the integrated three signal model, if the potential for CD28/B7 interactions is not limiting, the remaining critical parameters for the activation of any given antigen-specific T cell are: (a) the quantity of TCR signals, which is a function largely of peptide/MHC (pMHC) density on the APC; (b) the quality of TCR signals, which is a function of the affinity and duration of TCR/pMHC interactions; and (*c*) the level of expression and, perhaps more importantly, the cellular localization of CTLA-4.

It has been speculated that the threshold mechanism may also apply to responses primed by activated APC (101, 102, 104). If so, CTLA-4 most likely sets a threshold for the quantity and/or quality of TCR signals necessary for T cell activation and would affect clonal representation in the response by lowering the number of T cells bearing low-affinity TCRs. Thus, the enhanced T cell responses observed in these systems would be as a result of increased recruitment of T cells bearing low-affinity TCRs into the responding pool.

An alternative model is that CTLA-4 preferentially attenuates the expansion of T cells that have been strongly acivated (197). This notion is supported by the observation that proliferation of naïve CD4$^+$ TCR transgenic T cells stimulated by agonist peptide is most tightly regulated by CTLA-4 at high ligand density (37). Additionally it has been suggested that CTLA-4 preferentially regulates T cells bearing TCRs that bind pMHC with high stability/affinity (107). CTLA-4 would prevent this high-affinity population from dominating the primed pool by restricting proliferation early in the response. Engagement of CTLA-4 would then serve to broaden the pool of T cells by limiting clonal representation of the high-affinity population, thus allowing more equal representation of the cells bearing lower affinity TCRs in the early stages of the clonal evolution of the response.

Predictions of the threshold and attenuation models were tested in two in vivo systems under conditions where costimulation by B7 would not be limiting. Adoptive transfer experiments using CD4$^+$ TCR transgenic T cells were performed to examine the effects of CTLA-4-blockade on the proliferative capacity, or average number of daughter cells per responder, for cells primed with agonist or weak agonist peptides in adjuvant. Blockade significantly increased the proliferative capacity of T cells primed with the agonist ligand but had a minimal effect on the cells responding to the weak agonist peptide. In normal, unmanipulated mice, blockade of CTLA-4 increased not only the frequency, but also the overall affinity of a polyclonal population of antigen-specific CD4$^+$ T cells primed with peptide in adjuvant (MS Kuhns, PA Savage, JG Egen, MM Davis, JA Allison, manuscript in preparation). These results suggest that CTLA-4 preferentially regulates the proliferation of T cells receiving strong agonist signals.

A variety of mechanisms could explain the ability of CTLA-4 to preferentially act on the high-affinity population of T cell responders. The most straightforward of these mechanisms would be that CTLA-4 expression is upregulated to highest levels in those cells receiving the strongest TCR signal. While differential expression of CTLA-4 probably does impact a T cell response, there is no evidence that the absolute level of CTLA-4 expression correlates with function (108).

Another, more subtle mechanism that could explain preferential regulation of the high-affinity T cells by CTLA-4 would be a correlation between strength of TCR signal and the extent of CTLA-4 localization to sites of T cell contact with APC. Thus, a certain strength of TCR signal would be needed to achieve localization of critical levels of CTLA-4 at the immunological synapse. As previously discussed, the majority of intracellular CTLA-4 polarizes toward sites facing T cell contact (65). Recent studies indicate that this polarization can occur under conditions where the T cell receives either agonist or weak agonist signals. This is not an unexpected result, given that any TCR signal sufficient for MTOC reorganization will result in relocalization of associated intracellular membrane compartments (66). However, localization of CTLA-4 to the T cell–APC interface was not directly related to the polarization of intracellular stores of CTLA-4. Significantly, translocation of CTLA-4 to the immunological synapse primarily occurred when previously activated T cells were stimulated by strong agonist peptide, and to a much lesser extent when stimulated by weak agonist peptide. CD28 localization was comparable in response to both stimuli (JG Egen, JA Allison, manuscript in preparation). Thus, it appears that translocation of CTLA-4 into the synapse correlates with the strength of TCR signals.

The dynamic integration model of T cell activation originally proposed that T cell activation upregulated CTLA-4, which would then terminate the response when antigen was encountered again. As this model evolves in light of new data, it appears that increased CTLA-4 expression upon activation modulates T cell responses differentially and might serve to limit the burst size of responding T cells. Overall, these results suggest that the quality of the TCR signal is critical to determining if and/or how dramatically CTLA-4 regulates the proliferative capacity of any antigen-specific clone selected from the T cell repertoire. While the TCR and CD28 might primarily determine the range of T cells responding to antigen, CTLA-4 would limit clonal representation of those T cells with high-affinityTCRs. As discussed below, this may have implications for the type and ultimate outcome of a T cell response primed under inflammatory conditions.

CTLA-4 IN T HELPER SUBSET DIFFERENTIATION

It has been proposed that CD28 directs Th2 differentiation (2), whereas CTLA-4 serves to counter CD28 by preventing Th2 differentiation and thus promoting Th1 differentiation (38). The primary evidence linking CTLA-4 to the prevention of Th2 differentiation is that $CD4^+ TCR Tg^+ CTLA-4^{-/-}$ T cells produced IL-4, while CTLA-4 expressing littermate control cells produced IFN-γ upon secondary in vitro stimulation (38). Similarly, IL-4 was produced during secondary stimulation of $CD4^+$ T cells if CTLA-4 had been blocked by anti-CTLA-4 Fab fragments during priming, but production was limited if anti-CTLA-4 antibodies were used to cross-link CTLA-4 (109). In addition, blockade of CTLA-4 during activation by SEB in vivo resulted in enhanced Th2 responses (110). Likewise, Th2 responses to *Nippostrongylus brasiliensis* were enhanced by CTLA-4 blockade (111).

In contrast, blockade of CTLA-4 facilitated resistance to *Leishmania major* in susceptible Balb/c mice by enhancing Th1 responses (112). Th1 responses to the model antigen KLH were also enhanced by CTLA-4 blockade during priming, at least at a population level (113). Finally, as discussed above, CTLA-4 blockade enhanced Th1-mediated disease in EAE models (99, 100). Together, these data suggest that CTLA-4 engagement limits Th1 differentiation. The opposing results obtained in the different systems suggest that there is no inherent capacity for CTLA-4 to regulate Th1 vs. Th2 differentiation.

There are other ways in which CTLA-4 might influence the T helper responses. It has been suggested that the strength of TCR and costimulatory signals can have an effect on cytokine polarization (2, 114). CTLA-4 might influence polarization by affecting the overall strength of the integrated signals. It is also likely that CTLA-4 can influence the development of Th responses not at the single cell, but at the population level. A primed polyclonal $CD4^+$ T cell population contains mixed subsets of cells with different T helper functions and the relative ratios of these cells may dictate the overall T helper response. An analysis of cytokine production at the single cell level in an EAE system, for example, revealed that both IFN-γ and IL-4-producing cells were present in primed mice (107). The frequency of both subsets increased upon CTLA-4 blockade, but the IFN-γ-producing population was increased to a larger extent. These changes in the size of the primed population and T helper ratios corresponded with exacerbated disease under normal EAE-inducing conditions and amelioration of disease antagonism by an altered peptide ligand. These data argue that the disease differences upon CTLA-4 blockade occurred because of a shift in the relative proportions of T helper subsets in the population. Thus, CTLA-4 may not serve to directly regulate T helper differentiation but may shift the response at the level of the T cell population.

Additionally, CTLA-4 could regulate the response of a specific T helper subset after differentiation. However, both Th1 and Th2 cells express CTLA-4, and CTLA-4 engagement is known to inhibit the responses of both types of clones (108, 115). Clearly, regulation of T helper responses is complex. Altogether the data suggest that the regulation of Th1 or Th2 responses by CTLA-4 is dependent on the context under which T cell responses occur.

CTLA-4 AND PERIPHERAL TOLERANCE

The role of CD28 costimulation in the maintenance and loss of tolerance has been reviewed in (2). Recent data suggests that CTLA-4 /B7 interactions may also be very important in tolerance. This has been most effectively demonstrated in models of autoimmunity, graft rejection, and tumor rejection. One possible mechanism, the raising of the threshold of activation when B7 levels are limiting, has been discussed above. Additional mechanisms have been proposed, including a direct role in regulating T cell anergy, an indirect effect via the costimulation of secretion of inhibitory cytokines, and finally direct mediation of the suppressive activity of immunoregulatory T cells.

Anergy

The original characterization of the phenomenon of costimulation demonstrated that T cell clones activated solely by TCR engagement became anergic. The discovery that there was a second ligand for B7 molecules that could inhibit T cell activation raised the possibility that CTLA-4/B7 interactions may play a role in the induction of anergy in the presence of low B7. The requirement of CTLA-4/B7 interactions for anergy induction has been examined in a number of experimental models. The first study to examine this used adoptive transfer of CD4$^+$ T cells from OVA-specific DO11.10 TCR transgenic mice (116). Blockade of CTLA-4 prevented the induction of hyporesponsiveness when antigen was administered in tolerigenic (i.e. weak adjuvant) conditions. This was taken as evidence that engagement of the TCR when CTLA-4 could not be ligated was a neutral event and that CTLA-4 engagement was required for the induction of nonresponsiveness. Similar results were obtained when the peptide was administered intravenously, also shown to be a strongly tolerigenic route (117). A role for CTLA-4 ligation in superantigen-induced tolerance in vivo has also been reported (110). Finally, a requirement for CD4 was reported in the induction of T cell nonresponsiveness by CTLA in an in vitro system (41). However, in other systems CTLA-4 was not required for induction of hyporesponsiveness. In a study using the DO11.10 adoptive transfer system that examined the induction of anergy by intranasal administration of soluble peptide, CTLA-4 blockade had no effect (118). It has also been reported that stimulation of CTLA-4$^{-/-}$ T cells with anti-CD3 still resulted in anergy (119).

Overall, there may be a role for CTLA-4 in the induction of T cell anergy, but the data are obviously mixed. The experimental approaches used to examine the issue are very complicated and often suffer from an unclear definition of anergy. The line between hyporesponsiveness and anergy is often a quantitative rather than qualitative one, and results are often difficult to interpret.

CTLA-4 in the Induction of Inhibitory Cytokines

It has been reported that cross-linking of CTLA-4 may enhance production of TGFβ by activated T cells (48, 120). This raises the possibility that CTLA-4 does not directly inhibit T cell activation but does so by the active induction of this inhibitory cytokine. One observation taken as evidence for an indirect role for CTLA-4 in the inhibition of T cell responses was the failure of mixed bone marrow chimeric mice generated with CTLA-4$^{-/-}$ and wild-type bone marrow to develop a phenotype equivalent to the *ctla-4* null mice (121). It was proposed that there is no primary defect in CTLA-4$^{-/-}$ T cells but that the CTLA-4$^{-/-}$ phenotype is due to a failure of T cells to secrete inhibitory cytokines such as TGFβ.

Although the lack of an intrinsic defect is the most simplistic interpretation for the failure of mixed bone marrow chimeric mice to develop a phenotype resembling that of CTLA-4$^{-/-}$ mice, the results were clearly more complicated (121). The fact that mice reconstituted entirely with CTLA-4$^{-/-}$ bone marrow often failed to develop organ infiltration, and none showed signs of lymphoproliferative disease, although all eventually died, indicates that the situation is more complex. An alternative possibility is that there is an intrinsic defect in the cells that can be regulated by extrinsic factors. Still, the basis for the observed differences between the mixed bone marrow radiation chimeras and CTLA-4$^{-/-}$ mice are intriguing and need to be resolved.

Recent studies showed that CTLA-4 cross-linking resulted in the inhibition of proliferation of T cells from TGFβ $^{-/-}$ mice or of T cells from mice lacking Smad3, a critical downstream signaling molecule in the TGFβ pathway (122; and J Letterio, TJ Sullivan, CA Chambers, A van Elsas, JP Allison, manuscript in preparation). This suggests that neither TGFβ production nor its signaling pathway is required for CTLA-4-mediated inhibition of T cell responses. These studies also failed to show a role for CTLA-4 in regulating TGFβ production, since it was produced by CTLA-4 $^{-/-}$ T cells. Finally, CTLA-4 ligation failed to induce production of TGFβ by normal naïve T cells (122).

CTLA-4 and Regulatory T cells

Over the last several years, a considerable literature has documented a role for CD25$^+$CD45RB^{low}CD4$^+$ regulatory T cells (Treg) in the maintenance of peripheral tolerance to organ-specific self-antigens (123). The observation that these cells constitutively express CTLA-4 has raised the possibility that CTLA-4 may be directly involved in their function (42, 124–126). One interesting characteristic of Treg cells is a failure to secrete IL-2 or to proliferate in response to ligation of the TCR and CD28, despite a requirement of CD28 for their generation and homeostasis (124). The hyporesponsiveness might be attributed to the inhibitory properties of CTLA-4. However, to date, attempts to release the block on proliferation in response to TCR engagement by CTLA-4 blockade have not been successful (125, 127; B Metzler, JP Allison, unpublished data).

Perhaps a more relevant issue is the role of CTLA-4 in the suppressive function of these cells. Here the results are mixed. Administration of either anti-CTLA-4 antibodies or anti-TGFβ reversed the inhibitory effects of transferred CD25$^+$ Treg cells on the induction of colitis by transferred CD4$^+$ CD25$^-$ cells in SCID mice (126). This was taken as evidence for a blocking of the suppressive effects of Treg cells by preventing CTLA-4-mediated induction of TGFβ production. However, the results are correlative and do not exclude the possibility that the effect of anti-CTLA-4 was a result of enhancement of the effector T cells. In a separate study, depletion of CD25$^+$ Tregs or anti-CTLA-4 treatment alone failed to induced colitis in normal Balb/c mice. However, colitis was induced when CD25$^+$ Tregs were depleted and CTLA-4 was blocked (125). Some of the data in this report may in fact suggest that CTLA-4 and CD25$^+$ Tregs represent independent but complementary mechanisms of maintaining peripheral tolerance. For example, CD25$^+$CD4$^+$ T cells from CTLA-4$^{-/-}$ mice retained inhibitory activity in in vitro inhibition assays. This would suggest that CTLA-4 expression was not required for the function of CD25$^+$CD4$^+$ Treg cells.

A role for CTLA-4 in the function of Treg cells is also not supported by recent findings in a tumor immunotherapy system (128). Depletion of either CD4$^+$ T cells or CD25$^+$ T cells improved the effectiveness of a GM-CSF-producing tumor cell vaccine in the B16 melanoma system. This finding confirms a role for Treg cells in partially suppressing the T cell response in this system. However, depletion of CD4$^+$ T cells or CD25$^+$ cells also enhances, rather than diminishes, the effectiveness of anti-CTLA-4 in inducing both tumor rejection and the increase in T cells specific for a D^b-restricted peptide derived from the *trp-2* gene product. The effectiveness of CTLA-4 blockade was not reduced, but rather was considerably enhanced, by the removal of CD25$^+$ T cells, strongly suggesting that CTLA-4 is not directly involved in the function of Treg cells.

On balance, the evidence for a direct role of CTLA-4 in the function of Treg cells is indirect and not strongly supported by all results. It seems likely that CTLA-4 and Treg cells are independent mechanisms of regulating responses to self-antigen. This is an area that clearly needs further work.

MANIPULATION OF COSTIMULATORY SIGNALS IN TUMOR IMMUNOTHERAPY

The idea that one of the major roles of the immune system is to provide protection against constantly arising tumors is an old one, proposed by Ehrlich almost a century ago. While the experimental evidence for tumor immunosurveillance is mixed, considerable data support the notion that tumor cells can express antigens potentially capable of eliciting T cell responses. It is also clear that these responses may be largely ineffective. Still, the prospect of manipulating the immune system to obtain tumor rejection and protection against metastasis and recurrence is an attractive therapeutic approach, especially given the alternatives.

One of the reasons for the poor immunogenicity of tumors is a failure to express costimulatory ligands. Thus, despite expression of relevant antigens, a tumor may be invisible to the immune system until T cells are alerted by cross-priming by professional APC. The importance of costimulation to tumor immune responses was shown by the fact that in many cases introduction of B7 expression to tumor cells was sufficient not only to result in a rejection, but also to induce prophylactic immunity. This work demonstrated the relevance of costimulation to tumor immunity and offered a new strategy for immunotherapy. However, this approach was limited to application to inherently immunogenic tumors. And, while capable of inducing prophylactic immunity, B7$^+$ tumor cell vaccines were generally of limited effectiveness in treating established tumors (for review, see 129).

Given the demonstrated ability of CTLA-4 blockade to enhance T cell responses in a variety of settings, it was reasonable to determine whether it could also enhance anti-tumor responses. The importance of costimulation provided by host APC to anti-tumor responses was confirmed in experiments showing that the growth of relatively immunogenic transplanted tumors was accelerated by blockade of costimulation with anti- CD28 antibodies (130). CTLA-4 blockade, on the other hand, has been shown to lead to rejection of a number of immunogenic transplanted tumor cell lines, including colorectal carcinoma, renal carcinoma, lymphoma, and fibrocarcoma cell lines (131–134). In some experiments, administration of anti-CTLA-4 resulted in rejection even when treatment was delayed until weeks after tumor implantation and when there were sizable tumor masses (130). These results demonstrated that weak responses elicited by tumors could be converted into potent responses sufficient for tumor rejection by removal of the inhibitory effects of CTLA-4. In other tumor systems, CTLA-4 blockade was effective if given only during early stages of tumor growth (131). In some, but not all tumor models, CTLA-4 blockade was capable of reversing tumor-induced T cell hyporesponsiveness (133, 134).

While this work clearly demonstrated the potential of this approach as a strategy for tumor immunotherapy, CTLA-4 blockade by itself was not effective against all experimental tumors—susceptibility appears to correlate with the inherent immunogenicity of the tumor (for review, see 132). This led to an examination of the effectiveness of CTLA-4 blockade in combination with other strategies for therapy of poorly immunogenic tumors. One approach that appeared to be complementary to CTLA-4 blockade was the use of irradiated tumor cell vaccines engineered to express the cytokine GM-CSF (135). GM-CSF tumor cell vaccines were effective in stimulating responses to the poorly immunogenic melanoma B16 by a mechanism that involved enhancement of cross-priming by host APC (136). While effective in prophylaxis, the GM-CSF tumor cell vaccine by itself was not sufficient to obtain rejection of established tumors. When combined with CTLA-4 blockade, however, GM-CSF-producing tumor cell vaccines were effective in inducing rejection of the B16 melanoma and another poorly immunogenic tumor, mammary carcinoma SM-1 (103, 104). Similarly, CTLA-4 blockade in combination with a GM-CSF-vaccine has been effective in delaying and reducing the severity of primary adenocarcinoma in the TRAMP system, a transgenic model of prostate cancer (105). In each of these systems, therapeutic effectiveness is lost if initiated too late, which may be a result of the tumor passing a critical mass or inactivation of potentially reactive T cells. However, the potent synergy observed in these systems clearly demonstrates the potential of CTLA-4 as part of a combinatorial approach to tumor immunotherapy.

Use of CTLA-4 blockade in combinatorial strategies is not limited to conventional immunomodulators. Anti-CTLA-4 can synergize with low doses of chemotherapeutic drugs to achieve tumor rejection (137). CTLA-4 blockade initiated following surgical resection of transplanted prostatic adenocarcinoma at the primary site reduces the incidence of metastases in the draining lymph nodes (138).

Studies of the cellular requirements for the therapeutic effect of CTLA-4 blockade have provided insight into the mechanisms involved. The response elicited by the GM-CSF B16 cell vaccine is absolutely dependent on CD4$^+$ T cells (139). While CD8$^+$ T cells are involved in the response, their contribution is minimal. Tumor protection requires Th2 cytokines, and the effector cells for rejection of the tumor cells, which do not express MHC class II gene products, are probably eosinophils (139). In the combinatorial treatment with anti-CTLA-4, however, CD4$^+$ cells are totally dispensable—only CD8$^+$ T cells and NK1.1$^+$ cells are required (104). Indeed, the anti-tumor effect is even more vigorous in the absence of CD4$^+$ T cells. This finding has two important implications. The first is that CTLA-4 blockade may lower the threshold for activation of CD8$^+$ T cells by host APC, perhaps by eliminating the requirement for licensing by CD40L or other CD4$^+$ T cell–dependent mechanisms. Second, as discussed in more detail above, the mechanism by which CTLA-4 blockade enhances anti-tumor responses is at the level of the effector cell, and not inhibition of the suppressive effects of Treg cells.

An interesting consequence of the induction of tumor immunity in the B16 and TRAMP models is the development of tissue-specific autoimmunity. Mice that have rejected the B16 melanoma develop a progressive depigmentation as a result of elimination of normal melanocytes (104). This depigmentation has never been observed in mice treated with the GM-CSF producing B16 cell vaccine alone. Similarly, immunization of mice with the GM-CSF-producing TRAMP tumor cell line together with anti-CTLA-4 results in the development of autoimmune prostatitis, but not depigmentation. Together, these results suggest that the anti-tumor response enhanced by CTLA-4 blockade is in large part directed against normal tissue-derived gene products, rather than tumor-specific antigens. In support of this idea, the main target of T cells from mice cured of melanoma is a normal, unmutated peptide derived from the trp-2 gene, which is expressed in normal melanoma (A van Elsas, J Ziskin, N Restif, and JP Allison, unpublished results).

These findings suggest that the anti-tumor effect of CTLA-4 blockade in these models is a consequence of removal of constraints on T cells directed against normal tissue antigens, allowing the elaboration of a response that eliminates tumor cells on the basis of their tissue of origin. This has two important implications. First, this approach to therapy will not require knowledge of expression of individually specific tumor antigens and may be more generally useful in the clinic. However, this same feature might limit the usefulness of the approach to the treatment of tumors of nonessential tissues. Even with this limitation, the list would include many prevalent cancers, such as melanoma, prostate, testicular, ovarian, and mammary tumors.

SUMMARY AND CONCLUSION

Recent advances in our understanding of the mechanisms involved in costimulation have led to an appreciation of the importance of inhibition by CTLA-4 in the regulation of early stages of the T cell response. Although controversial areas require further inquiry for resolution, significant advances have been made in our understanding of CTLA-4 activity at the molecular, single cell, and population levels. Results demonstrating the effectiveness of CTLA-4 blockade in enhancing anti-tumor responses in experimental systems offer the exciting possibility of translating our basic knowledge of costimulatory regulation into new strategies for tumor therapy.

ACKNOWLEDGMENTS

The authors would like to thank Tim Sullivan for helpful discussions and critique of the manuscript. We would also like to thank Barbara Metzler, Peter Savage, and the remainder of the Allison Laboratory for thoughtful comments and discussions. CA Chambers is a recipient of the Worcester Foundation for Biomedical Research Scholar Award and is a Cancer Research Institute Investigator.

Visit the Annual Reviews home page at www.AnnualReviews.org

LITERATURE CITED

1. Mueller DL, Jenkins MK, Schwartz RH. 1989. Clonal expansion versus functional clonal inactivation: a costimulatory signalling pathway determines the outcome of T cell antigen receptor occupancy. *Annu. Rev. Immunol.* 7:445–80

2. Lenschow DJ, Walunas TL, Bluestone JA. 1996. CD28/B7 system of T cell costimulation. *Annu. Rev. Immunol.* 14:233–58

3. Martin PJ, Ledbetter JA, Morishita Y, June CH, Beatty PG, Hansen JA. 1986. A 44 kilodalton cell surface homodimer regulates interleukin 2 production by activated human T lymphocytes. *J. Immunol.* 136:3282–87

4. Jenkins MK, Taylor PS, Norton SD, Urdahl KB. 1991. CD28 delivers a costimulatory signal involved in antigen-specific IL-2 production by human T cells. *J. Immunol.* 147:2461–66

5. Harding F, McArthur JG, Gross JA, Raulet DH, Allison JP. 1992. CD28 mediated signalling costimulates murine T cells and prevents the induction of anergy in T cell clones. *Nature* 356:607–9

6. Sagerstrom CG, Kerr EM, Allison JP, Davis MM. 1993. Activation and differentiation requirments of primary T cells *in vitro. Proc. Natl. Acad. Sci. USA* 90:8987–91

7. Linsley PS, Brady W, Grosmaire L, Aruffo A, Damle NK, Ledbetter JA. 1991. Binding of the B cell activation antigen B7 to CD28 costimulates T cell proliferation and Interleukin 2 mRNA accumulation. *J. Exp. Med.* 173:721–30

8. Hathcock KS, Laszlo G, Dickler HB, Brad-

shaw J, Linsley P, Hodes RJ. 1993. Identification of an alternative CTLA-4 ligand costimulatory for T cell activation. *Science* 262:905–7

9. Lenshcow DJ, Bluestone JA. 1993. T cell co-stimulation and in vivo tolerance. *Curr. Opin. Immunol.* 5:747–52

10. Shahinian A, Pfeffer K, Lee KP, Kundig TM, Kishihara K, Wakeham A, Kawai K, Ohashi PS, Thompson CB, Mak T. 1993. Differential T cell costimulatory requirements in CD28-deficient mice. *Science* 261:609–12

11. Kundig TM, Shahinian A, Kawai K, Mittrucker HW, Sebzda E, Bachmann MF, Mak TW, Ohashi PS. 1996. Duration of TCR stimulation determines costimulatory requirement of T cells. *Immunity* 5:41–52

12. Borriello F, Sethna MP, Boyd SD, Schweitzer AN, Tivol EA, Jacoby D, Strom TB, Simpson EM, Freeman GJ, Sharpe AH. 1997. B7-1 and B7-2 have overlapping, critical roles in immunoglobulin class switching and germinal center formation. *Immunity* 6:303–13

13. Brunet JF, Denizot F, Luciani MF, Roux-Dosseto M, Suzan M, Mattei MF, Golstein P. 1987. A new member of the immunoglobulin superfamily CTLA-4. *Nature* 328:267–70

14. Linsley PS, Greene JL, Brady W, Bajorath J, Ledbetter JA, Peach R. 1994. Human B7-1 (CD80) and B7-2 (CD86) bind with similar avidities but distinct kinetics to CD28

and CTLA-4 receptors. *Immunity* 1:793–801

15. Linsley PS, Brady W, Urnes M, Grosmaire LS, Damle NK, Ledbetter JA. 1991. CTLA-4 is a second receptor for the B cell activation antigen B7. *J. Exp. Med.* 174:561–69

16. Greene JL, Leytze GM, Emswiler J, Peach R, Bajorath J, Cosand W, Linsley PS. 1996. Covalent Dimerization of CD28/CTLA-4 and oligomerization of CD80/86 regulate T cell costimulatory interactions. *J. Biol. Chem.* 271:26762–71

17. Thompson CB, Allison JP. 1997. The emerging role of CTLA-4 as an immune attenuator. *Immunity* 7:445–50

18. Walunas TL, Lenschow DJ, Bakker CY, Linsley PS, Freeman GJ, Green JM, Thompson CB, Bluestone JA. 1994. CTLA-4 can function as a negative regulator of T cell activation. *Immunity* 1:405–13

19. Krummel MF, Allison JP. 1995. CD28 and CTLA-4 have opposing effects on the response of T cells to stimulation. *J. Exp. Med.* 182:459–65

20. Kearney ER, Walunas TL, Karr RW, Morton PA, Loh DY, Bluestone JA, Jenkins MK. 1995. Antigen-dependent clonal expansion of a trace population of antigen-specific CD4+ T cells in vivo is dependent on CD28 costimulation and inhibited by CTLA-4. *J. Immunol.* 155:1033–36

21. Krummel MF, Sullivan TJ, Allison JP. 1996. Superantigen responses and costimulation: CD28 and CTLA-4 have opposing effects on T cell expansion *in vitro* and *in vivo*. *Int. Immunity* 8:519–23

22. Waterhouse P, Penninger JM, Timms E, Wakeham A, Shahinian A, Lee KP, Thompson CB, Griesser H, Mak TW. 1995. Lymphoproliferative disorders with early lethality in mice deficient in CTLA-4. *Science* 270:985–88

23. Tivol EA, Borriello F, Schweitzer AN, Lynch WP, Bluestone JA, Sharpe AH. 1995. Loss of CTLA-4 leads to massive lymphoproliferation and fatal multiorgan tissue destruction, revealing a critical negative regulatory role of CTLA-4. *Immunity* 3:541–47

24. Chambers CA, Cado D, Truong T, Allison JP. 1997. Thymocyte differentiation occurs normally in the absence of CTLA-4. *Proc. Natl. Acad. Sci. USA* 94:9296–9301

25. Nagata S, Golstein P. 1995. The Fas death factor. *Science* 267:1449–56

26. Lucas PJ, Kim SJ, Melby SJ, Gress RE. 2000. Disruption of T cell homeostasis in mice expressing a T cell-specific dominant negative transforming growth factor beta II receptor. *J. Exp. Med.* 191:1187–96

27. Gorelik L, Flavell RA. 2000. Abrogation of TGFβ signaling in T cells leads to spontaneous T cell differentiation and autoimmune disease. *Immunity* 12:171–81

28. Nishimura H, Nose M, Hiai H, Minato N, Honjo T. 1999. Development of lupus-like autoimmune diseases by disruption of the PD-1 gene encoding an ITIM motif-carrying immunoreceptor. *Immunity* 11:141–51

29. Chambers CA, Sullivan TJ, Allison JP. 1997. Lymphoproliferation in CTLA-4-deficient mice is mediated by costimulation-dependent activation of CD4+ T cells. *Immunity* 7:885–95

30. Lee K-M, Chuang E, Griffin M, Khattri R, Hong DK, Zhang W, Straus D, Samelson LE, Thompson CB, Bluestone JA. 1998. Molecular basis of T cell inactivation by CTLA-4. *Science* 282:2263–66

31. Marengere LEM, Waterhouse P, Duncan GS, Mittrucker HW, Feng GS, Mak TW. 1996. Regulation of T cell receptor signaling by tryosine phosphatase SYP association with CTLA-4. *Science* 272:1170–73

32. Tivol EA, Boyd SD, McKeon S, Borriello F, Nickerson P, Strom TB, Sharpe AH. 1997. CTLA4Ig prevents lymphoproliferation and fatal multiorgan tissue destruction in CTLA-4-deficient mice. *J. Immunol.* 158:5091–94

33. Mandelbrot DA, McAdam AJ, Sharpe AH.

1999. B7-1 or B7-2 is required to produce the lymphoproliferative phenotype in mice lacking cytotoxic T lymphocyte-associated antigen 4 (CTLA-4). *J. Exp. Med.* 189:435–40

34. Khattri R, Auger JA, Griffin MD, Sharpe AH, Bluestone JA. 1999. Lymphoproliferative disorder in CTLA-4 knockout mice is characterized by CD28-regulated activation of Th2 responses. *J. Immunol.* 162:5784–91

35. Waterhouse P, Bachmann MF, Penninger JM, Ohashi PS, Mak TW. 1997. Normal thymic selection, normal viability and decreased lymphoproliferation in T cell receptor-transgenic CTLA-4-deficient mice. *Eur. J. Immunol.* 27:1887–92

36. Chambers CA, Sullivan TJ, Truong T, Allison JP. 1998. Secondary but not primary T cell responses are enhanced in CTLA-4-deficient CD8+ T cells. *Eur. J. Immunol.* 28:3137–43

37. Chambers CA, Kuhns MS, Allison JP. 1999. Cytotoxic T lymphocyte antigen-4 (CTLA-4) regulates primary and secondary peptide-specific CD4(+) T cell responses. *Proc. Natl. Acad. Sci. USA* 96:8603–8

38. Oosterwegel MA, Mandelbrot DA, Boyd SD, Lorsbach RB, Jarrett DY, Abbas AK, Sharpe AH. 1999. The role of CTLA-4 in regulating Th2 differentiation. *J. Immunol.* 163:2634–39

39. Chambers CA, Allison JP. 1999. CTLA-4: The costimulatory molecule that doesn't: regulation of T cell responses by inhibition. *Cold Spring Harbor Symp. Quant. Biol.* 1999:303–127

40. Bachmann MF, Waterhouse P, Speiser DE, McKall-Faienza K, Mak TW, Ohashi PS. 1998. Normal responsiveness of CTLA-4-deficient anti-viral cytoxic T cells. *J. Immunol.* 160:95–100

41. Metz DP, Farber DL, Taylor T, Bottomly K. 1998. Differential role of CTLA-4 in regulation of resting memory versus naive CD4 T cell activation. *J. Immunol.* 161:5855–61

42. Metzler B, Burkhart C, Wraith DC. 1999. Phenotypic analysis of CTLA-4 and CD28 expression during transient peptide-induced T cell activation in vivo. *Int. Immunol.* 11:667–75

43. Gribben JG, Freeman GJ, Boussiotis VA, Rennert P, Jellis CL, Greenfield E, Barber M, Restivo VA, Ke X, Gray GS, Nadler LM. 1995. CTLA-4 mediates antigen-specific apoptosis of human T cells. *Proc. Natl. Acad. Sci. USA* 92:811–15

44. Scheipers P, Reiser H. 1998. Fas-independent death of activated CD4+ T lymphocytes induced by CTLA-4 crosslinking. *Proc. Natl. Acad. Sci. USA* 95:10083–88

45. Krummel MF, Allison JP. 1996. CTLA-4 engagement inhibits IL-2 accumulation and cell cycle progression upon activation of resting T cells. *J. Exp. Med.* 183:2533–40

46. Walunas TL, Bakker CY, Bluestone JA. 1996. CTLA-4 ligation blocks CD28-dependent T cell activation. *J. Exp. Med.* 183:2541–50

47. Calvo CR, Amsen D, Kruisbeek AM. 1997. Cytotoxic lymphocyte antigen 4 (CTLA-4) interferes with extracellular signal-regulated kinase (ERK) and Jun NH$_2$-terminal kinase (JNK) activation, but does not affect phophorylation of T cell receptor ζ and ZAP70. *J. Exp. Med.* 186:1645–53

48. Chen W, Jin W, Wahl SM. 1998. Engagement of cytotoxic T lymphocyte-associated antigen 4 (CTLA-4) induces transforming growth factor beta (TGF-beta) production by murine CD4(+) T cells. *J. Exp. Med.* 188:1849–57

49. Blair PJ, Riley JL, Levine BL, Lee KP, Craighead N, Francomano T, Perfetto SJ, Gray GS, Carreno BM, June CH. 1998. CTLA-4 ligation delivers a unique signal to resting human CD4 T cells that inhibits interleukin-2 secretion but allows Bcl-Xl induction. *J. Immunol.* 160:12–15

50. Van Parijs L, Refaeli Y, Lord JD, Nelson BH, Abbas AK, Baltimore D. 1999. Uncoupling IL-2 signals that regulate T cell

proliferation, survival, and Fas-mediated activation-induced cell death. *Immunity* 11:281–88

51. Fraser JD, Weiss A. 1992. Regulation of T-cell lymphokine gene transcription by the accessory molecule CD28. *Mol. Cell. Biol.* 12:4357–63

52. Lindsten T, June CH, Ledbetter JA, Stella G, Thompson CB. 1989. Regulation of lymphokine messenger RNA stability by a surface-mediated T cell activation pathway. *Science* 244:339–43

53. Brunner MC, Chambers CA, Chan FK, Hanke J, Winoto A, Allison JP. 1999. CTLA-4-mediated inhibition of early events of T cell proliferation. *J. Immunol.* 162:5813–20

54. Lindsten T, Lee KP, Harris ES, Petryniak B, Craighead N, Reynolds PJ, Lombard DB, Freeman GJ, Nadler LM, Gray GS, Thompson CB, June CH. 1993. Characterization of CTLA-4 structure and expression on human T cells. *J. Immunol.* 151:3489–99

55. Leung HT, Bradshaw J, Cleaveland JS, Linsley PS. 1995. Cytotoxic T lymphocyte-associated molecule-4, a high avidity receptor for CD80 and CD86, contains an intracellular localization motif in its cytoplasmic tail. *J. Biol. Chem.* 270:25107–14

56. Oki S, Kohsaka T, Azuma M. 1999. Augmentation of CTLA-4 expression by wortmannin: involvement of lysosomal sorting properties of CTLA-4. *Int. Immunol.* 11:1563–71

57. Schneider H, Martin M, Agarraberes FA, Yin L. Rapaport I, Kirchhausen T, Rudd CE. 1999. Cytolytic T lymphocyte-associated antigen-4 and the TCRζ/CD3 comples, but not CD28, interact with clathrin adaptor complexes AP-1 and AP-2. *J. Immunol.* 163:1868–79

58. Shiratori T, Miyatake S, Ohno H, Nakaseko C, Isono K, Bonifacino JS, Saito T. 1997. Tyrosine phosphorylation controls internalization of CTLA-4 by regulating its interaction with clathrin-associated adaptor complex AP-2. *Immunity* 6:583–89

59. Chuang E, Alegre ML, Duckett CS, Noel PJ, Vander Heiden MG, Thompson CB. 1997. Interaction of CTLA-4 with the clathrin-associated protein AP50 results in ligand-independent endocytosis that limits cell surface expression. *J. Immunol.* 159:144–51

60. Bradshaw JD, Lu P, Leytze G, Rodgers J, Schieven GL, Bennett KL, Linsley PS, Kurtz SE. 1997. Interaction of the cytoplasmic tail of CTLA-4 (CD152) with a clathrin- associated protein is negatively regulated by tyrosine phosphorylation. *Biochemistry* 36:15975–82

61. Zhang Y, Allison JP. 1997. Interaction of CTLA-4 with AP50, a clathrin-coated pit adaptor protein. *Proc. Natl. Acad. Sci. USA* 94:9273–78

62. Barrat FJ, Le Deist F, Benkerrou M, Bousso P, Feldmann J, Fischer A, De Saint Basile G. 1999. Defective CTLA-4 cycling pathway in Chediak-Higashi syndrome: a possible mechanism for deregulation of T lymphocyte activation. *Proc. Natl. Acad. Sci. USA* 96:8645–50

63. Cefai D, Schneider H, Matangkasombut O, Kang H, Brody J, Rudd CE. 1998. CD28 receptor endocytosis is targeted by mutations that disrupt phosphatidylinositol 3-kinase binding and costimulation. *J. Immunol.* 160:2223–30

64. Gross JA, St.John T, Allison JP. 1990. The murine homolog of the T lymphocyte antigen CD28: molecular cloning and cell surface expression. *J. Immunol.* 144:3201–10

65. Linsley PS, Bradshaw J, Greene J, Peach R, Bennett KL, Mittler RS. 1996. Intracellular trafficking of CTLA-4 and focal localization towards sites of TCR engagement. *Immunity* 4:535–43

66. Kupfer A, Swain SL, Singer SJ. 1987. The specific direct interaction of helper T cells and antigen-presenting B cells. II. Reorientation of the microtubule organizing

center and reorganization of the membrane-associated cytoskeleton inside the bound helper T cells. *J. Exp. Med.* 165:1565–80

67. Shapiro VS, Truitt KE, Imboden JB, Weiss A. 1997. CD28 mediates transcriptional upregulation of the interleukin-2 (IL-2) promoter through a composite element containing the CD28RE and NF-IL-2B AP-1 sites. *Mol. Cell. Biol.* 17:4051–58

68. Su B, Jacinto E, Hibi M, Kallunki T, Karin M, Ben-Neriah Y. 1994. JNK is involved in signal integration during costimulation of T lymphocytes. *Cell* 77:727–36

69. Monks CR, Kupfer H, Tamir I, Barlow A, Kupfer A. 1997. Selective modulation of protein kinase C-theta during T-cell activation. *Nature* 385:83–86

70. Wulfing C, Davis MM. 1998. A receptor/cytoskeletal movement triggered by costimulation during T cell activation. *Science* 282:2266–69

71. Grakoui A, Bromley SK, Sumen C, Davis MM, Shaw AS, Allen PM, Dustin ML. 1999. The immunological synapse: a molecular machine controlling T cell activation. *Science* 285:221–27

72. Viola A, Schroeder S, Sakakibara Y, Lanzavecchia A. 1999. T lymphocyte costimulation mediated by reorganization of membrane microdomains. *Science* 283:680–82

73. Langlet C, Bernard AM, Drevot P, He HT. 2000. Membrane rafts and signaling by the multichain immune recognition receptors. *Curr. Opin. Immunol.* 12:250–55

74. Hutchcroft JE, Bierer BE. 1996. Signaling through CD28/CTLA-4 family receptors: puzzling participation of phosphatidylinositol-3 kinase. *J. Immunol.* 156:4071–74

75. Vivier E, Daëron M. 1997. Immunoreceptor tyrosine-based inhibition motifs. *Immunol. Today* 18:286–91

76. Chambers CA, Allison JP. 1996. The role of tyrosine phosphorylation and PTP-1C in CTLA-4 signal transduction. *Eur. J. Immunol.* 26:3224–9

77. Chuang E, Lee KM, Robbins MD, Duerr JM, Alegre ML, Hambor JE, Neveu MJ, Bluestone JA, Thompson CB. 1999. Regulation of cytotoxic T lymphocyte-associated molecule-4 by Src kinases. *J. Immunol.* 162:1270–77

78. Schneider H, Rudd CE. 2000. Tyrosine phosphatase SHP-2 binding to CTLA-4: absence of direct YVKM/YFIP motif recognition. *Biochem. Biophys. Res. Commun.* 269:279–83

79. Chikuma S, Murakami M, Tanaka K, Uede T. 2000. Janus kinase 2 is associated with a box 1-like motif and phosphorylates a critical tyrosine residue in the cytoplasmic region of cytotoxic T lymphocyte associated molecule-4. *J. Cell. Biochem.* 78:241–50

80. Chuang E, Fisher TS, Morgan RW, Robbins MD, Duerr JM, Vander Heiden MG, Gardner JP, Hambor JE, Neveu MJ, Thompson CB. 2000. The CD28 and CTLA-4 receptors associated with the serine/threonine phosphatase PP2A. *Immunity* 13:313–22

81. Calvo CR, Amsen D, Kruisbeek AM. 1997. Cytotoxic T lymphocyte antigen 4 (CTLA-4) interferes with extracellular signal-regulated kinase (ERK) and Jun NH2-terminal kinase (JNK) activation, but does not affect phosphorylation of T cell receptor zeta and ZAP70. *J. Exp. Med.* 186:1645–53

82. Nakaseko C, Miyatake S, Iida T, Hara S, Abe R, Ohno H, Saito Y, Saito T. 1999. Cytotoxic T lymphocyte antigen 4 (CTLA-4) engagement delivers an inhibitory signal through the membrane-proximal region in the absence of the tyrosine motif in the cytoplasmic tail. *J. Exp. Med.* 190:765–74

83. Carreno BM, Bennett F, Chau TA, Ling V, Luxenberg D, Jussif J, Baroja ML, Madrenas J. 2000. CTLA-4 (CD152) can inhibit T cell activation by two different mechanisms depending on its level of cell surface expression. *J. Immunol.* 165:1352–56

84. Baroja ML, Luxenberg D, Chau T, Ling V, Strathdee CA, Carreno BM, Madrenas J. 2000. The inhibitory function of CTLA-4 does not require its tyrosine phosphorylation. *J. Immunol.* 164:49–55

85. Masteller EL, Chuang E, A.C. M, Reiner SL, Thompson CB. 2000. Structural analysis of CTLA-4 function in vivo. *J. Immunol.* 164:5319–27

86. Ikemizu S, Gilbert RJC, Fennelly JA, Collins AV, Harlos K, Jones EY, Stuart DI, Davis SJ. 2000. Structure and dimerization of a soluble form of B7-1. *Immunity* 12:51–60

87. Ostrov DA, Shi W, Schwartz J-CD, Almo SC, Nathenson SG. 2000. Structure of murine CTLA-4: a novel dimer modulating T cell responsiveness. *Science* 290:816–19

87a. Jenkins MK. 1994. The ups and downs of costimulation. *Immunity* 1:443–45

88. Chambers CA, Krummel MF, Boitel B, Hurwitz AA, Sullivan TJ, Fournier S, Cassell D, Brunner M, Allison JP. 1996. The role of CTLA-4 in the regulation and initiation of T cell responses. *Immunol. Rev.* 153:27–46

89. Luhder F, Hoglund P, Allison JP, Benoist C, Mathis D. 1997. CTLA-4 regulates the unfolding of autoimmune diabetes. *J. Exp. Med.* 187:427–32

90. Luhder F, Chambers CA, Allison JP, Benoist C, Mathis D. 2000. Pinpointing when CTLA-4 must be engaged to dampen diabetogenic T cells. *Proc. Natl. Acad. Sci. USA* 97:12204–9

91. van Oers NSC, Killeen N, Weiss A. 1994. ZAP-70 is constitutively associated with tyrosine-phosphoryated TCR z in murine thymocytes and lymph node cells. *Immunity* 1:675–85

92. Goldrath AW, Bevan MJ. 1999. Selecting and maintaining a diverse T-cell repertoire. *Nature* 402:255–62

93. Seddon B, Legname G, Tomlinson P, Zamoyska R. 2000. Long-term survival but impaired homeostatic proliferation of naive T cells in the absence of p56(lck). *Science* 290:127–31

94. Dorfman JR, Stefanova I, Yasutomo K, Germain RN. 2000. CD4$^+$ T cell survival is not directly linked to self-MHC-induced TCR signaling. *Nat. Immunol.* 1:329–35

95. Gozalo Sanmillan, McNally J, Lin M-Y, Chambers CA, Berg LJ. Two distinct mechanisms lead to impaired T cell homeostasis in JAK3- and CTLA-4-deficient mice. *J. Immunol.* In press

96. Martin WD, Hicks GG, Mendiratta SK, Leva HI, Ruley HE, Van Kaer L. 1996. H2-M mutant mice are defective in the peptide loading of class II molecules, antigen presentation, and T cell repertoire selection. *Cell* 84:543–50

97. Miyazaki T, Wolf P, Tourne S, Waltzinger C, Dierich A, Barois N, Ploegh H, Benoist C, Mathis D. 1996. Mice lacking H2-M complexes, enigmatic elements of the MHC class II peptide-loading pathway. *Cell* 84:531–41

98. Chambers CA, Kang J, Wu Y, Held W, Raulet D, Allison JP. 2000. The lymphoproliferative defect in CTLA-4-deficient mice is ameliorated by the inhibitory NK cell receptor Ly49A. Submitted

99. Karandikar NJ, Vanderlugt CL, Walunas TL, Miller SD, Bluestone JA. 1996. CTLA-4: A negative regulator of autoimmune disease. *J. Exp. Med.* 184:783–88

100. Perrin PJ, Maldonado JH, Davis TA, June CH, Racke MK. 1996. CTLA-4 blockade enhances clinical disease and cytokine production during experimental allergic encephalomyelitis. *J. Immunol.* 157:1333–36

101. Hurwitz AA, Sullivan TJ, Krummel MF, Sobel RA, Allison JP. 1997. Specific blockade of CTLA-4/B7 interactions results in exacerbated clinical and histologic disease in an actively-induced model of experimental allergic encephalomyelitis. *J. Neuroimmunol.* 73:57–62

102. Karandikar NJ, Eagar TN, Vanderlugt CL, Bluestone JA, Miller SD. 2000. CTLA-4 downregulates epitope spreading and mediates remission in relapsing experimental autoimmune encephalomyelitis. *J. Neuroimmunol.* 109:173–80

103. Hurwitz AA, Yu TF, Leach DR, Allison JP. 1998. CTLA-4 blockade synergizes with tumor-derived GM-CSF for treatment of an experimental mammary carcinoma. *Proc. Natl. Acad. Sci. USA* 95:10067–71

104. van Elsas A, Hurwitz AA, Allison JP. 1999. Combination immunotherapy of B16 melanoma using anti-CTLA-4 and GM-CSF producing vaccines induces rejection of subcutaneous and metastatic tumors accompanied by autoimmune depigmentation. *J. Exp. Med.* 190:355–66

105. Hurwitz AA, Foster BA, Kwon ED, Trong T, Choi EM, Greenberg NM, Burg MB, Allison JP. 2000. Combination immunotherapy of primary prostate cancer in a transgenic model using CTLA-4 blockade. *Cancer Res.* 60:2444–48

106. McCoy KD, Hermans IF, Fraser JH, Le Gros G, Ronchese F. 1999. Cytotoxic T lymphocyte-associated antigen 4 (CTLA-4) can regulate dendritic cell-induced activation and cytotoxicity of CD8+ T cells independently of CD4+ T cell help. *J. Exp. Med.* 189:1157–62

107. Kuhns MS, Epshteyn V, Sobel RA, Allison JP. 2000. CTLA-4 regulates the size, function, and reactivity of a primed pool of T cells. *Proc. Natl. Acad. Sci. USA* 97:12711–16

108. Alegre ML, Shiels H, Thompson CB, Gajewski TF. 1998. Expression and function of CTLA-4 in Th1 and Th2 cells. *J. Immunol.* 161:3347–56

109. Kato T, Nariuchi H. 2000. Polarization of naive CD4+ T cells toward the Th1 subset by CTLA-4 costimulation. *J. Immunol.* 164:3554–62

110. Walunas TL, Bluestone JA. 1998. CTLA-4 regulates tolerance induction and T cell differentiation in vivo. *J. Immunol.* 160:3855–60

111. McCoy K, Camberis M, Gros GL. 1997. Protective immunity to nematode infection is induced by CTLA-4 blockade. *J. Exp. Med.* 186:183–87

112. Saha B, Chattopadhyay S, Germond R, Harlan DM, Perrin PJ. 1998. CTLA4 (CD152) modulates the Th subset response and alters the course of experimental *Leishmania major* infection. *Eur. J. Immunol.* 28:4213–20

113. Piganelli JD, Poulin M, Martin T, Allison JP, Haskins K. 2000. Cytotoxic T lymphocyte antigen 4 (CD152) regulates self-reactive T cells in BALB/c but not in the autoimmune NOD mouse. *J. Autoimmun.* 14:123–31

114. Constant SL, Bottomly K. 1997. Induction of Th1 and Th2 CD4+ T cell responses: the alternative approaches. *Annu. Rev. Immunol.* 15:297–322

115. Freeman GJ, Lombard DB, Gimmi CD, Brod SA, Lee K, Laning JC, Hafler DA, Dorf ME, Gray GS, Reiser H, June CH, Thompson CB, Nadler LM. 1992. CTLA-4 and CD28 mRNA are coexpressed in most T cells after activation. *J. Immunol.* 149:3705–3801

116. Perez VL, Van Parijs L, Biuckians A, Zheng XX, Strom TB, Abbas AK. 1997. Induction of peripheral T cell tolerance in vivo requires CTLA-4 engagement. *Immunity* 6:411–17

117. Van Parijs L, Perez VL, Biuckians A, Maki RG, London CA, Abbas AK. 1997. Role of interleukin 12 and costimulation in T cell anergy in vivo. *J. Exp Med* 186:1119–28

118. Tsitoura DC, DeKruyff RH, Lamb JR, Umetsu DT. 1999. Intranasal exposure to protein antigen induces immunological tolerance mediated by functionally disabled CD4+ T cells. *J. Immunol.* 163:2592–2600

119. Frauwirth KA, Alegre M-L, Thompson CB. 2000. Induction of T cell anergy in

the absence of CTLA-4/B7 interaction. *J. Immunol.* 164:2987–93

120. Gomes NA, Gattass CR, Barreto-de-Souza V, Wilson ME, DosReis GA. 2000. TGF-β mediates CTLA-4 suppression of cellular immunity in murine kalaazar. *J. Immunol.* 164:2001–8

121. Bachmann MF, Köhler G, Ecabert B, Mak TW, Kopf M. 1999. Cutting edge: lymphoproliferative disease in the absence of CTLA-4 is not T cell autonomous. *J. Immunol.* 163:1128–31

122. Sullivan TJ. 2000. *Characterizing the Function of CTLA-4 In Vitro and In Vivo.* Berkeley, CA: Univ. Calif. Press. 148 pp.

123. Shevach EM. 2000. Regulatory T cells in autoimmmunity. *Annu. Rev. Immunol.* 18:423–49

124. Salomon B, Lenschow DJ, Rhee L, Ashourian N, Singh B, Sharpe A, Bluestone JA. 2000. B7/CD28 costimulation is essential for the homeostasis of the CD4$^+$CD25$^+$ immunoregulatory T cells that control autoimmune diabetes. *Immunity* 12:431–40

125. Takahashi T, Tagami T, Yamazaki S, Uede T, Shimizu J, Sakaguchi N, Mak TW, Sakaguchi S. 2000. Immunologic self-tolerance maintained by CD25($^+$)CD4($^+$) regulatory T cells constitutively expressing cytotoxic T lymphocyte-associated antigen 4. *J. Exp. Med.* 192:303–10

126. Read S, Malmstrom V, Powrie F. 2000. Cytotoxic T lymphocyte-associated antigen 4 plays an essential role in the function of CD25($^+$)CD4($^+$) regulatory cells that control intestinal inflammation. *J. Exp. Med.* 192:295–302

127. Thornton AM, Shevach EM. 1998. CD4$^+$CD25$^+$ immunoregulatory T cells suppress polyclonal T cell activation in vitro by inhibiting interleukin 2 production. *J. Exp. Med.* 188:287–96

128. Sutmuller RPM, van Duivenvoorde L, van Elsas A, Allison JP, Toes REM, Melief CJM, Offringa R. 2000. CTLA-4 and CD25 constitute independent mecha-nisms of inhibition of auto-reactive cyto-toxic T lymphocytes. Submitted

129. Allison JP, Hurwitz AA, Leach DR. 1995. Manipulation of costimulatory signals to enhance antitumor T-cell responses. *Curr. Opin. Immunol.* 7:682–86

130. Leach D, Krummel M, Allison JP. 1996. Enhancement of antitumor immunity by CTLA-4 blockade. *Science* 271:1734–36

131. Yang Y, Zou J, Mu J, Wijesuriya R, Ono S, Walunas T, Bluestone J, Fujiwara H, Hamaoka T. 1997. Enhanced induction of antitumor T-cell responses by cytotoxic T lymphocyte associated molecule-4 block-ade: the effect is manifested only at the restricted tumor-bearing stages. *Cancer Res.* 57:4036–41

132. Hurwitz AA, van Elsas A, Leach D, Ziskin J, Villasenor J, Truong T, Allison JP. 1999. Manipulation of T cell activa-tion to generate antitumor CTLs. In *Cyto-toxic Cells: Basic Mechanisms and Med-ical Applications*, ed. MV Sitovsky, PA Henkart, pp. 385–93. Philadelphia, PA: Lippincott Williams & Wilkins

133. Shrikant P, Khoruts A, Mescher MF. 1999. CTLA-4 blockade reverses CD8$^+$ T cell tolerance to tumor by a CD4$^+$T cell and IL-2 dependent mechanism. *Im-munity* 11:483–93

134. Sotomayor EM, Borrello IM, Tubb E, Al-lison JP, Levitsky HI. 1999. In vivo block-ade of CTLA-4 enhances the priming of responsive T-cells but fails to prevent the induction of tumor antigen-specific tolerance. *Proc. Natl. Acad. Sci. USA* 96:11476–81

135. Dranoff G, Jaffee E, Lazenby A, Golum-bek P, Levitsky H, Brose K, Jackson V, Hamada H, Pardoll D, Mulligan RC. 1993. Vaccination with irradiated tumor cells engineered to secrete GM-CSF stim-ulates potent, specific, and long lasting anti-tumor immunity. *Proc. Natl. Acad. Sci. USA* 90:3539–43

136. Huang AY, Golumbek P, Ahmadzadeh M,

Jaffee E, Pardoll D, Levitsky H. 1994. Role of bone marrow-derived cells in presenting MHC class I-restricted tumor antigens. *Science* 264:961–65

137. Mokyr MB, Kalinichenko T, Gorelik L, Bluestone JA. 1998. Realization of the therapeutic potential of CTLA-4 blockade in low-dose chemotherapy-treated tumor-bearing mice. *Cancer Res.* 58:5301–4

138. Kwon ED, Foster BA, Hurwitz AA, Madias C, Allison JP, Greenberg NM, Burg MB. 1999. Elimination of residual metastatic prostate cancer following surgery and adjuncitve CTLA-4 blockade immunotherapy. *Proc. Natl. Acad. Sci. USA* 96:15074–79

139. Hung K, Hayashi R, Lafond-Walker A, Lowenstein C, Pardoll D, Levitsky H. 1998. The central role of CD4$^+$ T cells in the antitumor immune response. *J. Exp. Med.* 188:2357–68

Annu. Rev. Immunol. 2001. 19:595–621

B CELL DEVELOPMENT PATHWAYS

Richard R. Hardy and Kyoko Hayakawa

*Institute for Cancer Research, Fox Chase Cancer Center, 7701 Burholme Ave.,
Philadelphia, Pennsylvania 19111; e-mail: rr_hardy@fccc.edu, k_hayakawa@fccc.edu*

Key Words   pre-BCR, selection, CD5+ B cells, B-1 B cells

■ **Abstract**   B cell development is a highly regulated process whereby functional peripheral subsets are produced from hematopoietic stem cells, in the fetal liver before birth and in the bone marrow afterward. Here we review progress in understanding some aspects of this process in the mouse bone marrow, focusing on delineation of the earliest stages of commitment, on pre-B cell receptor selection, and B cell tolerance during the immature-to-mature B cell transition. Then we note some of the distinctions in hematopoiesis and pre-B selection between fetal liver and adult bone marrow, drawing a connection from fetal development to B-1/CD5+ B cells. Finally, focusing on CD5+ cells, we consider the forces that influence the generation and maintenance of this distinctive peripheral B cell population, enriched for natural autoreactive specificities that are encoded by particular germline V_H-V_L combinations.

INTRODUCTION

In the mouse, B cells are generated from pluripotent hematopoietic stem cells in the liver during mid-to-late fetal development and in the bone marrow after birth. The intermediate stages of this developmental pathway have been very thoroughly investigated and characterized over the past ten years, revealing important growth factors and regulatory interactions (1–4). As our understanding has progressed, interesting differences between B cell development during fetal and adult stageshave become apparent (5–10). These differences are particularly intriguing when we consider cell transfer data suggesting that peripheral B cells characterized by CD5 expression (11) arise from precursors present early in life (12). This raises the question of how fetal B cell development differs from that occurring in the bone marrow of adult animals. Here we review progress over the past several years in delineating and characterizing stages of developing B cells, emphasizing genes critical in the early stages of this process, the central role of the pre-B cell receptor (pre-BCR), and elimination of self-reactive B cells. Next we consider how this process may differ during fetal development. Finally, we discuss novel

0732-0582/01/0407-0595$14.00

features relating to selection and maintenance of the CD5$^+$ B cell subset that may distinguish them from other peripheral B populations.

EARLIEST STAGES OF B CELL DEVELOPMENT

Phenotypic Delineation of Developmental Stages

Bone marrow in mouse contains B lineage cells at all stages of development, from earliest progenitors to mature B cells. Various approaches for identifying and isolating cells at defined stages have been described based on cell surface phenotype, and several different nomenclatures have been proposed for classifying these stages (13–15). The Weissman group has characterized a common lymphoid progenitor (CLP) subset, early in the pathway, immediately prior to B lineage commitment (16). While lacking cell surface expression of a set of lineage molecules (including the CD45R/B220 B lineage marker, the CD11b/Mac-1 and GR1 myeloid/granulocyte/macrophage lineage markers, and the Ter119 erythroid lineage marker), these cells are recognized by expression of c-kit and the IL-7 receptor α chain. Individual cells with this surface phenotype give rise to mixed B, T, and natural killer (NK) progeny, but not to other hematopoietic lineages (myeloid/erythroid)–conclusions reached using various clonal assays.

Immediately following the CLP stage, B lineage restriction can be recognized by expression of the B220 isoform of CD45 (17–19). Although there are several non-B lineage cell types (including some NK cells) in mouse bone marrow that also express this molecule (20), the use of multiparameter flow cytometry allows discrimination of CD45R$^+$ cells that lack surface molecules expressed on these non-B lineage cells. This earliest stage of B lineage development can readily be recognized as a CD45R/B220$^+$ subset that lacks CD19 (18, 19), a molecule whose expression characterizes all later B lineage stages. In addition, the monoclonal antibody AA4.1, expressed from early progenitor through the immature B cell stage, has been used to discriminate true B lineage precursors within the CD45R/B220$^+$CD19$^-$ cell subset in bone marrow (18). The expression pattern of many of the surface markers used in defining stages of B cell development in mouse bone marrow is diagrammed in Figure 1.

Early B lineage cells in the CD45R/B220$^+$ subset, prior to CD19 expression, also exhibit relatively low levels of CD24/HSA (as revealed by the 30F1 monoclonal antibody), similar to levels reported on CLP cells (16), and distinctively lower than expressed on most CD19$^+$ B lineage cells in bone marrow (13–18). It is important to note variation in this staining using different anti-CD24 monoclonal antibodies, such that analyses with some reagents or using different staining conditions may not reveal this difference (21). In particular, an excess of anti-HSA antibody can result in clumping of bone marrow cells and may also obscure the

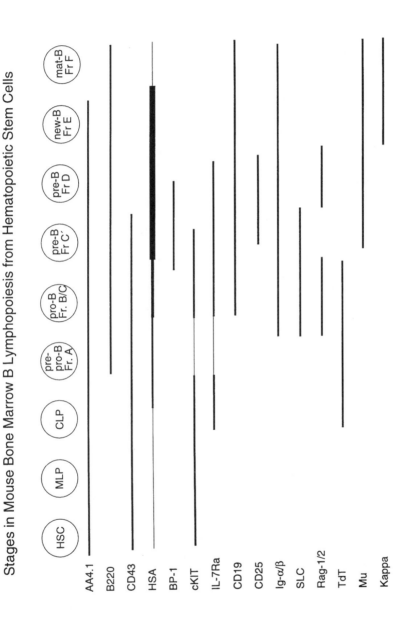

Figure 1 Diagram of B lineage development from hematopoietic stem cells (HSC) in mouse bone marrow through multilineage progenitor (MLP) and common lymphoid progenitor (CLP) to B cell committed stages (Fr. A to F) showing cell surface phenotype, expression of B-lineage genes and of mu heavy chain and kappa light chain. Relative expression levels are indicated by line thickness. Note that only Fr. C′ is pre-BCR^T. SLC, surrogate light chain.

useful distinctions in staining levels that allow discrimination of the HSA^{low} subset, referred to by us as "fraction A" (13, 17, 18). This subset was originally described within the B220$^+$CD43$^+$ subset of bone marrow early B lineage cells and was later delimited further as AA4.1$^+$, whereas the AA4.1$^-$ subset consists of non-B lineage cells (18). Recently, a portion of the AA4.1$^+$ Fr. A subset has been reported to express Ly-6C (21), and these cells appear to correspond to the CD4$^+$ portion of Fr. A (termed "A$_1$"). It seems likely that these are also non-B lineage cells, a likelihood based on poor cloning efficiency in B cell cultures (17) and the fact that Ly-6C is generally not associated with the B lineage (22).

The very early B-lineage-restricted cells in Fr. A (Fr. A2) have little or no immunoglobulin rearrangement and are referred to either as Pro-B (Basel) or pre-Pro-B (Philadelphia) stage cells (13, 15, 17–19). See Table 1 for a comparison of nomenclatures of early B lineage cells related to cell surface phenotype and also to immunoglobulin rearrangement. An intriguing observation is the diminished levels of IL-7Rα seen on this subset as compared to the levels detected on CLP and on later-stage B lineage cells (16, 23), although this is disputed in recent work from Kincade's group (21). It may seem surprising or unreasonable to some that an IL-7Rα low stage could be intermediate between two IL-7Rα high stages, but exit from proliferation may be a critical step in B lineage commitment. The finding that most cells in this IL-7Rα low stage are in G0/G1–a result based on DNA content analysis using propidium iodide staining–is consistent with this idea (RR Hardy et al, unpublished). Clearly more work is needed to address this issue.

Transcription Factors and Commitment

There is considerable interest in determining the transcriptional control of development and lineage restriction during hematopoiesis, and notable progress has been made over the past several years studying B cell development of various transcription factor in knockout mice. Thus, for example, inactivation of the E2A gene, already recognized as critical in initiating immunoglobulin gene rearrangement (24, 25), was shown to block B cell development very early, just at the stage where CD45R/B220 was being upregulated (26). In contrast, mice lacking the EBF

TABLE 1   Terms for early B cell stages and Ig rearrangement status

Phenotypic subset	Fr. A	Fr. B/C	Fr. C'	Fr. D	Fr. E
Philadelphia	Pre-	Pro-B	Early	Late	New-B
Nomenclature	Pro-B		Pre-B	Pre-B	
Basel Nomenclature	Pro-B	Pre-B-I	Pre-B-I	Pre-B-II	
IgH locus	GL	rearranging	VDJ	VDJ	VDJ
IgL locus	GL	GL	GL	rearranging	VJ

transcription factor (27) had more B lineage cells at the CD45R/B220$^+$ stage but still failed to progress to later stages, likely due to absence of Ig rearrangement. Interestingly, PU.1, with a recognized role in B lymphocyte development (28, 29), was critical at a much earlier stage of hematopoiesis, because PU.1 inactivation also affected development of T cells, granulocytes, and monocytes (30, 31).

Recent work from Busslinger's group revealed a critical role for the PAX-5/BSAP transcription factor (32) in maintaining B lineage restriction in developing B cells. His group showed that inactivation of Pax-5 allowed generation of multiple hematopoietic cell types from cells that would normally be B lineage restricted (33). In joint work with Melchers' group, they also found that even T cells could be generated from cultured pre-B cells when transferred into irradiated recipients (34). Thus, Pax-5 expression plays a key role in B lineage specification, probably by inhibiting differentiation along the monocyte/myeloid pathway. Increasing knowledge of gene regulation during hematopoiesis, including the induction and extinction of growth factor receptors, coupled with a clear understanding of the intermediate stages of developing B cells, will eventually lead to a complete picture of B lineage commitment and provide insights into how this process may be disrupted in immunodeficiencies.

REGULATION OF B CELL DEVELOPMENT BY THE PRE-BCR

Progression from early CD43$^+$ stages of B cell development to later CD43$^-$ stages is blocked in a number of immunodeficient mice, many of them engineered knockout lines. Thus, for example, SCID mice that have a defect in the DNA-PK repair complex and consequently fail to rejoin DNA efficiently during Ig heavy chain rearrangement (35) show a block in development at this stage (36). Likewise targeting of the Rag-1 and Rag-2 genes that normally generate double strand breaks in DNA during Ig rearrangement (37) results in a similar phenotype (38, 39). This block in SCID and Rag knockout mice can be overcome by introducing a rearranged heavy chain as a transgene (36, 40, 41). See Figure 2 for a diagram of Ig rearrangement during B cell development, highlighting the block due to the absence of heavy chain.

The function of heavy chain mu protein in B cell development can be understood by considering the role of two proteins, λ5 and VpreB, that together associate with mu in pre-B cells as a surrogate light chain (SLC), prior to rearrangement and expression of conventional light chain (42, 43). This pre-B cell receptor (pre-BCR) assembles with the Ig accessory proteins Igα and Igβ, similar to the B cell antigen receptor (BCR) on mature B cells, and, as with the BCR, plays a critical role in cell differentiation (14). Thus, absence of heavy chain protein due to defective rearrangement or direct targeting of the locus (the J$_H$ knockout) prevents assembly of the pre-BCR and results in a block in development at the

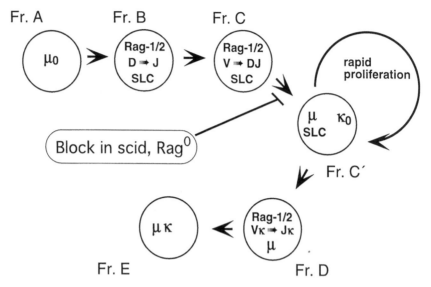

Figure 2 Relationship of Rag genes, Ig rearrangement and expression, cell proliferation, and B cell development seen in numerous mutant mice, such as SCID and Rag-deficient (Rag^0), that fail to generate a pre-BCR signal is indicated. Germline transcripts that precede rearrangement are also indicated (μ_0, κ_0)

CD43$^+$ stage. Elimination of other components of the pre-BCR complex, $\lambda5$ and Igβ, also blocks development at this stage (44, 45). It is interesting to note that this is precisely at the point in development where a proliferative burst occurs, likely dependent on assembly and signaling of the pre-BCR (13). This is shown as Fr. C′ in Figure 2.

A reasonable explanation for the dependence of pre-B cell clonal expansion on assembly of the pre-BCR is that this association acts as a screen for heavy chain V regions that have an appropriate structure for folding with light chain into an antibody combining site (14). In this model, SLC serves as a template for light chain, so that inability to complex with it tends to select against pre-B cells carrying heavy chains that will likely not form good BCRs. This screening process may be particularly important due to the action of terminal deoxynucleotidyl transferase (TdT) that adds nontemplated nucleotides at the V-D and D-J junctions of the heavy chain (46, 47), greatly increasing diversity in the third complementarity determining region (CDR3) of the antibody combining site. Pre-BCR selection is diagrammed in Figure 3.

Recognition of the role of the pre-BCR in signaling pre-B cell clonal expansion and progression to later stages of development has provided an explanation of a long-standing paradox in B cell biology: a certain V_H gene called 81X, while extremely abundant in transformed immature pre-B cell lines, is rare in B cell hybridomas made with mature peripheral B cells (48). It appears that most rearrangements of 81X result in heavy chain protein that assembles poorly with

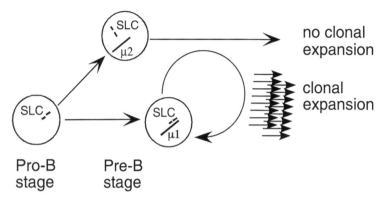

Figure 3 Bone marrow pre-BCR selection. Cells that contain heavy chains with V regions that associate efficiently with surrogate light chain components ($\lambda 5$ and VpreB) proliferate extensively at the early pre-B stage, while cells with heavy chains associating poorly (such as many $V_H 81X$ rearrangements) do not.

SLC (49, 50) and thus is inefficiently complexed into a competent pre-BCR. Pre-B cells with this incompetent pre-BCR will not signal effectively, will not clonally expand, and may not downregulate Rag expression (51), severely handicapping them. Analysis of the extent of 81X rearrangement in B lineage cells at different stages of development has confirmed this model, showing a profound decrease just at the stage of clonal expansion in bone marrow (52). However, the puzzle remains as to why early B cell development favors rearrangement of a V_H gene that usually generates incompetent pre-B cells. Furthermore, Melchers' group has suggested that rearrangements of many (perhaps most) of the VH7183 and Q52 family genes may similarly yield heavy chains that are nonfunctional in terms of pre-BCR signaling (53). Understanding differences in B cell development during fetal/neonatal life (see below) may eventually provide an explanation for conservation in the germline of so many nonfunctional V_H genes.

Another well-established example of distinctive pre-BCR selection is seen in Clarke's $V_H 12$ transgenic mouse model (54). $V_H 12$, when associated with $V_\kappa 4$, encodes a natural autoantibody enriched in the B cell subset expressing CD5 (55). Clarke's group has reported striking restriction of the CDR3 in $V_H 12$ heavy chains sequenced from autoantibody-producing hybridomas and from auto-antigen specific $CD5^+$ B cells (56). Interestingly, his group has recently found that similar restriction is already evident at the late pre-B cell stage in bone marrow (57). These investigators suggest that this restriction is due to pre-BCR interaction with a bone marrow–expressed ligand, although CDR3 restriction due to requirement for association with SLC is another possibility to be considered. Furthermore, it appears that only a limited set of light chains are capable of associating with $V_H 12$ μ chains (58), suggesting that the ability of heavy chain to associate with light chain is a critical checkpoint in B cell development prior to surface IgM expression, at least in this model.

REGULATION OF B CELL DEVELOPMENT BY THE BCR

The next checkpoint in B cell development occurs during progression from immature to mature B cell stages. This process has been examined in a number of autoreactive transgenic mouse models (59–77) that have shown that encounter of immature B cells with antigen capable of cross-linking their BCR typically leads to one of three results: (*a*) cells are eliminated (clonal deletion); (*b*) cells become nonresponsive and likely short lived (anergic); or (*c*) cells revise their BCR to eliminate self-reactivity (editing). It appears likely that high-affinity interactions with membrane-bound antigen result in deletion, whereas lower-affinity interactions and soluble antigens allow editing or result in anergy (59, 60, 62, 66, 69). Even very low-affinity interactions are usually considered to have a negative impact on developing B cells (66). On the other hand, recent studies with a natural autoreactive BCR transgenic model have revealed a positive role for antigen in generating and maintaining this pool of B cells (78).

Cells at this new-B immature stage can be recognized by expression of surface Ig, although this may be sharply downregulated by interaction with antigen (59). Various stages of development during the progression from immature to mature B cells can be recognized based on expression of surface molecules such as IgD, CD23, CD24/HSA, and CD21/35 (see Table 2). As the normal regulated expression of many of these molecules may be disrupted by activation or in transgenic animals, other surface markers such as 493 (79) and AA4.1 (80, 81) may also be helpful in defining stages of immature and mature B cells.

TABLE 2   Phenotypes of peripheral B cell subsets

	Peripheral B cell subset					
Surface marker	T1	T2	MR/B-2	B-1a	B-1b	MZ
IgM	+++	++	+	+++	+++	+++
IgD	+/−	+	+++	+/−	+/−	+/−
493/AA4.1	++	+	−	−	−	−
B220(6B2)	+	++	+++	+/++	+/++	++
CD21	+/−	+	++	+/−	+/−	+++
CD23	−	+	++	++/−[a]	++/−[a]	−
HSA(J11d/30F1)	+++	++	+	++	++	++
CD43	+/−	−	−	++/−[a]	++/−[a]	
CD5	−	−	−	+	−	−
CD11b/Mac-1	−	−	−	+[b]	+[b]	−

[a] part are ++ and part are −.

[b] Only in peritoneal cavity; B-1 cells are CD11b/Mac-1⁻ in spleen.

T1, T2 = transitional (maturing) B cells.

MR = mature recirculating B cells.

MZ = marginal zone B cells.

Just as pre-BCR signaling results in a transient downregulation of Rag genes (82), production of a BCR appears critical in final cessation of Rag expression, as well as in Ig light chain rearrangement. Hence, productive B cell development requires expression of a light chain that can efficiently pair with the cell's particular heavy chain to form a cell surface BCR. However, the resulting BCR must not signal above some critical threshold (66). Otherwise, it appears that Rag expression continues (66), allowing further light chain kappa V genes to rearrange and produce alternative light chains to effectively pair with heavy chain. In order to successfully generate a nonautoreactive BCR, this light chain editing process can continue on both alleles and eventually proceed to the second light chain locus if unsuccessful at kappa, resulting in lambda light chain expression (65). Besides increased usage of lambda light chains, another hallmark of light chain editing is excessive use of the downstream J_κ segments, $J_\kappa 4$ and $J_\kappa 5$ (71). The critical role of the BCR in regulating Rag expression may be at least part of the reason for Rag re-expression in germinal center cells (83, 84), where hypermutation could alter Ig chains so that they fail to assemble efficiently into a BCR (or even become nonfunctional). A conditional knockout of Ig heavy chain has revealed a critical role for continued BCR expression, and probably low level signaling, in maintenance of the mature B cell pool (85).

DIFFERENCES BETWEEN FETAL LIVER AND ADULT BONE MARROW B CELL DEVELOPMENT

Peripheral B cells can be divided into several subpopulations based on differential surface expression of a variety of molecules, including IgM/IgD, CD23, CD24/HSA, and CD21/35 (86–90). About 20 years ago we identified a normal B cell subset expressing the CD5 molecule, found on normal T cells and on certain malignant B cells (12). In addition to sharing the phenotype of a set of B lymphomas (11), cells in this subset were of interest due to their expansion in certain autoimmune mouse strains and their ability to secrete natural autoantibodies in normal mouse strains (91). A surprising observation made early in the study of this subset was the poor level of repopulation found in cell transfer experiments that used adult bone marrow as a source of hematopoietic stem cells (92). The difficulty was not that CD5$^+$ B cells could not be generated in irradiated adult hosts, because similar experiments using liver from fetal or newborn animals reconstituted normal levels of this subset.

Subsequently, transfer experiments from two groups using more carefully fractionated B cell precursors showed that the phenotype of B cells generated with fetal liver is quite distinct from that using comparable precursors isolated from adult bone marrow (6, 93). This difference in B lymphopoiesis could be compared to the developmental switch in fetal to adult type hemoglobin (94–96) and raises the question of whether there are any other differences in hematopoiesis between fetal and adult development. In the T cell lineage, Weissman's group found that $V\gamma 3$ expressing $\gamma\delta$ cells could be generated from fetal liver hematopoietic stem cells (HSC) in fetal thymic organ culture, but not from HSC isolated from adult bone marrow (5).

More recently, work from Busslinger's group studying a Pax5/BSAP knockout mouse has also demonstrated differences between hematopoietic development in fetal liver and adult bone marrow (9). B cell development in Pax5/BSAP-deficient bone marrow proceeded to the $B220^+CD43^+$ stage and normal levels of D_H to J_H rearrangement were observed, although V_H to D_HJ_H rearrangement was severely depressed. In contrast, B lymphoid precursors were undetectable in fetal liver, suggesting a different (and critical) function for the Pax5/BSAP transcription factor during fetal hematopoiesis as compared to adult bone marrow.

Another difference between fetal and adult B cell development is that fetal B cell precursors express little or no TdT during the D-J and V-DJ stages of heavy chain rearrangement in fetal liver (7), and consequently precursors exhibit decreased (or absent) nontemplated nucleotide addition (N-regions) at these junctions (7, 46). As a further consequence of this lack, Feeney's group has reported that D-J and V-D junctions with one homology to several nucleotide homologies at the ends of adjacent coding segments are predominant (8, 97, 98). This homology-directed recombination, together with the absence of N-regions, serves to greatly restrict the diversity of the fetal/neonatal heavy chain V_H region repertoire. Interestingly, based on their germline sequences, homology-directed recombination will favor in frame (productive) rearrangements of V_H7183 and Q52 genes, but out-of-frame (nonproductive) rearrangements of the large J558 gene family (98). Wu's group has also found altered D_H frame usage as a consequence of TdT expression (99). Interestingly, enforced expression of TdT during fetal life in a transgenic mouse eliminated the well-characterized T15 anti-PC B cell subset that is protective against pneumococcal infection, and these animals were susceptible to such infection (100).

Besides these mechanisms that alter the heavy chain repertoire between fetal and adult B lymphopoiesis, there is also evidence for a difference in selection early in development, prior to the immature B cell stage. Careful analysis of the frequency of V_H81X utilization in cultures initiated with progenitors derived either from fetal liver or adult bone marrow revealed that V_H81X rearrangement decreased with length of culture; however, unlike bone marrow cultures, fetal progenitor cultures exhibited increased frequency of productive V_H81X rearrangements (101, 102). As mentioned above, heavy chains with V_H81X rearrangements often assemble poorly with surrogate light chain (49, 50), so these data may indicate that productive V_H81X rearrangements are more functional in fetal development. Poor assembly with SLC is also seen with a V_H11 heavy chain, and analysis of a V_H11 transgenic mouse showed expression biased toward fetal development (10). The well-known association of V_H11 with $CD5^+$ B cells (103, 104) makes this observation particularly intriguing.

A possible explanation for these unusual findings comes from analysis of the effect of pre-BCR assembly/signaling on the proliferation of pre-B cells in stromal cell culture (10). Curiously, although expression of a heavy chain transgene (capable of associating well with SLC) results in similar or even greater proliferation of adult bone marrow B lineage precursors (compared with precursors from Rag-deficient mice), comparable experiments using fetal liver cells showed that heavy chain expression inhibited proliferation. Similar experiments with a V_H11 heavy chain had much less suppressive effect on fetal proliferation, consistent with the hypothesis that pre-BCR assembly/signaling, rather than enhancing proliferation as in bone marrow, instead induces exit from cell cycle in fetal liver pre-B cells. In this model, V_H81X or V_H11 heavy chains that associate poorly with SLC would signal weakly, allow greater pre-B cell expansion, and so contribute more to the fetal Ig repertoire. Further suggestion of a differential response to pre-BCR signaling between fetal liver and bone marrow comes from analysis of SCID mice bearing the M54 transgene, where pre-BCR progression occurred in bone marrow, but not in fetal liver (105).

An underlying mechanism for a difference in cell proliferation (more rapid cell division versus exit from cycle) remains to be determined. The underlying reason why cells should behave in this fashion is also unclear. There has been speculation that the fetal/neonatal B cell Ig repertoire is skewed toward multireactive antibodies binding branched carbohydrate determinants present on common pathogens that also cross-react with self-determinants, promoting selection of such B cells into a long-lived pool (106–108). The heavy chains for such antibodies could be selected over evolutionary time for favorable expression during fetal development (by appropriate homologous regions flanking the V, D, and J elements). Furthermore, if surrogate light chain serves as a template for an average light chain structure in pre-BCR selection (see above), then failure to associate efficiently with SLC might imply a preference for atypical light chain V regions (as has been reported with V_H12; 58). Should this be the case, the particular heavy chain V region might require a specific light chain V region to complement it and thereby a novel antibody would be "hard-wired" into the repertoire. This could provide a mechanism for ensuring the expression of useful specificities, prior to emergence of the adaptive immune system. Table 3 summarizes known distinctions between fetal and adult hematopoiesis.

SELECTION AND MAINTENANCE OF PERIPHERAL CD5$^+$ B-1 B CELLS

B cells in the peripheral tissues can be subdivided into various subsets based on differences in surface phenotype (see Table 2). One can broadly discriminate mature recirculating CD5$^-$ B cells from CD5$^+$ B cells, and these are often referred to as "B-2" versus "B-1" B cells, respectively. This nomenclature, based on surface phenotype, was introduced to take account of a subset of B cells that has a similar phenotype to CD5$^+$ B cells but lacks CD5. Thus, B-1 phenotype B cells are further subdivided into B-1a (CD5$^+$) and B-1b (CD5$^-$). However, given that CD5 can be induced on "B-2" phenotype cells (109) and also that several of the phenotypic distinctions of B-1 cells are also shared with activated B cells, we caution that

TABLE 3   Distinctions in hematopoiesis between fetal and adult life

Aspect of development	Fetal liver	Bone marrow
HSC FTOC	Many $V\beta3^+$ $\gamma\delta$ T cells	No $V\beta3^+$ $\gamma\delta$ T cells
Pro-B cell transfer	Predominant B-1 B cells	Predominant B-2 B cells
TdT expression	Absent or low; little N-addition at heavy chain junctions	High in pro-B; N-addition at heavy chain junctions
Homology-directed recombination	Predominant— limits repertoire	Minimal- diverse repertoire
Pax-5 knockout	Absence of B220$^+$ cells	B cells blocked at Fr. C
Pre-BCR signaling	Exit from cell cycle— selection against strong SLC association	Proliferative burst— selection for SLC association

interpretation of data based purely on cell surface phenotype may be complex. Considering the fetal origin of the majority of CD5$^+$ B cells and the distinctions between fetal and adult development, it may be more appropriate to use B-1 to refer to fetal development (and progeny) and B-2 to describe adult bone marrow development (and progeny). In the following sections we review progress in our understanding of the processes regulating the generation and maintenance of B-1 B cells. Although a recent conditional knockout experiment showed that persistence of most peripheral B cells requires continued expression of the BCR (85), it remains to be determined whether this reflects a requirement for interaction of the BCR with external ligands, or instead whether simple expression of the BCR results in a level of signaling necessary for cell survival. On the other hand, considerable data suggest a strong connection between BCR-signaling and B-1 B cells (110, 111). Mice with alterations in B cell subsets are summarized in Table 4.

Role of BCR Signaling

B-1 cell development and maintenance appear to depend critically on BCR signaling, because a reduction of B-1 cell numbers occurs if there is insufficient BCR signaling. This may be caused by either a lack of antigen or a defect in the signaling machinery. In terms of defective BCR signaling, genetically engineered mutant mice defective in (or overexpressing) BCR signaling components are informative, although interpretation is not always straightforward. That is, whereas most analysis is done with B cell populations established in the adult, a BCR signaling defect may act at several stages: pre-BCR expansion, immature B cell selection, mature B cell activation, or mature B cell survival/persistence. It is important to recognize

TABLE 4 Mutations that alter CD5$^+$/B-1a, B-1b, or B2 B cell frequency

Type of alteration	Mutation	Effect
Weaken BCR signal	CD19 knockout	Decrease CD5$^+$ B cells
	BLNK/SLP-65 knockout	Decrease CD5$^+$ B cells
	CD21 knockout	Decrease CD5$^+$ B cells
	vav knockout	Decrease CD5$^+$ B cells
	PI3-kinase	Decrease CD5$^+$ B cells
	btk knockout (and xid)	Decrease CD5$^+$ B cells
Cell cycle progression	Cyclin D2 knockout	Decrease CD5$^+$ B cells
Strengthen BCR signal	SHP-1 mutant (me)	Increase CD5$^+$ B cells
	CD19-TG	Increase CD5$^+$ B cells
	CD22 knockout	Increase B-1b B cell
	lyn knockout	Increase B-1b B cells
	PD-1 knockout	Increase B-1b B cells
Restrict BCR specificity	3H9μ-TG	Decrease CD5$^+$ B cells
	M54μ-TG	Decrease CD5$^+$ B cells
	3-83$\mu\delta$-TG	Decrease CD5$^+$ B cells
	VH11μ-TG	Increase CD5$^+$ B cells
	VH12μ-TG	Increase CD5$^+$ B cells
	VH3609μ-TG	Increase CD5$^+$ B cells
Anti-apoptotic	BCL-2-TG	Increase B-2 B cells
Unknown gene	bcmd mutant	Decrease B-2 B cells

that the normal adult B cell populations are generated through the interplay of all of these processes in a dynamic fashion.

These considerations notwithstanding, it is generally found that mutations in positive regulators of BCR signaling, including deficiency of the CD19 BCR costimulatory transmembrane protein (112), the BLNK/SLP-65 adapter protein (113), the *Cr2* gene-encoded CD21 molecule that complexes with CD19 (114), vav (115, 116), the PI3-kinase p85α (117, 118), the Btk tyrosine kinase (119), and the Oct-2 transcription factor (120), all result in a greater reduction of B-1 cells compared to other peripheral B cells. Since most of these factors are known to play roles in BCR mediated activation, the decrease in CD5$^+$ B cells has usually been attributed to disruption of activation-mediated upregulation of CD5 expression. However, it is important to note that at least some of these signaling components may play a role in cell survival as well. Btk, in particular, acts to prevent BCR-mediated apoptosis (121). A role for signaling mediators in selection during B cell development is also likely, as in the case of vav in thymocyte selection (122). Finally, the well-characterized BCR/CD19/vav/PI3K pathway (123) may also be involved in selection/survival of B cells. Thus a decrease in CD5$^+$ B cells may reflect not a direct disruption of activation-induced CD5 expression, but rather altered recruitment/selection or maintenance/persistence of CD5$^+$ B cells.

BCR-mediated signaling is also controlled by negative regulators, such as the CD22 BCR adapter molecule (124, 125). The src family kinase, Lyn, has been recently suggested as a negative regulator of BCR signaling based on its capacity to phosphorylate the inhibitory receptors $Fc\gamma RIIb$ or CD22 (126). PD-1, an Ig superfamily member with an ITIM motif, was also reported recently as a negative regulator (127, 128). Tolerance induction is likely affected by altered BCR signaling thresholds. $Fc\gamma RIIb$, CD22, and PD-1 can all recruit SHP-1 protein tyrosine phosphatase that can play a major role in negative signaling. While SHP-1 mutant motheaten (Me) mice show increased CD5$^+$ B cells (129), mice lacking CD22, lyn, or PD-1 all show an increase of CD5$^-$ B-1b phenotype cells (rather than CD5$^+$ B-1a cells) together with splenomegaly and autoantibody production (130–132). We speculate that the Me mouse may represent excessive promotion of positive selection in B-1 precursors because analysis can only be carried out in young animals before they die prematurely; thus the B cells analyzed are mostly the progeny of B-1 development. The increase in B-1b-like cells in CD22-, lyn-, or PD-1-deficient adult animals might be due to a breakdown in tolerance during B-2 development, since adult bone marrow cells can generate B-1b type cells (93). As the autoreactive repertoire rescued by such defective B-2 development (of cells normally tolerized) likely differs from that of B-1, CD5 upregulation does not occur, and so one obtains the B-1b phenotype. The CD5$^+$ B cell increase in the spleen of transgenic mice that overexpress CD19 (133) is more difficult to understand, due either to enhanced positive selection or to defective negative regulation or activation.

Role of BCR Specificity

Transgenic mice with BCRs characteristic of CD5$^+$ B cells typically develop increased numbers of this subset, often to the exclusion of CD5$^-$ B cells (54, 134), demonstrating the importance of particular BCR specificities in generating these cells. If B-1 cell development requires BCR signaling, then the lack of appropriate antigen may diminish their generation. This possibility is supported by the observation of reduced numbers of CD5$^+$ B cells (B-1a) in most transgenic mouse lines with a non-selecting specificity such as toward irrelevant anti-H-2 (134) or with a privileged specificity such as that to antigens expressed in isolated sites, such as brain anti-myelin/oligodendrocyte glycoprotein (135). In contrast, B-2 cell generation is intact in these mice.

Recently the role of antigen in selecting CD5$^+$ B-1 B cells has been demonstrated definitively (78). Assessing whether CD5$^+$ B cells have an absolute requirement for self-antigen, by elimination of self-antigen, has been difficult because such antigens are typically glycosylations of proteins or lipids that are critical cellular constituents and thus cannot be eliminated in live cells. This was overcome recently by utilizing a CD5$^+$ B cell–derived specificity reactive to a carbohydrate epitope of the Thy-1/CD90 glycoprotein (136), encoded by $V_H3609/V_\kappa21C$ germline genes (137). Introducing $V_H3609\mu$ as a transgene resulted in an increase of CD5$^+$ B cells reactive with anti-thymocyte autoantigen (ATA), generated through pairing of the transgene with endogenous $V_\kappa 21C$, and resulting in high ATA levels in serum (78). Importantly, accumulation of these ATA B cells and increased ATA Ig serum titer did not occur when the self-antigen was eliminated in Thy-1 gene knockout mice. Thus, self-antigen is clearly critical for the generation of natural autoreactive B cells and of serum natural autoantibody. Also this study demonstrates that the Thy-1 glycoprotein can serve as a major source of physiologic self-antigen ligand for natural autoreactive B cells.

BCR specificities characteristic of B-1a ($CD5^+$) B cells, selected and maintained throughout life, appear to be encoded by distinctive germline genes, often in combination with particular light chain genes, constituting a restricted hard-wired antibody repertoire. This suggests that B-1 cell generation is a part of innate immunity, genetically selected for reactivity to self/natural antigens, and there is, therefore, no necessity for affinity maturation normally associated with immune responses. However, if B-1 precursors are genetically engineered not to express such appropriate inherited specificities, then cells in this population may continue to attempt to express specificities favoring positive selection. This may explain the common finding of a failure of allelic exclusion in peritoneal cavity B-1 cells from Ig transgenic mice and also the continuing Rag expression in B-1a cell from anti-NP V-region knockin mice (138).

Non-BCR Related Mediators

Overexpression of anti-apoptosis genes such as *Bcl-2* or *Bcl-xL* in transgenic mice can rescue negative selection in B-2 B cell development. In contrast, such overexpression did not increase B-1a B cells (RR Hardy, K Hayakawa, unpublished), suggesting that positive selection is not further promoted as long as self-antigen is present, though these cells likely require Bcl-2 for baseline survival (139). Other than this requirement for Bcl-2 family genes (probably shared with B-1), the question arises as to whether B-2 cells possess alternative survival mechanisms in place of the positive selection–based B-1 survival.

Intriguingly, the Hays and Cancro groups found that in A/WySnJ mice, defective for the *bcmd* gene (140, 141), B-2 B cells have a reduced life span (142); while primary antibody response is intact, the memory response is defective. In contrast, B-1 cell frequency is normal in these mice. This segregation of B-2 and B-1 in A/WySn mice may provide a clue in understanding distinctive B cell development and may aid in determining their independent functions. Solvason and colleagues (143) noted that $CD5^+$ B cells were uniquely decreased in animals lacking cyclin D2, which may indicate that generation of a long-lived population of these cells requires cyclin D2-dependent cell cycle progression (in contrast to long-lived subsets of $CD5^-$ B cells).

Possible Role of CD5

Analysis of cell activation using B cells isolated from CD5-deficient mice, by Bondada and colleagues, suggested that this molecule plays a direct role in modulating the response to BCR cross-linking, acting as a negative regulator (144).

Further work from this group suggests that this is due to the capacity of CD5 to recruit SHP-1, a cytosolic protein tyrosine phosphatase, to the BCR (145). Direct evidence for the function of CD5 in a B cell tolerance model has been reported by Behrens (146), who found that HEL-Ig mice on the soluble HEL Tg background had increased levels of anti-HEL antibody on a CD5-deficient background. B cells in these mice also showed enhanced proliferation in response to Ig cross-linking, compared to cells from mice on a CD5 wild-type background. However, the significance of the CD5 molecule in B-1 cell positive selection is not clear because anti-PtC or ATA B cell accumulation and natural serum secretion occur in CD5 knockout mice at levels comparable to wild type (78).

It seems likely that CD5 induction has significance in the self-regulation of autoreactivity after B-1 cells mature, such as an elimination of B-1 cells rendered overactive, as previously suggested by prevention of apoptosis induced by anti-IgM (extra BCR signaling) in CD5 knockout mice (144). Understanding of the CD5 glycoprotein as an antigen receptor adapter protein functioning as a positive or negative regulator has progressed in recent years, now including aspects of CD5 structure (147–149), CD5 ligands (150, 151), and signaling initiated either indirectly by antigen receptor or directly by CD5 cross-linking (145, 152–158). This information mostly derives from work with T cells expressing high levels of CD5 (152–155). In considering the relevance of CD5 on B cells, NFAT seems to be involved in BCR-induced upregulation of CD5 on B cells (159). The cytoplasmic portion of CD5 has been found to interact with Tctex-1 (a light chain component of the dynein motor complex) and the Ca^{2+}/calmodulin-dependent kinase IIδ, which may be involved in the BCR internalization and the subsequent negative regulatory role of CD5 (156). CD5 internalization and subsequent control of signaling is an interesting ongoing area of research.

Importance of Location: Peritoneal Cavity and Autoreactive B Cells

Honjo and associates provided a series of experiments demonstrating the pathogenic role of peritoneal cavity B cells with an anti-erythrocyte autoreactivity in a transgenic mouse model (160). In contrast to the deletion of B cells in the spleen, B cells are present in the peritoneal cavity. They show B-1b phenotype, with a potential to secrete anti-erythrocyte autoantibody following either LPS, IL-5, or IL-10 administration. Overexpression of IL-5 increases their frequency and differentiation into antibody secreting cells. Furthermore, such cells are decreased in the absence of the IL-5R, a scenario similar to normal B-1a in the peritoneal cavity. However, unlike B-1, whose development is essentially independent of T cell help (11), these anti-erythrocyte B cells in the peritoneal cavity are not generated on a Rag$-/-$ background and thus appear to be dependent on T cells for IL-10/IL-5 secretion (161, 162).

A critical issue is whether such cells are representative of normal CD5$^+$ B-1 cells. The peritoneal cavity may provide a unique site to protect B cells normally deleted. Since both B-1 and B-2 development can generate B cells in the peritoneal cavity with a similar B-1b phenotype, cells with such a phenotype may be derived from either pathway and by a variety of mechanisms. It may be that this pathogenic, presumably non-germline encoded, anti-erythrocyte autoantibody BCR may not model normal B-1 cell development, but rather may provide a key to understanding pathogenic processes not restricted to either B-1 or B-2. Developing B-1 and B-2 cells are both subject to deletion when strong BCR cross-linking occurs, and this deletion may be rescued by a distinctive cytokine milieu (T cell derived in this case) provided by the peritoneal cavity microenvironment. Initially, these investigators considered the presence of B-1b cells in the peritoneal cavity as due to the absence of antigen. However, their recent data suggest that antigenic exposure is involved at some level, since mice homozygous for the Tg with higher Tg Ig levels on the surface were more completely deleted in the spleen than were heterozygous mice (as expected), whereas peritoneal B-1b cells were instead increased (163). This may imply a unique feature of the peritoneal cavity environment to rescue antigen-induced apoptosis. As a recent report shows, overexpression of IL-9, known as tumor promoting factor, results in a dramatic increase of B-1b cells but not B-1a cells (164). This IL-9-induced proliferative effect does not depend on IL-5. These data may indicate a mixed origin of B-1b phenotype cell in which B-1b generation from B-2 may depend on T cells and cytokines with a higher potential for pathogenesis. In this regard, it will be interesting to determine whether the inability to induce plasmacytomas in *btk*-deficient Xid mice (165) reflects a specific deficiency in B-1 cells or of peritoneal cavity localized B-2 cells.

CONCLUDING REMARKS

B cell development progresses through several critical stages involving commitment, initial establishment of the Ig repertoire, and cellular selection. Evidence is accumulating that at least some of these processes differ with ontogeny, resulting in the generation of distinctive Ig repertoires at different ages. B-1 represents fetal/neonatal B cell development in mice, whose development and maintenance appears to depend critically on positive selection, possibly in contrast to B-2 in the adult. This positive selection may explain several characteristics previously associated with the established B-1 cell pool: their autoreactive repertoire, distinctive phenotype, and preferential peritoneal cavity localization. Consideration of B-1 as encompassing the entire fetal developmental process, involving surface alteration including the CD5$^-$ to CD5$^+$ stages, may help to avoid some of the confusion of a classification based solely on surface phenotype criteria. Further elucidation of ontogenically distinctive B cell developmental mechanisms in mice is an important subject of further research, with implications for understanding the evolution (phylogeny) of the immune system and age-related changes in the immune response.

ACKNOWLEDGMENTS

We would like to thank Drs. K Campbell, D Kappes, and D Wiest for critical reading of this manuscript.

Visit the Annual Reviews home page at www.AnnualReviews.org

LITERATURE CITED

1. Lee G, Namen AE, Gillis S, Ellingsworth LR, Kincade PW. 1989. Normal B cell precursors responsive to recombinant murine IL-7 and inhibition of IL-7 activity by transforming growth factor-beta. *J. Immunol.* 142:3875–83

2. Ishihara K, Medina K, Hayashi S,Pietrangeli C, Namen AE, Miyake K, Kincade PW. 1991. Stromal-cell and cytokine-dependent lymphocyte clones which span the pre-B- to B-cell transition. *Dev. Immunol.* 1:149–61

3. Winkler TH, Melchers F, Rolink AG. 1995. Interleukin-3 and interleukin-7 are alternative growth factors for the same B-cell precursors in the mouse. *Blood* 85:2045–51

4. Rolink A, Ghia P, Grawunder U, Haasner D, Karasuyama H, Kalberer C, Winkler T, Melchers F. 1995. In-vitro analyses of mechanisms of B-cell development. *Semin. Immunol.* 7:155–67

5. Ikuta K, Kina T, MacNeil I, Uchida N, Peault B, Chien YH, Weissman IL. 1990. A developmental switch in thymic lymphocyte maturation potential occurs at the level of hematopoietic stem cells. *Cell* 62:863–74

6. Hardy RR, Hayakawa K. 1991. A developmental switch in B lymphopoiesis. *Proc. Natl. Acad. Sci. USA* 88:11550–54

7. Li YS, Hayakawa K, Hardy RR. 1993. The regulated expression of B lineage associated genes during B cell differentiation in bone marrow and fetal liver. *J. Exp. Med.* 178:951–60

8. Feeney AJ. 1992. Predominance of VH-D-JH junctions occurring at sites of short sequence homology results in limited junctional diversity in neonatal antibodies. *J. Immunol.* 149:222–29

9. Nutt SL, Urbanek P, Rolink A, Busslinger M. 1997. Essential functions of Pax5 (BSAP) in pro-B cell development: difference between fetal and adult B lymphopoiesis and reduced V-to-DJ. recombination at the IgH locus. *Genes Dev.* 11:476–91

10. Wasserman R, Li YS, Shinton SA, Carmack CE, Manser T, Wiest DL, Hayakawa K, Hardy RR. 1998. A novel mechanism for B cell repertoire maturation based on response by B cell precursors to pre-B receptor assembly. *J. Exp. Med.* 187:259–64

11. Hayakawa K, Hardy RR. 1988. Normal, autoimmune, and malignant CD5+ B cells:the Ly-1 B lineage? *Annu. Rev. Immunol.* 6:197–218

12. Hayakawa K, Hardy RR, Parks DR, Herzenberg LA. 1983. The "Ly-1 B" cell subpopulation in normal, immunodefective, and autoimmune mice. *J. Exp. Med.* 157:202–18

13. Hardy RR, Carmack CE, Shinton SA, Kemp JD, Hayakawa K. 1991. Resolution and characterization of pro-B and pre-pro-B cell stages in normal mouse bone marrow. *J. Exp. Med.* 173:1213–25

14. Karasuyama H, Rolink A, Melchers F. 1996. Surrogate light chain in B cell development. *Adv. Immunol.* 63:1–41

15. Osmond DG, Rolink A, Melchers F. 1998. Murine B lymphopoiesis: towards a unified model. *Immunol. Today* 19:65–68

16. Kondo M, Weissman IL, Akashi K. 1997.

Identification of clonogenic common lymphoid progenitors in mouse bone marrow. *Cell* 91:661–72

17. Allman D, Li J, Hardy RR. 1999. Commitment to the B lymphoid lineage occurs before DH-JH recombination. *J. Exp. Med.* 189:735–40

18. Li YS, Wasserman R, Hayakawa K, Hardy RR. 1996. Identification of the earliest B lineage stage in mouse bone marrow. *Immunity* 5:527–35

19. Ogawa M, ten Boekel E, Melchers F. 2000. Identification of CD19($-$)B220($^+$)c-Kit($^+$)Flt3/Flk-2($^+$)cells as early B lymphoid precursors before pre-B-I cells in juvenile mouse bone marrow. *Int. Immunol.* 12:313–24

20. Rolink A, ten Boekel E, Melchers F, Fearon DT, Krop I, Andersson J. 1996. A subpopulation of B220$^+$ cells in murine bone marrow does not express CD19 and contains natural killer cell progenitors. *J. Exp. Med.* 183:187–94

21. Tudor KS, Payne KJ, Yamashita Y, Kincade PW. 2000. Functional assessment of precursors from murine bone marrow suggests a sequence of early B lineage differentiation events. *Immunity* 12:335–45

22. Schlueter AJ, Malek TR, Hostetler CN, Smith PA, deVries P, Waldschmidt TJ. 1997. Distribution of Ly-6C on lymphocyte subsets: I. Influence of allotype on T lymphocyte expression. *J. Immunol.* 158:4211–22

23. Loffert D, Schaal S, Ehlich A, Hardy RR, Zou YR, Muller W, Rajewsky K. 1994. Early B-cell development in the mouse: insights from mutations introduced by gene targeting. *Immunol. Rev.* 137:135–53

24. Zhuang Y, Cheng P, Weintraub H. 1996. B-lymphocyte development is regulated by the combined dosage of three basic helix-loop-helix genes, E2A, E2-2, and HEB. *Mol. Cell. Biol.* 16:2898–2905

25. Jacobs Y, Xin XQ, Dorshkind K, Nelson C. 1994. Pan/E2A expression precedes immunoglobulin heavy-chain expression during B lymphopoiesis in nontransformed cells, and Pan/E2A proteins are not detected in myeloid cells. *Mol. Cell. Biol.* 14:4087–96

26. Bain G, Robanus Maandag EC, te Riele HP, Feeney AJ, Sheehy A, Schlissel M, Shinton SA, Hardy RR, Murre C. 1997. Both E12 and E47 allow commitment to the B cell lineage. *Immunity* 6:145–54

27. Lin H, Grosschedl R. 1995. Failure of B-cell differentiation in mice lacking the transcription factor EBF. *Nature* 376:263–67

28. Eisenbeis CF, Singh H, Storb U. 1993. PU.1 is a component of a multiprotein complex which binds an essential site in the murine immunoglobulin lambda 2-4 enhancer. *Mol. Cell. Biol.* 13:6452–61

29. Klemsz MJ, McKercher SR, Celada A, Van Beveren C, Maki RA. 1990. The macrophage and B cell-specific transcription factor PU.1 is related to the ets oncogene. *Cell* 61:113–24

30. Scott EW, Simon MC, Anastasi J, Singh H. 1994. Requirement of transcription factor PU.1 in the development of multiple hematopoietic lineages. *Science* 265:1573–77

31. McKercher SR, Torbett BE, Anderson KL, Henkel GW, Vestal DJ, Baribault H, Klemsz M, Feeney AJ, Wu GE, Paige CJ, Maki RA. 1996. Targeted disruption of the PU.1 gene results in multiple hematopoietic abnormalities. *Embo J.* 15:5647–58

32. Barberis A, Widenhorn K, Vitelli L, Busslinger M. 1990. A novel B-cell lineage-specific transcription factor present at early but not late stages of differentiation. *Genes Dev.* 4:849–59

33. Nutt SL, Heavey B, Rolink AG, Busslinger M. 1999. Commitment to the B-lymphoid lineage depends on the transcription factor Pax5. *Nature* 401:556–62

34. Rolink AG, Nutt SL, Melchers F, Busslinger M. 1999. Long-term in vivo reconstitution of T-cell development by Pax5- deficient B-cell progenitors. *Nature* 401:603–6

35. Blunt T, Finnie NJ, Taccioli GE, Smith GC, Demengeot J, Gottlieb TM, Mizuta R, Varghese AJ, Alt FW, Jeggo PA, 1995. Defective DNA-dependent protein kinase activity is linked to V(D)J. recombination and DNA repair defects associated with the murine scid mutation. *Cell* 80:813–23

36. Reichman-Fried M, Hardy RR, Bosma MJ. 1990. Development of B-lineage cells in the bone marrow of scid/scid mice following the introduction of functionally rearranged immunoglobulin transgenes. *Proc. Natl. Acad. Sci. USA* 87:2730–34

37. Oettinger MA, Schatz DG, Gorka C, Baltimore D. 1990. RAG-1 and RAG-2, adjacent genes that synergistically activate V(D)J. recombination. *Science* 248:1517–23

38. Shinkai Y, Rathbun G, Lam KP, Oltz EM, Stewart V, Mendelsohn M, Charron J, Datta M, Young F, Stall AM, 1992. RAG-2-deficient mice lack mature lymphocytes owing to inability to initiate V(D)J. rearrangement. *Cell* 68:855–67

39. Mombaerts P, Iacomini J, Johnson RS, Herrup K, Tonegawa S, Papaioannou VE. 1992. RAG-1-deficient mice have no mature B and T lymphocytes. *Cell* 68:869–77

40. Spanopoulou E, Roman CA, Corcoran LM, Schlissel MS, Silver DP, Nemazee D, Nussenzweig MC, Shinton SA, Hardy RR, Baltimore D. 1994. Functional immunoglobulin transgenes guide ordered B-cell differentiation in Rag-1-deficient mice. *Genes Dev.* 8:1030–42

41. Young F, Ardman B, Shinkai Y, Lansford R, Blackwell TK, Mendelsohn M, Rolink A, Melchers F, Alt FW. 1994. Influence of immunoglobulin heavy- and light-chain expression on B-cell differentiation [published erratum appears in *Genes Dev.* 1995 Dec 15;9(24):3190]. *Genes Dev.* 8:1043–57

42. Karasuyama H, Kudo A, Melchers F. 1990. The proteins encoded by the VpreB and lambda 5 pre-B cell-specific genes can as-

sociate with each other and with mu heavy chain. *J. Exp. Med.* 172:969–72

43. Karasuyama H, Rolink A, Melchers F. 1993. A complex of glycoproteins is associated with VpreB/lambda 5 surrogate light chain on the surface of mu heavy chain-negative early precursor B cell lines. *J. Exp. Med.* 178:469–78

44. Kitamura D, Kudo A, Schaal S, Muller W, Melchers F, Rajewsky K. 1992. A critical role of lambda 5 protein in B cell development. *Cell* 69:823–31

45. Gong S, Nussenzweig MC. 1996. Regulation of an early developmental checkpoint. in the B cell pathway by Ig beta. *Science* 272:411–14

46. Gilfillan S, Dierich A, LemEur M, Benoist C, Mathis D. 1993. Mice lacking TdT: mature animals with an immature lymphocyte repertoire [published erratum appears in *Science* 1993 Dec 24;262(5142):1957]. *Science* 261:1175–78

47. Komori T, Okada A, Stewart V, Alt FW. 1993. Lack of N regions in antigen receptor variable region genes of TdT-deficient lymphocytes. *Science* 261:1171–75

48. Yancopoulos GD, Desiderio SV, Paskind M, Kearney JF, Baltimore D, Alt FW. 1984. Preferential utilization of the most JH-proximal VH gene segments in pre-B-cell lines. *Nature* 311:727–33

49. Keyna U, Beck-Engeser GB, Jongstra J, Applequist SE, Jack HM. 1995. Surrogate light chain-dependent selection of Ig heavy chain V regions. *J. Immunol.* 155:5536–42

50. Kline GH, Hartwell L, Beck-Engeser GB, Keyna U, Zaharevitz S, Klinman NR, Jack HM. 1998. Pre-B cell receptor-mediated selection of pre-B cells synthesizing functional mu heavy chains. *J. Immunol.* 161:1608–18

51. Karasuyama H, Nakamura T, Nagata K, Kuramochi T, Kitamura F, Kuida K. 1997. The roles of preB cell receptor in early B cell development and its signal transduction. *Immunol. Cell Biol* 75:209–16

52. Decker DJ, Kline GH, Hayden TA, Zaharevitz SN, Klinman NR. 1995. Heavy chain V gene-specific elimination of B cells during the pre-B cell to B cell transition. *J. Immunol.* 154:4924–35

53. ten Boekel E, Melchers F, Rolink AG. 1997. Changes in the V(H) gene repertoire of developing precursor B lymphocytes in mouse bone marrow mediated by the pre-B cell receptor. *Immunity* 7:357–68

54. Arnold LW, Pennell CA, McCray SK, Clarke SH. 1994. Development of B-1 cells: segregation of phosphatidyl choline-specific B cells to the B-1 population occurs after immunoglobulin gene expression. *J. Exp. Med.* 179:1585–95

55. Pennell CA, Sheehan KM, BrodEur PH, Clarke SH. 1989. Organization and expression of VH gene families preferentially expressed by Ly-1$^+$ (CD5) B cells. *Eur. J. Immunol.* 19:2115–21

56. Clarke SH, McCray SK. 1993. VH CDR3-dependent positive selection of murine VH12-expressing B cells in the neonate. *Eur. J. Immunol.* 23:3327–34

57. Ye J, McCray SK, Clarke SH. 1996. The transition of pre-BI to pre-BII cells is dependent on the VH structure of the mu/surrogate L chain receptor. *Embo J.* 15:1524–33

58. Tatu C, Ye J, Arnold LW, Clarke SH. 1999. Selection at multiple checkpoints focuses V(H)12 B cell differentiation toward a single B-1 cell specificity. *J. Exp. Med.* 190:903–14

59. Goodnow CC, Crosbie J, Adelstein S, Lavoie TB, Smith GSJ, Brink RA, Pritchard BH, Wotherspoon JS, Loblay RH, Raphael K, Trent RJ, Basten A. 1988. Altered immunoglobulin expression and functional silencing of self-reactive B lymphocytes in transgenic mice. *Nature* 334:676–82

60. Hartley SB, Crosbie J, Brink R, Kantor AB, Basten A, Goodnow CC. 1991. Elimination from peripheral lymphoid tissues of self-reactive B lymphocytes recognizing membrane-bound antigens. *Nature* 353:765–69

61. Hartley SB, Cooke MP, Fulcher DA, Harris AW, Cory S, Basten A, Goodnow CC. 1993. Elimination of self-reactive B lymphocytes proceeds in two stages: arrested development and cell death. *Cell* 72:325–35

62. Hartley SB, Goodnow CC. 1994. Censoring of self-reactive B cells with a range of receptor affinities in transgenic mice expressing heavy chains for a lysozyme-specific antibody. *Int. Immunol.* 6:1417–25

63. Nemazee DA, Burki K. 1989. Clonal deletion of B lymphocytes in a transgenic mouse bearing anti-MHC class I antibody genes. *Nature* 337:562–66

64. Russell DM, Dembic Z, Morahan G, Miller JF, Burki K, Nemazee D. 1991. Peripheral deletion of self-reactive B cells. *Nature* 354:308–11

65. Tiegs SL, Russell DM, Nemazee D. 1993. Receptor editing in self-reactive bone marrow B cells. *J. Exp. Med.* 177:1009–20

66. Lang J, Jackson M, Teyton L, Brunmark A, Kane K, Nemazee D. 1996. B cells are exquisitely sensitive to central tolerance and receptor editing induced by ultralow affinity, membrane-bound antigen. *J. Exp. Med.* 184:1685–97

67. Pelanda R, Schwers S, Sonoda E, Torres RM, Nemazee D, Rajewsky K. 1997. Receptor editing in a transgenic mouse model: site, efficiency, and role in B cell tolerance and antibody diversification. *Immunity* 7:765–75

68. Retter MW, Nemazee D. 1998. Receptor editing occurs frequently during normal B cell development. *J. Exp. Med.* 188:1231–38

69. Benschop RJ, Melamed D, Nemazee D, Cambier JC. 1999. Distinct signal thresholds for the unique antigen receptor-linked gene expression programs in mature and immature B cells. *J. Exp. Med.* 190:749–56

70. Erikson J, Radic MZ, Camper SA, Hardy

RR, Carmack C, Weigert M. 1991. Expression of anti-DNA immunoglobulin transgenes in non-autoimmune mice. *Nature* 349:331–34

71. Radic MZ, Erikson J, Litwin S, Weigert M. 1993. B lymphocytes may escape tolerance by revising their antigen receptors. *J. Exp. Med.* 177:1165–73

72. Gay D, Saunders T, Camper S, Weigert M. 1993. Receptor editing: an approach by autoreactive B cells to escape tolerance. *J. Exp. Med.* 177:999–1008

73. Chen C, Radic MZ, Erikson J, Camper SA, Litwin S, Hardy RR, Weigert M. 1994. Deletion and editing of B cells that express antibodies to DNA. *J. Immunol.* 152:1970–82

74. Chen C, Nagy Z, Radic MZ, Hardy RR, Huszar D, Camper SA, Weigert M. 1995. The site and stage of anti-DNA B-cell deletion. *Nature* 373:252–55

75. Prak EL, Weigert M. 1995. Light chain replacement: a new model for antibody gene rearrangement. *J. Exp. Med.* 182:541–48

76. Chen C, Prak EL, Weigert M. 1997. Editing disease-associated autoantibodies. *Immunity* 6:97–105

77. Xu H, Li H, Suri-Payer E, Hardy RR, Weigert M. 1998. Regulation of anti-DNA B cells in recombination-activating gene-deficient mice. *J. Exp. Med.* 188:1247–54

78. Hayakawa K, Shinton SA, Asano M, Hardy RR. 2000. B-1 cell definition. *Curr. Top. Microbiol. Immunol.* In press

79. Rolink AG, Andersson J, Melchers F. 1998. Characterization of immature B cells by a novel monoclonal antibody, by turnover and by mitogen reactivity. *Eur. J. Immunol.* 28:3738–48

80. McKearn JP, Baum C, Davie JM. 1984. Cell surface antigens expressed by subsets of pre-B cells and B cells. *J. Immunol.* 132:332–39

81. Petrenko O, Beavis A, Klaine M, Kittappa R, Godin I, Lemischka IR. 1999. The molecular characterization of the fetal stem cell marker AA4. *Immunity* 10:691–700

82. Grawunder U, Leu TM, Schatz DG, Werner A, Rolink AG, Melchers F, Winkler TH. 1995. Down-regulation of RAG1 and RAG2 gene expression in preB cells after functional immunoglobulin heavy chain rearrangement. *Immunity* 3:601–8

83. Hikida M, Ohmori H. 1998. Rearrangement of lambda light chain genes in mature B cells in vitro and in vivo. Function of reexpressed recombination-activating gene (RAG) products. *J. Exp. Med.* 187:795–99

84. Han S, Dillon SR, Zheng B, Shimoda M, Schlissel MS, Kelsoe G. 1997. V(D)J recombinase activity in a subset of germinal center B lymphocytes. *Science* 278:301–5

85. Lam KP, Rajewsky K. 1998. Rapid elimination of mature autoreactive B cells demonstrated by Cre- induced change in B cell antigen receptor specificity in vivo. *Proc. Natl. Acad. Sci. USA* 95:13171–75

86. Hardy RR, Hayakawa K, Haaijman J, Herzenberg LA. 1982. B cell subpopulations identified by two-color fluorescence analysis. *Nature* 297:589–91

87. Waldschmidt TJ, Conrad DH, Lynch RG. 1988. The expression of B cell surface receptors. I. The ontogeny and distribution of the murine B cell IgE Fc receptor. *J. Immunol.* 140:2148–54

88. Allman DM, Ferguson SE, Cancro MP. 1992. Peripheral B cell maturation. I. Immature peripheral B cells in adults are heat-stable antigenhi and exhibit unique signaling characteristics. *J. Immunol.* 149:2533–40

89. Allman DM, Ferguson SE, Lentz VM, Cancro MP. 1993. Peripheral B cell maturation. II. Heat-stable antigen(hi) splenic B cells are an immune developmental intermediate in the production of long-lived marrow-derived B cells. *J. Immunol.* 151:4431–44

90. Takahashi K, Kozono Y, Waldschmidt TJ, Berthiaume D, Quigg RJ, Baron A, Holers VM. 1997. Mouse complement receptors type 1 (CR1;CD35) and type 2 (CR2;CD21): expression on normal B cell

subpopulations and decreased levels during the development of autoimmunity in MRL/lpr mice. *J. Immunol.* 159:1557–69

91. Hayakawa K, Hardy RR, Honda M, Herzenberg LA, Steinberg AD, Herzenberg LA. 1984. Ly-1 B cells: functionally distinct lymphocytes that secrete IgM autoantibodies. *Proc. Natl. Acad. Sci. USA* 81:2494–98

92. Hayakawa K, Hardy RR, Herzenberg LA, Herzenberg LA. 1985. Progenitors for Ly-1 B cells are distinct from progenitors for other B cells. *J. Exp. Med.* 161:1554–68

93. Kantor AB, Stall AM, Adams S, Herzenberg LA, Herzenberg LA. 1992. Differential development of progenitor activity for three B-cell lineages. *Proc. Natl. Acad. Sci. USA* 89:3320–24

94. Enver T, Raich N, Ebens AJ, Papayannopoulou T, Costantini F, Stamatoyannopoulos G. 1990. Developmental regulation of human fetal-to-adult globin gene switching in transgenic mice. *Nature* 344:309–13

95. Whitelaw E, Tsai SF, Hogben P, Orkin SH. 1990. Regulated expression of globin chains and the erythroid transcription factor GATA-1 during erythropoiesis in the developing mouse. *Mol. Cell. Biol.* 10:6596–6606

96. Wong PMC, Chung S-W, Reicheld SM, Chui DHK. 1986. Hemoglobin switching during murine embryonic development: evidence for two populations of embryonic erythropoietic progenitor cells. *Blood* 67:716–21

97. Chukwuocha RU, Feeney AJ. 1993. Role of homology-directed recombination: predominantly productive rearrangements of Vh81X in newborns but not in adults. *Mol. Immunol.* 30:1473–79

98. Chukwuocha RU, Nadel B, Feeney AJ. 1995. Analysis of homology-directed recombination in VDJ. junctions from cytoplasmic Ig- pre-B cells of newborn mice. *J. Immunol.* 154:1246–55

99. Marshall AJ, Doyen N, Bentolila LA,

Paige CJ, Wu GE. 1998. Terminal deoxynucleotidyl transferase expression during neonatal life alters D(H) reading frame usage and Ig-receptor-dependent selection of V regions. *J. Immunol.* 161:6657–63

100. Benedict CL, Kearney JF. 1999. Increased junctional diversity in fetal B cells results in a loss of protective antiphosphorylcholine antibodies in adult mice. *Immunity* 10:607–17

101. Marshall AJ, Wu GE, Paige GJ. 1996. Frequency of VH81x usage during B cell development: initial decline in usage is independent of Ig heavy chain cell surface expression. *J. Immunol.* 156:2077–84

102. Marshall AJ, Paige CJ, Wu GE. 1997. V(H) repertoire maturation during B cell development in vitro: differential selection of Ig heavy chains by fetal and adult B cell progenitors. *J. Immunol.* 158:4282–91

103. Carmack CE, Shinton SA, Hayakawa K, Hardy RR. 1990. Rearrangement and selection of VH11 in the Ly-1 B cell lineage. *J. Exp. Med.* 172:371–74

104. Hardy RR, Carmack CE, Shinton SA, Riblet RJ, Hayakawa K. 1989. A single VH gene is utilized predominantly in anti-BrMRBC hybridomas derived from purified Ly-1 B cells. Definition of the VH11 family. *J. Immunol.* 142:3643–51

105. Bosma GC, Chang Y, Karasuyama H, Bosma MJ. 1999. Differential effect of an Ig mu transgene on development of pre-B cells in fetal and adult SCID mice. *Proc. Natl. Acad. Sci. USA* 96:11952–57

106. Teale JM, Kearney JF. 1986. Clonotypic analysis of the fetal B cell repertoire:evidence for an early and predominant expression of idiotypes associated with the VH 36- 60 family. *J. Mol. Cell. Immunol.* 2:283–92

107. Vakil M, Sauter H, Paige C, Kearney JF. 1986. In vivo suppression of perinatal multispecific B cells results in a distortion of the adult B cell repertoire. *Eur. J. Immunol.* 16:1159–65

108. Kearney JF, Won WJ, Benedict C, Moratz C, Zimmer P, Oliver A, Martin F, Shu F. 1997. B cell development in mice. *Int. Rev. Immunol.* 15:207–41

109. Cong YZ, Rabin E, Wortis HH. 1991. Treatment of murine CD5- B cells with anti-Ig, but not LPS, induces surface CD5:two B-cell activation pathways. *Int. Immunol.* 3:467–76

110. Su I, Tarakhovsky A. 2000. B-1 cells:-orthodox or conformist? *Curr. Opin. Immunol.* 12:191–94

111. Hayakawa K, Hardy RR. 2000. Development and function of B-1 cells. *Curr. Opin. Immunol.* 12:346–53

112. Inaoki M, Sato S, Weintraub BC, Goodnow CC, Tedder TF. 1997. CD19-regulated signaling thresholds control peripheral tolerance and autoantibody production in B lymphocytes. *J. Exp. Med.* 186:1923–31

113. Xu S, Tan JE, Wong EP, Manickam A, Ponniah S, Lam KP. 2000. B cell development and activation defects resulting in xid-like immunodeficiency in BLNK/SLP-65-deficient mice. *Int. Immunol.* 12:397–404

114. Carroll MC. 1998. The role of complement and complement receptors in induction and regulation of immunity. *Annu. Rev. Immunol.* 16:545–68

115. Tarakhovsky A, Turner M, Schaal S, Mee PJ, Duddy LP, Rajewsky K, Tybulewicz VL. 1995. Defective antigen receptor-mediated proliferation of B and T cells in the absence of Vav. *Nature* 374:467–70

116. Zhang R, Alt FW, Davidson L, Orkin SH, Swat W. 1995. Defective signalling through the T- and B-cell antigen receptors in lymphoid cells lacking the vav proto-oncogene. *Nature* 374:470–73

117. Suzuki H, Terauchi Y, Fujiwara M, Aizawa S, Yazaki Y, Kadowaki T, Koyasu S. 1999. Xid-like immunodeficiency in mice with disruption of the p85alpha subunit of phosphoinositide 3-kinase. *Science* 283:390–92

118. Fruman DA, Snapper SB, Yballe CM, Davidson L, Yu JY, Alt FW, Cantley LC. 1999. Impaired B cell development and proliferation in absence of phosphoinositide 3-kinase p85alpha. *Science* 283:393–97

119. Khan WN, Alt FW, Gerstein RM, Malynn BA, Larsson I, Rathbun G, Davidson L, Muller S, Kantor AB, Herzenberg LA, Rosen FS, Sideras P. 1995. Defective B cell development and function in *Btk*-deficient mice. *Immunity* 3:283

120. Humbert PO, Corcoran LM. 1997. oct-2 gene disruption eliminates the peritoneal B-1 lymphocyte lineage and attenuates B-2 cell maturation and function. *J. Immunol.* 159:5273–84

121. Anderson JS, Teutsch M, Dong Z, Wortis HH. 1996. An essential role for Bruton's tyrosine kinase in the regulation of B-cell apoptosis. *Proc. Natl. Acad. Sci. USA* 93:10966–71

122. Kong YY, Fischer KD, Bachmann MF, Mariathasan S, Kozieradzki I, Nghiem MP, Bouchard D, Bernstein A, Ohashi PS, Penninger JM. 1998. Vav regulates peptide-specific apoptosis in thymocytes. *J. Exp. Med.* 188:2099–2111

123. O'Rourke LM, Tooze R, Turner M, Sandoval DM, Carter RH, Tybulewicz VL, Fearon DT. 1998. CD19 as a membrane-anchored adaptor protein of B lymphocytes: costimulation of lipid and protein kinases by recruitment of Vav. *Immunity* 8:635–45

124. Cyster JG, Goodnow CC. 1997. Tuning antigen receptor signaling by CD22: integrating cues from antigens and the microenvironment. *Immunity* 6:509–17

125. O'Keefe TL, Williams GT, Davies SL, Neuberger MS. 1996. Hyperresponsive B cells in CD22-deficient mice. *Science* 274:798–801

126. Nishizumi H, Horikawa K, Mlinaric-Rascan I, Yamamoto T. 1998. A double-edged kinase Lyn: a positive and negative

regulator for antigen receptor-mediated signals. *J. Exp. Med.* 187:1343–48

127. Nishimura H, Nose M, Hiai H, Minato N, Honjo T. 1999. Development of lupus-like autoimmune diseases by disruption of the PD-1 gene encoding an ITIM motif-carrying immunoreceptor. *Immunity* 11:141–51

128. Nishimura H, Honjo T, Minato N. 2000. Facilitation of beta selection and modification of positive selection in the thymus of PD-1-deficient mice. *J. Exp. Med.* 191:891–98

129. Sidman CL, Shultz LD, Hardy RR, Hayakawa K, Herzenberg LA. 1986. Production of immunoglobulin isotypes by Ly-1$^+$ B cells in viable motheaten and normal mice. *Science* 232:1423–25

130. Chan VW, Meng F, Soriano P, DeFranco AL, Lowell CA. 1997. Characterization of the B lymphocyte populations in Lyn-deficient mice and the role of Lyn in signal initiation and down-regulation. *Immunity* 7:69–81

131. Nishizumi H, Taniuchi I, Illic D, Mori S, Watanabe T. 1995. Impaired proliferation of peripheral B cells and indication of autoimmune disease in *lyn*-deficient mice. *Immunity* 3:549–60

132. Wang J, Koizumi T, Watanabe T. 1996. Altered antigen receptor signaling and impaired Fas-mediated apoptosis of B cells in Lyn-deficient mice. *J. Exp. Med.* 184:831–38

133. Sato S, Ono N, Steeber DA, Pisetsky DS, Tedder TF. 1996. CD19 regulates B lymphocyte signaling thresholds critical for the development of B-1 lineage cells and autoimmunity. *J. Immunol.* 157:4371–78

134. Chumley MJ, Dal Porto JM, Kawaguchi S, Cambier JC, Nemazee D, Hardy RR. 2000. A VH11V kappa 9 B cell antigen receptor drives generation of CD5$^+$ B cells both in vivo and in vitro. *J. Immunol.* 164:4586–93

135. Litzenburger T, Fassler R, Bauer J, Lassmann H, Linington C, Wekerle H, Iglesias A. 1998. B lymphocytes producing demyelinating autoantibodies: development and function in gene-targeted transgenic mice. *J. Exp. Med.* 188:169–80

136. Gui M, Wiest DL, Li J, Kappes D, Hardy RR, Hayakawa K. 1999. Peripheral CD4$^+$ T cell maturation recognized by increased expression of Thy-1/CD90 bearing the 6C10 carbohydrate epitope. *J. Immunol.* 163:4796–4804

137. Hayakawa K, Carmack CE, Hyman R, Hardy RR. 1990. Natural autoantibodies to thymocytes: origin, VH genes, fine specificities, and the role of Thy-1 glycoprotein. *J. Exp. Med.* 172:869–78

138. Qin XF, Schwers S, Yu W, Papavasiliou F, Suh H, Nussenzweig A, Rajewsky K, Nussenzweig MC. 1999. Secondary V(D)J. recombination in B-1 cells. *Nature* 397:355–59

139. Veis DJ, Sorenson CM, Shutter JR, Korsmeyer SJ. 1993. Bcl-2-deficient mice demonstrate fulminant lymphoid apoptosis, polycystic kidneys, and hypopigmented hair. *Cell* 75:229–40

140. Miller DJ, Hayes CE. 1991. Phenotypic and genetic characterization of a unique B lymphocyte deficiency in strain A/WySnJ. mice. *Eur. J. Immunol.* 21:1123–30

141. Miller DJ, Hanson KD, Carman JA, Hayes CE. 1992. A single autosomal gene defect severely limits IgG but not IgM responses in B lymphocyte-deficient A/WySnJ mice. *Eur. J. Immunol.* 22:373–79

142. Lentz VM, Hayes CE, Cancro MP. 1998. Bcmd decreases the life span of B-2 but not B-1 cells in A/WySnJ mice. *J. Immunol.* 160:3743–47

143. Solvason N, Wu WW, Parry D, Mahony D, Lam EW, Glassford J, Klaus GG, Sicinski P, Weinberg R, Liu YJ, Howard M, Lees E. 2000. Cyclin D2 is essential for BCR-mediated proliferation and CD5 B cell development. *Int. Immunol.* 12:631–38

144. Bikah G, Carey J, Ciallella JR, Tarakhovsky A, Bondada S. 1996. CD5-mediated negative regulation of antigen receptor-induced growth signals in B-1 B cells. *Science* 274:1906–9

145. Sen G, Bikah G, Venkataraman C, Bondada S. 1999. Negative regulation of antigen receptor-mediated signaling by constitutive association of CD5 with the SHP-1 protein tyrosine phosphatase in B-1 B cells. *Eur. J. Immunol.* 29:3319–28

146. Hippen KL, Tze LE, Behrens TW. 2000. CD5 maintains tolerance in anergic B cells. *J. Exp. Med.* 191:883–90

147. Calvo J, Padilla O, Places L, Vigorito E, Vila JM, Vilella R, Mila J, Vives J, Bowen MA, Lozano F. 1999. Relevance of individual CD5 extracellular domains on antibody recognition, glycosylation and co-mitogenic signalling. *Tissue Antigens* 54:16–26

148. McAlister MS, Brown MH, Willis AC, Rudd PM, Harvey DJ, Aplin R, Shotton DM, Dwek RA, Barclay AN, Driscoll PC. 1998. Structural analysis of the CD5 antigen-expression, disulphide bond analysis and physical characterisation of CD5 scavenger receptor superfamily domain 1. *Eur. J. Biochem.* 257:131–41

149. Rudd PM, Wormald MR, Harvey DJ, Devasahayam M, McAlister MS, Brown MH, Davis SJ, Barclay AN, Dwek RA. 1999. Oligosaccharide analysis and molecular modeling of soluble forms of glycoproteins belonging to the Ly-6, scavenger receptor, and immunoglobulin superfamilies expressed in Chinese hamster ovary cells. *Glycobiology* 9:443–58

150. Bikah G, Lynd FM, Aruffo AA, Ledbetter JA, Bondada S. 1998. A role for CD5 in cognate interactions between T cells and B cells, and identification of a novel ligand for CD5. *Int. Immunol.* 10:1185–96

151. Calvo J, Places L, Padilla O, Vila JM, Vives J, Bowen MA, Lozano F. 1999. Interaction of recombinant and natural soluble CD5 forms with an alternative cell surface ligand. *Eur. J. Immunol.* 29:2119–29

152. Perez-Villar JJ, Whitney GS, Bowen MA, Hewgill DH, Aruffo AA, Kanner SB. 1999. CD5 negatively regulates the T-cell antigen receptor signal transduction pathway: involvement of SH2-containing phosphotyrosine phosphatase SHP-1. *Mol. Cell. Biol.* 19:2903–12

153. Gringhuis SI, de LeiJ. LF, Coffer PJ, Vellenga E. 1998. Signaling through CD5 activates a pathway involving phosphatidylinositol 3-kinase, Vav, and Rac1 in human mature T lymphocytes. *Mol. Cell. Biol.* 18:1725–35

154. Calvo J, Vilda JM, Places L, Simarro M, Padilla O, Andreu D, Campbell KS, Aussel C, Lozano F. 1998. Human CD5 signaling and constitutive phosphorylation of C-terminal serine residues by casein kinase II. *J. Immunol.* 161:6022–29

155. Raman C, Kimberly RP. 1998. Differential CD5-dependent regulation of CD5-associated CK2 activity in mature and immature T cells:implication on TCR/CD3-mediated activation. *J. Immunol.* 161:5817–20

156. Bauch A, Campbell KS, Reth M. 1998. Interaction of the CD5 cytoplasmic domain with the Ca^{2+}/calmodulin-dependent kinase IIdelta. *Eur. J. Immunol.* 28:2167–77

157. Simarro M, Calvo J, Vila JM, Places L, Padilla O, Alberola-Ila J, Vives J, Lozano F. 1999. Signaling through CD5 involves acidic sphingomyelinase, protein kinase C-zeta, mitogen-activated protein kinase kinase, and c-Jun NH2-terminal kinase. *J. Immunol.* 162:5149–55

158. Pers JO, Jamin C, Le Corre R, Lydyard PM, Youinou P. 1998. Ligation of CD5 on resting B cells, but not on resting T cells, results in apoptosis. *Eur. J. Immunol.* 28:4170–76

159. Berland R, Wortis HH. 1998. An NFAT-dependent enhancer is necessary for anti-IgM-mediated induction of murine CD5

expression in primary splenic B cells. *J. Immunol.* 161:277–85

160. Murakami M, Tsubata T, Okamoto M, Shimizu A, Kumagai S, Imura H, Honjo T. 1992. Antigen-induced apoptotic death of Ly-1 B cells responsible for autoimmune disease in transgenic mice. *Nature* 357:77–80

161. Sakiyama T, Ikuta K, Nisitani S, Takatsu K, Honjo T. 1999. Requirement of IL-5 for induction of autoimmune hemolytic anemia in anti-red blood cell autoantibody transgenic mice. *Int. Immunol.* 11:995–1000

162. Nisitani S, Sakiyama T, Honjo T. 1998. Involvement of IL-10 in induction of autoimmune hemolytic anemia in anti-

erythrocyte Ig transgenic mice. *Int. Immunol.* 10:1039–47

163. Watanabe N, Nisitani S, Ikuta K, Suzuki M, Chiba T, Honjo T. 1999. Expression levels of B cell surface immunoglobulin regulate efficiency of allelic exclusion and size of autoreactive B-1 cell compartment. *J. Exp. Med.* 190:461–70

164. Vink A, Warnier G, Brombacher F, Renauld JC. 1999. Interleukin 9-induced in vivo expansion of the B-1 lymphocyte population. *J. Exp. Med.* 189:1413–23

165. Potter M, Wax JS, Hansen CT, Kenny JJ. 1999. BALB/c.CBA/N mice carrying the defective Btk(xid) gene are resistant to pristane-induced plasmacytomagenesis. *Int. Immunol.* 11:1059–64

Annu. Rev. Immunol. 2001. 19:623–55

IRF Family of Transcription Factors as Regulators of Host Defense

Tadatsugu Taniguchi, Kouetsu Ogasawara, Akinori Takaoka, and Nobuyuki Tanaka

Department of Immunology, Graduate School of Medicine and Faculty of Medicine, University of Tokyo, Hongo 7-3-1, Bunkyo-ku, Tokyo 113-0033, Japan; e-mail: tada@m.u-tokyo.ac.jp

Key Words interferon, cytokine, interferon regulatory factor, transcriptional regulation, oncogenesis

■ **Abstract** Interferon regulatory factors (IRFs) constitute a family of transcription factors that commonly possess a novel helix-turn-helix DNA-binding motif. Following the initial identification of two structurally related members, IRF-1 and IRF-2, seven additional members have now been reported. In addition, virally encoded IRFs, which may interfere with cellular IRFs, have also been identified. Thus far, intensive functional analyses have been done on IRF-1, revealing a remarkable functional diversity of this transcription factor in the regulation of cellular response in host defense. Indeed, IRF-1 selectively modulates different sets of genes, depending on the cell type and/or the nature of cellular stimuli, in order to evoke appropriate responses in each. More recently, much attention has also been focused on other IRF family members. Their functional roles, through interactions with their own or other members of the family of transcription factors, are becoming clearer in the regulation of host defense, such as innate and adaptive immune responses and oncogenesis.

INTRODUCTION

Prompt and regulated cellular response is central to host defense and is coordinated by a genetic regulatory network in which a given transcription factor controls the expression of a diverse set of target genes depending on the cell type and/or the nature of cellular stimuli. The functional diversity of such a transcription factor is dependent on its modification (e.g., phosphorylation) and/or interaction with other transcription factors that are co-expressed and/or activated in the cell (1, 2). In fact, such regulatory networks are critical for host defense against extracellular pathogens as they rapidly alter the expression of relevant genes.

0732-0582/01/0407-0623$14.00

Interferons (IFNs), the first series of cytokines to be molecularly characterized, have been extensively studied in the context of host defense against viral infection. There are two types of IFNs, i.e., type I IFNs (IFN-αs and IFN-β), and type II IFN (IFN-γ): The former are produced by a variety of cells upon viral infection, while the latter is produced by activated T lymphocytes (T cells) and natural killer (NK) cells (3–7). Like many other cytokines, these two types of IFNs show multiple biological activities, but both commonly evoke an antiviral response in their target cells through the stimulation of homologous receptors (3–10).

The IRF-1 transcription factor was originally identified as a regulator of virus-inducible enhancer-like elements of the human *IFN-β* gene (11). Subsequently, another factor that is structurally related to IRF-1 was also identified and termed IRF-2 (12). In fact, these factors constitute a family of transcription factors, termed the IRF family, which has now expanded to nine members (Figure 1, see color insert). In addition, viral members of this family, vIRFs, encoded by human herpes virus 8 (HHV-8), were also identified (13). In this review, we first describe briefly the historical background of each IRF family member and their cardinal features; we then try to incorporate them in the context of salient biological systems that operate during host defense. Review articles documenting the roles of IRF members were also published previously (14–16).

IDENTIFICATION OF THE IRF MEMBERS AND THEIR CARDINAL FEATURES

IRF-1 and IRF-2: The Inception

The induction of the *IFN-β* gene by a virus is due primarily to transcriptional activation that requires virus-inducible enhancer-like elements of its gene promoter (4, 17, 18). During the study on the regulation of the *IFN-β* gene, a factor(s) was found to bind to these elements and was tentatively termed IRF-1 (19). Subsequently, cDNA encoding mouse IRF-1 was cloned and its structure elucidated (11). IRF-1 was also characterized in several other contexts (20–22). Subsequently, a cDNA encoding a molecule structurally related to IRF-1 was isolated by cross-hybridization with IRF-1 cDNA, and the molecule was termed IRF-2 (12). In fact, the deduced primary structures of IRF-1 and IRF-2 showed 62% homology in their amino-terminal regions, spanning the first 154 residues, whereas the rest of the molecules showed only 25% homology (12). DNA-binding site selection studies revealed that these two factors bind to the same DNA element, termed IRF-E (consensus sequence: G(A)AAA$^G/_C$$^T/_C$GAAA$^G/_C$$^T/_C$) (23), which is almost indistinguishable from the interferon-stimulated response element (ISRE; consensus sequence: $^A/_G$NGAAANNGAAACT) (24) activated by IFN signaling (see below). Mutational analysis of IRF-1 and IRF-2 revealed that DNA-binding activity resides in the amino-terminal region, with some strictly conserved amino acids, particularly the five tryptophan repeats (Figure 1, see color insert) (12). On the one hand, the carboxyl-terminal region of IRF-1 is characterized by the abundance of acidic amino acids and serine-threonine residues, and this region constitutes the transcriptional activation domain (12). On the other hand, the corresponding region of IRF-2 is relatively rich in basic amino acids (Figure 1, see color insert), suggesting the distinct function of this factor (see below).

IRF-1 and IRF-2 mRNAs are both expressed in a variety of cell types, and their expression levels, particularly IRF-1 mRNA, are dramatically upregulated upon viral infection or IFN stimulation (11, 12). A series of cDNA transfection experiments revealed that IRF-1 can activate IFN-α/β promoters (12, 25). In fact, a high-level expression of IRF-1 cDNA resulted in the induction of endogenous *IFN-α* and *IFN-β* genes in a variety of cell lines, albeit at low efficiency (25, 26). Unlike IRF-1, IRF-2 had no such effect; rather, it repressed IRF-1-induced transcriptional activation (25, 27). IRF-1 protein is very unstable (half-life, $\sim$30 min), whereas IRF-2 protein is apparently stable (half-life, $\sim$8 hours) (28). These initial observations were suggestive that IRF-1 and IRF-2 function as a transcriptional activator and repressor, respectively, for the *IFN-α/β* genes. In addition, evidence has also been provided that IRF-2 functions as a transcriptional activator for *vascular cell adhesion molecule-1 (VCAM-1)* (29) and cell-cycle-regulated *histone H4* genes (30). As documented more thoroughly below, subsequent genetic analyses of *IRF-1* and *IRF-2* genes have provided a different vista of the functions of these factors.

IRF-3 and IRF-7

IRF-3 and IRF-7 are closely related to each other in terms of their primary structures (Figure 1, see color insert) (14–16). IRF-3 was identified through a search of an EST database for IRF-1 and IRF-2 homologs (31). IRF-3 was also characterized as a component of the virus-inducible dsRNA-activated factor 1 (DRAF1) complex (32). One IRF family member found in chicken was originally termed IRF-3 (33), but its relationship with mammalian IRF-3 is somewhat unclear. IRF-3 mRNA is expressed constitutively in all tissues and is not induced by viral infection or IFN treatment (31). IRF-7 was first identified as a new member of the IRF family and directly submitted to the GeneBank database (accession numbers U73036, U73037). Subsequently, IRF-7 cDNA was cloned as a factor that binds to the Epstein-Barr virus Qp promoter region using the yeast one-hybrid system (34). The expression of IRF-7 is ubiquitous (34); however, it is totally dependent on IFN-α/β signaling, whereas IRF-3 expression is constitutive and remains essentially unaffected by virus and IFNs (35, 36). IRF-3 contains an activation domain that includes the nuclear export signal (NES) and the IRF association domain (IAD) (Figure 1, see color insert) (37, 38). Evidence has been provided that this domain is flanked by two autoinhibitory domains that interact with each other; in virally infected cells, this interaction is relieved by virus-induced phosphorylation, thereby unmasking both IAD and DNA-binding domains (38). As described below, recent studies have established the essential and distinct roles of these two factors in the induction of *IFN-α/β* genes.

IRF-4

IRF-4 has been characterized in several different contexts with different terminologies: (i) Pip, a binding factor to the murine immunoglobulin light chain enhancer $E_{\lambda 2-4}$, in concert with PU.1 (39); (ii) LSIRF, a new IRF family member expressed only in lymphoid cells (40); and (iii) ICSAT, a factor that binds to the promoter region of the human *interleukin-5* gene (41). The expression of IRF-4 is restricted to T and B cell lineages and is not induced by IFNs (39–41). In fact, the critical role of IRF-4 in lymphocyte development and function is underscored by its abnormalities found in mice lacking IRF-4 (see below).

IRF-5 and IRF-6

The cDNA sequences of IRF-5 and IRF-6 were directly submitted to the GeneBank database (accession numbers: human IRF-5, U51127; human IRF-6, AF027292). These two factors are structurally related to each other (Figure 1, see color insert), but information has been scarce regarding their functions. Interestingly, the expression of IRF-5 is induced by IFN-α/β stimulation (T Nakaya, T Taniguchi, unpublished observation), suggesting its participation in the IFN system. A Xenopus gene reported to encode a protein highly similar to mouse IRF-6, termed xIRF-6, is expressed in the posterior mesoderm during the early development of *Xenopus laevis* (42); its function, however, remains unclear.

IRF-8/ICSBP

Interferon consensus sequence binding protein (ICSBP)/IRF-8 was originally identified as a protein that binds to the ISRE motif in the promoter region of the MHC class I gene, $H-2L^D$ (43, 44). The expression of IRF-8 is restricted to myeloid and lymphoid cell lineages and is induced by IFN-γ, but not by IFN-α/β (43, 45). The DNA-binding activity of IRF-8 per se is very weak but is dramatically increased by interaction with IRF-1 and IRF-2 (46, 47). The interaction is mediated by IAD, which is conserved among several IRF members (Figure 1, see color insert) (48). IRF-8 also binds with the Ets-family transcription factor PU.1, which is required for development along the lymphoid and myeloid lineages of the cells. A multiprotein complex composed of IRF-8, IRF-1, and PU.1 functions as a transcriptional activator (49). This factor is apparently critical for the regulation of the immune system and oncogenesis, as described below.

IRF-9/p48/ISGF3γ

IRF-9 was originally discovered as a DNA-binding subunit of the transcription factor ISGF3 (interferon stimulated gene factor 3), and termed p48/ISGF3γ (50–53). In fact, ISGF3 was originally identified as a transcriptional factor specifically induced in IFN-α-stimulated cells and was subsequently found to consist of three components: signal transducers and activators of transcription (Stat) 1, Stat2, and IRF-9 (51–56). Like IRF-1 and IRF-2, IRF-9 is expressed in a variety of tissues and shown to be essential for the antiviral response by IFN-α/β and IFN-γ (16, 24, 57) (see below).

vIRF

HHV-8 is thought to be the viral etiologic agent of Kaposi's sarcoma and primary effusion lymphoma. This virus, also termed Kaposi's sarcoma–associated herpes virus (KSHV), encodes four IRF homologs (viral IRFs; vIRFs) (13). ORF K9 (vIRF-1) encodes a hypothetical 449 amino acid protein with 13.4% amino acid identity to human IRF-8 protein and partial conservation of the IRF DNA-binding domain (13). vIRF-1 binds with several cellular IRFs, including IRF-1, and inhibits IRF-mediated transcriptional activation (58–60), suggesting its role in escaping from IFN action and other immune systems. Moreover, expression of an antisense RNA for vIRF-1 results in the repression of several HHV-8 lytic genes, including viral IL-6 (60), suggesting that vIRF-1 also positively regulates gene expression. Regarding the two other vIRFs, vIRF-2 interacts with IRF-1, IRF-2, and ICSBP in vitro (61), and vIRF-3 may inhibit both IRF-3 and IRF-7 activities, resulting in the inhibition of the virus-mediated synthesis of IFN-α/β (62).

Structural Basis of IRFs for Their Interaction with DNA

The crystal structure of the DNA-binding domain of IRF-1 bound to DNA was determined (63). The IRF-1 DNA-binding region has an α/β architecture containing three α-helices, four-stranded antiparallel β-sheets, and three long loops. This structure is similar to the helix–turn–helix (HTH)-containing DNA-binding domains. However, its mode of DNA interaction is distinct from those of other HTH-containing proteins and revealed a new HTH motif. The third α-helix contacts the major groove of the GAAA sequence, and several other segments, including the three loops and the three α-helices, contact its surrounding sequence. The crystal structure of the DNA-binding domain of IRF-2 was also determined. The structure of the DNA-binding domain bound to DNA indicates its recognition sequence, <u>AANNGAAA</u> (recognized bases are underlined), and shows cooperative binding to a tandem repeat of the GAAA core sequence induced by DNA structural distortions (64). The secondary structure of the DNA-binding domain for other IRF family members is similar to that of IRF-1 and IRF-2, suggesting that these

IRF members recognize similar, if not identical, DNA sequences; e.g., IRF-E, ISRE, ICS (interferon consensus sequence) (43, 65), or PRD (positive regulatory domain) (66, 67).

CELLULAR SIGNALING EVENTS AFFECTING IRF ACTIVITIES

Role of IRF and Stat Transcription Factors in IFN Signaling

Ligand-induced activation of type I and type II IFN receptors, IFNAR and IFNGR, results in the activation or induction of similar transcription factors of the IRF and Stat families (Figure 2, see color insert). IFNAR stimulation results in the activation of Janus family protein tyrosine kinases, Tyk2 and Jak1, which are associated with subcomponents IFNAR1 and IFNAR2, respectively. This activation is followed by the site-specific tyrosine phosphorylations of Stat1 (residue 701 for mouse Stat1) and Stat2 (residue 688 for mouse Stat2) (24, 68–70). These two phosphorylated Stats, in combination with IRF-9, form a heterotrimeric transcription factor complex, ISGF3, which translocates into the nucleus and binds to ISRE to activate IFN-inducible genes (24, 57). The carboxyl-terminal domain of IRF-9 was demonstrated to mediate the formation of the ISGF3 complex through direct association with Stat1 and Stat2 (Figure 1, see color insert) (71, 72). Additionally, the phosphorylated Stat1 also undergoes homodimerization and is converted into its transcriptionally active form, termed IFN-γ-activated factor/IFN-α-activated factor (GAF/AAF), which binds to the IFN-γ-activated site (GAS; consensus sequence TTCNNNGAA) and activates its target genes (Figure 2, see color insert) (24, 57).

In the case of IFNGR signaling, IFNGR1, the ligand-binding subunit that interacts with Jak1, and IFNGR2, which interacts with Jak2, associate upon binding of the dimeric form of the ligand, resulting in the activation of these Jak PTKs (68). Like IFNAR stimulation, IFNGR stimulation also results in the efficient activation of Stat1 (Figure 2, see color insert) (24). Furthermore, Stat2 is also tyrosine-phosphorylated by IFN-γ stimulation, albeit at much lower levels than IFN-α/β stimulation, leading to the formation of ISGF3 (73, 74). The formation of a trimeric complex, termed Stat1-p48, which consists of Stat1 dimer and IRF-9, was also reported in a monkey kidney cell line, Vero (75) (Figure 2, see color insert).

The activation of the Stats during IFN signaling requires their recruitment to the receptors (76–78). Recent study offers a mechanism by which IFN-γ stimulation results in the activation of ISGF3. In fact, a novel form of cross-talk occurs between IFN-α/β and IFN-γ signalings, in which IFN-γ signaling is dependent on a weak IFNAR stimulation by spontaneously produced IFN-α/β (74). Further evidence was provided for the physical association between IFNAR1 and IFNGR2 receptor subunits. In view of the report demonstrating the Stat2-docking site within the intracellular domain of IFNAR1 (77, 78), which is physically associated with IFNGR2 at the caveolar membrane domain (74), this docking site may be utilized for IFN-γ-induced activation of the ISGF3 complex. IRF-1 is expressed at low levels in unstimulated cells but is induced by many cytokines such as IFNs (-α,-β,-γ), TNF-α, IL-1, IL-6, and LIF, and by viral infection (11, 22, 79). The analysis of the *IRF*-1 promoter region revealed that this induction is mediated by Stat and NF-κB transcription factors, the binding sites for which are found within this region (80, 81). In fact, IFN-induced expression of IRF-1 mRNA was completely abolished in *Stat1*-deficient (*Stat1$^{-/-}$*) cells (82, 83). As described above, the recognition sequence of IRF-1 (IRF-E) overlaps with that of ISRE, which binds ISGF3. These observations suggest that IRF-1 functions as a regulator of cellular responses to IFNs by affecting a set of IFN-inducible genes (see below). In contrast, IRF-2 is inducible by IFN-α/β, albeit with slower kinetics of induction than IRF-1 (12). This induction is mediated by ISGF3, the binding site for which is found within the *IRF*-2 promoter region (81). As described below, recent genetic study has revealed that IRF-2 acts as a transcriptional attenuator of ISGF3.

Other IRF members induced by IFN signaling include IRF-5, IRF-7, and IRF-8 (35, 36, 43; T Nakaya, T Taniguchi, unpublished data). The biological significance of IFN-induced IRF-7 has become clearer and is discussed below in the context of *IFN-α/β* gene regulation.

Modification of IRFs and Their Cooperation with Other Transcription Factors

IRF-1 protein undergoes posttranslational modifications such as phosphorylation. IRF-1 was reported to be serine-phosphorylated by protein kinase A (PKA), protein kinase C (PKC), and casein kinase II (CKII) at two clustered sites (amino acids 138-150 and amino acids 219-231) (84). The mutation of these tyrosine residues inhibited the transactivation of IRF-1, suggesting the possible role of phosphorylation by these kinases in the regulation of IRF-1 transcriptional activity (84–86). There is also evidence for the interaction of IRF-1 with other transcription factors; a multimeric complex, termed enhanceosome, is formed in virally infected cells, in which the interaction of NF-κB with IRF-1 is critical for synergistic promoter activation (87–89). In addition, IRF-1 protein is stabilized in γ-irradiated MEFs and cooperates with the tumor suppressor p53 to induce the *p21$^{WAF1/CIP1}$* gene (90). It is unknown, however, if and how IRF-1 undergoes modification so that it can interact with these transcription factors.

The carboxyl-terminus of IRF-2 contains a repression domain, the deletion of which converts IRF-2 to a transcriptional activator (91). With regard to the regulatory modifications of IRF-2 protein, IRF-2 undergoes inducible proteolytic processing. IRF-2 is cleaved in the carboxyl-terminal region following viral infection or double-stranded RNA treatment, resulting in its conversion to either an activator or a strong repressor (92–94). As other types of posttranslational modifications, IRF-2 is phosphorylated and PKA, PKC, and CKII phosphorylate serine residues of IRF-2 (86).

The modification and cooperation of IRF-3 and IRF-7 have been studied most extensively in the context of *IFN-α/β* gene regulation in virally infected cells. In normally growing cells, most if not all of these factors reside in the cytoplasm, and they are activated and undergo nuclear translocation upon viral infection (35–37, 95–98). IRF-3 is activated through the specific phosphorylation of serine residues in its carboxyl-terminal region, leading to an association with the general co-activator p300/CBP (37, 38, 95–97, 99). The prominent phosphorylation sites have been mapped to Ser385, Ser386, and the distal region; the mutations of these residues abolish virus-induced activation (37, 96). Similarly, IRF-7 also undergoes serine phosphorylation in its carboxyl-terminal region, which is highly homologous to the corresponding region of IRF-3. In fact, mutation or deletion in this region also results in the inactivation of this factor (35, 36). There is also evidence that IRF-3 and IRF-7 form homo- or hetero-dimers, and that each of the three different combinations of dimers may selectively affect the *IFN-α* gene subfamilies and the *IFN-β* gene (35, 38, 97, 100). These factors may also undergo modification in response to other types of stimuli (14, 15).

Of all the members of the IRF family, IRF-4 and IRF-8 are predominantly expressed in lymphoid cells. IRF-4, together with PU.1, a hematopoietic-specific member of the Ets family, is known to form a transcriptional assembly implicated in the regulation of the expression of B cell–specific genes, such as the *immunoglobulin light chain* (*IgL*) gene (101, 102) or the *CD20* gene (103). The PU.1-IRF-4 interaction requires PU.1 binding to DNA with subsequent recruitment of IRF-4 via a phosphorylated serine residue (Ser-148) in the PEST region of PU.1 (104, 105). A carboxyl-terminal regulatory domain within IRF-4 is required not only for ternary complex assembly (105) but also for autoinhibition of the DNA binding of IRF-4 by masking the DNA-binding domain of IRF-4 in the absence of PU.1 (106). IRF-4 can also form ternary complexes on an Ets-IRF composite element (EICE) with Spi-B, a closely related factor to PU.1, in a manner similar to IRF-1-PU.1 interaction (107, 108). Recently, it was reported that IRF-4 is posttranslationally regulated by the immunophilin FK506-binding protein 52 (FKBP52). IRF-4 is associated with FKBP52, and this association inhibits the DNA-binding activity of IRF-4 (109). IRF-4 and IRF-8 also form a complex that represses the expression of the *interferon-stimulated gene-15* in macrophages (110).

Although not extensively pursued yet, the fact that several tyrosines within the DNA-binding domains of the IRF family members are conserved may raise an issue that, like Stats, tyrosine phosphorylation may modulate their biological activities (47). One such example was reported for IRF-8; its DNA-binding activity is modulated by tyrosine phosphorylation (47). Tyrosine phosphorylation of IRF-8 inhibits the DNA-binding activity of IRF-8 per se but facilitates its association with IRF-1 or IRF-2 and enhances DNA binding through the formation of a heterocomplex (47).

IRF-8 also forms transcriptional complexes on EICE in a PU.1- or Spi-B-dependent manner by serine phosphorylation (39, 107, 108). However, unlike the case of IRF-4, the PU.1-IRF-8 complex is less active in transactivation due to the lack of an activation domain within IRF-8 (48, 105). Evidence has been provided that $IRF\text{-}8^{-/-}$ macrophages are defective in inducing certain IFN-γ-responsive genes, such as *iNOS* and *FcγRI*, and further that IRF-8 is recruited to a transcriptional complex on the GAS element (111). Thus, IRF-8, in addition to being a repressor of the ISRE-dependent transcription by IFN-α/β, also serves as an activator of the GAS-dependent transcription by IFN-γ.

REGULATION OF THE IFN SYSTEM BY IRFS

IFN-α/β Gene Induction by IRFs; A Retrospective View

The induction of IFN-α/β gene transcription in virus-infected cells is an event central to innate immunity (112). This induction is primarily due to transcriptional activation requiring sequences in the 5' region of the *IFN-α* and *IFN-β* genes, termed virus-inducible enhancers (4, 17, 18). Through the analysis of these promoter regions, IRF recognition sequences were found to be essential elements for induction by a virus (19, 66, 113, 114). Although IRF-1 was originally a candidate factor for the positive regulator of *IFN-α/β* genes, two independently performed gene targeting studies commonly pointed to the existence of an IRF-1-independent mechanism of the gene induction in virally infected cells. In fact, the induction of both *IFN-α* and *IFN-β* genes by double-stranded RNA was suppressed in primary mouse embryonic fibroblasts (MEFs) from $IRF\text{-}1^{-/-}$ mice; however, it occurred normally in cells infected by Newcastle disease virus (NDV) (115, 116).

Subsequently, virus-induced expression of the *IFN-α* gene was shown to be dramatically reduced in $IFNAR1^{-/-}$ or $IRF\text{-}9^{-/-}$ MEFs (117). In contrast, virus-induced expression of the *IFN-β* gene is only slightly suppressed. These results may provide an insight into a unique feature of the IFN induction mechanism. First, upon viral infection, small amounts of IFN-β are initially produced through the activation of unidentified factor(s). Thus produced, IFN-β then stimulates IFNAR to activate ISGF3. In this stage, ISGF3 per se or factor(s) induced by ISGF3 can efficiently activate *IFN-α/β* genes. In fact, there is evidence that ISGF3 binds to the IFN-β promoter (118, 119). This two-step induction model is also supported by subsequent experiments showing that *IFN-α* gene induction by a virus is clearly suppressed in MEFs from $IFN\text{-}\beta^{-/-}$ mice (120). Subsequent study provided strong evidence that ISGF3 participates indirectly through IRF-7 induction (100).

Distinct and Essential Roles of IRF-3 and IRF-7 in the Biphasic Induction of IFN-α/β Genes

More recently, two structurally related IRF family members, IRF-3 and IRF-7, were found to be involved in *IFN-α/β* gene induction. It was first shown that IRF-3, which resides in the cytoplasm in the latent form, translocates to the nucleus upon viral infection (37, 95–97). The nuclear IRF-3 is phosphorylated predominantly, if not exclusively, in its carboxyl-terminal region, interacts with the transcriptional co-activator CBP/p300, and binds specifically to IFN-β IRF-E (or PRDI element) (37, 38, 95–97). Furthermore, overexpression of IRF-3 leads to a marked increase in virus-induced IFN-β mRNA expression (95).

Subsequently, the *IRF-7* gene (and IRF-7 protein) was expressed at a very low level in MEFs, and it was strongly induced by IFNs through the activation of ISGF3, pointing to the involvement of IRF-7 in ISGF3-dependent gene induction, as described above. Like IRF-3, IRF-7 also undergoes virus-induced nuclear translocation (35, 36, 98). Interestingly, ectopic expression of IRF-7 can activate both *IFN-α* and *IFN-β* genes, whereas IRF-3 mainly affects the *IFN-β* gene (36). The importance of these two factors was also underscored by the observation that IRF-3 and IRF-7 form a complex, termed virus-activated factor (VAF), which binds to the *IFN-β* promoter in vivo (97). Thus, it was important to clarify further to what extent and how these two factors contribute to the induction of *IFN-α/β* genes in response to viral infection.

In fact, the essential and distinct roles of IRF-3 and IRF-7 in *IFN-α/β* gene induction became clearer by a recent gene disruption/introduction study. Mice carrying a null mutation in the IRF-3 alleles were highly vulnerable to viral infection, and IFN-α/β mRNA expression levels, induced by NDV, were found to be dramatically diminished in *IRF-3$^{-/-}$* MEFs (100). Furthermore, in MEFs and splenocytes from mice doubly deficient for IRF-3 and IRF-9 (DKO mice), in which IRF-7 mRNA induction is totally abolished, IFN-α/β mRNA induction was completely abolished. In addition, the induction of IFN-α/β mRNA expression by three different types of viruses, i.e., encephalomyocarditis virus (EMCV; picornaviridae), vesicular stomatitis virus (VSV; rhabdoviridae), and herpes simplex virus (HSV; herpesviridae) is also not observed in DKO MEFs, indicating the general importance of IRF-3 and IRF-7 in antiviral response (100). In these cells, the ectopic expression of either IRF-3 or IRF-7 cannot restore the normal induction profiles of IFN-α/β mRNAs, unless these factors are co-expressed. These results demonstrated the essential and distinct roles of IRF-3 and IRF-7, which together ensure the transcriptional efficiency and diversity of *IFN-α/β* genes for the antiviral response. These results, together with previous results (35, 36), indicate the operation of a positive feedback regulation of *IFN-α/β* gene induction, in which IRF-3 is critical for both early and late phases of the *IFN-α/β* gene induction (Figure 3, see color insert). In the early phase, which is mostly IFN-independent, IRF-3 functions mainly for the *IFN-β* gene induction. On the other hand, in the late phase, IRF-3 is also critical for two reasons: for the potentiation of the overall IFN-α/β mRNA induction and for full procurement of the normal mRNA induction profile for IFN-α subspecies by cooperating with IRF-7 (100). Clearly, IRF-7 is more critical for the late induction phase than for the early phase (35, 36). In effect, the biphasic *IFN-α/β* gene induction mechanism, regulated by IRF-3 and IRF-7, ensures the transcriptional efficiency and diversity of the genes for efficient antiviral response (Figure 3, see color insert).

In retrospect, the previous result that *IFN-α/β* gene induction is significantly upregulated in *IRF-2⁻/⁻* MEFs (40) can be explained as follows. IRF-7 expression is upregulated in these cells, due to the absence of the interference (transcriptional attenuation; see below) of ISGF3, by IRF-2 (27, 115). In addition, IRF-2 represses the IFN-β gene induction by invading the virus-activated enhansosome (121).

It is interesting to note that the IFN-induced IRF-7 has a very short half-life (0.5 ~ 1 hr), suggesting that this labile nature of IRF-7 represents a mechanism that is critical to make the whole *IFN* gene induction process transient (100). The detailed mechanism by which IRF-3 and IRF-7 undergo nuclear translocation by phosphorylation remains to be fully elucidated, particularly the identification of kinase(s) responsible for the phosphorylation of these IRFs.

Regulation of IFN-Induced Antiviral Activities by IRFs

The fact that IRF family members recognize the ISRE suggests that those that are activated or induced by IFNs are critical to IFN-mediated cellular responses. To assess the role of IRF-1 and IRF-9 (in the context of ISGF3) in IFN-mediated antiviral response, MEFs from mice carrying null mutations in one or both of these genes were examined. Establishment of the maximum antiviral state against a variety of viruses is impaired in cells lacking either of the two IRF members, indicating that they perform nonredundant functions in the establishment of the antiviral response by IFN-α or IFN-γ (122, 123), and implying that one or both are required for IFN induction of a set of target genes critical to the full-range antiviral response. In fact, IFN-γ receptor stimulation, which evokes activation of Jak1 and Jak2, also results in the formation of trimeric complexes consisting of either IRF-9:Stat1:Stat1 or IRF-9:Stat1:Stat2 (Figure 2, see color insert) (24, 57, 73). IFN-inducible genes can be divided into distinct classes according to their dependence on IRF-1, IRF-9, or both for proper expression, as revealed by analyzing MEFs lacking either IRF-1 or IRF-9 or both. It is likely that this requirement for one or both transcription factors is determined by the promoter context, i.e., the presence or absence of additional factor(s) that cooperate with these different IRF family members on a given promoter (2, 16). The role of IRF family members in other aspects of the IFN responses in immune system regulation is described below.

REGULATION OF OTHER IMMUNE RESPONSES

In view of the findings that expression and/or function of IRF family members are regulated by immunomodulatory cytokines and that some members are selectively expressed in cells of hematopoietic lineage, it is likely that they participate in the regulation of the development and function of the immune system, in addition to antiviral response. In fact, gene targeting studies have revealed a remarkable functional diversity of IRF-1 (Table 1) and of other IRF family members in the regulation of innate and adaptive immune systems. The overall involvement of the

TABLE 1   Potential target genes of IRF-1 and their role in host defense

Target gene	Expression pattern	Role	Reference
IFN-α/β	Most cell types	Anti-viral response	(25, 115)
GBP	Most cell types	Anti-viral response?	(122)
iNOS	Macrophages	Anti-bacterial response	(130)
IL-12p40	Macrophages	Th1 type immune responses	(125, 132)
Cox2	Macrophages	Inflammation	(134)
IL-15	Bone-marrow stroma cells	NK cell differentiation	(127)
CIITA	Macrophages, dendritic cells	MHC class II expression	(137)
TAP1, LMP2	Most cell types	MHC class I expression	(135)
PA28α, PA28β, β2-microglobulin	Most cell types	MHC class I expression	(M Matsumoto and T Taniguchi, unpublished)
gp91^{phox}	Myelomonocytic cells	Anti-bacterial response	(49)
p21$^{WAF1/CIP1}$	Fibroblasts	Induction of cell cycle arrest	(90)
Caspase 1	T lymphocytes	Induction of apoptosis	(155)
Caspase 7	T lymphocytes	Induction of apoptosis	(K Ishiodori and T Taniguchi, unpublished)
Lysyl oxidase	Fibroblasts	Inhibition of cell transformation	(161)

IRFs in the regulation of the immune system is depicted in Figure 4 (see color insert).

NK Cell Development and Function

NK cells can produce IFN-γ when stimulated with IL-12, a cytokine critical for inducing T helper (Th) 1-type immune response (124). Initially, it was found that unlike wild-type (WT) mice, *IRF-1$^{-/-}$* mice failed to induce IL-12 upon intraperitoneal administration of IL-12. In addition, NK cell–mediated cytolytic activity was not observed in cells from $IRF\text{-}1^{-/-}$ spleen and liver (125), and $IRF\text{-}1^{-/-}$ mice were unable to eliminate syngenic, MHC class I-negative tumor cells in vivo (126). Consistently, the number of NK (NK1.1$^+$ TCRα/β^-) cells was dramatically reduced in both spleen and liver of $IRF\text{-}1^{-/-}$ mice (125; K Ogasawara, T Taniguchi, unpublished observation). These results indicate that NK cell development is impaired in $IRF\text{-}1^{-/-}$ mice. Furthermore, the lack of IRF-1 selectively affects radioresistant (stroma) cells that constitute the microenvironment for NK cell development, but not for NK cell progenitors (127); $IRF\text{-}1^{-/-}$ bone marrow (BM) cells can generate functional NK cells when transplanted into irradiated WT mice. $IRF\text{-}1^{-/-}$ BM cells can also give rise to mature, functional NK cells in vitro, when cultured with IL-15, suggesting that the $IL\text{-}15$ gene is transcriptionally regulated by IRF-1 (127). Promoter analysis of the $IL\text{-}15$ gene revealed that this is, in fact, the case (127). In addition, the numbers of NK-T (NK1.1$^+$ TCRα/β^+) cells and $\gamma\delta$T cells were also shown to be reduced in $IRF\text{-}1^{-/-}$ mice (128). These observations suggest the presence of additional target gene(s) affecting the development of these cell lineages.

Recently, $IRF\text{-}2^{-/-}$ mice were shown to carry defects in NK cell development and/or function (129). $IRF\text{-}2^{-/-}$ splenocytes displayed a larger decrease in NK cell cytotoxic activity than did $IRF\text{-}2^{+/-}$ splenocytes stimulated with Poly (I):(C) in vivo. A notable defect in NK cell activity was also noted in vivo in a tumor rejection model using the NK sensitive cell line. Furthermore, the number of NK cells (NK1.1$^+$TCRα/β^-) was dramatically decreased in $IRF\text{-}2^{-/-}$ mice. Unlike $IRF\text{-}1^{-/-}$ BM cells, $IRF\text{-}2^{-/-}$ BM cells could not generate NK cells when cultured with IL-15 (129). Interestingly, although the number of NK-T cells was reduced in $IRF\text{-}1^{-/-}$ mice, that in $IRF\text{-}2^{-/-}$ mice was normal (129). It is currently unknown how IRF-2 contributes to these phenomena.

It has been also suggested that IRF-1 and IRF-9 (in the context of ISGF3) are essential for IL-12-induced and IFN-α/β-induced activation of NK cells, respectively (K Ogasawara, unpublished data).

Macrophage Function

The inducible nitric oxide synthetase ($iNOS$) gene is induced by IFN-β and/or lipopolysaccharide (LPS) in WT macrophages, but not in $IRF\text{-}1^{-/-}$ macrophages (130, 131). The enzyme encoded by the $iNOS$ gene catalyzes the production of nitric oxide, a short-lived volatile gas that plays a major role in the effector phase of Th1 immune response; i.e., macrophage cytotoxicity against tumor cells, bacteria, and other targets. Indeed, this may explain the observation that $IRF\text{-}1^{-/-}$ mice develop severe symptoms resembling military cutaneous tuberculosis when infected with *Mycobacterium bovis* (130). In addition, the induction of the gene encoding the p40 subunit of IL-12, the cytokine essential for Th1-type differentiation of the immune system, is totally dependent on IRF-1 (125, 132).

Neutrophils and macrophages play an important role in restricting bacterial replication (e.g., *Listeria monocytogenes* infection) in the early phase of primary infection in mice, and cytokines IFN-γ and TNF-α are essential for protection. *IRF-2$^{-/-}$* and *IRF-8$^{-/-}$* mice are highly susceptible to *Listeria* infection compared with *IRF-1$^{-/-}$* mice. Therefore, IRF-8 and IRF-2 are critical for IFN-γ mediated protection against *Listeria*, which may affect the production of reactive oxygen intermediates (ROIs) and possibly others in macrophages (133).

Cyclooxygenase (Cox)-2 is upregulated by proinflammatory agents, initiating many prostanoid-mediated pathological aspects of inflammation. IRF-1 and IRF-2 are shown to regulate IFN-γ dependent Cox-2 expression (134).

Regulation of MHC Expression

IFN-α/β and IFN-γ are known to enhance the expression of MHC class I and class II molecules. CD8$^+$ T cell population is significantly reduced in *IRF-1$^{-/-}$* mice, which may be due to the low level of expression of MHC class I molecules (115). This may be a consequence of the reduced expression of a transporter associated with antigen processing-1 (TAP-1) and the low molecular weight protein-2 (LMP-2) (135). In fact, IFN-γ induces *TAP*-1 and *LMP*-2 gene expression through IRF-1 (135). IRF-1 may also be involved in the IFN-γ-induced expression of *PA28α*, *PA28β* and *β2-microglobulin* gene in MEFs (16). On the other hand, IRF-9 (ISGF3) and IRF-1 may both contribute to the induction of MHC class I molecules, TAP1, LMP2, and β2-microglobulin by IFN-α/β stimulation (16).

The expression of MHC class II (e.g., MHC II, Ii, HLA-DM) molecules is also uniquely regulated by IRF-1, via an indirect mechanism: The expression of CIITA, a critical transcription factor for *MHC class II* gene induction by IFN-γ, requires Stat1 and IRF-1 (136). In fact, the induction of CIITA mRNA was reduced in *IRF-1$^{-/-}$* mice (137).

IRF-8 was originally identified as a transcription factor binding to the ISRE motif in the promoter region of the *MHC class I* gene (43). Since IRF-8 is induced by IFN-γ, but not IFN-α/β (43), IRF-8 may contribute to IFN-γ-dependent MHC upregulation. Although IRF-8 is known to affect the activity of *MHC class I* and *β2-microglobulin* promoters (138), no significant alterations were detected in their mRNA levels or the surface expression of MHC class I on *IRF-8$^{-/-}$* lymphoid cells (139), pointing to an alternative pathway of gene expression.

Regulation of Development and Function of T and B Cells

IRF-1$^{-/-}$ mice carry lineage-specific defects in thymocyte development; immature T cells (i.e., double-positive TCR$\alpha\beta^+$CD4$^+$CD8$^+$) were able to develop into mature CD4$^+$ but not efficiently into CD8$^+$ T cells. In fact, a marked reduction in the number of CD8$^+$ T cells (10-fold) was evident in peripheral blood, spleen, and lymph node by flow cytometric analysis (115). Further studies revealed that IRF-1 may control the positive and negative selection of CD8$^+$ thymocytes. In fact, positive and negative T cell selection is impaired in $IRF\text{-}1^{-/-}$ H-Y and $IRF\text{-}1^{-/-}$ P14 transgenic mice (140). Although the cell surface expression of MHC class I is low on $IRF\text{-}1^{-/-}$ thymocytes and thymic stromal cells, the defect in $CD8^+$T cell development does not reside in the thymic environment; $IRF\text{-}1^{-/-}$ stromal cells can fully support the development of $CD8^+$ thymocytes in in vivo bone marrow chimeras and in vitro reaggregation cultures (140). Moreover, $IRF\text{-}1^{-/-}$ thymocytes displayed impaired TCR-mediated signal transduction, and the induction of negative selection in TCR transgenic thymocytes from $IRF\text{-}1^{-/-}$ mice required a 1000-fold higher level of the selecting peptide than that for $IRF\text{-}1^{+/-}$ mice. Thus, IRF-1 may regulate the expression of gene(s) in developing thymocytes, which is required for lineage commitment and selection of $CD8^+$ thymocytes (140).

$CD8^+$ T cells have cytotoxic effector functions. Cytotoxic T lymphocyte (CTL) response to LCMV (lymphocytic choriomeningitis virus)-infected target cells was significantly reduced in $IRF\text{-}1^{-/-}$ mice. In contrast, $IRF\text{-}2^{-/-}$ mice showed normal CTL activity against LCMV-infected target cells, although some nonspecific cytotoxicity was detected (115). $IRF\text{-}4^{-/-}$ mice after LCMV infection showed no CTL activity against target cells (141). In $IRF\text{-}8^{-/-}$ mice, analysis of CTL responses after VSV and VV (vaccinia virus) infection revealed a three- to tenfold reduction of CTL activity (139). These results collectively indicate that IRF-1, IRF-2, IRF-4, and IRF-8 all contribute to the induction of CTL activity.

IRF-4 is expressed in all stages of B cell development as well as in mature T cells, and the expression is also inducible in these lymphocytes in a primary culture stimulated by concanavalin A, CD3 cross-linking, anti-IgM and PMA (phorbol myristate acetate) treatment (40). Lymph nodes and spleen of $IRF\text{-}4^{-/-}$ mice showed normal lymphocyte distribution and cellularity at 4 to 5 weeks of age (141). At 10 to 15 weeks, although the thymus of $IRF\text{-}4^{-/-}$ mice was normal, the spleen was enlarged three to five times and lymph nodes were enlarged 10 times those of control mice, due to an increase in the number of $CD4^+$ and $CD8^+$ T cells and B cells. In addition, late-stage B cell maturation was blocked in the spleen from $IRF\text{-}4^{-/-}$ mice. $IRF\text{-}4^{-/-}$ mice exhibited a marked reduction in serum immunoglobulin level and could not produce antibodies against T cell-dependent and -independent antigen stimulations. B cell activation and proliferation were also impaired in $IRF\text{-}4^{-/-}$ mice (141). Moreover, T cell functions, such as cytokine production, cytotoxic activity, and proliferation, were also abrogated in $IRF\text{-}4^{-/-}$ mice. Thus, IRF-4 is essential for the function and homeostasis of both mature B and T cells (141).

Regulation of $CD8^+$ T Cell Response by IRF-2 and IRF-9 (ISGF3)

Cytokines are not always beneficial to the host because many cytokines are multifunctional and often invoke antigen-nonspecific response of the cell. In this context, regulatory mechanisms have been reported for other cytokine systems, downregulating their signaling events (reviewed in 142–145). Recently, $IRF\text{-}2^{-/-}$

mice in C57BL/6 background spontaneously were found to have developed an inflammatory skin disease resembling psoriasis (27, 115). The pathogenic involvement of CD8$^+$, but not CD4$^+$, T cells is evident, as skin disease development is suppressed upon the selective depletion of these T cells. CD8$^+$ T cells exhibit in vitro hyper-responsiveness to antigen stimulation, accompanied with a notable upregulation of the expression of genes induced by IFN-α/β (27). Furthermore, both disease development and CD8$^+$ T cell abnormality are suppressed by the introduction of nullizygosity to the genes that positively regulate the IFN-α/β signaling pathway (27).

Thus, IRF-2 may represent a unique negative regulator, attenuating IFN-α/β-induced gene transcription, which is necessary for balancing the beneficial and harmful effects of IFN-α/β signaling in the immune system (Figure 4, see color insert) (27). On the other hand, CD8$^+$ T cells lacking a functional IFN-α/β receptor or IRF-9 show hypo-responsiveness to stimulation by allogeneic MHC class I molecules, whereas CD4$^+$ T cells show normal response to class II molecules (K Ogasawara. T Taniguchi, unpublished data). These studies may provide a new link between the IFN-α/β system and the CD8$^+$ T cell-mediated adaptive immune system.

Regulation of Th1/Th2 Differentiation

IRF-1 is required for the development of Th1-type immune response, and its absence leads to the induction of Th2-type immune response instead (125, 132). This compromised differentiation into Th1 cells was associated with multiple defects as described below. In fact, $IRF-1^{-/-}$ mice were vulnerable to *Listeria monocytogenes* and *Leishmania major*, but resistant to *Nippostrongylus brasiliensis* (125, 132).

As described above, $IRF-1^{-/-}$ macrophage is defective for the induction of the *IL-12p40* gene. In addition, *IRF*-1 deficiency also affects the response of CD4$^+$ T cells to IL-12; the undifferentiated CD4$^+$ T cells from $IRF-1^{-/-}$ mice fail to properly respond to WT antigen-producing cells to differentiate into Th1 cells (125). Further studies revealed that IL-12-induced upregulation of IRF-1 is mediated by Stat4, which binds to the GAS sequence in the promoter region of the *IRF*-1 gene (146, 147). Thus, *IRF-1* may be a target gene of IL-12, which is critical to induce the onset of Th1 cell differentiation by affecting the expression of as-yet-unidentified gene(s).

IRF-2 was originally described as an antagonist of the IRF-1-mediated transcriptional regulation of IFN-inducible genes (25). Since Th1 cell development and NK cell development are impaired in $IRF-1^{-/-}$ mice, one would have expected that $IRF-2^{-/-}$ mice might manifest opposite phenotypes. However, IL-12 production is suppressed in $IRF-2^{-/-}$ macrophages (129), and $IRF-2^{-/-}$ mice are susceptible to *Leishmania major* infection due to a defect in Th1 cell differentiation (129). Thus, rather than functioning as negative regulator, IRF-2 may contribute to *IL-12* gene expression in cooperation with other factors, such as IRF-8, in activated macrophages.

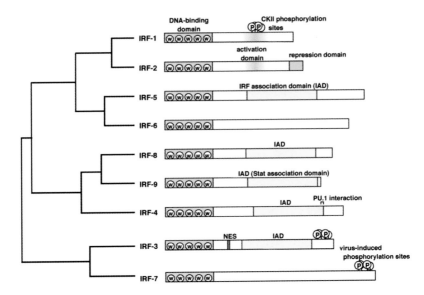

Figure 1 Members of the human IRF family; phylogenetic relationships and their functional domains. Protein sequences were aligned by the unweighted pair group method with arithmetic mean (UPGMA) using the GeneWorks program (left). Members of the IRF family show significant homology of the 115 amino acids in the animo-terminal region, which comprises the DNA-binding domain. Five tryptophan (W) repeats are conserved among these family members. It was determined that 177 amino acids in the carboxyl-terminal region of IRF-8 comprise the association domain with IRF-1 or IRF-2 (IRF association domain; IAD; (48). This domain shows significant homology with those of IRF-9 and IRF-4, and little homology with those of IRF-5 and IRF-3 (48). The IAD-like domain in IRF-9 mediates its interaction with Stat1 and Stat2 (189). The association domain of IRF-4 with PU.1 was determined (39, 106). Phosphorylation sites of IRFs were also determined (see text). NES: nuclear export signal.

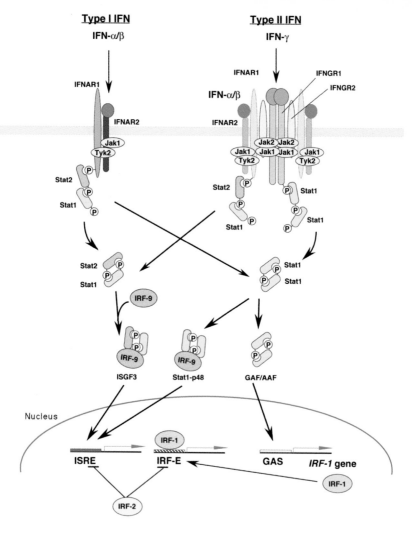

Figure 2 Role of IRF transcriptional factors in IFN signaling. In the type I IFN system ligand binding to IFNAR results in the activation of Jak1 and Tyk2, which tyrosine-phosphorylates IFNAR1 at residue 455 (Y455 for mouse IFNAR1) of its intracellular domain. Subsequently, Stat2 recruits to this Y455 via its SH2 domain, followed by tyrosine phosphorylation of this factor, while Stat1 is recruited by IFNAR1, through its interaction with phosphorylated Stat2 (77, 78). These two Stat factors, together with IRF-9, form a heterotrimeric complex, which in turn leads to the activation of IFN-inducible genes via ISRE (24, 57). IRF-2 functions as a transcriptional attenuator of both IRF-E-mediated and ISRE-mediated transcriptional activation, that is, IRF-2 does not suppress IFN-α/β responses completely but to control the chronic, weak IFN-α/β signaling by attenuating the ISGF3-mediated gene induction. In the type II IFN system, it was shown that constitutive

Figure 2 *continued*

subthreshold IFN-α/β signaling, which is triggered by a low concentration of spontaneously produced IFN-α/β, is required for the full procurement of IFN-γ signaling for two
reasons (74). First, the constitutive subthreshold IFN-α/β signaling leads to the enhancement of the otherwise weak association between the two non-ligand-binding components,
IFNAR1 and IFNGR2. Second, this signaling maintains IFNAR1 in the phosphorylated
form in order to provide docking sites for Stat1/Stat2. Upon stimulation by IFN-γ, which
is known to function as a dimer, both Jak1 and Jak2 are activated, followed by the phosphorylation of tyrosine residue 423 (Y423 for mouse IFNGR1) intracellular region of
IFNGR1. Stat1 recruits to this Y423 via its SH2 domain and is tyrosine-phosphorylated.
During the process of Stat dimerization, IFNAR1 provides docking sites for ISGF3 complex formation as well as for efficient dimerization of Stat1. Dimerization of Stat1 forms
GAF complex, which subsequently binds to GAS and activates IFN-inducible genes. IRF-
1 gene is induced via GAS which is found within the IRF-1 promoter. IRF-1 then bind to
IRF-E, leading to the activation of IFN-inducible genes.

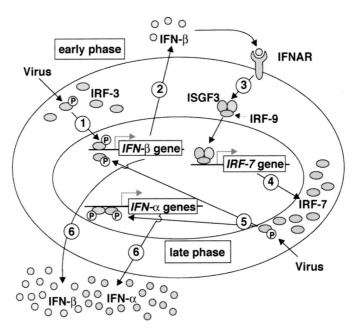

Figure 3 Schematic representation of the biphasic mechanism for IFN-α/β gene induction,
mediated by IRF-3 and IRF-7. In the early phase, constitutively expressed IRF-3 is activated by viral infection, resulting in the weak activation of the IFN-β gene. In this phase,
IRF-7 is expressed only at very low levels by spontaneous IFN-α/β signaling. This initially produced IFN-β strongly induces IRF-7 expression through activation of the ISGF3. In
the late phase, IRF-3 and IRF-7 cooperate with each other to amplify IFN-α/β gene induction, resulting in the full procurement of the normal mRNA induction profile of the IFN-α
gene subfamily (100). Circled numbers indicate the sequence of events.

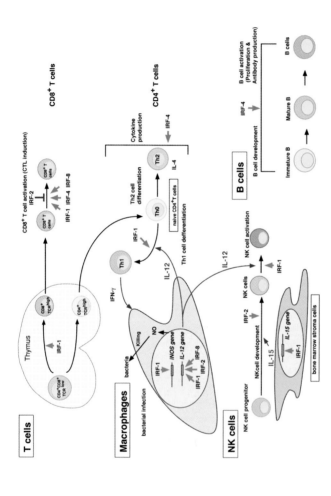

Figure 4 Regulation of the immune system by IRF family members. IRFs regulate lymphocyte development and function. Only known target genes in this system are shown. IRF-1, IRF-2 and IRF-8 contribute to IL-12p40 gene induction and have crucial roles in Th1-type immune response. IRF-1 regulates NK cell development through the induction of the IL-15 gene in bone marrow stroma cells. The iNOS gene is induced by IFN-γ through IRF-1 in macrophages for anti bacterial infection. Although critical target genes are unclear, the other processes regulated by IRFs are indicated by red arrows. It was shown that IRF-2 is involved in activation (red arrow) or repression (blue line) in these processes. See text for the details.

In fact, *IRF-8$^{-/-}$* spleen cells are also defective in IL-12 production when stimulated with LPS plus IFN-γ (139). Compared with WT mice, *IRF-8$^{-/-}$* mice after *Toxoplasma gondii* infection exhibited unchecked parasite replication and rapidly succumbed due to a defect in Th1 cell differentiation (148). Similar results were obtained in *IRF-8$^{-/-}$* mice after *Leishmania major* infection (149). Thus, IRF-8 is essential for Th1 cell development through its role in regulating *IL-12* gene expression. In view of the report on the multimeric complex formation of IRF-8 with IRF-1/IRF-2, it is possible that the IL-12p40 promoter requires such a complex for its activation (148).

IRFs in Autoimmunity

Evidence has been provided for the role played by IRF-1 in autoimmunity. The incidence and severity of type II collagen-induced arthritis (CIA) and synovial inflammation were significantly decreased in *IRF-1$^{-/-}$* mice compared with those in control mice (150). Furthermore, the incidence of experimental allergic encephalomyelitis (EAE) in *IRF-1$^{-/-}$* mice was also decreased compared with that in *IRF-1$^{+/-}$* mice (150). In *IRF-1$^{+/-}$* mice, the expression of IRF-1 mRNA was upregulated in the spinal cord with EAE, and the expression of iNOS was also detected in inflamed spinal cords (151). Therefore, IRF-1 appears to play a key role in promoting inflammation and autoimmunity.

As described above, the development of CD8$^+$ T cell–mediated inflammatory skin disease in *IRF-2$^{-/-}$* mice may be another example of the involvement of this IRF family member in autoimmunity. Little is known regarding the involvement of other IRF family members in the regulation of autoimmunity.

INVOLVEMENT OF IRF-1 AND OTHER IRF FAMILY MEMBERS IN ONCOGENESIS

Regulation of Cell Cycle and Apoptosis by IRF-1

The expression of IRF-1 is regulated throughout the cell cycle; IRF-1 mRNA expression is markedly elevated in NIH 3T3 cells subjected to serum starvation, but following the addition of serum, its expression rapidly declines, to be followed again by a gradual increase prior to and during DNA synthesis, suggesting its involvement in cell cycle regulation (152). Subsequently, *IRF-1$^{-/-}$* MEFs were found deficient in their ability to undergo DNA damage-induced cell cycle arrest, a phenotype similar to that observed in MEFs lacking the tumor suppressor p53 (90). Furthermore, transcriptional induction of the gene encoding the CDK inhibitor, p21$^{WAF1/CIP1}$, by γ-irradiation was dependent on both IRF-1 and p53. In these cells, IRF-1 mRNA was not upregulated, but IRF-1 protein level was augmented, presumably due to its stabilization, so as to act on the *p21* promoter region, containing the IRF-1- and p53-binding sites (90). Thus, these two transcription factors cooperate to prevent the accumulation of mutations following DNA damage by activating a common target gene that regulates the cell cycle.

In contrast to normal MEFs, those carrying an activated form of c-Ha-*ras* oncogene undergo apoptosis upon noxious stresses such as γ-irradiation, and this DNA damage-induced apoptosis is dependent on IRF-1 and p53 (153). In addition, DNA damage-induced apoptosis in mitogenically activated mature T lymphocytes, which is known to be p53-independent (154), is dependent on IRF-1 (155). The target gene(s) of IRF-1 critical for apoptotic response are not known but may include *caspase 1 and 7* genes (155, 156; K Ishiodori, T Taniguchi, unpublished data). These results collectively demonstrate that IRF-1 functions not only in immune system regulation, but also in the regulation of cell cycle and apoptosis (Table 1).

IRF-1 as Tumor Susceptibility Gene

The above observations suggest a potential tumor suppressor-like function of IRF-1. In fact, oncogene-transformed cultured cell lines can be reverted to their normal phenotype by ectopic expression of IRF-1 (157). The tumor suppressor-like function of IRF-1 was further demonstrated in oncogenic transformation assays using *IRF-1$^{-/-}$* MEFs. Transformation of WT MEFs normally requires at least two oncogenes. For example, the activated form of the c-Ha-*ras* gene will not transform MEFs unless introduced together with another oncogene such as *c-myc* or polyoma large-T antigen (158, 159). Introduction of the *c-H-ras* gene alone is sufficient to transform *IRF-1$^{-/-}$* MEFs (153).

More recently, the loss of *IRF-1* alleles per se has been shown to have no effect on spontaneous tumor development in the mouse, but it dramatically exacerbates previous tumor predispositions caused by *c-Ha-ras* transgene or nullizygosity for *p53* (160). This accelerated tumor development may not be due to several immunological disorders as mentioned above, because in *IRF-1$^{-/-}$ p53$^{-/-}$* (*IRF-1, p53* double-deficient) $\leftrightarrow$ *p53$^{-/-}$* chimeric mice, generated by the aggregation of their respective embryos, most tumors originated from *IRF-1$^{-/-}$ p53$^{-/-}$* cells (160). In addition, notable alterations in the tumor spectrum in *IRF-1$^{-/-}$ p53$^{-/-}$* mice indicated that IRF-1 is not hypostatic to p53. Furthermore, *IRF-1$^{-/-}$ p53$^{-/-}$* MEFs were more sensitive to drug-induced mutagenesis and exhibited hyperactive proliferation as compared to single-null cells. Thus, IRF-1 may regulate a new pathway(s) that suppresses tumorigenesis in the absence of p53; *IRF-1* is a new member of the tumor susceptibility genes.

In order to clarify the mechanism underlying accelerated tumor susceptibility in the absence of IRF-1, the *lysyl oxidase* gene was identified (161). *Lysyl oxidase*, the product of which plays a critical role in the biogenesis of connective tissue matrices, was identified as being identical to the mouse *ras* recision gene (rrg), and it was implicated in the reversion of *ras*-transformed NIH 3T3 cells (162, 163). However, the phenotype observed in *IRF-1$^{-/-}$* mice, especially its relationship with p53, could not be completely explained by the loss of expression of this gene as well as it was for the case of the *p21* gene (90). Therefore, more as yet unknown target gene(s) may exist.

Involvement of IRF-1 in Human Cancer

In addition to the functional analyses described above, clinical studies have also indicated that the loss of IRF-1 may affect the development of some forms of human leukemia. This was initially suggested by the mapping of the *IRF-1* gene to the chromosomal region 5q31.1 (164, 165). The deletion of this region is one of the most frequently observed cytogenetic abnormalities in patients suffering from leukemia or preleukemic myelodysplastic syndrome (MDS) (166). In a study of 13 patients with leukemia or MDS who exhibited cytogenetic abnormalities in the 5q region, *IRF-1* was the only gene found to be consistently deleted or rearranged in either or both alleles (165). Thus, the loss of IRF-1 function may be a critical event in the development of human leukemias. On the other hand, in some patients with MDS/AML associated with 5q abnormalities, while one allele of the *IRF-1* gene is deleted, the other remains intact (167). In addition to its association with hematopoietic malignancies, several reports have indicated that the loss of an *IRF-1* allele is also frequent in esophageal and gastric cancers (168, 169) and, in one out of four cases of gastric cancers examined, the deletion was accompanied by an inactivating point mutation in the other allele (170).

Two alternative mechanisms that lead to the loss-of-function of IRF-1 were reported. Nucleophosmin (NPM), a putative ribosome assembly factor often over-expressed in leukemic cells, binds to IRF-1 and inhibits its function (171). Other studies suggested that splicing aberrations in the *IRF-1* gene also account for the loss of IRF-1 expression. The human *IRF-1* gene is highly prone to exon-skipping, which generates mRNAs lacking exon 2 or exons 2 and 3, with consequent loss of the correct AUG initiator codon. Interestingly, in 6 out of 20 AML/MDS patients, no productive IRF-1 mRNA could be detected at all by RT-PCR (172), suggesting that subtle alteration of the splicing machinery (173) may selectively affect "error-prone" genes such as *IRF-1*. Recently, another mechanism for inactivation of IRF-1 by human papilloma virus (HPV) 16-encoded E7 oncoprotein has been reported (174a).

Tumor Suppressive Function of IRF-8

As described above, IRF-8 is expressed in hematopoietic cells. $IRF-8^{-/-}$ mice develop a pathological syndrome similar to human chronic myelogenous leukemia (CML) (139). Moreover, about 30% of $IRF-8^{-/-}$ mice transit from a chronic stage to acute blast crisis characterized by the clonal expansion of leukemic cells. These findings indicate that IRF-8 functions as a tumor suppressor in the mouse system. Expression of IRF-8 is downregulated in a Bcr-Abl-induced murine chronic myelogenous leukemia-like disease, and forced coexpression of IRF-8 inhibits the development of Bcr-Abl-induced myeloproliferative disorder (174). At present, only a few reports are available that suggest the involvement of IRF-8 in human cancers. For example, the IRF-8 mRNA expression level is reduced in several human CML and acute myeloid leukemia cases (175).

Oncogenic Potential of IRF-2 and IRF-4

Unlike IRF-1, IRF-2 functions as a transcriptional attenuator, critical in balancing IFN action in vivo (27). In NIH 3T3 cells, the overexpression of IRF-2 causes oncogenic transformation, and concomitant constitutive expression of IRF-1 causes these cells to revert to the nontransformed phenotype (152). Although the exact mechanism underlying this cell transformation is still unknown, it is possible that IRF-2 exerts its oncogenic function via the mediation of IRF-1 and/or other IRF family members that bind to the same IRF-E. This possibility is supported by the finding that NIH 3T3 cells expressing only the DNA-binding domain of IRF-2 were also transformed (176). On the other hand, IRF-2 activates gene(s) involved in oncogenesis, such as *Histone 4* (30, 177).

Several experiments also suggested the existence of a relationship between IRF-4 and oncogenesis. In human T cells, the expression of IRF-4 mRNA is induced by PMA or infection by the human T cell leukemia virus-1 (HTLV-1) (41). Moreover, overexpression of the HTLV-1 oncoprotein Tax induces IRF-4 mRNA expression in Jurkat cells, suggesting the involvement of IRF-4 in HTLV-1-induced leukemogenesis. Interestingly, in some patients with multiple myeloma and cell lines derived from this tumor, a chromosomal translocation t(6;14) × (p25;q32) juxtaposes the immunoglobulin heavy-chain locus to the *MUM1* (multiple myeloma 1) locus, which is virtually identical to *IRF-4*, resulting in the overexpression of IRF-4 (178). This chromosomal translocation is likely to be responsible for the leukemogenesis, since, like IRF-2, IRF-4 has oncogenic activity in vitro (178). However, the overexpression of IRF-4 alone is not sufficient for leukemogenesis in transgenic mice overexpressing IRF-4 in lymphocytes (179), suggesting that, unlike *c-myc*-induced leukemogenesis (180), additional factors are required for the oncogenic activity of IRF-4 in vivo.

vIRF

As inIRF-2 and IRF-4, the overexpression of vIRF-1 leads to oncogenic transformation of NIH 3T3 cells (58). At present, the precise nature of involvement of vIRFs in the pathogenesis of Kaposi's sarcoma and other cancers remains unclear because HHV-8 encodes several other proteins that may function as an oncogene (181). Therefore, it would be interesting to analyze the functions of viral oncogenic IRFs to gain more insight into the role of IRF family members in oncogenesis.

Other IRFs

Even though the role of IRF-9 in the IFN system has been extensively analyzed, its role in oncogenesis has not yet been established. The importance of IRF-9 in cancer has been analyzed in the context of IFN-α/β-mediated suppression of tumor cell growth (182). In contrast, it was reported that the *IRF-9* gene is directly activated by *c-myc*, and that cells lacking IRF-9 expression are highly susceptible to the cytocidal action of anticancer drugs (183). These findings suggest the involvement of IRF-9 in cell cycle regulation, although further work is required to clarify this point.

Recently, HPV 16 E6 oncoprotein has been shown to bind to IRF-3 and to inhibit its transcriptional activity (184). Although this inhibition may be advantageous for viral replication, it was also demonstrated that IRF-3 is activated by UV or anticancer drugs (185). These results suggest the possibility that IRF-3 also functions in tumor suppression.

CONCLUSIONS AND PERSPECTIVES

The expansion and functional analyses of the IRF family of transcription factors have provided new insights into the regulation mechanisms operating in host defense. In fact, gene disruption studies in mouse revealed that these factors seem not to affect the normal development of these animals but are essential to maintain their homeostasis through regulation of the immune system and oncogenesis. Thus, as stated elsewhere (186), one could rephrase "it is not just interferon regulatory factors any more."

Most notably, studies on IRF-1 revealed the remarkable functional diversity of this transcription factor in the regulation of cellular responses in host defense. These include host response to viral and bacterial infections, regulation of IFN-inducible genes, development of functional lymphocytes, susceptibility to oncogenic transformation, regulation of the cell cycle, and induction of growth arrest and programmed cell death (Table 1). IRF-1 may thus provide clues to reveal hitherto unnoticed connections among these diverse host defense mechanisms. From a mechanistic point of view, an interesting question is how a single transcription factor can be involved in all of these different responses. The function of IRF-1 apparently differs with cell type, presumably due to the presence or absence of cell-type-specific factors that direct IRF-1 to a particular set of promoters or that require IRF-1 for their own function (16, 46, 48). Secondly, the different levels of IRF-1 expression seem to dictate how it functions; the expression of the *IRF-1* gene is rapidly induced following stimulation by IFNs, and these high IRF-1 expression levels are required for the induction of a set of IFN-inducible genes for an efficient antiviral response (12, 122). On the other hand, the basal IRF-1 expression level appears to be sufficient for its antitumor function (153). Higher intracellular concentrations of IRF-1 may be required for antiviral response in order to interact with other factors whose concentrations are normally limited. Posttranslational modification of IRF-1 may also influence its function (47, 84). Finally, it is possible that the expression of IRF-1 target genes is dependent on its accessibility on chromatins. Our future study will focus on the intriguing possibility of IRF-1 affecting chromatin remodeling.

The induction of *IFN-α/β* genes in virally infected cells has been extensively studied in many laboratories as a paradigm of gene regulation in mammalian cells (2, 4, 17, 18). The identification of IRF-3 and IRF-7 and their functional analyses have finally revealed the essential and distinct roles of these factors in the biphasic gene induction, which may have evolved to make the host defense against viruses more efficient (35–37, 95–98, 100). It will be important to study the activation mechanism of IRF-3 and IRF-7, particularly the identification of the responsible kinase(s). It is also interesting to explore the roles of these factors in other aspects of host defense, in view of the reports suggesting their potential involvement in other genes (188, 189).

Obviously, we will learn much more about the host defense mechanisms through functional studies on these and other IRF family members.

ACKNOWLEDGMENTS

The work in our laboratory was supported in part by a special grant for Advanced Research on Cancer from the Ministry of Education, Science, Sports and Culture of Japan.

Visit the Annual Reviews home page at www.AnnualReviews.org

LITERATURE CITED

1. Ptashne M. 1992. *A Genetic Switch*. Cambridge, MA: Cell Press & Blackwell Sci.
2. Tjian R, Maniatis T. 1994. Transcriptional activation: a complex puzzle with few easy pieces. *Cell* 77:5–8
3. Lengyel P. 1982. Biochemistry of interferons and their actions. *Annu. Rev. Biochem.* 51:251–82
4. Weissmann C, Weber H. 1986. The interferon genes. *Prog. Nucleic Acid Res. Mol. Biol.* 33:251–300
5. Pestka S, Langer JA, Zoon KC, Samuel CE. 1987. Interferons and their actions. *Annu. Rev. Biochem.* 56:727–77
6. De Maeyer E, De Maeyer-Guignard J. 1988. *Interferons and Other Regulatory Cytokines*. New York: Wiley
7. Vilcek J, Sen GS. 1996. Interferons and other cytokines. In *Fields Virology*, ed. DM Fields, PM Knipe, PM Howley, pp. 375–99. Philadelphia: Lippincott-Raven. 3rd ed.
8. Paul WE, Seder RA. 1994. Lymphocyte responses and cytokines. *Cell* 76:241–51
9. Billiau A. 1996. Interferon-gamma: biology and role in pathogenesis. *Adv. Immunol.* 62:61–130
10. Bach EA, Aguet M, Schreiber RD. 1997. The IFNγ receptor: a paradigm for cytokine receptor signaling. *Annu. Rev. Immunol.* 15:563–91
11. Miyamoto M, Fujita T, Kimura Y, Maruyama M, Harada H, Sudo Y, Miyata T, Taniguchi T. 1988. Regulated expression of a gene encoding a nuclear factor, IRF-1, that specifically binds to IFN-β gene regulatory elements. *Cell* 54:903–13
12. Harada H, Fujita T, Miyamoto M, Kimura Y, Maruyama M, Furia A, Miyata T, Taniguchi T. 1989. Structurally similar but functionally distinct factors, IRF-1 and IRF-2, bind to the same regulatory elements of IFN and IFN-inducible genes. *Cell* 58:729–39

13. Moore PS, Boshoff C, Weiss RA, Chang Y. 1996. Molecular mimicry of human cytokine and cytokine response pathway genes by KSHV. *Science* 274:1739–44

14. Nguyen H, Hiscott J, Pitha PM. 1997. The growing family of interferon regulatory factors. *Cytokine Growth Factor Rev.* 8:293–312

15. Mamane Y, Heylbroeck C, Genin P, Algarte M, Servant MJ, LePage C, DeLuca C, Kwon H, Lin R, Hiscott J. 1999. Interferon regulatory factors: the next generation. *Gene* 237:1–14

16. Taniguchi T, Tanaka N, Ogasawara K, Taki S, Sato M, Takaoka A. 2000. The transcription factor IRF-1 and its family members in the regulation of host defense. *Cold Spring Harbor Symp. Quant. Biol.* 64:465–72

17. Taniguchi T. 1988. Regulation of cytokine gene expression. *Annu. Rev. Immunol.* 6:439–64

18. Maniatis T, Whittermore LA, Du W, Fan CM, Keller A, Palmobella V, Thanos D. 1992. Positive and negative control of human interferon-β gene expression. In *Transcriptional Regulation, Part 2*, ed. SL McKnight, KR Yamamoto, pp. 1193–1220. Cold Spring Harbor, NY: Cold Spring Harbor Lab. Press

19. Fujita T, Sakakibara J, Sudo Y, Miyamoto M, Kimura Y, Taniguchi T. 1988. Evidence for a nuclear factor(s), IRF-1, mediating induction and silencing properties to human IFN-β gene regulatory elements. *EMBO J.* 7:3397–3405

20. Pine R, Decker T, Kessler DS, Levy DE, Darnell JE Jr. 1990. Purification and cloning of interferon-stimulated gene factor 2 (ISGF2): ISGF2 (IRF-1) can bind to the promoters of both beta interferon- and interferon-stimulated genes but is not a primary transcriptional activator of either. *Mol. Cell. Biol.* 10:2448–57

21. Yu-Lee L-Y, Hrachovy JA, Stevens AM, Schwarz LA. 1990. Interferon-regulatory factor 1 is an immediate-early gene under transcriptional regulation by prolactin in Nb2 T cells. *Mol. Cell. Biol.* 10:3087–94

22. Abdollahi A, Lord KA, Hoffman-Liebermann B, Liebermann D. 1991. Interferon regulatory factor 1 is a myeloid differentiation primary response gene induced by interleukin 6 and leukemia inhibitory factor: role in growth inhibition. *Cell Growth Differ.* 2:401–7

23. Tanaka N, Kawakami T, Taniguchi T. 1993. Recognition DNA sequences of interferon regulatory factor 1 (IRF-1) and IRF-2, regulators of cell growth and the interferon system. *Mol. Cell. Biol.* 13:4531–38

24. Darnell JE Jr, Kerr IM, Stark GR. 1994. Jak-STAT pathways and transcriptional activation in response to IFNs and other extracellular signaling proteins. *Science* 264:1415–21

25. Harada H, Willison K, Sakakibara J, Miyamoto M, Fujita T, Taniguchi T. 1990. Absence of the type I IFN system in EC cells: transcriptional activator (IRF-1) and repressor (IRF-2) genes are developmentally regulated. *Cell* 63:303–2

26. Fujita T, Kimura Y, Miyamoto M, Barsoumian EL, Taniguchi T. 1989. Induction of endogenous IFN-α and IFN-β genes by a regulatory transcription factor, IRF-1. *Nature* 337:270–72

27. Hida S, Ogasawara K, Sato K, Abe M, Takayanagi H, Yokochi T, Sato T, Hirose S, Shirai T, Taki S, Taniguchi T. 2000. CD8$^+$ T cell mediated skin disease in mice lacking IRF-2, the transcriptional attenuator of interferon-α/β signalling. *Immunity.* 13:643–55

28. Watanabe N, Sakakibara J, Hovanessian A, Taniguchi T, Fujita T. 1991. Activation of IFN-β promoter element by IRF-1 requires a post-translational event in addition to IRF-1 synthesis. *Nucleic Acids Res.* 16:4421–28

29. Jesse TL, LaChance R, Iademarco MF, Dean DC. 1998. Interferon regulatory factor-2 is a transcriptional activator in muscle where it regulates expression of

vascular cell adhesion molecule-1. *J. Cell Biol.* 140:1265–76

30. Vaughan PS, Aziz F, van Wijnen AJ, Wu S, Harada H, Taniguchi T, Soprano KJ, Stein JL, Stein GS. 1995. Activation of a cell-cycle-regulated histone gene by the oncogenic transcription factor IRF-2. *Nature* 377:362–65

31. Au WC, Moore PA, Lowther W, Juang YT, Pitha PM. 1995. Identification of a member of the interferon regulatory factor family that binds to the interferon-stimulated response element and activates expression of interferon-induced genes. *Proc. Natl. Acad. Sci. USA* 92:11657–61

32. Weaver BK, Kumar KP, Reich NC. 1998. Interferon regulatory factor 3 and CREB-binding protein/p300 are subunits of double-stranded RNA-activated transcription factor DRAF1. *Mol. Cell. Biol.* 18:1359–68

33. Grant CE, Vasa MZ, Deeley RG. 1995. cIRF-3, a new member of the interferon regulatory factor (IRF) family that is rapidly and transiently induced by dsRNA. *Nucleic Acids Res.* 23:2137–46

34. Zhang L, Pagano JS. 1997. IRF-7, a new interferon regulatory factor associated with Epstein-Barr virus latency. *Mol. Cell. Biol.* 17:5748–57

35. Marie I, Durbin JE, Levy DE. 1998. Differential viral induction of distinct interferon-α genes by positive feedback through interferon regulatory factor-7. *EMBO J.* 17:6660–69

36. Sato M, Hata N, Asagiri M, Nakaya T, Taniguchi T, Tanaka N. 1998. Positive feedback regulation of type I IFN genes by the IFN-inducible transcription factor IRF-7. *FEBS Lett.* 441:106–10

37. Yoneyama M, Suhara W, Fukuhara Y, Fukuda M, Nishida E, Fujita T. 1998. Direct triggering of the type I interferon system by virus infection: activation of a transcription factor complex containing IRF-3 and CBP/p300. *EMBO J.* 17:1087–95

38. Lin R, Mamane Y, Hiscott J. 1999. Structural and functional analysis of interferon regulatory factor 3: localization of the transactivation and autoinhibitory domains. *Mol. Cell. Biol.* 19:2465–74

39. Eisenbeis CF, Singh H, Storb U. 1995. Pip, a novel IRF family member, is a lymphoid-specific, PU.1-dependent transcriptional activator. *Genes Dev.* 9:1377–87

40. Matsuyama T, Grossman A, Mittrücker HW, Siderovski DP, Kiefer F, Kawakami T, Richardson CD, Taniguchi T, Yoshinaga SK, Mak TW. 1995. Molecular cloning of LSIRF, a lymphoid-specific member of the interferon regulatory factor family that binds the interferon-stimulated response element (ISRE). *Nucleic Acids Res.* 23:2127–36

41. Yamagata T, Nishida J, Tanaka S, Sakai R, Mitani K, Yoshida M, Taniguchi T, Yazaki Y, Hirai H. 1996. A novel interferon regulatory factor family transcription factor, IC-SAT/Pip/LSIRF, that negatively regulates the activity of interferon-regulated genes. *Mol. Cell. Biol.* 16:1283–94

42. Hatada S, Kinoshita M, Takahashi S, Nishihara R, Sakumoto H, Fukui A, Noda M, Asashima M. 1997. An interferon regulatory factor-related gene (xIRF-6) is expressed in the posterior mesoderm during the early development of Xenopus laevis. *Gene* 203:183–88

43. Driggers PH, Ennist DL, Gleason SL, Mak W-H, Marks MS, Levi B-Z, Flanagan JR, Appella E, Ozato K. 1990. An interferon γ-regulated protein that binds the interferon-inducible enhancer element of major histocompatibility complex class I genes. *Proc. Natl. Acad. Sci. USA* 87:3743–47

44. Weisz A, Marx P, Sharf R, Appella E, Driggers PH, Ozato K, Levi BZ. 1992. Human interferon consensus sequence binding protein is a negative regulator of enhancer elements common to interferon-inducible genes. *J. Biol. Chem.* 267:25589–96

45. Nelson N, Kanno Y, Hong C, Contursi C, Fujita T, Fowlkes BJ, O'Connell E, Hu-Li

J, Paul WE, Jankovic D, Sher AF, Coligan JE, Thornton A, Appella E, Yang Y, Ozato K. 1996. Expression of IFN regulatory factor family proteins in lymphocytes. Induction of Stat-1 and IFN consensus sequence binding protein expression by T cell activation. *J. Immunol.* 156:3711–20

46. Bovolenta C, Driggers PH, Marks MS, Medin JA, Politis AD, Vogel SN, Levy DE, Sakaguchi K, Appella E, Coligan JE, Ozato K. 1994. Molecular interactions between interferon consensus sequence binding protein and members of the interferon regulatory factor family. *Proc. Natl. Acad. Sci. USA* 91:5046–5050

47. Sharf R, Meraro D, Azriel A, Thornton AM, Ozato K, Petricoin EF, Larner AC, Schaper F, Hauser H, Levi BZ. 1997. Phosphorylation events modulate the ability of interferon consensus sequence binding protein to interact with interferon regulatory factors and to bind DNA. *J. Biol. Chem.* 272:9785–92

48. Sharf R, Azriel A, Lejbkowicz F, Winograd SS, Ehrlich R, Levi BZ. 1995. Functional domain analysis of interferon consensus sequence binding protein (ICSBP) and its association with interferon regulatory factors. *J. Biol. Chem.* 270:13063–69

49. Eklund EA, Jalava A, Kakar R. 1998. PU.1, interferon regulatory factor 1, and interferon consensus sequence-binding protein cooperate to increase gp91(phox) expression. *J. Biol. Chem.* 273:13957–65

50. Veals SA, Schindler C, Leonard D, Fu XY, Aebersold R, Darnell JE Jr, Levy DE. 1992. Subunit of an alpha-interferon-responsive transcription factor is related to interferon regulatory factor and Myb families of DNA-binding proteins. *Mol. Cell. Biol.* 12:3315–24

51. Levy DE, Kessler DS, Pine R, Darnell JE Jr. 1989. Cytoplasmic activation of ISGF3, the positive regulator of interferon-alpha-stimulated transcription, reconstituted in vitro. *Genes Dev.* 3:1362–71

52. Kessler DS, Veals SA, Fu XY, Levy DE.

1990. Interferon-alpha regulates nuclear translocation and DNA-binding affinity of ISGF3, a multimeric transcriptional activator. *Genes Dev.* 4:1753–65

53. Fu XY, Kessler DS, Veals SA, Levy DE, Darnell JE Jr. 1990. ISGF3, the transcriptional activator induced by interferon alpha, consists of multiple interacting polypeptide chains. *Proc. Natl. Acad. Sci. USA* 87:8555–59

54. Schindler C, Fu XY, Improta T, Aebersold R, Darnell JE Jr. 1992. Proteins of transcription factor ISGF-3: one gene encodes the 91-and 84-kDa ISGF-3 proteins that are activated by interferon alpha. *Proc. Natl. Acad. Sci. USA* 89:7836–39

55. Fu XY, Schindler C, Improta T, Aebersold R, Darnell JE Jr. 1992. The proteins of ISGF-3, the interferon alpha-induced transcriptional activator, define a gene family involved in signal transduction. *Proc. Natl. Acad. Sci. USA* 89:7840–43

56. Fu XY. 1992. A transcription factor with SH2 and SH3 domains is directly activated by an interferon alpha-induced cytoplasmic protein tyrosine kinase(s). *Cell* 70:323–35

57. Bluyssen AR, Durbin JE, Levy DE. 1996. ISGF3γ p48, a specificity switch for interferon activated transcription factors. *Cytokine Growth Factor Rev.* 7:11–17

58. Gao SJ, Boshoff C, Jayachandra S, Weiss RA, Chang Y, Moore PS. 1997. KSHV ORF K9 (vIRF) is an oncogene which inhibits the interferon signaling pathway. *Oncogene* 15:1979–85

59. Zimring JC, Goodbourn S, Offermann MK. 1998. Human herpesvirus 8 encodes an interferon regulatory factor (IRF) homolog that represses IRF-1-mediated transcription. *J. Virol.* 72:701–7

60. Li M, Lee H, Guo J, Neipel F, Fleckenstein B, Ozato K, Jung JU. 1998. Kaposi's sarcoma-associated herpesvirus viral interferon regulatory factor. *J. Virol.* 72:5433–40

61. Burysek L, Yeow WS, Pitha PM. 1999.

Unique properties of a second human herpesvirus 8-encoded interferon regulatory factor (vIRF-2). *J. Hum. Virol.* 2:19–32

62. Lubyova B, Pitha PM. 2000. Characterization of a novel human herpesvirus 8-encoded protein, vIRF-3, that shows homology to viral and cellular interferon regulatory factors. *J. Virol.* 74:8194–8201

63. Escalante CR, Yie J, Thanos D, Aggarwal AK. 1998. Structure of IRF-1 with bound DNA reveals determinants of interferon regulation. *Nature* 391:103–6

64. Fujii Y, Shimizu T, Kusumoto M, Kyogoku Y, Taniguchi T, Hakoshima T. 1999. Crystal structure of an IRF-DNA complex reveals novel DNA recognition and cooperative binding to a tandem repeat of core sequences. *EMBO J.* 18:5028–5041

65. Sugita K, Miyazaki J, Appella E, Ozato K. 1987. Interferons increase transcription of a major histocompatibility class I gene via a 5′ interferon consensus sequence. *Mol. Cell. Biol.* 7:2625–30

66. Goodbourn S, Zinn K, Maniatis T. 1985. Human β-interferon gene expression is regulated by an inducible enhancer element. *Cell* 41:509–20

67. Goodbourn S, Maniatis T. 1988. Overlapping positive and negative regulatory domains of the human β-interferon gene. *Proc. Natl. Acad. Sci. USA* 85:1447–51

68. Ihle JN, Kerr IM. 1995. Jaks and Stats in signaling by the cytokine receptor superfamily. *Trends Genet.* 11:69–74

69. Taniguchi T. 1995. Cytokine signaling through nonreceptor protein tyrosine kinases. *Science* 268:251–55

70. Stark GR, Kerr IM, Williams BR, Silverman RH, Schreiber RD. 1998. How cells respond to interferons. *Annu. Rev. Biochem.* 67:227–64

71. Horvath CM, Darnell JE Jr. 1996. The antiviral state induced by alpha interferon and gamma interferon requires transcriptionally active Stat1 protein. *J. Virol.* 70:647–50

72. Martinez-Moczygemba M, Gutch MJ, French DL, Reich NC. 1997. Distinct STAT structure promotes interaction of STAT2 with the p48 subunit of the interferon-alpha-stimulated transcription factor ISGF3. *J. Biol. Chem.* 272:20070–76

73. Matsumoto M, Tanaka N, Harada H, Kimura T, Yokochi T, Kitagawa M, Schindler C, Taniguchi T. 1999. Activation of the transcription factor ISGF3 by interferon-γ. *Biol. Chem.* 380:699–703

74. Takaoka A, Mitani Y, Suemori H, Sato M, Yokochi T, Noguchi S, Tanaka N, Taniguchi T. 2000. Cross talk between interferon-γ and -α/β signaling components in caveolar membrane domains. *Science* 288:2357–60

75. Bluyssen HA, Muzaffar R, Vlietstra RJ, van der Made AC, Leung S, Stark GR, Kerr IM, Trapman J, Levy DE. 1995. Combinatorial association and abundance of components of interferon-stimulated gene factor 3 dictate the selectivity of interferon responses. *Proc. Natl. Acad. Sci. USA* 92:5645–49

76. Greenlund AC, Morales MO, Viviano BL, Yan H, Krolewski J, Schreiber RD. 1995. Stat recruitment by tyrosine-phosphorylated cytokine receptors: an ordered reversible affinity-driven process. *Immunity* 2:677–87

77. Yan H, Krishnan K, Greenlund AC, Gupta S, Lim JT, Schreiber RD, Schindler CW, Krolewski JJ. 1996. Phosphorylated interferon-alpha receptor 1 subunit (IFNαR1) acts as a docking site for the latent form of the 113 kDa STAT2 protein. *EMBO J.* 15:1064–74

78. Li X, Leung S, Kerr IM, Stark GR. 1997. Functional subdomains of STAT2 required for preassociation with the α interferon receptor and for signaling. *Mol. Cell. Biol.* 17:2048–56

79. Fujita T, Reis LF, Watanabe N, Kimura Y, Taniguchi T, Vilcek J. 1989. Induction of the transcription factor IRF-1 and interferon-beta mRNAs by cytokines and

activators of second-messenger pathways. *Proc. Natl. Acad. Sci. USA* 86:9936–40

80. Pine R, Canova A, Schindler C. 1994. Tyrosine phosphorylated p91 binds to a single element in the ISGF2/IRF-1 promoter to mediate induction by IFN alpha and IFN gamma, and is likely to autoregulate the p91 gene. *EMBO J.* 13:158–67

81. Harada H, Takahashi E, Itoh S, Harada K, Hori TA, Taniguchi T. 1994. Structure and regulation of the human interferon regulatory factor 1 (IRF-1) and IRF-2 genes: implications for a gene network in the interferon system. *Mol. Cell. Biol.* 14:1500–9

82. Meraz MA, White JM, Sheehan KC, Bach EA, Rodig SJ, Dighe AS, Kaplan DH, Riley JK, Greenlund AC, Campbell D, Carver-Moore K, DuBois RN, Clark R, Aguet M, Schreiber RD. 1996. Targeted disruption of the Stat1 gene in mice reveals unexpected physiologic specificity in the JAK-STAT signaling pathway. *Cell* 84:431–42

83. Durbin JE, Hackenmiller R, Simon MC, Levy DE. 1996. Targeted disruption of the mouse Stat1 gene results in compromised innate immunity to viral disease. *Cell* 84:443–50

84. Lin R, Hiscott J. 1999. A role for casein kinase II phosphorylation in the regulation of IRF-1 transcriptional activity. *Mol. Cell. Biochem.* 191:169–80

85. Lin R, Mustafa A, Nguyen H, Gewert D, Hiscott J. 1994. Mutational analysis of interferon (IFN) regulatory factors 1 and 2. Effects on the induction of IFN-β gene expression. *J. Biol. Chem.* 269:17542–49

86. Birnbaum MJ, van Zundert B, Vaughan PS, Whitmarsh AJ, van Wijnen AJ, Davis RJ, Stein GS, Stein JL. 1997. Phosphorylation of the oncogenic transcription factor interferon regulatory factor 2 (IRF2) in vitro and in vivo. *J. Cell. Biochem.* 66:175–83

87. Thanos D, Maniatis T. 1992. The high mobility group protein HMG I(Y) is required for NF-κB-dependent virus induction of the human IFN-β gene. *Cell* 71:777–89

88. Du W, Thanos D, Maniatis T. 1993. Mechanisms of transcriptional synergism between distinct virus-inducible enhancer elements. *Cell* 74:887–98

89. Merika M, Williams AJ, Chen G, Collins T, Thanos D. 1998. Recruitment of CBP/p300 by the IFNβ enhanceosome is required for synergistic activation of transcription. *Mol. Cell* 1:277–87

90. Tanaka N, Ishihara M, Lamphier MS, Nozawa H, Matsuyama T, Mak TW, Aizawa S, Tokino T, Oren M, Taniguchi T. 1996. Cooperation of the tumor suppressors IRF-1 and p53 in response to DNA damage. *Nature* 382:816–18

91. Yamamoto H, Lamphier MS, Fujita T, Taniguchi T, Harada H. 1994. he oncogenic transcription factor IRF-2 possesses a transcriptional repression and a latent activation domain. *Oncogene* 9:1423–28

92. Palombella VJ, Maniatis T. 1992. Inducible processing of interferon regulatory factor-2. *Mol. Cell. Biol.* 12:3325–36

93. Cohen L, Hiscott J. 1992. Characterization of TH3, an induction-specific protein interacting with the interferon β promoter. *Virology* 191:589–99

94. Whiteside ST, King P, Goodbourn S. 1994. A truncated form of the IRF-2 transcription factor has the properties of a postinduction repressor of interferon-β gene expression. *J. Biol. Chem.* 269:27059–65

95. Sato M, Tanaka N, Hata N, Oda E, Taniguchi T. 1998. Involvement of the IRF family transcription factor IRF-3 in virus-induced activation of the IFN-β gene. *FEBS Lett.* 425:112–116

96. Lin R, Heylbroeck C, Pitha PM, Hiscott J. 1998. Virus-dependent phosphorylation of the IRF-3 transcription factor regulates nuclear translocation, transactivation potential, and proteasome-mediated degradation. *Mol. Cell. Biol.* 18:2986–96

97. Wathelet MG, Lin CH, Parekh BS,

Ronco LV, Howley PM, Maniatis T. 1998. Virus infection induces the assembly of coordinately activated transcription factors on the IFN-β enhancer in vivo. *Mol. Cell.* 1:507–18

98. Au WC, Moore PA, LaFleur DW, Tombal B, Pitha PM. 1998. Characterization of the interferon regulatory factor-7 and its potential role in the transcription activation of interferon A genes. *J. Biol. Chem.* 273:29210–17

99. Navarro L, David M. 1999. p38-dependent activation of interferon regulatory factor 3 by lipopolysaccharide. *J. Biol. Chem.* 274:35535–38

100. Sato M, Suemori S, Hata N, Asagiri M, Ogasawara K, Nakao K, Nakaya T, Katsuki M, Noguchi S, Tanaka N, Tadatsugu Taniguchi T. 2000. Distinct and essential roles of transcription factors IRF-3 and IRF-7 in response to viruses for IFN-α/β gene induction. *Immunity* 13:539–48

101. Pongubala JM, Nagulapalli S, Klemsz MJ, McKercher SR, Maki RA, Atchison ML. 1992. PU.1 recruits a second nuclear factor to a site important for immunoglobulin κ 3' enhancer activity. *Mol. Cell. Biol.* 12:368–78

102. Eisenbeis CF, Singh H, Storb U. 1993. PU.1 is a component of a multiprotein complex which binds an essential site in the murine immunoglobulin λ_{2-4} enhancer. *Mol. Cell. Biol.* 13:6452–61

103. Himmelmann A, Riva A, Wilson GL, Lucas BP, Thevenin C, Kehrl JH. 1997. PU.1/Pip and basic helix loop helix zipper transcription factors interact with binding sites in the CD20 promoter to help confer lineage- and stage-specific expression of CD20 in B lymphocytes. *Blood* 90:3984–95

104. Pongubala JM, Van Beveren C, Nagulapalli S, Klemsz MJ, McKercher SR, Maki RA, Atchison ML. 1993. Effect of PU.1 phosphorylation on interaction with NF-EM5 and transcriptional activation. *Science* 259:1622–25

105. Brass AL, Kehrli E, Eisenbeis CF, Storb U, Singh H. 1996. Pip, a lymphoid-restricted IRF, contains a regulatory domain that is important for autoinhibition and ternary complex formation with the Ets factor PU.1. *Genes Dev.* 10:2335–47

106. Brass AL, Zhu AQ, Singh H. 1999. Assembly requirements of PU.1-Pip (IRF-4) activator complexes: inhibiting function in vivo using fused dimers. *EMBO J.* 18:977–91

107. Ray D, Bosselut R, Ghysdael J, Mattei MG, Tavitian A, Moreau-Gachelin F. 1992. Characterization of Spi-B, a transcription factor related to the putative oncoprotein Spi-1/PU.1. *Mol. Cell. Biol.* 12:4297–4304

108. Su GH, Ip HS, Cobb BS, Lu MM, Chen HM, Simon MC. 1996. The Ets protein Spi-B is expressed exclusively in B cells and T cells during development. *J. Exp. Med.* 184:203–14

109. Mamane Y, Sharma S, Petropoulos L, Lin R, Hiscott J. 2000. Posttranslational regulation of IRF-4 activity by the immunophilin FKBP52. *Immunity* 12:129–40

110. Rosenbauer F, Waring JF, Foerster J, Wietstruk M, Philipp D, Horak I. 1999. Interferon consensus sequence binding protein and interferon regulatory factor-4/Pip form a complex that represses the expression of the interferon-stimulated gene-15 in macrophages. *Blood* 94:4274–81

111. Contursi C, Wang IM, Gabriele L, Gadina M, O'Shea J, Morse HC, 3rd, Ozato K. 2000. IFN consensus sequence binding protein potentiates STAT1-dependent activation of IFNgamma-responsive promoters in macrophages. *Proc. Natl. Acad. Sci. USA* 97:91–96

112. Janeway CA, Travers P, Walport M, Capra JD. 1999. *Immunobiology: The Immune System in Health and Disease.* New York: Garland. 4th ed.

113. Ryals J, Dierks P, Ragg H, Weissmann C. 1985. A 46-nucleotide promoter segment

from an IFN-alpha gene renders an unrelated promoter inducible by virus. *Cell* 41:497–507

114. Fujita T, Ohno S, Yasumitsu H, Taniguchi T. 1985. Delimitation and properties of DNA sequences required for the regulated expression of human interferon-β gene. *Cell* 41:489–96

115. Matsuyama T, Kimura T, Kitagawa M, Pfeffer K, Kawakami T, Watanabe N, Kündig TM, Amakawa R, Kishihara K, Wakeham A, Potter J, Furlonger CL, Narendran A, Suzuki H, Ohashi PS, Paige CJ, Taniguchi T, Mak TW. 1993. Targeted disruption of IRF-1 or IRF-2 results in abnormal type I IFN gene induction and aberrant lymphocyte development. *Cell* 75:83–97

116. Reis LF, Ruffner H, Stark G, Aguet M, Weissmann C. 1994. Mice devoid of interferon regulatory factor 1 (IRF-1) show normal expression of type I interferon genes. *EMBO J.* 13:4798–4806

117. Harada H, Matsumoto M, Sato M, Kashiwazaki Y, Kimura T, Kitagawa M, Yokochi T, Tan RS, Takasugi T, Kadokawa Y, Schindler C, Schreiber RD, Noguchi S, Taniguchi T. 1996. Regulation of IFN-α/β genes: evidence for a dual function of the transcription factor complex ISGF3 in the production and action of IFN-α/β. *Genes Cells* 1:995–1005

118. Kawakami T, Matsumoto M, Sato M, Harada H, Taniguchi T, Kitagawa M. 1995. Possible involvement of the transcription factor ISGF3 gamma in virus-induced expression of the IFN-β gene. *FEBS Lett.* 358:225–29

119. Yoneyama M, Suhara W, Fukuhara Y, Sato M, Ozato K, Fujita T. 1996. Autocrine amplification of type I interferon gene expression mediated by interferon stimulated gene factor 3 (ISGF3). *J. Biochem. (Tokyo)* 120:160–69

120. Erlandsson L, Blumenthal R, Eloranta ML, Engel H, Alm G, Weiss S, Leanderson T. 1998. Interferon-β is required for interferon-alpha production in mouse fibroblasts. *Curr. Biol.* 8:223–26

121. Senger K, Merika M, Agaloti T, Tie J, Excalante CR, Chen G, Aggarwal AK, Thanos D. 2000. Gene repression by coactivator repulsion. *Mol. Cell* 6:931–37

122. Kimura T, Nakayama K, Penninger J, Kitagawa M, Harada H, Matsuyama T, Tanaka N, Kamijo R, Vilcek J, Mak TW, Taniguchi T. 1994. Involvement of the IRF-1 transcription factor in antiviral responses to interferons. *Science* 264:1921–24

123. Kimura T, Kadonaga Y, Harada H, Matsumoto M, Sato M, Kashiwazaki Y, Tarutani M, Tan RS-P, Takasugi T, Matsuyama T, Mak TW, Noguchi S, Taniguchi T. 1996. Essential and non-redundant roles of p48 (ISGF3γ) and IRF-1 in both type I and type II interferon responses, as revealed by gene targeting studies. *Genes Cells* 1:115–24

124. Trinchieri G. 1989. Biology of natural killer cells. *Adv. Immunol.* 47:187–376

125. Taki S, Sato T, Ogasawara K, Fukuda T, Sato M, Hida S, Suzuki G, Mitsuyama M, Shin EH, Kojima S, Taniguchi T, Asano Y. 1997. Multistage regulation of Th1-type immune responses by the transcription factor IRF-1. *Immunity* 6:673–79

126. Duncan GS, Mittrucker HW, Kagi D, Matsuyama T, Mak TW. 1996. The transcription factor interferon regulatory factor-1 is essential for natural killer cell function in vivo. *J. Exp. Med.* 184:2043–48

127. Ogasawara K, Hida S, Azimi N, Tagaya Y, Sato T, Yokochi-Fukuda T, Waldmann TA, Taniguchi T, Taki S. 1998. Requirement for IRF-1 in the microenvironment supporting development of natural killer cells. *Nature* 391:700–3

128. Ohteki T, Yoshida H, Matsuyama T, Duncan GS, Mak TW, Ohashi PS. 1998. The transcription factor interferon regulatory factor 1 (IRF-1) is important during the maturation of natural killer 1.1$^+$ T cell

receptor-α/β^+ (NK1$^+$ T) cells, natural killer cells, and intestinal intraepithelial T cells. *J. Exp. Med.* 187:967–72

129. Lohoff M, Duncan GS, Ferrick D, Mittrucker HW, Bischof S, Prechtl S, Rollinghoff M, Schmitt E, Pahl A, Mak TW. 2000. Deficiency in the transcription factor interferon regulatory factor (IRF)-2 leads to severely compromised development of natural killer and T helper type 1 cells. *J. Exp. Med.* 192:325–36

130. Kamijo R, Harada H, Matsuyama T, Bosland M, Gerecitano J, Shapiro D, Le J, Koh SI, Kimura T, Green SJ, Mak TW, Taniguchi T, Vlicek J. 1994. Requirement for transcription factor IRF-1 in NO synthase induction in macrophages. *Science* 263:1612–15

131. Martin E, Nathan C, Xie QW. 1994. Role of interferon regulatory factor 1 in induction of nitric oxide synthase. *J. Exp. Med.* 180:977–84

132. Lohoff M, Ferrick D, Mittrucker HW, Duncan GS, Bischof S, Rollinghoff M, Mak TW. 1997. Interferon regulatory factor-1 is required for a T helper 1 immune response *in vivo*. *Immunity* 6:681–89

133. Fehr T, Schoedon G, Odermatt B, Holtschke T, Schneemann M, Bachmann MF, Mak TW, Horak I, Zinkernagel RM. 1997. Crucial role of interferon consensus sequence binding protein, but neither of interferon regulatory factor 1 nor of nitric oxide synthesis for protection against murine listeriosis. *J. Exp. Med.* 185:921–31

134. Blanco JC, Contursi C, Salkowski CA, DeWitt DL, Ozato K, Vogel SN. 2000. Interferon regulatory factor (IRF)-1 and IRF-2 regulate interferon γ-dependent cyclooxygenase 2 expression. *J. Exp. Med.* 191:2131–44

135. White LC, Wright KL, Felix NJ, Ruffner H, Reis LFL, Pine R, Ting JP-Y. 1996. Regulation of LMP2 and TAP1 genes

by IRF-1 explains the paucity of CD8 T cells in IRF-1 mice. *Immunity* 5:247–53

136. Muhlethaler-Mottet A, Di Berardino W, Otten LA, Mach B. 1998. Activation of the MHC class II transactivator CIITA by interferon-γ requires cooperative interaction between Stat1 and USF-1. *Immunity* 8:157–66

137. Hobart M, Ramassar V, Goes N, Urmson J, Halloran PF. 1997. IFN regulatory factor-1 plays a central role in the regulation of the expression of class I and II MHC genes in vivo. *J. Immunol.* 158:4260–69

138. Nelson N, Marks MS, Driggers PH, Ozato K. 1993. Interferon consensus sequence-binding protein, a member of the interferon regulatory factor family, suppresses interferon-induced gene transcription. *Mol. Cell. Biol.* 13:588–99

139. Holtschke T, Löhler J, Kanno Y, Fehr T, Giese N, Rosenbauer F, Lou J, Knobeloch K-P, Gabriele L, Waring JF, Bachmann MF, Zinkernagel RM, Morse III HC, Ozato K, Horak I. 1996. Immunodeficiency and chronic myelogenous leukemia-like syndrome in mice with a targeted mutation of the ICSBP gene. *Cell* 87:307–17

140. Penninger JM, Sirard C, Mittrucker HW, Chidgey A, Kozieradzki I, Nghiem M, Hakem A, Kimura T, Timms E, Boyd R, Taniguchi T, Matsuyama T, Mak TW. 1997. The interferon regulatory transcription factor IRF-1 controls positive and negative selection of CD8$^+$ thymocytes. *Immunity* 7:243–54

141. Mittrücker HW, Matsuyama T, Grossman A, Kündig TM, Potter J, Shahinian A, Wakeham A, Patterson B, Ohashi PS, Mak TW. 1997. Requirement for the transcription factor LSIRF/IRF4 for mature B and T lymphocyte function. *Science* 275:540–43

142. Ihle JN. 1995. The Janus protein tyrosine

kinases in hematopoietic cytokine signaling. *Semin. Immunol.* 7:247–54

143. Naka T, Fujimoto M, Kishimoto T. 1999. Negative regulation of cytokine signaling: STAT-induced STAT inhibitor. *Trends Biochem. Sci.* 24:394–98

144. Yasukawa H, Sasaki A, Yoshimura A. 2000. Negative regulation of cytokine signaling pathways. *Annu. Rev. Immunol.* 18:143–64

145. Miyazono K. 2000. TGF-β signaling by Smad proteins. *Cytokine Growth Factor Rev.* 11:15–22

146. Coccia EM, Passini N, Battistini A, Pini C, Sinigaglia F, Rogge L. 1999. Interleukin-12 induces expression of interferon regulatory factor-1 via signal transducer and activator of transcription-4 in human T helper type 1 cells. *J. Biol. Chem.* 274:6698–6703

147. Galon J, Sudarshan C, Ito S, Finbloom D, O'Shea JJ. 1999. IL-12 induces IFN regulating factor-1 (IRF-1) gene expression in human NK and T cells. *J. Immunol.* 162:7256–62

148. Scharton-Kersten T, Contursi C, Masumi A, Sher A, Ozato K. 1997. Interferon consensus sequence binding protein-deficient mice display impaired resistance to intracellular infection due to a primary defect in interleukin 12 p40 induction. *J. Exp. Med.* 186:1523–34

149. Giese NA, Gabriele L, Doherty TM, Klinman DM, Tadesse-Heath L, Contursi C, Epstein SL, Morse HC III. 1997. Interferon (IFN) consensus sequence-binding protein, a transcription factor of the IFN regulatory factor family, regulates immune responses in vivo through control of interleukin 12 expression. *J. Exp. Med.* 186:1535–46

150. Tada Y, Ho A, Matsuyama T, Mak TW. 1997. Reduced incidence and severity of antigen-induced autoimmune diseases in mice lacking interferon regulatory factor-1. *J. Exp. Med.* 185:231–38

151. Shiraishi A, Dudler J, Lotz M. 1997. The role of IFN regulatory factor-1 in synovitis and nitric oxide production. *J. Immunol.* 159:3549–54

152. Harada H, Kitagawa M, Tanaka N, Yamamoto H, Harada K, Ishihara M, Taniguchi T. 1993. Anti-oncogenic and oncogenic potentials of interferon regulatory factors-1 and -2. *Science* 259:971–74

153. Tanaka N, Ishihara M, Kitagawa M, Harada H, Kimura T, Matsuyama T, Lamphier MS, Aizawa S, Mak TW, Taniguchi T. 1994. Cellular commitment to oncogene-induced transformation or apoptosis is dependent on the transcription factor IRF-1. *Cell* 77:829–39

154. Strasser A, Harris AW, Jacks T, Cory S. 1994. DNA damage can induce apoptosis in proliferating lymphoid cells via p53-independent mechanisms inhibitable by Bcl-2. *Cell* 79:329–39

155. Tamura T, Ishihara M, Lamphier MS, Tanaka N, Oishi I, Aizawa S, Matsuyama T, Mak TW, Taki S, Taniguchi T. 1995. An IRF-1-dependent pathway of DNA damage-induced apoptosis in mitogen-activated T lymphocytes. *Nature* 376:596–99

156. Sanceau J, Hiscott J, Delattre O, Wietzerbin J. 2000. IFN-β induces serine phosphorylation of Stat-1 in Ewing's sarcoma cells and mediates apoptosis via induction of IRF-1 and activation of caspase-7. *Oncogene* 19:3372–83

157. Tanaka N, Ishihara M, Taniguchi T. 1994. Suppression of c-*myc* or *fosB*-induced cell transformation by the transcription factor IRF-1. *Cancer Lett.* 83:191–96

158. Weinberg RA. 1985. The action of oncogenes in the cytoplasm and nucleus. *Science* 230:770–76

159. Weinberg RA. 1989. Oncogenes, antioncogenes, and the molecular basis of multistep carcinogenesis. *Cancer Res.* 49:3713–21

160. Nozawa H, Oda E, Nakao K, Ishihara M, Ueda S, Yokochi T, Ogasawara K, Nakatsuru Y, Shimizu S, Ohira Y, Hioki K,

Aizawa S, Ishikawa T, Katsuki M, Muto T, Taniguchi T, Tanaka N. 1999. Loss of transcription factor IRF-1 affects tumor susceptibility in mice carrying the Ha-*ras* transgene or nullizygosity for *p53*. *Genes Dev.* 13:1240–45

161. Tan RS, Taniguchi T, Harada H. 1996. Identification of the *lysyl oxidase* gene as target of the antioncogenic transcription factor, IRF-1, and its possible role in tumor suppression. *Cancer Res.* 56:2417–21

162. Contente S, Kenyon K, Rimoldi D, Friedman RM. 1990. Expression of gene rrg is associated with reversion of NIH 3T3 transformed by LTR-c-H-*ras*. *Science* 249:796–98

163. Kenyon K, Contente S, Trackman PC, Tang J, Kagan HM, Friedman RM. 1991. Lysyl oxidase and rrg messenger RNA. *Science* 253:802

164. Itoh S, Harada H, Nakamura Y, White R, Taniguchi T. 1991. Assignment of the human interferon regulatory factor-1 (IRF1) gene to chromosome 5q23-q31. *Genomics* 10:1097–99

165. Willman CL, Sever CE, Pallavicini MG, Harada H, Tanaka N, Slovak ML, Yamamoto H, Harada K, Meeker TC, List AF, Taniguchi T. 1993. Deletion of *IRF-1*, mapping to chromosome 5q31.1, in human leukemia and preleukemic myelodysplasia. *Science* 259:968–71

166. Van den Berghe H, Vermaelen K, Mecucci C, Barbieri D, Tricot G. 1985. The 5q-anomaly. *Cancer Genet. Cytogenet.* 17:189–255

167. Boultwood J, Fidler C, Lewis S, MacCarthy A, Sheridan H, Kelly S, Oscier D, Buckle VJ, Wainscoat JS. 1993. Allelic loss of IRF1 in myelodysplasia and acute myeloid leukemia: retention of IRF1 on the 5q- chromosome in some patients with the 5q- syndrome. *Blood* 82:2611–16

168. Ogasawara S, Tamura G, Maesawa C, Suzuki Y, Ishida K, Satoh N, Uesugi

N, Saito K, Satodate R. 1996. Common deleted region on the long arm of chromosome 5 in esophageal carcinoma. *Gastroenterology* 110:52–57

169. Tamura G, Ogasawara S, Nishizuka S, Sakata K, Maesawa C, Suzuki Y, Terashima M, Saito K, Satodate R. 1996. Two distinct regions of deletion on the long arm of chromosome 5 in differentiated adenocarcinomas of the stomach. *Cancer Res.* 56:612–15

170. Nozawa H, Oda E, Ueda S, Tamura G, Maesawa C, Muto T, Taniguchi T, Tanaka N. 1998. Functionally inactivating point mutation in the tumor-suppressor IRF-1 gene identified in human gastric cancer. *Int. J. Cancer* 77:522–27

171. Kondo T, Minamino N, Nagamura-Inoue T, Matsumoto M, Taniguchi T, Tanaka N. 1997. Identification and characterization of nucleophosmin/B23/numatrin which binds the anti-oncogenic transcription factor IRF-1 and manifests oncogenic activity. *Oncogene* 15:1275–81

172. Harada H, Kondo T, Ogawa S, Tamura T, Kitagawa M, Tanaka N, Lamphier MS, Hirai H, Taniguchi T. 1994. Accelerated exon skipping of IRF-1 mRNA in human myelodysplasia/leukemia; a possible mechanism of tumor suppressor inactivation. *Oncogene* 9:3313–20

173. Mayeda A, Helfman DM, Krainer AR. 1993. Modulation of exon skipping and inclusion by heterogeneous nuclear ribonucleoprotein A1 and pre-mRNA splicing factor SF2/ASF. *Mol. Cell. Biol.* 13:2993–3001

174. Hao SX, Ren R. 2000. Expression of interferon consensus sequence binding protein (ICSBP) is downregulated in Bcr-Abl-induced murine chronic myelogenous leukemia-like disease, and forced coexpression of ICSBP inhibits Bcr-Abl-induced myeloproliferative disorder. *Mol. Cell. Biol.* 20:1149–61

174a. Park JS, Kim EJ, Kwon HJ, Hwang ES, Namkoong SE, Um SE. 2000. Inactivation of interferon regulatory factor-1 tumor suppressor protein by HPV E7 oncoprotein. Implication for the E7-mediated immune evasion mechanism in cervical carcinogenesis. *J. Biol. Chem.* 275:6764–69

175. Schmidt M, Nagel S, Proba J, Thiede C, Ritter M, Waring JF, Rosenbauer F, Huhn D, Wittig B, Horak I, Neubauer A. 1998. Lack of interferon consensus sequence binding protein (ICSBP) transcripts in human myeloid leukemias. *Blood* 91:22–29

176. Nguyen H, Mustafa A, Hiscott J, Lin R. 1995. Transcription factor IRF-2 exerts its oncogenic phenotype through the DNA binding/transcription repression domain. *Oncogene* 11:537–44

177. Vaughan PS, van der Meijden CM, Aziz F, Harada H, Taniguchi T, van Wijnen AJ, Stein JL, Stein GS. 1998. Cell cycle regulation of histone H4 gene transcription requires the oncogenic factor IRF-2. *J. Biol. Chem.* 273:194–99

178. Iida S, Rao PH, Butler M, Corradini P, Boccadoro M, Klein B, Chaganti RS, Dalla-Favera R. 1997. Deregulation of MUM1/IRF4 by chromosomal translocation in multiple myeloma. *Nat. Genet.* 17:226–30

179. Saito T, Yamagata T, Takahashi T, Honda H, Hirai H. 1999. ICSAT overexpression is not sufficient to cause adult T-cell leukemia or multiple myeloma. *Biochem. Biophys. Res. Commun.* 260:329–31

180. Felsher DW, Bishop JM. 1999. Reversible tumorigenesis by MYC in hematopoietic lineages. *Mol. Cell.* 4:199–207

181. Moore PS, Chang Y. 1998. Antiviral activity of tumor-suppressor pathways: clues from molecular piracy by KSHV. *Trends Genet.* 14:144–50

182. Matikainen S, Ronni T, Lehtonen A, Sareneva T, Melen K, Nordling S, Levy DE, Julkunen I. 1997. Retinoic acid induces signal transducer and activator of transcription (STAT) 1, STAT2, and p48 expression in myeloid leukemia cells and enhances their responsiveness to interferons. *Cell Growth Differ.* 8: 687–98

183. Weihua X, Lindner DJ, Kalvakolanu DV. 1997. The interferon-inducible murine p48 (ISGF3γ) gene is regulated by protooncogene c-myc. *Proc. Natl. Acad. Sci. USA* 94:7227–32

184. Ronco LV, Karpova AY, Vidal M, Howley PM. 1998. Human papillomavirus 16 E6 oncoprotein binds to interferon regulatory factor-3 and inhibits its transcriptional activity. *Genes Dev.* 12:2061–72

185. Kim T, Kim TY, Song YH, Min IM, Yim J, Kim TK. 1999. Activation of interferon regulatory factor 3 in response to DNA-damaging agents. *J. Biol. Chem.* 274:30686–89

186. Vaughan PS, van Wijnen AJ, Stein JL, Stein GS. 1997. Interferon regulatory factors: growth control and histone gene regulation—it's not just interferon anymore. *J. Mol. Med.* 75:348–59

187. Lin R, Heylbroeck C, Genin P, Pitha PM, Hiscott J. 1999. Essential role of interferon regulatory factor 3 in direct activation of RANTES chemokine transcription. *Mol. Cell. Biol.* 19:959–66

188. Heylbroeck C, Balachandran S, Servant MJ, DeLuca C, Barber GN, Lin R, Hiscott J. 2000. The IRF-3 transcription factor mediates Sendai virus-induced apoptosis. *J. Virol.* 74:3781–92

189. Veals SA, Santa Maria T, Levy DE. 1993. Two domains of ISGF3γ that mediate protein-DNA and protein-protein interactions during transcription factor assembly contribute to DNA-binding specificity. *Mol. Cell. Biol.* 13:196–206

Annu. Rev. Immunol. 2001. 19:657–82

X-Linked Lymphoproliferative Disease: A Progressive Immunodeficiency

Massimo Morra, Duncan Howie, Maria Simarro Grande, Joan Sayos, Ninghai Wang, Chengbin Wu, Pablo Engel* and Cox Terhorst

Division of Immunology, RE-204, Beth Israel Deaconess Medical Center, Harvard Medical School, 330 Brookline Ave, Boston, Massachusetts 02215; e-mail: terhorst@caregroup.harvard.edu
*Immunology Unit, Department of Cellular Biology and Pathology, ID1B APS, Medical School, University of Barcelona, Spain

Key Words XLP, SAP/SH2D1A, SLAM, EBV, lymphocyte

■ **Abstract** Our understanding of the X-linked lymphoproliferative syndrome (XLP) has advanced significantly in the last two years. The gene that is altered in the condition (SAP/SH2D1A) has been cloned and its protein crystal structure solved. At least two sets of target molecules for this small SH2 domain-containing protein have been identified: A family of hematopoietic cell surface receptors, i.e. the SLAM family, and a second molecule, which is a phosphorylated adapter. A SAP-like protein, EAT-2, has also been found to interact with this family of surface receptors. Several lines of evidence, including structural studies and analyses of missense mutations in XLP patients, support the notion that SAP/SH2D1A is a natural inhibitor of SH2-domain-dependent interactions with members of the SLAM family. However, details of its role in signaling mechanisms are yet to be unravelled. Further analyses of the SAP/SH2D1A gene in XLP patients have made it clear that the development of dysgammaglobulinemia and B cell lymphoma can occur without evidence of prior EBV infection. Moreover, preliminary results of virus infections of a mouse in which the SAP/SH2D1A gene has been disrupted suggest that EBV infection is not per se critical for the development of XLP phenotypes. It appears therefore that the SAP/SH2D1A gene controls signaling via the SLAM family of surface receptors and thus may play a fundamental role in T cell and APC interactions during viral infections.

INTRODUCTION

A familial disorder affecting males with a rapidly fatal course in response to Epstein-Barr virus (EBV) infection was first reported by David Purtilo more than 25 years ago (1). Six male maternal cousins out of 18, who were born in one generation, died of fulminant infectious mononucleosis, while none of their sisters were

0732-0582/01/0407-0657$14.00

657

affected. The disease was characterized by proliferation of lymphocytes and histiocytes, variable hepatic abnormalities and alterations in serum immunoglobulins ranging from agammaglobulinemia to polyclonal hypergammaglobulinemia. Two of the cousins, who were half-brothers from separate fathers, had lymphomas of the ileum and central nervous system. The disease was initially called X-linked recessive progressive combined variable immunodeficiency, or Duncan's disease after the family's name. Subsequently, the possibility of a lymphoproliferative disorder was entertained, and it was speculated that a cytotoxic effect of EBV on B-cells or an abnormal T cell response to transformation of B-cells by EBV might lead to B-cell dysfunction and agammaglobulinemia. In the ensuing years the disease syndrome became known as X-linked lymphoproliferative disease (XLP) (2, 3).

XLP is clinically characterized by three major phenotypes: fulminant infectious mononucleosis (FIM) (50%), B cell lymphomas (20%), or dys-gammaglobulinemia (30%) (2, 4). Additionally, aplastic anemia, vasculitis, and pulmonary lymphomatoid granulomatosis are often associated with the syndrome. The majority of the malignant lymphomas are extra-nodal non-Hodgkin lymphomas, usually of the Burkitt type, and most involve the ileocaecal region of the intestine. Uncontrolled lymphocyte proliferation, organ infiltration, and T cell cytotoxic activity lead to multiorgan failure: hepatic necrosis and bone marrow failure constitute the most common events that determine death in these patients. XLP mortality is 100% by the age of 40. An XLP registry was established in 1978 and has approximately 300 patients registered from over 80 families (2).

EPSTEIN-BARR VIRUS AND XLP

Although EBV is carried by a vast majority of individuals, the percentage of individuals who develop clinical evidence of infectious mononucleosis is remarkably low. Similarly, the percentage is small of immunosuppressed individuals (transplant patients or AIDS patients) who develop immunoproliferative diseases that may turn into monoclonal lymphoma or a malignant tumor of the lymph nodes. This is most likely due to a finely tuned equilibrium between the regulation of viral gene expression and the immune system, in particular T cell responses (5–7). T cell responses to EBV are thought to be dominated by primary and memory CTL responses directed toward MHC/peptide complexes derived from the EBNA3A, 3B, and 3C latent proteins. Responses to other latent proteins (EBNA1, 2, -LP and LMP1, 2) and to lytic cycle proteins are not dominant and therefore less well studied (8, 9).

In spite of the potential immune responses against EBV-infected cells, during infectious mononucleosis the CTL responses may last from two to three months before the number of B cell blasts has been reduced to a manageable size (10). This may be because of the daunting task for CTLs to control as many as 10% of all B cells in the human body. Whereas the XLP gene is affected in fulminant infectious mononucleosis (FIM), there is no indication that a genetic predisposition exists for infectious mononucleosis itself.

Studies of the immune-responses in XLP patients with FIM suggest that abnormal T and B cell proliferation occurs in response to EBV-induced lymphoblasts (11, 12). This impressive polyclonal T cell and B cell proliferation infiltrates many organs, leading to fulminant hepatitis and bone marrow failure with a hemophagocytic component.

The cellular mechanisms that lead to the B cell expansion are not understood. The B lymphocytes of XLP males do not appear to be resistant to T cell–mediated immunity. XLP-derived EBV-transformed B cells resemble normal lymphoblastoid cell lines (LCLs) with respect to induction of EBV-specific cytotoxic T cells, the ability to present EBV antigens, and the susceptibility to MHC-restricted, CTL-mediated lysis. Thus, the failure to eliminate EBV-transformed B cells in XLP does not seemed to be caused by a B cell–specific defect (13).

Variable defects in both T and NK cells have been reported (11). In some cases NK cell numbers are low, and in other patients have normal numbers of NK cells but have lost the ability to lyse the appropriate target cells (14–16; and A Etzioni, personal communication). Although dysgammaglobinemia and B cell lymphomas have been detected after an EBV infection, a causal relationship between the virus and these XLP phenotypes has not been established. Immunoglobulin deficiencies and B cell non-Hodgkin's lymphomas have now been observed in XLP patients who were sero- and/or PCR-negative for EBV (R Sorensen, personal communication) (17–19). Because XLP diagnosis is at times difficult, the role of EBV can only be assessed with more certainty now that the XLP gene has been identified. The development of dysgammaglobulinemia and lymphoma without evidence of prior EBV infection has made it clear that SAP/SH2D1A, the gene that is altered in XLP, has a more fundamental role in T/B cell homeostasis.

THE XLP GENE

In 1998, two groups independently reported the cloning of the gene responsible for the XLP disease. Identification of the gene stemmed from two different approaches, namely a classical positional cloning effort and an indirect approach.

Coffey et al (20) employed a multistep positional cloning strategy starting with the construction of a YAC contig based upon a patient (IARC739) whose X-chromosome lacked two thirds of Xq25, in addition to two other patients with deletions (21–25). A specific marker (DXS739) was found absent in all three deletions (26). Information from YAC and bacterial contigs was then integrated in a physical map of approximately 3 Mb located between DXS6791 and DXS100, 2.3 Mb of which were sequenced. With sequence analysis and exon-trapping, only four genes could be identified within the DNA segment. Two genes were immediately excluded because they were located outside of the deleted Xq25 region of the referral patient (21), while Tenascin-M (TNM) and an SH2-domain containing gene, termed SH2D1A, were entirely within the region. Full-length coding cDNAs and exon-intron boundary sequences were obtained for both genes.

Subsequently, the SH2D1A gene was proven to be responsible for XLP by analysis of 16 unrelated XLP patients. Mutations interfering with transcription or translation were found in nine of these patients. No sequence alterations were detected in any of the samples derived from healthy individuals. Consequently, the SH2D1A gene was identified as the gene altered in XLP.

Sayos et al (27) cloned the XLP gene serendipitously, while focusing their studies on the characterization of biochemical pathways induced by engagement of a recently identified lymphocyte cell surface co-receptor termed SLAM (signaling lymphocytic-activation molecule) (28). A cDNA encoding a novel SLAM-associated protein (SAP) was isolated in a yeast two-hybrid system by virtue of its specific binding to the cytoplasmic tail of SLAM. SAP, identical to SH2D1A, is a 128-amino acid protein consisting of an SH2 domain and a 24-amino acid tail (Figure 1, see color insert). Since the protein was primarily expressed in T lymphocytes and also bound to SLAM with high selectivity, mouse genomic SAP was isolated to facilitate in-depth functional analyses. A BAC clone, which contained all four exons of mouse SAP, was mapped within band A5.1 of the murine X chromosome. Synteny between this mouse chromosome region and the human Xq25 locus prompted an analysis of the integrity of the SAP gene in XLP patients. Moreover, as the major clinical phenotype of XLP is uncontrolled B and T lymphoproliferation and dysglobulinemia, and because SAP binds to a glycoprotein SLAM that functions on the interface of T and B lymphocytes, the possibility that SAP was the product of the XLP gene was appealing. Next, two brothers in an XLP family were found to have a deleted SAP gene, whereas the gene was present in a healthy sibling (27). A third patient with clinical features that were consistent with XLP, had a CG mutation in the intron sequence adjacent to the exon 2 splice acceptor site, a substitution that leads to a partial skipping of exon 2. The possibility that this nucleotide alteration represented a genetic polymorphism was excluded by the analysis of 108 healthy individuals, definitively proving the involvement of SAP in XLP pathogenesis. We thus refer to the XLP gene as the SAP/SH2D1A gene and to its product as SAP.

Organization and Regulation of Expression of SAP/SH2D1A

Human and mouse SAP/SH2D1A consist of four exons and three introns spanning approximately 25 kb (20, 29). As indicated in Figure 1, the SH2 domain of SAP is encoded by the first three exons, whereas exon 4 encodes part of the tail sequence and all of the 3'UT (20, 29). Sequences immediately upstream of exon 1 include putative binding sites for transcription factors that are important for T lymphocyte development and function, and these include multiple GR (glucocorticoid receptor) binding sites, c-Ets-1, and IRF-1 (20, 29). Human SAP/SH2D1A is highly homologous to monkey and murine SAP (Figure 1).

Northern blotting experiments and isolated cDNAs show that human SAP/SH2D1A exists as two RNA species of 2.5 kb and 0.9 kb (27). SAP/SH2D1A is highly expressed in the thymus: at a low level in double-negative thymocytes and at a high level in double-positive thymocytes. Expression is moderately high in single-positive thymocytes, with a slightly higher level in $CD8^+$ cells than in $CD4^+$ cells (29). In the peripheral compartment, SAP/SH2D1A is expressed in T cells, including $CD8^+$, $CD4^+$ single-positive T cells (27, 29). Its expression is prevalent in Th1 cells, but Th2 cells also contain the transcript (29).

Interestingly, SAP expression is downregulated upon anti-CD3 stimulation of both $CD4^+$ and $CD8^+$ single positive T cells, whereas SLAM expression is markedly augmented upon activation (29). A similar observation has been made with antigen-specific mouse Th1 cells (29) and in human T cells using cytoplasmic staining with a monoclonal antibody (D Howie, unpublished). The rapid down-regulation is the result of the presence of AUUUA in the $3'$UT region of both the long and the short mRNA species (29). The importance of this finding is that the variable ratio between SAP/SLAM in different stages of activation may have a functional role in this pathway's regulation.

Mouse SAP/SH2D1A mRNA was found at low levels in resting NK cells, but increases upon infection with MCMV or LCMV. Kinetics of SAP expression in cultured murine NK cells differed from that in T lymphocytes because SAP expression increased upon activation in the presence of IL-2 (29a). Taken together, the expression data are consistent with the notion that SAP is a highly regulated gene and that it acts predominantly in T cells and NK cells. The latter observation is relevant to the disease because some XLP patients have an impaired NK cell function (11, 15, 16). Whether SAP is expressed in a subset of normal B cells remains uncertain. Significantly, the gene is not expressed in EBV transformed lymphoblastoid cell lines, and only a small number of B cell tumors express SAP/SH21DA (30, 27, 31). Although its presence in human lymph nodes has been reported (31; E Clark, personal communication), SAP was not found in the B cells isolated from mutant mice that lack T cells and NK cells (tgε26) (C Gullo, unpublished).

SAP/SH2D1A in XLP Patients

Different SAP/SH2D1A mutations have been identified in XLP patients (19, 20, 27, 32, 33): (*a*) micro/macro-deletions; (*b*) mutations interfering with mRNA transcription or splicing; (*c*) nonsense or missense mutations leading to premature stop codons or amino acid substitutions. No correlation between mutation and clinical phenotype has been found for this disease. Identical mutations manifest different phenotypes within the same family (20, 27, 31, 32), and no significant differences are detectable in phenotypes or severity of the disease based on type (deletion, truncation, missense) or location of mutations (32).

The percentage of patients originally diagnosed with the XLP syndrome that have a mutation in SAP/SH2D1A is relatively low (50%–60%) (20, 27, 31). The possibility of a mutation in an undetected critical *cis*-regulatory element distal from the gene or in one of the introns cannot be excluded. In a large study by Sumegi et al (32) of 35 individuals with two or more maternally related male family members that manifest an XLP phenotype, 34 had a mutation in SAP/SH2D1A. By contrast, no mutations were found in 25 males with sporadic XLP (32). In our own studies 11/11 patients had a SAP/SH2D1A mutation in 5 families that were analyzed. However, no SAP/SH2D1A mutations were found in patients with an XLP-like syndrome but without family history. Therefore, a positive familiar history is key in determining whether SAP is altered in patients with a clinical presentation compatible with XLP.

As discussed previously, patients with XLP clinically present with a variable combination of at least three major phenotypes (2, 4). Sometimes the XLP presentation is totally polarized toward a clinical situation as variable degrees of immunoglobulin deficiencies associated with chronic respiratory infections. Therefore, some XLP patients may clinically resemble CVID (common variable immuno deficiency), in a clinical heterogeneous syndrome that recognizes a multifactorial/multigene origin (34). Indeed, two groups found mutations in the SAP/SH2D1A gene in some patients previously reported as CVID (M Morra, unpublished) (36).

SAP/SH2D1A AND EAT-2 ARE MEMBERS
OF A GENE FAMILY

The mouse and human EAT-2 genes encode a 132-amino acid protein that, like SAP, consists of a single SH2 domain followed by a short C-terminal sequence (Figure 1) (Human EAT-2 GenBank Accession Number: AF256653) (37). Like SAP/SH2D1A, the human EAT-2 gene consists of four exons that are distributed in the same pattern as the SAP exons (M Morra, Poy F, Martin M, Sayos J, Gullo C, Thompson AD, Denny C, Jaffe M, Engel P, Eck M, Terhorst C, submitted). Human EAT-2 is located on the long arm of chromosome1 (1q23) approximately 700 kb from the SLAM gene (37; Wang N, Morra M, Wu C, Engel P, Howie D, Terhorst C submitted).

The mouse EAT-2 gene was first identified as a transcript induced by transformation of NIH3T3 mouse fibroblasts by the EWS/FLI1 oncogene (37). A 1.5-kb long mouse EAT-2 transcript is detected in murine spleen and lung. And a 1.2 kb transcript is found in liver, skeletal muscle, and kidney (37). Using PCR and cell separation techniques starting with spleens from immunodeficient mice, we found that mouse EAT-2 is expressed in macrophages and B cells but not in thymus-derived lymphocytes (M Morra et al, submitted).

Thus, it appears that the SAP/SH2D1A and EAT-2 genes represent the first two identified members of a new family of genes, which are expressed in different tissues. It is conceivable that similar genes exist that play a role in regulating signal transduction in different cell types.

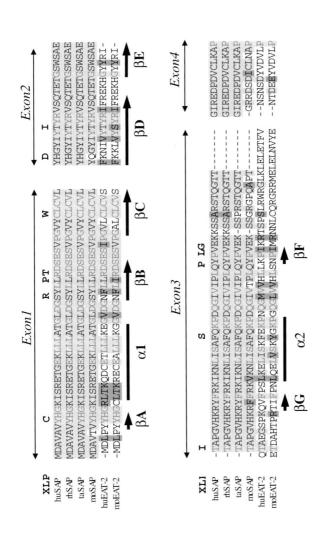

Figure 1 Amino acid sequences of members of the SAP family.

Blocks of colors indicate different levels of similarity or identity among the different proteins according to Vector NTI analysis (Yellow areas = residues' identity; Green areas = blocks of similarity; Blue areas = conserved positions). The highest degree of similarity is observed for the first three exons that encode the SH2 domain. The borders between each of the four exons are indicated by introduction of spaces between them. Elements of secondary structure based on the crystal structure are indicated at the bottom. In the top row amino acid residue substitutions found in XLP patients are indicated.

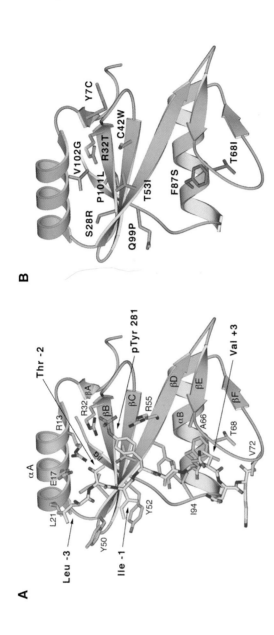

Figure 2 Crystal structure of SAP and location of missense mutations identified in XLP patients.

(*A*) Ribbon diagram showing the SAP/SLAM pY281 peptide complex. The phospho-peptide is shown in a stick representation (yellow). Selected SAP residues that form the binding site are shown in blue.

(*B*) Point mutations identified in XLP patients cluster along the peptide binding site and at the back of the SH2 domain. Residue's colors identify different classes of mutations according to crystal structure predictions (green = disruption of phosphotyrosine binding pocket; magenta = disruption of C-terminal interactions; gold = possible structure destabilization).

(Reproduced with permission from Poy et al, 1999, Mol. Cell 4: 555-61).

```
hu-SLAM    -MDPKGLLSIIFVLFL LAFGAS GTGGRM NCPKIL QLGSKVLLPLTYERINKSMN SIHIVV MAKSLE SVENKI SLDPSEAG
hu-2B4     ------ML QVVTLILLLKV QGKGCQ SADHVV VLSGVPL LQPNS------IQ KVDSIA KKLLPS NGFHHIIKWE-NG L
hu-Ly-9    ICTAQNPVSQ SSLPVH GQFCTD GASRGG TGETVV VLGEPV LPIALP----AC DTEKVV LFNTSLISKEREEATADPLIK
hu-CD84    -------MA HHIWILILCIQTW EAAGKD EIFTVN IIGESV FPVNIQ-----EP QVKIIA TSKISVAYVTPGD ETAPVV V
hu-19A     -------MA SPTCLTIYLWQLIGSAAS PVKELV SVGGAV FPLKS-----KV QVDSIV TFNTPLVIIQ-- EGG-TIIV
hu-BCM1-L  ------MVMRPIWSLIIW ALLPIT TGACVL KVGGSVLIVAARP-----PG QVREAI RSLWPS ELLATF RGSLETLY
hu-CD48    ---MCSRGW SCLALEILLPLSLLVTSIQ HLVHMT VSGSNV LNISES-----LP NYKQLT FYTFDQ NEWDS KSK----Y


hu-SLAM    PPRYLGDRYK YLENLTLGIRESR EDEGWIMTLEKN S--VQR CLQLRLVEQVSTP IKVLNK QENG---TCTLILGCTVEK -
hu-2B4     PSNISNDRFS IVKNLSLLIKAAQ QDSGLY LEVTSI G-KVQTATFGVFEDKVEKP LQGQGKILDRG---RCQVALSCLVSR-D
hu-Ly-9    SRDFYKNRVW SSQDCSLKISQIKTEAGPY AYVCSEASSVISM HVTLLIVRRLRKP ITWSLR SEDG---ICRISLTCSVED G
hu-CD84    THRNYERIHALGPNVNLVISDLR EDAGDY ADINTQADPYTTT RYNLQIYRRLGKP ITQSLMASVNS---TCNVTLTCSVEK E
hu-19A     TQNRNREVD PDGGYSLKLSKIK NSGIY VGTYSS LQQPST EXVLHVEHLSKP VTLGLQ NKNG---TCVTNLTCCMEH E
hu-BCM1-L  HSR LGR--A LHSNLSLELGPLE GDSGNF VLMVDT GQ-PWT TLQLKV DAVPRP VQUFIA ERDACP KTCQVFLSCWAPN-I
hu-CD48    FES FKGRVRLDPQSGA YISKVQ EDNSTYIMRVLKK G-NEQE KIKLQVLDPVRKP IKIEKI DMDDN---CYLKLSCVIPG--


hu-SLAM    DHVAYSNS A ---- L A S LLSL L A I I S ISN-NSCTFS                          S
hu-2B4     GNVSYANYRG ------KLIQTA NLTYLD EVDING HTYTCN SNPVSW-ESHTINLTQDCQNAHQEFRF ----
hu-Ly-9    NTVMAWT L ----- A S SL SS L AS SR-SSHQFL I S
hu-CD84    KNVTYNWSPL ------ IFQT--PEDQ LTYTCTAQNPVSN-NSDSISARQLCADIAMGFRT HTG---
hu-19A     EDVIYTWKAL ------ AANESH GSILPI WRWGES MTFICVARNPVSRNFSSPILARKLCEGAADDPDS M-----
hu-BCM1-L  SETTYSNR              SL          LSI L A S I S SW-DLATVT S AA A ----
hu-CD48    ESVNYTNYGD R------PFFPKEL NSVLET LMPHNY RCYTCQ SNSVSS-KNGTVCLSPCTLARSFGVE IASWLV TVPTIL L
```

Figure 4 (*A*) Alignment of the amino acid sequences of the extracellular domains of the SLAM family members. Blocks of colors indicate different levels of similarity or identity among the different genes according to Vector NTI analysis (Yellow areas = residues' identity; Green areas = blocks of similarity; Blue areas = conserved positions). Yellow vertical lanes identify extremely conserved residues of critical function in the architecture of the Immunoglobulin-like domains. The sequence of the human Ly-9 protein was aligned starting by position 190.

SAP IS A NATURAL INHIBITOR OF SH2 DOMAIN DEPENDENT INTERACTIONS

Based on its structure comprising an SH2 domain with a short N-terminal tail and its known properties, SAP has been postulated to be a natural blocker of events involving its binding site (27). It is also conceivable that SAP is an adapter if a second protein could bind specifically to its tail. Whereas no evidence exists for an adapter function, the notion of SAP as a blocking molecule has found considerable support from biochemical assay, physico-chemical studies, and analysis of SAP mutations found in XLP patients.

Details of the SAP/SLAM Interaction

Because the SAP/SLAM interaction involves a free SH2 domain and because it was discovered in yeast in which no phosphotyrosine residues are found, the contact area between the two proteins was investigated in greater detail. SAP (and not its tail) bound to a 14 amino acid peptide in the proximity of Y281 cytoplasmic tail of SLAM in the absence of phosphorylation (27). Further studies indicated that amino acids N- and C-terminal to the Y281 are important for stabilizing the in vitro interaction. In vivo, in transiently transfected COS-7 cells or in T lymphocytes, SAP bound to the cytoplasmic tail of SLAM without detectable phosphorylation (27). Importantly, a mutation in R32 of the SAP molecule eliminated the binding of SAP to the non-phospho SLAM. SAP binds to a second sequence motif in the cytoplasmic tail of SLAM, Y327, in a phosphotyrosine-dependent manner (D Howie, Terhorst C, manuscript in preparation).

The SAP Crystal Stucture

SAP has the overall characteristics of an SH2 domain fold, which includes a central sheet with helices packed against either side (Figure 2, see color insert) (38). The uniqueness of the SAP/SLAM binding lies in the fact that, in addition to the classical "two-pronged" interaction between an SH2 domain and its ligand peptide, a third contact point is formed (38–40). Specific features include

1. Phosphorylated and nonphosphorylated SLAM Y281 peptides bind in the same manner in a pocket of the central β sheet. The pY281 coordinates a set of hydrogen bonds with residues R32, S34, E35, S36, and R55 in a manner similar to that observed in the N-terminal SH2 domain of SHP-2. In spite of its nonphosphorylated state, the hydroxyl group of Y281 organizes an extensive network of hydrogen bonds;

2. Val +3 is buried in a mostly hydrophobic cleft, similar to other SH2 domain interactions (38, 39);

3. A third interaction involves three residues N terminal to Y281. The SLAM N-terminal residues at positions pY-1, and pY-3 intercalate with

hydrophobic residues in β strand D of the SAP SH2 domain. Of particular interest, however, is Thr-2 (Thr 279 of SLAM), which hydrogen bonds with Glu 17 and a buried water molecule that also involves R32.

These N-terminal interactions provide the additional binding energy that explains the extremely high affinity of the SAP/SLAM binding as judged by fluorescence polarization (38). Detailed peptide binding studies confirmed the important contributions of the amino acids N and C terminal to the pY281.

The three pronged interaction between SAP and the SLAM peptide predicted that the affinity would be highest in the case of the binding to the phosphorylated form of SLAM. Indeed, fluorescence polarization studies support that view. A binding constant of 600–700 nM for SAP with the nonphosphorylated SLAM Y281 peptide and 180 nM for SAP with the pY281 peptide (38; M Morra, submitted). These values indicate a high affinity of SAP for its binding site compared with other SH2 domains and their peptide motifs (41). The high-affinity interactions of the Src SH2 domain and the p85N SH2 domain with their optimal peptides are recognized with dissociation constants in the order of 500 nM (41). Thus, the high affinity between SAP and phospho-SLAM strongly supports the idea that SAP functions as a blocker of recruitment of signal transduction molecules to the Y281 site in the cytoplasmic tail of SLAM.

SAP Blocks Recruitment of SHP-2 to the Cytoplasmic Tail of SLAM

Because the protein tyrosine phosphatase SHP-2 had been shown to bind tyrosine-phosphorylated SLAM in the absence of SAP, the blocking hypothesis could be tested. Indeed, in COS-7 cells SAP completely blocks binding of SHP-2 to phospho-SLAM (27). Although this provided formal proof for the concept of SAP as a natural blocker, the number of molecules that bind to this site is as yet unclear. Nevertheless, the experiments suggest that two states of SLAM signal transduction exist: one with SAP and another without SAP. This is plausible because of the downregulation of expression of the SAP gene in the early phases of T cell activation followed by a re-expression late in T cell activation.

Maximum levels of catalysis by the SHP-2 phosphatase (PTPase) are dependent upon occupation of both of its SH2 domains (42) because regulation of SHP-2 is controlled by the N-terminal SH2 domain (43–45). Either it binds to the PTPase domain and blocks its active site or it binds a phosphotyrosine residue (46–48). The C-terminal SH2 domain, although not directly involved in this regulation, contributes affinity and specificity to the target interaction. SHP-2 binds to pY281 and pY327 of the SLAM cytoplasmic tail, the same site that SAP binds. Because of its high affinity, SAP will block recruitment of SHP-2 completely, provided a sufficient number of SAP molecules are present. If not, blocking by SAP of one of the sites might only recruit an inactive or less active enzyme.

It is conceivable that although SLAM binds SHP-2, it itself is not a substrate of the PTPase. Thus, SLAM may provide a scaffold for SHP-2 to act at the immune synapse, where multiple targets such as TCR, Fyn, Lck, and ZAP-70 are phosphorylated immediately following TCR engagement (49–51). In this fashion, by blocking PTPase recruitment, SAP could function indirectly to prolong phosphorylation of important substrates during TCR triggering.

Further Analysis of SAP Mutations in XLP Patients Provides Support for the Natural Inhibitor Model

Eleven missense mutations identified in XLP families were analyzed in vitro and in vivo. (M Morra, Simarro Grande M, Chen A, Lanyi A, Sayos J, Silander O, Sumegi J, Eck M, Pawson T, Li SC, Terhorst C, submitted) These studies further support the model of SAP as a natural blocker rather than as a signal amplifying adapter molecule. The missense mutations that are distributed throughout the three dimensional structure of SAP (Figure 1 and 2b, see color insert) (38; M Morra et al, submitted) fall under three categories:

1. Instability of the protein as judged by a substantially decreased half-life (*e.g.* mutants Y7C, S28R, Q99P, P101L, V102G and Stop codon129 R (M Morra et al, submitted);

2. Disruption of the specific interactions with both phosphorylated and nonphosphorylated SLAM forms. R32Q, C42W affect interactions with the classical phosphotyrosine binding pocket as well as with the threonine residue in the −2 position of the SLAM Y281 motif. T68I disrupts the binding of V284 to the hydrophobic cleft. Thus, binding to both phospho- and nonphospho SLAM is affected;

3. in mutant T53I only the nonphospho interaction appears to be disrupted (M Morra et al, submitted).

The notion that limited amounts of a wild-type protein may lead to the pathogenesis of a fatal disease is particularly remarkable. The mutant proteins in category 1 are all in principle capable of binding to the SLAM motif via a three-pronged interaction. The type 1 mutations are functionally similar to those with partial transcriptional defect, an example of which is the patient with a mutation in the second exon's splice acceptor area in intron 1 (27). This XLP patient still produces 5%–10% of wild-type SAP protein (27). The mutation of the stop codon (129R) suggested at first that the SAP tail might have a significant functional role. Pulse chase labeling experiments showed, however, that the additional 12 amino acids provide a degradation signal resulting in a short half-life of the protein.

Of particular interest is the group three mutant T53I. Binding studies indicate its inability to bind normally to nonphospho-SLAM (dissociation constant 8–9 mM), while it preserves unaffected binding features when the SLAM Tyr is phosphorylated (KD $\sim$180 nM). Analysis of the SAP crystal structure indicates that the isoleucine replacing the T53 eliminates the binding pocket for Thr (-2) of SLAM. This prevents the interaction of Thr-2 with the buried water molecule and with E17 (M Morra et al, submitted), thus blocking interactions of one of the amino acids located N terminal to Y281. This suggests that the nonphospho interactions involving SAP play a major role in XLP.

The unique ability of the SH2 domain of SAP to bind the nonphosphorylated Y281 of SLAM suggests several modes in which SAP might function. Firstly, it is clear that SAP blocks SHP-2 binding to SLAM. It is likely that if there are other proximal signaling molecules capable of binding the peptide segment around Y281 of SLAM, they too will be prevented from binding by SAP. Secondly, by binding to nonphosphorylated Y281 of SLAM, SAP may block src kinase-mediated phosphorylation of this site, further reducing the chance of other SH2 molecules binding at this position. Thirdly, a role for SAP as a scaffold or adapter protein to coordinate larger signaling complexes following SLAM triggering cannot be excluded.

SAP AND OTHER PROTEINS

SAP and the SLAM Family

Screening of a phospho-peptide library of random peptides indicated an optimal SAP binding motif (T/S.I.pY.x.x.V/I) (38). Because the same or a very similar motif is also present in other members of the SLAM family, i.e. 2B4, Ly-9 and CD84, they were tested for SAP binding (Figure 3). As the SAP/SLAM association had originally been discovered in a two-hybrid system, the same method was used to examine binding of SAP to these other cell surface structures. Whereas none of the cytoplasmic tails interacted with SAP/SH2D1A in a classical yeast two hybrid system, 2B4, CD84, and Ly-9 did bind to SAP if a mutated form of the src-kinase *c-fyn* was cointroduced into the yeast cell. This altered two-hybrid system therefore showed that the interactions between SAP and SLAM are different from those between SAP and the other proteins (Figure 3) (27).

This principle was then confirmed in lymphoid cells where SAP binds to human 2B4 in transfected BaF3 cells (52), and in an NK cell line YT (29a). SAP also binds to Ly-9 in mouse thymocytes and to CD84 in transfected Jurkat or in Raji cells, which express CD84 (J Sayos et al, submitted). In all of these cases, phosphorylation of the cytoplasmic tail tyrosine residues with either pervanadate pretreatment or with receptor-specific monoclonal antibody was required for binding. SHP-2 binds to phosphorylated 2B4, Ly-9, and CD84, but blocking of SHP-2 recruitment by SAP in a COS-7 cell assay proved to be less efficient than in the case of SLAM (52; J Sayos et al, submitted).

These distinctions in terms of SAP binding between SLAM and the other cell surface proteins are somewhat surprising, given the homology of the consensus motifs in these receptors. The SAP/SLAM interaction is unique because it occurs in the absence of tyrosine phosphorylation. Nevertheless, interactions of SAP with these SLAM family members are thought to be of significance for their function on the interface between activated T and B cells. It is likely, however, that following

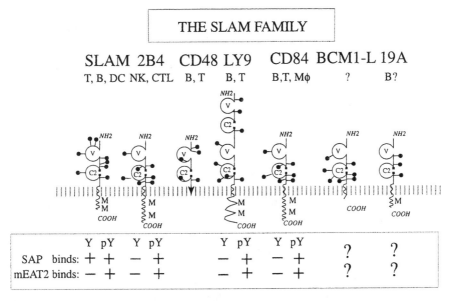

Figure 3 Interaction of SLAM and related molecules with SAP and EAT-2 proteins. A summary of the interactions between SAP or EAT-2 and the cytoplasmic tails of the members of the SLAM family as tested in an altered yeast two hybrid system. Tyrosines are phosphorylated by a mutant of the src-kinase *c-fyn* (Sayos J, Martin M, Chen A, Simarro Grande M, Howie D, Morra M, Engel P, Terhorst C, submitted; M Morra et al, submitted). The + or − symbols respectively indicate the presence or absence of interaction between the different molecules. The SAP-SLAM interaction is unique because it takes place in either the presence or the absence of phosphorylation. The 19A molecule was not tested for interaction but contains at least one SAP binding motif. Prevalent cell expression of the SLAM related molecules is also indicated (T, T lymphocytes; B, B lymphocytes; DC, dendritic cells; NK, natural killer cells; CTL, cytotoxic T lymphocytes; Mo, macrophages; and M, SAP binding motif).

TCR triggering, 2B4, Ly-9, and CD84 are rapidly tyrosine phosphorylated, thus recruiting SAP to the T/B cell contact site.

SAP and p62^{dok}

Recently, SAP has been shown to bind to a 62-kDa phosphoprotein that serves as an adapter molecule, p62^{dok}, in a number of hematopoietic cells (53). p62^{dok} was cloned as a constitutively tyrosine phosphorylated molecule associated with p120 RAS-GTPase activating protein (p120 RAS-GAP) (54–56).

SAP binds specifically to a phosphorylated site in p62^{dok}, ALY$_{449}$SQVQK, which is similar to the SAP binding site in SLAM (TIY$_{281}$AQVQK). Sylla et al hypothesize that SAP might serve to block SHP-2 binding to p62^{dok}, thus prolonging the inhibition induced by p62^{dok} of the Ras pathway by maintaining tyrosine phosphorylation of p62^{dok}. Alternatively, SAP may block the binding of the Src kinase inhibitor Csk to Y_{449} of $p62^{dok}$, thus inhibiting Csk recruitment to the plasma membrane. The role of the negative signaling of $p62^{dok}$ of B cells has been well characterized (54, 57, 58) Studies with the $p62^{dok}$ null mouse support the role of $p62^{dok}$ in inhibition of the Ras pathway in B cells (54). The role of $p62^{dok}$ in T cells needs to be investigated further.

THE SLAM GENE FAMILY

Sequence comparisons suggest that SLAM, 2B4, Ly-9, CD84, and 19A belong to a small subfamily of the Ig superfamily (Figure 4A and Figure 4B). In fact two other genes, CD48 and BCM1-L appear to share similar sequences and have the same basic exon/intron organization (Figure 4A, and Figure 4B, see color insert) (59; N Wang et al, submitted). The SLAM, 2B4, Ly-9, CD84, CD48, and 19A genes are located in a 260-kb fragment on chromosome 1 (1q23), which was mapped using a number of finished and unfinished genomic sequences. The basis of the mapping was provided by the completed segment AL121985.13 (GI:7161187) of 195976 bp of length (Figure 5) (N Wang et al, submitted). Their location, in addition to their sequence similarities, suggests that these receptors arose via successive duplications of a common ancestral gene (52, 59–70). Sequence comparisons have revealed that the seven members of this SLAM family are more closely related to each other than to CD2 as suggested previously (61).

In addition to sharing binding of SAP to specific recognition sites in their cytoplasmic tails, a number of SLAM gene family members form homo-and heterotypic receptor-ligand pairs (Figure 6). SLAM (71, 72), Ly-9 and CD84 (P Engel, personal communication) are homophilic adhesion molecules. Furthermore CD48 is the ligand for 2B4. Whereas some insights have been obtained about the signal transduction event that triggers SLAM, CD48 and 2B4, little is known about the others.

Human **SLAM (CD150)** is found on $CD45RO^{high}$ memory T cells, immature thymocytes, a small fraction of B cells and dendritic cells; it is rapidly upregulated upon activation of T, B and dendritic cells (28, 73, 74). In mice, SLAM is normally expressed on all thymocytes and T and B cells and is also upregulated after activation (75; D Howie, personal communication).

Anti-SLAM antibodies are also particularly effective at inducing IFN-γ by both Th 1 clones and mitogen-activated human or mouse T lymphocytes (28, 75; D Howie, personal communication). Furthermore, polarized Th2 populations from either rheumatoid arthritis or atopic dermatitis patients are reverted to a Th0 phenotype in the presence of mAbs to anti-SLAM (76, 77). These mAbs promote proliferation of human and mouse T cells in a CD28 and IL-2-independent fashion (28, 71; D Howie, personal communication).

SLAM is a heavily N-glycosylated type I glycoprotein (mol wt,–70 to 95 Kda) (28, 75; N Wang et al, submitted). That SLAM self-associates is readily detected upon transfection of SLAM or SLAM-GFP into cells that do not express the molecule, resulting in a dramatic increase in cell adhesion. In vitro plasmon

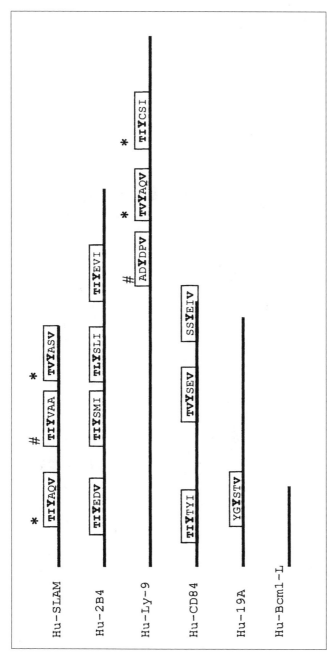

Figure 4B Cytoplasmic domains of the SLAM family members. Lines indicate the cytoplasmic domain of the SLAM family members, while blocks represents real (*) or putative SAP binding motifs. Blocks labeled as # are putative motifs proven to be incapable of SAP's binding. The Bcm1-L gene doesn't contain any SAP putative binding site.

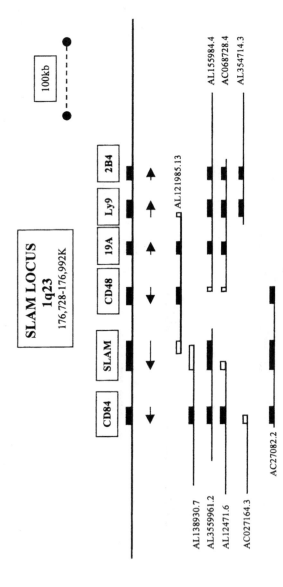

Figure 5 Genomic organization of the SLAM locus in chromosome 1q23. Six genes belonging to the SLAM family are clustered in a genomic segment of approximately 260 kb. The genomic map reflects information derived by the analysis of a number of BAC clones. Filled boxes represent blocks of sequence containing a complete set of exons of a gene, whereas empty boxes indicate partial gene segments (from N Wang et al, submitted).

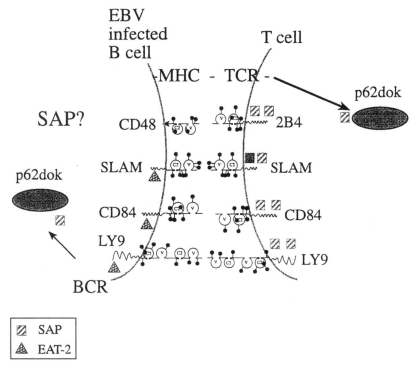

Figure 6   A model summarizing interactions between the SAP-associated molecules at the interface between T lymphocytes and EBV-infected B cells. Homo- and heterophilic interactions between the SLAM family members are indicated. The homophilic interactions involving Ly-9 and CD84 are not certain. While SAP is prevalently expressed in T cells, EAT-2 expression is prevalent in B lymphocytes. As discussed in the text, the presence of SAP in B cells is uncertain. Interplay between SAP-p62dok in BCR or TCR cell activation is also indicated.

resonance studies confirm this self-association, although the observed dissociation constants differ widely. These discrepancies could be caused by the aggregation of the soluble SLAM ecto-domains (71, 72, 78). Because antibodies to SLAM cause the formation of a SLAM plaque on the surface of human peripheral blood T cells, this membrane protein might play a role in the immune synapse (D Howie, personal communication). This could explain the function of SLAM as a co-stimulator (28, 75).

Curiously, mAbs against SLAM fail to enhance human B cell proliferation but seem to potentiate CD95-mediated apoptosis in some B cell lines (79, 80). Nevertheless, some studies have shown that sSLAM and mSLAM increase B cell proliferation and production of IgM, IgG, and IgA normally induced by CD40 mAb or other costimuli (78, 81). Based on these observations, it appears that ligating SLAM in human B cells triggers different events from those in T lymphocytes.

CDw150 on B cells associates with the Src-family kinase Fgr and the SH2-containing inositol polyphosphate 5′-phosphatase SHIP (79). Both Fgr and SHIP interact with phosphorylated tyrosines in CDw150 cytoplasmic tail. Ligation of CDw150 induces the rapid dephosphorylation of both SHIP and CDw150 as well as the association of Lyn and Fgr with SHIP (79). It was recently discovered that SLAM serves as a receptor for Measles virus (81a). Because the tissue distribution of SLAM is restricted to lymphoid and dendritic cells, it may play a major role in the suppression of the immune response after viral infection.

2B4 is an N-glycosylated protein of relative molecular mass, 66 to 80 kDa (70, 82). As is common among the SLAM related proteins, murine 2B4 is expressed as more than one isoform. In this case there are two alternately spliced variants, a long (-L) and a short (-S) one, which differ in their cytoplasmic tails (65, 70, 83, 84). The cytoplasmic tail of mouse and human 2B4-L contains six tyrosines; four are embedded in a potential SAP motif (Figure 4B). The shorter form is missing the three distal tyrosine-based motifs at the C-terminal (83). The high affinity between 2B4 and its ligand CD48 (85–87) is of importance for our thinking about XLP, because CD48 is one of the major receptors that is upregulated on B cells following EBV transformation (Figure 6).

Murine and human 2B4 are expressed on all NK cells, $\gamma\delta$ T cells, monocytes, some CD8$^+$ thymocytes, and on a subset of CD8$^+$ peripheral T cells (88–91). Expression of 2B4 is upregulated on CD8$^+$ and CD4$^+$ T cells after activation. Expression of 2B4 is also upregulated in NK and CD8$^+$ cells after infection with LCMV or MCMV (29a).

2B4 regulates NK cell activation independently of MHC class I (92). Ligation of m2B4 with mAb triggered cell-mediated cytotoxicity, IFN-γ and IL-2 secretion (88, 91), granule exocytosis (88), and proliferation of resting $\gamma\delta$ T cells (91). In humans, cross-linking of 2B4 on NK cells triggers redirected lysis of FcR+ cells in cytotoxic assays and cytokine secretion (IFN-γ, IL-8, and TNF-α) (89, 90, 93). Similarly, 2B4 activates NK-mediated lysis upon binding CD48 on target cells (89). In a recent study, Parolini et al observe that the failure of NK cells from XLP patients to kill EBV(+) B cell lines is the consequence of inhibitory signals generated by the interaction between 2B4 and CD48, as the antibody-mediated disruption of the 2B4-CD48 interaction restored lysis of EBV(+) target cells (15).

The function of 2B4 in human CD8$^+$ T cells is unknown. Preliminary data on human CD8$^+$ T cells indicate that 2B4 induces modest lytic activity and no proliferation or cytokine production (89). Interaction between 2B4 on CD8$^+$ T cells and CD48 on target or antigen-presenting cells (APC) may increase cell-cell adhesion, rather than directly activating T cells. Therefore, 2B4/CD48 interactions may enhance the recruitment of rafts into the immune synapse, as has been demonstrated for interactions between T cell surface CD2 and APC surface CD48 (94).

CD48 is widely expressed on lymphocytes and upregulated on B cells after EBV-mediated transformation (95) (Figure 6). CD48 null mice are severely impaired in

CD4$^+$ T cell activation: proliferative responses to mitogens, anti-CD3 mAb, and alloantigen are all reduced. In line with its tissue distribution, CD48's effect on TCR driven responses depends on its function in both T and antigen-presenting cells. It is likely that the disruption of the 2B4 gene will result in an overlapping phenotype.

Murine and human *LY-9* expression is restricted to mature T cells, B cells, and thymocytes (96). There are two murine allelic variants Ly-9.1 and Ly-9.2 (62, 97, 98). Ly-9 is a 100-kDa glycosylated protein (62, 66, 96). The cytoplasmic tail of Ly-9 contains two SAP binding motifs (Figure 4B), in addition to another motif that lacks Thr-2.

CD84 is predominantly expressed by B cells, platelets, and myeloid cells. It is also expressed at low levels on T cells (60, 99, 100). CD84 is a glycosylated protein ranging from 70 to 95 kDa in size (60, 61). The cytoplasmic tail of CD84 contains three putative SAP binding motif (Figure 4B) (61, 101).

INTERACTIONS BETWEEN SLAM FAMILY MEMBERS AND EAT-2

Fluorescence polarization assays indicate that EAT-2 binds to the phosphorylated Y281 SLAM peptide with an affinity comparable to that of SAP. But no binding is detected to the unphosphorylated peptide (M Morra et al, submitted). This observation was confirmed and extended in the altered yeast two hybrid system, where EAT-2 binds to the cytoplasmic tails of SLAM, 2B4, Ly-9 and CD84 after co-expression of *c-fyn* only (Figure 3). Preliminary in vivo results in COS-7 cells and B cells are in agreement with this finding (M Morra et al, submitted).

EAT-2 is expressed in different tissues than SAP, but often co-expresses with members of the SLAM family. We conclude that SAP and EAT-2 control signal transduction through members of the SLAM family in other tissues as well as T and B cells. Thus, the two SAP family members may control functions of the SLAM family of hematopoietic cells in a variety of ways, independent of XLP.

The interactions of SAP with the SLAM family members are summarized in Figure 6. As discussed previously, it remains to be determined whether SAP is expressed in human B cells, and if so, in which subsets. Nevertheless this model predicts that in spite of the unique interaction between SAP and SLAM, disruption of the SAP gene will provide a more complex phenotype than that of SLAM alone. Perhaps more importantly, preliminary data show that SLAM and SAP are present in the immune synapse formed between antigen specific CTL clones and antigen pulsed B lymphoblastoid cells as APCs (D Howie et al, unpublished observations). Thus, SAP is introduced into the immune synapse at high concentrations via SLAM and perhaps via Ly9, CD84 or 2B4 to ensure its presence at the T cell/APC interface. EAT-2 may serve a similar role in other hematopoietic cells.

TOWARD A MOUSE MODEL FOR XLP

Preliminary analyses of a SAP^{null} mouse have shed some light on the complex phenotypes of XLP. As there is no direct murine equivalent of EBV, mice with a disrupted SAP gene were infected with two strains of LCMV, the hepatotropic strain LCMV-WE and LCMV-ARM (102). Infection with LCMV-WE resulted in increased mortality and accelerated time to death in SAP^{null} mice versus wild type. SAP^{null} mice responded to LCMV-ARM infection with increased numbers of CD8$^+$ and CD4$^+$ IFN-γ producing cells in liver and spleen. SAP^{null} T cells also have an inherent deficiency in IL-4 gene activation and increased IFN-γ production following TCR triggering (Wu C, Nguyeng KB, Pien GC, Wang N, Gullo C, Howie D, Rodriguez Sosa M, Edwards MJ, Borrow P, Satoskar AR, Sharpe AH, Biron CA, Terhorst C, submitted).

To examine the in vivo responses to a strong mitogen SAP, null mice and wild-type littermates were injected with 20 μg of purified anti-CD3 (103). This induced severe depletion of T cells in spleen and lymph nodes within 24 h to 48 h. In wild-type mice the remaining T cells were rendered refractory to in vitro stimulation with anti-CD3 and the co-stimulator anti-CD28, even though they still express high levels of TCR/CD3. However, this nonresponsive state could not be induced in SAP null mice. Taken together, these data support the notion that disruption of the mouse SAP gene results in abnormally aggressive T cell proliferation upon infection with the LCMV virus or injection with anti-CD3. Importantly, this effect can be caused by a virus that is quite different from EBV.

A disrupted SAP gene may therefore render the animal more susceptible to a variety of viral infections. It is conceivable that repeated infections with viruses other than EBV may have a cumulative effect on XLP patients, which may influence the other XLP phenotypes. Thus, XLP must be seen as a progressive immunodeficiency. Similarly, the NK cell defect observed in some but not all XLP patients could develop with cumulative immunological insults. This can be tested in the SAP null mouse because it does not have an NK cell defect at young age. It has become clear that further studies of the SAP null mouse will provide insights into the role of this gene and of the SLAM family genes in normal immune responses.

CONCLUSIONS

In the past two years, there have been a number of exciting advances in the study of X-linked lymphoproliferative disease. Most importantly, the gene that is defective in this condition, SAP/SH2D1A, was identified. The observations made thus far support a model in which XLP is likely to be an immunodeficiency that is manifested progressively after viral infections. However, the ubiquitous thread of EBV accelerates the clinical situation in the case of the fulminant infectious mononucleosis.

Initial data on the function of this small tailed-SH2 domain protein suggest that it serves to block critical events in T and NK cell signal transduction and perhaps in B cells. Moreover, SAP binds to four members of the SLAM family and to p62^{dok1}. Despite those important breakthrough, there are a number of important issues remaining to be resolved that concern the function of SAP in T/B cell homeostasis during viral infection. To unravel the role of SAP in this complicated process, it will be necessary to answer fundamental questions about the signaling pathways in which SAP participates. In what way is SAP involved in the SLAM/TCR-mediated amplification of T cell proliferation and IFN-γ production in response to antigen? Does SAP control the threshold of sensitivity of T (or B) cells to FAS-induced apoptosis via SLAM? In addition to these questions, it remains to be demonstrated which T cell subsets are most affected by mutations in SAP. It is tempting to speculate that disruption of SAP's function in suppressor cells such as the recently described Tr1 cells might lead to loss of T cell homeostasis following clearance of viral infections. Mice in which genes of the SLAM and the SAP family members are disrupted will shed light on these questions. But further studies of the process in which the immune responses of XLP patients deviate are of equal importance. In further studies, we will learn not only about the molecular etiology of XLP, but about more fundamental issues of T cell activation and interactions between T cells and APCs.

ACKNOWLEDGMENTS

The authors wish to thank Drs. C Biron, R Buckley, E Clarke, M Eck, A Etzioni, H Oettgen, and R Sorensen for sharing data and Drs. Y de Jong, M Exley, C Gullo, and H Oettgen for a critical review of the manuscript. This work was supported by grants from the NIH (AI-35714) and from the National March of Dimes Foundation.

Visit the Annual Reviews home page at www.AnnualReviews.org

LITERATURE CITED

1. Purtilo DT, Cassel CK, Yang JP, Harper R. 1975. X-linked recessive progressive combined variable immunodeficiency (Duncan's disease). *Lancet* 1:935–40

2. Hamilton JK, Paquin LA, Sullivan JL, Maurer HS, Cruzi FG, Provisor AJ, Steuber CP, Hawkins E, Yawn D, Cornet JA, Clausen K, Finkelstein GZ, Landing B, Grunnet M, Purtilo DT. 1980. X-linked lymphoproliferative syndrome registry report. *J. Pediatr.* 96:669–73

3. IUIS Scientific Committee. 1999. Primary immunodeficiency diseases. Report of an IUIS Scientific Committee. International Union of Immunological Societies. *Clin. Exp. Immunol.* 118:1–28

4. Howie D, Sayos J, Terhorst C, Morra M. 2000. The gene defective in X-linked lymphoproliferative disease controls T cell dependent immune surveillance against Epstein-Barr virus. *Curr. Opin. Immunol.* 12:474–78

5. Rickinson AB, Moss DJ. 1997. Human cytotoxic T lymphocyte responses to Epstein-Barr virus infection. *Annu. Rev. Immunol.* 1997:405–31

6. Tan LC, Gudgeon N, Annels NE, Hansasuta P, O'Callaghan CA, Rowland-Jones S, McMichael AJ, Rickinson AB, Callan MF. 1999. A re-evaluation of the frequency of CD8+ T cells specific for EBV in healthy virus carriers. *J. Immunol.* 162:1827–35

7. Tomkinson BE, Wagner DK, Nelson DL, Sullivan JL. 1987. Activated lymphocytes during acute Epstein-Barr virus infection. *J. Immunol.* 139:3802–7

8. Klein G. 1994. Epstein-Barr virus strategy in normal and neoplastic B cells. *Cell* 77:791–93

9. Lee SP, Tierney RJ, Thomas WA, Brooks JM, Rickinson AB. 1997. Conserved CTL epitopes within EBV latent membrane protein 2:a potential target for CTL-based tumor therapy. *J. Immunol.* 158:3325–34

10. Callan MF, Tan L, Annels N, Ogg GS, Wilson JD, O'Callaghan CA, Steven N, McMichael AJ, Rickinson AB. 1998. Direct visualization of antigen-specific CD8+ T cells during the primary immune response to Epstein-Barr virus in vivo. *J. Exp. Med.* 187:1395–402

11. Sullivan JL, Byron KS, Brewster FE, Purtilo DT. 1980. Deficient natural killer cell activity in X-linked lymphoproliferative syndrome. *Science* 210:543–45

12. Sullivan JL, Byron KS, Brewster FE, Baker SM, Ochs HD. 1983. X-linked lymphoproliferative syndrome. Natural history of the immunodeficiency. *J. Clin. Invest.* 71:1765–78

13. Jager M, Benninger-Doring G, Prang N, Sylla BS, Laumbacher B, Wank R, Wolf H, Schwarzmann F. 1988. Epstein-Barr virus-infected B cells of males with the X-linked lymphoproliferative syndrome stimulate and are susceptible to T-cell-mediated lysis. *Int. J. Cancer* 76(5):694–701

14. Rousset F, Souillet G, Roncarolo MG, Lamelin JP. 1986. Studies of EBV-lymphoid cell interactions in two patients with the X-linked lymphoproliferative syndrome: normal EBV-specific HLA-restricted cytotoxicity. *Clin. Exp. Immunol.* 63:280–89

15. Parolini S, Bottino C, Falco M, Augugliaro R, Giliani IS, Franceschini R, Ochs H, Wolf H, Bonnefoy JY, Biassoni R, Moretta L, Notarangelo LD, Moretta A. 2000. X-linked lymphoproliferative disease: 2B4 molecules displaying inhibitory rather than activating function killer cells to kill Epstein-Barr virus-infected cells. *J. Exp. Med.* 3:337–46

16. Benoit L, Wang X, Pabst HF, Dutz J, Tan R. 2000. Defective natural killer cell activation in X-linked lymphoproliferative disease. *J. Immunol.* 465:3549–53

17. Grierson HL, Skare J, Hawk J, Pauza M, Purtilo DT. 1991. Immunoglobulin class and subclass deficiencies prior to Epstein-Barr virus infection in males with X-linked lymphoproliferative disease. *Am. J. Med. Genet.* 40:294–97

18. Strahm B, Rittweiler K, Duffner U, Brandau O, Orlowska-Volk M, Karajannis MA, Stadt Uz, Tiemann M, Reiter A, Brandis M, Meindl A, Niemeyer CM. 2000. Recurrent B-cell non-Hodgkin's lymphoma in two brothers with X-linked lymphoproliferative disease without evidence for Epstein-Barr virus infection. *Br. J. Haematol.* 108:377–82

19. Brandau O, Schuster V, Weiss M, Hellebrand H, Fink FM, Kreczy A, Friedrich W, Strahm B, Niemeye C, Belohradsky BH, Meindl A. 1999. Epstein-Barr virus-negative boys with non-Hodgkin lymphoma are mutated in the SH2D1A gene, as are patients with X-linked lymphoproliferative disease (XLP). *Hum. Mol. Genet.* 8:2407–13

20. Coffey AJ, Brooksbank RA, Brandau O, Oohashi T, Howell GR, Bye JM, Cahn AP, Durham J, Heath P, Wray P, Pavitt R, Wilkinson J, Leversha M, Huckle E,

Shaw-Smith CJ, Dunham A, Rhodes S, Schuster V, Porta G, Yin L, Serafini P, Sylla B, Zollo M, Franco B, Bentley DR, et al. 1998. Host response to EBV infection in X-linked lymphoproliferative disease results from mutations in an SH2-domain encoding gene. *Nat. Genet.* 20:129–35

21. Skare J, Wu BL, Madan S, Pulijaal V, Purtilo D, Haber D, Nelson D, Sylla B, Grierson H, Nitowsky H, et al. 1993. Characterization of three overlapping deletions causing X-linked lymphoproliferative disease. *Genomics* 16:254–55

22. Wyandt HE, Grierson HL, Sanger WG, Skare JC, Milunsky A, Purtilo DT. 1989. Chromosome deletion of Xq25 in an individual with X-linked lymphoproliferative disease. *Am. J. Med. Genet.* 33:426–30

23. Skare JC, Sullivan JL, Milunsky A. 1989. Mapping the mutation causing the X-linked lymphoproliferative syndrome in relation to restriction fragment length polymorphisms on Xq. *Hum Genet.* 82:349–53

24. Skare JC, Milunsky A, Byron KS, Sullivan JL. 1987. Mapping the X-linked lymphoproliferative syndrome. *Proc. Natl. Acad. Sci. USA* 84:2015–18

25. Sylla BS, Wang Q, Hayoz D, Lathrop GM, Lenoir GM. 1989. Multipoint linkage mapping of the Xq25–q26 region in a family affected by the X-linked lymphoproliferative syndrome. *Clin. Genet.* 36:459–62

26. Wu BL, Milunsky A, Nelson D, Schmeckpeper B, Porta G, Schlessinger D, Skare J. 1993. High-resolution mapping of probes near the X-linked lymphoproliferative disease (XLP) locus. *Genomics* 17:163–70

27. Sayos J, Wu C, Morra M, Wang N, Zhang X, Allen D, van Schaik S, Notarangelo L, Geha R, Roncarolo MG, Oettgen H, De Vries JE, Aversa G, Terhorst C. 1998. The X-linked lymphoproliferative-disease gene product SAP regulates signals induced through the co-receptor SLAM. *Nature* 395:462–69

28. Cocks BG, Chang CC, Carballido JM, Yssel H, de Vries JE, Aversa G. 1995. A novel receptor involved in T-cell activation. *Nature* 376:260–63

29. Wu C, Sayos J, Wang N, Howie D, Coyle A, Terhorst C. 2000. Genomic organization and characterization of murine SAP: the gene coding for X-linked lymphoproliferative disease. *Immunogenetics* 51:805–15

29a. Sayos J, Nguyen KB, Wu C, Stepp SE, Howie D, Schatzle JD, Kumar V, Biron CA, Terhorst C. 2000. Potential pathways for regulation of NK and T cell responses: differential XLP gene product SAP interactions with SLAM and 2B4. *Int. Immunol.* In press

30. Nagy N, Cerboni C, Mattsson K, Maeda A, Gogolak P, Sumegi J, Lanyi A, Szekely L, Carbone E, Klein E, Klein G. 2000. SH2D1A and SLAM expression in human lymphocytes and derived cell lines. *Int. J. Cancer* 88:439–47

31. Nichols KE, Harkin DP, Levitz S, Krainer M, Kolquist KA, Genovese C, Bernard A, Ferguson M, Zuo L, Snyder E, Buckler AJ, Wise C, Ashley J, Lovett M, Valentine MB, Look AT, Gerald W, Housman DE, H. DA. 1998. Inactivating mutations in an SH2 domain-encoding gene in X-linked lymphoproliferative syndrome. *Proc. Natl. Acad. Sci. USA* 95:13765–70

32. Sumegi J, Huang D, Lanyi A, Davis JD, Seemayer TA, Maeda A, Klein G, Seri M, Wakiguchi H, Purtilo DT, Gross TG. 2000. Correlation of mutations of the SH2D1A gene and Epstein-Barr virus (EBV) infection with clinical phenotype and outcome in X-linked lymphoproliferative disease (XLP). *Blood* 96:3118–25

33. Yin L, Ferrand V, Lavoue MF, Hayoz D, Philippe N, Souillet G, Seri M, Giacchino R, Castagnola E, Hodgson S, Sylla BS, Romeo G. 1999. SH2D1A mutation analysis for diagnosis of XLP in typical and atypical patients. *Hum. Genet.* 105:501–5

34. Cunningham-Rundles C, Bodian C. 1999. Common variable immunodeficiency:

clinical and immunological features of 248 patients. *Clin. Immunol.* 92:34–48

35. Buckley RH, Sidbury JB. 1968. Hereditary alterations in the immune response: coexistence of "agammaglobulinemia", acquired hypogammaglobulinemia and selective immunoglobulin deficiency in a sibship. *Pediatr. Res.* 2:72–84

36. Gilmour KC, Cranston T, Jones A, Davies EG, Goldblatt D, Thrasher A, Kinnon C, Nichols KE, G. HB. 2000. Diagnosis of X-linked lymphoproliferative disease by analysis of SLAM-associated protein expression. *Eur. J. Immunol.* 30:1691–97

37. Thompson AD, Braun BS, Arvand A, Stewart SD, May WA, Chen E, Korenberg J, Denny C. 1996. EAT-2 is a novel SH2 domain containing protein that is up regulated by Ewing's sarcoma EWS/FLI1 fusion gene. *Oncogene.* 13:2649–58

38. Poy F, Yaffe MB, Sayos J, Saxena K, Morra M, Sumegi J, Cantley LC, Terhorst C, Eck MJ. 1999. Crystal structures of the XLP protein SAP reveal a class of SH2 domains with extended, phosphotyrosine-independent sequence recognition. *Mol. Cell* 4:555–61

39. Li SC, Gish G, Yang D, Coffey AJ, Forman-Kay JD, Ernberg I, Kay LE, Pawson T. 1999. Novel mode of ligand binding by the SH2 domain of the human XLP disease gene product SAP/SH2D1A. *Curr. Biol.* 9:1355–62

40. Scott D, Pawson T. 2000. Cell communication: the inside story. *Sci. Am.* June:72–79

41. Ladbury JE, Lemmon MA, Zhou M, Green J, Botfield MC, Schlessinger J. 1995. Measurement of the binding of tyrosyl phosphopeptides to SH2 domains: a reappraisal. *Proc. Natl. Acad. Sci.* 92:3199–203

42. Pluskey S, Wandless TJ, Walsh CT, Shoelson SE. 1995. Potent stimulation of SH-PTP2 phosphatase activity by simultaneous occupancy of both SH2 domains. *J. Biol. Chem.* 270:2897–900

43. Barford D, Neel BG. 1998. Revealing mechanisms for SH2 domain mediated regulation of the protein tyrosine phosphatase SHP-2. *Structure* 6:249–54

44. Dechert U, Adam M, Harder KW, Clark-Lewis I, Jirik F. 1994. Characterization of protein tyrosine phosphatase SH-PTP2. Study of phosphopeptide substrates and possible regulatory role of SH2 domains. *J. Biol. Chem.* 269:5602–11

45. Feng GS, Pawson T. 1994. Phosphotyrosine phosphatases with SH2 domains: regulators of signal transduction. *Trends. Genet.* 10:54–58

46. Hof P, Pluskey S, Dhe-Paganon S, Eck MJ, Shoelson SE. 1998. Crystal structure of the tyrosine phosphatase SHP-2. *Cell* 92:441–50

47. Neel BG. 1993. Structure and function of SH2-domain containing tyrosine phosphatases. *Semin. Cell Biol.* 4:419–32

48. Neel BG, Tonks NK. 1997. Protein tyrosine phosphatases in signal transduction. *Curr. Opin. Cell Biol.* 9:193–204

49. Kane LP, Lin J, Weiss A. 2000. Signal transduction by the TCR for antigen. *Curr. Opin. Immunol.* 12:242–49

50. Feng GS, Hui CC, Pawson T. 1993. SH2-containing phosphotyrosine phosphatase as a target of protein-tyrosine kinases. *Science* 259:1607–11

51. Vogel W, Lammers R, Huang J, Ullrich A. 1993. Activation of a phosphotyrosine phosphatase by tyrosine phosphorylation. *Science* 259:1611–14

52. Tangye SG, Lazetic S, Woollatt E, Sutherland GR, Lanier LL, Phillips JH. 1999. Human 2B4, an activating NK cell receptor, recruits the protein tyrosine phosphatase SHP-2 and the adaptor signaling protein SAP. *J. Immunol.* 162:6981–85

53. Sylla BS, Murphy K, Cahir-McFarland E, Lane WS, Mosialos G, Kieff E. 2000. The X-linked lymphoproliferative syndrome gene product SH2D1A associates with p62dok (Dok1) and activates NF-kappa B. *Proc. Natl. Acad. Sci. USA* 97:7470–75

54. Yamanashi Y, Tamura T, Kanamori T, Yamane H, Nariuchi H, Yamamoto T, Baltimore D. 2000. Role of the rasGAP-associated docking protein p62(dok) in negative regulation of B cell receptor-mediated signaling. *Genes. Dev.* 14:11–16

55. Carpino N, Wisniewski D, Strife A, Marshak D, Kobayashi R, Stillman B, Clarkson B. 1997. p62(dok): a constitutively tyrosine-phosphorylated, GAP-associated protein in chronic myelogenous leukemia progenitor cells. *Cell* 88:197–204

56. Ellis C, Moran M, McCormick F, Pawson T. 1990. Phosphorylation of GAP and GAP-associated proteins by transforming and mitogenic tyrosine kinases. *Nature* 343:377–81

57. Tamir I, Stolpa JC, Helgason CD, Nakamura K, Bruhns P, Daeron M, Cambier JC. 2000. The RasGAP-binding protein p62dok is a mediator of inhibitory FcgammaRIIB signals in B cells. *Immunity* 12:347–58

58. Kashige N, Carpino N, Kobayashi R. 2000. Tyrosine phosphorylation of p62dok by p210bcr-abl inhibits RasGAP activity. *Proc. Natl. Acad. Sci. USA* 97:2093–98

59. Wong YW, Williams AF, S Kingsmore, Seldin MF. 1990. Structure, expression, and genetic linkage of the mouse BCM1 (OX45 or Blast-1) antigen. Evidence for genetic duplication giving rise to the BCM1 region on mouse chromosome 1 and the CD2/LFA3 region on mouse chromosome 3. *J. Exp. Med.* 171:2115–30

60. De la Fuente MA, Pizcueta P, Nadal M, Bosch J, Engel P. 1997. CD84 leukocyte antigen is a new member of the Ig superfamily. *Blood* 90:2398–405

61. De la Fuente MA, Tovar V, Pizcueta P, Nadal M, Bosch J, Engel P. 1999. Molecular cloning, characterization, and chromosomal localization of the mouse homologue of CD84, a member of the CD2 family of cell surface molecules. *Immunogenetics* 49:249–55

62. Hogarth PM, Graig J, McKenzie IF. 1980. A monoclonal antibody detecting the Ly-9.2 (Lgp-100) cell-membrane alloantigen. *Immunogenetics* 11:65–74

63. Kingsmore SF, Souryal CA, Watson ML, Patel DD, Seldin MF. 1995. Physical and genetic linkage of the genes encoding Ly-9 and CD48 on mouse and human chromosomes 1. *Immunogenetics* 42:59–62

64. Kubota K, Katoh H, Muguruma K, Koyama K. 1999. Characterization of a surface membrane molecule expressed by natural killer cells in most inbred mouse strains: monoclonal antibody C9.1 identifies an allelic form of the 2B4 antigen. *Immunology.* 96:491–97

65. Mathew PA, Garni-Wagner BA, Land K, Takashima A, Stoneman E, Bennett M, Kumar V. 1993. Cloning and characterization of the 2B4 gene encoding a molecule associated with non-MHC-restricted killing mediated by activated natural killer cells and T cells. *J. Immunol.* 151:5328–37

66. Sandrin MS, Henning MM, Lo MF, Baker E, Sutherland GR, McKenzie IF. 1996. Isolation and characterization of cDNA clones for Humly9: the human homologue of mouse Ly9. *Immunogenetics* 43:13–19

67. Staunton DE, Fisher RC, Le Beau MM, Lawrence JB, Barton DE, Francke U, Dustin M, Thorley-Lawson DA. 1989. Blast-1 possesses a glycosyl-phosphatidylinositol (GPI) membrane anchor, is related to LFA3 and OX-45, maps to chromosome 1q21–23. *J. Exp. Med.* 169:1087–99

68. Tangye SG, Phillips JH, Lanier LL. 2000. The CD2-subset of the Ig superfamily of cell surface molecules:receptor-ligand pairs expressed by NK and other immune cells. *Semin. Immunol.* 12:149–57

69. Callanan MB, Le Baccon P, Mossuz P, Duley S, Bastard C, Hamoudi R, Dyer MJ, Klobeck G, Rimokh R, Sotto JJ, Leroux D. 2000. The IgG Fc receptor, FcgammaRIIB, is a target for deregulation by chromosomal translocation in malignant lymphoma.

Proc. Natl. Acad. Sci. USA 97:309–14

70. Nakajima H, Colonna M. 2000. 2B4: an NK cell activating receptor with unique specificity and signal transduction mechanism. *Hum. Immunol.* 61:39–43

71. Aversa G, Carballido J, Punnonen J, Chang CC, Hauser T, Cocks BG, De Vries JE. 1997. SLAM and its role in T cell activation and Th responses. *Immunol. Cell Biol.* 75:202–5

72. Mavaddat N, Mason DW, Atkinson PD, Evans EJ, Gilbert RJC, Stuart DI, Fennelly JA, Barclay AN, Davis SJ, Brown MH. 2000. Signaling lymphocytic activation molecule (SLAM, CDw150) is homophilic but self-associates with very low affinity. *J. Biol. Chem.* 275:28100–9

73. Sidorenko SP, Clark EA. 1993. Characterization of a cell surface glycoprotein IPO-3, expressed on activated human B and T lymphocytes. *J. Immunol.* 151:4614–24

74. Polacino PS, Pinchuk LM, Sidorenko SP, Clark EA. 1996. Immunodeficiency virus cDNA synthesis in resting T lymphocytes is regulated by T cell activation signals and dendritic cells. *J. Med. Primatol.* 25:201–9

75. Castro AG, Hauser TM, Cocks BG, Abrams J, Zurawski S, Churakova T, Zonin F, Robinson D, Tangye SG, Aversa G, Nichols KE, de Vries JE, Lanier LL, O'Garra A. 1999. Molecular and functional characterization of mouse signaling lymphocytic activation molecule (SLAM): differential expression and responsiveness in Th1 and Th2 cells. *J. Immunol.* 163:5860–70

76. Carballido JM, A. G., Kaltoft K, Cocks BG, Punnonen J, Yssel H, Thestrup-Pedersen K, de Vries JE. 1997. Reversal of human allergic T helper 2 responses by engagement of signaling lymphocytic activation molecule. *J. Immunol.* 159:4316–21

77. Isomaki P, Aversa G, Cocks BG, Luukkainen, Saario R, Toivanen P, de Vries JE, Punnonen J. 1997. Increased expression of signaling lymphocytic activation

molecule in patients with rheumatoid arthritis and its role in the regulation of cytokine production in rheumatoid synovium. *J. Immunol.* 159:2986–93

78. Punnonen J, Cocks BG, Carballido JM, Bennett B, Peterson D, Aversa G, de Vries JE. 1997. Soluble and membrane-bound forms of signaling lymphocytic activation molecule (SLAM) induce proliferation and Ig synthesis by activated human B lymphocytes. *J. Exp. Med.* 185:555–61

79. Mikhalap SV, Shlapatska LM, Berdova AG, Law CL, Clark EA, Sidorenko SP. 1999. CDw150 associates with src-homology 2-containing inositol phosphatase and modulates CD95-mediated apoptosis. *J. Immunol.* 162:5719–27

80. Liu Q, Olivera-Dos-Santos AJ, Mariathasans, Bouchard D, Jones J, Sarao R, Kozieradzki I, Ohashi PS, Penninger JM, Dumont DJ. 1998. The inositol polyphosphate 5-phosphatase ship is a crucial negative regulator of B cell antigen receptor signaling. *J. Exp. Med.* 188:1333–42

81. Isomaki P, Aversa G, Chang CC, Luukkainen R, Nikkari S, Toivanen P, de Vries JE, Punnonen J. 1999. Expression of soluble human signaling lymphocytic activation molecule in vivo. *J. Allergy Clin. Immunol.* 103:114–18

81a. Tatsuo H, Ono N, Tanaka T, Yanagi Y. 2000. SLAM (CDw150) is a cellular receptor for measles virus. *Nature* 406:893–97

82. Sivori S, Parolini S, Falco M, Marcenaro E, Biassoni R, Bottino C, Moretta L, Moretta A. 2000. 2B4 functions as a co-receptor in human NK cell activation. *Eur. J. Immunol.* 30:787–93

83. Stepp SE, Schatzle JD, Bennett M, Kumar V, Mathew PA. 1999. Gene structure of the murine NK cell receptor 2B4: presence of two alternatively spliced isoforms with distinct cytoplasmic domains. *Eur. J. Immunol.* 29:2392–99

84. Schatzle JD, Sheu S, Stepp SE, Mathew PA, Bennett M, Kumar V. 1999.

Characterization of inhibitory and stimulatory forms of the murine natural killer cell receptor 2B4. *Proc. Natl. Acad. Sci. USA* 96:3870–975

85. Brown MH, Boles K, van der Merwe PA, Kumar V, Mathew PA, Barclay AN. 1998. 2B4, the natural killer and T cell immunoglobulin superfamily surface protein, is a ligand for CD48. *J. Exp. Med.* 188:2083–90

86. Kubin MZ, Parshley DL, Din W, Waugh JY, Davis-Smith T, Smith CA, Macduff BM, Armitage RJ, Chin W, Cassiano L, Borges L, Petersen M, Trinchieri G, Goodwin RG. 1999. Molecular cloning and biological characterization of NK cell activation-inducing ligand, a counterstructure for CD48. *Eur. J. Immunol.* 29:3466–77

87. Latchman Y, McKay PF, Reiser H. 1998. Identification of the 2B4 molecule as a counter-receptor for CD48. *J. Immunol.* 161:5809–12

88. Garni-Wagner BA, Purohit A, Mathew PA, Bennett M, Kumar V. 1993. A novel function-associated molecule related to non-MHC-restricted cytotoxicity mediated by activated natural killer cells and T cells. *J. Immunol.* 151:60–70

89. Nakajima H, Cella M, Langen H, Friedlein A, Colonna M. 1999. Activating interactions in human NK cell recognition: the role of 2B4-CD48. *Eur. J. Immunol.* 29:1676–83

90. Valiante NM, Trinchieri G. 1993. Identification of a novel signal transduction surface molecule on human cytotoxic lymphocytes. *J. Exp. Med.* 178:1397–1406

91. Schuhmachers G, Ariizumi K, Mathew PA, Bennett M, Kumar V, Takashima A. 1995. 2B4, a new member of the immunoglobulin gene superfamily, is expressed on murine dendritic epidermal T cells and plays a functional role in their killing of skin tumors. *J. Invest Dermatol.* 105:592–96

92. Lanier LL. 1998. NK cell receptors. *Annu. Rev. Immunol.* 16:359–93

93. Boles KS, Nakajima H, Colonna M, Chuang SS, Stepp SE, Bennett M, Kumar V, Mathew PA. 1999. Molecular characterization of a novel human natural killer cell receptor homologous to mouse 2B4. *Tissue Antigens* 54:27–34

94. Moran M, Miceli MC. 1998. Engagement of GPI-linked CD48 contributes to TCR signals and cytoskeletal reorganization: a role for lipid rafts in T cell activation. *Immunity* 9:799–806

95. Fisher RC, Thorley-Lawson DA. 1991. Characterization of the Epstein-Barr virus-inducible gene encoding the human leukocyte adhesion and activation antigen BLAST-1 (CD48). *Mol. Cell Biol.* 11:1614–23

96. Sandrin MS, Gumley TP, Henning MM, Vaughan HA, Gonez LJ, Trapani JA, M. IF. 1992. Isolation and characterization of cDNA clones for mouse Ly-9. *J. Immunol.* 149:1636–41

97. Ledbetter JA, Goding JW, Tsu TT, Herzenberg LA. 1979. A new mouse lymphoid alloantigen (Lgp100) recognized by a monoclonal rat antibody. *Immunogenetics* 8:347–60

98. Mathieson BJ, Sharrow SO, Bottomly K, Fowlkes BJ. 1980. Ly-9, an alloantigen maker of lymphocyte differentiation. *J. Immunol.* 125:2127–36

99. Tedder TF, Wagner N, Engel P. 1995. B-cell antigens section report. Oxford, UK: *Oxford Univ. Press.* 1:483–504

100. Krause SW, Rehli M, Heinz S, Ebner R, Andreesen R. 2000. Characterization of MAX.3 antigen, a glycoprotein expressed on mature macrophages, dendritic cells and blood platelets: identity with CD84. *Biochem. J.* 346:729–36

101. Palou E, Pirotto F, Sole J, Freed JH, Peral B, Vilardell C, Vilella R, Vives J, Gaya A. 2000. Genomic characterization of CD84 reveals the existence of five isoforms

differing in their cytoplasmic domains. *Tissue Antigens* 55:118–27

102. Biron CA, Nguyen KB, Pien GC, Cousens LP, Salazar-Mather TP. 1999. Natural killer cells in antiviral defense: function and regulation by innate cytokines. *Annu. Rev. Immunol.* 17:189–220

103. Muraille E, Andris F, Pajak B, Wissing KM, De Smedt T, Desalle F, Goldman M, Alegre ML, Urbain J, Moser M, Leo O. 1999. Downregulation of antigen-presenting cell functions after administration of mitogenic anti-CD3 monoclonal antibodies in mice. *Blood* 94:4347–57

Annu. Rev. Immunol. 2001. 19:683–765

INTERLEUKIN-10 AND THE INTERLEUKIN-10 RECEPTOR

Kevin W. Moore[1], Rene de Waal Malefyt[2], Robert L. Coffman[3], and Anne O'Garra[3]

Departments of [1]Molecular Biology, [2]Pharmacology, and [3]Immunology, DNAX Research Institute of Molecular and Cellular Biology Inc., Palo Alto, California 94304; e-mail: robert.coffman@dnax.org; rene.de.waal.malefyt@dnax.org; kevin.moore@dnax.org; anne.o'garra@dnax.org

Key Words interferon, inflammation, tolerance, infectious disease, dendritic cell, monocyte, macrophage, T cell, T regulatory cell

■ **Abstract** Interleukin-10 (IL-10), first recognized for its ability to inhibit activation and effector function of T cells, monocytes, and macrophages, is a multifunctional cytokine with diverse effects on most hemopoietic cell types. The principal routine function of IL-10 appears to be to limit and ultimately terminate inflammatory responses. In addition to these activities, IL-10 regulates growth and/or differentiation of B cells, NK cells, cytotoxic and helper T cells, mast cells, granulocytes, dendritic cells, keratinocytes, and endothelial cells. IL-10 plays a key role in differentiation and function of a newly appreciated type of T cell, the T regulatory cell, which may figure prominently in control of immune responses and tolerance in vivo. Uniquely among hemopoietic cytokines, IL-10 has closely related homologs in several virus genomes, which testify to its crucial role in regulating immune and inflammatory responses. This review highlights findings that have advanced our understanding of IL-10 and its receptor, as well as its in vivo function in health and disease.

INTRODUCTION

Interleukin-10 (IL-10) was first described as cytokine synthesis inhibitory factor (CSIF) (1), an activity produced by mouse Th2 cells that inhibited activation of and cytokine production by Th1 cells. Mouse and human IL-10 (mIL-10, hIL-10) cDNAs were reported a short while later, along with the discovery of IL-10's counterpart Epstein-Barr virus gene, BCRF1 (viral IL-10, vIL-10) (2–4). The ability of IL-10 to inhibit cytokine production by both T cells and NK cells was found to be indirect, via inhibition of accessory cell (macrophage/monocyte) function (5–8). These studies were soon extended to show that IL-10 profoundly inhibited a broad spectrum of activated macrophage/monocyte functions, including

0732-0582/01/0407-0683$14.00

monokine synthesis, NO production, and expression of class II MHC and costimulatory molecules such as IL-12 and CD80/CD86 (9–16).

In vitro and in vivo studies with recombinant cytokine and neutralizing antibodies revealed pleiotropic activities of IL-10 on B, T, and mast cells (17–22) and provided evidence for in vivo significance of several of IL-10s in vitro activities (23–25). Inflammatory bowel disease and other exaggerated inflammatory responses exhibited by IL-10 deficient (IL-10-/-) mice (26–28) indicated that a critical in vivo function of IL-10 is to limit inflammatory responses. Clinical studies of IL-10 in normal subjects and several human inflammatory and autoimmune settings are well underway (29).

This is being written at the tenth anniversary of IL-10's discovery. Our database searches reveal nearly 4200 reports of research involving IL-10. This chapter emphasizes more recent developments illuminating the role of IL-10 in normal and pathological immune responses in vivo, as well as IL-10 and IL-10 receptor (IL-10R) structure and signalling.

IL-10 PROTEIN, GENE, AND EXPRESSION

Protein

IL-10 amino acid sequences have been derived from cloned cDNAs. The Genbank database contains entries for the human (4), pig-tailed macaque, mangabey, rhesus, and owl monkeys, lemur, mouse (2), rat (30), guinea pig, Syrian hamster, rabbit, woodchuck, gerbil, opossum, cat, dog, cow, sheep, red deer, pig, horse, and killer whale cytokines. The open reading frames (ORF) encode secreted proteins of $\sim$178 amino acids with rather well conserved sequences—mIL-10 and hIL-10 are $\sim$73% identical—consistent with an α-helical bundle structure similar to interferons and hemopoietic cytokines (31).

Recombinant hIL-10 and vIL-10 are 17–18 kDa polypeptides that are not N-glycosylated. Both recombinant and T cell–derived mIL-10 appear to be heterogeneously N-glycosylated at a site near the N-terminus (2, 32); glycosylation of mIL-10 has no known influence on biological activity. At least one rat monoclonal antibody (Mab) cross-reacts with m- and hIL-10 (33). hIL-10 is active on both mouse and human cells, whereas mIL-10 is effective only on mouse cells.

Early studies suggested that IL-10 is dimeric (1, 34, 35). Biochemical (36) and X-ray crystallographic analyses of hIL-10 (37–39) and vIL-10 (40) demonstrated that IL-10 is an acid-sensitive, noncovalent homodimer of two interpenetrating polypeptide chains, similar to interferon-γ (IFNγ) (41). An engineered hIL-10 altered to favor monomer formation bound to the IL-10 receptor (IL-10R) and retained biological activity, although with reduced (60-fold) affinity and 10-fold lower specific activity in a biological assay compared to the wild-type cytokine (42).

Synthetic peptides derived from the IL-10 amino acid sequence were described that appear to mimic certain IL-10 activities in vitro and in vivo (43, 44). A peptide consisting of the 9 C-terminal amino acids of hIL-10 was reported to inhibit IL-8 production and HLA-DR expression by human monocytes and TNF production by $CD8^+$ T cells, enhance IL-1RA production by monocytes, chemoattract $CD8^+$ T cells, and enhance proliferation of a murine mast cell line (MC/9) in response to IL-4. A second peptide corresponding to hIL-10 amino acids #8–#16 also stimulated MC/9 cells but did not exhibit any other IL-10-like activities (43). Administration of the former peptide in a rabbit model of acute lung injury reportedly reduced mortality and inhibited development of acute lung injury (44). These results imply provocatively that IL-10 actions can be mimicked by small fragments of the cytokine. As no information is yet available regarding direct interaction of such peptides with IL-10R or induction of IL-10R-dependent signaling pathways, it remains to be determined whether they act as genuine IL-10 mimics or function indirectly, for example by facilitating endogenous IL-10 expression or release.

The IL-10 Gene and Its Expression

The mIL-10 and hIL-10 genes are encoded by five exons on the respective chromosomes 1 (45, 46). Activation of IL-10 gene expression results in ∼2 kb (hIL-10) and ∼1.4 kb (mIL-10) mRNAs; a ∼1 kb mRNA was also seen in a mouse Th2 clone (2, 4). IL-10 can be expressed by a variety of cells, usually in response to an activation stimulus; clearly its expression is regulated by different mechanisms in different cell types, such as T cells and monocytes/macrophages (reviewed in 47). Recent work has shown that, in contrast to many other cytokines, IL-10 transcription can be regulated by transcription factors Sp1 and Sp3, which are expressed constitutively by many different cell types (48, 49). Combined with control of IL-10 mRNA stability at the posttranscriptional level (50), this suggests that the IL-10 gene is transcribed to some degree constitutively and subject to control by alteration of posttranscriptional RNA degradation mechanisms. This situation under some circumstances may facilitate more rapid control of IL-10 expression than can be achieved just by activation of transcription. In this regard we note that a transient, massive IL-10 release attributed to liver macrophages was reported during liver transplantation (51).

Several polymorphisms have been noted in the human IL-10 gene 5′-flanking sequence. They include two areas of multiple (CA)n repeat microsatellite polymorphisms ∼1.2 kb and ∼4 kb upstream of the transcription start site and three linked point mutations at −1082(G/A), −819(C/T), and −592(C/A) (52, 53). Although the IL-10 promoter has not been completely defined, these polymorphisms are presumed to lie within the promoter region. Indeed, a correlation of particular microsatellite polymorphisms with LPS-induced IL-10 secretion by PBMC in vitro (presumably mostly from monocytes) was reported (54); the −1082(G) allele was associated with higher ConA-induced IL-10 production (likely both T cells and monocytes) (55). While individual variation was considerable, these trends were statistically significant.

Possible linkage of IL-10 promoter haplotypes to disease susceptibility or severity has been reported. Perhaps the strongest association is for systemic lupus erythematosus (SLE), where high IL-10 expression (56, 57), and the corresponding IL-10 alleles (58), have been suggested to play a causal or exacerbatory role (59–61). To what extent high IL-10 expression actually contributes to or is just a consequence of the disease is unclear. However, healthy relatives of lupus patients also exhibit elevated IL-10 expression (57, 62), suggesting that high IL-10 levels may predispose to disease and precede onset. A recent study also indicated a 40-fold increased risk for developing SLE in individuals who have particular alleles of both the IL-10 and bcl-2 genes (63). One of the lupus susceptibility loci in the New Zealand mouse is near IL-10 on chromosome 1 (64), and an IL-10 promoter polymorphism in this strain has been noted (65).

Genetic predisposition to high IL-10 expression is also associated with a higher rate of mortality in meningococcal disease (66). Chronically infected hepatitis C patients who are genetically predisposed to high IL-10 production were reportedly less likely to benefit from IFNα therapy (67).

Genes Related to IL-10

Recent studies identified cellular genes encoding proteins with weak (<30%) homology but unmistakeable structural relationship to IL-10. A Herpesvirus saimiri-induced gene, AK155, is encoded on human chromosome 12q15 near the IFNγ locus and is also expressed at low levels by uninfected T cells (68). Mouse T cells also express an IL-9-inducible cytokine-like molecule, IL-TIF (69), the human version of which (70) has also been termed IL-22 (71). The mouse mob-5 gene is induced by oncogenic ras expression (72) and encodes a secreted protein related to IL-10 and to the rat C49a (73) and human mda-7 (74–76) proteins.

The biological activities of these IL-10-related proteins are not well characterized. AK155 has no known function. IL-TIF/IL-22 activated Stat1, Stat3, and Stat5 in mesangial and neuronal cell lines (69), a renal carcinoma, and colon, and it may inhibit to some degree IL-4 production by Th2-polarized human T cells (71). IL-TIF/IL-22 enhanced production of acute-phase reactants in the HepG2 cell line and in mouse liver in response to IL-TIF/IL-22 injection (70). The receptor for IL-TIF/"IL-22" appears to consist of IL-10R2/CRF2-4 and a novel IFNR family member termed "IL-22R;" both subunits are required for signal transduction (70, 71). Although both receptor subunits detectably bind IL-TIF/IL-22, the relative ligand affinities of these IL-22R subunits and their combination are not yet known (71).

Mob-5 may be the mouse homolog of rat C49a and human mda-7, and as such it could share the latter's reported ability to inhibit growth of and induce apoptosis in certain tumor cells and cell lines by an unknown mechanism (74–76). However mob-5 is a secreted protein, whereas mda-7 was reportedly expressed intracellularly. The biological functions of these and potentially other relatives of IL-10 thus remain to be established.

Viral IL-10 Genes

IL-10 gene homologs have been found in the Epstein-Barr virus (EBV), equine herpes virus type 2 (EHV2), poxvirus Orf, and human cytomegalovirus genomes (2, 4, 77–79). Except for cytomegalovirus IL-10 (cmvIL-10), conservation of amino acid sequence between the viral and host cellular IL-10 (cIL-10) proteins is striking: the mature hIL-10 and EBV viral IL-10 (vIL-10) amino acid sequences are 84% identical, and most differences occur in the N-terminal 20 amino acids. Not unexpectedly, nearly all anti-hIL-10 antibodies–and ELISA assays utilizing them–cross-react with vIL-10 (10, 80, 81). Likewise, the EHV2 and Orf IL-10 homologs differ most from cellular IL-10s in the N-terminal region. vIL-10 is a 17-kDa nonglycosylated polypeptide that is expressed during the lytic phase of virus infection (82, 83) and exhibits only a subset of cIL-10 activities in vitro and in vivo (4, 5, 18, 19, 47, 81, 84–86), which as discussed later, implies the existence of distinct IL-10R complexes and/or signal transduction mechanisms on vIL-10-responsive and vIL-10-nonresponsive cells.

cmvIL-10 has several unique features among viral IL-10s. First, it is only 27% identical to hIL-10, in contrast to the much closer similarity exhibited by EBV vIL-10. Nonetheless, cmvIL-10 binds to and signals via the IL-10R complex (79). In addition, the cmvIL-10 gene has conserved the positions of introns 1 and 3 of hIL-10, while the other vIL-10s lack intervening sequences. These observations support the notion that vIL-10s represent captured cIL-10 genes, which then evolved to suit requirements of each particular virus' interaction with the host.

THE IL-10 RECEPTOR AND IL-10 SIGNALING

IL-10R Structure and Expression

The IL-10 receptor is composed of at least two subunits that are members of the interferon receptor (IFNR) family.

IL-10R1   The ligand-binding subunit (IL-10Rα, IL-10R1) binds cIL-10 with high affinity (K_d ~35–200 pM) (33, 34, 81, 87). Its affinity for vIL-10 is at least 1000-fold lower (42, 81, 88). Cross-linking studies with ^{35}S-Met- or ^{125}I-hIL-10 and immunoprecipitation data indicated a molecular size of 90–120 kDa for IL-10R1 (33, 34, 81, 87), consistent with N-glycosylated hIL-10R1 and mIL-10R1 proteins of 578 and 576 amino acids, respectively (60% homologous). Consistent with the observed species-specificity of IL-10, mIL-10R1 binds both mIL-10 and hIL-10, while hIL-10R1 does not bind mIL-10. mIL-10R1 encoded by mast cell and macrophage-derived cDNAs were identical, even though these cells respond differently to cIL-10 and vIL-10 (87). IL-10R1 mRNA was detected in all IL-10-responsive cells tested, and neutralizing anti-IL-10R1 monoclonal antibodies (Mabs) blocked all known cIL-10 and vIL-10 activities (33, 81, 87, 89); thus IL-10R1 is required for responses to both cIL-10 and vIL-10. The hIL-10R1 gene maps to chromosome 11q23.3 (33, 90).

Although there are no reports of detection of soluble IL-10R1 (sIL-10R1) in vivo, recombinant sIL-10R1 has been expressed (81, 89, 91). High shIL-10R1 concentrations relative to ligand exhibited antagonist activity in vitro (81, 91). hIL-10/shIL-10R1 complexes can be multimeric, consisting of up to two ligand dimers bound to as many as four shIL-10R1 molecules (42, 91). Consistent with this, we have observed that at low sIL-10R1:IL-10 ratios, sIL-10R1 can potentiate, rather than inhibit IL-10 activity (Y Liu, S H-Y Wei, & KW Moore, unpublished).

Model studies (39) based on the likely related structure of the IFNγ/sIFNγR1 complex (41) suggested that the regions of IL-10 likely involved in contact with IL-10R1 were the N-terminus, helix A, the AB loop, part of helix B, and the C-terminal helices E/F. Epitope and peptide mapping data generally supported this picture (92). The altered sequence and structure of the vIL-10 N-terminus (40) suggest impaired IL-10R1 interaction in this region and are consistent with the dramatically lower affinity of vIL-10 for IL-10R1 (81).

IL-10R1 is expressed by most hemopoietic cells, although generally at measured levels of only a few hundred per cell (33, 34, 81, 87, 93). IL-10R1 expression on T cells is downregulated by activation at both the mRNA (33) and protein levels; in contrast, activation of monocytes is associated with upregulation of IL-10R1 expression (R dW Malefyt, KW Moore, unpublished), consistent with IL-10's role as an inhibitory factor for these cells.

IL-10R1 expression has been observed on nonhemopoietic cells as well, although it is more often induced rather than constitutive. For example, IL-10R1 expression was induced in fibroblasts by LPS (94), and in epidermal cells or keratinocytes by glucocorticoids, a leflunomide metabolite, or dihyroxy-vitamin D3 (95–97). Constitutive IL-10R1 expression by placental cytotrophoblasts (98) and colonic epithelium (99, 100) has been described.

IL-10R2   Like IFNγR (101) and IFN$\alpha\beta$R (102), IL-10R utilizes an accessory subunit for signaling, IL-10R2 (IL-10Rβ). IL-10R2 was originally described as orphan IFNR family member CRFB4/CRF2-4 located in the IFNR gene complex on chromosome 21 (human) and 16 (mouse) (103–105). Several lines of evidence support IL-10R2's role in the IL-10R complex. First, hIL-10R2 complements defective hIL-10R1 signaling in transfected hamster cell lines and can be cross-linked to and coprecipitated with IL-10/IL-10R1 in IL-10-responsive cells (106). Moreover, IL-10R2$-/-$ mice, like IL-10$-/-$ animals, develop chronic severe enterocholitis, and cells from these mice are unresponsive to IL-10 (107) (however, presumably IL-TIF/IL-22 functions are also impaired in IL-10R2 $-/-$ mice). Finally, anti-hIL-10R2 Mabs block IL-10 responses (Y Liu, KW Moore, R dW Malefyt, unpublished). IL-10R2 contributes little to IL-10-binding affinity; its principal function appears to be recruitment of a Jak kinase (Tyk2) into the signaling complex (106, 107) (see below). Thus, in studies utilizing IFNγ as ligand and a hybrid receptor containing the extracellular domain of IFNγR1 and cytoplasmic signaling domain of IL-10R1, the accessory subunit functions required to generate the expected array of "IL-10" responses could be provided by IFNγR2 (108).

IL-10R2 is constitutively expressed in most cells and tissues examined (103, 105), and we have found no evidence for significant activation-associated regulation of IL-10R2 expression in immune cells (KW Moore, R dW Malefyt, unpublished). Thus, any stimulus activating IL-10R1 expression should suffice to render most cells responsive to IL-10.

IL-10R Signal Transduction

IL-10 and the Jak/stat System   Because of widespread interest and reagent availability, the best characterized IL-10 signaling pathway is the Jak/stat system. The IL-10/IL-10R interaction engages the Jak family tyrosine kinases Jak1 and Tyk2 (109, 110), which are constitutively associated with IL-10R1 (A Mui, HY Wei, KW Moore, unpublished) and IL-10R2 (106) respectively. IL-10 induces tyrosine phosphorylation and activation of the latent transcription factors stat3, stat1, and in nonmacrophage cells, stat5 (109, 111–113).

Recent studies, both in vitro and in gene-deficient mice, have linked the biology of IL-10 to IL-10 signaling molecules and pathways. Macrophages from Jak1$-/-$ mice do not respond to IL-10 (114), which indicates that Jak1 plays an obligatory early role in IL-10 signaling. Stat3 is also implicated strongly as a key mediator of IL-10 responses. Stat3 is recruited directly to the IL-10/IL-10R complex via either of two tyrosine residues in the IL-10R1 cytoplasmic domain that become phosphorylated in response to IL-10 (113) and are required for IL-10 signalling (89, 108, 110). Overexpression of a dominant negative stat3 mutant or an inducibly active form of stat3 demonstrated that stat3 activation was both necessary and sufficient to mediate inhibition of macrophage proliferation by IL-10 (89), at least in part via enhancement of expression of the cell cycle inhibitors p19^{INK4D} and p21^{CIP1} (115). In contrast, the stat3 mutant did not detectably impair IL-10's ability to inhibit LPS-induced monokine production (the "anti-inflammatory" activity of IL-10), nor did the inducibly active form of stat3 itself effect inhibition of acitivation-induced monokine synthesis. These observations suggest that inhibition of macrophage proliferation and monokine production by IL-10 are governed by two distinct signaling pathways, the former requiring stat3 (89).

Recent data refined this picture. "Conditional knockout" mice, in which stat3 expression was abolished in macrophages and neutrophils, develop chronic enterocholitis, and their macrophages are completely refractory to the effects of IL-10 (108, 116). These observations seem to conflict with those of O'Farrell et al. (89), however the latter's "dominant negative" stat3 mutant likely lacks only the transcription factor activity of stat3, while other possible functions, such as that of a docking molecule that could recruit other proteins to the IL-10R complex, may remain intact. Moreover, it appears that activation of stat3, while necessary for the anti-inflammatory action of IL-10, is not sufficient: a C-terminal ~15 amino acid segment of IL-10R1, along with stat3, plays a key functional role in inhibition of macrophage activation by IL-10, but not in other IL-10 functions (108). Thus, the current picture regards stat3 as indispensible for IL-10 signaling in all IL-10-responsive cells, but one or more additional pathway(s) must be activated to effect inhibition of macrophage activation by IL-10.

In contrast to stat3, the roles of stat1 and stat5 in IL-10 biology and signal transduction remain unclear. Stat1 and stat5 do not appear to interact directly with the IL-10/IL-10R complex (113), and overexpression of dominant negative stat1 or stat5 did not block IL-10's effects on a macrophage cell line (89). Moreover, macrophages from stat1$-/-$ mice remain responsive to IL-10 (117), although a detailed characterization of their IL-10 responses has not been reported. Furthermore, since the bulk of IL-10 signaling studies have been carried out using monocytes/macrophages, T cells, and B cells, it is possible that less understood IL-10 signaling pathways play prominent roles in other cells. For example, IL-10 has a number of effects on neutrophils but induces little FcγRI expression or detectable stat1 or stat3 activation in these cells (118, 119).

How does IL-10 signaling via the Jak/stat pathway result in inhibition of macrophage activation? A recent report (120) showed that IL-10's inhibition of IFN-induced gene transcription (IP-10, ISG54, ICAM-1) in human monocytes correlates with an observed inhibition by IL-10 of IFN-induced stat1 activation and tyrosine phosphorylation (120, 121). The latter inhibition diminished at higher IFN concentrations relative to IL-10, suggesting competing or interacting IL-10- and IFN-induced intracellular mechanisms, the relative strengths of which determine the degree of stat1 activation and IFN-induced gene transcription. Moreover, IL-10 rapidly induced transcription of SOCS3 (120, 122), which in some cells is a stat3-regulated gene (123). Whether IL-10-induced SOCS3 provides mainly negative feedback regulation of IL-10 signaling itself or also contributes significantly to IL-10's inhibition of the IFN response remains to be determined.

Other IL-10 Signaling Pathways   Consistent with its ability to inhibit macrophage activation and monokine production, IL-10 inhibits NFκB activation in response to stimuli in vitro (124–128). Inhibition of NFκB activation in CD3$^+$ T cells was also reported although it appears to be indirect, via the accessory cell (129). The in vitro data correlated with in vivo observations (130, 131), although in vivo effects may be direct or indirect. Mechanism studies revealed that IL-10 inhibits NFκB activation at least two different ways: by inhibiting activation of IκB kinase–similar to salicylate (132)–and by inhibiting NFκB DNA binding activity (the latter mechanism is not understood) (125).

However, it was also reported that IL-10 activates AP-1 and NFκB in CD8$^+$ T cells (133). This finding, while in contrast to IL-10's effects on macrophages and CD4$^+$ T cells, is nonetheless consistent with IL-10's ability to promote growth, differentiation, and cytotoxic activity of both $CD8^+$ T cells and NK cells (8, 21, 134–139), and it suggests significant differences in the responses of $CD4^+$ and $CD8^+$ T cells to IL-10.

IL-10 induced Bcl-2 expression in $CD34^+$ progenitors and germinal center B cells (140, 141), consistent with its growth-cofactor activity on such cells. IL-10 also activated c-fos expression in human B cells (142). In monocytes, IL-10 activated p85 PI3- and p70 S6 kinases, although specific blockade of these pathways affected only the proliferation-regulating but not anti-inflammatory activities of IL-10 (143).

Activation of the raf/ras/MAP kinase cascade does not occur in response to IL-10 and may be inhibited in some cases (144–146). In this light it is unlikely that IL-10 on its own could sustain long-term cellular proliferation; rather it would act as a viability-enhancing or growth cofactor cytokine (110).

BIOLOGICAL ACTIVITIES OF IL-10

Effects of IL-10 on Monocytes, Macrophages, and Dendritic Cells

IL-10 modulates expression of cytokines, soluble mediators and cell surface molecules by cells of myeloid origin, with important consequences for their ability to activate and sustain immune and inflammatory responses. The effects of IL-10 on cytokine production and function of human macrophages are generally similar to those on monocytes, although less pronounced (147–153).

IL-10 potently inhibits production of IL-1α, IL-1β, IL-6, IL-10 itself, IL-12, IL-18, GM-CSF, G-CSF, M-CSF, TNF, LIF and PAF by activated monocytes/macrophages (10, 11, 154–156). The inhibitory effects of IL-10 on IL-1 and TNF production are crucial to its anti-inflammatory activities, because these cytokines often have synergistic activities on inflammatory pathways and processes, and amplify these responses by inducing secondary mediators such as chemokines, prostaglandins, and PAF.

IL-10 also inhibits production of both CC (MCP1, MCP-5, Mip-1α, Mip-1β, Mip-3α, Mip-3β, Rantes, MDC) and CXC chemokines (IL-8, IP-10, MIP-2, KC (Gro-α) by activated monocytes (152,157–159). These chemokines are implicated in the recruitment of monocytes, dendritic cells, neutrophils, and T cells. Thus, IL-10 inhibits expression of most inducible chemokines that are involved in inflammation. Moreover, IL-10 thereby has the ability to affect both Th1 and Th2 responses: IP-10 is induced by IFNγ and attracts Th1 cells, and MDC is induced by IL-4 and attracts Th2 cells. IL-10 upregulates expression of the fMLP receptor, the PAF receptor, CCR1, CCR2, and CCR5 on monocytes, making these cells more responsive to chemotactic factors (160–162) and monocytes more susceptible to HIV infection (160, 161). In contrast, IL-12 inhibits CCR5 expression by monocytes (163).

IL-10 not only inhibits production of these effectors, but in addition, enhances expression of their natural antagonists. IL-10 enhanced production of interleukin-1 receptor antagonist (IL-1RA) and soluble p55 and p75 TNFR (164–167), and it inhibited expression of IL-1RI and IL-1RII (10, 168, 169) by activated monocytes, indicating that IL-10 not only deactivates monocytes but also induces production of anti-inflammatory molecules. In addition, the chemokine HCC4 is strongly upregulated by IL-10 in monocytes and is a chemoattractant for monocytes (170). This would suggest that HCC4 has an anti-inflammatory role, possibly by recruitment of monocytes and macrophages in the resolving phase of an inflammatory response. Moreover, pretreatment of monocytes with MCP1–4 suppressed production of IL-12p70 by inducing endogenous IL-10 production, providing further evidence for interactions between IL-10 and chemokines to regulate inflammation (171). These findings fit with a novel paradigm in which chemokines and chemokine receptors are oppositely regulated by pro- and anti-inflammatory mediators, including IL-10 and TGFβ (161, 172).

Both transcriptional and posttranscriptional mechanisms have been implicated in the inhibitory effects of IL-10 on cytokine and chemokine production (9, 127, 173, 174). IL-10 regulates production of certain cytokines, such as Gro-α (KC), by destabilizing mRNA via AU-rich elements in the 3′-UTR of sensitive genes (175, 176). IL-10 also enhances IL-1RA expression via inhibition of mRNA degradation (177).

IL-10 inhibited production of prostaglandin E2 (PGE2), through downregulation of cyclooxygenase 2 (COX-2) expression (178–180). This also affected expression of matrix metalloproteinases, which are regulated by a PGE-cAMP pathway (180). Consequently, IL-10 inhibited the ability of monocytes/macrophages to modulate extracellular matrix turnover through its inhibitory effects on the production of gelatinase and collagenase (MMP2/MMP9), and also its ability to enhance production of tissue inhibitor of metalloproteinases (TIMP) and hyaluronectin, which binds and inhibits angiogenic- and migration-promoting activities of hyaluronic acid (180–184).

IL-10 inhibited expression of MHC class II antigens, CD54 (ICAM-1), CD80 (B7), and CD86 (B7.2) on monocytes, even following induction of these molecules by IL-4 or IFNγ (5, 12, 185, 186), through a posttranscriptional mechanism involving inhibition of transport of mature, peptide loaded MHC class II molecules to the plasma membrane (187). Downregulated expression of these molecules significantly affected the T cell–activating capacity of monocyte APC (5–7).

IL-10 enhanced expression of CD16 and CD64 FcγR on monocytes (154, 188, 189) but downregulated the expression of IL-4-induced CD23 (FcεRII) (190). Upregulation of CD64 correlated with enhanced antibody-dependent cell-mediated cytotoxicity (ADCC) (188). Upregulation of FcγR expression by IL-10 correlated with an enhanced capacity of monocytes/macrophages to phagocytose opsonized particles, bacteria, or fungi (191, 192), although IL-10 reduced the ability of the cells to kill the ingested organisms by decreasing the generation of superoxide anion ($O_2{}^-$) and nitric oxide (NO) (9, 13, 193–198). The inhibitory effects of IL-10 on production of NO by mouse macrophages occurred by an indirect mechanism involving inhibition of endogenous cytokine (TNF, IFNγ) synthesis (14, 199). Interestingly, ligation of CD23 or CD64 induced expression of IL-10 by monocytes, which was active in suppressing inflammation (200, 201). These results suggest that a regulatory loop exists whereby IL-10 (or IFNγ) upregulates CD64 expression and subsequent CD64 ligation leads to enhanced IL-10 production, which inhibits the inflammatory response. This has indeed been demonstrated by induction of peripheral tolerance to an aggregated encephalitogenic proteolipid protein–Ig fusion in a model of EAE, resulting in IL-10 production and amelioration of disease (202).

Thus, IL-10 inhibits cytokine, chemokine, and PGE2 production (178, 179), and antigen presentation. IL-10 also downregulates expression of TLR4, the signal-transducing receptor for LPS (203), and enhances expression of CD14, CD16, CD64, and CD163, a scavenger receptor that is downregulated by LPS, IFNγ and TNF (204). Collectively these observations indicate that IL-10 induces differentiation of a macrophage-like cell that limits ongoing immune responses and inflammation, and contributes to clearance of the infection via enhanced phagocytosis.

Effects of IL-10 on Dendritic Cells

Mouse and human dendritic cells (DC) are defined by their ability to activate and prime naïve resting T cells and initiate an immune response. However, different DC subsets have been described, and in vitro culture methods to obtain cells with characteristics closely resembling their in vivo counterparts were developed using either human CD34$^+$ stem cells or monocytes or rodent bone marrow (205).

When considering the effects of IL-10 on DC, it is important to note that mouse and human DC populations are not necessarily equivalent between species. Earlier work showed that IL-10 inhibited production of IL-12 and expression of costimulatory molecules by various types of DC (206–210), which correlated with its ability to inhibit primary alloantigen-specific T cell responses (211, 212). Recently, these observations have been extended and, in general, have shown that IL-10 treatment of DC can induce or contribute to a state of anergy in allo-antigen- or peptide-antigen- activated T cells (213–218). In addition, treatment of DC/T cell cocultures with glucocorticosteroids, vitamin D3, prostaglandins, or IFNα resulted in IL-10-producing T cell populations with either Th2 or Tr1 characteristics (219–224). Whether in these experiments such agents act on DC, on the T cell, or both remains unclear.

Culture of human monocytes with GM-CSF and IL-4 for 6 days induces a population of immature DC that can be activated by LPS, CD40 ligand, or TNF to mature into highly efficient APC that secrete IL-12 and induce differentiation of naïve T cells to Th1 cells. Addition of IL-10 during culture with GM-CSF and IL-4 or at the activation step inhibits generation and maturation of monocyte-derived DC. Instead, as observed with monocytes cultured in the absence of GM-CSF and IL-4, IL-10 induced differentiation of these immature DC into macrophage-like cells that expressed reduced levels of costimulatory molecules and MHC class II, did not produce IL-12, and exhibited enhanced phagocytosis (225–227). Increased expression of MCSF and MCSFR, as well as defined effects on expression of signal-transducing molecules, accompany these changes (145, 228). In contrast, IL-10 did not affect mature monocyte-derived DC; these cells may have lost IL-10R1 expression (KW Moore, R deW Malefyt, unpublished) in a way similar to fully differentiated DC from rheumatoid synovium (229).

IL-10 also affects lymphoid or plasmacytoid DC, defined in the human system by expression of IL-3R, CD4, and lack of CD11c. These cells produce large amounts of IFNα following activation by virus, and they differentiate in vitro with IL-3 and CD40L into "DC2" cells that can support differentiation of Th2 cells producing IL-10. IL-10 induced apoptosis of freshly isolated or cultured plasmacytoid DC (230), which could account for reduced production of IFNα observed following treatment of virus-activated PBMC with IL-10 (231). Interestingly, this DC population is enhanced in GCSF- or Flt-3 ligand-mobilized blood and, through its priming capacity for IL-10-producing Th2 cells, could contribute to prevention of GvHD and graft acceptance in peripheral blood stem cell transplantation (232, 233). The mouse DC population that has been designated lymphoid DC is defined by expression of CD8α. Interestingly, these cells produce IL-10 and can efficiently inhibit tumor antigen-specific responses induced by CD8- DC (234).

Different DC populations producing IL-10 have been identified from Peyer's patches and liver; these populations are associated with development of either Th2 responses or hyporesponsiveness (235, 236). In contrast, human DC derived from CD34$^+$ stem cells as well as mature Langerhans cells do not produce IL-10, although CD14$^+$ DC that are equivalent to CD11c positive cells do produce IL-10 (237–240). In general, the effects of IL-10 on DC are consistent with inhibition of Th1 inflammatory responses and can be achieved by inhibitory effects on "inflammation-inducing DC" or by induction of anti-inflammatory T cell populations by IL-10-producing DC.

Effects of IL-10 on Neutrophils

LPS, LPS plus IFNγ or TNF, opsonized yeast, or the MP-F2 manno-protein fraction of *Candida albicans* variously induce production of TNF, IL-1α/β, IL-8, IL-12p40, GROα, MIP1α/β, MIG, ITAC and IP10 by neutrophils; this cytokine and chemokine production is inhibited by IL-10 (177, 241–245). The inhibitory effects of IL-10 on cytokine and chemokine production were delayed, observed only from 2 h post-stimulation onward, and at least for LPS-induced production of chemokines were dependent on the inhibitory effects of IL-10 on endogenous TNF and IL-1β production (119, 241, 242). IL-10 also attenuated production of other inflammatory mediators such as platelet activating factor (PAF) (246).

Contradictory findings have been reported concerning the effects of IL-10 on prostaglandin (PG) production by PMN. LPS, TNF, and IL-1β induce expression of cyclooxygenase 2 (COX-2). Niiro et al. reported a reduction of COX-2 expression by IL-10, but others failed to confirm this (247, 248). In the same studies, Niiro et al. described effects of endogenously produced IL-10 by PMN, whereas others failed to demonstrate IL-10 production by human neutrophils (249, 250). It is possible that PMN populations used by Niiro were contaminated by monocytes. It is also controversial whether IL-10 can directly inhibit generation of superoxide anion production and the respiratory burst or whether it regulates the enhancing effects of IFNγ on these processes (119, 251, 252).

However, in vivo, IL-10 suppressed killing of phagocytosed bacteria, and neutralization of endogenous IL-10 led to enhanced survival in murine models of *Klebsiella pneumoniae, Streptococcus pneumoniae*, and *Mycobacterium avium* infections (253–255). Furthermore, IL-10 inhibited phagocytosis of *E. coli* and attenuated neutrophil microbicidal activity toward internalized bacteria (256), which correlated with a reduction in CR3 expression. Interestingly, in contrast to human monocytes, IL-10 did not induce expression of CD64 (FcγRI) on neutrophils and did not modify ingestion of IgG-coated SRBC, C3-coated zymosan particles, or *Candida*, although inhibition of ADCC by IL-10 has been described (118, 252). As noted above, the absence of CD64 modulation correlated with the lack of stat1 and stat3 phosphorylation in freshly isolated neutrophils by IL-10 (118, 122).

As for monocytes, IL-10 enhanced production of IL-1RA by neutrophils (177, 257). Together with the inhibitory effects on IL-1α/β production, this resulted in a significant shift in the IL-1α/β:IL-1RA ratio and diminished the proinflammatory effects of IL-1. These inhibitory effects of IL-10 on cytokine and chemokine production are responsible for the observed reduction of neutrophil migration in IgG complex-induced lung injury and LPS- or antigen-induced pulmonary inflammation (258–262).

IL-10 does not directly affect the spontaneous rate of human neutrophil apoptosis (263). However, whether LPS- or cytokine-induced survival of neutrophils and eosinophils is inhibited by IL-10 is controversial (245, 249, 260, 264).

Inhibition by IL-10 of production of chemokines, proinflammatory cytokines, and mediators of granulocyte survival no doubt helps to limit the duration and harmful pathology of inflammatory responses.

Effects of IL-10 on B Cells and Immunoglobulin Production

IL-10 enhanced expression of MHC class II antigens and survival of resting mouse B cells (18), and it inhibited motility and IL-5-induced antibody production against thymus-independent type I and II antigens (produced by B-1 cells) (265–267); serum immunoglobulin levels and development of B-1 cells were nonetheless normal in IL-10$-/-$ mice (26). Furthermore, inflammatory bowel disease (IBD) that develops in IL-10$-/-$ mice is not dependent on B cells (268), as the incidence and severity of the disease is not altered in IL-10$-/- \times$ Ig$\mu-/-$ mice. Studies involving administration of IL-10 protein, IL-10 gene delivery, IL-10 transgenic mice, or inhibition of IL-10 production by neutralizing mAbs or gene targeted animals all suggest that the in vivo role of IL-10 in murine B cell function is limited (269–271). A notable exception is the delayed onset of autoimmunity in lupus-prone NZB mice treated with anti-IL-10 Mab (25); however, it is not clear whether IL-10 directly affects B cells or instead acts on underlying autoimmune mechanisms that induce disease onset.

IL-10's effects on survival, proliferation, and differentiation of human B cells have been more extensively studied. IL-10 enhanced survival of normal human B cells (depending on their activation state), which correlated with increased expression of the anti-apoptotic protein bcl-2 (140, 272). IL-10 also induced hTERT expression and upregulated telomerase activity in B cells activated by anti-IgM (273). IL-10 is a potent cofactor for proliferation of human B cell precursors and mature B cells activated by anti-IgM, SAC, or CD40 cross-linking (20, 274). This IL-10-induced proliferation of activated B cells was further enhanced by both IL-2 and IL-4, which in the case of IL-2 correlated with IL-10-enhanced expression of the high-affinity IL-2 receptor on B cells (275).

B cell–derived and exogenous IL-10 affected B cell differentiation and isotype switching (276). Isotype-committed B cells, activated by SAC or anti-CD40 Mabs, produced large amounts of IgM, IgG1-3, and IgA in the presence of IL-10, and of IgG4 and IgE in the presence of both IL-10 and IL-4 (20, 277–280). Anti-CD40 and IL-10 stimulation of sIgD$^+$ naive B cells also resulted in production of IgD, IgM, IgG1-3, and IgA (281–283), and it was shown that IL-10 is a switch factor for IgG1, IgG3 (284), and in combination with TGFβ, for IgA1 and IgA2 (281, 285). Interestingly, in PBMC cultures, IL-10 enhanced IgG4 production, possibly by potentiating IL-4-induced IgG4 switching, and inhibited IgE production when added at the onset of culture, providing evidence that under certain conditions, it can differentiatially modulate IgG4 and IgE responses (277, 286). Long-term culture of B cells stimulated by either anti-CD40, activated T cells or follicular dendritic cells, and IL-10 resulted in differentiation of B cells into plasma cells (287–289) and IL-10 acted synergistically with CD27/CD70 signals to induce plasma cell differentiation from CD27$^+$ memory B cells (290).

The effects of IL-10 on B cell function suggest its therapeutic use in at least two indications. IL-10 may enhance Ig production or isotype switching in patients suffering from common variable immunodeficiencies (CVI). IL-10 induced production of IgA by anti-CD40 activated B cells of patients suffering from IgA-deficiency, although no defects in IL-10 production were observed in these patients (291). In addition, IL-10 and CD40 activation induced IgG production by X-linked hyper-IgM-syndrome patients (292). Secondly, antagonists of IL-10 could be useful in treatment of antibody-mediated autoimmune diseases such as systemic lupus erythematosus (SLE). Indeed, positive correlations were demonstrated between serum IL-10 levels and severity of disease, and between the production of IL-10 and auto-antibodies by SLE patients' B cells (56, 293–296); anti-IL-10 treatment of SLE patients ameliorated disease in a pilot trial (297).

Direct Effects of IL-10 on T Cells

IL-10 strongly inhibited cytokine production and proliferation of CD4$^+$ T cells and T cell clones via its downregulatory effects on APC function (5, 6). IL-10 also directly affects the function of T cells and inhibits IL-2, TNF, and IL-5 production depending on activation conditions (17, 298, 299) as well as expression of CXCR4 and chemotaxis in response to the CXCR4 ligand SDF1 (300). In contrast, IL-10 has stimulatory effects on $CD8^+$ T cells and induces their recruitment, cytotoxic activity, and proliferation (135, 136, 138, 301). Stimulatory activities of IL-10 on mouse T cells were also described where it acts as a thymocyte growth factor and augments outgrowth of cytotoxic T cell precursors (19, 21).

Interestingly, activation of T cells in the presence of IL-10 can induce nonresponsiveness/anergy, which cannot be reversed by IL-2 or stimulation by anti-CD3 and anti-CD28 (213). A role for IL-10 in induction and maintenance of nonresponsiveness or anergy was suggested by studies of anti-tumor cell responses, uv-induced tolerance, hapten-specific tolerance, parasitic and HIV infections, and superantigen-induced hyporesponsiveness (86, 302–309); such anergy can be induced by specifc immunotherapy (310) or by continuous antigenic challenge in vivo (311). IL-10-mediated anergy can be associated with induction of a population of regulatory T cells that produce high levels of IL-10 and can suppress antigen-specific responses in vivo and in vitro (312–320) as is discussed later.

Biological Functions of EBV vIL-10

EBV vIL-10 mimics several activities of IL-10, including CSIF/macrophage deactivating factor activity on mouse and human cells (3–5, 8, 10, 178, 194) and mouse and human B cell stimulatory activities (18, 20, 281). However, the ability of vIL-10 to manifest several other IL-10 activities on mouse and human cells is markedly reduced. vIL-10 did not enhance class II MHC expression on mouse B cells (18) or effectively costimulate mouse thymocyte or mast cell proliferation (4, 19). Similarly, vIL-10 had greatly reduced ($\sim$1000-fold) ability to inhibit IL-2 production by an activated human $CD4^+$ T cell clone, consistent with 3-log lower binding affinity for IL-10R1 (81). Nonetheless, sufficiently high vIL-10 concentrations did exhibit this latter activity.

These in vitro observations are consistent with animal model studies involving mIL-10 or vIL-10 gene transfer into immunogenic and allogeneic mouse tumor cells (84, 86). mIL-10-expressing tumors were more rapidly rejected compared to controls, but vIL-10-transduced tumor cells were either not rejected at all, or their mean survival time was significantly enhanced. Rejection of mouse heart allografts expressing vIL-10 was also inhibited (85). The results of such studies indicate that (a) vIL-10 has retained some—but not all—cIL-10 activities, and (b) by engaging only a subset of IL-10-responsive cells, vIL-10 can have a profoundly different effect on the outcome of an in vivo immune response than that of cIL-10.

What is the molecular basis for the different activity profiles of cIL-10 and vIL-10? That vIL-10 and cIL-10 differ most in sequence and structure in the N-terminal $\sim$20 amino acids (4, 40) suggests that this region should be important. However, an isoleucine/alanine interchange at position 87 of hIL-10/vIL-10 had significant effects on the proteins' activities (88). hIL-10 and mIL-10 when substituted at position 87 with alanine (cIL-10 I87A) lost most or all ability to stimulate proliferation of mouse thymocytes and a murine mast cell line, while retaining the CSIF activities of cIL-10. Likewise vIL-10 substituted at position 87 with isoleucine (vIL-10 A87I) acquired significant mast cell stimulating activity. Moreover, hIL-10 (I87A), like vIL-10, exhibited substantially (~100-fold) lower binding affinity for IL-10R1, whereas vIL-10 (A87I) was only ~30-fold reduced in its receptor-binding ability compared to hIL-10. These in vitro biological activities of mutant c,vIL-10 were paralleled by survival kinetics of mouse heart allografts transfected to express wild-type and mutant c,vIL-10s: hIL-10 (I87A), similar to vIL-10, enhanced survival compared to wild-type hIL-10, while vIL-10 (A87I) was significantly less able to prolong graft survival than vIL-10. While other sequence differences between cIL-10 and vIL-10 are doubtless important, the significance of position 87 is striking and awaits clarification via structural studies.

It is not yet certain if the restricted activities of vIL-10 developed via evolutionary drift or are of actual benefit to EBV. However, since vIL-10 is expressed during the lytic phase (82, 83), presumably the target cells for which it retains specificity–dendritic cells, macrophages/monocytes, B cells–are those specifically relevant to that portion of the EBV life cycle. vIL-10's ability to inhibit dendritic cell/macrophage/monocyte activation probably suppresses an anti-viral immune response, thus allowing the virus to establish latency. This idea was supported by studies showing that cells infected with a vIL-10-deleted EBV were, unlike wild-type virus-infected cells, unable to block IFNγ production by autologous human peripheral blood cells (321). In addition, the B cell growth and differentiation promoting activity could enhance the numbers and susceptibility to infection of EBV's principal host cell. However, in the absence of good animal models of EBV infection, it has proven difficult to confirm such notions. Whether vIL-10 plays any part in EBV-induced B cell transformation is controversial (321–323). Low IL-10 receptor (IL-10R1) binding affinity may restrict vIL-10 to local effects in the vicinity of the infected cell, as suggested by in vivo studies (85, 86). In any case, because it has been so highly conserved, vIL-10 likely confers a number of adaptive advantages upon EBV in its interaction with the immune system. Moreover, capture of an IL-10 gene by the ancestor of EBV was likely an important event in the development of the virus as a sophisticated, mostly benign parasite.

SYSTEMIC AND LOCALIZED ACUTE INFLAMMATION

A systemic inflammatory response can occur following septicemia or endotoxemia, as well as after non-infectious events such as severe trauma, burn, or ischemia-reperfusion injuries. A cascade of events including pro-inflammatory cytokine production, cell trafficking, extravasation, mediator production, coagulation, fibrinolysis, and changes in hemodynamic parameters and microvascular permeability can ultimately lead to disseminated intravascular coagulation (DIC), multiple organ failure, and death. It is important to note that the initial systemic inflammatory response syndrome (SIRS), which includes production of TNF and IL-1, can be followed by a state of immunosuppression or immunoparalysis (324).

TNF and IL-1 play a central role in the initiation and propagation of these events, since their administration can mimic–and inhibition of their production can prevent and ameliorate–this inflammatory response. The inhibitory effects of IL-10 on proinflammatory cytokine production and physiology of individual cell types suggest that it could have potent anti-inflammatory activities in vivo. Indeed, a protective role of IL-10 in experimental endotoxemia has been demonstrated. IL-10 rescued Balb/c mice from LPS-induced toxic shock, which correlated with reduced serum levels of TNF (325, 326). Inhibition of TNF production in experimental endotoxemia was also observed following IL-10 administration in baboons and humans (327, 328). Both IL-10 protein and intratracheal IL-10 gene transfer protected mice from a lethal intra-peritoneal endotoxin challenge and furthermore reduced pulmonary TNF levels and neutrophil infiltration following LPS challenge (329).

Administration of endotoxin induced IL-10 production in mice, chimpanzees, baboons, and humans (328, 330–332). This endogenous IL-10 confers significant protection from the harmful effects of endotoxin challenge and reduces TNF, IFNγ, and MIP-2 levels (333, 334) as well as regulates hemodynamic parameters, leukocyte-endothelial cell interactions, and microvascular permeability (335). Its protective role in endotoxemia is also clearly observed in mice treated from birth with anti-IL-10 Mabs and in IL-10$-/-$ mice, which are killed by 20-fold lower doses of LPS than kill wild-type mice (24, 28). IL-10$-/-$ mice were also extremely vulnerable to a generalized Schwartzmann reaction in which prior exposure to a small amount of LPS primes the host for a lethal response to a subsequent, otherwise sublethal dose (28). IL-10 is implicated in in vitro induction of endotoxin tolerance (336) and is involved in impaired antigen presentation observed under these conditions (337, 338). Interestingly, reduced expression of HLA-DR antigens on monocytes can be used as a prognostic marker for identification of patients with high risk of infection (339). As in endotoxin challenge models, IL-10 has shown efficacy in ischemia reperfusion and burn models (340–342).

The effects of IL-10 have also been assessed in infectious sepsis models using live microorganisms. In a model of septic peritonitis in which mice undergo cecal ligation and puncture, endogenous IL-10 was protective (334, 343, 344), and IL-10 protected neonatal mice from lethal streptococcal B infections (345). Furthermore, IL-10 prevented lethality due to SEB-induced shock, which is dependent on IL-2 and IFNγ production by T cells (346, 347).

Human IL-10 production during septicaemia and septic shock correlated with intensity of the inflammatory response, severity of injury (348–353), and with clinical outcome. This was especially evident in patients suffering from septic shock associated with meningococcal infections (354–356). In addition, many strategies that are used to intervene in sepsis affect IL-10 production (357–359), indicating an important role for this cytokine in controlling systemic inflammatory responses.

Similarly, IL-10 exhibited protective effects in several experimental models of local inflammation, such as pancreatitis (360), uveitis (361–364), keratitis (365), hepatitis (366), peritonitis (334, 343, 344), lung injury (259, 261, 367, 368), and brain or spinal cord injury (369, 370).

IL-10 IN INFECTIOUS DISEASE

The challenge faced by the immune system of an infected host is to respond with sufficient intensity and duration to control and eliminate the infection while minimizing nonspecific injury to host tissue. IL-10 plays a central role in striking a balance between pathology and protection; indeed, the phenotype of IL-10−/− mice suggests that this is the most essential of its many functions.

Certain aspects of IL-10 biology can be studied in vitro by measuring the effect of IL-10 on the responses of individual cell types to microorganisms or microbial products. However, host-pathogen interactions typically are complex, varying in time and location according to the life cycle of the pathogen and the evolution of the host response. Most of what has been learned about IL-10 in infectious disease derives from animal model (principally mouse) experiments in which pathology, protection, or both are altered by manipulating levels of IL-10 in vivo.

Innate and Specific Immune Responses to Intracellular Bacterial, Fungal and Protozoan Infections

Many of the inflammatory responses triggered by infectious microorganisms and regulated by IL-10 have been described in the previous section. The central features of the innate and adaptive immune responses against most intracellular pathogens are shown in Figure 1. A key concept in this scheme is the integral link between innate and adaptive immunity (371). Experimental support derives primarily from a few well-studied infections in mice, including *L. monocytogenes* (372, 373), *C. albicans* (374, 375), *L. major* (376), and *T. gondii* (377). However, a large body of data now confirms the generality of these mechanisms in humans and experimental animals, with, of course, many individual variations.

This "typical" response (Figure 1) to infection with a wide range of bacterial, fungal, and protozoan pathogens can be expressed as a sequence of distinct intercellular interactions leading to induction of an array of microbiocidal effector functions:

1. Recognition of the microbe or specific microbial products by macrophages, neutrophilic granulocytes, and/or dendritic cells. Many types of receptors can be involved in this recognition, and our understanding of this "primitive" form of immunity is far from complete. Many recognize molecules and chemical structures common to groups of microorganisms, such as bacterial endotoxin (recognized by Toll-like receptor 4) or cell-wall polysaccharides (recognized by a variety of lectins).

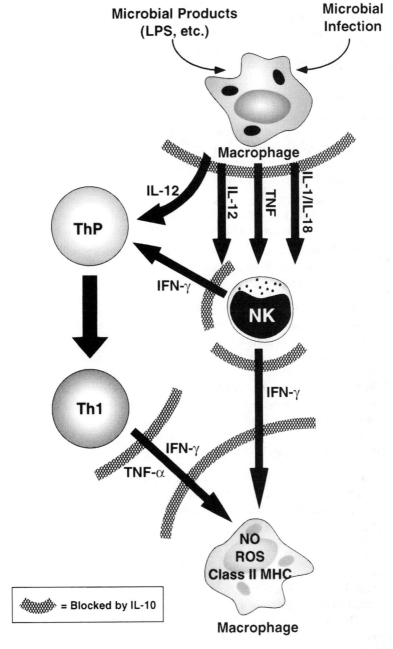

Figure 1 A schematic depiction of IL-10's roles in regulating the innate and adaptive immune responses to infection.

2. Recognition of microbial structures leads to production of multiple cytokines, especially IL-12, IL-18, TNF, and IL-1 by macrophages and monocytes. The combination of IL-12, IL-1, and TNF is particularly efficient in stimulating rapid production of IFNγ by NK cells. For fungal pathogens, such as *Candida*, neutrophils can be the major cell type producing IL-12 at this stage (119, 378).

3. NK-produced IFNγ induces multiple microbiocidal functions in macrophages, such as phagocytosis and production of nitric oxide and reactive oxygen intermediates, and stimulates cell infiltration by both macrophages and neutrophils. These mechanisms, in aggregate, can be very effective in controlling infections, even in the absence of subsequent specific T cell responses.

4. T cells responding to microbial antigens in a microenvironment dominated by this set of cytokines, especially IL-12 and IFNγ, preferentially differentiate into Th1 cells.

5. Th1 cells, largely through the production of IFNγ and TNF, continue to mediate essentially the same effector functions as the innate response, but with increased specificity and memory.

IL-10 inhibits many of the individual steps in this pathway of antimicrobial immunity (Figure 1). The inhibitory effect on some individual processes, even under optimized conditions, is often no more than 3- to 10-fold. However, this modest inhibition can be multiplied at sequential steps in the pathway, resulting in profound inhibition of the ultimate effector functions. Thus, the differences in response to infection between IL-10-overexpressing and IL-10-nonexpressing mice (Table 1) can sometimes be quite dramatic, greater than would be expected from a single in vitro analysis.

IL-10 in Animal Models of Infectious Disease

The overall role of IL-10 in animal models (principally mouse) of infectious disease has been determined by experimentally elevating or reducing IL-10 during the course of infection. In virtually all cases, elevated IL-10 levels have been produced by frequent injections of recombinant IL-10 or by the use of IL-10 transgenic mice. Likewise, reduction or elimination of IL-10 is effected either by treatment with neutralizing anti-IL-10 Mab or via the use of IL-10−/− mice. In general, these experiments are structured to produce mice with either little or no IL-10, or with high IL-10 levels effecting full IL-10R occupancy, thus defining the maximum range of IL-10 effects in these infections.

The effects of manipulating IL-10 in bacterial, fungal, and protozoan infections are summarized in Table 1, in terms of the effect on control or clearance of the infectious agents itself. Despite model-specific variations in treatment regimens and readouts, it is clear that resistance to infection can nearly always be improved by reducing IL-10 levels. Thus, even normal IL-10 levels tend to limit the effectiveness of the immune response to most pathogens. The inhibition imposed by endogenous IL-10 is far from complete, however, as administration of exogenous IL-10 nearly always further impairs an anti-pathogen response.

Based on the known effects of IL-10 on inflammatory responses (Figure 1), both innate and adaptive immune responses should be enhanced or impaired by experimental depletion or elevation, respectively, of IL-10 in vivo. This has been confirmed in mouse models in which the two forms of immune response can be clearly distinguished. For example, elevated IL-10 severely compromises resistance to *Listeria* in *scid* mice, which are deficient in the T and B cells required for adaptive immunity, but retain normal innate immunity (379, 380). Similarly, the enhanced innate response to *Listeria* in IL-10−/− (381) and anti-IL-10-treated (382) mice leads to rapid control of *Listeria* within the first few days of infection. Similar enhancement of early innate responses has been reported in *C. albicans* (383), *T. gondii* (384, 385), and *T. cruzi* (386) infections.

The effects of altering IL-10 levels in viral infection models have not been included in Table 1, as there are very few reports in which viral titers have been measured. IL-10−/− mice have more severe pathology and morbidity than do wild-type mice in a neurotropic mouse hepatitis virus model, but do not clear the virus more effectively (387). Similarly, rIL-10 reduced lesion formation and mortality in a viral myocarditis model, but did not lead to increased virus titers (388). The relative lack of influence of IL-10 on these antiviral responses may reflect the greater involvement of CD8$^+$ T cells in most antiviral responses. In contrast, Vaccinia virus replication is significantly impaired in IL-10−/− mice (389), perhaps reflecting a greater contribution of CD4$^+$ T cells to this response.

Modulation of Immunopathology by IL-10

The effects of IL-10 on pathogen control are only part of a complete view of IL-10 in infectious disease. The potent antimicrobial effector mechanisms induced via the pathway illustrated in Figure 1 can also cause significant collateral damage to the host that is often more harmful than the infection itself. This damage can range from localized destruction of infected cells to widespread tissue necrosis, from transient cellular infiltration to chronic granuloma formation with fibrosis and replacement of normal tissue. Moreover, destruction of small areas of critical tissues, such as cardiac muscle or myelin sheath, can have serious consequences. A sufficiently strong systemic response to microbes or their products can also lead to septic/toxic shock resulting in death from multiple organ failure. These consequences can occur in a host that is, paradoxically, controlling or clearing the primary infection quite effectively.

Thus, the critical role of IL-10 in infectious disease appears to be modulation of the pathological consequences of inflammatory responses to microbial pathogens. As described above for viral infections, this protection from immunopathology can occasionally involve minimal inhibition of the antimicrobial response by IL-10. More frequently, decreased immunopathology is at the expense of less efficient

TABLE 1   Low IL-10 increases resistance and high IL-10 increases susceptibility to intracellular pathogens in mouse models

Organism	Enhanced disease susceptibility when IL-10 increased by:			Enhanced disease resistance when IL-10 decreased by:		
	Method	Result	References	Method	Result	References
Bacteria						
Listeria monocytogenes	rIL-10	Yes	(379)	Anti-IL-10	Yes	(382)
	IL-10 TG	Yes	(269)	IL-10 KO	Yes	(381)
	induced IL-10	Yes	(380)	—	—	
Salmonella choleraesuis	—	—		Anti-IL-10	Yes	(644)
Klebsiella pneumoniae	—	—		Anti-IL-10	Yes	(254, 645)
Streptococcus pneumoniae	rIL-10	Yes	(255)	Anti-IL-10	Yes	(255)
Staphylococcus aureus	—	—		Anti-IL-10	Yes	(646)
Borrelia burgdorferi	—	—		IL-10 KO	Yes	(394)
Chlamydia trachomatis	—	—		Anti-IL-10	Yes	(647)
				IL-10 KO	Yes	(648)

Mycobacteria						
Mycobacterium avium	Anti-IL-10	Yes	(253, 649)	—	—	—
M. tuberculosis	IL-10 KO	No	(650)	—	—	—
M. bovis BCG	IL-10 KO	Yes	(652)	IL-10 TG	Yes	(651)
Fungi						
Candida albicans	Anti-IL-10	Yes	(654)	rIL-10	Yes	(653)
Cryptococcus neoformans	IL-10 KO	Yes	(383, 655)	—	—	—
Coccidioides immitis	IL-10 KO	Yes	(656)	—	—	—
Aspergillus fumigatus	IL-10 KO	Yes	(657)	—	—	—
	Anti-IL-10	Yes	(658)	—	—	—
	IL-10 KO	Yes	(655)	—	—	—
Protozoa						
Leishmania major	Anti-IL-10	No	(659)	rIL-10	No	(659)
	IL-10 KO	Yes	Coffman, unpublished	IL-10 TG	Yes/No	(269, 507)
Trypanosoma cruzi	Anti-IL-10	Yes	(660)	rIL-10	Yes	(386)
	IL-10 KO	Yes	(386, 391, 392)	—	—	—
Trypanosoma congolese	Anti-IL-10	Yes	(661)	—	—	—
Toxoplasma gondii	IL-10 KO	Yes (*scid* mice)	(384)	—	—	—

control or clearance of the infection. Experiments (Table 1) exploring extremes of high or low IL-10 demonstrate the consequences of inappropriate balance between inflammation and IL-10. IL-10−/− mice infected with *T. gondii* (384, 385), *P. chaubudi* (390), or certain strains of *T. cruzi* (391, 392) have greatly elevated IFNγ, IL-12 and TNF levels and reduced parasitemia, but a substantially increased risk of death from a toxic shock-like syndrome, compared to wild-type controls.

Similarly, infection of IL-10−/− mice with *H. hepaticus* leads to enterocolitis (393), and infection with *B. burgdorferi* leads to more severe Lyme arthritis in IL-10−/−, compared to wild-type mice (394). To the viral infection models mentioned previously can be added the model of herpes simplex virus–induced keratitis, which can be substantially inhibited by topical administration of IL-10 (365, 395, 396). In these examples, immunopathology is dependent upon Th1 (CD4$^+$) or Tc1 (CD8$^+$) T cells, but IL-10 also inhibits Th2-mediated granulomas and fibrosis in mouse models of schistomiasis (397–400).

The clinical promise of IL-10 in treating viral immunopathology was shown by a recent study in which hIL-10 reversed liver fibrosis without increasing viral titers in patients with chronic hepatitis C infection (401).

Evidence for a Role of IL-10 in Human Infectious Disease

As experimental tests of IL-10 in vivo of the sort that have been so informative in mouse models are not feasible in humans, it is necessary to rely upon correlative evidence in vivo and experimental evidence in vitro to show similarities or differences in IL-10 function between human and mouse.

Strong correlation exists between IL-10 protein or mRNA levels and a number of chronic or progressive human infectious diseases, including visceral leishmaniasis, (402–405), malaria (406, 407), filariasis (408–410), leprosy (411), tuberculosis (412, 413), candidiasis (414), and *M. avium* infection (415). In some diseases, IL-10 levels decreased upon successful resolution of the infection by drug therapy. Thus, much of the human data corresponds to data obtained, often with the same pathogens, in mouse models. However, correlative data do not allow one to distinguish whether high pathogen burdens are the cause of elevated IL-10 or vice versa. In actuality, it is likely that both scenarios occur.

The second type of evidence that IL-10 inhibits protective immunity in human, as in mouse, comes from experiments in which anti-IL-10 Mabs restore responses of pathogen-specific T cells from infected patients in vitro. This has been demonstrated in a number of chronic diseases, including visceral leishmaniasis, (403, 416), filariasis (409, 410), schistosomiasis (307), leprosy (417), and tuberculosis (418). Typically, PBL from such patients make little or no recall response in vitro to the pathogen or to antigenic fractions thereof. In most of these diseases, patients have been deemed "anergic" or "unresponsive" to the pathogen, despite quite high microbial burdens. However, neutralization of IL-10 during a 2–3-day culture period usually reveals a significant response of the Th1 or Th2 type, demonstrating active suppression by IL-10. The combination of elevated

IL-10 in vivo and IL-10-mediated unresponsiveness to antigen in vitro in many of these chronic diseases suggests strongly that IL-10 is a major cause of ineffective antipathogen immune responses. Such correspondence between mouse and human infections with the same or closely related organisms suggests that extrapolation from animal models is valid.

IL-10 has been studied extensively in HIV infection as well. Asymptomatic HIV[+] individuals frequently have defective responses not only to HIV proteins, but also to common antigens such as influenza and tetanus toxoid (419). As in the above examples, responses of blood lymphocytes from these patients can be enhanced in vitro by neutralization of IL-10 (420–422). It is not clear whether IL-10 plays a similar role in AIDS patients with low CD4[+] T cell counts, however. Understanding the role of IL-10 in AIDS is complicated by evidence that IL-10 has direct effects on virus production by infected cells. The significance of these in vitro observations is not yet clear, especially as IL-10 has been reported to either stimulate (423–425) or inhibit (426–428) HIV production by monocytic cells in vitro.

In summary, there is now extensive evidence in the mouse, and significant confirmation in human, that IL-10 production usually imposes some limits on the effectiveness of antipathogen immune responses, especially innate immunity and adaptive Th1 responses. This cost is often outweighed by the ability of IL-10 to protect the host from collateral damage by antimicrobial cytokines and effector molecules. A successful response must strike a balance between protection and pathology, and IL-10 appears central to the establishment of this balance. Thus, both IL-10 and IL-10 inhibitors may offer therapeutic promise in the treatment of either infectious diseases or infection-related immunopathologies.

THE ROLE OF IL-10 IN PROTECTION FROM ORGAN-SPECIFIC AUTOIMMUNITY

IL-10 plays a very important role in limiting the immune response to pathogens to eradicate the pathogen with minimum immunopathology to the host. Likewise, IL-10 has been suggested to play a role in peripheral tolerance and in protection against autoimmunity. In chronic autoimmune diseases, such as experimental autoimmune encephalomyelitis (EAE), diabetes, insulin-dependent diabetes mellitus (IDDM), and rheumatoid arthritis (RA), pathogenic roles have been ascribed to Th1 cells, due to their production of cytokines such as IFNγ, lymphotoxin, and TNF (429–433). In contrast, a protective role was attributed initially to Th2 cells because of their ability to produce the cytokines IL-4 and IL-10. However, this latter notion may not be accurate, since IL-10 is produced by a wide variety of cells. In this context CD4[+] T cell regulatory populations producing high levels of IL-10 have been described that can inhibit the proliferation of naive CD4[+] T cells and/or the induction of pathology by mucosal antigens, such as in inflammatory bowel disease (213, 312, 317, 434, 435). IL-10, as well as IL-4 and TGFβ, may play an essential role in tolerance to self antigens (436–440) and to mucosal antigens (312, 317, 434, 440, 441). However, TGFβ−/− mice develop a *multi-organ* autoimmune syndrome (442), whereas IL-4 and IL-10-deficient mice do not. IL-10-deficient mice do spontaneously develop inflammatory bowel disease (26, 443), which appears due to a defect in IL-10-producing regulatory T cells that moderate responsiveness to intestinal flora (317).

In this section the possible role of IL-10 in regulation of responses to auto- as well as mucosal antigens is discussed, as well as the potential use of IL-10 as a therapeutic in autoimmune and other inflammatory diseases. Regulatory T cells as a source of IL-10 and their potential in regulating both Th1 and Th2-mediated pathologies are discussed, as well as factors that induce IL-10 production.

IL-10 and Regulation of Experimental Autoimmune Encephalomyelitis (EAE)

Initial studies showed that spontaneous recovery of rats and mice from EAE correlated with expansion of Th2-like cells producing IL-4 and/or IL-10 (444–446). Furthermore, low IL-10 production was observed in chronic relapsing EAE (447), suggesting that endogenous IL-10 may regulate such pathologies of the central nervous system (CNS). IFNβ, which has been used with some success to treat MS patients, can induce expression of IL-10 in peripheral blood mononuclear cells (448), suggesting that one mechanism for protection involves IL-10 production.

Direct support for a role of IL-10 in regulating CNS autoimmune pathologies was provided by studies showing that neutralization of endogenous IL-10 increased the severity and incidence of SEB- or TNF-induced EAE relapse (449) and that disease is more severe in IL-10−/− than in wild-type mice (450–452).

Attempts to treat EAE with recombinant IL-10 yielded contradictory results. Systemic treatment of rats or mice with IL-10 partially inhibited disease progression in EAE induced by active immunization with CNS antigens, but only if treatment was begun at the time of initial immunization (453, 454). In this study, the initial use of site-directed delivery of IL-10 to the CNS at first yielded conflicting results. Intracranial injection of IL-10 or of plasmids expressing IL-10 cDNA under the control of a retroviral promoter 12 days after active immunization did not suppress EAE (455), nor did adoptive transfer of a myelin basic protein (MBP)-specific hybridoma transduced with IL-10 (456). This lack of effect could also reflect the timing of IL-10 expression. In contrast, IL-10 administration exacerbated disease in an adoptive transfer model of EAE (457). This latter result might have been obtained because (*a*) appropriate levels of IL-10 in the CNS were not attained, and/or (*b*) IL-10 may be necessary to inhibit development and/or migration of pathogenic encephalitogenic Th1 cells.

However, several other reports showed that IL-10 can effect virtually complete inhibition of EAE. Antigen-inducible IL-10 expressed under control of the IL-2 promoter in proteolipid protein (PLP)-specific T memory cells suppressed EAE when T cells were adoptively transferred to PLP-immunized mice one day prior to expected disease onset (458). Transgenic FVB X SJLF1 mice expressing murine IL-10 under control of the CD2 promoter were resistant to EAE induced by PLP immunization (450). Similarly, mice transgenic for human IL-10 (hIL-10-Tg) expressed under the control of the MHC class-II promoter were completely protected from induced EAE (459).

In hIL-10Tg mice several mechanisms are possible for the regulatory effect of hIL-10 in EAE: inhibition of the initial development of autoreactive Th1 cells; inhibition of Th1 effector function by IL-10; immune deviation toward a Th2-type response; or development of T regulatory populations which themselves produce IL-10. Generation of Th1 autoantigen was not impaired in hIL-10Tg mice, nor was there evidence of immune deviation to a Th2 response. IL-10-producing regulatory T cells were not implicated, as protection did not require T-cell-derived endogenous mIL-10. Furthermore, pathogenic Th1 populations passively transferred to hIL-10Tg mice caused no disease, whereas they did in nontransgenic controls. These observations suggested that the principal action of transgenic hIL-10 was inhibition of the effector stage of the autoimmune response (459). Such an effect of IL-10 on effector functions induced by Th1 cytokines, rather than on the Th1 cells themselves, was also evidenced by the ability of a replication-defective adenovirus vector expressing hIL-10 (hIL-10-rAdV), delivered intracranially, to completely inhibit EAE when given only 2–4 days prior to the onset of symptoms (460). Additionally, this treatment halted progression and accelerated remission when given to mice with active disease and prevented relapses when given during the first remission in a relapsing-remitting disease model.

The importance of the site and timing of IL-10 administration to therapeutic success was also demonstrated in experiments with hIL-10-rAdV (460). Intravenous injection of hIL-10-rAdV produced approximately the same systemic hIL-10 levels as intracranial injection, but was undetectable hIL-10 in the CNS and poor protection from EAE. Similarly, daily intracranial injection of hIL-10 protein could protect from EAE, but protection was rapidly lost when injections ceased. This need for sustained high hIL-10 levels at the site of potential inflammation indicates that IL-10 acts primarily by blocking entry and/or activity of pathogenic T cells in the CNS.

How Does IL-10 Affect Insulin-Dependent Diabetes Mellitus in the Nonobese Diabetic Mouse?

The nonobese diabetic (NOD) mouse is an animal model of human insulin-dependent diabetes mellitus (IDDM) which develops spontaneous clinical disease at 4–7 months with destruction of the β cells of the islets and elevations in blood glucose (432, 461, 462). The disease is both $CD4^+$ and $CD8^+$ T cell dependent (463) and a role for macrophages (464) has been described. Th1 cells are clearly implicated in the pathology of diabetes (429–431), thus suggesting that IL-10 might inhibit the onset or severity of IDDM in NOD mice.

However, the effects of IL-10 on diabetes in this model are surprisingly complex. Some experiments support the predicted role of IL-10 as an immunosuppressive factor in IDDM. Daily subcutaneous treatment of 9–10-week-old NOD mice delayed onset of diabetes and significantly reduced disease incidence (465). Treatment with IL-10 also reduced the severity of insulitis and prevented cellular infiltration of islet cells. Furthermore, systemic administration with a noncytolytic IL-10/Fc fusion protein in mice from 5 to 25 weeks of age completely prevented the occurrence of diabetes in NOD female mice and appeared to confer lasting protection following cessation of therapy (466). Passive transfer of splenic leukocytes from IL-10/Fc-treated NOD mice inhibited disease caused by simultaneous transfer of splenic leukocytes from acutely diabetic mice into irradiated, prediabetic NOD recipients (466). Moreover, adoptive transfer of islet-specific T cell clones transduced with IL-10 cDNA also prevented diabetes (467).

In contrast to these immunosuppressive effects of IL-10, expression of an IL-10 transgene by insulin-producing pancreatic β cells led to an accelerated onset of diabetes in NOD mice (468, 469), with no inhibition of immune-mediated destruction of islets (470). NOD mice expressing an IL-10 transgene in glucagon-producing pancreatic α cells also developed accelerated diabetes (471). This apparently contradictory effect of IL-10 on IDDM depended upon transgene expression in early life and was accompanied by enhanced leukocyte extravasation into the pancreatic tissue (468). Consistent with the notion that it is the timing of IL-10 expression that is important for its immunostimulatory effects in IDDM, neutralization of endogenous IL-10 in female NOD mice at three weeks of age inhibited development of insulitis in NOD mice (472), whereas treatment at a later age with anti-IL-10 had no effect on the onset of diabetes (465).

Protective Effects of IL-10 in Models of Rheumatoid Arthritis

IL-10 is also expressed at inflammatory foci in other autoimmune diseases where Th1 cytokines are believed to play a pathogenic role, such as in the joints of rheumatoid arthritis (RA) patients (293, 473–475). Endogenous IL-10 produced in the joint by synovial macrophages and T cells (473, 474), inhibited production of inflammatory cytokines by synovial cells, suggesting that IL-10 may have a protective role in vivo (474). Although IL-10 expression in RA has been linked to increased autoantibody production and B cell activation (476), IL-10 was protective in animal models of RA. When administered to animals before and/or after induction of disease, IL-10 reduced joint swelling, infiltration, cytokine production, and cartilage degradation in collagen- and streptococcal cell wall–induced arthritis (477–483).

IL-10 in the Pathogenesis of Systemic Lupus Erythematosis (SLE)

SLE is a complex autoimmune disorder characterized in part by polyclonal B cell activation, high levels of serum autoantibodies and glomerular immune complex deposition. Both B cells and macrophages from SLE patients spontaneously produce high levels of IL-10 in vitro (484), and several studies have shown a correlation between serum levels of IL-10 and disease activity (57, 294, 485, 486). Studies in both a mouse model of SLE (25) and in *scid* mice reconstituted with PBL from SLE patients (56) showed that autoantibody production and immune complex pathology could be substantially inhibited by treatment with anti-IL-10 antibodies. These studies suggested that IL-10 stimulation of immunoglobulin production by B cells plays a major role in the pathogenesis of SLE. More recently, treatment of 6 SLE patients with a mouse anti-hIL-10 Mab achieved a long-lasting reduction of most disease parameters in 5/6 patients (297). As noted, overproduction of IL-10 in SLE patients may have a genetic basis.

IL-10 Modulates Allergic Responses

Airway infiltration by inflammatory cells, particularly eosinophils, basophils, and mast cells, along with production of IgE, plays an important role in the pathology of asthma and other allergic diseases (487–489). Th2 cells secreting IL-4, IL-5, and IL-13 induce, prolong, and amplify the allergic response by enhancing production of IgE and the recruitment, growth, and differentiation of eosinophils and mast cells; and themselves directly cause airway hyperreactivity (487–491). Therapies for asthma have thus focused on eliminating eosinphils, lymphocytes, or IgE, or on directly antagonizing pathology-inducing mediators such as histamine or leukotrienes (487, 488).

It has been suggested that Th2-mediated allergic diseases such as asthma result from inadequate Th1 cytokine production (487, 492). However, allergen-specific Th1 cells are not prominent in the lungs of normal, nonasthmatic individuals, suggesting other mechanisms for regulation of responses to allergens. Furthermore, the presence of activated Th1 cells in the lung can also lead to inflammatory pathologies (487).

A role for IL-10 in regulation of immune responses to allergens was first suggested by studies showing that IL-10 could inhibit survival of and cytokine production by eosinophils stimulated with LPS (264). Later it was shown that IL-10 could also inhibit production of cytokines such as TNF and IL-6 by stimulated mast cells (493, 494). These in vitro findings were corroborated by in vivo studies in which a single intranasal dose of IL-10 concurrent with antigen challenge in previously sensitized mice specifically inhibited airway neutrophilia and eosinophilia and TNF production induced by antigenic challenge (258).

Expression of IL-10 via gene transfer in mouse lung also inhibited mucosal sensitization to aerosolized ovalbumin (OVA) in the context of nasal administration of a replication-deficient adenovirus carrying the GM-CSF gene (Ad/GM-CSF) (270). Cotransfer of the IL-10 gene (Ad/IL-10) inhibited the marked Th2 cytokine profile and eosinophilia otherwise observed, decreased the number of mononuclear cells, neutrophils, and eosinophils in the BALF, and reduced antigen-specific IgE levels. These effects were not mediated by IFNγ, indicating that a Th2 to Th1 switch was not involved. Mice exposed to OVA in the context of Ad/GM-CSF or the vector control were hyperresponsive to methacholine (McH) when re-exposed to aerosolized OVA 6 months later. However, responsiveness of IL-10-treated mice to McH was similar to that of naive mice. An IL-10-induced decrease in grain dust-induced airway inflammation and hyperreactivity was also observed (495). In contrast, other studies showed that, although IL-10 can indeed inhibit a pulmonary inflammatory response, it can also in some cases enhance airway hyperreactivity in allergen-sensitized mice and actually appears to be required for airway hyperresponsiveness (496, 497). This difference may reflect the timing of IL-10 administration relative to allergen sensitization and/or the time after administration that the mice were examined.

Consistent with a role for IL-10 in allergic inflammation is the observation that significantly less IL-10 is found in the lungs of asthmatic patients (498, 499). Thus, IL-10 production in lungs of nonasthmatic patients may play a role in limiting pathology-inducing inflammatory Th2 responses. The anergic state arising in peripheral T cells after allergen (bee-venom)-specific immunotherapy (BV-SIT) results from increased production of IL-10 (310), initially by activated $CD4^+$ $CD25^+$ allergen-specific T cells, later by B cells and monocytes. Neutralization of IL-10 in PBMC from patients undergoing BV-SIT fully reconstituted allergen-specific proliferative and cytokine responses. A role for endogenous IL-10 in the regulation of Th2 responses was also demonstrated in a murine model of allergic bronchopulmonary aspergillosis (500). Lung cells and BALF obtained from IL-10$-/-$ mice after repeated *Aspergillus fumigatus* inhalation produced highly elevated levels of IL-4, IL-5, and IFNγ. IL-10$-/-$ animals exhibited exaggerated airway inflammation compared to wild-type control mice (500).

IL-10 in Inflammatory Bowel Disease

Crohn's disease and ulcerative colitis are complex chronic diseases of the gut, the etiology and pathogenesis of which are poorly understood. $CD4^+$ T cells are responsible for much of the disease pathogenesis, but subsets of $CD4^+$ T cells also play a role in normal regulation of responses to mucosal antigens (501, 502). That IL-10 plays an important role in mucosal immune regulation was demonstrated by the observation that IL-10$-/-$ mice develop enterocolitis (26). Development and persistence of colitis in IL-10$-/-$ mice is dependent on IL-12 (503) and requires the presence of resident enteric bacteria (504). Transfer of CD45RB^{high} $CD4^+$ T cells from normal donors into C.B-17 SCID mice also led to development of a severe inflammatory response in the colon (505, 506) that is IFNγ- and TNF-dependent (505). Administration of mIL-10 prevented colitis in SCID mice reconstituted with CD45RB^{high} $CD4^+$ T cells (505). Furthermore, CD45RB^{high} $CD4^+$ T cells isolated from transgenic mice expressing IL-10 under control of the IL-2 promoter failed to transfer colitis but, rather, were able to inhibit colitis induced by wild-type CD45RB^{high} $CD4^+$ T cells (507). Oral administration to mice of *Lactococcus lactis* secreting mIL-10 reduced dextran sulfate sodium-induced colitis and prevented colitis onset in IL-10−/− mice (508). Taken together, these studies provide evidence that IL-10 is an important regulator of intestinal immune responses.

IL-10-Producing Regulatory T Cell Subsets Distinct from Th1 and Th2 cells

Multiple studies now suggest that regulatory T cell populations exist that are distinct from Th2 cells. Regulatory CD4$^+$ T cell subsets have been described that inhibit cell-mediated immune responses and/or inflammatory pathologies (312, 434, 436–441, 509–511). These T regulatory cell subsets have been isolated under different conditions and exhibit different cytokine expression profiles. It is yet uncertain whether they represent one or multiple distinct CD4$^+$ T cell subsets capable of regulating both Th1- and Th2-mediated responses. Many of the characterized populations are heterogeneous, and the molecular mechanisms for their derivation and full effector function have not been clearly defined.

CD45Rb^{low} CD4$^+$ T cells contain a regulatory population that can inhibit CD45RB^{high} CD4$^+$ T cell–mediated colitis; this suppression of colitis is inhibited by anti-TGFβ and/or anti-IL-10R1 mAbs (317, 441), suggesting a role for both cytokines in regulation of mucosal inflammation. A role for TGFβ has also been demonstrated for a number of T regulatory populations, including Th3 and T regulatory 1 (Tr1) cells, in inhibition of autoimmune pathologies, gut inflammation, and/or proliferation of antigen-specific T cells (312, 434, 437, 438, 440, 512). Asseman et al. (317) implicated both TGFβ and IL-10 as key factors in the ability of CD45RB^{low}CD4$^+$ T cells to inhibit CD45RB^{high}CD4$^+$ T cell–mediated colitis.

The relationship between these two cytokines in regulating inflammatory pathologies is unclear. It is unlikely that IL-10 is required for production of TGFβ because IL-10−/− mice show inflammatory pathology only of the intestine (26), whereas TGFβ−/− mice develop inflammatory diseases of multiple organs (442). However, TGFβ induces production of IL-10 by APC (513), suggesting that these molecules may act in concert to influence development and function of regulatory T cells, which is favored by chronic stimulation in the presence of IL-10 (213, 312, 434). These cells are reminiscent of CD4$^+$ T cells previously isolated from peripheral blood of SCID-reconstituted patients, in whom high levels of IL-10 were associated with successful allogeneic stem cell transplantation (514). Whether IL-10 induces development of these IL-10-producing T cells by acting on APC and/or directly on the T cell is as yet unclear. However, in view of (*a*) IL-10's inhibitory effects on DC and macrophage function, and (*b*) the observation that IL-10-treated DC induce tolerance (214, 217), an effect of IL-10 on APC is likely required. Additional studies are necessary to clarify mechanisms involved in development and function of T regulatory cells, and the respective roles of IL-10, TGFβ and other mediators.

Factors Inducing IL-10 Production and Conditions Under Which IL-10 Acts as a Regulatory Molecule In Vivo

Regimens of antigen administration that have been suggested to generate anergy/tolerance in vivo induce production of IL-10. For example, influenza hemagglutinin (HA)-specific CD4$^+$ T cells rendered anergic in vivo in mice expressing HA under the control of the Igκ promoter produced 100-fold higher levels of IL-10 than did naive or recently activated T cells (311). These anergic HA-specific T cells exhibited an impaired ability to cause diabetes in vivo compared to naive counterparts when transferred into immunodeficient recipients expressing HA under the control of the insulin promoter (311). Similar findings were obtained with CD8$^+$ T cells specific for the male antigen H-Y, which were rendered anergic in vivo (313). These T cells did not proliferate or mobilize calcium upon activation, and they failed to express IL-2 or IL-2R but secreted IL-10 and survived for extended periods in vivo. A potential role of IL-10 in tolerance was also demonstrated in a model involving multiple injections of superantigen A (SEA) into TCR-Vβ transgenic mice. IL-10 production was detected after the second injection of SEA, and it dominated the response after the third (309). Coadministration of anti-IL-10 Mab with SEA prevented suppression of in vivo IFNγ, TNF, and IL-4 responses but had no effect on IL-2 production. That repeated administration of superantigen generates a regulatory population of CD4$^+$ T cells has been suggested by experiments using a viral superantigen (515, 516) that generated a population of CD25$^+$CD4$^+$ T cells resistant to clonal deletion and producing high amounts of IL-10. These cells were IL-2 dependent and could not be induced in IL-2$-/-$ mice (515, 516).

Immune responses to antigens in the eye are regulated by the ocular environment and can induce systemic alterations in the immune response referred to as immune deviation (517). The eye itself contributes to immune deviation, in part via immunoregulatory molecules present in aqueous humor and/or expressed by ocular cells. When T cells encounter antigen in the eye, they become anergic, undergo apoptosis, and/or secrete cytokines such as TGFβ that suppress subsequent inflammatory responses, thus avoiding inflammatory injury. Apoptosis of inflammatory cells is required for induction of immune deviation via antigen presentation in the eye (518). Thus, Fas-mediated apoptosis of lymphoid cells was accompanied by rapid production of IL-10 and subsequent inhibition of APC function and Th1 responses (518). Whereas apoptotic cells from wild-type mice "fed" to APC in vitro promoted Th2 development with production of IL-4 and IL-10, those obtained from IL-10$-/-$ mice favored development of Th1 cells. However, immune deviation could be induced in IL-10$-/-$ mice when IL-10-containing apoptotic cells were presented in the eye.

A connection between the DNA damage that occurs in apoptotic cells and IL-10 production has been demonstrated (519). Induction of IL-10 expression was linked to pyrimidine dimer formation in keratinocytes in UV-exposed skin. Furthermore, IL-10 mediates at least some of the suppressive effects of UV-irradiation on cell-mediated immunity (520). UV-induced apoptosis is mediated by Fas (521), consistent with a link between Fas-mediated death and IL-10 production. This association is strengthened by detection of monocyte IL-10 expression induced by exposure to UVB-irradiated apoptotic PBL (522).

Collectively, these observations demonstrate an antiinflammatory component of apoptosis, mediated by IL-10, that helps control potentially harmful immune responses. However, a comprehensive pathway linking induction of DNA damage, apoptosis, production of IL-10, and induction of tolerance by repeated exposure to self/neo-antigen or superantigen as described earlier remains to be elucidated.

CANCER AND TRANSPLANTATION

The profound immunosuppressive effects of IL-10 have prompted numerous studies of its expression and function in association with cancers and both bone marrow and solid organ transplantation. A thorough perspective on this large and seemingly contradictory literature is beyond the scope of this review. Because of its multiple activities, the ultimate consequences of IL-10 expression or therapy are a net outcome of many variables, including IL-10 levels, systemic vs. local expression/therapy, effects during induction vs. effector stages of an immune response, and growth-inhibitory or -cofactor activity for tumor or graft cells.

Cancer

IL-10 Expression in Cancer   Several reports have described association of elevated IL-10 expression levels with certain cancers, for example ovarian (523–525), various carcinomas (526–532), melanoma (529, 533–538), and lymphoma/ myeloma (reviewed by 539; 540–545). We note that elevated IL-10 expression can occur for multiple reasons with very different implications. IL-10 can be expressed by tumor cells themselves, possibly suppressing antitumor responses. In other cases, IL-10 could be produced by activated cells involved in a host antitumor reaction, and thus it could be an indicator of a potent inflammatory response rather than immunosuppression. Thus, in the absence of expression data for a broader panel of cytokines and other immune response parameters, it is difficult to interpret the significance of elevated IL-10 expression in many such studies.

IL-10 Expression as a Prognostic Indicator in Cancer   A more specific issue is whether elevated IL-10 expression correlates with favorable or adverse patient outcomes. Elevated IL-10 serum levels have been reported as a negative prognostic factor for survival or response to treatment in Hodgkin's and non-Hodgkin's lymphoma (546–551), although evidence suggested (550) that such "correlation" may be due to EBV vIL-10 (which is also detected by most hIL-10 ELISA assays) rather than to hIL-10. Detectable IL-10 in serum was also described as a negative indicator for clinical outcome in hepatocellular carcinoma (526), lung cancer

(528, 552), renal carcinoma (532), gastric or colorectal carcinoma (553), and other solid tumors (527). The presence of strongly staining IL-10-producing cells of undetermined origin correlated with a poor outcome in one group's studies of patients with oral, oropharyngeal, and nasopharyngeal (NPC) carcinomas (530, 554), although EBV vIL-10 and hIL-10 again were not distinguished, an issue of particular relevance to NPC. In contrast, serum IL-10 levels did not correlate with prognosis in a study of diffuse large cell lymphoma (555), and an assessment of IL-10 mRNA in B-CLL indicated association of *favorable* prognosis with higher IL-10 mRNA expression (556).

How might the presence of IL-10 contribute to a poor prognosis for some cancers? One possibility is growth-factor or -cofactor activity for tumor cells. IL-10 stimulates growth and differentiation of B cells (20), and exogenously provided IL-10 enhances growth of some B cell tumor cells in vitro (275, 557–559). Experiments involving neutralization of IL-10 activity or expression have suggested a possible role as an autocrine growth (co)factor for certain types of B-lymphoma (545, 558, 560). Similar data were also reported for melanoma (537). IL-10 stimulated proliferation of myeloma cells (557), although the effect appeared to be indirect, via induction of autocrine oncostatin M growth factor expression (542, 561). However, in contrast, IL-10 inhibited production of the autocrine growth factor GM-CSF by myelogenous leukemic blast cells (562–564). Thus, while IL-10 may contribute to growth of B cell tumors, there is little evidence supporting a general role for IL-10 as a tumor growth factor.

A second possibility is that IL-10 produced by or in the vicinity of a tumor could hinder induction or effector function of an antitumor immune response. As already discussed, IL-10 inhibits dendritic cell (DC) function, which could blunt induction of a response against tumor cells (207, 212, 214–218, 565–567). At least one in vivo model suggests that this notion is plausible: A Lewis lung carcinoma cell line grows more rapidly in a transgenic mouse expressing IL-10 under control of an IL-2 promoter than in nontransgenic control mice (507, 568).

However, the impact of this activity of IL-10 cannot be assessed or predicted outside the context of its other relevant functions, such as leukocyte recruitment via both chemotaxis (138, 161, 170, 569) and induction of endothelial cell adhesion molecule expression (468, 570, 571), stimulation of the growth and function of cytotoxic cells (8, 21, 137, 572), ability to increase the sensitivity of target cells to NK-mediated lysis (573, 574), and enhancement of antibody-mediated immunity (20, 134, 575). In contrast to an inhibitory effect on DC function, these latter activities would likely contribute to inhibition of tumor establishment, growth, or even metastasis.

Effects of cIL-10 and vIL-10 Protein or Gene Therapy in Animal Models of Cancer   The ultimate effect of IL-10 in vivo has been addressed by a number of studies of IL-10 protein administration or IL-10 gene therapy in animal models of tumor establishment and growth. In mastocytoma (576), breast cancer (134, 573, 577–580), melanoma (84, 139, 534, 581, 582), prostate cancer

(583–585), and colon carcinoma (84, 586) models, IL-10 expressed by gene transfer into tumor cells, or administered as protein, effected a profound inhibition of tumor establishment, growth, and metastasis. Much of this process occurred in SCID or nude mouse tumor recipients (139, 183, 534, 582–585), suggesting that an important component of the response is T cell–independent. Consistent with this notion, intratumor cellular infiltrates in the presence of IL-10 include not only T cells, but macrophages, NK cells, and neutrophils (139, 581, 586, 587). In addition, several studies utilizing non-immunodeficient mice as hosts demonstrated that effective and prolonged anti-tumor immune responses were established in the presence of IL-10 (84, 134, 581, 586, 588). Inhibition of tumor angiogenesis was also implicated (183, 534, 582, 585).

The above observations indicate that in these in vivo tumor model systems the pleiotropic (i.e., non-CSIF) activities of IL-10 exert a dominant influence on the outcome of IL-10 expression or protein therapy. Consistent with this idea are the strikingly different results obtained when EBV vIL-10, the pleiotropic activities of which are substantially impaired (4, 18, 19, 81, 88), was used instead of cIL-10. In contrast to the accelerated tumor rejection and induced antitumor immunity obtained with cIL-10, when vIL-10 expression was employed in melanoma, colorectal carcinoma, or sarcoma models, prolonged or indefinite tumor growth was observed, accompanied by a locally impaired immune response (84, 86). Similar results were observed in a mastocytoma model (589, 590), although some rejection phenomena were observed, perhaps due to apparently 10- to 20-fold higher levels of vIL-10 expression achieved in these latter studies.

Collectively, studies of IL-10 expression and function in cancer present a complex picture of varied outcomes that can be obtained depending on level, source, timing, and duration of IL-10 expression during tumor development. The well-characterized immunosuppressive CSIF activity of IL-10 clearly functions in vivo, most likely during induction of an immune response, but under some conditions it can be overshadowed by alternate mechanisms engaged by IL-10 that induce an anti-tumor response.

Transplantation

The ability of IL-10 to inhibit induction and effector function of T cell-mediated- and inflammatory immune responses led to numerous studies of its expression, function, and potential utility in bone marrow and organ transplantation. The current picture is complex but is, in our opinion, amenable to a few general conclusions.

IL-10 Pretreatment of, or Pre-existing Elevated Spontaneous IL-10 Expression by Graft Recipients Is Associated with Improved Graft Acceptance In studies of vascularized heart allografts in mice, IL-10 treatment of recipient animals prior to grafting enhanced graft survival (390, 591), whereas providing IL-10 at or after the time of grafting had little beneficial effect or even enhanced rejection

(592–594). Similar results were also obtained for rat liver allografts (595). Studies of bone marrow transplantation (BMT) and graft-vs-host disease (GVHD) also support this idea: Patients exhibiting elevated levels of IL-10 production prior to BMT have lower incidence of GVHD and improved survival (514, 596, 597). Taken together, such observations suggest a key inhibitory/tolerogenic role for IL-10 prior to and during the initial priming events in organ transplantation and BMT. As noted earlier, this presumably reflects IL-10's ability to inhibit the function of DC and other accessory cells and to influence subsequent development of the T cells that they stimulate (213, 218, 434).

IL-10 Treatment or Expression at the Time of or Posttransplantation Can Enhance Graft Rejection or GVHD   In contrast to pre-BMT patients discussed above, high IL-10 levels in post-BMT GVHD patients indicate a poor prognosis for survival (598). Furthermore, posttransplant administration of IL-10 protein to mice in models of BMT/GVHD was generally deleterious, resulting in unimproved or increased mortality (599–561).

However, when given to mice in small amounts, 10^{-3}–10^{-4} of the amount that increased mortality, IL-10 protected against GVHD-associated lethality (602), suggesting that low in vivo IL-10 concentrations preferentially induce the immunosuppressive effects of IL-10. Consistent with this notion, we have observed that IL-10 is about 10-fold more potent in vitro in assays measuring its immunosuppressive activity than in assays measuring other activities such as costimulation of mast cell and thymocyte proliferation (KW Moore, R deW Malefyt, unpublished).

Organ transplantation studies have been carried out utilizing IL-10 protein, IL-10 gene transfer, and IL-10 transgenic mice. Some of these reports described prolongation of graft survival time due to IL-10 protein treatment (595) or IL-10 expression via gene transfer (603–605) in liver transplant models. In this connection, it was noted that liver allografts tend to be less immunogenic than other organs (604), an observation that could be related to transient but massive IL-10 release attributed to liver-resident macrophages during transplantation (51). As noted above, lower doses of exogenous IL-10 protein tended to be protective, while a higher dose exacerbated rejection (595). This aspect is more difficult to evaluate in gene transfer studies because the amounts of bioavailable IL-10 are a complex function of vector delivery efficiency, expression levels in infected cells and their physical location in vivo, how quickly their expression or viability is compromised by host reactions, and the half-life of IL-10 in vivo. A recent study of rat cardiac allografts utilizing rat IL-10 adenovirus also described a modest prolongation of graft survival in association with IL-10 expression (606).

In contrast, a number of studies have reported neutral or unfavorable effects of IL-10 expression in allograft models. Expression of transgenic IL-10 in pancreatic β-cells enhanced accumulation of leukocytes, did not impair induction of autoimmune diabetes, and did not inhibit rejection of transgenic islets transplanted to MHC-disparate mice (468, 470). Likewise an IL-10-Fc fusion protein accelerated islet allograft rejection in mice (607). Posttransplant injection of IL-10 protein in mouse cardiac allograft recipients enhanced rejection and arterial disease (593, 594, 608) and inhibited the therapeutic effects of cyclosporine treatment (594). Antagonism of IL-10 via administration of anti-IL-10 Mab also prolonged cardiac and liver allograft acceptance in mice (609). IL-10 treatment did not enhance acceptance of corneal allografts (610).

Clearly the effects of IL-10 on BMT and organ allografts are a complex outcome of multiple factors including timing, kinetics, and amounts of cytokine, as well as the relative impact of the different activities of IL-10 in each particular experimental scheme and model system. We also emphasize that in most such studies the experimental endpoint ("rejection") is defined by necrosis or loss of function; little attention has been devoted to defining potentially significant cellular and mechanistic differences leading to rejection in the presence or absence of IL-10, as pointed out by others (611, 612). Thus, in models where IL-10 protein or expression enhances rejection, it may be that completely different rejection mechanisms elicited by IL-10 are at work compared to those active in its absence. As discussed below, a somewhat clearer picture has developed via use of natural (vIL-10) and more recently artificial (88) IL-10 variants with a more restricted biological activity profile.

Viral IL-10 Expression, in Contrast to cIL-10, Is Consistently Beneficial for Graft Acceptance and Survival   As observed in in vivo tumor models, gene transfer-mediated vIL-10 expression by vIL-10-transduced graft cells or by cells in the vicinity of the graft enhanced graft acceptance, although to varying extents in different allograft models (85, 88, 589, 613–618). These results are paralleled by experiments involving human (619) and rat (620) cells showing that vIL-10 expression by graft cells or by DC (215) inhibited alloreactivity in vitro. Moreover Nast et al. (621) described a kidney transplant patient with transplant-associated lymphoproliferation who exhibited prolonged graft acceptance, with minimal immunosuppressive therapy, which was associated with intragraft vIL-10 expression. These data collectively indicate that vIL-10, with its restricted bioactivity profile favoring the CSIF or immunosuppressive activities of IL-10 and ability to effectively engage only a limited subset of IL-10-responsive cells in vivo, is in contrast to cIL-10 a potent and consistent immunosuppressive cytokine in in vivo models of organ transplantation.

CLINICAL STUDIES

IL-10 has been considered an attractive candidate for therapeutic use based on its potent in vitro immunomodulating activities and proven effects in animal models of acute and chronic inflammation, autoimmunity, cancer and infectious disease. Phase I and II clinical trials investigating safety, tolerance, pharmacokinetics, pharmacodynamics, immunological and hematological effects of single or multiple doses of IL-10 administered by intravenous (iv) or subcutaneous (sc) route have been performed in various settings on healthy volunteers and specific patient populations (622–624). These studies showed that IL-10 is well tolerated without serious side effects at doses up to 25 μg/kg; mild to moderate flu-like symptoms were observed in a fraction of recipients at doses up to 100 μg/kg.

In vivo administration of IL-10 inhibited the ex vivo LPS-induced production of IL-6, IL-1, and TNF in whole blood cell assays and decreased proliferative responses and IFNγ production following PHA stimulation of PBMC, indicating that IL-10 retains immunomodulatory activities when administered in vivo. The doses required to effect 50% of maximal inhibition (IC_{50}) of TNF and IL-1β production and a maximal fraction of inhibition (I_{max}) indicated that IL-10 inhibited production of proinflammatory mediators in vivo at concentrations similar to those used in in vitro experiments (625).

Single intravenous (iv) or subcutaneous (sc) doses of IL-10 resulted in transient dose-dependent changes in white blood cell populations, including increases in total white blood cells and neutrophils. A reduction was observed in the number of $CD3^+CD4^+$ and $CD3^+CD8^+$ lymphocytes accompanied by an increase in the percentage of $CD14^+$ $HLA-DR^+$ monocytes. Furthermore, transient decreases in expression levels of CD11a (LFA1) on $CD3^+$ T cells, which may account for some of the observed changes in lymphocyte circulation, and a decrease in the expression levels of HLA-DR on $CD14^+$ monocytes, but not on $CD20^+$ B cells, were measured following a single iv dose of IL-10 in healthy volunteers (626, 627). Downregulation of HLA-DR expression on monocytes but not B cells correlates well with in vitro effects of IL-10 and is associated with inhibition of antigen presentation.

In addition to transient neutrophilia, lymphocytopenia, and monocytosis, a delayed decrease in platelet counts was observed following a single sc dose of IL-10 (624). Decreases in platelet counts were also reported following multiple dose regimens in a proportion of patients receiving 10–20 μg/kg doses (628, 629). Platelet counts reached nadirs of 20–50% of baseline generally at day 7 of treatment, but they did not attain clinically compromising levels and either stabilized or returned to normal during or following cessation of IL-10 therapy.

Because several of IL-10's potential indications are chronic inflammatory diseases for which steroid treatment is an accepted therapy, its interaction with such drugs was studied. Single doses of IL-10 resulted in statistically significant but clinically insignificant 20% increases in 24 h plasma cortisol area under serum concentration–time curve (AUC). However, coadministration of IL-10 and prednisolone did not result in pharmacokinetic alterations of either drug and showed net responses that were similar to or greater than effects produced by the more strongly acting agent (630, 631). In addition, IL-10 administration did not significantly alter cytochrome P450 (CYP)-mediated drug metabolism as characterized by CYP1A2, CYP2C9, and CYP2D6 activities and by a 12% reduction of CYP3A-mediated biotransformation (632).

Pharmacokinetic parameters of IL-10 clearance were determined following iv or sc administration of doses ranging from 0.1 to 100 μg/kg. Following iv administration, IL-10 serum levels initially declined fairly rapidly but yielded a less steep terminal phase with a $t_{1/2}$ of 2–3 h. Mean exposure parameters (maximum serum concentration, C_{max}, and AUC) were linearly related to dosage, and IL-10 tended to remain in the vascular compartment. Because hIL-10 is nonglycosylated, it is cleared mainly through the kidney, as indicated by the increased $t_{1/2}$ and AUC of IL-10 in patients with moderate to severe renal insufficiencies. Administration of IL-10 did not produce adverse effects in this patient population (633). Subcutaneous administration of IL-10 resulted in slow absorption from the IL-10 depot formed at the injection site, which reached C_{max} at 2–6.5 h post injection. The slower absorption of IL-10 following sc versus iv administration led to prolonged but lower AUC with a mean terminal $t_{1/2}$ of 2.7—4.5 h and so resulted in a prolonged immunosuppressive effect. Mean exposure parameters were also linearly related to dosage (625). Production of neutralizing antibodies was not observed in any of the studies.

IL-10 administered iv at 25 μg/kg inhibited LPS-induced rises in temperature and release of TNF, IL-6, IL-8, and IL-1RA in healthy human volunteers, when given 2 min before but not 1 h after endotoxin (328). Such "pretreatment" with IL-10 also reduced endotoxin-induced granulocyte accumulation in the lungs, granulocyte degranulation, cortisol levels, activation of the fibrinolytic system, inhibition of fibrinolysis, activation of the coagulation system, and inhibition of expression of the CC chemokines Mip1α, Mip1β and MCP1 (634, 635). Delay in administration of IL-10 for 1 h only reduced IL-6 and Mip1β production, cortisol levels, inhibition of fibrinolysis, and activation of the coagulation system, indicating that timing of IL-10 administration is important for its full anti-inflammatory activity during experimental endotoxemia. However, IL-10 failed to alter proinflammatory cytokine production or physiological changes associated with the Jarisch-Herxheimer reaction, an acute systemic inflammatory response that follows antibiotic treatment of *Borrelia recurrentis* infection (636). In addition, the effects of IL-10 on systemic production of proinflammatory cytokines in renal transplant patients who received OKT3 as induction therapy (575) were investigated. Pretreatment with IL-10 reduced release of TNF induced by OKT3, but high IL-10 doses may have promoted early sensitization to OKT3 and exerted reversible adverse effects on graft acceptance.

IL-10 has been tested in specific patient populations including those with Crohn's disease, RA, psoriasis, and patients suffering from chronic hepatitis C infections. Administration of IL-10 (7 days iv) reduced the Crohn's disease activity index (CDAI) score in patients with steroid-refractory Crohn's disease and showed some clinical benefit in a larger 28-day sc safety and efficacy study in patients with chronic active Crohn's disease (CACD) (628, 637). Similarly, a trend towards efficacy and a good safety profile was observed when IL-10 was administered for 28 days to RA patients (629). Both Crohn's disease and RA are heterogeneous diseases, and IL-10 alone or in combination with other therapies, such as low dose steroid or therapeutic anti-TNF Mab (638, 639), may yet benefit a significant patient population.

An open label phase II trial on ten psoriasis patients indicated that sc IL-10 treatment for seven weeks was well tolerated and efficacious: significant decreases of psoriatic area and severity index were observed in 9/10 patients (640, 641). IL-10 likely affects monocytes and T cells rather than keratinocytes in this disease that is characterized by Th1-mediated IFNγ production (642).

Two recent trials investigated use of IL-10 to suppress pathology associated with chronic hepatitis C (HCV) infection (401, 643). IL-10 was administered sc at 4 or 8 μg/kg for 28 or 90 days in patients who had not received any therapy or who did not respond to interferon-based therapy, the current standard of care. IL-10 normalized serum levels of alanine aminotransferase, a marker for hepatic inflammation, improved liver histology and reduced liver fibrosis in over 50% of treated patients. However, IL-10 did not reduce serum HCV RNA levels, indicating that it did not affect viral load, but instead limited pathogen-induced pathology as discussed earlier. The safety profile and biological activities of IL-10 suggest its potential utility as a therapeutic, and results from several early clinical trials are encouraging. It is not easy to predict which condition will benefit most from IL-10 therapy, but IL-10–cIL-10 or vIL-10–either alone or in combination with other agents may hold significant promise.

CONCLUSIONS

IL-10 is a pleiotropic cytokine that regulates a variety of functions of hemopoietic cells. Its principal everyday function seems to be containment and eventual termination of inflammatory responses; by doing so, IL-10 facilitates elimination of infectious organisms with minimal damage to host tissues. In addition, IL-10 plays important roles in immune tolerance, T cell and DC development, and growth and differentiation of B cells. Early clinical trials suggest that IL-10 has a good safety profile and possible utility in treatment of autoimmune and inflammatory conditions. In addition, IL-10 antagonists–perhaps anti-IL-10 or anti-IL-10R Mabs–may find application in treatment of SLE and a number of infectious diseases.

What important issues remain to be addressed about IL-10's function? First, our understanding of IL-10R structure and signaling is not complete. That certain cells (e.g. monocytes, B cells) respond comparably to cIL-10 and vIL-10 whereas others are comparatively insensitive to vIL-10 suggests differences in IL-10R subunit composition or its signal transduction machinery in the former. Furthermore, the molecular basis for the different effects of IL-10 on different cell types remains to be clarified. Why IL-10 generally inhibits monocyte/macrophage and CD4$^+$ T cell function, yet stimulates development of B cells and CD8$^+$ T cells despite outwardly similar signaling responses in all cells is not understood.

What determines which of IL-10's activities will dominate in an immune response? As discussed, studies of IL-10 in vivo in models of autoimmunity, cancer, and transplantation have revealed that IL-10 can effect very different outcomes depending on timing, dose, and location of expression; in some scenarios the expected immunosuppressive activities are observed, while in others IL-10 enhances immune or inflammatory responses. The cellular mechanisms underlying these phenomena are unclear, and their elucidation is of particular importance for the successful use of IL-10 in the clinic. Valuable understanding in this area may come from further studies of IL-10's effects on DC and renewed efforts to understand its activity on other hemopoietic cells.

Understanding the role of IL-10 in differentiation and function of T regulatory cells—in their various manifestations—is crucial for attaining a complete understanding of these cells and their in vivo significance in immune tolerance. The most helpful advance in this area would be an improved method of growing and maintaining such cells in vitro. The potential utility of these cells in treating autoimmune disorders and in organ transplantation cannot be ignored.

Finally, the clinical potential of IL-10 requires further evaluation. It is possible that IL-10 or anti-IL-10 may synergize with existing suboptimal therapies (e.g., cyclosporine, steroids, anti-microbials) to effect a superior therapeutic outcome with fewer undesirable side effects. Moreover, because of the restricted bioactivity profile of vIL-10, the viral cytokine or a modified hIL-10 with impaired pleiotropic activities (88) may in fact be the preferred therapeutic entity in a number of IL-10 protein or gene therapy applications.

In this area, the emerging field of pharmacogenomics may offer the ability to determine in advance which patient subsets are most likely to respond to IL-10 or anti-IL-10 therapy. A foundation for this already exists in knowledge derived from IL-10 promoter genotype studies. It is also plausible that similar studies of the IL-10R1 and/or IL-10R2 loci may reveal polymorphisms that correlate with the ability of patients to respond to such therapies.

We are confident that the second decade of research on IL-10 will be as productive as the first.

ACKNOWLEDGMENTS

We thank colleagues who have worked in our laboratories during the last ten years for their participation in the work reviewed herein. We also are grateful to Dr. Paul Grint and Dr. Marco Cassatella for their critical review of this manuscript.

Visit the Annual Reviews home page at www.AnnualReviews.org

LITERATURE CITED

1. Fiorentino DF, Bond MW, Mosmann TR. 1989. Two types of mouse helper T cell. IV. Th2 clones secrete a factor that inhibits cytokine production by Th1 clones. *J. Exp. Med.* 170:2081–95

2. Moore KW, Vieira P, Fiorentino DF, Trounstine ML, Khan TA, Mosmann TR. 1990. Homology of cytokine synthesis inhibitory factor (IL-10) to the Epstein Barr virus gene BCRFI. *Science* 248:1230–34

3. Hsu D-H, de Waal Malefyt R, Fiorentino DF, Dang M-N, Vieira P, de Vries J, Spits H, Mosmann TR, Moore KW. 1990. Expression of IL-10 activity by Epstein-Barr virus protein BCRFI. *Science* 250:830–32

4. Vieira P, de Waal-Malefyt R, Dang M-N, Johnson KE, Kastelein R, Fiorentino DF, de Vries JE, Roncarolo M-G, Mosmann TR, Moore KW. 1991. Isolation and expression of human cytokine synthesis inhibitory factor (CSIF/IL10) cDNA clones: homology to Epstein-Barr virus open reading frame BCRFI. *Proc. Natl. Acad. Sci. USA* 88:1172–76

5. de Waal Malefyt R, Haanen J, Spits H, Roncarolo M-G, te Velde A, Figdor C, Johnson K, Kastelein R, Yssel H, de Vries JE. 1991. IL-10 and viral IL-10 strongly reduce antigen-specific human T cell proliferation by diminishing the antigen-presenting capacity of monocytes via downregulation of class II MHC expression. *J. Exp. Med.* 174:915–24

6. Fiorentino DF, Zlotnik A, Vieira P, Mosmann TR, Howard M, Moore KW, O'Garra A. 1991. IL-10 acts on the antigen-presenting cell to inhibit cytokine production by Th1 cells. *J. Immunol.* 146:3444–51

7. Ding L, Shevach EM. 1992. IL-10 inhibits mitogen-induced T cell proliferation by selectively inhibiting macrophage costimulatory function. *J. Immunol.* 148:3133–39

8. Hsu D-H, Moore KW, Spits H. 1992. Differential effects of interleukin-4 and -10 on interleukin-2-induced interferon-γ synthesis and lymphokine-activated killer activity. *Int. Immunol.* 4:563–69

9. Bogdan C, Vodovotz Y, Nathan C. 1991. Macrophage deactivation by interleukin 10. *J. Exp. Med.* 174:1549–55

10. de Waal Malefyt R, Abrams J, Bennett B, Figdor C, de Vries J. 1991. IL-10 inhibits cytokine synthesis by human monocytes: an autoregulatory role of IL-10 produced by monocytes. *J. Exp. Med.* 174:1209–20

11. Fiorentino DF, Zlotnik A, Mosmann TR, Howard MH, O'Garra A. 1991. IL-10 inhibits cytokine production by activated macrophages. *J. Immunol.* 147:3815–22

12. Ding L, Linsley PS, Huang L-Y, Germain RN, Shevach EM. 1993. IL-10 inhibits macrophage costimulatory activity by selectively inhibiting the up-regulation of B7 expression. *J. Immunol.* 151:1224–34

13. Gazzinelli RT, Oswald IP, James SL, Sher A. 1992. IL-10 inhibits parasite killing and nitric oxide production by IFN-γ-activated macrophages. *J. Immunol.* 148:1792–96

14. Oswald IP, Gazzinelli RT, Sher A, James SL. 1992. IL-10 synergizes with IL-4 and TGF-beta to inhibit macrophage cytotoxic activity. *J. Immunol.* 148:3578–82

15. Ralph P, Nakoinz I, Sampson-Johannes A, Fong S, Lowe D, Min H-Y, Lin L. 1992. IL-10, T lymphocyte inhibitor of human blood cell production of IL-1 and tumor necrosis factor. *J. Immunol.* 148:808–14

16. Murphy EE, Terres G, Macatonia SE, Hsieh C-S, Mattson J, Lanier L, Wysocka M, Trinchieri G, Murphy K, O'Garra A. 1994. B7 and interleukin-12 cooperate for proliferation and IFNγ production by mouse Th1 clones that are unresponsive to B7 costimulation. *J. Exp. Med.* 180:223–31

17. de Waal Malefyt R, Yssel H, de Vries JE. 1993. Direct effects of IL-10 on subsets of human CD4+ T cell clones and resting T cells. *J. Immunol.* 150:4754–65

18. Go NF, Castle BE, Barrett R, Kastelein R, Dang W, Mosmann TR, Moore KW, Howard M. 1990. Interleukin 10 (IL-10), a novel B cell stimulatory factor: unresponsiveness of X chromosome-linked immunodeficiency B cells. *J. Exp. Med.* 172:1625–31

19. MacNeil I, Suda T, Moore KW, Mosmann TR, Zlotnik A. 1990. IL-10: a novel cytokine growth cofactor for mature and immature T cells. *J. Immunol.* 145:4167–73

20. Rousset F, Garcia E, Defrance T, Peronne C, Hsu D-H, Kastelein R, Moore KW, Banchereau J. 1992. IL-10 is a potent

growth and differentiation factor for activated human B lymphocytes. *Proc. Natl. Acad. Sci. USA* 89:1890–93

21. Chen W-F, Zlotnik A. 1991. Interleukin 10: A novel cytotoxic T cell differentiation factor. *J. Immunol.* 147:528–34

22. Thompson-Snipes L, Dhar V, Bond MW, Mosmann TR, Moore KW, Rennick D. 1991. Interleukin-10: a novel stimulatory factor for mast cells and their progenitors. *J. Exp. Med.* 173:507–10

23. Ishida H, Hastings R, Kearny J, Howard M. 1992. Continuous anti-IL-10 antibody administration depletes mice of CD5 B cells but not conventional B cells. *J. Exp. Med.* 175:1213–20

24. Ishida H, Hastings R, Snipes L, Howard M. 1993. Modified immunological status of anti-IL-10 treated mice. *Cell. Immunol.* 148:371–84

25. Ishida H, Muchamuel T, Sakaguchi S, Andrade S, Menon S, Howard M. 1994. Continuous administration of anti-IL-10 antibodies delays onset of autoimmunity in NZB/W F1 mice. *J. Exp. Med.* 179:305–10

26. Kuhn R, Lohler J, Rennick D, Rajewsky K, Muller W. 1993. Interleukin-10 deficient mice develop chronic enterocholitis. *Cell* 75:263–74

27. Berg DJ, Leach MW, Kuhn R, Rajewsky K, Muller W, Davidson NJ, Rennick D. 1995. Interleukin 10 but not interleukin 4 is a natural suppressant of cutaneous inflammatory responses. *J. Exp. Med.* 182:99–108

28. Berg DJ, Kuhn R, Rajewsky K, Muller W, Menon S, Davidson N, Grunig G, Rennick D. 1995. Interleukin-10 is a central regulator of the response to LPS in murine models of endotoxic shock and the Shwartzman reaction but not endotoxin tolerance. *J. Clin. Invest.* 96:2339–47

29. Opal SM, Wherry JC, Grint P. 1998. Interleukin-10: potential benefits and possible risks in clinical infectious diseases. *Clin. Infect. Dis.* 27:1497–1507

30. Goodman RE, Oblak J, Bell RG. 1992. Synthesis and characterization of rat interleukin-10 (IL-10) cDNA clones from the RNA of cultured OX8- OX22- thoracic duct T cells. *Biochem. Biophys. Res. Commun.* 189:1–7

31. Sprang SR, Bazan JF. 1993. Cytokine structural taxonomy and mechanisms of receptor engagement. *Curr. Opin. Struct. Biol.* 3:815–27

32. Mosmann TR, Schumacher J, Fiorentino DF, Leverah J, Moore KW, Bond MW. 1990. Isolation of monoclonal antibodies specific for IL4, IL5, IL6, and a new Th2-specific cytokine (IL-10), cytokine synthesis inhibitory factor, by using a solid phase radioimmunoadsorbent assay. *J. Immunol.* 145:2938–45

33. Liu Y, Wei SH-Y, Ho AS-Y, de Waal Malefyt R, Moore KW. 1994. Expression cloning and characterization of a human interleukin-10 receptor. *J. Immunol.* 152:1821–29

34. Tan JC, Indelicato S, Narula SK, Zavodny PJ, Chou C-C. 1993. Characterization of interleukin-10 receptors on human and mouse cells. *J. Biol. Chem.* 268:21,053–59

35. Windsor WT, Syto R, Tsarbopoulos A, Zhang R, Durkin J, Baldwin S, Paliwal S, Mui PW, Pramanik B, Trotta PP, Tindall SH. 1993. Disulfide bond assignments and secondary structure analysis of human and murine interleukin 10. *Biochemistry (Mosc).* 32:8807–15

36. Syto R, Murgolo NJ, Braswell EH, Mui P, Huang E, Windsor WT. 1998. Structural and biological stability of the human interleukin 10 homodimer. *Biochemistry (Mosc)* 37:16943–51

37. Walter MR, Nagabhushan TL. 1995. Crystal structure of interleukin 10 reveals an interferon γ-like fold. *Biochemistry (Mosc).* 34:12118–25

38. Zdanov A, Schalk-Hihi C, Gustchina A, Tsang M, Weatherbee J, Wlodawer A. 1995. Crystal structure of interleukin-10

reveals the functional dimer with an unexpected topological similarity to interferon γ. *Structure* 3:591–601

39. Zdanov A, Schalk-Hihi C, Wlodawer A. 1996. Crystal of human interleukin-10 at 1.6 A resolution and a model of a complex with its soluble receptor. *Protein Sci.* 5:1955–62

40. Zdanov A, Schalk-Hihi C, Menon S, Moore KW, Wlodawer A. 1997. Crystal structure of Epstein-Barr virus protein BCRF1, a homolog of cellular interleukin-10. *J. Mol. Biol.* 268:460–67

41. Walter MR, Windsor WT, Nagabhushan TL, Lundell DJ, Lunn CA, Zavodny PJ, Narula SK. 1995. Crystal structure of a complex between interferon-γ and its soluble high affinity receptor. *Nature* 376:230–35

42. Josephson K, DiGiacomo R, Indelicato SR, Ayo AH, Nagabhushan TL, Parker MH, Walter MR. 2000. Design and analysis of an engineered human interleukin-10 monomer. *J. Biol. Chem.* 275:13552–57

43. Gesser B, Leffers H, Jinquan T, Vestergaard C, Kirstein N, Sindet-Pedersen S, Jensen SL, Thestrup-Pedersen K, Larsen CG. 1997. Identification of functional domains on human interleukin 10. *Proc. Natl. Acad. Sci. USA* 94:14620–25

44. Osman MO, Jacobsen NO, Kristensen JU, Deleuran B, Gesser B, Larsen CG, Jensen SL. 1998. IT 9302, a synthetic interleukin-10 agonist, diminishes acute lung injury in rabbits with acute necrotizing pancreatitis. *Surgery* 124:584–92

45. Kim JM, Brannan CI, Copeland NG, Jenkins NA, Khan TA, Moore KW. 1992. Structure of the mouse interleukin-10 gene and chromosomal localization of the mouse and human genes. *J. Immunol.* 148:3618–23

46. de Waal Malefyt R, de Vries J. 1996. In *Interleukin-10*, ed. B. Aggarwal, J. Gutterman, pp. 19–42. Cambridge MA: Blackwell Sci.

47. de Waal Malefyt R, Moore KW. 1998. In *Interleukin-10*, ed. A. Thomson, pp. 333–64. San Diego, CA: Academic Press

48. Brightbill HD, Plevy SE, Modlin RL, Smale ST. 2000. A prominent role for Sp1 during lipopolysaccharide-mediated induction of the IL-10 promoter in macrophages. *J. Immunol.* 164:1940–51

49. Tone M, Powell MJ, Tone Y, Thompson SA, Waldmann H. 2000. IL-10 gene expression is controlled by the transcription factors Sp1 and Sp3. *J. Immunol.* 165:286–91

50. Powell MJ, Thompson SA, Tone Y, Waldmann H, Tone M. 2000. Posttranscriptional regulation of IL-10 gene expression through sequences in the 3'-untranslated region. *J. Immunol.* 165:292–96

51. Le Moine O, Marchant A, Durand F, Ickx B, Pradier O, Belghiti J, Abramowicz D, Gelin M, Goldman M, Deviere J. 1994. Systemic release of interleukin-10 during orthotopic liver transplantation. *Hepatology* 20:889–92

52. Eskdale J, Kube D, Tesch H, Gallagher G. 1997. Mapping of the human IL10 gene and further characterization of the 5' flanking sequence. *Immunogenetics* 46:120–28

53. Hurme M, Lahdenpohja N, Santtila S. 1998. Gene polymorphisms of interleukins 1 and 10 in infectious and autoimmune diseases. *Ann. Med.* 30:469–73

54. Eskdale J, McNicholl J, Wordsworth P, Jonas B, Huizinga T, Field M, Gallagher G. 1998. Interleukin-10 microsatellite polymorphisms and IL-10 locus alleles in rheumatoid arthritis susceptibility [letter]. *Lancet* 352:1282–83

55. Turner DM, Williams DM, Sankaran D, Lazarus M, Sinnott PJ, Hutchinson IV. 1997. An investigation of polymorphism in the interleukin-10 gene promoter. *Eur. J. Immunogenet.* 24:1–8

56. Llorente L, Zou W, Levy Y, Richaud-Patin Y, Wijdenes J, Alcocer-Varela J, Morel-Fourrier B, Brouet JC, Alarcon-Segovia D, Galanaud P. 1995. Role of interleukin 10 in the B lymphocyte hyperactivity and

autoantibody production of systemic lupus erythematosus. *J. Exp. Med.* 181:839–44

57. Llorente L, Richaud-patin Y, Couderc J, Alarcon-Segovia D, Ruiz-Soto R, Alcocer-Castillejos N, Alcocer-Varela J, Granados J, Bahena S, Galanaud P, Emilie D. 1997. Dysregulation of interleukin-10 production in relatives of patients with systemic lupus erythematosus. *Arthritis Rheum.* 40:1429–35

58. Eskdale J, Wordsworth P, Bowman S, Field M, Gallagher G. 1997. Association between polymorphisms at the human IL-10 locus and systemic lupus erythematosus [published erratum appears in *Tissue Antigens* 1997 Dec;50(6):699]. *Tissue Antigens* 49:635–39

59. Lazarus M, Hajeer AH, Turner D, Sinnott P, Worthington J, Ollier WE, Hutchinson IV. 1997. Genetic variation in the interleukin 10 gene promoter and systemic lupus erythematosus. *J. Rheumatol.* 24:2314–17

60. Gonzalez-Amaro R, Portales-Perez D, Baranda L, Abud-Mendoza C, Llorente L, Richaud-Patin Y, Alcocer-Varela J, Alarcon-Segovia D. 1998. Role of IL-10 in the abnormalities of early cell activation events of lymphocytes from patients with systemic lupus erythematosus. *J. Autoimmun.* 11:395–402

61. Rood MJ, Keijsers V, van der Linden MW, Tong TQ, Borggreve SE, Verweij CL, Breedveld FC, Huizinga TW. 1999. Neuropsychiatric systemic lupus erythematosus is associated with imbalance in interleukin 10 promoter haplotypes. *Ann. Rheum. Dis.* 58:85–89

62. Grondal G, Kristjansdottir H, Gunnlaugsdottir B, Arnason A, Lundberg I, Klareskog L, Steinsson K. 1999. Increased number of interleukin-10-producing cells in systemic lupus erythematosus patients and their first-degree relatives and spouses in Icelandic multicase families. *Arthritis Rheum,* 42:1649–54

63. Mehrian R, Quismorio FP Jr, Strassmann G, Stimmler MM, Horwitz DA, Kitridou RC, Gauderman WJ, Morrison J, Brautbar C, Jacob CO. 1998. Synergistic effect between IL-10 and bcl-2 genotypes in determining susceptibility to systemic lupus erythematosus. *Arthritis Rheum.* 41:596–602

64. Kono DH, Burlingame RW, Owens DG, Kuramochi A, Balderas RS, Balomenos D, Theofilopoulos AN. 1994. Lupus susceptibility loci in New Zealand mice. *Proc. Natl. Acad. Sci. USA* 91:10168–72

65. Morse HR, Bidwell JL, Raveche ES. 1999. A poly(C) repeat polymorphism in the promoter of the IL-10 gene in NZB mice. *Eur. J. Immunogenet.* 26:377–78

66. Westendorp RG, Langermans JA, Huizinga TW, Elouali AH, Verweij CL, Boomsma DI, Vandenbroucke JP, Vandenbrouke JP. 1997. Genetic influence on cytokine production and fatal meningococcal disease [published erratum appears in *Lancet* 1997 Mar 1;349(9052):656]. *Lancet* 349:170–73

67. Edwards-Smith CJ, Jonsson JR, Purdie DM, Bansal A, Shorthouse C, Powell EE. 1999. Interleukin-10 promoter polymorphism predicts initial response of chronic hepatitis C to interferon alfa. *Hepatology* 30:526–30

68. Knappe A, Hor S, Wittmann S, Fickenscher H. 2000. Induction of a novel cellular homolog of interleukin-10, AK155, by transformation of T lymphocytes with herpesvirus saimiri. *J. Virol.* 74:3881–87

69. Dumoutier L, Louahed J, Renauld JC. 2000. Cloning and characterization of IL-10-related T cell-derived inducible factor (IL-TIF), a novel cytokine structurally related to IL-10 and inducible by IL-9. *J. Immunol.* 164:1814–9

70. Dumoutier L, Van Roost E, Colau D, Renauld JC. 2000. Human interleukin-10-related T cell-derived inducible factor: molecular cloning and functional characterization as an hepatocyte-stimulating factor. *Proc. Natl. Acad. Sci. USA* 97:10144–49

71. Xie M-H, Aggarwal S, Ho W-H, Foster J, Zhang Z, Stinson J, Wood WI, Goddard AD, Gurney AL. 2000. IL-22, a novel human cytokine that signals through the interferon receptor related proteins CRF2-4 and IL-22R. *J. Biol. Chem.* 275:31335–39

72. Zhang R, Tan Z, Liang P. 2000. Identification of a novel ligand-receptor pair constitutively activated by ras oncogenes. *J. Biol. Chem.* 275:24436–43

73. Soo C, Shaw WW, Freymiller E, Longaker MT, Bertolami CN, Chiu R, Tieu A, Ting K. 1999. Cutaneous rat wounds express c49a, a novel gene with homology to the human melanoma differentiation associated gene, mda-7. *J. Cell. Biochem.* 74:1–10

74. Jiang H, Lin JJ, Su Z-Z, Goldstein NI, Fisher PB. 1995. Subtraction hybridization identifies a novel melanoma differentiation associated gene, mda-7, modulated during human melanoma differentiation, growth, and progression. *Oncogene* 11:2477–86

75. Jiang H, Su Z-Z, Lin JJ, Goldstein NI, Young CSH, Fisher PB. 1996. The melanoma differentiation associated gene mda-7 suppresses cancer cell growth. *Proc. Natl. Acad. Sci. USA* 93:9160–65

76. Su Z-Z, Madireddi MT, Lin JJ, Young CSH, Kitada S, Reed JC, Goldstein NI, Fisher PB. 1998. The cancer growth suppressor gene mda-7 selectively induces apoptosis in human breast cancer cells and inhibits tumor growth in nude mice. *Proc. Natl. Acad. Sci. USA* 95:14,400–5

77. Rode H-J, Janssen W, Rosen-Wolff A, Bugert JJ, Thein P, Becker Y, Darai G. 1993. The genome of equine herpesvirus type 2 harbors an interleukin-10 (IL-10)-like gene. *Virus Genes* 7:111–16

78. Fleming SB, McCaughan CA, Andrews AE, Nash AD, Mercer AA. 1997. A homolog of interleukin-10 is encoded by the poxvirus Orf virus. *J. Virol.* 71:4857–61

79. Kotenko SV, Saccani S, Izotova LS, Mirochnitchenko OV, Pestka S. 2000. Human cytomegalovirus harbors its own unique IL-10 homolog (cmvIL-10). *Proc. Natl. Acad. Sci. USA* 97:1695–1700

80. Ho AS-Y, Moore KW. 1994. Interleukin-10 and its receptor. *Ther. Immunol.* 1:173–85

81. Liu Y, de Waal Malefyt R, Briere F, Parham C, Bridon J-M, Banchereau J, Moore KW, Xu J. 1997. The Epstein-Barr virus interleukin-10 (IL-10) homolog is a selective agonist with impaired binding to the IL-10 receptor. *J. Immunol.* 158:604–13

82. Hudson GS, Bankier AT, Satchwell SC, Barrell BG. 1985. The short unique region of the B95-8 Epstein-Barr virus genome. *Virology* 147:81–98

83. Stewart JP, Behm FG, Arrand JR, Rooney CM. 1994. Differential expression of viral and human interleukin-10 (IL-10) by primary B cell tumors and B cell lines. *Virology* 200:724–32

84. Berman RM, Suzuki T, Tahara H, Robbins PD, Narula SK, Lotze MT. 1996. Systemic administration of cellular IL-10 induces an effective, specific, and long-lived immune response against established tumors in mice. *J. Immunol.* 157:231–38

85. Qin L, Chavin KD, Ding Y, Tahara H, Favaro JP, Woodward JE, Suzuki T, Robbins PD, Lotze MT, Bromberg JS. 1996. Retrovirus-mediated transfer of viral IL-10 gene prolongs murine cardiac allograft survival. *J. Immunol.* 156:2316–23

86. Suzuki T, Tahara H, Narula S, Moore KW, Robbins PD, Lotze MT. 1995. Viral interleukin 10 (IL-10), the human herpes virus 4 cellular IL-10 homologue, induces local anergy to allogeneic and syngeneic tumors. *J. Exp. Med.* 182:477–86

87. Ho AS-Y, Liu Y, Khan TA, Hsu D-H, Bazan JF, Moore KW. 1993. A receptor for interleukin-10 is related to interferon receptors. *Proc. Natl. Acad. Sci. USA* 90:11267–71

88. Ding Y, Qin L, Kotenko SV, Pestka S, Bromberg JS. 2000. A single amino acid

determines the immunostimulatory activity of interleukin 10. *J. Exp. Med.* 191:213–24

89. O'Farrell A-M, Liu Y, Moore KW, Mui AL-F. 1998. IL-10 inhibits macrophage activation and proliferation by distinct signalling mechanisms: evidence for stat3-dependent and -independent pathways. *EMBO J.* 17:1006–18

90. Taniyama T, Takai S, Miyazaki E, Fukumura R, Sato J, Kobayashi Y, Hirakawa T, Moore KW, Yamada K. 1995. The human interleukin-10 receptor gene maps to chromosome 11q23.3. *Hum. Genet.* 95:99–101

91. Tan JC, Braun S, Rong H, DiGiacomo R, Dolphin E, Baldwin S, Narula SK, Zavodny PJ, Chou C-C. 1995. Characterization of recombinant extracellular domain of human interleukin-10 receptor. *J. Biol. Chem.* 270:12906–11

92. Reineke U, Sabat R, Volk H-D, Schneider-Mergener J. 1998. Mapping of the interleukin-10/interleukin-10 receptor combining site. *Protein Sci.* 7:951–60

93. Carson WE, Lindemann MJ, Baiocchi R, Linett M, Tan JC, Chou C-C, Narula S, Caligiuri MA. 1995. The functional characterization of interleukin-10 receptor expression on human natural killer cells. *Blood* 85:3577–85

94. Weber-Nordt RM, Meraz MA, Schreiber RD. 1994. LPS-dependent induction of IL-10 receptor expression on murine fibroblasts. *J. Immunol.* 153:3734–44

95. Michel G, Mirmohammadsadegh A, Olasz E, Jarzebska-Deussen B, Muschen A, Kemeny L, Abts HF, Ruzicka T. 1997. Demonstration and functional analysis of IL-10 receptors in human epidermal cells: decreased expression in psoriatic skin, down- modulation by IL-8, and up-regulation by an antipsoriatic glucocorticosteroid in normal cultured keratinocytes. *J. Immunol.* 159:6291–97

96. Michel G, Gailis A, Jarzebska-Deussen B, Muschen A, Mirmohammadsadegh A, Ruzicka T. 1997. 1,25-(OH)2-vitamin D3 and calcipotriol induce IL-10 receptor gene expression in human epidermal cells. *Inflamm. Res.* 46:32–34

97. Mirmohammadsadegh A, Homey B, Abts HF, Kohrer K, Ruzicka T, Michel G. 1998. Differential modulation of pro- and antiinflammatory cytokine receptors by N-(4-trifluoromethylphenyl)-2-cyano-3-hydroxy-crotonic acid amide (A77 1726), the physiologically active metabolite of the novel immunomodulator leflunomide. *Biochem. Pharmacol.* 55:1523–29

98. Roth I, Fisher SJ. 1999. IL-10 is an autocrine inhibitor of human placental cytotrophoblast MMP- 9 production and invasion. *Dev. Biol.* 205:194–204

99. Bourreille A, Segain JP, Raingeard de la Bletiere D, Siavoshian S, Vallette G, Galmiche JP, Blottiere HM. 1999. Lack of interleukin 10 regulation of antigen presentation-associated molecules expressed on colonic epithelial cells. *Eur. J. Clin. Invest.* 29:48–55

100. Denning TL, Campbell NA, Song F, Garofalo RP, Klimpel GR, Reyes VE, Ernst PB. 2000. Expression of IL-10 receptors on epithelial cells from the murine small and large intestine. *Int. Immunol.* 12:133–39

101. Bach EA, Aguet M, Schreiber RD. 1997. The IFN gamma receptor: a paradigm for cytokine receptor signaling. *Annu. Rev. Immunol.* 15:563–91

102. Mogensen KE, Lewerenz M, Reboul J, Lutfalla G, Uze G. 1999. The type I interferon receptor: structure, function, and evolution of a family business. *J. Interferon Cytokine Res.* 19:1069–98

103. Lutfalla G, Gardiner K, Uze G. 1993. A new member of the cytokine receptor gene family maps on chromosome 21 at less than 35 kb from IFNAR. *Genomics* 16:366–73

104. Cheng S, Lutfalla G, Uze G, Chumakov IM, Gardiner K. 1993. GART, SON, IFNAR, and CRF2-4 genes cluster on

human chromosome 21 and mouse chromosome 16. *Mamm. Genome* 4:338–42

105. Gibbs VC, Pennica D. 1997. CRF2-4: isolation of cDNA clones encoding the human and mouse proteins. *Gene* 186:97–101

106. Kotenko SV, Krause CD, Izotova LS, Pollack BP, Wu W, Pestka S. 1997. Identification and functional characterization of a second chain of the interleukin-10 receptor complex. *EMBO J.* 16:5894–5903

107. Spencer SD, Di Marco F, Hooley J, Pitts-Meek S, Bauer M, Ryan AM, Sordat B, Gibbs VC, Aguet M. 1998. The orphan receptor CRF2-4 is an essential subunit of the interleukin 10 receptor. *J. Exp. Med.* 187:571–78

108. Riley JK, Takeda K, Akira S, Schreiber RD. 1999. Interleukin-10 receptor signaling through the JAK-STAT pathway. *J. Biol. Chem.* 274:16513–21

109. Finbloom DS, Winestock KD. 1995. IL-10 induces the tyrosine phosphorylation of tyk2 and Jak1 and the differential assembly of STAT1α and STAT3 complexes in human T cells and monocytes. *J. Immunol.* 155:1079–90

110. Ho AS-Y, Wei SH-Y, Mui AL-F, Miyajima A, Moore KW. 1995. Functional regions of the mouse IL-10 receptor cytoplasmic domain. *Mol. Cell. Biol.* 15:5043–53

111. Lai C-F, Ripperger J, Morella KK, Jurlander J, Hawley TS, Carson WE, Kordula T, Caligiuri MA, Hawley RG, Fey GH, Baumann H. 1996. Receptors for interleukin (IL)-10 and IL-6-type cytokines use similar signaling mechanisms for inducing transcription through IL-6 response elements. *J. Biol. Chem.* 271:13968–75

112. Wehinger JW, Gouilleux F, Groner B, Finke J, Mertelsmann R, Weber-Nordt RM. 1996. IL-10 induces DNA binding activity of three STAT proteins (Stat1, Stat3, and Stat5) and their distinct combinatorial assembly in the promoters of selected genes. *FEBS Lett.* 394:365–70

113. Weber-Nordt RM, Riley JK, Greenlund AC, Moore KW, Darnell JE, Schreiber RD. 1996. Stat3 recruitment by two distinct ligand-induced tyrosine phosphorylated docking sites in the IL-10 receptor intracellular domain. *J. Biol. Chem.* 271:27954–61

114. Rodig SJ, Meraz MA, White JM, Lampe PA, Riley JK, Arthur CD, King KL, Sheehan KC, Yin L, Pennica D, Johnson EM Jr, Schreiber RD. 1998. Disruption of the Jak1 gene demonstrates obligatory and nonredundant roles of the Jaks in cytokine-induced biologic responses. *Cell* 93:373–83

115. O'Farrell AM, Parry DA, Zindy F, Roussel MF, Lees E, Moore KW, Mui AL-F. 2000. Stat3-dependent induction of p19INK4D by IL-10 contributes to inhibition of macrophage proliferation. *J. Immunol.* 164:4607–15

116. Takeda K, Clausen BE, Kaisho T, Tsujimura T, Terada N, Forster I, Akira S. 1999. Enhanced Th1 activity and development of chronic enterocholitis in mice devoid of Stat3 in macrophages and neutrophils. *Immunity* 10:39–49

117. Meraz MA, White JM, Sheehan KCF, Bach EA, Rodig SJ, Dighe AS, Kaplan DH, Riley JK, Greenlund AC, Campbell D, Carver-Moore K, DuBois RN, Clark R, Aguet M, Schreiber RD. 1996. Targeted disruption of the Stat1 gene in mice reveals unexpected physiologic specificity in the JAK-STAT signaling pathway. *Cell* 84:431–42

118. Bovolenta C, Gasperini S, McDonald PP, Cassatella MA. 1998. High affinity receptor for IgG (Fc gamma RI/CD64) gene and STAT protein binding to the IFN-gamma response region (GRR) are regulated differentially in human neutrophils and monocytes by IL-10. *J. Immunol.* 160:911–19

119. Cassatella MA. 1998. The neutrophil: one of the cellular targets of interleukin-10. *Int. J. Clin. Lab. Res.* 28:148–61

120. Ito S, Ansari P, Sakatsume M, Dickensheets H, Vazquez N, Donnelley RP, Larner AC, Finbloom DS. 1999. Interleukin-10 inhibits expression of both interferon α- and interferon γ-induced genes by suppressing tyrosine phosphorylation of STAT1. *Blood* 93:1456–63

121. Yamaoka K, Otsuka T, Niiro H, Nakashima H, Tanaka Y, Nagano S, Ogami E, Niho Y, Hamasaki N, Izuhara K. 1999. Selective DNA-binding activity of interleukin-10-stimulated STAT molecules in human monocytes. *J. Interferon Cytokine Res.* 19:679–85

122. Cssatella MA, Gasperini S, Bovolenta C, Calzetti F, Vollebregt M, Scapini P, Marchi M, Suzuki R, Suzuki A, Yoshimura A. 1999. Interleukin-10 (IL-10) selectively enhances CIS3/SOCS3 mRNA expression in human neutrophils: evidence for an IL-10-induced pathway that is independent of STAT protein activation. *Blood* 94:2880–89

123. Auernhammer CJ, Bousquet C, Melmed S. 1999. Autoregulation of pituitary corticotroph SOCS-3 expression: characterization of the murine SOCS-3 promoter. *Proc. Natl. Acad. Sci. USA* 96:6964–69

124. Wang P, Wu P, Siegel MI, Egan RW, Billah MM. 1995. Interleukin (IL)-10 inhibits nuclear factor kappa B (NF kappa B) activation in human monocytes. IL-10 and IL-4 suppress cytokine synthesis by different mechanisms. *J. Biol. Chem.* 270:9558–63

125. Schottelius AJ, Mayo MW, Sartor RB, Baldwin AS, Jr. 1999. Interleukin-10 signaling blocks inhibitor of kappaB kinase activity and nuclear factor kappaB DNA binding. *J. Biol. Chem.* 274:31868–74

126. Ehrlich LC, Hu S, Peterson PK, Chao CC. 1998. IL-10 down-regulates human microglial IL-8 by inhibition of NF-kappaB activation. *Neuroreport* 9:1723–26

127. Clarke CJ, Hales A, Hunt A, Foxwell BM. 1998. IL-10-mediated suppression of TNF-alpha production is independent of its ability to inhibit NF kappa B activity. *Eur. J. Immunol.* 28:1719–26

128. Dokter WHA, Koopmans SB, Vellenga E. 1996. Effects of IL-10 and IL-4 on LPS-induced transcription factors (AP-1, NF-IL6 and NF-kappa B) which are involved in IL-6 regulation. *Leukemia* 10:1308–16

129. Romano MF, Lamberti A, Petrella A, Bisogni R, Tassone PF, Formisano S, Venuta S, Turco MC. 1996. IL-10 inhibits nuclear factor-kappa B/Rel nuclear activity in CD3-stimulated human peripheral T lymphocytes. *J. Immunol.* 156:2119–23

130. Lentsch AB, Shanley TP, Sarma V, Ward PA. 1997. In vivo suppression of NF-kappa B and preservation of I kappa B alpha by interleukin-10 and interleukin-13. *J. Clin. Invest.* 100:2443–48

131. Yoshidome H, Kato A, Edwards MJ, Lentsch AB. 1999. Interleukin-10 suppresses hepatic ischemia/reperfusion injury in mice: implications of a central role for nuclear factor kappaB. *Hepatology* 30:203–8

132. Yin M-J, Yamamoto Y, Gaynor RB. 1998. The anti-inflammatory agents aspirin and salicylate inhibit the activity of IκB kinase-β. *Nature* 396:77–80

133. Hurme M, Henttinen T, Karppelin M, Varkila K, Matikainen S. 1994. Effect of interleukin-10 on NF-kB and AP-1 activities in interleukin-2 dependent CD8 T lymphoblasts. *Immunol. Lett.* 42:129–33

134. Giovarelli M, Musiani P, Modesti A, Dellabona P, Casorati G, Allione A, Consalvo M, Cavallo F, di Pierro F, De Giovanni C, et al. 1995. Local release of IL-10 by transfected mouse mammary adenocarcinoma cells does not suppress but enhances antitumor reaction and elicits a strong cytotoxic lymphocyte and antibody-dependent immune memory. *J. Immunol.* 155:3112–23

135. Groux H, Bigler M, de Vries JE, Roncarolo MG. 1998. Inhibitory and stimulatory effects of IL-10 on human CD8+ T cells. *J. Immunol.* 160:3188–93

136. Santin AD, Hermonat PL, Ravaggi A, Bellone S, Pecorelli S, Roman JJ, Parham GP, Cannon MJ. 2000. Interleukin-10 increases Th1 cytokine production and cytotoxic potential in human papillomavirus-specific CD8(+) cytotoxic T lymphocytes. *J. Virol.* 74:4729–37

137. Schwarz MA, Hamilton LD, Tardelli L, Narula SK, Sullivan LM. 1994. Stimulation of cytolytic activity by interleukin-10. *J. Immunother.* 16:95–104

138. Jinquan T, Larsen CG, Gesser B, Matsushima K, Thestrup-Pedersen K. 1993. Human interleukin 10 is a chemoattractant for CD8+ T lymphocytes and an inhibitor of IL-8-induced CD4+ T lymphocyte migration. *J. Immunol.* 151:4545–51

139. Zheng LM, Ojcius DM, Garaud F, Roth C, Maxwell E, Li Z, Rong H, Chen J, Wang XY, Catino JJ, King I. 1996. Interleukin-10 inhibits tumor metastasis through an NK cell-dependent mechanism. *J. Exp. Med.* 184:579–84

140. Levy Y, Brouet JC. 1994. Interleukin-10 prevents spontaneous death of germinal center B cells by induction of the bcl-2 protein. *J. Clin. Invest.* 93:424–28

141. Weber-Nordt RM, Henschler R, Schott E, Wehinger J, Behringer D, Mertelsmann R, Finke J. 1996. Interleukin-10 increases Bcl-2 expression and survival in primary human CD34+ hematopoietic progenitor cells. *Blood* 88:2549–58

142. Bonig H, Korholz D, Pafferath B, Mauz-Korholz C, Burdach S. 1996. Interleukin 10 induced c-fos expression in human B cells by activation of divergent protein kinases. *Immunol. Invest.* 25:115–28

143. Crawley JB, Williams LM, Mander T, Brennan FM, Foxwell BMJ. 1996. Interleukin-10 stimulation of phosphatidylinositol 3-kinase and p70 S6 kinase is required for the proliferative but not the antiinflammatory effects of the cytokine. *J. Biol. Chem.* 271:16357–62

144. Geng Y, Gulbins E, Altman A, Lotz M. 1994. Monocyte deactivation by interleukin 10 via inhibition of tyrosine kinase activity and the Ras signaling pathway. *Proc. Natl. Acad. Sci. USA* 91:8602–6

145. Sato K, Nagayama H, Tadokoro K, Juji T, Takahashi TA. 1999. Extracellular signal-regulated kinase, stress-activated protein kinase/c-Jun N-terminal kinase, and p38mapk are involved in IL-10-mediated selective repression of TNF-alpha-induced activation and maturation of human peripheral blood monocyte-derived dendritic cells. *J. Immunol.* 162:3865–72

146. Tan J, Town T, Saxe M, Paris D, Wu Y, Mullan M. 1999. Ligation of microglial CD40 results in p44/42 mitogen-activated protein kinase-dependent TNF-alpha production that is opposed by TGF-beta1 and IL-10. *J. Immunol.* 163:6614–21

147. Wilkes DS, Neimeier M, Mathur PN, Soliman DM, Twigg HLr, Bowen LK, Heidler KM. 1995. Effect of human lung allograft alveolar macrophages on IgG production: immunoregulatory role of interleukin-10, transforming growth factor-beta, and interleukin-6. *Am. J. Respir. Cell Mol. Biol.* 13:621–28

148. Armstrong L, Jordan N, Millar A. 1996. Interleukin 10 (IL-10) regulation of tumour necrosis factor alpha (TNF-alpha) from human alveolar macrophages and peripheral blood monocytes. *Thorax* 51:143–49

149. Park DR, Skerrett SJ. 1996. IL-10 enhances the growth of Legionella pneumophila in human mononuclear phagocytes and reverses the protective effect of IFN-gamma: differential responses of blood monocytes and alveolar macrophages. *J. Immunol.* 157:2528–38

150. Thomassen MJ, Divis LT, Fisher CJ. 1996. Regulation of human alveolar macrophage inflammatory cytokine production by interleukin-10. *Clin. Immunol. Immunopathol.* 80:321–24

151. Zissel G, Schlaak J, Schlaak M, Muller-Quernheim J. 1996. Regulation of cytokine release by alveolar macrophages treated with interleukin-4, interleukin-10, or transforming growth factor beta. *Eur. Cytokine Netw.* 7:59–66

152. Berkman N, John M, Roesems G, Jose PJ, Barnes PJ, Chung KF. 1995. Inhibition of macrophage inflammatory protein-1 alpha expression by IL-10. Differential sensitivities in human blood monocytes and alveolar macrophages. *J. Immunol.* 155:4412–18

153. Nicod LP, el Habre F, Dayer JM, Boehringer N. 1995. Interleukin-10 decreases tumor necrosis factor alpha and beta in alloreactions induced by human lung dendritic cells and macrophages. *Am. J. Respir. Cell Mol. Biol.* 13:83–90

154. de Waal Malefyt R, Figdor CG, Huijbens R, Mohan PS, Bennett B, Culpepper J, Dang W, Zurawski G, de VJ. 1993. Effects of IL-13 on phenotype, cytokine production, and cytotoxic function of human monocytes. Comparison with IL-4 and modulation by IFN-gamma or IL-10. *J. Immunol.* 151:6370–81

155. D'Andrea A, Aste AM, Valiante NM, Ma X, Kubin M, Trinchieri G. 1993. Interleukin 10 (IL-10) inhibits human lymphocyte interferon gamma-production by suppressing natural killer cell stimulatory factor/IL-12 synthesis in accessory cells. *J. Exp. Med.* 178:1041–48

156. Gruber MF, Williams CC, Gerrard TL. 1994. Macrophage-colony-stimulating factor expression by anti-CD45 stimulated human monocytes is transcriptionally up-regulated by IL-1 beta and inhibited by IL-4 and IL-10. *J. Immunol.* 152:1354–61

157. Rossi DL, Vicari AP, Franz-Bacon K, McClanahan TK, Zlotnik A. 1997. Identification through bioinformatics of two new macrophage proinflamatory human chemokines MIP-3α and MIP-3β. *J. Immunol.* 158:1033–36

158. Marfaing-Koka A, Maravic M, Humbert M, Galanaud P, Emilie D. 1996. Contrasting effects of IL-4, IL-10 and corticosteroids on RANTES production by human monocytes. *Int. Immunol.* 8:1587–94

159. Kopydlowski KM, Salkowski CA, Cody MJ, van Rooijen N, Major J, Hamilton TA, Vogel SN. 1999. Regulation of macrophage chemokine expression by lipopolysaccharide in vitro and in vivo. *J. Immunol.* 163:1537–44

160. Andrew DP, Chang MS, McNinch J, Wathen ST, Rihanek M, Tseng J, Spellberg JP, Elias CG, 3rd. 1998. STCP-1 (MDC) CC chemokine acts specifically on chronically activated Th2 lymphocytes and is produced by monocytes on stimulation with Th2 cytokines IL-4 and IL-13. *J. Immunol.* 161:5027–38

161. Sozzani S, Ghezzi S, Iannolo G, Luini W, Borsatti A, Polentarutti N, Sica A, Locati M, Mackay C, Wells TN, Biswas P, Vicenzi E, Poli G, Mantovani A. 1998. Interleukin 10 increases CCR5 expression and HIV infection in human monocytes. *J. Exp. Med.* 187:439–44

162. Thivierge M, Parent JL, Stankova J, Rola-Pleszczynski M. 1999. Modulation of formyl peptide receptor expression by IL-10 in human monocytes and neutrophils. *J. Immunol.* 162:3590–95

163. Wang J, Guan E, Roderiquez G, Norcross MA. 1999. Inhibition of CCR5 expression by IL-12 through induction of beta-chemokines in human T lymphocytes. *J. Immunol.* 163:5763–69

164. Hart PH Hunt EK, Bonder CS, Watson CJ, Finlay-Jones JJ. 1996. Regulation of surface and soluble TNF receptor expression on human monocytes and synovial fluid macrophages by IL-4 and IL-10. *J. Immunol.* 157:3672–80

165. Joyce DA, Steer JH. 1996. IL-4, IL-10 and IFN-gamma have distinct, but interacting, effects on differentiation-induced changes in TNF-alpha and TNF receptor

release by cultured human monocytes. *Cytokine* 8:49–57

166. Linderholm M, Ahlm C, Settergren B, Waage A, Tarnvik A. 1996. Elevated plasma levels of tumor necrosis factor (TNF)-alpha, soluble TNF receptors, interleukin (IL)-6, and IL-10 in patients with hemorrhagic fever with renal syndrome. *J. Infect. Dis.* 173:38–43

167. Dickensheets HL, Freeman SL, Smith MF, Donnelly RP. 1997. Interleukin-10 upregulates tumor necrosis factor receptor type-II (p75) gene expression in endotoxin-stimulated human monocytes. *Blood* 90:4162–71

168. Jenkins JK, Malyak M, Arend WP. 1994. The effects of interleukin-10 on interleukin-1 receptor antagonist and interleukin-1 beta production in human monocytes and neutrophils. *Lymphokine Cytokine Res.* 13:47–54

169. Dickensheets HL, Donnelly RP. 1997. IFN-gamma and IL-10 inhibit induction of IL-1 receptor type I and type II gene expression by IL-4 and IL-13 in human monocytes. *J. Immunol.* 159:6226–33

170. Hedrick JA, Helms A, Vicari A, Zlotnik A. 1998. Characterization of a novel CC chemokine, HCC-4, whose expression is increased by interleukin-10. *Blood* 91:4242–47

171. Braun MC, Lahey E, Kelsall BL. 2000. Selective suppression of IL-12 production by chemoattractants. *J. Immunol.* 164:3009–17

172. Sato K, Kawasaki H, Nagayama H, Enomoto M, Morimoto C, Tadokoro K, Juji T, Takahashi TA. 2000. TGF-beta 1 reciprocally controls chemotaxis of human peripheral blood monocyte-derived dendritic cells via chemokine receptors. *J. Immunol.* 164:2285–95

173. Aste-Amezaga M, Ma X, Sartori A, Trinchieri G. 1998. Molecular mechanisms of the induction of IL-12 and its inhibition by IL-10 [published erratum appears in *J. Immunol.* 2000

May 15;164(10):5330]. *J. Immunol.* 160:5936–44

174. Brown CY, Lagnado CA, Vadas MA, Goodall GJ. 1996. Differential regulation of the stability of cytokine mRNAs in lipopolysaccharide-activated blood monocytes in response to interleukin-10. *J. Biol. Chem.* 271:20108–12

175. Kim HS, Armstrong D, Hamilton TA, Tebo JM. 1998. IL-10 suppresses LPS-induced KC mRNA expression via a translation-dependent decrease in mRNA stability. *J. Leukocyte Biol.* 64:33

176. Kishore R, Tebo JM, Kolosov M, Hamilton TA. 1999. Cutting edge: clustered AU-rich elements are the target of IL-10-mediated mRNA destabilization in mouse macrophages. *J. Immunol.* 162:2457–61

177. Cassatella MA, Meda L, Gasperini S, Calzetti F, Bonora S. 1994. Interleukin 10 (IL-10) upregulates IL-1 receptor antagonist production from lipopolysaccharide-stimulated human polymorphonuclear leukocytes by delaying mRNA degradation. *J. Exp. Med.* 179:1695–99

178. Niiro H, Otsuka T, Kuga S, Nemoto Y, Abe M, Hara N, Nakano T, Ogo T, Niho Y. 1994. IL-10 inhibits prostaglandin E2 production by lipopolysaccharide-stimulated monocytes. *Int. Immunol.* 6:661–64

179. Niiro H, Otsuka T, Tanabe T, Hara S, Kuga S, Nemoto Y, Tanaka Y, Nakashima H, Kitajima S, Abe M, et al. 1995. Inhibition by interleukin-10 of inducible cyclooxygenase expression in lipopolysaccharide-stimulated monocytes: its underlying mechanism in comparison with interleukin-4. *Blood* 85:3736–45

180. Mertz PM, DeWitt DL, Stetler-Stevenson WG, Wahl LM. 1994. Interleukin 10 suppression of monocyte prostaglandin H synthase-2. Mechanism of inhibition of prostaglandin-dependent matrix metalloproteinase production. *J. Biol. Chem.* 269:21322–29

181. Lacraz S, Nicod LP, Chicheportiche R, Welgus HG, Dayer JM. 1995. IL-10 inhibits metalloproteinase and stimulates TIMP-1 production in human mononuclear phagocytes. *J. Clin. Invest.* 96:2304–10

182. Stearns ME, Wang M, Stearns M. 1995. IL-10 blocks collagen IV invasion by "invasion stimulating factor" activated PC-3 ML cells: upregulation of TIMP-1 expression. *Oncol. Res.* 7:157–63

183. Stearns ME, Rhim J, Wang M. 1999. Interleukin 10 (IL-10) inhibition of primary human prostate cell-induced angiogenesis: IL-10 stimulation of tissue inhibitor of metalloproteinase-1 and inhibition of matrix metalloproteinase (MMP)-2/MMP-9 secretion. *Clin. Cancer Res.* 5:189–96

184. Girard N, Maingonnat C, Bertrand P, Vasse M, Delpech B. 1999. Hyaluronectin secretion by monocytes: downregulation by IL-4 and IL-13, upregulation by IL-10. *Cytokine* 11:579–84

185. Kubin M, Kamoun M, Trinchieri G. 1994. Interleukin-12 synergizes with B7/CD28 interaction in inducing efficient proliferation and cytokine production by human T cells. *J. Exp. Med.* 180:263–74

186. Willems F, Marchant A, Delville JP, Gerard C, Delvaux A, Velu T, de Boer M, Goldman M. 1994. Interleukin-10 inhibits B7 and intercellular adhesion molecule-1 expression on human monocytes. *Eur. J. Immunol.* 24:1007–9

187. Koppelman B, Neefjes JJ, de Vries JE, de Waal Malefyt R. 1997. Interleukin-10 downregulates MHC Class II ab peptide complexes at the plasma membrane of monocytes by affecting arrival and recycling. *Immunity* 7:861–71

188. te Velde AA, de Waal Malefijt R, Huijbens RJ, de Vries JE, Figdor CG. 1992. IL-10 stimulates monocyte Fc gamma R surface expression and cytotoxic activity. Distinct regulation of antibody-dependent cellular cytotoxicity by IFN-gamma, IL-4, and IL-10. *J. Immunol.* 149:4048–52

189. Calzada-Wack JC, Frankenberger M, Ziegler-Heitbrock HW. 1996. Interleukin-10 drives human monocytes to CD16 positive macrophages. *J. Inflamm.* 46:78–85

190. Morinobu A, Kumagai S, Yanagida H, Ota H, Ishida H, Matsui M, Yodoi J, Nakao K. 1996. IL-10 suppresses cell surface CD23/Fc epsilon RII expression, not by enhancing soluble CD23 release, but by reducing CD23 mRNA expression in human monocytes. *J. Clin. Immunol.* 16:326–33

191. Capsoni F, Minonzio F, Ongari AM, Carbonelli V, Galli A, Zanussi C. 1995. IL-10 up-regulates human monocyte phagocytosis in the presence of IL-4 and IFN-gamma. *J. Leukoc. Biol.* 58:351–58

192. Spittler A, Schiller C, Willheim M, Tempfer C, Winkler S, Boltz-Nitulescu G. 1995. IL-10 augments CD23 expression on U937 cells and down-regulates IL-4-driven CD23 expression on cultured human blood monocytes: effects of IL-10 and other cytokines on cell phenotype and phagocytosis. *Immunology* 85:311–17

193. Cunha FQ, Moncada S, Liew FY. 1992. Interleukin-10 (IL-10) inhibits the induction of nitric oxide synthase by interferon-g in murine macrophages. *Biochem. Biophys. Res. Commun.* 182:1155–59

194. Niiro H, Otsuka T, Abe M, Satoh H, Ogo T, Nakano T, Furukawa Y, Niho Y. 1992. Epstein-Barr virus BCRF1 gene product (viral interleukin 10) inhibits superoxide anion production by human monocytes. *Lymphokine Cytokine Res.* 11:209–14

195. Wu J, Cunha FQ, Liew FY, Weiser WY. 1993. IL-10 inhibits the synthesis of migration inhibitory factor and migration inhibitory factor-mediated macrophage activation. *J. Immunol.* 151:4325–32

196. Cenci E, Romani L, Mencacci A, Spaccapelo R, Schiaffella E, Puccetti P, Bistoni F. 1993. Interleukin-4 and

interleukin-10 inhibit nitric oxide-dependent macrophage killing of Candida albicans. *Eur. J. Immunol.* 23:1034–38

197. Kuga S, Otsuka T, Niiro H, Nunoi H, Nemoto Y, Nakano T, Ogo T, Umei T, Niho Y. 1996. Suppression of superoxide anion production by interleukin-10 is accompanied by a downregulation of the genes for subunit proteins of NADPH oxidase. *Exp. Hematol.* 24:151–57

198. Roilides E, Dimitriadou A, Kadiltsoglou I, Sein T, Karpouzas J, Pizzo PA, Walsh TJ. 1997. IL-10 exerts suppressive and enhancing effects on antifungal activity of mononuclear phagocytes against Aspergillus fumigatus. *J. Immunol.* 158:322–29

199. Flesch IE, Hess JH, Oswald IP, Kaufmann SH. 1994. Growth inhibition of Mycobacterium bovis by IFN-gamma stimulated macrophages: regulation by endogenous tumor necrosis factor-alpha and by IL-10. *Int. Immunol.* 6:693–700

200. Dugas N, Vouldoukis I, Becherel P, Arock M, Debre P, Tardieu M, Mossalayi DM, Delfraissy JF, Kolb JP, Dugas B. 1996. Triggering of CD23b antigen by anti-CD23 monoclonal antibodies induces interleukin-10 production by human macrophages. *Eur. J. Immunol.* 26:1394–98

201. Sutterwala FS, Noel GJ, Salgame P, Mosser DM. 1998. Reversal of proinflammatory responses by ligating the macrophage Fcgamma receptor type I. *J. Exp. Med.* 188:217–22

202. Legge KL, Min B, Bell JJ, Caprio JC, Li L, Gregg RK, Zaghouani H. 2000. Coupling of peripheral tolerance to endogenous interleukin 10 promotes effective modulation of myelin-activated T cells and ameliorates experimental allergic encephalomyelitis. *J. Exp. Med.* 191:2039–52

203. Muzio M, Bosisio D, Polentarutti N, D'Amico G, Stoppacciaro A, Mancinelli R, van't Veer C, Penton-Rol G, Ruco LP,

Allavena P, Mantovani A. 2000. Differential expression and regulation of toll-like receptors (TLR) in human leukocytes: selective expression of TLR3 in dendritic cells. *J. Immunol.* 164:5998–6004

204. Buechler C, Ritter M, Orso E, Langmann T, Klucken J, Schmitz G. 2000. Regulation of scavenger receptor CD163 expression in human monocytes and macrophages by pro- and antiinflammatory stimuli. *J. Leukoc. Biol.* 67:97–103

205. Banchereau J, Briere F, Caux C, Davoust J, Lebecque S, Liu YJ, Pulendran B, Palucka K. 2000. Immunobiology of dendritic cells. *Annu. Rev. Immunol.* 18:767–811

206. Macatonia SE, Doherty TM, Knight SC, O'Garra A. 1993. Differential effect of interleukin 10 on dendritic cell-induced T cell proliferation and IFN-γ production. *J. Immunol.* 150:3755–65

207. Peguet-Navarro J, Moulon C, Caux C, Dalbiez-Gauthier C, Banchereau J, Schmitt D. 1994. Interleukin-10 inhibits the primary allogeneic T cell response to human epidermal Langerhans cells. *Eur. J. Immunol.* 24:884–91

208. Mitra RS, Judge TA, Nestle FO, Turka LA, Nickoloff BJ. 1995. Psoriatic skin-derived dendritic cell function is inhibited by exogenous IL-10. Differential modulation of B7-1 (CD80) and B7-2 (CD86) expression. *J. Immunol.* 154:2668–77

209. Ludewig B, Graf D, Gelderblom HR, Becker Y, Kroczek RA, Pauli G. 1995. Spontaneous apoptosis of dendritic cells is efficiently inhibited by TRAP (CD40-ligand) and TNF-alpha, but strongly enhanced by interleukin-10. *Eur. J. Immunol.* 25:1943–50

210. Buelens C, Willems F, Pierard G, Delvaux A, Velu T, Goldman M. 1995. IL-10 inhibits the primary allogeneic T cell response to human peripheral blood dendritic cells. *Adv. Exp. Med. Biol.* 378:363–65

211. Bejarano M-T, de Waal Malefyt R,

Abrams JS, Bigler M, Bacchetta R, de Vries JE, Roncarolo M-G. 1992. IL-10 inhibits allogeneic proliferative and cytotoxic T cell responses generated in primary MLC. *Int. Immunol.* 4:1389–97

212. Caux C, Massacrier C, Vanbervliet B, Barthelemy C, Liu YJ, Banchereau J. 1994. Interleukin 10 inhibits T cell alloreaction induced by human dendritic cells. *Int. Immunol.* 6:1177–85

213. Groux H, Bigler M, de Vries JE, Roncarolo MG. 1996. Interleukin-10 induces a long-term antigen-specific anergic state in human CD4+ T cells [see comments]. *J. Exp. Med.* 184:19–29

214. Steinbrink K, Wolfl M, Jonuleit H, Knop J, Enk AH. 1997. Induction of tolerance by IL-10-treated dendritic cells. *J. Immunol.* 159:4772–80

215. Takayama T, Nishioka Y, Lu L, Lotze MT, Tahara H, Thomson AW. 1998. Retroviral delivery of viral interleukin-10 into myeloid dendritic cells markedly inhibits their allostimulatory activity and promotes the induction of T-cell hyporesponsiveness. *Transplantation* 66:1567–74

216. Enk AH, Jonuleit H, Saloga J, Knop J. 1997. Dendritic cells as mediators of tumor-induced tolerance in metastatic melanoma. *Int. J. Cancer* 73:309–16

217. Steinbrink K, Jonuleit H, Muller G, Schuler G, Knop J, Enk AH. 1999. Interleukin-10-treated human dendritic cells induce a melanoma-antigen-specific anergy in CD8(+) T cells resulting in a failure to lyse tumor cells. *Blood* 93:1634–42

218. Zeller JC, Panoskaltsis-Mortari A, Murphy WJ, Ruscetti FW, Narula S, Roncarolo MG, Blazar BR. 1999. Induction of CD4+ T cell alloantigen-specific hyporesponsiveness by IL-10 and TGF-beta. *J. Immunol.* 163:3684–91

219. Liu L, Rich BE, Inobe J, Chen W, Weiner HL. 1998. Induction of Th2 cell differentiation in the primary immune response: dendritic cells isolated from adherent cell culture treated with IL-10 prime naive CD4+ T cells to secrete IL-4. *Int. Immunol.* 10:1017–26

220. de Jong EC, Vieira PL, Kalinski P, Kapsenberg ML. 1999. Corticosteroids inhibit the production of inflammatory mediators in immature monocyte-derived DC and induce the development of tolerogenic DC3. *J. Leukoc. Biol.* 66:201–4

221. Rea D, van Kooten C, van Meijgaarden KE, Ottenhoff TH, Melief CJ, Offringa R. 2000. Glucocorticoids transform CD40-triggering of dendritic cells into an alternative activation pathway resulting in antigen-presenting cells that secrete IL-10. *Blood* 95:3162–67

222. Penna G, Adorini L. 2000. 1 Alpha,25-dihydroxyvitamin D3 inhibits differentiation, maturation, activation, and survival of dendritic cells leading to impaired alloreactive T cell activation. *J. Immunol.* 164:2405–11

223. Matyszak MK, Citterio S, Rescigno M, Ricciardi-Castagnoli P. 2000. Differential effects of corticosteroids during different stages of dendritic cell maturation. *Eur. J. Immunol.* 30:1233–42

224. Vieira PL, Kalinski P, Wierenga EA, Kapsenberg ML, de Jong EC. 1998. Glucocorticoids inhibit bioactive IL-12p70 production by in vitro-generated human dendritic cells without affecting their T cell stimulatory potential. *J. Immunol.* 161:5245–51

225. Allavena P, Piemonti L, Longoni D, Bernasconi S, Stoppacciaro A, Ruco L, Mantovani A. 1998. IL-10 prevents the differentiation of monocytes to dendritic cells but promotes their maturation to macrophages. *Eur. J. Immunol.* 28:359–69

226. Kalinski P, Schuitemaker JH, Hilkens CM, Kapsenberg ML. 1998. Prostaglandin E2 induces the final maturation of IL-12-deficient CD1a+CD83+ dendritic cells: the levels of IL-12 are determined during the final dendritic cell

maturation and are resistant to further modulation. *J. Immunol.* 161:2804–9

227. Fortsch D, Rollinghoff M, Stenger S. 2000. IL-10 converts human dendritic cells into macrophage-like cells with increased antibacterial activity against virulent Mycobacterium tuberculosis. *J. Immunol.* 165:978–87

228. Rieser C, Ramoner R, Bock G, Deo YM, Holtl L, Bartsch G, Thurnher M. 1998. Human monocyte-derived dendritic cells produce macrophage colony-stimulating factor: enhancement of c-fms expression by interleukin-10. *Eur. J. Immunol.* 28:2283–88

229. MacDonald KP, Pettit AR, Quinn C, Thomas GJ, Thomas R. 1999. Resistance of rheumatoid synovial dendritic cells to the immunosuppressive effects of IL-10. *J. Immunol.* 163:5599–5607

230. Rissoan MC, Soumelis V, Kadowaki N, Grouard G, Briere F, de Waal Malefyt R, Liu YJ. 1999. Reciprocal control of T helper cell and dendritic cell differentiation. *Science* 283:1183–86

231. Payvandi F, Amrute S, Fitzgerald-Bocarsly P. 1998. Exogenous and endogenous IL-10 regulate IFN-alpha production by peripheral blood mononuclear cells in response to viral stimulation. *J. Immunol.* 160:5861–68

232. Arpinati M, Green CL, Heimfeld S, Heuser JE, Anasetti C. 2000. Granulocyte-colony stimulating factor mobilizes T helper 2-inducing dendritic cells. *Blood* 95:2484–90

233. Pulendran B, Banchereau J, Burkeholder S, Kraus E, Guinet E, Chalouni C, Caron D, Maliszewski C, Davoust J, Fay J, Palucka K. 2000. Flt3-ligand and granulocyte colony-stimulating factor mobilize distinct human dendritic cell subsets in vivo. *J. Immunol.* 165:566–72

234. Grohmann U, Bianchi R, Belladonna ML, Vacca C, Silla S, Ayroldi E, Fioretti MC, Puccetti P. 1999. IL-12 acts selectively on CD8 alpha- dendritic cells to enhance presentation of a tumor peptide in vivo. *J. Immunol.* 163:3100–5

235. Iwasaki A, Kelsall BL. 1999. Freshly isolated Peyer's patch, but not spleen, dendritic cells produce interleukin 10 and induce the differentiation of T helper type 2 cells. *J. Exp. Med.* 190:229–39

236. Khanna A, Morelli AE, Zhong C, Takayama T, Lu L, Thomson AW. 2000. Effects of liver-derived dendritic cell progenitors on Th1- and Th2-like cytokine responses in vitro and in vivo. *J. Immunol.* 164:1346–54

237. de Saint-Vis B, Fugier-Vivier I, Massacrier C, Gaillard C, Vanbervliet B, Ait-Yahia S, Banchereau J, Liu YJ, Lebecque S, Caux C. 1998. The cytokine profile expressed by human dendritic cells is dependent on cell subtype and mode of activation. *J. Immunol.* 160:1666–76

238. Geissmann F, Revy P, Regnault A, Lepelletier Y, Dy M, Brousse N, Amigorena S, Hermine O, Durandy A. 1999. TGF-beta 1 prevents the noncognate maturation of human dendritic Langerhans cells. *J. Immunol.* 162:4567–75

239. Tazi A, Moreau J, Bergeron A, Dominique S, Hance AJ, Soler P. 1999. Evidence that Langerhans cells in adult pulmonary Langerhans cell histiocytosis are mature dendritic cells: importance of the cytokine microenvironment. *J. Immunol.* 163:3511–15

240. Caux C, Massacrier C, Dubois B, Valladeau J, Dezutter-Dambuyant C, Durand I, Schmitt D, Saeland S. 1999. Respective involvement of TGF-beta and IL-4 in the development of Langerhans cells and non-Langerhans dendritic cells from CD34+ progenitors. *J. Leukoc. Biol.* 66:781–91

241. Cassatella MA, Meda L, Bonora S, Ceska M, Constantin G. 1993. Interleukin 10 (IL-10) inhibits the release of proinflammatory cytokines from human polymorphonuclear leukocytes. Evidence for an autocrine role of tumor necrosis factor and

IL-1 beta in mediating the production of IL-8 triggered by lipopolysaccharide. *J. Exp. Med.* 178:2207–11

242. Kasama T, Strieter RM, Lukacs NW, Burdick MD, Kunkel SL. 1994. Regulation of neutrophil-derived chemokine expression by IL-10. *J. Immunol.* 152:3559–69

243. Wang P, Wu P, Anthes JC, Siegel MI, Egan RW, Billah MM. 1994. Interleukin-10 inhibits interleukin-8 production in human neutrophils. *Blood* 83:2678–83

244. Cassatella MA, Gasperini S, Calzetti F, Bertagnin A, Luster AD, McDonald PP. 1997. Regulated production of the interferon-gamma-inducible protein-10 (IP-10) chemokine by human neutrophils. *Eur. J. Immunol.* 27:111–15

245. Gasperini S, Marchi M, Calzetti F, Laudanna C, Vicentini L, Olsen H, Murphy M, Liao F, Farber J, Cassatella MA. 1999. Gene expression and production of the monokine induced by IFN-gamma (MIG), IFN-inducible T cell alpha chemoattractant (I-TAC), and IFN-gamma-inducible protein-10 (IP-10) chemokines by human neutrophils. *J. Immunol.* 162:4928–37

246. Bussolati B, Mariano F, Montrucchio G, Piccoli G, Camussi G. 1997. Modulatory effect of interleukin-10 on the production of platelet-activating factor and superanions by human leucocytes. *Immunology* 90:440–44

247. Niiro H, Otsuka T, Izuhara K, Yamaoka K, Oshima K, Tanabe T, Hara S, Nemoto Y, Tanaka Y, Nakashima H, Niho Y. 1997. Regulation by interleukin-10 and interleukin-4 of cyclooxygenase-2 expression in human neutrophils. *Blood* 89:1621–28

248. Maloney CG, Kutchera WA, Albertine KH, McIntyre TM, Prescott SM, Zimmerman GA. 1998. Inflammatory agonists induce cyclooxygenase type 2 expression by human neutrophils. *J. Immunol.* 160:1402–10

249. Keel M, Ungethum U, Stecholzer U,

Niederer E, Hartung T, Trenz O, Ertel W. 1997. Interleukin-10 counterregulates proinflammatory cytokine-induced inhibition of neutrophil apoptosis during severe sepsis. *Blood* 90:3356–61

250. Reglier H, Arce-Vicioso M, Fay M, Gougerot-Pocidalo MA, Chollet-Martin S. 1998. Lack of IL-10 and IL-13 production by human polymorphonuclear neutrophils. *Cytokine* 10:192–98

251. Chaves MM, Silvestrini AA, Silva-Teixeira DN, Nogueira-Machado JA. 1996. Effect in vitro of gamma interferon and interleukin-10 on generation of oxidizing species by human granulocytes. *Inflamm. Res.* 45:313–15

252. Capsoni F, Minonzio F, Ongari AM, Carbonelli V, Galli A, Zanussi C. 1997. IL-10 down-regulates oxidative metabolism and antibody-dependent cellular cytotoxicity of human neutrophils. *Scand. J. Imunol.* 45:269–76

253. Denis M, Ghadirian E. 1993. IL-10 neutralization augments mouse resistance to systemic Mycobacterium avium infections. *J. Immunol.* 151:5425–30

254. Greenberger MJ, Strieter RM, Kunkel SL, Danforth JM, Goodman RE, Standiford TJ. 1995. Neutralization of IL-10 increases survival in a murine model of Klebsiella pneumonia. *J. Immunol.* 155:722–29

255. van der Poll T, Marchant A, Keogh CV, Goldman M, Lowry SF. 1996. Interleukin-10 impairs host defense in murine pneumococcal pneumonia. *J. Infect. Dis.* 174:994–1000

256. Laichalk LL, Danforth JM, Standiford TJ. 1996. Interleukin-10 inhibits neutrophil phagocytic and bactericidal activity. *FEMS Immunol. Med. Microbiol.* 15:181

257. Marie C, Pitton C, Fitting C, Cavaillon JM. 1996. IL-10 and IL-4 synergize with TNF-alpha to induce IL-1ra production by human neutrophils. *Cytokine* 8:147–51

258. Zuany-Amorim C, Haile S., Leduc D., Dunarey C., Huerre M., Vargaftig BB, Pretolani M. 1995. Interleukin-10 inhibits antigen-induced cellular recruitment into the airways of sensitized mice. *J. Clin. Invest.* 95:2644–51

259. Shanley TP, Schmal H, Friedl HP, Jones ML, Ward PA. 1995. Regulatory effects of intrinsic IL-10 in IgG immune complex-induced lung injury. *J. Immunol.* 154:3454–60

260. Cox G. 1996. IL-10 enhances resolution of pulmonary inflammation in vivo by promoting apoptosis of neutrophils. *Am. J. Physiol.* 271:L566–L71

261. Steinhauser ML, Hogaboam CM, Kunkel SL, Lukacs NW, Strieter RM, Standiford TJ. 1999. IL-10 is a major mediator of sepsis-induced impairment in lung antibacterial host defense. *J. Immunol.* 162:392–99

262. Shanley TP, Vasi N, Denenberg A. 2000. Regulation of chemokine expression by Il-10 in lung inflammation. *Cytokine* 12:1054–64

263. Ward P Murray J, Bruce L, Farrow S, Chilvers ER, Hannah S, Haslett C, Rossi AG. 1997. Interleukin-10 does not directly affect the constitutive rate of human neutrophil or eosinophil apoptosis. *Biochem. Soc. Trans.* 25:245S

264. Takanashi S, Nonaka R., Xing Z., O'Byrne P., Dolovich J., and Jordana M. 1994. Interleukin 10 inhibits lipopolysaccharide-induced survival and cytokine production by human peripheral blood eosinophils. *J. Exp. Med.* 180:711–15

265. Pecanha LM, Snapper CM, Lees A, Mond JJ. 1992. Lymphokine control of type 2 antigen response. IL-10 inhibits IL-5- but not IL-2-induced Ig secretion by T cell-independent antigens. *J. Immunol.* 148:3427–32

266. Pecanha LM, Snapper CM, Lees A, Yamaguchi H, Mond JJ. 1993. IL-10 inhibits T cell-independent but not T cell-dependent

responses in vitro. *J. Immunol.* 150:3215–23

267. Clinchy B, Bjorck P, Paulie S, Moller G. 1994. Interleukin-10 inhibits motility in murine and human B lymphocytes. *Immunology* 82:376–82

268. Davidson NJ, Leach MW, Fort MM, Thompson-Snipes L, Kuhn R, Muller W, Berg DJ, Rennick DM. 1996. T helper cell 1-type CD4+ T cells, but not B cells, mediate colitis in interleukin 10-deficient mice. *J. Exp. Med.* 184:241–51

269. Groux H, Cottrez F, Rouleau M, Mauze S, Antonenko S, Hurst S, McNeil T, Bigler M, Roncarolo MG, Coffman RL. 1999. A transgenic model to analyze the immunoregulatory role of IL-10 secreted by antigen-presenting cells. *J. Immunol.* 162:1723–29

270. Stampfli MR, Cwiartka M, Gajewska BU, Alvarez D, Ritz SA, Inman MD, Xing Z, Jordana M. 1999. Interleukin-10 gene transfer to the airway regulates allergic mucosal sensitization in mice. *Am. J. Respir. Cell Mol. Biol.* 21:586–96

271. Tournoy KG, Kips JC, Pauwels RA. 2000. Endogenous interleukin-10 suppresses allergen-induced airway inflammation and nonspecific airway responsiveness. *Clin. Exp. Allergy* 30:775–83

272. Itoh K, Hirohata S. 1995. The role of IL-10 in human B cell activation, proliferation, and differentiation. *J. Immunol.* 154:4341–50

273. Hu BT, Insel RA. 1999. Up-regulation of telomerase in human B lymphocytes occurs independently of cellular proliferation and with expression of the telomerase catalytic subunit. *Eur. J. Immunol.* 29:3745–53

274. Saeland S, Duvert V, Moreau I, Banchereau J. 1993. Human B cell precursors proliferate and express CD23 after CD40 ligation. *J. Exp. Med.* 178:113–20

275. Fluckiger AC, Garrone P, Durand I, Galizzi JP, Banchereau J. 1993. Interleukin 10

(IL-10) upregulates functional high affinity IL-2 receptors on normal and leukemic B lymphocytes. *J. Exp. Med.* 178:1473–81

276. Burdin N, Van Kooten C, Galibert L, Abrams JS, Wijdenes J, Banchereau J, Rousset F. 1995. Endogenous IL-6 and IL-10 contribute to the differentiation of CD40-activated human B lymphocytes. *J. Immunol.* 154:2533–44

277. Punnonen J, de Waal Malefyt R, van Vlasselaer P, Gauchat J-F, de Vries JE. 1993. IL-10 and viral IL-10 prevent IL-4-induced IgE synthesis by inhibiting the accessory cell function of monocytes. *J. Immunol.* 151:1280–89

278. Nonoyama S, Hollenbaugh D, Aruffo A, Ledbetter JA, Ochs HD. 1993. B cell activation via CD40 is required for specific antibody production by antigen-stimulated human B cells. *J. Exp. Med.* 178:1097–1102

279. Garrone P, Galibert L, Rousset F, Banchereau J. 1994. Regulatory effects of prostaglandin E2 on the growth and differentiation of human B lymphocytes activated through their CD40 antigen. *J. Immunol.* 152:82–90

280. Uejima Y, Takahashi K, Komoriya K, Kurozumi S, Ochs HD. 1996. Effect of interleukin-10 on anti-CD40- and interleukin-4-induced immunoglobulin E production by human lymphocytes. *Int. Arch. Allergy Immunol.* 110:225–32

281. Defrance T, Vanbervliet B, Briere F, Durand I, Rousset F, Banchereau J. 1992. Interleukin 10 and transforming growth factor β cooperate to induce anti-CD40-activated naive human B cells to secrete immunoglobulin A. *J. Exp. Med.* 175:671–82

282. Briere F, Servet-Delprat C, Bridon J-M, Saint-Remy J-M, Banchereau J. 1994. Human interleukin 10 induces naive sIgD+ B cells to secrete IgG1 and IgG3. *J. Exp. Med.* 179:757–62

283. Levan-Petit I, Lelievre E, Barra A, Limosin A, Gombert B, Preud'homme JL, Lecron JC. 1999. T(h)2 cytokine dependence of IgD production by normal human B cells. *Int. Immunol.* 11:1819–28

284. Malisan F, Briere F, Bridon JM, Harindranath N, Mills FC, Max EE, Banchereau J, Martinez-Valdez H. 1996. Interleukin-10 induces immunoglobulin G isotype switch recombination in human CD40-activated naive B lymphocytes. *J. Exp. Med.* 183:937–47

285. Zan H, Cerutti A, Dramitinos P, Schaffer A, Casali P. 1998. CD40 engagement triggers switching to IgA1 and IgA2 in human B cells through induction of endogenous TGF-beta: evidence for TGF-beta but not IL-10-dependent direct S mu→S alpha and sequential S mu→S gamma, S gamma→S alpha DNA recombination. *J. Immunol.* 161:5217–25

286. Jeannin P, Lecoanet S, Delneste Y, Gauchat JF, Bonnefoy JY. 1998. IgE versus IgG4 production can be differentially regulated by IL-10. *J. Immunol.* 160:3555–61

287. Merville P, Dechanet J, Grouard G, Durand I, Banchereau J. 1995. T cell-induced B cell blasts differentiate into plasma cells when cultured on bone marrow stroma with IL-3 and IL-10. *Int. Immunol.* 7:635–43

288. Rousset F, Peyrol S, Garcia E, Vezzio N, Andujar M, Grimaud JA, Banchereau J. 1995. Long-term cultured CD40-activated B lymphocytes differentiate into plasma cells in response to IL-10 but not IL-4. *Int. Immunol.* 7:1243–53

289. Choe J, Choi YS. 1998. IL-10 interrupts memory B cell expansion in the germinal center by inducing differentiation into plasma cells. *Eur. J. Immunol.* 28:508–15

290. Agematsu K, Nagumo H, Oguchi Y, Nakazawa T, Fukushima K, Yasui K, Ito S, Kobata T, Morimoto C, Komiyama A. 1998. Generation of plasma cells

from peripheral blood memory B cells: synergistic effect of interleukin-10 and CD27/CD70 interaction. *Blood* 91:173–80

291. Briere F, Bridon JM, Chevet D, Souillet G, Bienvenu F, Guret C, Martinez-Valdez H, Banchereau J. 1994. Interleukin 10 induces B lymphocytes from IgA-deficient patients to secrete IgA. *J. Clin. Invest.* 94:97–104

292. Agematsu K, Nagumo H, Shinozaki K, Hokibara S, Yasui K, Terada K, Kawamura N, Toba T, Nonoyama S, Ochs HD, Komiyama A. 1998. Absence of IgD-CD27(+) memory B cell population in X-linked hyper-IgM syndrome. *J. Clin. Invest.* 102:853–60

293. Llorente L, Richaud-Patin Y, Fior R, Alcocer-Varela J, Wijdenes J, Fourrier BM, Galanaud P, Emilie D. 1994. In vivo production of interleukin-10 by non-T cells in rheumatoid arthritis, Sjogren's syndrome, and systemic lupus erythematosus: a potential mechanism of B lymphocyte hyperactivity and autoimmunity. *Arthritis Rheum.* 37:1647–55

294. Houssiau FA, Lefebvre C, Vanden Berghe M, Lambert M, Devogelaer JP, Renauld JC. 1995. Serum interleukin 10 titers in systemic lupus erythematosus reflect disease activity. *Lupus* 4:393–95

295. Hagiwara E, Gourley MF, Lee S, Klinman DK. 1996. Disease severity in patients with systemic lupus erythematosus correlates with an increased ratio of interleukin-10:interferon-gamma-secreting cells in the peripheral blood. *Arthritis Rheum.* 39:379–85

296. al-Janadi M, al-Dalaan A, al-Balla S, al-Humaidi M, Raziuddin S. 1996. Interleukin-10 (IL-10) secretion in systemic lupus erythematosus and rheumatoid arthritis: IL-10-dependent CD4+CD45RO+ T cell-B cell antibody synthesis. *J. Clin. Immunol.* 16:198–207

297. Llorente L, Richaud-Patin Y, Garcia-Padilla C, Claret E, J. J.-O, Cardiel MH, Alco-cer-Varela J, Grangeot-Keros L, Alarcon-Segovia D, Wijdenes J, Galanaud P, Emilie D. 2000. Clinical and biological effects of anti-interleukin-10 monoclonal antibody administration in systemic lupus erythematosus. *Arthritis Rheum.* 43:1790–1800

298. Taga K, Mostowski H, Tosato G. 1993. Human interleukin-10 can directly inhibit T-cell growth. *Blood* 81:2964–71

299. Schandene L, Alonso-Vega C, Willems F, Gerard C, Delvaux A, Velu T, Devos R, de Boer M, Goldman M. 1994. B7/CD28-dependent IL-5 production by human resting T cells is inhibited by IL-10. *J. Immunol.* 152:4368–74

300. Jinquan T, Quan S, Jacobi HH, Madsen HO, Glue C, Skov PS, Malling HJ, Poulsen LK. 2000. CXC chemokine receptor 4 expression and stromal cell-derived factor-1alpha-induced chemotaxis in CD4+ T lymphocytes are regulated by interleukin-4 and interleukin-10. *Immunology* 99:402–10

301. Rowbottom AW, Lepper MW, Garland RJ, Cox CV, Corley EG, Oakhill A, Steward CG. 1999. IL-10 induced CD8 cell proliferation. *Immunology* 98:80–89

302. Enk AH, Angeloni VL, Udey MC, Katz SI. 1993. Inhibition of Langerhans cell antigen-presenting function by IL-10. A role for IL-10 in induction of tolerance. *J. Immunol.* 151:2390–98

303. Enk AH, Saloga J, Becker D, Madzadeh M, Knop J. 1994. Induction of hapten-specific tolerance by interleukin 10 in vivo. *J. Exp. Med.* 179:1397–1402

304. Flores-Villanueva PO, Chikunguwo SM, Harris TS, Stadecker MJ. 1993. Role of IL-10 on antigen-presenting cell function for Schistosomal egg-specific monoclonal T helper cell responses in vitro and in vivo. *J. Immunol.* 151:3192–98

305. Flores Villanueva PO, Reiser H, Stadecker MJ. 1994. Regulation of T helper cell responses in experimental murine schistosomiasis by IL-10. Effect

on expression of B7 and B7-2 costim-
ulatory molecules by macrophages. *J. Immunol.* 153:5190–99

306. Becker JC, Czerny C, Brocker EB. 1994. Maintenance of clonal anergy by endoge-nously produced IL-10. *Int. Immunol.* 6:1605–12

307. King CL, Medhat A, Malhotra I, Nafeh M, Helmy A, Khaudary J, Ibrahim S, El-Sherbiny M, Zaky S, Stupi RJ, Brustoski K, Shehata M, Shata MT. 1996. Cytokine control of parasite-specific anergy in hu-man urinary schistosomiasis. IL-10 mod-ulates lymphocyte reactivity. *J. Immunol.* 156:4715–21

308. Schols D, De Clercq E. 1996. Human im-munodeficiency virus type 1 gp120 in-duces anergy in human peripheral blood lymphocytes by inducing interleukin-10 production. *J. Virol.* 70:4953–60

309. Sundstedt A, Holden I, Rosendahl A, Kalland T, van Rooijen N, Dohlsten M. 1997. Immunoregulatory role of IL-10 during superantigen-induced hy-poresponsiveness in vivo. *J. Immunol.* 158:180–86

310. Akdis CA, Blesken Akdis M, Wuthrich B, Blaser K. 1998. Role of interleukin 10 in specific immunotherapy. *J. Clin. Invest.* 102:98–106

311. Buer J, Lanoue A, Franzke A, Garcia C, von Boehmer Harald, Sarukan A. 1998. Interleukin 10 secretion and impaired ef-fector function of major histocompatibil-ity complex class II-restricted T cells an-ergized in vivo. *J. Exp. Med.* 187:177–83

312. Groux H, O'Garra A, Bigler M, Rouleau M, Antonenko S, de Vries JE, Roncarolo MG. 1997. A CD4+ T-cell subset inhibits antigen-specific T-cell responses and pre-vents colitis. *Nature* 389:737–42

313. Tanchot C, Guillaume S., Delon J., Bour-geois C., Franzke A., Sarukhan A., Traut-man A., Rocha B. 1998. Modifications of CD8+ T cell function during in vivo memory or tolerance induction. *Immunity* 8:581–90

314. Shreedhar VK, Pride MW, Sun Y, Kripke ML, Strickland FM. 1998. Origin and characteristics of ultraviolet-B radiation-induced suppressor T lymphocytes. *J. Im-munol.* 161:1327–35

315. Cobbold S, Waldmann H. 1998. Infec-tious tolerance. *Curr. Opin. Immunol.* 10:518–24

316. Seo N, Tokura Y, Takigawa M, Egawa K. 1999. Depletion of IL-10- and TGF-beta-producing regulatory gamma delta T cells by administering a daunomycin-conjugated specific monoclonal antibody in early tumor lesions augments the ac-tivity of CTLs and NK cells. *J. Immunol.* 163:242–49

317. Asseman C, Mauze S, Leach MW, Coff-man RL, Powrie F. 1999. An essential role for interleukin 10 in the function of reg-ulatory T cells that inhibit intestinal in-flammation. *J. Exp. Med.* 190:995–1004

318. Kitani A, Chua K, Nakamura K, Strober W. 2000. Activated self-MHC-reactive T cells have the cytokine phenotype of Th3/T regulatory cell 1 T cells. *J. Im-munol.* 165:691–702

319. Doetze A, Satoguina J, Burchard G, Rau T, Loliger C, Fleischer B, Hoerauf A. 2000. Antigen-specific cellular hypore-sponsiveness in a chronic human helminth infection is mediated by T(h)3/T(r)1-type cytokines IL-10 and transforming growth factor-beta but not by a T(h)1 to T(h)2 shift. *Int. Immunol.* 12:623–30

320. Cavani A, Nasorri F, Prezzi C, Sebastiani S, Albanesi C, Girolomoni G. 2000. Hu-man CD4+ T lymphocytes with remark-able regulatory functions on dendritic cells and nickel-specific Th1 immune re-sponses. *J. Invest. Dermatol.* 114:295–302

321. Swaminathan S, Hesselton R, Sullivan J, Kieff E. 1993. Epstein-Barr virus recom-binants with specifically mutated BCRF1 genes. *J. Virol.* 67:7406–13

322. Burdin N, Peronne C, Banchereau J, Rousset F. 1993. Epstein-Barr virus

transformation induces B lymphocytes to produce human interleukin-10. *J. Exp. Med.* 177:295–304

323. Miyazaki I, Cheung RK, Dosch H-M. 1993. Viral interleukin 10 is critical for the induction of B cell growth transformation by Epstein-Barr virus. *J. Exp. Med.* 178:439–47

324. Volk HD, Reinke P, Krausch D, Zuckermann H, Asadullah K, Muller JM, Docke WD, Kox WJ. 1996. Monocyte deactivation–rationale for a new therapeutic strategy in sepsis. *Intensive Care Med.* 22 Suppl 4:S474–81

325. Howard M, Muchamuel T, Andrade S, Menon S. 1993. Interleukin 10 protects mice from lethal endotoxemia. *J. Exp. Med.* 177:1205–8

326. Gerard C, Bruyns C, Marchant A, Abramowicz D, Vandenabeele P, Delvaux A, Fiers W, Goldman M, Velu T. 1993. Interleukin 10 reduces the release of tumor necrosis factor and prevents lethality in experimental endotoxemia. *J. Exp. Med.* 177:547–50

327. van der Poll T, Jansen PM, Montegut WJ, Braxton CC, Calvano SE, Stackpole SA, Smith SR, Swanson SW, Hack CE, Lowry SF, Moldawer LL. 1997. Effects of IL-10 on systemic inflammatory responses during sublethal primate endotoxemia. *J. Immunol.* 158:1971–75

328. Pajkrt D, Camoglio L, Tiel-van Buul MC, de Bruin K, Cutler DL, Affrime MB, Rikken G, van der Poll T, ten Cate JW, van Deventer SJ. 1997. Attenuation of proinflammatory response by recombinant human IL-10 in human endotoxemia: effect of timing of recombinant human IL-10 administration. *J. Immunol.* 158:3971–77

329. Rogy MA, Auffenberg T, Espat NJ, Philip R, Remick D, Wollenberg GK, Copeland EMr, Moldawer LL. 1995. Human tumor necrosis factor receptor (p55) and interleukin 10 gene transfer in the mouse reduces mortality to lethal endotoxemia

and also attenuates local inflammatory responses. *J. Exp. Med.* 181:2289–93

330. Durez P, Abramowicz D, Gerard C, Van Mechelen M, Amraoui Z, Dubois C, Leo O, Velu T, Goldman M. 1993. In vivo induction of interleukin 10 by anti-CD3 monoclonal antibody or bacterial lipopolysaccharide: differential modulation by cyclosporin A. *J. Exp. Med.* 177:551–55

331. van der Poll T, Jansen J, Levi M, ten Cate H, ten Cate JW, van Deventer SJ. 1994. Regulation of interleukin 10 release by tumor necrosis factor in humans and chimpanzees. *J. Exp. Med.* 180:1985–88

332. Jansen PM, van der Pouw Kraan TC, de Jong IW, van Mierlo G, Wijdenes J, Chang AA, Aarden LA Taylor FBJr, Hack CE. 1996. Release of interleukin-12 in experimental Escherichia coli septic shock in baboons: relation to plasma levels of interleukin-10 and interferon-gamma. *Blood* 87:5144–51

333. Marchant A, Bruyns C, Vandenabeele P, Abramowicz D, Gerard C, Delvaux A, Ghezzi P, Velu T, Goldman M. 1994. The protective role of interleukin-10 in endotoxin shock. *Prog. Clin. Biol. Res.* 388:417–23

334. Standiford TJ, Strieter RM, Lukacs NW, Kunkel SL. 1995. Neutralization of IL-10 increases lethality in endotoxemia. Cooperative effects of macrophage inflammatory protein-2 and tumor necrosis factor. *J. Immunol.* 155:2222–29

335. Hickey MJ, Issekutz AC, Reinhardt PH, Fedorak RN, Kubes P. 1998. Endogenous interleukin-10 regulates hemodynamic parameters, leukocyte-endothelial cell interactions, and microvascular permeability during endotoxemia. *Circ. Res.* 83:1124–31

336. Randow F, Syrbe U, Meisel C, Krausch D, Zuckermann H, Platzer C, Volk HD. 1995. Mechanism of endotoxin desensitization: involvement of interleukin 10 and

transforming growth factor beta. *J. Exp. Med.* 181:1887–92

337. Wolk K, Docke W, von Baehr V, Volk H, Sabat R. 1999. Comparison of monocyte functions after LPS- or IL-10-induced reorientation: importance in clinical immunoparalysis. *Pathobiology* 67:253–56

338. Wolk K, Docke WD, von Baehr V, Volk HD, Sabat R. 2000. Impaired antigen presentation by human monocytes during endotoxin tolerance. *Blood* 96:218–23

339. Asadullah K, Woiciechowsky C, Docke WD, Egerer K, Kox WJ, Vogel S, Sterry W, Volk HD. 1995. Very low monocytic HLA-DR expression indicates high risk of infection–immunomonitoring for patients after neurosurgery and patients during high dose steroid therapy. *Eur. J. Emerg. Med.* 2:184–90

340. Hess PJ, Seeger JM, Huber TS, Welborn MB, Martin TD, Harward TR, Duschek S, Edwards PD, Solorzano CC, Copeland EM, Moldawer LL. 1997. Exogenously administered interleukin-10 decreases pulmonary neutrophil infiltration in a tumor necrosis factor-dependent murine model of acute visceral ischemia. *J. Vasc. Surg.* 26:113–18

341. Engles RE, Huber TS, Zander DS, Hess PJ, Welborn MB, Moldawer LL, Seeger JM. 1997. Exogenous human recombinant interleukin-10 attenuates hindlimb ischemia-reperfusion injury. *J. Surg. Res.* 69:425–28

342. Lyons A, Goebel A, Mannick JA, Lederer JA. 1999. Protective effects of early interleukin-10 antagonism on injury-induced immune dysfunction. *Arch. Surg.* 134:1317–24

343. Kato T, Murata A, Ishida H, Toda H, Tanaka N, Hayashida H, Monden M, Matsuura N. 1995. Interleukin 10 reduces mortality from severe peritonitis in mice. *Antimicrob. Agents Chemother.* 39:1336–40

344. van der Poll T, Marchant A, Buurman WA, Berman L, Keogh CV, Lazarus DD, Nguyen L, Goldman M, Moldawer LL, Lowry SF. 1995. Endogenous IL-10 protects mice from death during septic peritonitis. *J. Immunol.* 155:5397–5401

345. Cusumano V, Genovese F, Mancuso G, Carbone M, Fera MT, Teti G. 1996. Interleukin-10 protects neonatal mice from lethal group B streptococcal infection. *Infect. Immun.* 64:2850–52

346. Florquin S, Amraoui Z, Abramowicz D, Goldman M. 1994. Systemic release and protective role of IL-10 in staphylococcal enterotoxin B-induced shock in mice. *J. Immunol.* 153:2618–23

347. Bean AGD, Freiberg RA, Andrade S, Menon S, Zlotnik A. 1993. Interleukin 10 protects mice against staphylococcal enterotoxin B-induced lethal shock. *Infect. Immun.* 61:4937–39

348. Marchant A, Bruyns C, Vandenabeele P, Ducarme M, Gerard C, Delvaux A, De Groote D, Abramowicz D, Velu T, Goldman M. 1994. Interleukin-10 controls interferon-gamma and tumor necrosis factor production during experimental endotoxemia. *Eur. J. Immunol.* 24:1167–71

349. Marchant A, Alegre ML, Hakim A, Pierard G, Marecaux G, Friedman G, De Groote D, Kahn RJ, Vincent JL, Goldman M. 1995. Clinical and biological significance of interleukin-10 plasma levels in patients with septic shock. *J. Clin. Immunol.* 15:266–73

350. Gomez-Jimenez J, Martin MC, Sauri R, Segura RM, Esteban F, Ruiz JC, Nuvials X, Boveda JL, Peracaula R, Salgado A. 1995. Interleukin-10 and the monocyte/macrophage-induced inflammatory response in septic shock. *J. Infect. Dis.* 171:472–75

351. Sherry RM, Cue JI, Goddard JK, Parramore JB, DiPiro JT. 1996. Interleukin-10 is associated with the development of sepsis in trauma patients. *J. Trauma* 40:613–16; discussion 6–7

352. van der Poll T, de Waal Malefyt R, Coyle

SM, Lowry SF. 1997. Antiinflammatory cytokine responses during clinical sepsis and experimental endotoxemia: sequential measurements of plasma soluble interleukin (IL)-1 receptor type II, IL-10, and IL-13. *J. Infect. Dis.* 175:118–22

353. Neidhardt R, Keel M, Steckholzer U, Safret A, Ungethuem U, Trentz O, Ertel W. 1997. Relationship of interleukin-10 plasma levels to severity of injury and clinical outcome in injured patients. *J. Trauma* 42:863–70; discussion 70–71

354. Frei K, Nadal D, Pfister HW, Fontana A. 1993. Listeria meningitis: identification of a cerebrospinal fluid inhibitor of macrophage listericidal function as interleukin 10. *J. Exp. Med.* 178:1255–61

355. Derkx B, Marchant A, Goldman M, Bijlmer R, van Deventer S. 1995. High levels of interleukin-10 during the initial phase of fulminant meningococcal septic shock. *J. Infect. Dis.* 171:229–32

356. Lehmann AK, Halstensen A, Sornes S, Rokke O, Waage A. 1995. High levels of interleukin 10 in serum are associated with fatality in meningococcal disease. *Infect. Immun.* 63:2109–12

357. Bourrie B, Bouaboula M, Benoit JM, Derocq JM, Esclangon M, Le Fur G, Casellas P. 1995. Enhancement of endotoxin-induced interleukin-10 production by SR 31747A, a sigma ligand. *Eur. J. Immunol.* 25:2882–87

358. Mengozzi M, Fantuzzi G, Faggioni R, Marchant A, Goldman M, Orencole S, Clark BD, Sironi M, Benigni F, Ghezzi P. 1994. Chlorpromazine specifically inhibits peripheral and brain TNF production, and up-regulates IL-10 production, in mice. *Immunology* 82:207–10

359. Suberville S, Bellocq A, Fouqueray B, Philippe C, Lantz O, Perez J, Baud L. 1996. Regulation of interleukin-10 production by beta-adrenergic agonists. *Eur. J. Immunol.* 26:2601–5

360. Van Laethem JL, Marchant A, Delvaux A, Goldman M, Robberecht P, Velu T, Deviere J. 1995. Interleukin 10 prevents necrosis in murine experimental acute pancreatitis. *Gastroenterology* 108:1917–22

361. Li Q, Sun B, Dastgheib K, Chan CC. 1996. Suppressive effect of transforming growth factor beta1 on the recurrence of experimental melanin protein-induced uveitis: upregulation of ocular interleukin-10. *Clin. Immunol. Immunopathol.* 81:55–61

362. Rosenbaum JT, Angell E. 1995. Paradoxical effects of IL-10 in endotoxin-induced uveitis. *J. Immunol.* 155:4090–94

363. Rizzo LV, Xu H, Chan CC, Wiggert B, Caspi RR. 1998. IL-10 has a protective role in experimental autoimmune uveoretinitis. *Int. Immunol.* 10:807–14

364. Okada AA, Keino H, Suzuki J, Sakai J, Usui M, Mizuguchi J. 1998. Kinetics of intraocular cytokines in the suppression of experimental autoimmune uveoretinitis by type I IFN. *Int. Immunol.* 10:1917–22

365. Tumpey TM, Elner VM, Chen SH, Oakes JE, Lausch RN. 1994. Interleukin-10 treatment can suppress stromal keratitis induced by herpes simplex virus type 1. *J. Immunol.* 153:2258–65

366. Arai T, Hiromatsu K, Kobayashi N, Takano M, Ishida H, Nimura Y, Yoshikai Y. 1995. IL-10 is involved in the protective effect of dibutyryl cyclic adenosine monophosphate on endotoxin-induced inflammatory liver injury. *J. Immunol.* 155:5743–49

367. Mulligan MS, Jones ML, Vaporciyan AA, Howard MC, Ward PA. 1993. Protective effects of IL-4 and IL-10 against immune complex-induced lung injury. *J. Immunol.* 151:5666–74

368. Mulligan MS, Warner RL, Foreback JL, Shanley TP, Ward PA. 1997. Protective effects of IL-4, IL-10 , IL-12 and IL-13 in IgG immune complex induced lung injury: role of endogenous IL-12. *J. Immunol.* 159:3483–89s

369. Bethea JR, Nagashima H, Acosta MC, Briceno C, Gomez F, Marcillo AE, Loor K, Green J, Dietrich WD. 1999. Systemically administered interleukin-10 reduces tumor necrosis factor-alpha production and significantly improves functional recovery following traumatic spinal cord injury in rats. *J. Neurotrauma* 16:851–63

370. Woiciechowsky C, Asadullah K, Nestler D, Eberhardt B, Platzer C, Schoning B, Glockner F, Lanksch WR, Volk HD, Docke WD. 1998. Sympathetic activation triggers systemic interleukin-10 release in immunodepression induced by brain injury. *Nat. Med.* 4:808–13

371. Fearon DT, Locksley RM. 1996. The instructive role of innate immunity in the acquired immune response. *Science* 272:50–53

372. Milon G. 1997. Listeria monocytogenes in laboratory mice: a model of short-term infectious and pathogenic processes controllable by regulated protective immune responses. *Immunol. Rev.* 158:37–46

373. Unanue ER. 1997. Studies in listeriosis show the strong symbiosis between the innate cellular system and the T-cell response. *Immunol. Rev.* 158:11–25

374. Mencacci A, Cenci E, Bistoni F, Bacci A, Del Sero G, Montagnoli C, Fe d'Ostiani C, Romani L. 1998. Specific and nonspecific immunity to Candida albicans: a lesson from genetically modified animals. *Res. Immunol.* 149:352–61; discussion 517–19

375. Romani L, Bistoni F, Puccetti P. 1997. Initiation of T-helper cell immunity to Candida albicans by IL-12: the role of neutrophils. *Chem. Immunol.* 68:110–35

376. Scott P, Farrell JP. 1998. Experimental cutaneous leishmaniasis: induction and regulation of T cells following infection of mice with Leishmania major. *Chem. Immunol.* 70:60–80

377. Yap GS, Sher A. 1999. Cell-mediated immunity to Toxoplasma gondii: initiation, regulation and effector function. *Immunobiology* 201:240–47

378. Romani L, Mencacci A, Cenci E, Del Sero G, Bistoni F, Puccetti P. 1997. An immunoregulatory role for neutrophils in CD4+ T helper subset selection in mice with candidiasis. *J. Immunol.* 158:2356–62

379. Kelly JP, Bancroft GJ. 1996. Administration of interleukin-10 abolishes innate resistance to Listeria monocytogenes. *Eur. J. Immunol.* 26:356–64

380. Tripp CS, Beckerman KP, Unanue ER. 1995. Immune complexes inhibit antimicrobial responses through interleukin-10 production. Effects in severe combined immunodeficient mice during Listeria infection. *J. Clin. Invest.* 95:1628–34

381. Dai WJ, Kohler G, Brombacher F. 1997. Both innate and acquired immunity to Listeria monocytogenes infection are increased in IL-10-deficient mice. *J. Immunol.* 158:2259–67

382. Wagner RD, Maroushek NM, Brown JF, Czuprynski CJ. 1994. Treatment with anti-interleukin-10 monoclonal antibody enhances early resistance to but impairs complete clearance of Listeria monocytogenes infection in mice. *Infect. Immun.* 62:2345–53

383. Vazquez-Torres A, Jones-Carson J, Wagner RD, Warner T, Balish E. 1999. Early resistance of interleukin-10 knockout mice to acute systemic candidiasis. *Infect. Immun.* 67:670–74

384. Neyer LE, Grunig G, Fort M, Remington JS, Rennick D, Hunter CA. 1997. Role of interleukin-10 in regulation of T-cell-dependent and T-cell-independent mechanisms of resistance to Toxoplasma gondii. *Infect. Immun.* 65:1675–82

385. Gazzinelli RT, Wysocka M, Hieny S, Scharton-Kersten T, Cheever A, Kuhn R, Muller W, Trinchieri G, Sher A. 1996. In the absence of endogenous IL-10, mice acutely infected with Toxoplasma gondii succumb to a lethal immune response

dependent on CD4+ T cells and accompanied by overproduction of IL-12, IFN-gamma and TNF-alpha. *J. Immunol.* 157:798–805

386. Abrahamsohn IA, Coffman RL. 1996. Trypanosoma cruzi: IL-10, TNF, IFN-gamma, and IL-12 regulate innate and acquired immunity to infection. *Exp. Parasitol.* 84:231–44

387. Lin MT, Hinton DR, Parra B, Stohlman SA, van der Veen RC. 1998. The role of IL-10 in mouse hepatitis virus-induced demyelinating encephalomyelitis. *Virology* 245:270–80

388. Nishio R, Matsumori A, Shioi T, Ishida H, Sasayama S. 1999. Treatment of experimental viral myocarditis with interleukin-10. *Circulation* 100:1102–8

389. van Den Broek M, Bachmann MF, Kohler G, Barner M, Escher R, Zinkernagel R, Kopf M. 2000. IL-4 and IL-10 antagonize IL-12-mediated protection against acute vaccinia virus infection with a limited role of IFN-gamma and nitric oxide synthetase 2. *J. Immunol.* 164:371–78

390. Li C, Corraliza I, Langhorne J. 1999. A defect in interleukin-10 leads to enhanced malarial disease in plasmodium chabaudi chabaudi infection in mice. *Infect. Immun.* 67:4435–42

391. Holscher C, Mohrs M, Dai WJ, Kohler G, Ryffel B, Schaub GA, Mossmann H, Brombacher F. 2000. Tumor necrosis factor alpha-mediated toxic shock in trypanosoma cruzi-infected interleukin 10-deficient mice. *Infect. Immun.* 68: 4075–83

392. Hunter CA, Ellis-Neyes LA, Slifer T, Kanaly S, Grunig G, Fort M, Rennick D, Araujo FG. 1997. IL-10 is required to prevent immune hyperactivity during infection with Trypanosoma cruzi. *J. Immunol.* 158:3311–16

393. Kullberg MC, Ward JM, Gorelick PL, Caspar P, Hieny S, Cheever A, Jankovic D, Sher A. 1998. Helicobacter hepaticus triggers colitis in specific-pathogen-

free interleukin-10 (IL-10)-deficient mice through an IL-12- and gamma interferon-dependent mechanism. *Infect. Immun.* 66:5157–66

394. Brown JP, Zachary JF, Teuscher C, Weis JJ, Wooten RM. 1999. Dual role of interleukin-10 in murine Lyme disease: regulation of arthritis severity and host defense. *Infect. Immun.* 67:5142–50

395. Boorstein SM, Elner SG, Meyer RF, Sugar A, Strieter RM, Kunkel SL, Elner VM. 1994. Interleukin-10 inhibition of HLA-DR expression in human herpes stromal keratitis. *Ophthalmology* 101:1529–35

396. Daheshia M, Kuklin N, Kanangat S, Manickan E, Rouse BT. 1997. Suppression of ongoing ocular inflammatory disease by topical administration of plasmid DNA encoding IL-10. *J. Immunol.* 159:1945–52

397. Flores-Villanueva PO, Zheng XX, Strom TB, Stadecker MJ. 1996. Recombinant IL-10 and IL-10/Fc treatment down-regulate egg antigen-specific delayed hypersensitivity reactions and egg granuloma formation in schistosomiasis. *J. Immunol.* 156:3315–20

398. Hoffmann KF, Cheever AW, Wynn TA. 2000. IL-10 and the dangers of immune polarization: excessive type 1 and type 2 cytokine responses induce distinct forms of lethal immunopathology in murine schistosomiasis. *J. Immunol.* 164:6406–16

399. Wynn TA, Morawetz R, Scharton-Kersten T, Hieny S, Morse HC, 3rd, Kuhn R, Muller W, Cheever AW, Sher A. 1997. Analysis of granuloma formation in double cytokine-deficient mice reveals a central role for IL-10 in polarizing both T helper cell 1- and T helper cell 2-type cytokine responses in vivo. *J. Immunol.* 159:5014–23

400. Wynn TA, Cheever AW, Williams ME, Hieny S, Caspar P, Kuhn R, Muller W, Sher A. 1998. IL-10 regulates liver

pathology in acute murine Schistosomiasis mansoni but is not required for immune down-modulation of chronic disease. *J. Immunol.* 160:4473–80

401. Nelson DR, Lauwers GY, Lau JY, Davis GL. 2000. Interleukin 10 treatment reduces fibrosis in patients with chronic hepatitis C: a pilot trial of interferon nonresponders. *Gastroenterology* 118:655–60

402. Gasim S, Elhassan AM, Khalil EA, Ismail A, Kadaru AM, Kharazmi A, Theander TG. 1998. High levels of plasma- IL-10 and expression of IL-10 by keratinocytes during visceral leishmaniasis predict subsequent development of post-kala-azar dermal leishmaniasis [published erratum appears in *Clin. Exp. Immunol.* 1998 Jun;112(3):547]. *Clin. Exp. Immunol.* 111:64–69

403. Ghalib HW, Piuvezam MR, Skeiky YA, Siddig M, Hashim FA, el-Hassan AM, Russo DM, Reed SG. 1993. Interleukin 10 production correlates with pathology in human Leishmania donovani infections. *J. Clin. Invest.* 92:324–29

404. Holaday BJ, Pompeu MM, Jeronimo S, Texeira MJ, Sousa AdA, Vasconcelos AW, Pearson RD, Abrams JS, Locksley RM. 1993. Potential role for interleukin-10 in the immunosuppression associated with kala azar. *J. Clin. Invest.* 92:2626–32

405. Karp CL, el-Safi SH, Wynn TA, Satti MM, Kordofani AM, Hashim FA, Hag-Ali M, Neva FA, Nutman TB, Sacks DL. 1993. In vivo cytokine profiles in patients with kala-azar. Marked elevation of both interleukin-10 and interferon-gamma. *J. Clin. Invest.* 91:1644–48

406. Peyron F, Burdin N, Ringwald P, Vuillez JP, Rousset F, Banchereau J. 1994. High levels of circulating IL-10 in human malaria. *Clin. Exp. Immunol.* 95:300–3

407. Wenisch C, Parschalk B, Narzt E, Looareesuwan S, Graninger W. 1995. Elevated serum levels of IL-10 and IFN-gamma in patients with acute Plasmodium falciparum malaria. *Clin. Immunol. Immunopathol.* 74:115–17

408. Mahanty S, Mollis SN, Ravichandran M, Abrams JS, Kumaraswami V, Jayaraman K, Ottesen EA, Nutman TB. 1996. High levels of spontaneous and parasite antigen-driven interleukin-10 production are associated with antigen-specific hyporesponsiveness in human lymphatic filariasis. *J. Infect. Dis.* 173:769–73

409. Mahanty S, Ravichandran M, Raman U, Jayaraman K, Kumaraswami V, Nutman TB. 1997. Regulation of parasite antigen-driven immune responses by interleukin-10 (IL-10) and IL-12 in lymphatic filariasis. *Infect. Immun.* 65:1742–47

410. King CL, Mahanty S, Kumaraswami V, Abrams JS, Regunathan J, Jayaraman K, Ottesen EA, Nutman TB. 1993. Cytokine control of parasite-specific anergy in human lymphatic filariasis. Preferential induction of a regulatory T helper type 2 lymphocyte subset. *J. Clin. Invest.* 92:1667–73

411. Yamamura M, Uyemura K, Deans RJ, Weinberg K, Rea TH, Bloom BR, Modlin RL. 1991. Defining protective responses to pathogens: cytokine profiles in leprosy lesions [published erratum appears in *Science* 1992 Jan 3;255(5040):12]. *Science* 254:277–79

412. Zhang M, Gong J, Iyer DV, Jones BE, Modlin RL, Barnes PF. 1994. T cell cytokine responses in persons with tuberculosis and human immunodeficiency virus infection. *J. Clin. Invest.* 94:2435–42

413. Gerosa F, Nisii C, Righetti S, Micciolo R, Marchesini M, Cazzadori A, Trinchieri G. 1999. CD4(+) T cell clones producing both interferon-gamma and interleukin-10 predominate in bronchoalveolar lavages of active pulmonary tuberculosis patients. *Clin. Immunol.* 92:224–34

414. Roilides E, Sein T, Schaufele R, Chanock SJ, Walsh TJ. 1998. Increased serum concentrations of interleukin-10 in patients

with hepatosplenic candidiasis. *J. Infect. Dis.* 178:589–92

415. Muller F, Aukrust P, Lien E, Haug CJ, Froland SS. 1998. Enhanced interleukin-10 production in response to Mycobacterium avium products in mononuclear cells from patients with human immunodeficiency virus infection. *J. Infect. Dis.* 177:586–94

416. Carvalho EM, Bacellar O, Brownell C, Regis T, Coffman RL, Reed SG. 1994. Restoration of IFN-gamma production and lymphocyte proliferation in visceral leishmaniasis. *J. Immunol.* 152:5949–56

417. Sieling PA, Abrams JS, Yamamura M, Salgame P, Bloom BR, Rea TH, Modlin RL. 1993. Immunosuppressive roles for IL-10 and IL-4 in human infection. In vitro modulation of T cell responses in leprosy. *J. Immunol.* 150:5501–10

418. Gong JH, Zhang M, Modlin RL, Linsley PS, Iyer D, Lin Y, Barnes PF. 1996. Interleukin-10 downregulates Mycobacterium tuberculosis-induced Th1 responses and CTLA-4 expression. *Infect. Immun.* 64:913–18

419. Clerici M, Lucey DR, Berzofsky JA, Pinto LA, Wynn TA, Blatt SP, Dolan MJ, Hendrix CW, Wolf SF, Shearer GM. 1993. Restoration of HIV-specific cell-mediated immune responses by interleukin-12 in vitro. *Science* 262:1721–24

420. Clerici M, Wynn TA, Berzofsky JA, Blatt SP, Hendrix CW, Sher A, Coffman RL, Shearer GM. 1994. Role of interleukin-10 (IL-10) in T helper cell dysfunction in asymptomatic individuals infected with human immunodeficiency virus (HIV-1). *J. Clin. Inv.* 93:768–75

421. Clerici M, Sarin A, Berzofsky JA, Landay AL, Kessler HA, Hashemi F, Hendrix CW, Blatt SP, Rusnak J, Dolan MJ, Coffman RL, Henkart PA, Shearer GM. 1996. Antigen-stimulated apoptotic T-cell death in HIV infection is selective for CD4+ T cells, modulated by cytokines and effected by lymphotoxin. *AIDS* 10:603–11

422. Landay AL, Clerici M, Hashemi F, Kessler H, Berzofsky JA, Shearer GM. 1996. In vitro restoration of T cell immune function in human immunodeficiency virus-positive persons: effects of interleukin (IL)-12 and anti-IL-10. *J. Infect. Dis.* 173:1085–91

423. Finnegan A, Roebuck KA, Nakai BE, Gu DS, Rabbi MF, Song S, Landay AL. 1996. IL-10 cooperates with TNF-alpha to activate HIV-1 from latently and acutely infected cells of monocyte/macrophage lineage. *J. Immunol.* 156:841–51

424. Rabbi MF, Finnegan A, Al-Harthi L, Song S, Roebuck KA. 1998. Interleukin-10 enhances tumor necrosis factor-alpha activation of HIV-1 transcription in latently infected T cells. *J. Acquir. Immune Defic. Syndr. Hum. Retrovirol.* 19:321–31

425. Weissman D, Poli G, Fauci AS. 1995. IL-10 synergizes with multiple cytokines in enhancing HIV production in cells of monocytic lineage. *J. Acquir. Immune Defic. Syndr. Hum. Retrovirol.* 9:442–49

426. Akridge RE, Oyafuso LK, Reed SG. 1994. IL-10 is induced during HIV-1 infection and is capable of decreasing viral replication in human macrophages. *J. Immunol.* 153:5782–89

427. Chang J, Naif HM, Li S, Jozwiak R, Ho-Shon M, Cunningham AL. 1996. The inhibition of HIV replication in monocytes by interleukin 10 is linked to inhibition of cell differentiation. *AIDS Res. Hum. Retroviruses* 12:1227–35

428. Goletti D, Weissman D, Jackson RW, Collins F, Kinter A, Fauci AS. 1998. The in vitro induction of human immunodeficiency virus (HIV) replication in purified protein derivative-positive HIV-infected persons by recall antigen response to Mycobacterium tuberculosis is the result of a balance of the effects of endogenous interleukin-2 and proinflammatory and antiinflammatory cytokines. *J. Infect. Dis.* 177:1332–38

429. Powrie F, Coffman RL. 1993. Cytokine regulation of T-cell function: potential for therapeutic intervention. *Immunol. Today.* 14:270–74

430. Liblau R, Singer S, McDevitt H. 1995. Th1 and Th2 CD4+ T cells in the pathogenesis of organ-specific autoimmune diseases. *Immunol. Today* 16:34–38

431. O'Garra A, Steinman L., and Gijbels K. 1997. CD4+ T-cell subsets in autoimmunity. *Curr. Opin. Immunol.* 9:872–83

432. Tisch R, and McDevitt H. 1996. Insulin-dependent diabetes mellitus. *Cell* 85:291–97

433. Miller SD, and Karpus WJ. 1994. The immunopathogenesis and regulation of T-cell-mediated demyelinating diseases. *Immunol. Today* 15:356–61

434. Groux H, Powrie F. 1999. Regulatory T cells and inflammatory bowel disease. *Immunol. Today* 20:442–45

435. Chai JG, Bartok I, Chandler P, Vendetti S, Antoniou A, Dyson J, Lechler R. 1999. Anergic T cells act as suppressor cells in vitro and in vivo. *Eur. J. Immunol.* 29:686–92

436. Seddon B, Mason D. 1999. Regulatory T cells in the control of autoimmunity: the essential role of transforming growth factor b and interleukin 4 in the prevention of autoimmune thryroiditis in rats by peripheral CD4+ CD45RC- cells and CD4+ CD8- thymocytes. *J. Exp. Med.* 189:279–88

437. Seddon B, and Mason D. 2000. The third function of the thymus. *Immunol. Today* 21:95–99

438. Bridoux F, Badou A, Saoudi A, Bernard I, Druet E, Pasquier R, Druet P, Pelletier L. 1997. Transforming growth factor β (TGFβ)-dependent inhibition of T helper 2 (Th2)-induced autoimmunity by self-major histocompatibility complex (MHC) class II-specific, regulatory CD4+ T cell lines. *J. Exp. Med.* 185:1769–75

439. Han HS, Jun HS, Utsugi T, Yoon JW. 1996. A new type of CD4+ suppressor T cell completely prevents spontaneous autoimmune diabetes and recurrent diabetes in syngeneic islet-transplanted NOD mice. *J. Autoimmun.* 9:331–39

440. Weiner HL. 1997. Oral tolerance for the treatment of autoimmune diseases. *Annu. Rev. Med.* 48:341–51

441. Powrie F, Carlino J, Leach MW, Mauze S, Coffman RL. 1996. A critical role for transforming growth factor-β but not interleukin 4 in the suppression of T helper type 1-mediated colitis by CD45RB^{low} CD4+ T cells. *J. Exp. Med.* 183:2669–74

442. Shull MM, Ormsby I, Kier AB, Pawlowski S, Diebold RJ, Yin M, Allen R, Sidman C, Proetzel G, Calvin D, Annunziata N, Doetschman T. 1992. Targeted disruption of the mouse transforming growth factor-b1 gene results in multifocal inflammatory disease. *Nature* 359:693–99

443. Berg DJ, Davidson N, Kuhn R, Muller W, Menon S, Holland G, Thompson-Snipes L, Leach MW, Rennick D. 1996. Enterocolitis and colon cancer in interleukin-10-deficient mice are associated with aberrant cytokine production and CD4(+) TH1-like responses. *J. Clin. Invest.* 98:1010–20

444. Khoury SJ, Hancock WW, Weiner HL. 1992. Oral tolerance to myelin basic protein and natural recovery from experimental autoimmune encephalomyelitis are associated with downregulation of inflammatory cytokines and differential upregulation of transforming growth factor β, interleukin 4 and prostaglandin E expression in the brain. *J. Exp. Med.* 176:1355–64

445. Kennedy M, K., Torrance D, S., Picha K, S., Mohler K.M. 1992. Analysis of cytokine mRNA expression in the central nervous system of mice with experimental autoimmune encephalomyelitis reveals that IL-10 mRNA expression

correlates with recovery. *J. Immunol.* 149:2496–2505

446. Issazadeh S, Ljungdahl A, Hojeberg B, Mustafa M, Olsson T. 1995. Cytokine production in the central nervous system of Lewis rats with experimental autoimmune encephalomyelitis: dynamics of mRNA expression for interleukin-10, interleukin-12, cytolysin, tumor necrosis factor α and tumor necrosis β. *J. Neuroimmunol.* 61:205–12

447. Issazadeh S, Lorentzen JC, Mustafa MI, Hojeberg B, Mussener A, Olsson T. 1996. Cytokines in relapsing experimental autoimmune encephalomyelitis in DA rats: persistent mRNA expression of proinflammatory cytokines and absent expression of interleukin-10 and transforming growth factor-β. *J. Neuroimmunol.* 69:103–15

448. Navikas V, Link J, Palasik W, Soderstrom M, Fredrikson S, Olsson T, Link H. 1995. Increased mRNA expression of IL-10 in mononuclear cells in multiple sclerosis and optic neuritis. *Scand. J. Immunol.* 41:171–78

449. Crisi GM, Santambrogio L, Hochwald GM, Smith SR, Carlino JA, Thorbecke GJ. 1995. Staphylococcal enterotoxin B and tumor necrosis factor-alpha-induced relapses of experimental allergic encephalomyelitis: protection by transforming growth factor-beta and interleukin-10. *Eur. J. Immunol.* 23:3035–40

450. Bettelli E, Das MP, Howard ED, Weiner HL, Sobel RA, Kuchroo VK. 1998. IL-10 is critical in the regulation of autoimmune encephalomyelitis as demonstrated by studies of IL-10- and IL-4-deficient and transgenic mice. *J. Immunol.* 161:3299–3306

451. Samilova EB, Horton JL, Chen Y. 1988. Acceleration of experimental autoimmune encephalomyelitis in interleukin-10-deficient mice: roles of interleukin-10 in disease progression and recovery. *Cellular Immunol.* 188:118–24

452. Segal BM, Dwyer BK, Shevach EM. 1998. An interleukin (IL)-10/IL-12 immunoregulatory circuit controls susceptibility to autoimmune disease. *J. Exp. Med.* 187:537–46

453. Rott O, Fleischer B, Cash E. 1994. Interleukin-10 prevents experimental allergic encephalomyelitis in rats. *Eur. J. Immunol.* 24:1434–40

454. Nagelkerken L, Blauw B, Tielmans M. 1997. IL-4 abrogates the inhibitory effect of IL-10 on the development of experimental allergic encephalomyelitis in SJL mice. *Int. Immunol.* 9:1243–51

455. Croxford JL, Triantaphyllopuolos K, Podhajeer OL, Feldman M, Baker D, Chernajovsky Y. 1998. Cytokine gene therapy in experimental allergic encephalomyelitis by injection of plasmid DNA-cationic liposome complex into the central nervous system. *J. Immunol.* 160:5181–87

456. Shaw MK, Lorens JB, Dhawan A, Dal-Canto R, Tse HY, Tran AB, Bonpane C, Eswaran SL, Brocke S, Sarvetnik S, et al. 1997. Local delivery of interleukin 4 by retrovirus-transduced T lymphocytes ameliorates experimental autoimmune encephalomyelitis. *J. Exp. Med.* 185:1711–14

457. Cannella B, Gao YL, Brosnan C, Raine CS. 1996. IL-10 fails to abrogate experimental autoimmune encephalomyelitis. *J. Neuroscience Res.* 45:735–46

458. Mathisen PM, Yu M, Johnson JM, Drazba JA, Tuohy VK. 1997. Treatment of experimental autoimmune encephalomyelitis with genetically modified memory T cells. *J. Exp. Med.* 186:159–64

459. Cua DJ, Groux H, Hinton DR, Stohlman SA, Coffman RL. 1999. Transgenic interleukin 10 prevents induction of experimental autoimmune encephalomyelitis. *J. Exp. Med.* 189:1005–10

460. Cua D, Hutchins B, LaFace DM, Stohlman S, Coffman RL. 2001. Central nervous system expression of IL-10

inhibits autoimmune encephalomyelitis. *J. Immunol.* In press

461. Castano L, Eisenbarth GS. 1990. Type-I diabetes: A chronic autoimmune disease of human, mouse and rat. *Annu. Rev. Immunol.* 8:647–79

462. Kikutani H, Makino S. 1992. The murine autoimmune diabetes model: NOD and related strains. *Adv. Immunol.* 51:285–322

463. Bendelac A, Carnaud C, Boitard C, Bach JF. 1987. Syngeneic transfer of autoimmune diabetes from diabetic NOD mice to healthy neonates. Requirement for both L3T4+ and Lyt-2+ T cells. *J. Exp. Med.* 166:823–32

464. Hutchings P, Rosen H, O'Reilly L, Simpson E, Gordon S, Cooke A. 1990. Transfer of diabetes in mice prevented by blockade of adhesion-promoting receptor on macrophages. *Nature* 348:639–42

465. Pennline KJ, Roque-Gaffney E, Monahan M. 1994. Recombinant human IL-10 prevents the onset of diabetes in the nonobese diabetic (NOD) mouse. *Clin. Immunol. Immunopathol.* 71:169–75

466. Zheng XX, Steele AW, Hancock WW, Stevens AC, Nickerson PW, Roy-Chaudhury P, Tian Y, Strom TB. 1997. A noncytolytic IL-10/Fc fusion protein prevents diabetes, blocks autoimmunity, and promotes suppressor phenomena in NOD mice. *J. Immunol.* 158:4507–13

467. Moritani M, Yoshimoto K, Ii S, Kondo M, Iwahana H, Yamaoka T, Sano T, Nakano N, Kikutani H, Itakura M. 1996. Prevention of adoptively transferred diabetes in nonobese diabetic mice with IL-10-transduced islet-specific Th1 lymphocytes. A gene therapy model for autoimmune diabetes. *J. Clin. Invest.* 98:1851–59

468. Wogensen L, Huang X, Sarvetnick N. 1993. Leukocyte extravasation into the pancreatic tissue in transgenic mice expressing interleukin 10 in the islets of Langerhans. *J. Exp. Med.* 178:175–85

469. Wogensen L, Lee MS, Sarvetnick N. 1994. Production of interleukin 10 by islet cells accelerates immune-mediated destruction of beta cells in nonobese diabetic mice. *J. Exp. Med.* 179:1379–84

470. Lee MS, Wogensen L, Shizuru J, Oldstone MB, Sarvetnick N. 1994. Pancreatic islet production of murine interleukin-10 does not inhibit immune-mediated tissue destruction. *J. Clin. Invest.* 93:1332–38

471. Moritani M, Yoshimoto K, Tashiro F, Hashimoto C, Miyazaki J-i, Setsuko I, Iwahana H, Hayashi Y, Sano T, Itakura M. 1994. Transgenic expression of IL-10 in pancreatic islet A cells accelerates autoimmune insulitis and diabetes in non-obese diabetic mice. *Int. Immunol.* 6:1927–36

472. Lee MS, Mueller R, Wicker LS, Peterson LB, Sarvetnick N. 1996. IL-10 is necessary and sufficient for autoimmune diabetes in conjunction with NOD MHC homozygosity. *J. Exp. Med.* 183:2663–68

473. Cohen SB, Katsikis PD, Chu CQ, Thomssen H, Webb LM, Maini RN, Londei M, Feldmann M. 1995. High level of interleukin-10 production by the activated T cell population within the rheumatoid synovial membrane. *Arthritis Rheum.* 38:946–52

474. Katsikis PD, Chu CQ, Brennan FM, Maini RN, Feldmann M. 1994. Immunoregulatory role of interleukin 10 in rheumatoid arthritis. *J. Exp. Med.* 179:1517–27

475. Cush JJ, Splawski JB, Thomas R, McFarlin JE, Schulze-Koops H, Davis LS, Fujita K, Lipsky PE. 1995. Elevated interleukin-10 levels in patients with rheumatoid arthritis. *Arthrit. Rheum.* 38:96–104

476. Perez L, Orte J, Brieva JA. 1995. Terminal differentiation of spontaneous rheumatoid factor-secreting B cells from rheumatoid arthritis patients depends on endogenous interleukin-10. *Arthritis Rheum.* 38:1771–76

477. Kasama T, Strieter RM, Lukacs NW,

Lincoln PM, Burdick MD, Kunkel SL. 1995. Interleukin-10 expression and chemokine regulation during the evolution of murine type II collagen-induced arthritis. *J. Clin. Invest.* 95:2868–76

478. Persson S, Mikulowska A, Narula S, O'Garra A, Holmdahl R. 1996. Interleukin-10 suppresses the development of collagen type II-induced arthritis and ameliorates sustained arthritis in rats. *Scand. J. Immunol.* 44:607–14

479. Tanaka Y, Otsuka T, Hotokebuchi T, Miyahara H, Nakashima H, Kuga S, Nemotos Y, Niiro H. Niho Y. 1996. Effect of IL-10 on collagen-induced arthritis in mice. *Inflamm. Res.* 45:283–88

480. van Roon JA, van Roy JL, Gmelig-Meyling FH, Lafeber FP, Bijlsma JW. 1996. Prevention and reversal of cartilage degradation in rheumatoid arthritis by interleukin-10 and interleukin-4. *Arthritis Rheum.* 39:829–35

481. Walmsley M, Katsikis PD, Abney E, Parry S, Williams RO, Maini RN, Feldmann M. 1996. Interleukin-10 inhibition of the progression of established collagen-induced arthritis. *Arthritis Rheum.* 39:495–503

482. Whalen JD, Lechman EL, Carlos CA, Weiss K, Kovesdi I, Glorioso JC, Robbins PD, Evans CH. 1999. Adenoviral transfer of the viral IL-10 gene periarticularly to mouse paws suppresses development of collagen-induced arthritis in both injected and uninjected paws. *J. Immunol.* 16:3625–32

483. Joosten LA, Lubberts E, Durez P, Helsen MM, Jacobs MJ, Goldman M, van den Berg W.B. 1997. Role of interleukin-4 and interleukin-10 in murine collagen-induced arthritis. Protective effect of interleukin-4 and interleukin-10 treatment in cartilage destruction. *Arthritis Rheum.* 40:249–60

484. Llorente L, Richaud-Patin Y, Wijdenes J, Alcocer-Varela J, Maillot MC, Durand-Gasselin I, Fourrier BM, Galanaud P, Emilie D. 1993. Spontaneous production of interleukin-10 by B lymphocytes and monocytes in systemic lupus erythematosus. *Eur. Cytokine Netw.* 4:421–27

485. Liu TF, Jones BM. 1998. Impaired production of IL-12 in system lupus erythematosus. II: IL-12 production in vitro is correlated negatively with serum IL-10, positively with serum IFN-gamma and negatively with disease activity in SLE. *Cytokine* 10:148–53

486. Lacki JK, Samborski W, Mackiewicz SH. 1997. Interleukin-10 and interleukin-6 in lupus erythematosus and rheumatoid arthritis, correlations with acute phase proteins. *Clin. Rheumatol.* 16:275–78

487. Umetsu DT, DeKruyff RH. 1997. Th1 and Th2 CD4+ T cells in human allergic diseases. *J. Allergy. Clin. Immunol.* 100:1–6

488. Umetsu D, and DeKruyff R.H. 1999. Interleukin-10: the missing link in asthma regulation. *Am. J. Respir. Cell. Mol. Biol.* 21:562–63

489. Romagnani S. 1994. Lymphokine production by human T cells in disease states. *Annu. Rev. Immunol.* 12:227–57

490. Sher A, Coffman RL. 1992. Regulation of immunity to parasites by T cells and T cell-derived cytokines. *Annu. Rev. Immunol.* 10:385–409

491. Robinson DS, Hamid Q, Ying S, Tsicopoulos A, Barkans J, Bentley AM, Corrigan CJ, Durham SR, Kay AB. 1992. Evidence for a predominant "Th2-type" bronchoalveolar lavage T-lymphocyte population in atopic asthma. *New. Engl. J. Med.* 326:298–304

492. Shirakawa T, Enomoto T, Shimazu S, Hopkin JM. 1997. The inverse association between tuberculin responses and atopic. *Science* 275:77–79

493. Arock M, Zuany-Amorim C, Singer M, Benhamou M, Pretolani M. 1996. Interleukin 10 inhibits cytokine generation from mast cells. *Eur. J. Immunol.* 26:166–70

494. Marshall JS, Leal-Berumen I, Nielsen L,

Glibetic M, Jordana M. 1996. Interleukin (IL)-10 inhibits long-term IL-6 production but not preformed mediator release from rat peritoneal mast cells. *J. Clin. Invest.* 97:1122–28

495. Quinn TJ, Taylor S, Wohlford-Lenane CL, Schwartz DA. 2000. IL-10 reduces grain dust-induced airway inflammation and airway hyperreactivity. *J. Appl. Physiol.* 88:173–79

496. Makela MJ, Kanehiro A, Borish L, Dakhama A, Loader J, Joetham A, Xing Z, Jordana M, Larsen GL, Gelfand EW. 2000. IL-10 is necessary for the expression of airway hyperresponsiveness but not pulmonary inflammation after allergic sensitization. *Proc. Natl. Acad. Sci. USA* 97:6007–12

497. van Scott MR, Justice JP, Bradfield JF, Enright E, Sigounas A, Sur S. 2000. IL-10 reduces Th2 cytokine production and eosinophilia but augments airway reactivity in allergic mice. *Am. J. Physiol. Lung Cell Mol. Physiol.* 278:L667–74

498. Borish L. 1998. IL-10: evolving concepts. *J. Allergy Clin.* 101:293–97

499. John M, Lim S, Seybold J, Jose P, Robichaud A, O'Connor B, Barnes PJ, Chung KF. 1998. Inhaled corticosteroids increase interleukin-10 but reduce macrophage inflammatory protein-1a, granulocyte-macrophage stimulating factor and Interferon-γ release from alveolar macrophages in asthma. *Am. J. Respir. Crit. Care Med.* 157:256–62

500. Grunig G, Corry DB, Leach MW, Seymour BWP, Kurup VP, Rennick DR. 1997. Interleukin-10 is a natural suppressor of cytokine production and inflammation in a murine model of allergic bronchopulmonary aspergillosis. *J. Exp. Med.* 185:1089–99

501. Elson CO, Sartor RB, Tennyson GS, Riddell RH. 1995. Experimental models of inflammatory bowel disease. *Gastroenterology* 109:1344–67

502. Powrie F. 1995. T cells in inflammatory bowel disease: protective and pathologic roles. *Immunity* 3:171–74

503. Davidson NJ, Hudak SA, Lesley RE, Menon S, Leach MW, Rennick DM. 1998. IL-12, but not IFN-γ, plays a major role in sustaining the chronic phase of colitis in IL-10-deficient mice. *J. Immunol.* 161:3143–49

504. Sellon RK, Tonkonogy S, Schultz M, Dieleman LA, Grenther W, Balish E, Rennick DM, Sartor RB. 1998. Resident enteric bacteria are necessary for development of spontaneous colitis and immune system activation in interleukin-10 deficient mice. *Infect. Immunity* 66:5224–1

505. Powrie F, Leach MW, Mauze S, Menon S, Caddle LB, Coffman RL. 1994. Inhibition of Th1 responses prevents inflammatory bowel disease in scid mice reconstituted with CD45RBhi CD4+ T cells. *Immunity* 1:553–2

506. Morrissey PJ, Charrier K, Braddy S, Liggitt D, Watson JD. 1993. CD4+ T cells that express high levels of CD45RB induce wasting disease when transferred into congenic severe combined immunodeficient mice. Disease is prevented by cotransfer of purified CD4+ T cells. *J. Exp. Med.* 178:237–4

507. Hagenbaugh A, Sharma S, Dubinett SM, Wei SHY, Aranda R, Cheroutre H, Fowell DJ, Binder S, Tsao B, Locksley RM, Moore KW, Kronenberg M. 1997. Altered immune responses in interleukin 10 transgenic mice. *J. Exp. Med.* 185:2101–0

508. Steidler L, Hans W, Schotte L, Neirynck S, Obermeier F, Falk W, Fiers W, Remaut E. 2000. Treatment of murine colitis by lactococcus lactis secreting interleukin-10. *Science* 289:1352–5

509. Mason D, Fowell D. 1992. T-cell subsets in autoimmunity. *Curr. Opin. Immunol.* 4:728–2

510. Sakaguchi S. 2000. Regulatory T cells: key controllers of immunologic self-tolerance. *Cell* 101:455–5

511. Shevach EM. 2000. Regulatory T cells

in autoimmmunity. *Annu. Rev. Immunol.* 18:423–9

512. Chen Y, Kuchroo VK, Inobe J-I, Hafler DA, Weiner HL. 1994. Regulatory T cell clones induced by oral tolerance: suppression of autoimmune encephalytis. *Science* 265:1237–40

513. Maeda H, Kuwahara H, Ichimura Y, Ohtsuki M, Kurakata S, Shiraishi A. 1995. TGF-β enhances macrophage ability to produce IL-10 in normal and tumor-bearing mice. *J. Immunol.* 155:4962–32

514. Bacchetta R, Bigler M, Touraine JL, Parkman R, Tovo PA, Abrams J, de Waal Malefyt R, de Vries JE, Roncarolo MG. 1994. High levels of interleukin 10 production in vivo are associated with tolerance in SCID patients transplanted with HLA mismatched hematopoietic stem cells. *J. Exp. Med.* 179:493–502

515. Papiernik M, do Carmo Leite-de-Moraes M, Pontoux C, Joret AM, Rocha B, Penit C, Dy M. 1997. T cell deletion induced by chronic infection with mouse mammary tumor virus spares a CD25-positive, IL-10-producing T cell population with infectious capacity. *J. Immunol.* 158:4642–53

516. Papiernik M, Leite de Moraes, Pontoux C., Vasseur F., Penit C. 1998. Regulatory CD4 T cells: expression of IL-2Ra chain, resistance to clonal deletion and IL-2 dependency. *Int. Immunol.* 10:371–78

517. Streilein JW, Ksander BR, Taylor AW. 1997. Immune deviation in relation to ocular immune privilege. *J. Immunol.* 158:3557–60

518. Gao Y, Herndon JM, Zhang H, Griffith TS, Ferguson TA. 1998. Antiinflammmatory effects of CD95 ligand (FasL)-induced apoptosis. *J. Exp. Med.* 188:887–96

519. Nishigori C, Yarosh DB, Ullrich SE, Vink AA, Bucana CD, Roza L, Kripke ML. 1996. Evidence that DNA damage triggers interleukin 10 cytokine production in UV-irradiated murine keratinocytes.

Proc. Natl. Acad. Sci. USA 93:10354–59

520. Rivas JM, Ullrich S.E. 1992. Systemic suppression of delayed-type hypersensitivity by supernatants from UV-irradiated keratinocytes. An essential role for keratinocyte-derived IL-10. *J. Immunol.* 149:3865–71

521. Leverkus M, Yaar M, Gilchrest BA. 1997. Fas/Fas ligand interaction contributes to UV-induced apoptosis in human keratinocytes. *Exp. Cell Res.* 232:255–62

522. Voll RE, Herrmann M, Roth EA, Stach C, Kalden JR, Girkonttaite I. 1997. Immunosuppressive effects of apoptotis cells. *Nature* 390:350–51

523. Pisa P, Halapi E, Pisa EK, Gerdin E, Hising C, Bucht A, Gerdin B, Kiessling R. 1992. Selective expression of interleukin 10, interferon gamma, and granulocyte-macrophage colony-stimulating factor in ovarian cancer biopsies. *Proc. Natl. Acad. Sci. USA* 89:7708–12

524. Gotlieb WH, Abrams JS, Watson JM, Velu TJ, Berek JS, Martinez-Maza O. 1992. Presence of interleukin 10 (IL-10) in the ascites of patients with ovarian and other intra-abdominal cancers. *Cytokine* 4:385–90

525. Loercher AE, Nash MA, Kavanagh JJ, Platsoucas CD, Freedman RS. 1999. Identification of an IL-10-producing HLA-DR-negative monocyte subset in the malignant ascites of patients with ovarian carcinoma that inhibits cytokine protein expression and proliferation of autologous T cells. *J. Immunol.* 163:6251–60

526. Chau GY, Wu CW, Lui WY, Chang TJ, Kao HL, Wu LH, King KL, Loong CC, Hsia CY, Chi CW. 2000. Serum interleukin-10 but not interleukin-6 is related to clinical outcome in patients with resectable hepatocellular carcinoma. *Ann. Surg.* 231:552–58

527. De Vita F, Orditura M, Galizia G, Romano C, Lieto E, Iodice P, Tuccillo C, Catalano G. 2000. Serum interleukin-10 is an

independent prognostic factor in advanced solid tumors. *Oncol. Rep.* 7:357–61

528. De Vita F, Orditura M, Galizia G, Romano C, Roscigno A, Lieto E, Catalano G. 2000. Serum interleukin-10 levels as a prognostic factor in advanced non-small cell lung cancer patients. *Chest* 117:365–73

529. Fortis C, Foppoli M, Gianotti L, Galli L, Citterio G, Consogno G, Gentilini O, Braga M. 1996. Increased interleukin-10 serum levels in patients with solid tumours. *Cancer Lett.* 104:1–5

530. Fujieda S, Sunaga H, Tsuzuki H, Fan GK, Saito H. 1999. IL-10 expression is associated with the expression of platelet-derived endothelial cell growth factor and prognosis in oral and oropharyngeal carcinoma. *Cancer Lett.* 136:1–9

531. Smith DR, Kunkel SL, Burdick MD, Wilke CA, Orringer MB, Whyte RI, Strieter RM. 1994. Production of interleukin-10 by human bronchogenic carcinoma. *Am. J. Pathol.* 145:18–25

532. Wittke F, Hoffmann R, Buer J, Dallmann I, Oevermann K, Sel S, Wandert T, Ganser A, Atzpodien J. 1999. Interleukin 10 (IL-10): an immunosuppressive factor and independent predictor in patients with metastatic renal cell carcinoma. *Br. J. Cancer* 79:1182–84

533. Dummer W, Becker JC, Schwaaf A, Leverkus M, Moll T, Brocker EB. 1995. Elevated serum levels of interleukin-10 in patients with metastatic malignant melanoma. *Melanoma Res.* 5:67–68

534. Huang S, Ullrich SE, Bar-Eli M. 1999. Regulation of tumor growth and metastasis by interleukin-10: the melanoma experience. *J. Interferon Cytokine Res.* 19:697–703

535. Kruger-Krasagakes S, Krasagakis K, Garbe C, Schmitt E, Huls C, Blankenstein T, Diamantstein T. 1994. Expression of interleukin 10 in human melanoma. *Br. J. Cancer* 70:1182–85

536. Sato T, McCue P, Masuoka K, Salwen S, Lattime EC, Mastrangelo MJ, Berd D. 1996. Interleukin 10 production by human melanoma. *Clin. Cancer Res.* 2:1383–90

537. Yue FY, Dummer R, Geertsen R, Hofbauer G, Laine E, Manolio S, Burg G. 1997. Interleukin-10 is a growth factor for human melanoma cells and down-regulates HLA class-I, HLA class-II and ICAM-1 molecules. *Int. J. Cancer* 71:630–37

538. Ekmekcioglu S, Okcu MF, Colome-Grimmer MI, Owen-Schaub L, Buzaid AC, Grimm EA. 1999. Differential increase of Fas ligand expression on metastatic and thin or thick primary melanoma cells compared with interleukin-10. *Melanoma Res.* 9:261–72

539. Khatri VP, Caligiuri MA. 1998. A review of the association between interleukin-10 and human B-cell malignancies. *Cancer Immunol. Immunother.* 46:239–44

540. Asadullah K, Docke WD, Haeussler A, Sterry W, Volk HD. 1996. Progression of mycosis fungoides is associated with increasing cutaneous expression of interleukin-10 mRNA. *J. Invest. Dermatol.* 107:833–37

541. Boulland ML, Meignin V, Leroy-Viard K, Copie-Bergman C, Briere J, Touitou R, Kanavaros P, Gaulard P. 1998. Human interleukin-10 expression in T/natural killer-cell lymphomas: association with anaplastic large cell lymphomas and nasal natural killer-cell lymphomas. *Am. J. Pathol.* 153:1229–37

542. Klein B, Lu ZY, Gu ZJ, Costes V, Jourdan M, Rossi JF. 1999. Interleukin-10 and Gp130 cytokines in human multiple myeloma. *Leuk. Lymphoma* 34:63–70

543. Denizot Y, Turlure P, Bordessoule D, Trimoreau F, Praloran V. 1999. Serum IL-10 and IL-13 concentrations in patients with haematological malignancies. *Cytokine* 11:634–35

544. Salmaggi A, Eoli M, Corsini E, Gelati M,

Frigerio S, Silvani A, Boiardi A. 2000. Cerebrospinal fluid interleukin-10 levels in primary central nervous system lymphoma: a possible marker of response to treatment? [letter]. *Ann. Neurol.* 47:137–38

545. Jones KD, Aoki Y, Chang Y, Moore PS, Yarchoan R, Tosato G. 1999. Involvement of interleukin-10 (IL-10) and viral IL-6 in the spontaneous growth of Kaposi's sarcoma herpesvirus-associated infected primary effusion lymphoma cells. *Blood* 94:2871–79

546. Blay JY, Burdin N, Rousset F, Lenoir G, Biron P, Philip T, Banchereau J, Favrot MC. 1993. Serum interleukin-10 in non-Hodgkin's lymphoma: a prognostic factor. *Blood* 82:2169–74

547. Bohlen H, Kessler M, Sextro M, Diehl V, Tesch H. 2000. Poor clinical outcome of patients with Hodgkin's disease and elevated interleukin-10 serum levels. Clinical significance of interleukin-10 serum levels for Hodgkin's disease. *Ann. Hematol.* 79:110–13

548. Viviani S, Notti P, Bonfante V, Verderio P, Valagussa P, Bonadonna G. 2000. Elevated pretreatment serum levels of IL-10 are associated with a poor prognosis in Hodgkin's disease, the Milan Cancer Institute experience. *Med. Oncol.* 17:59–63

549. Sarris AH, Kliche KO, Pethambaram P, Preti A, Tucker S, Jackow C, Messina O, Pugh W, Hagemeister FB, McLaughlin P, Rodriguez MA, Romaguera J, Fritsche H, Witzig T, Duvic M, Andreeff M, Cabanillas F. 1999. Interleukin-10 levels are often elevated in serum of adults with Hodgkin's disease and are associated with inferior failure-free survival. *Ann. Oncol.* 10:433–40

550. Cortes J, Kurzrock R. 1997. Interleukin-10 in non-Hodgkin's lymphoma. *Leuk. Lymphoma* 26:251–59

551. Stasi R, Zinzani L, Galieni P, Lauta VM, Damasio E, Dispensa E, Dammacco F, Tura S, Papa G. 1994. Detection of soluble interleukin-2 receptor and interleukin-10 in the serum of patients with aggressive non-Hodgkin's lymphoma. Identification of a subset at high risk of treatment failure. *Cancer* 74:1792–800

552. Wojciechowska-Lacka A, Matecka-Nowak M, Adamiak E, Lacki JK, Cerkaska-Gluszak B. 1996. Serum levels of interleukin-10 and interleukin-6 in patients with lung cancer. *Neoplasma* 43:155–58

553. De Vita F, Orditura M, Galizia G, Romano C, Infusino S, Auriemma A, Lieto E, Catalano G. 1999. Serum interleukin-10 levels in patients with advanced gastrointestinal malignancies. *Cancer* 86:1936–43

554. Fujieda S, Lee K, Sunaga H, Tsuzuki H, Ikawa H, Fan GK, Imanaka M, Takenaka H, Saito H. 1999. Staining of interleukin-10 predicts clinical outcome in patients with nasopharyngeal carcinoma. *Cancer* 85:1439–45

555. Cortes JE, Talpaz M, Cabanillas F, Seymour JF, Kurzrock R. 1995. Serum levels of interleukin-10 in patients with diffuse large cell lymphoma: lack of correlation with prognosis. *Blood* 85:2516–20

556. Sjoberg J, Aguilar-Santelises M, Sjogren AM, Pisa EK, Ljungdahl A, Bjorkholm M, Jondal M, Mellstedt H, Pisa P. 1996. Interleukin-10 mRNA expression in B-cell chronic lymphocytic leukaemia inversely correlates with progression of disease. *Br. J. Haematol.* 92:393–400

557. Lu ZY, Zhang XG, Rodriguez C, Wijdenes J, Gu ZJ, Morel-Fournier B, Harousseau JL, Bataille R, Rossi JF, Klein B. 1995. Interleukin-10 is a proliferation factor but not a differentiation factor for human myeloma cells. *Blood* 85:2521–27

558. Masood R, Zhang Y, Bond MW, Scadden DT, Moudgil T, Law RE, Kaplan MH, Jung B, Espina BM, Lunardi-Iskandar

Y, et al. 1995. Interleukin-10 is an autocrine growth factor for acquired immunodeficiency syndrome-related B-cell lymphoma. *Blood* 85:3423–30

559. Voorzanger N, Touitou R, Garcia E, Delecluse HJ, Rousset F, Joab I, Favrot MC, Blay JY. 1996. Interleukin (IL)-10 and IL-6 are produced in vivo by non-Hodgkin's lymphoma cells and act as cooperative growth factors. *Cancer Res.* 56:5499–5505

560. Beatty PR, Krams SM, Martinez OM. 1997. Involvement of IL-10 in the autonomous growth of EBV-transformed B cell lines. *J. Immunol.* 158:4045–51

561. Gu ZJ, Costes V, Lu ZY, Zhang XG, Pitard V, Moreau JF, Bataille R, Wijdenes J, Rossi JF, Klein B. 1996. Interleukin-10 is a growth factor for human myeloma cells by induction of an oncostatin M autocrine loop. *Blood* 88:3972–86

562. Bruserud O, Tore Gjertsen B, Terje Brustugun O, Bassoe CF, Nesthus I, Espen Akselsen P, Buhring HJ, Pawelec G. 1995. Effects of interleukin 10 on blast cells derived from patients with acute myelogenous leukemia. *Leukemia* 9:1910–20

563. Geissler K, Ohler L, Fodinger M, Virgolini I, Leimer M, Kabrna E, Kollars M, Skoupy S, Bohle B, Rogy M, Lechner K. 1996. Interleukin 10 inhibits growth and granulocyte/macrophage colony-stimulating factor production in chronic myelomonocytic leukemia cells. *J. Exp. Med.* 184:1377–84

564. Westermann F, Kube D, Haier B, Bohlen H, Engert A, Zuehlsdorf M, Diehl V, Tesch H. 1996. Interleukin 10 inhibits cytokine production of human AML cells. *Ann. Oncol.* 7:397–404

565. Gao JX, Madrenas J, Zeng W, Cameron MJ, Zhang Z, Wang JJ, Zhong R, Grant D. 1999. CD40-deficient dendritic cells producing interleukin-10, but not interleukin-12, induce T-cell hyporesponsiveness in vitro and prevent acute allograft rejection. *Immunology* 98:159–70

566. Faulkner L, Buchan G, Baird M. 2000. Interleukin-10 does not affect phagocytosis of particulate antigen by bone marrow-derived dendritic cells but does impair antigen presentation. *Immunology* 99:523–31

567. Beissert S, Ullrich SE, Hosoi J, Granstein RD. 1995. Supernatants from UVB radiation-exposed keratinocytes inhibit Langerhans cell presentation of tumor-associated antigens via IL-10 content. *J. Leukoc. Biol.* 58:234–40

568. Sharma S, Stolina M, Lin Y, Gardner B, Miller PW, Kronenberg M, Dubinett SM. 1999. T cell-derived IL-10 promotes lung cancer growth by suppressing both T cell and APC function. *J. Immunol.* 163:5020–28

569. Houle M, Thivierge M, Le Gouill C, Stankova J, Rola-Pleszczynski M. 1999. IL-10 up-regulates CCR5 gene expression in human monocytes. *Inflammation* 23:241–51

570. Fiehn C, Paleolog EM, Feldmann M. 1997. Selective enhancement of endothelial cell VCAM-1 expression by interleukin-10 in the presence of activated leucocytes. *Immunology* 91:565–71

571. Vora M, Romero LI, Karasek MA. 1996. Interleukin-10 induces E-selectin on small and large blood vessel endothelial cells. *J. Exp. Med.* 184:821–29

572. Ebert EC. 2000. IL-10 enhances IL-2-induced proliferation and cytotoxicity by human intestinal lymphocytes. *Clin. Exp. Immunol.* 119:426–32

573. Kundu N, Fulton AM. 1997. Interleukin-10 inhibits tumor metastasis, downregulates MHC class I, and enhances NK lysis. *Cell. Immunol.* 180:55–61

574. Petersson M, Charo J, Salazar-Onfray F, Noffz G, Mohaupt M, Qin Z, Klein G, Blankenstein T, Kiessling R. 1998. Constitutive IL-10 production accounts for the high NK sensitivity, low MHC class I expression, and poor transporter associated with antigen processing (TAP)-1/2

function in the prototype NK target YAC-1. *J. Immunol.* 161:2099–2105

575. Wissing KM, Morelon E, Legendre C, De Pauw L, LeBeaut A, Grint P, Maniscalki M, Ickx B, Vereerstraeten P, Chatenoud L, Kreis H, Goldman M, Abramowicz D. 1997. A pilot trial of recombinant human interleukin-10 in kidney transplant recipients receiving OKT3 induction therapy. *Transplantation* 64:999–1006

576. Grohmann U, Silla S, Belladonna ML, Bianchi R, Orabona C, Puccetti P, Fioretti MC. 1997. Circulating levels of IL-10 are critically related to growth and rejection patterns of murine mastocytoma cells. *Cell. Immunol.* 181:109–19

577. Allione A, Consalvo M, Nanni P, Lollini PL, Cavallo F, Giovarelli M, Forni M, Gulino A, Colombo MP, Dellabona P, et al. 1994. Immunizing and curative potential of replicating and nonreplicating murine mammary adenocarcinoma cells engineered with interleukin (IL)-2, IL-4, IL-6, IL-7, IL-10, tumor necrosis factor alpha, granulocyte-macrophage colony-stimulating factor, and gamma-interferon gene or admixed with conventional adjuvants. *Cancer Res.* 54:6022–26

578. Kundu N, Beaty TL, Jackson MJ, Fulton AM. 1996. Antimetastatic and antitumor activities of interleukin 10 in a murine model of breast cancer [see comments]. *J. Natl. Cancer Inst.* 88:536–41

579. Kundu N, Dorsey R, Jackson MJ, Guiterrez P, Wilson K, Fu S, Ramanujam K, Thomas E, Fulton AM. 1998. Interleukin-10 gene transfer inhibits murine mammary tumors and elevates nitric oxide. *Int. J. Cancer* 76:713–19

580. Sun H, Gutierrez P, Jackson MJ, Kundu N, Fulton AM. 2000. Essential role of nitric oxide and interferon-gamma for tumor immunotherapy with interleukin-10. *J. Immunother.* 23:208–14

581. Gerard CM, Bruyns C, Delvaux A, Baudson N, Dargent JL, Goldman M, Velu T. 1996. Loss of tumorigenicity

and increased immunogenicity induced by interleukin-10 gene transfer in B16 melanoma cells. *Hum. Gene Ther.* 7:23–31

582. Huang S, Xie K, Bucana CD, Ullrich SE, Bar-Eli M. 1996. Interleukin 10 suppresses tumor growth and metastasis of human melanoma cells: potential inhibition of angiogenesis. *Clin. Cancer Res.* 2:1969–79

583. Stearns ME, Fudge K, Garcia F, Wang M. 1997. IL-10 inhibition of human prostate PC-3 ML cell metastases in SCID mice: IL-10 stimulation of TIMP-1 and inhibition of MMP-2/MMP-9 expression. *Invasion Metastasis* 17:62–74

584. Stearns ME, Wang M. 1998. Antimetastatic and antitumor activities of interleukin 10 in transfected human prostate PC-3 ML clones: Orthotopic growth in severe combined immunodeficient mice. *Clin. Cancer Res.* 4:2257–63

585. Stearns ME, Garcia FU, Fudge K, Rhim J, Wang M. 1999. Role of interleukin 10 and transforming growth factor beta1 in the angiogenesis and metastasis of human prostate primary tumor lines from orthotopic implants in severe combined immunodeficiency mice. *Clin. Cancer Res.* 5:711–20

586. Adris S, Klein S, Jasnis M, Chuluyan E, Ledda M, Bravo A, Carbone C, Chernajovsky Y, Podhajcer O. 1999. IL-10 expression by CT26 colon carcinoma cells inhibits their malignant phenotype and induces a T cell-mediated tumor rejection in the context of a systemic Th2 response. *Gene Ther.* 6:1705–12

587. Huang DR, Zhou YH, Xia SQ, Liu L, Pirskanen R, Lefvert AK. 1999. Markers in the promoter region of interleukin-10 (IL-10) gene in myasthenia gravis: implications of diverse effects of IL-10 in the pathogenesis of the disease. *J. Neuroimmunol.* 94:82–87

588. Barth RJJr, Coppola MA, Green WR. 1996. In vivo effects of locally secreted

IL-10 on the murine antitumor immune response. *Ann. Surg. Oncol.* 3:381–86

589. Muller A, Schmitt L, Raftery M, Schonrich G. 1998. Paralysis of B7 costimulation through the effect of viral IL-10 on T cells as a mechanism of local tolerance induction. *Eur. J. Immunol.* 28:3488–98

590. Muller A, Raftery M, Schonrich G. 1999. T cell stimulation upon long-term secretion of viral IL-10. *Eur. J. Immunol.* 29:2740–47

591. Li W, Fu F, Lu L, Narula SK, Fung JJ, Thomson AW, Qian S. 1999. Recipient pretreatment with mammalian IL-10 prolongs mouse cardiac allograft survival by inhibition of anti-donor T cell responses. *Transplant. Proc.* 31:115

592. Li W, Lu L, Li Y, Fu F, Fung JJ, Thomson AW, Qian S. 1997. High-dose cellular IL-10 exacerbates rejection and reverses effects of cyclosporine and tacrolimus in Mouse cardiac transplantation. *Transplant. Proc.* 29:1081–82

593. Qian S, Li W, Li Y, Fu F, Lu L, Fung JJ, Thomson AW. 1996. Systemic administration of cellular interleukin-10 can exacerbate cardiac allograft rejection in mice. *Transplantation* 62:1709–14

594. Li W, Fu F, Lu L, Narula SK, Fung JJ, Thomson AW, Qian S. 1999. Differential effects of exogenous interleukin-10 on cardiac allograft survival: inhibition of rejection by recipient pretreatment reflects impaired host accessory cell function. *Transplantation* 68:1402–9

595. Zou XM, Yagihashi A, Hirata K, Tsuruma T, Matsuno T, Tarumi K, Asanuma K, Watanabe N. 1998. Downregulation of cytokine-induced neutrophil chemoattractant and prolongation of rat liver allograft survival by interleukin-10. *Surg. Today* 28:184–91

596. Baker KS, Roncarolo MG, Peters C, Bigler M, DeFor T, Blazar BR. 1999. High spontaneous IL-10 production in unrelated bone marrow transplant recipients is associated with fewer transplant-related complications and early deaths. *Bone Marrow Transplant.* 23:1123–29

597. Holler E, Roncarolo MG, Hintermeier-Knabe R, Eissner G, Ertl B, Schulz U, Knabe H, Kolb HJ, Andreesen R, Wilmanns W. 2000. Prognostic significance of increased IL-10 production in patients prior to allogeneic bone marrow transplantation. *Bone Marrow Transplant.* 25:237–41

598. Hempel L, Korholz D, Nussbaum P, Bonig H, Burdach S, Zintl F. 1997. High interleukin-10 serum levels are associated with fatal outcome in patients after bone marrow transplantation. *Bone Marrow Transplant.* 20:365–68

599. Blazar BR, Taylor PA, Smith S, Vallera DA. 1995. Interleukin-10 administration decreases survival in murine recipients of major histocompatibility complex disparate donor bone marrow grafts. *Blood* 85:842–51

600. Krenger W, Snyder K, Smith S, Ferrara JL. 1994. Effects of exogenous interleukin-10 in a murine model of graft-versus-host disease to minor histocompatibility antigens. *Transplantation* 58:1251–57

601. Emmanouilides CE, Luo J, Baldwin G, Buckley D, Lau P, Lopez E, Tabibzadeh S, Yu J, Wolin M, Rigor R, Territo M, Black AC. 1996. Murine IL-10 fails to reduce GVHD despite inhibition of alloreactivity in vitro. *Bone Marrow Transplant.* 18:369–75

602. Blazar BR, Taylor PA, Panoskaltsis-Mortari A, Narula SK, Smith SR, Roncarolo MG, Vallera DA. 1998. Interleukin-10 dose-dependent regulation of CD4+ and CD8+ T cell-mediated graft-versus-host disease. *Transplantation* 66:1220–29

603. Fabrega AJ, Fasbender AJ, Struble S, Zabner J. 1996. Cationic lipid-mediated transfer of the hIL-10 gene prolongs

survival of allogeneic hepatocytes in Nagase analbuminemic rats. *Transplantation* 62:1866–71

604. Shinozaki K, Yahata H, Tanji H, Sakaguchi T, Ito H, Dohi K. 1999. Allograft transduction of IL-10 prolongs survival following orthotopic liver transplantation. *Gene Ther.* 6:816–22

605. Shinozaki K, Yahata H, Hayamizu K, Tashiro H, Fan X, Okimoto T, Tanji H, Sakaguchi T, Ito H, Asahara T. 2000. Adenovirus-mediated allograft transduction of interleukin-10: role in the induction phase of liver allograft acceptance. *Transplant. Proc.* 32:247–48

606. David A, Chetritt J, Guillot C, Tesson L, Heslan JM, Cuturi MC, Soulillou JP, Anegon I. 2000. Interleukin-10 produced by recombinant adenovirus prolongs survival of cardiac allografts in rats. *Gene Ther.* 7:505–10

607. Zheng XX, Steele AW, Nickerson PW, Steurer W, Steiger J, Strom TB. 1995. Administration of noncytolytic IL-10/Fc in murine models of lipopolysaccharide-induced septic shock and allogeneic islet transplantation. *J. Immunol.* 154:5590–5600

608. Furukawa Y, Becker G, Stinn JL, Shimizu K, Libby P, Mitchell RN. 1999. Interleukin-10 (IL-10) augments allograft arterial disease: paradoxical effects of IL-10 in vivo. *Am. J. Pathol.* 155:1929–39

609. Li W, Fu F, Lu L, Narula SK, Fung JJ, Thomson AW, Qian S. 1998. Systemic administration of anti-interleukin-10 antibody prolongs organ allograft survival in normal and presensitized recipients. *Transplantation* 66:1587–96

610. Torres PF, de Vos AF, Martins B, Kijlstra A. 1999. Interleukin 10 treatment does not prolong experimental corneal allograft survival. *Ophthalmic Res.* 31:297–303

611. Chan SY, DeBruyne LA, Goodman RE, Eichwald EJ, Bishop DK. 1995. In vivo depletion of CD8+ T cells results in Th2

cytokine production and alternate mechanisms of allograft rejection. *Transplantation* 59:1155–61

612. Bromberg JS. 1995. IL-10 immunosuppression in transplantation. *Curr. Opin. Immunol.* 7:639–43

613. Qin L, Chavin KD, Ding Y, Favaro JP, Woodward JE, Lin J, Tahara H, Robbins P, Shaked A, Ho DY, et al. 1995. Multiple vectors effectively achieve gene transfer in a murine cardiac transplantation model. Immunosuppression with TGF-beta 1 or vIL-10. *Transplantation* 59:809–16

614. Qin L, Ding Y, Pahud DR, Robson ND, Shaked A, Bromberg JS. 1997. Adenovirus-mediated gene transfer of viral interleukin-10 inhibits the immune response to both alloantigen and adenoviral antigen. *Hum. Gene Ther.* 8:1365–74

615. Brauner R, Nonoyama M, Laks H, Drinkwater DC Jr, McCaffery S, Drake T, Berk AJ, Sen L, Wu L. 1997. Intracoronary adenovirus-mediated transfer of immunosuppressive cytokine genes prolongs allograft survival. *J. Thorac. Cardiovasc. Surg.* 114:923–33

616. Wang CK, Zuo XJ, Carpenter D, Jordan S, Nicolaidou E, Toyoda M Czer LS, Wang H, Trento A. 1999. Prolongation of cardiac allograft survival with intracoronary viral interleukin-10 gene transfer. *Transplant. Proc.* 31:951–52

617. DeBruyne LA, Li K, Chan SY, Qin L, Bishop DK, Bromberg JS. 1998. Lipid-mediated gene transfer of viral IL-10 prolongs vascularized cardiac allograft survival by inhibiting donor-specific cellular and humoral immune responses. *Gene Ther.* 5:1079–87

618. DeBruyne LA, Li K, Bishop DK, Bromberg JS. 2000. Gene transfer of virally encoded chemokine antagonists vMIP-II and MC148 prolongs cardiac allograft survival and inhibits donor-specific immunity. *Gene Ther.* 7:575–82

619. Benhamou PY, Mullen Y, Shaked A, Bahmiller D, Csete ME. 1996. Decreased

alloreactivity to human islets secreting recombinant viral interleukin 10. *Transplantation* 62:1306–12

620. Drazan KE, Wu L, Olthoff KM, Jurim O, Busuttil RW, Shaked A. 1995. Transduction of hepatic allografts achieves local levels of viral IL-10 which suppress alloreactivity in vitro. *J. Surg. Res.* 59:219–23

621. Nast CC, Moudgil A, Zuo XJ, Toyoda M, Jordan SC. 1997. Long-term allograft acceptance in a patient with posttransplant lymphoproliferative disorder: correlation with intragraft viral interleukin-10. *Transplantation* 64:1578–82

622. Chernoff AE, Granowitz EV, Shapiro L, Vannier E, Lonnemann G, Angel JB, Kennedy JS, Rabson AR, Wolff SM, Dinarello CA. 1995. A randomized, controlled trial of IL-10 in humans. Inhibition of inflammatory cytokine production and immune responses. *J. Immunol.* 154:5492–99

623. Huhn RD, Radwanski E, O'Connell SM, Sturgill MG, Clarke L, Cody RP, Affrime MB, Cutler DL. 1996. Pharmacokinetics and immunomodulatory properties of intravenously administered recombinant human interleukin-10 in healthy volunteers. *Blood* 87:699–705

624. Huhn RD, Radwanski E, Gallo J, Affrime MB, Sabo R, Gonyo G, Monge A, Cutler DL. 1997. Pharmacodynamics of subcutaneous recombinant human interleukin-10 in healthy volunteers. *Clin. Pharmacol. Ther.* 62:171–80

625. Radwanski E, Chakraborty A, Van Wart S, Huhn RD, Cutler DL, Affrime MB, Jusko WJ. 1998. Pharmacokinetics and leukocyte responses of recombinant human interleukin-10. *Pharm. Res.* 15:1895–901

626. Fuchs AC, Granowitz EV, Shapiro L, Vannier E, Lonnemann G, Angel JB, Kennedy JS, Rabson AR, Radwanski E, Affrime MB, Cutler DL, Grint PC, Dinarello CA. 1996. Clinical, hematologic, and immunologic effects of interleukin-10 in humans. *J. Clin. Immunol.* 16:291–303

627. Huhn RD, Pennline K, Radwanski E, Clarke L, Sabo R, Cutler DL. 1999. Effects of single intravenous doses of recombinant human interleukin-10 on subsets of circulating leukocytes in humans. *Immunopharmacology* 41:109–17

628. Schreiber S, Fedorak FN, Nielsen OH, Wild G, Williams NC, Jacyna M, Lashner BA, Cohard M, Kilian A, Lebeaut A, Hanauer SB. 1998. *A safety and efficacy study of recombinant human interleukin-10 (rHuIL-10) treatment in 329 patients with chronic active Crohn's disease (CACD).* Presented at the Annual mtg of AGA and AASLD, New Orleans 1998

629. Keystone E, Wherry J, Grint P. 1998. IL-10 as a therapeutic strategy in the treatment of rheumatoid arthritis. *Rheum. Dis. Clin. North Am.* 24:629–39

630. Chakraborty A, Blum RA, Mis SM, Cutler DL, Jusko WJ. 1999. Pharmacokinetic and adrenal interactions of IL-10 and prednisone in healthy volunteers. *J. Clin. Pharmacol.* 39:624–35

631. Chakraborty A, Blum RA, Cutler DL, Jusko WJ. 1999. Pharmacoimmunodynamic interactions of interleukin-10 and prednisone in healthy volunteers. *Clin. Pharmacol. Ther.* 65:304–18

632. Gorski JC, Hall SD, Becker P, Affrime MB, Cutler DL, Haehner-Daniels B. 2000. In vivo effects of interleukin-10 on human cytochrome P450 activity. *Clin. Pharmacol. Ther.* 67:32–43

633. Andersen SR, Lambrecht LJ, Swan SK, Cutler DL, Radwanski E, Affrime MB, Garaud JJ. 1999. Disposition of recombinant human interleukin-10 in subjects with various degrees of renal function. *J. Clin. Pharmacol.* 39:1015–20

634. Pajkrt D, van der Poll T, Levi M, Cutler DL, Affrime MB, van den Ende A, ten Cate JW, van Deventer SJ. 1997. Interleukin-10 inhibits activation of

coagulation and fibrinolysis during human endotoxemia. *Blood* 89:2701–5

635. Olszyna DP, Pajkrt D, Lauw FN, van Deventer SJ, van Der Poll T. 2000. Interleukin 10 inhibits the release of CC chemokines during human endotoxemia. *J. Infect. Dis.* 181:613–20

636. Cooper PJ, Fekade D, Remick DG, Grint P, Wherry J, Griffin GE. 2000. Recombinant human interleukin-10 fails to alter proinflammatory cytokine production or physiologic changes associated with the Jarisch-Herxheimer reaction. *J. Infect. Dis.* 181:203–9

637. van Deventer SJ, Elson CO, Fedorak RN. 1997. Multiple doses of intravenous interleukin 10 in steroid-refractory Crohn's disease. Crohn's Disease Study Group. *Gastroenterology* 113:383–89

638. Maini RN, Taylor PC. 2000. Anticytokine therapy for rheumatoid arthritis. *Annu. Rev. Med.* 51:207–29

639. Papadakis KA, Targan SR. 2000. Role of cytokines in the pathogenesis of inflammatory bowel disease. *Annu. Rev. Med.* 51:289–98

640. Asadullah K, Sterry W, Stephanek K, Jasulaitis D, Leupold M, Audring H, Volk HD, Docke WD. 1998. IL-10 is a key cytokine in psoriasis. Proof of principle by IL-10 therapy: a new therapeutic approach. *J. Clin. Invest.* 101:783–94

641. Asadullah K, Docke WD, Ebeling M, Friedrich M, Belbe G, Audring H, Volk HD, Sterry W. 1999. Interleukin 10 treatment of psoriasis: clinical results of a phase 2 trial. *Arch. Dermatol.* 135:187–92

642. Seifert M, Sterry W, Effenberger E, Rexin A, Friedrich M, Haeussler-Quade A, Volk HD, Asadullah K. 2000. The antipsoriatic activity of IL-10 is rather caused by effects on peripheral blood cells than by a direct effect on human keratinocytes. *Arch. Dermatol. Res.* 292:164–72

643. McHutchison JG, Giannelli G, Nyberg L, Blatt LM, Waite K, Mischkot P, Pianko S, Conrad A, Grint P. 1999. A pilot study of daily subcutaneous interleukin-10 in patients with chronic hepatitis C infection. *J. Interferon Cytokine Res.* 19:1265–70

644. Arai T, Hiromatsu K, Nishimura H, Kimura Y, Kobayashi N, Ishida H, Nimura Y, Yoshikai Y. 1995. Endogenous interleukin 10 prevents apoptosis in macrophages during Salmonella infection. *Biochem. Biophys. Res. Commun.* 213:600–7

645. Wang M, Jeng KC, Ping LI. 1999. Exogenous cytokine modulation or neutralization of interleukin-10 enhance survival in lipopolysaccharide-hyporesponsive C3H/HeJ mice with Klebsiella infection. *Immunology* 98:90–97

646. Sasaki S, Nishikawa S, Miura T, Mizuki M, Yamada K, Madarame H, Tagawa YI, Iwakura Y, Nakane A. 2000. Interleukin-4 and interleukin-10 are involved in host resistance to Staphylococcus aureus infection through regulation of gamma interferon. *Infect. Immun.* 68:2424–30

647. Yang X, HayGlass KT, Brunham RC. 1996. Genetically determined differences in IL-10 and IFN-gamma responses correlate with clearance of Chlamydia trachomatis mouse pneumonitis infection. *J. Immunol.* 156:4338–44

648. Yang X, Gartner J, Zhu L, Wang S, Brunham RC. 1999. IL-10 gene knockout mice show enhanced Th1-like protective immunity and absent granuloma formation following Chlamydia trachomatis lung infection. *J. Immunol.* 162:1010–17

649. Bermudez LE, Champsi J. 1993. Infection with Mycobacterium avium induces production of interleukin-10 (IL-10), and administration of anti-IL-10 antibody is associated with enhanced resistance to infection in mice. *Infect. Immun.* 61:3093–97

650. North RJ. 1998. Mice incapable of making IL-4 or IL-10 display normal resistance to infection with Mycobacterium

tuberculosis. *Clin. Exp. Immunol.* 113: 55–58

651. Murray PJ, Wang L, Onufryk C, Tepper RI, Young RA. 1997. T cell-derived IL-10 antagonizes macrophage function in mycobacterial infection. *J. Immunol.* 158:315–21

652. Murray PJ, Young RA. 1999. Increased antimycobacterial immunity in interleukin-10-deficient mice. *Infect. Immun.* 67:3087–95

653. Tonnetti L, Spaccapelo R, Cenci E, Mencacci A, Puccetti P, Coffman RL, Bistoni F, Romani L. 1995. Interleukin-4 and -10 exacerbate candidiasis in mice. *Eur. J. Immunol.* 25:1559–65

654. Romani L, Puccetti P, Mencacci A, Cenci E, Spaccapelo R, Tonnetti L, Grohmann U, Bistoni F. 1994. Neutralization of IL-10 up-regulates nitric oxide production and protects susceptible mice from challenge with Candida albicans. *J. Immunol.* 152:3514–21

655. Del Sero G, Mencacci A, Cenci E, d'Ostiani CF, Montagnoli C, Bacci A, Mosci P, Kopf M, Romani L. 1999. Antifungal type 1 responses are upregulated in IL-10-deficient mice. *Microbes Infect* 1:1169–80

656. Fierer J, Walls L, Eckmann L, Yamamoto T, Kirkland TN. 1998. Importance of interleukin-10 in genetic susceptibility of mice to Coccidioides immitis. *Infect. Immun.* 66:4397–402

657. Blackstock R, Buchanan KL, Adesina AM, Murphy JW. 1999. Differential regulation of immune responses by highly and weakly virulent Cryptococcus neoformans isolates. *Infect. Immun.* 67:3601–9

658. Cenci E, Mencacci A, Fe d'Ostiani C, Del Sero G, Mosci P, Montagnoli C, Bacci A, Romani L. 1998. Cytokine- and T helper-dependent lung mucosal immunity in mice with invasive pulmonary aspergillosis. *J. Infect. Dis.* 178:1750–60

659. Chatelain R, Mauze S, Coffman RL. 1999. Experimental Leishmania major infection in mice: role of IL-10. *Parasite Immunol.* 21:211–18

660. Reed SG, Brownell CE, Russo DM, Silva JS, Grabstein KH, Morrissey PJ. 1994. IL-10 mediates susceptibility to Trypanosoma cruzi infection. *J. Immunol.* 153:3135–40

661. Uzonna JE, Kaushik RS, Gordon JR, Tabel H. 1998. Immunoregulation in experimental murine Trypanosoma congolense infection: anti-IL-10 antibodies reverse trypanosome-mediated suppression of lymphocyte proliferation in vitro and moderately prolong the lifespan of genetically susceptible BALB/c mice. *Parasite Immunol.* 20:293–302

Subject Index

CUMULATIVE INDEXES

CONTRIBUTING AUTHORS, VOLUMES 1–19

CHAPTER TITLES, VOLUMES 1–19

Prefatory Chapters

Antigen Structure

Immunoglobulins and B Cell Receptors

T Lymphocyte and NK Cell Receptors

Major Histocompatibility Complex and Antigen Processing and Presentation

Lymphocyte Surface Antigens and Activation Mechanisms

Lymphocyte Development and Differentiation

Tolerance

Cytotoxic Cells

Phagocytosis and Inflammation

Autoimmunity

Immunodeficiency

Allergy

HIV, AIDS and Other Retroviral Infections

Transplantation Immunology